Cardiac Ultrasound

This title is a self-contained work entitled *Cardiac Ultrasound*. Additionally, it forms an integral part of *CLINICAL ULTRASOUND a comprehensive text* together with its companion titles, *Abdominal and General Ultrasound* and *Ultrasound in Obstetrics and Gynaecology*, each of which may be purchased separately.

For Churchill Livingstone

Publisher: Simon Fathers
Project Editor: Clare Wood-Allum
Indexer: Michele Clarke
Production Control: Neil Dickson
Sales Promotion Executive: Caroline Boyd

For Longman Malaysia

Production Co-ordination: Shirley Kerk

CLINICAL ULTRASOUND a comprehensive text

Cardiac Ultrasound

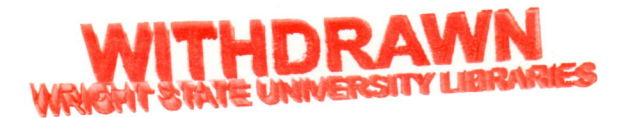

Edited by

Peter Wilde BSc MRCP FRCR
Consultant Cardiac Radiologist, Royal Infirmary and Royal
Hospital for Sick Children, Bristol, UK

Foreword by
Celia M. Oakley MD FRCP
Professor of Cardiology, Department of Clinical Cardiology,
Royal Postgraduate Medical School, London, UK

CHURCHILL LIVINGSTONE
EDINBURGH LONDON MADRID MELBOURNE NEW YORK AND TOKYO 1993

CHURCHILL LIVINGSTONE
Medical Division of Longman Group UK Limited

Distributed in the United States of America by Churchill Livingstone Inc., 650 Avenue of the Americas, New York, N.Y. 10011, and by associated companies, branches and representatives throughout the world.

© Longman Group UK Limited 1993

All rights reserved. No part of this publication may be reproduced, stored in a retrieval system, or transmitted in any form or by any means, electronic, mechanical, photocopying, recording or otherwise, without either the prior written permission of the publishers (Churchill Livingstone, Robert Stevenson House, 1–3 Baxter's Place, Leith Walk, Edinburgh EH1 3AF), or a licence permitting restricted copying in the United Kingdom issued by the Copyright Licensing Agency Ltd, 90 Tottenham Court Road, London W1P 9HE.

First published 1993

ISBN 0-443-04280-2

British Library Cataloguing in Publication Data
A catalogue record for this book is available from the British Library.

Library of Congress Cataloging in Publication Data
A catalog record for this book is available from the Library of Congress.

The publisher's policy is to use paper manufactured from sustainable forests

Printed and bound in Great Britain by
William Clowes Limited, Beccles and London

Foreword

At a meeting of the British Cardiac Society in 1967 after the first paper on cardiac ultrasound had been given to that Society, the late Cornelio Papp, a doyen of electrocardiography, predicted that one day cardiac ultrasound would be as important to cardiologists as the electrocardiogram. His forecast probably seemed unlikely to many who heard it at the time but the echocardiogram outstripped the electrocardiogram some years ago and now its importance in cardiac diagnosis can hardly be exaggerated, it being an essential part of clinical cardiology. It has made many a cardiac catheterisation and angiocardiography procedure redundant with these techniques being reserved for specific problems such as the imaging of coronary arteries. It is also an important research tool which is still developing. It is therefore with both pleasure and pride that I write the foreword to this text book on cardiac ultrasound with its wide range of authors from Britain and overseas.

Echocardiography now provides the main means of determining the anatomy and pathophysiology of the heart in congenital and acquired disease. Many of the advances in cardiac ultrasound over the twenty-five years that it has been in use have resulted from technical advances such as Doppler measurements of velocity allowing computation of flows and gradients, colour flow imaging which captivates even our surgical colleagues, trans-oesophageal and intra-operative visualisation and now exercise and pharmacological stress studies. Future sophisticated ultrasound methods of tissue characterisation may allow recognition of hibernating myocardium, rejection after transplantation and even of disarray of muscle fibres compared with secondary hypertrophy.

After so many rapid advances, progress in technical development must surely slow in the immediate future but the introduction of intravascular probes of ever diminishing diameter may be the next big step forward. These already allow atheroma to be 'visualised' and flow to be measured even in the smaller coronary arteries. They may even be used to guide angioplasty and to assess the results.

In spite of new methods having the greatest appeal the simple lessons of the past should not be forgotten. As emphasised by several authors, the most accurate ultrasound measurements are obtained from an M-mode trace and much functional information is deduced from alteration in structure. Echocardiography is still not a total diagnostic panacea and the information obtained must be tempered with clinical acumen. The echocardiographer does not hold all the cards. The velocity of blood flow through a stenosed aortic valve will be reduced by impaired left ventricular function and lower stroke volume. The velocity measured may not be the true maximum because of the difficulty in some cases of aligning the probe correctly with the maximum jet velocity at the same time as avoiding obstructions to measurement such as air in the lungs.

It is important to ensure that echocardiographic parameters make sense and when they are out of concert with other ultrasound measurements and clinical findings, to determine which is correct. While echocardiography may be used to discover unsuspected aortic stenosis in the elderly or a left atrial tumour, cardiac ultrasound remains relatively insensitive to the recognition of constrictive pericarditis and is notoriously poor at quantitating the severity of mitral regurgitation.

Although the problem of obtaining good ultrasound images from stressed and overbreathing patients delayed the application of stress echo, advances in technology have largely solved the problem. Using digitised data the chosen cardiac cycles can be compared before and after exercise or pharmacological stress to provide a highly specific means of recognising regional wall motion abnormalities.

Each advance in technology tends to be added to the existing routine to produce a further burden to both patient and taxpayer. The clinician should always select only the tests which are required to gain necessary information. Nowadays this may frequently result in the carefully appraised echocardiogram standing alone with the clinical findings, leaving cardiac catheterisation or other techniques as unnecessary additional investigations.

This fine textbook of cardiac ultrasound is one in a series of four volumes on clinical ultrasound. In itself it is the complete text for cardiologists and cardiac radiologists but with the other three volumes it will, I am sure, become the Bible on clinical ultrasound and the first of many editions to come.

C.M.O.

Preface

There are many authoritative text books on echocardiography available and careful thought was necessary before undertaking the production of another volume. The original stimulus for this work was the development of a large and comprehensive textbook on the whole range of clinical ultrasound applications, particularly in the field of diagnostic imaging.

During the planning of this project some aspects of clinical ultrasound appeared to stand distinctly, obstetric and cardiac ultrasound being the most obvious examples of this. It is for this reason that separate volumes have been devoted to obstetric and cardiac ultrasound. This allows convenient reference for those concerned with the field but equally allows a full reference text to be available for those individuals or libraries who wish to have a comprehensive reference source.

Whilst cardiac ultrasound has traditionally remained rather distinct from the remainder of ultrasound imaging, it is becoming increasingly common for equipment and operators to share their skills. This is partly due to financial pressures but equally is due to cross-fertilisation of interests, particularly within the field of radiology.

This volume aims to give a comprehensive review of the current state of cardiac ultrasound. In many instances considerable detail is given about techniques, particularly quantitation. It is important to realise, however, that in many of the subjects covered there is a far greater body of knowledge than can be represented even in a substantial volume of this size. The references in each chapter are thus intended to direct the reader to further work if they wish. It is hoped that the style of the book will be appropriate for both reference and study, with attention being given to a readable style and elimination of too much complex data. Much attention has been given to producing good quality illustrations, but of course it will never be possible to illustrate every clinical condition.

The chapter authors come from a wide range of institutions and backgrounds. Both radiologists and cardiologists are well represented and this is entirely intentional. Both these disciplines have much to offer in diagnostic cardiac ultrasound and in many cases the disciplines have much to learn from one another. Although the majority of authors are based in the United Kingdom, our overseas contributors are welcomed and I am particularly pleased to include the section on echocardiography in the developing world.

I am very grateful to all those who have been supportive in the production of this volume, most particularly the authors who have worked hard on their chapters, but also the secretaries who have typed out the manuscripts, the publishers who have worked with them and of course the families of all the authors who have no doubt suffered in the production of the work!

1992   P.W.

Orientation and labelling of illustrations

The cross-sectional cardiac images presented in this volume are taken from a wide range of transducer positions and many of the sections are taken in modified views in order to demonstrate anatomical and pathological features in the best possible way. In addition to this, different authors present the images in varying orientations according to the custom in their own institution. These orientations are discussed in Chapters 4 and 19. It was considered both impractical and illogical to modify all the illustrations to a standardised format. The cross-sectional imaging data presented here is therefore an accurate representation of work being carried out in many important echocardiographic centres.

In order to facilitate clear understanding of these varied presentations, the illustrations have been annotated wherever appropriate with labelled arrows indicating major orthogonal image planes and their orientation. Abbreviations used in this labelling are listed below.

Most of the images have been annotated to demonstrate relevant features as clearly as possible. In many cases the abbreviations are unique to an individual or to a small number of images. There are, however, many commonly used abbreviations that occur repeatedly throughout the volume.

These are listed below and will not be repeated with each figure. Descriptive abbreviations not appearing on this list will be defined with the legend of each individual illustration.

Orientation abbreviations

S, s	superior
I, i	inferior
A, a	anterior
P, p	posterior
L, l	left
R, r	right

Descriptive abbreviations

LA, la	left atrium
LV, lv	left ventricle
RA, ra	right atrium
RV, rv	right ventricle
AO, ao	aorta
PA, pa	pulmonary artery
SVC, svc	superior vena cava
IVC, ivc	inferior vena cava
MV, mv	mitral valve
TV, tv	tricuspid valve
AV, av	aortic valve
PV, pv	pulmonary valve

Contributors

Peter Bloomfield MD MRCP FACC
Consultant Cardiologist, Royal Infirmary, Edinburgh, UK

Duncan F. Ettles MB ChB MRCP
Radiologist, Bristol Royal Infirmary, Bristol, UK

Alan G. Fraser BSc MB ChB MRCP
Senior Lecturer in Cardiology and Honorary Consultant Cardiologist, University of Wales College of Medicine, Cardiff, UK

John L. Gibbs MRCP
Consultant Paediatric Cardiologist, Killingbeck Hospital, Leeds; Senior Lecturer, Department of Medicine, University of Leeds, UK

Derek G. Gibson MA MB FRCP
Consultant Cardiologist, Royal Brompton National Heart and Lung Hospital, London, UK

Michael J. Godman MB ChB FRCP (Ed)
Consultant Paediatric Cardiologist, Royal Hospital for Sick Children; Senior Lecturer, Department of Child Life and Health, University of Edinburgh, Edinburgh, UK

Vanda M. Gooch BSc (Hons)
Technician in Charge, Echocardiography Department, The Hospitals for Sick Children, London, UK

Michael Halliwell BSc PhD
Head of Clinical Engineering, United Bristol Healthcare Trust, Bristol General Hospital, Bristol, UK

George Hartnell MRCP FRCR
Director, Cardiac Radiology, New England Deaconess Hospital; Associate Professor of Radiology, Harvard Medical School, Boston, USA

Alan Houston MD FRCP(Glas) DCH
Consultant Paediatric Cardiologist, Royal Hospital for Sick Children, Glasgow, UK

Stewart Hunter MB ChB FRCP(E&G) DCH
Consultant Paediatric Cardiologist, Regional Department of Paediatric Cardiology, Freeman Hospital, Newcastle-upon-Tyne, UK

Robin P. Martin MB ChB MRCP
Consultant Paediatric Cardiologist, Bristol Royal Hospital for Sick Children, Bristol, UK

Paula Murphy MB BCh MRCPI FFR(RCSi) FRCR
Consultant Cardiovascular Radiologist, Bristol Royal Infirmary, Bristol, UK

Petros Nihoyannopoulos MD FESC FACC
Senior Lecturer and Consultant Cardiologist, Royal Postgraduate Medical School, Hammersmith Hospital, London, UK

James Nolan MB ChB MRCP
Research Fellow, Department of Cardiography, Royal Infirmary, Edinburgh, UK

Robert L. Parry MRCP FRCR
Lecturer in Cardiovascular Radiology, Bristol Royal Infirmary, Bristol, UK

Andrew N. Redington MD MRCP
Consultant Paediatric Cardiologist and Senior Lecturer, Royal Brompton National Heart and Lung Hospital, London, UK

Iain A. Simpson MD MRCP
Consultant Cardiologist, Southampton General Hospital, Southampton, UK

George Strang BSc FRCP (London)
Consultant Physician, Cecilia Makiwane Hospital, Mdantsane, Ciskei; Honorary Lecturer, Department of Medicine, University of Cape Town, South Africa

Ian D. Sullivan BMedSc MB ChB FRACP
Consultant Cardiologist, The Hospitals for Sick Children, London, UK

Graham Thirsk MIBiol
Technical Marketing Manager, Advanced Technology Laboratories, Munich, Germany

Thierry Touche MD
Cardiologist, Echocardiography Laboratory, Centre Cardiologique du Nord, Saint-Denis, Paris, France

Jamie Weir MB BS DMRD FRCP(Ed) FRCR
Consultant Radiologist, Aberdeen Teaching Hospitals; Clinical Professor of Radiology, University of Aberdeen, UK

Peter N. T. Wells PhD DSc FEng
Chief Physicist, United Bristol Healthcare Trust; Honorary Professor in Clinical Radiology, University of Bristol, Bristol, UK

Peter Wilde BSc MRCP FRCR
Consultant Cardiac Radiologist, Royal Infirmary and Royal Hospital for Sick Children, Bristol, UK

Neil Wilson MB BS DCH MRCP (UK)
Consultant Paediatric Cardiologist, King Faisal Specialist Hospital, Riyadh, Saudi Arabia

Contents

SECTION 1
Introduction to cardiac ultrasound

1. History 3
   Peter N. T. Wells

2. Physics and principles 9
   Michael Halliwell

3. Equipment 27
   Graham Thirsk

4. Examination technique 41
   Peter Wilde, Robert L. Parry

5. Left ventricular function 65
   Jamie Weir

6. Doppler quantitation – pressure drop estimation 79
   Iain A. Simpson

7. Doppler quantitation – pulmonary artery pressure 105
   Thierry Touche

8. Doppler quantitation – volume flow estimation 113
   Thierry Touche

9. Transoesophageal examination 129
   Duncan F. Ettles

SECTION 2
Acquired heart disease

10. Valvular disease 151
    Paula Murphy

11. Ischaemic heart disease 179
    Jamie Weir

12. Cardiomyopathy 191
    Petros Nihoyannopoulos

13. Infective endocarditis 209
    Petros Nihoyannopoulos

14. Prosthetic valves 223
    James Nolan, Peter Bloomfield

15. Cardiac masses 243
    Petros Nihoyannopoulos

16. Pericardium 259
    George Hartnell

17. Thoracic aorta 275
    George Hartnell

18. Echocardiography in the developing world 289
    George Strang

SECTION 3
Congenital heart disease

19. Segmental approach 307
    Ian D. Sullivan, Vanda M. Gooch

20. Left to right shunts 341
    John L. Gibbs, Neil Wilson

21. Left sided obstruction 387
    Alan Houston

22. Abnormalities of ventriculo-arterial connection 407
    Robin P. Martin

23. Right sided obstructions and malformations 429
    Michael J. Godman

24. Univentricular atrioventricular connection 447
    Stewart Hunter

25. Venous anomalies 455
    Ian D. Sullivan, Vanda M. Gooch

26. Cardiomyopathy in childhood 473
    Robin P. Martin

27. Great arterial anomalies 489
    John L. Gibbs

28. Coronary artery anomalies 495
    Alan Houston

SECTION 4
Echocardiography in perspective

29. The clinical view 511
    Andrew N. Redington, Derek G. Gibson

30. Recent advances 519
    Robert L. Parry, Alan G. Fraser

Index

Note: These plates are reproduced in black and white in the appropriate position within the text.

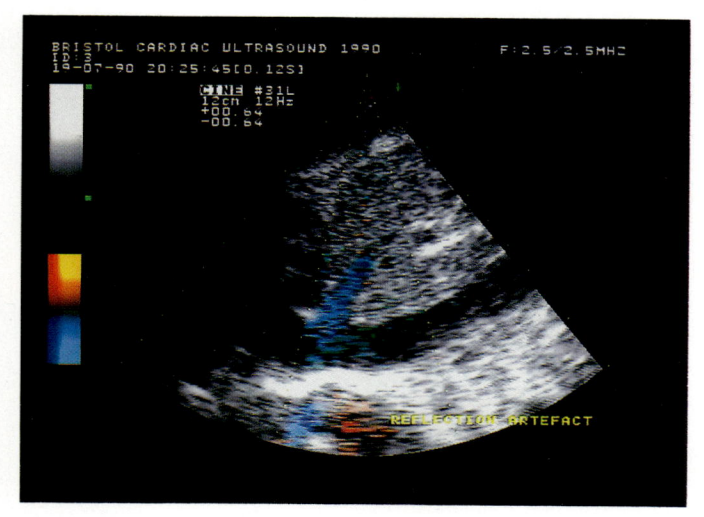

Ch. 2
Plate 1 Colour flow mapping image of a hepatic vein draining to the inferior vena cava. Note the artefactual flow image produced by mirror-like reflection of the beam in the posterior wall of the inferior vena cava.

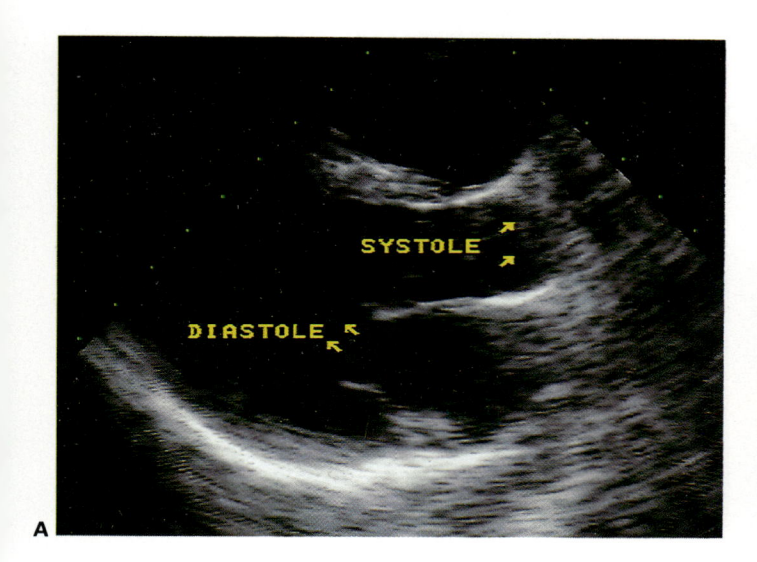

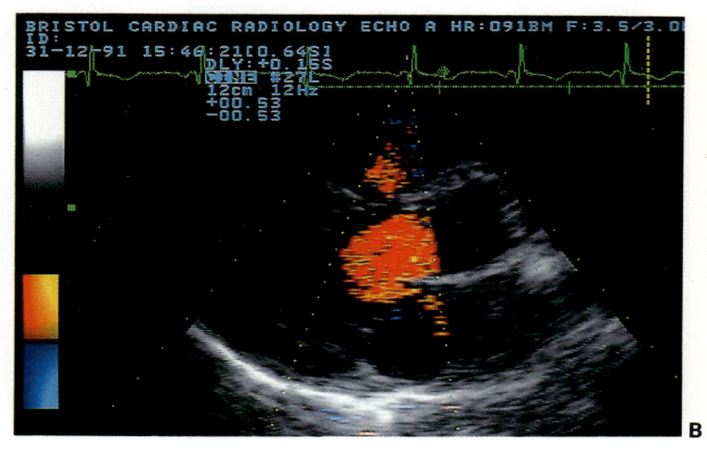

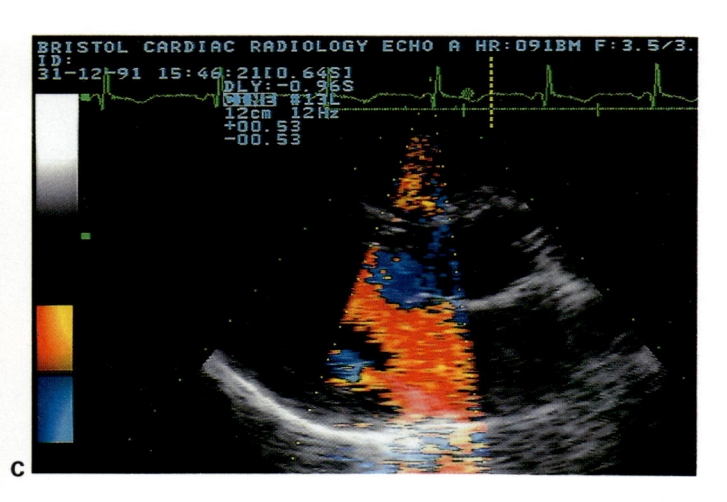

Ch. 4
Plate 1 A: Parasternal long axis view showing the direction of mitral inflow and of outflow towards the aortic valve. The precise direction of flow will vary from examination to examination. **B:** Colour flow mapping of the same study as Plate 1A taken in systole and showing flow towards the aortic valve in red as it is slightly towards the transducer. Note that the colour map is only shown over a limited sector. **C:** Diastolic frame taken from the same study as Plates 1A and B showing mitral inflow in red as it is slightly towards the transducer.

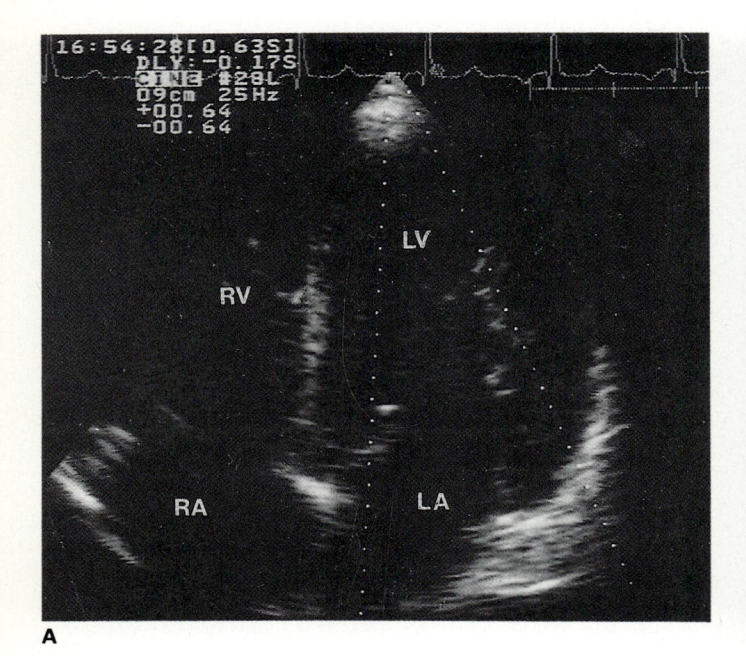

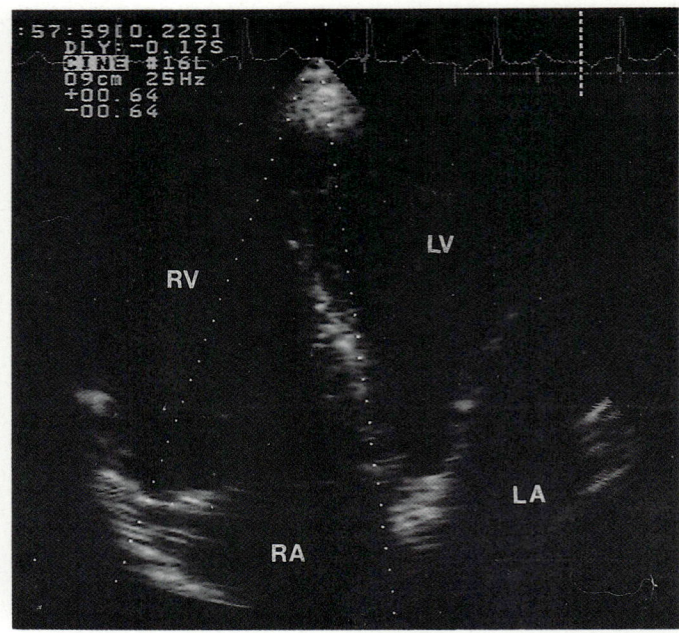

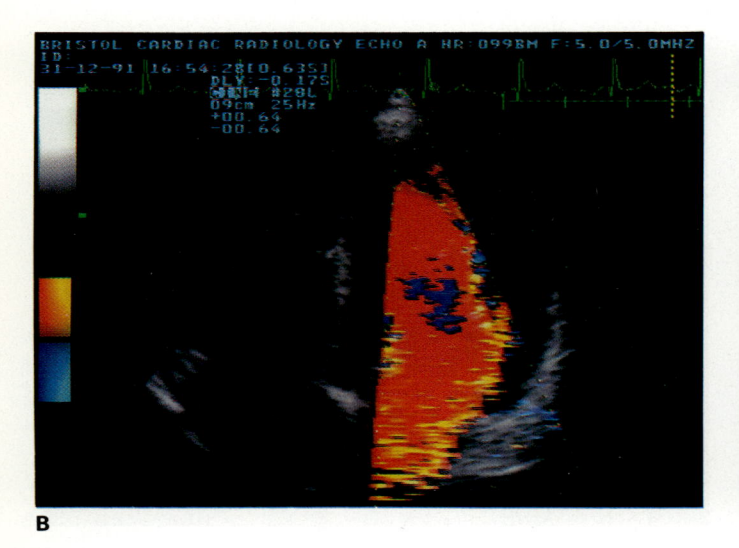

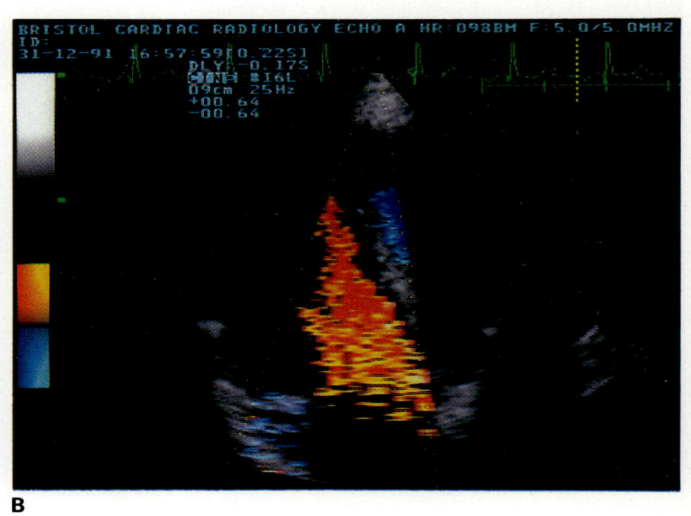

Ch. 4
Plate 2 A: Apical four chamber view showing the mitral valve open in diastole. B: Colour flow image corresponding to Plate 2A showing mitral inflow towards the transducer in red. The central part of the flow shows aliasing (blue).

Ch. 4
Plate 3 A: Apical view of the tricuspid valve taken from the same study as Plate 2A. B: Colour flow image corresponding to Plate 3A showing diastolic tricuspid inflow in red but there is no aliasing present as the velocity is lower than that of mitral inflow.

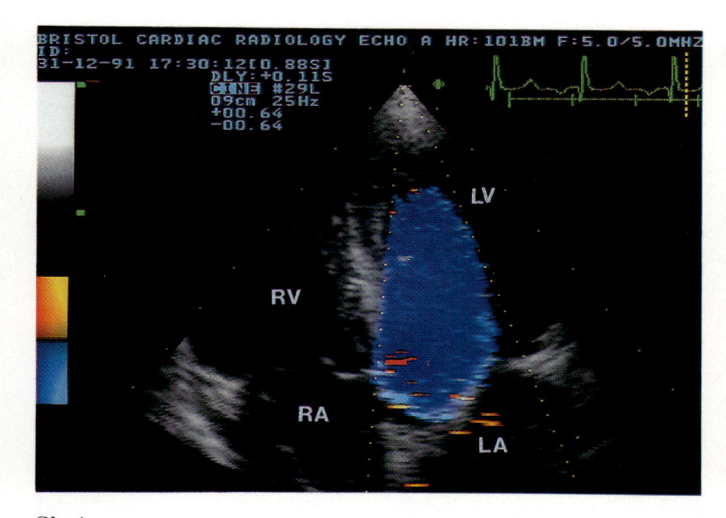

Ch. 4

Plate 4 Apical four chamber view angled upwards towards the left ventricular outflow tract. Colour flow mapping shows flow away from the transducer in blue.

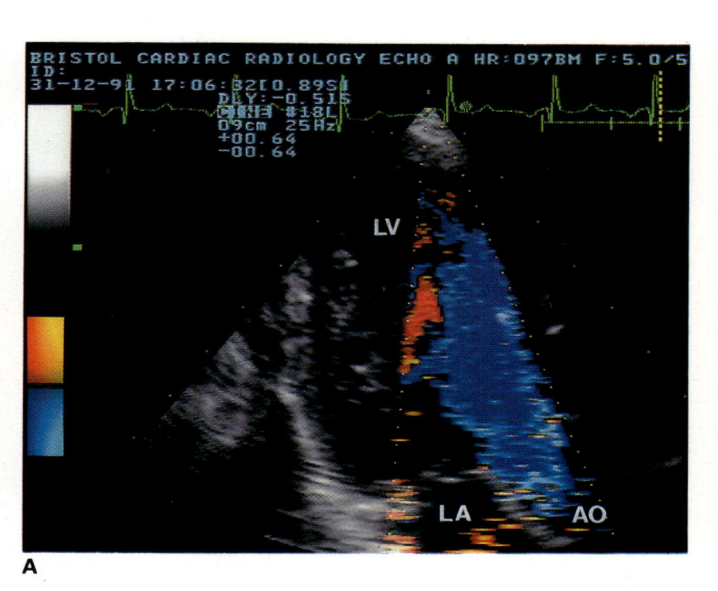

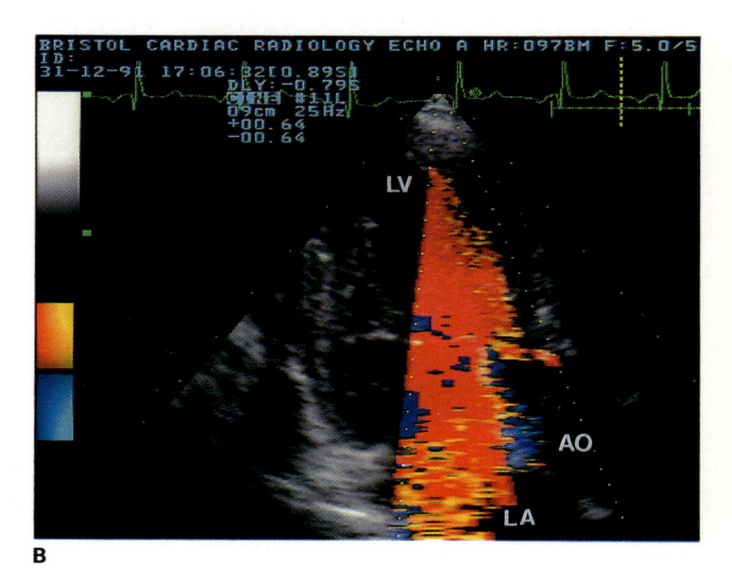

Ch. 4

Plate 5 A: Apical long axis view with the colour sector placed over the left ventricular outflow tract. Systolic flow through the aortic valve is shown in blue (compare with Fig. 25). **B:** Apical long axis view showing diastolic mitral inflow in red.

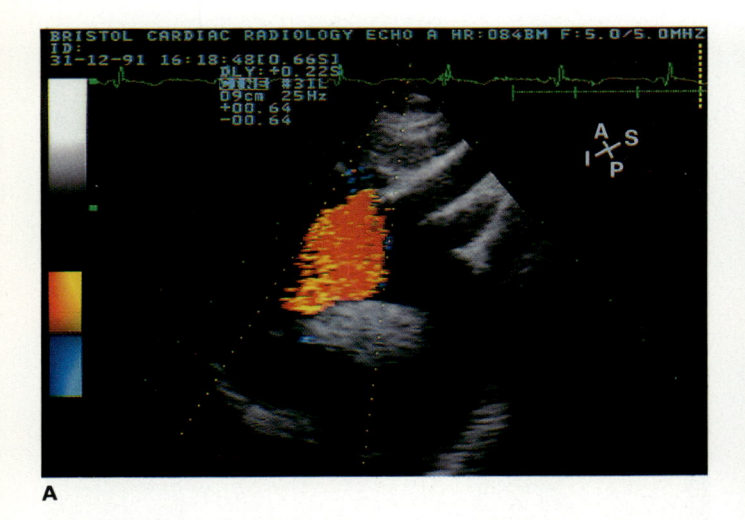

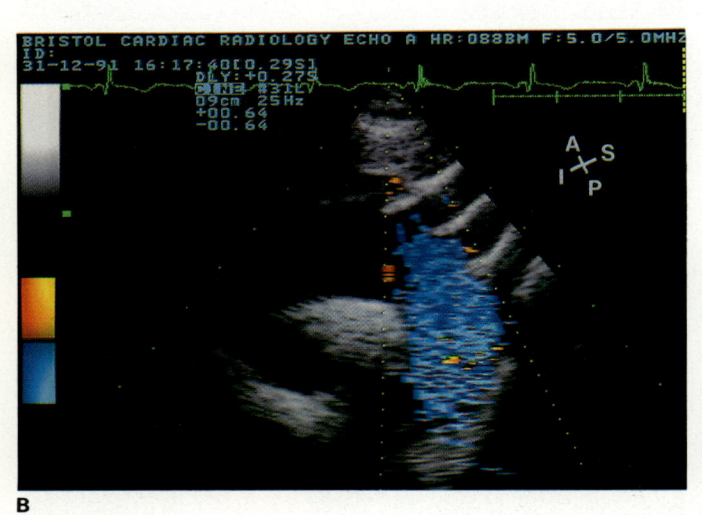

Ch. 4
Plate 6 A: Suprasternal view of the aortic arch. The colour sector has been placed over the ascending aorta and shows the flow towards the transducer in red. **B:** Similar view to Plate 6A with the colour sector placed over the descending aorta, showing the flow away from the transducer in blue.

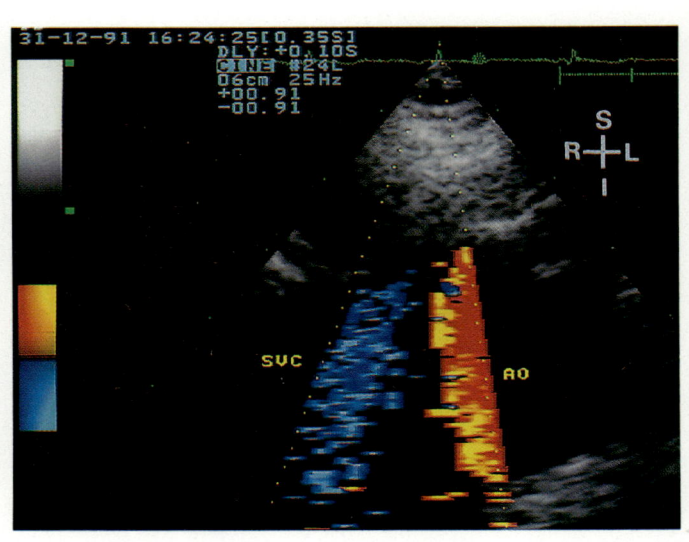

Ch. 4
Plate 7 Coronal suprasternal view in the same orientation as Fig. 22 showing flow in the superior vena cava away from the transducer in blue and flow in the ascending aorta towards the transducer in red.

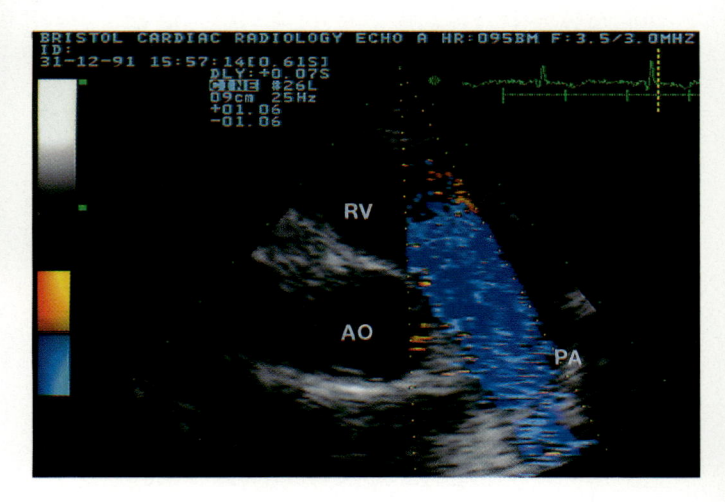

Ch. 4
Plate 8 Left parasternal short axis view showing flow in the right ventricular outflow tract and pulmonary artery. Flow away from the transducer is shown in blue (compare with Fig. 29).

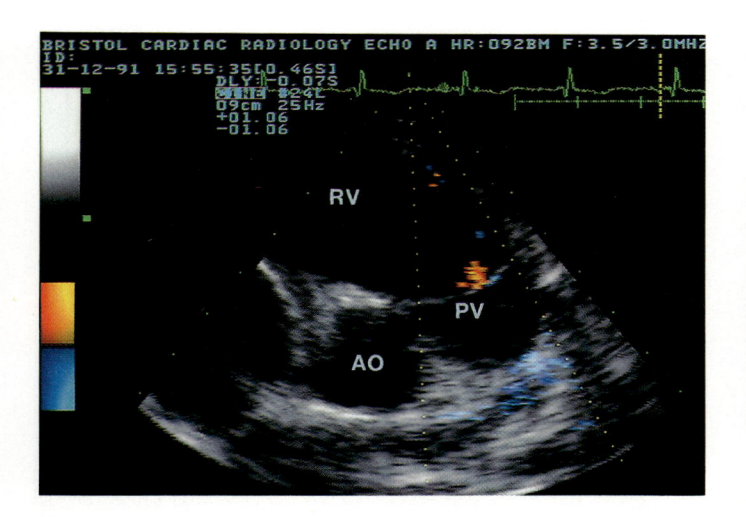

Ch. 4
Plate 9   Diastolic frame from the same examination as Plate 8. A small orange jet of physiological pulmonary regurgitation is seen just proximal to the pulmonary valve.

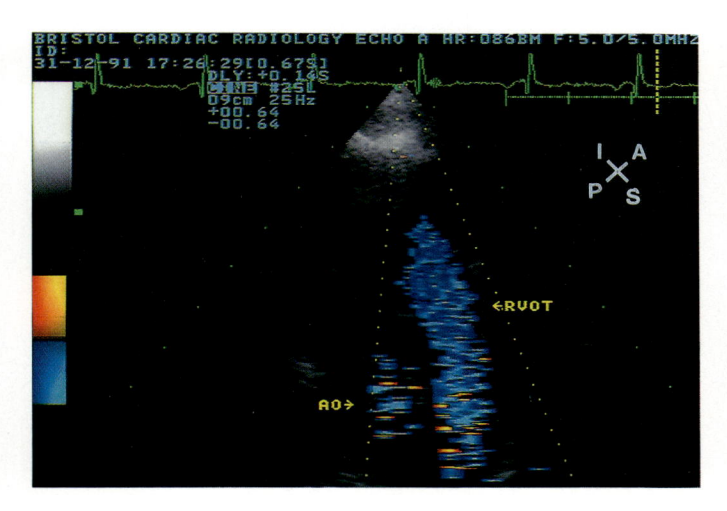

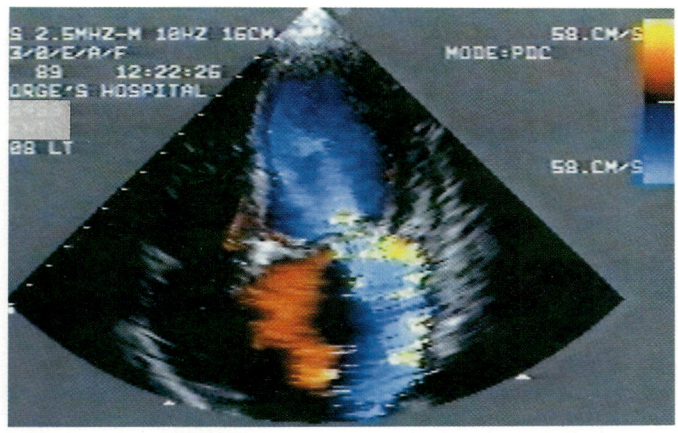

Ch. 6
Plate 1   Colour Doppler flow map image of mitral regurgitation showing that the jet is directed posteriorly within the left atrium rather than centrally. This information can be used to aid alignment of the continuous wave Doppler beam.

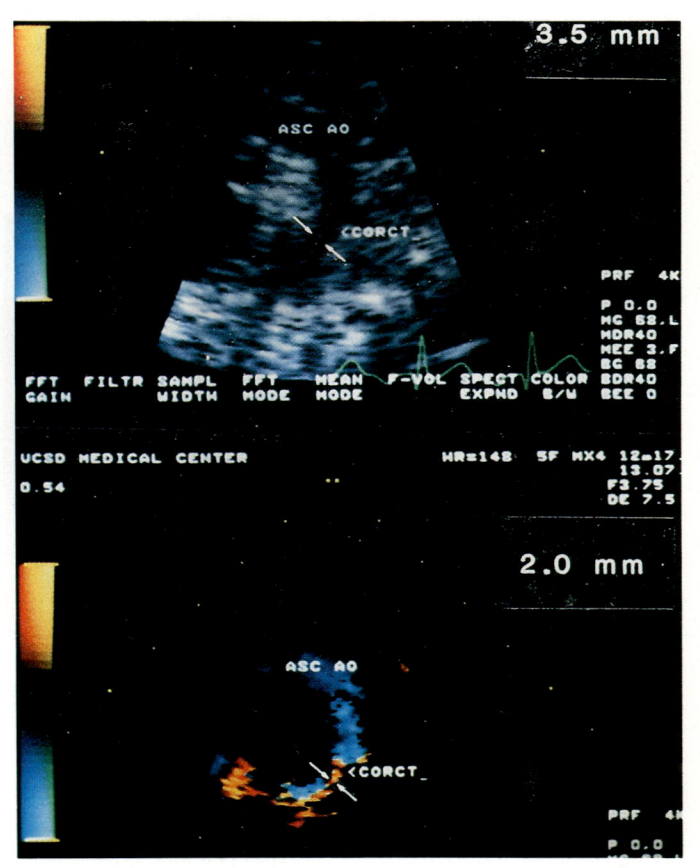

Ch. 4
Plate 10   Subcostal short axis view taken in systole showing systolic flow (in blue) in both the aortic root and the right ventricular outflow tract (compare Fig. 20).

Ch. 6
Plate 2   Two dimensional echo image (top) and colour Doppler flow map image (bottom) from a patient with coarctation of the aorta. The colour flow diameter was identical to that measured on magnetic resonance imaging and at surgery but two-dimensional imaging alone significantly underestimated the anatomical severity of the lesion. (Reproduced from Simpson et al. Circulation 1988; 77: 736–744, by permission of the American Heart Association.)

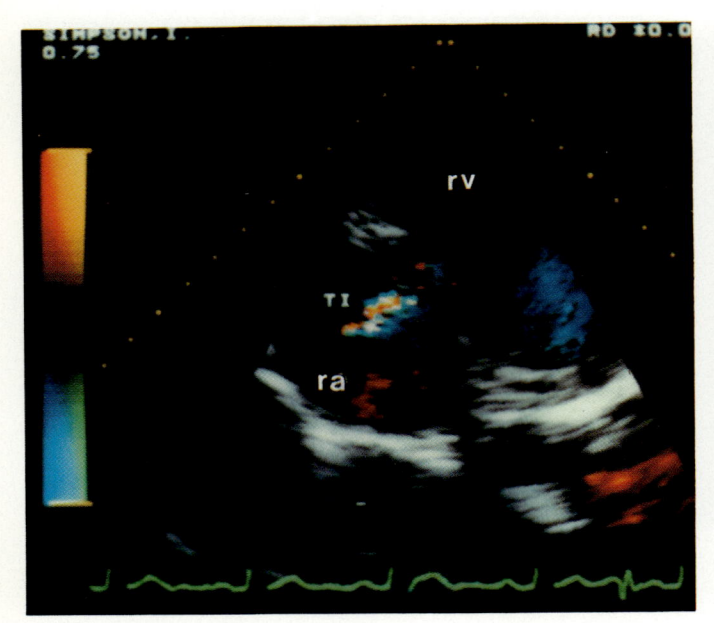

Ch. 6
Plate 3 Colour Doppler flow map image of the author's own physiological tricuspid regurgitation. Note the colour calibration bar at the left of the image with a Nyquist velocity limit for both red (towards) and blue (away) flow of 0.75 m/s (displayed above the colour bar).

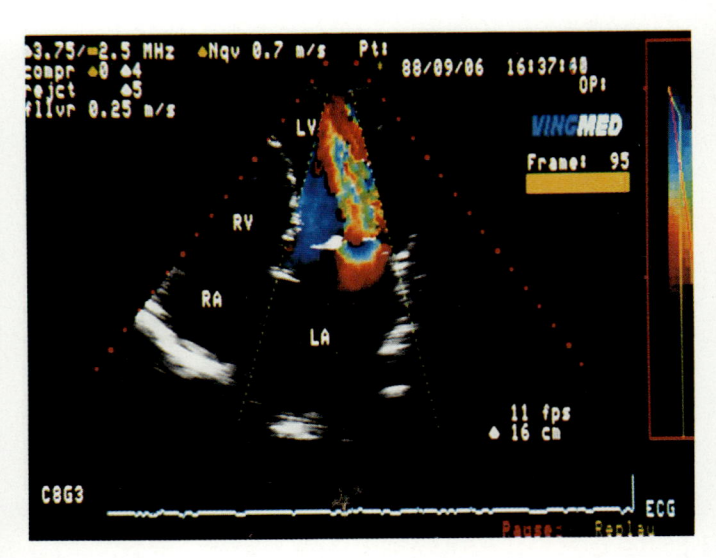

Ch. 6
Plate 5 Apical colour Doppler flow map image of mitral stenosis imaged using a velocity-variance colour flow map algorithm. Green is added to one side of the colour calibration bar such that high velocity, turbulent flow has green added to the red and blue velocity assignment. Distal to the mitral stenosis within the left ventricle, there is a considerable display of green rapidly identifying the presence and spatial distribution of abnormal flow. The region of acceleration towards the stenotic valve is clearly seen in the left atrium.

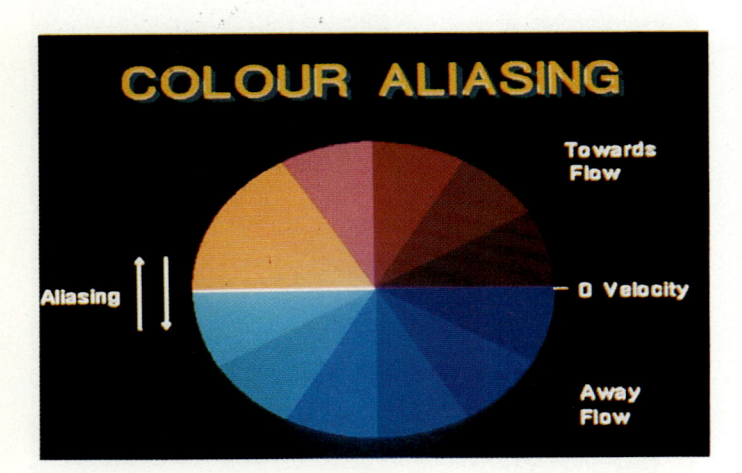

Ch. 6
Plate 4 Diagram to illustrate the effect of colour aliasing. As flow velocities away from the transducer (display as increasing colour intensities of blue) exceed the Nyquist velocity limit an alias to the highest red value will occur producing apparent directionally opposite colour encoding. Similarly flow towards the transducer which exceeds the maximum velocity limit will alias from increasing colours of red to the highest blue value with further velocity increases towards the transducer being displayed as decreasing colours of blue eventually aliasing again back to increasing colours of red.

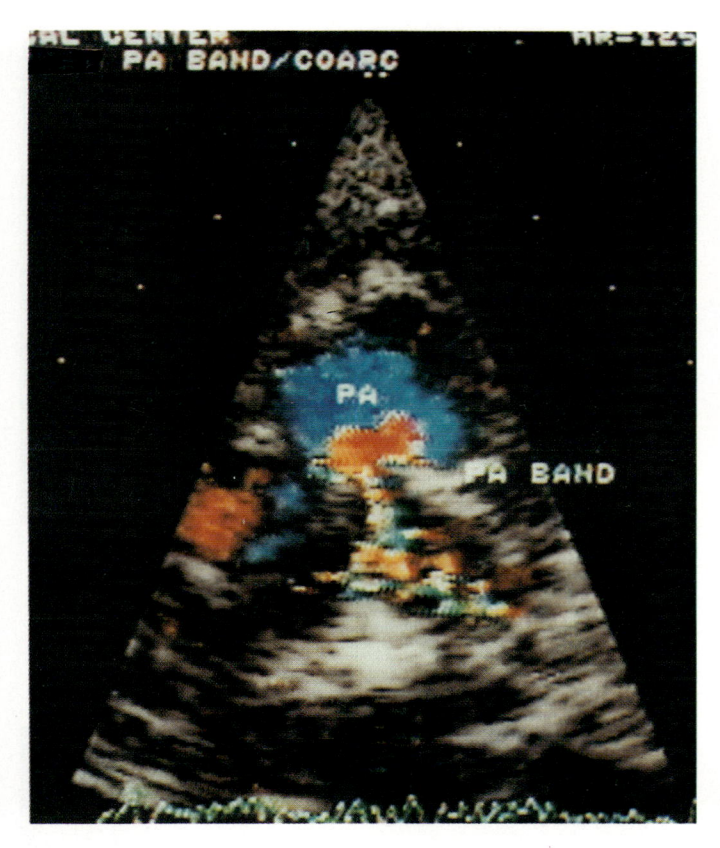

Ch. 6
Plate 6   Colour Doppler flow map image from a patient with a pulmonary artery band. As flow accelerates away from the transducer towards the band in the main pulmonary artery, this spatial acceleration is identified by a rational sequence of colour changes. Increasing colours of blue alias to the highest red value with decreasing values of red nearer the orifice indicating continued spatial acceleration. Distal to the obstruction a multi-colour mosaic pattern with high green values indicates the presence of high velocity, turbulent flow.

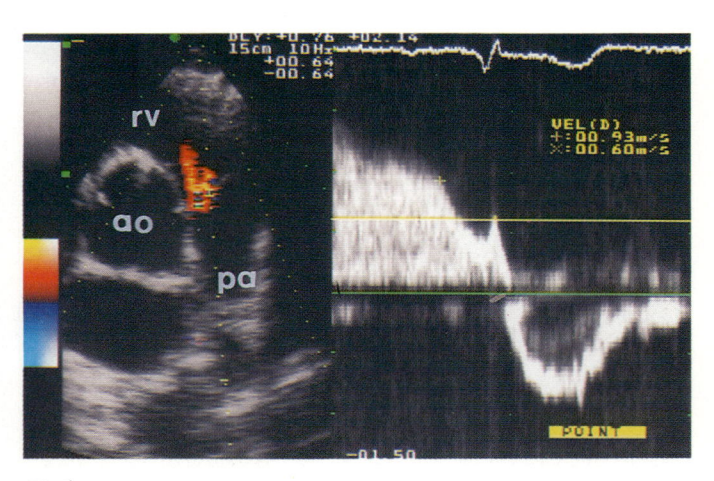

Ch. 7
Plate 1   Colour flow Doppler illustration of pulmonary regurgitation (left) with an accompanying pulsed Doppler recording from the left parasternal position.

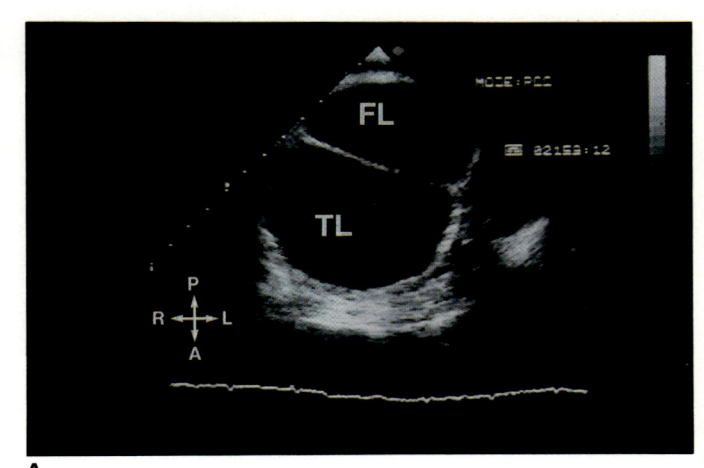

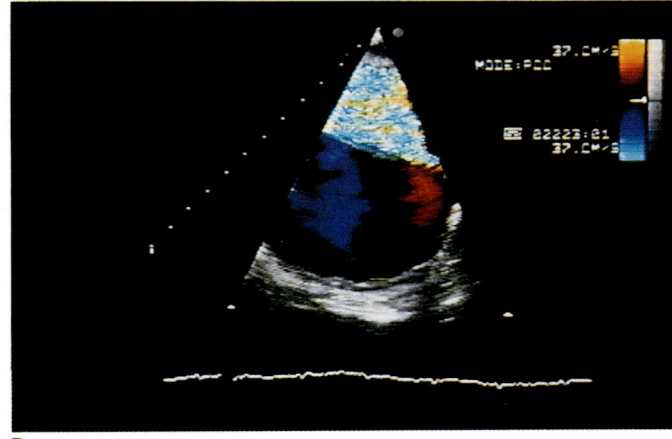

Ch. 9
Plate 1   A: True (TL) and false lumina (FL) are clearly identified in the ascending aorta in this case of Type I dissection. The transducer is directed anteriorly. **B:** Colour flow mapping shows a normal pattern of flow within the true lumen while a jet of turbulent flow is demonstrated in the false lumen.

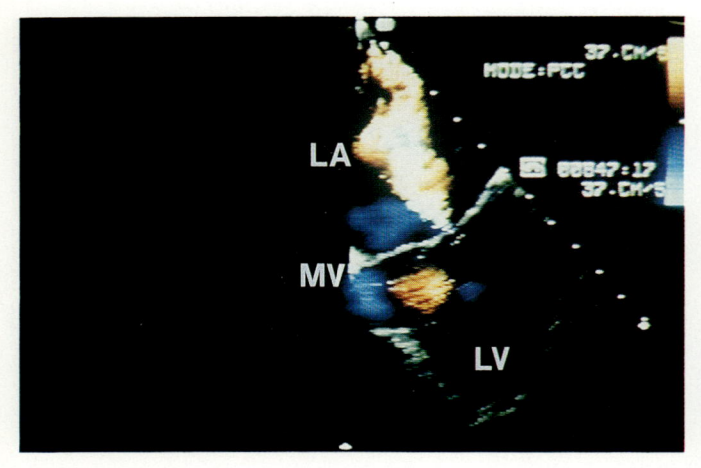

Ch. 9
Plate 2 Four chamber view. Colour flow mapping shows a 'candle flame' jet of regurgitation in an elderly subject with angiographically mild mitral regurgitation.

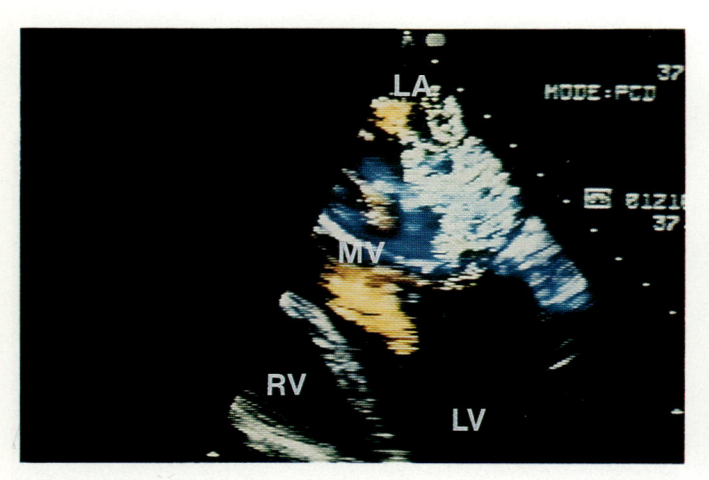

Ch. 10
Plate 1 Colour flow Doppler image of mitral stenosis from the apex showing turbulence and aliasing as the maximum velocity which can be recorded with colour flow Doppler examination is limited.

Ch. 9
Plate 3 Four chamber view. Mitral regurgitation in the presence of mitral valve prolapse. A widely based regurgitant flow jet is seen within the atrium and angiography confirmed the severity of regurgitation.

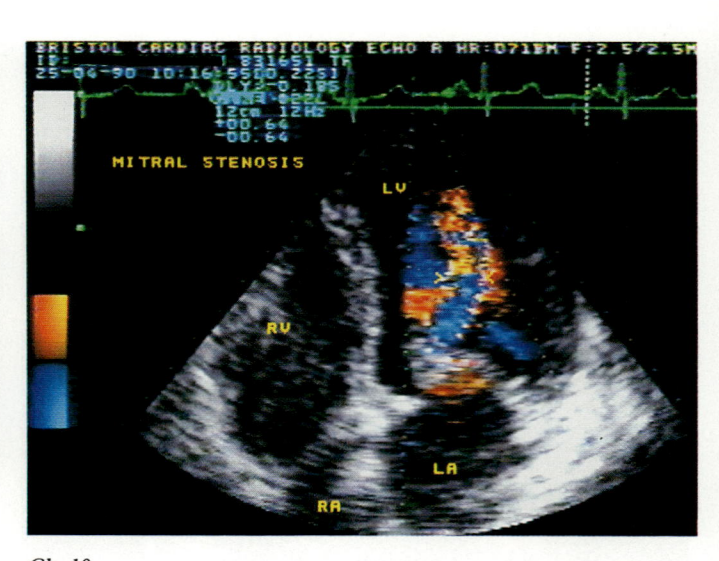

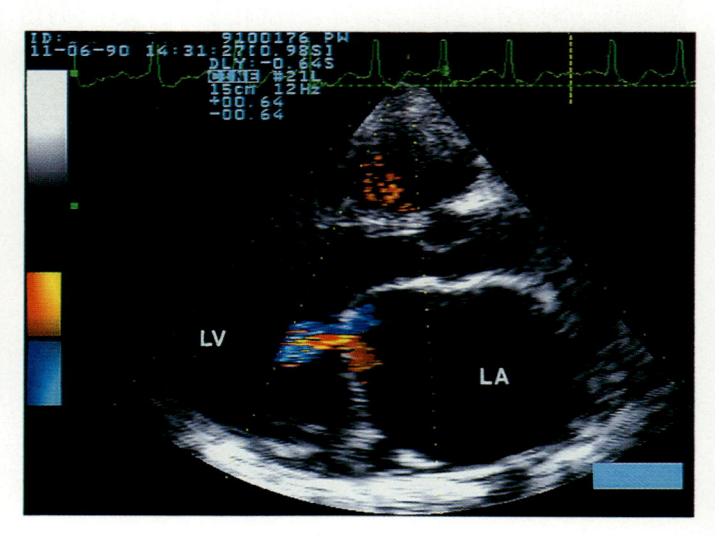

Ch. 10
Plate 2 Parasternal long axis view in a case of mitral stenosis. Colour flow mapping shows blood flow accelerating through the narrow orifice.

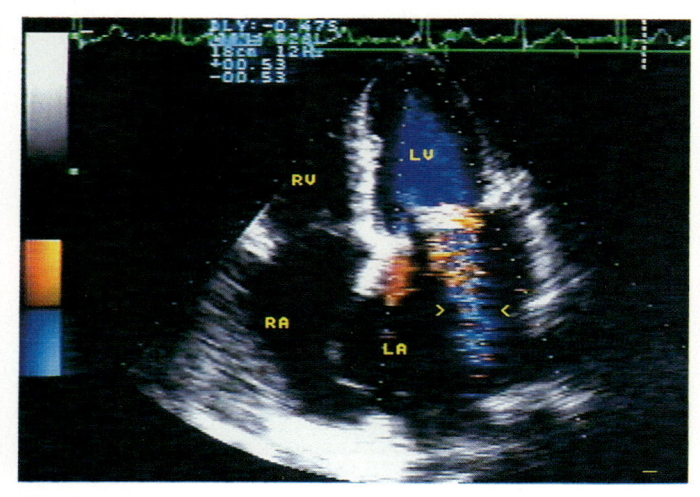

Ch. 10

Plate 3   Apical colour flow Doppler image of mitral regurgitation showing a blue jet (arrowed) away from the probe within the left atrium. There is aliasing and a mosaic pattern within the jet.

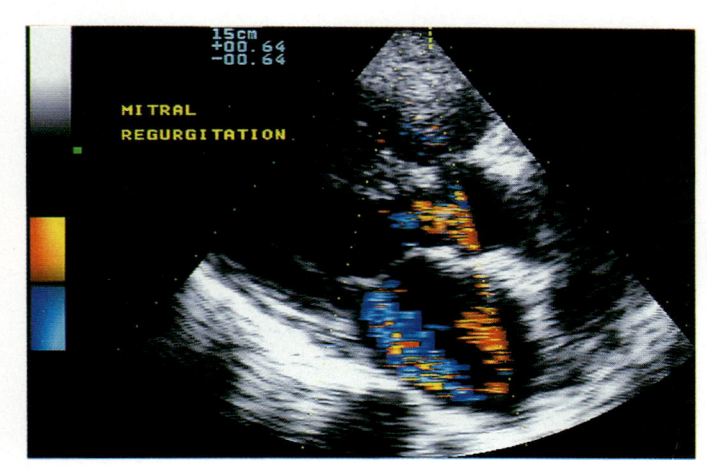

Ch. 10

Plate 4   Long axis left parasternal view showing mitral regurgitation as a blue jet into the left atrium. There is aliasing and a mosaic pattern in the jet.

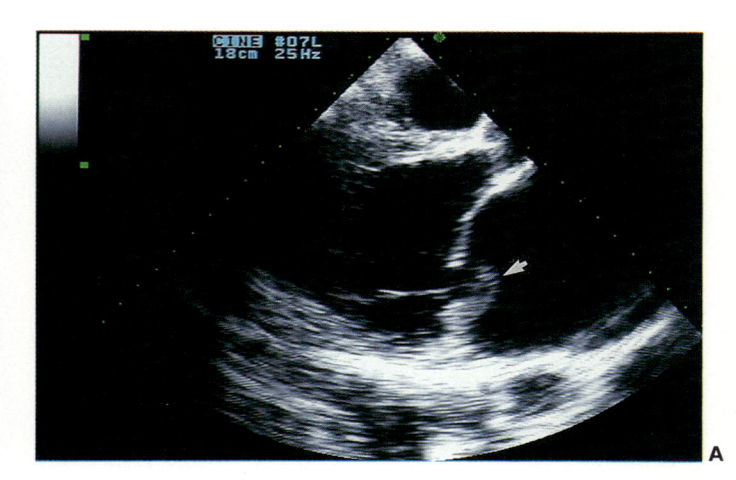

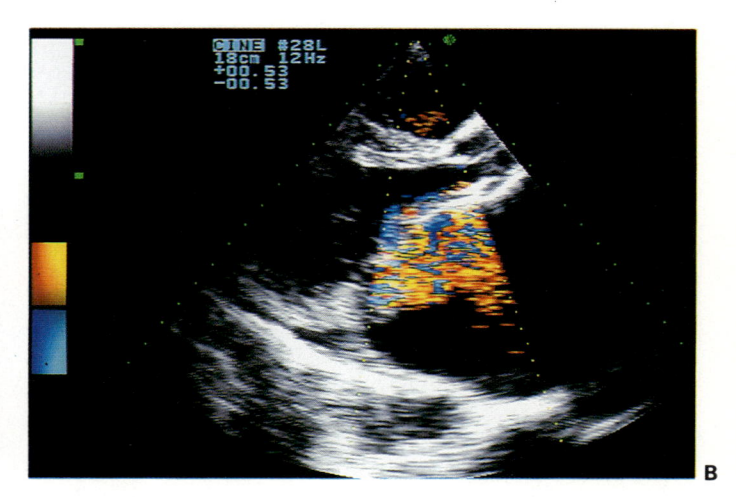

Ch. 10

Plate 5   A: Parasternal long axis view showing prolapse of the posterior mitral leaflet arrowed. **B:** Colour flow image simultaneously with **A** showing an intense mosaic jet of mitral regurgitation directed superiorly in the left atrium.

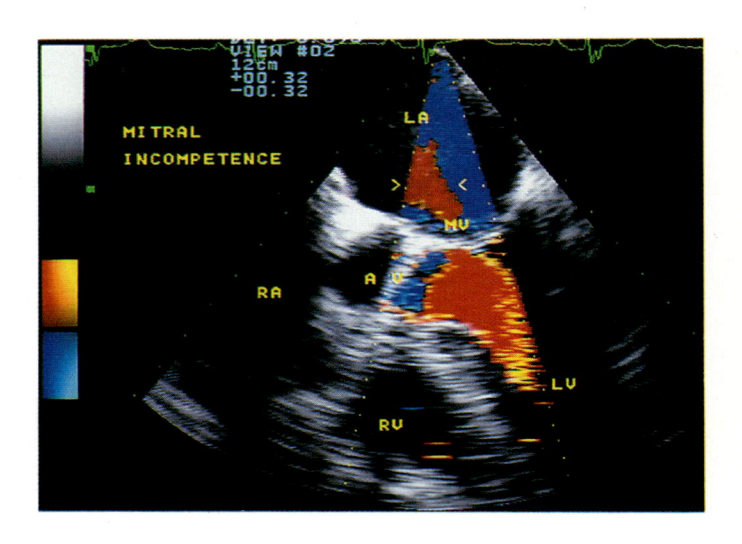

Ch. 10

Plate 6   Trans-oesophageal colour flow echocardiogram of mitral regurgitation showing a red jet (arrowed) extending posteriorly from the mitral valve into the left atrium towards the probe in the oesophagus. There is also an intense red signal in the left ventricular outflow tract indicating normal flow towards the mitral valve.

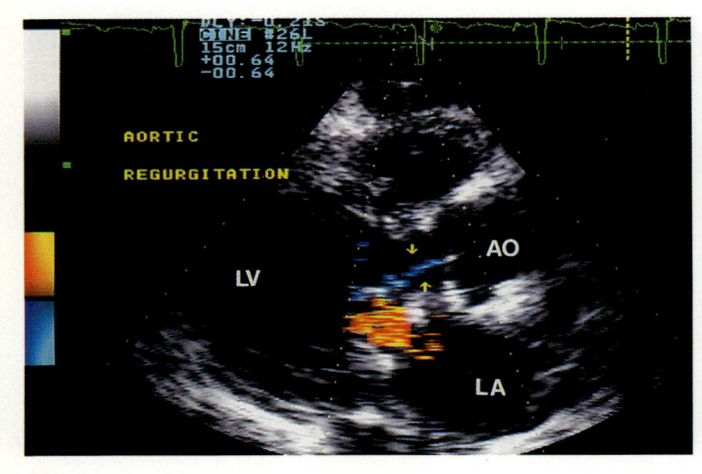

Ch. 10
Plate 7 Parasternal long axis view with colour flow Doppler mapping showing a tiny physiological jet of aortic regurgitation (arrowed).

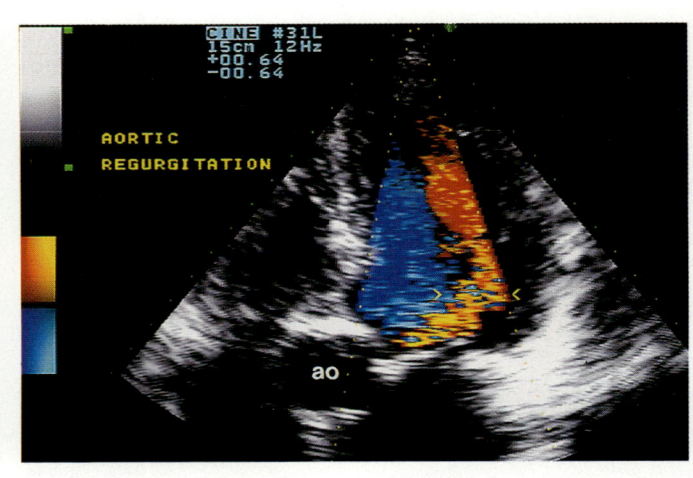

Ch. 10
Plate 9 Apical colour flow Doppler image of aortic regurgitation. In this apical four chamber view the regurgitant jet is red towards the probe but shows aliasing and a mosaic pattern.

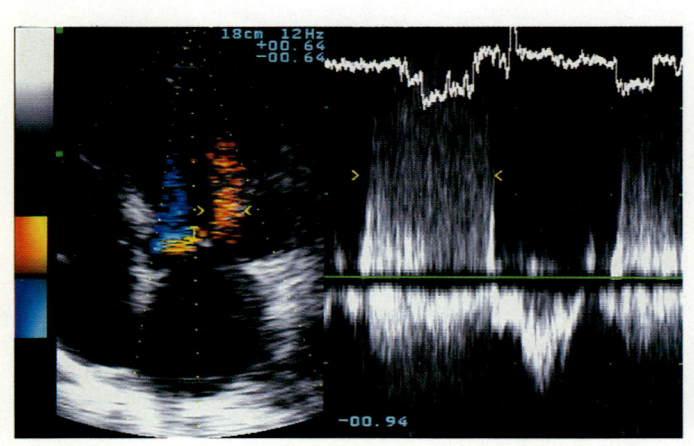

Ch. 10
Plate 8 Pulsed Doppler trace of aortic regurgitation (right) with accompanying colour flow image (left). The cursor is placed in the left ventricular outflow tract and mapping of the regurgitant jet can be performed by tracing the cursor back into the left ventricle.

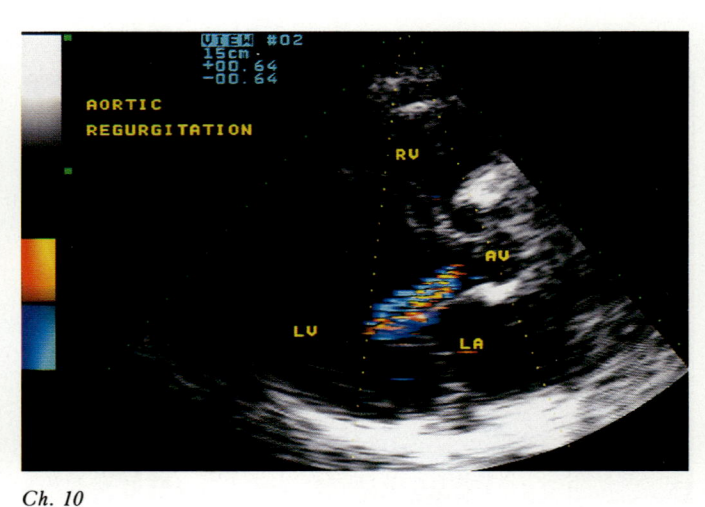

Ch. 10
Plate 10 Left parasternal long axis view showing aortic regurgitation as an aliasing blue jet directed towards the anterior mitral leaflet.

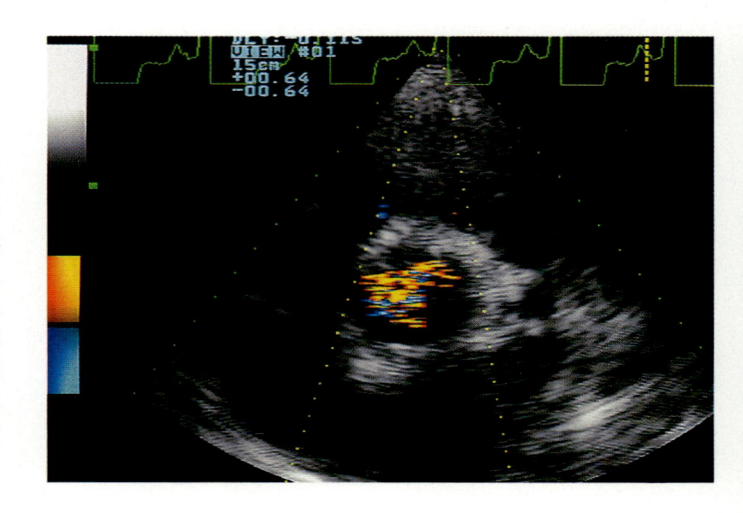

Ch. 10
Plate 11 Parasternal short axis colour flow image showing a moderately large jet of aortic regurgitation in the left ventricular outflow tract.

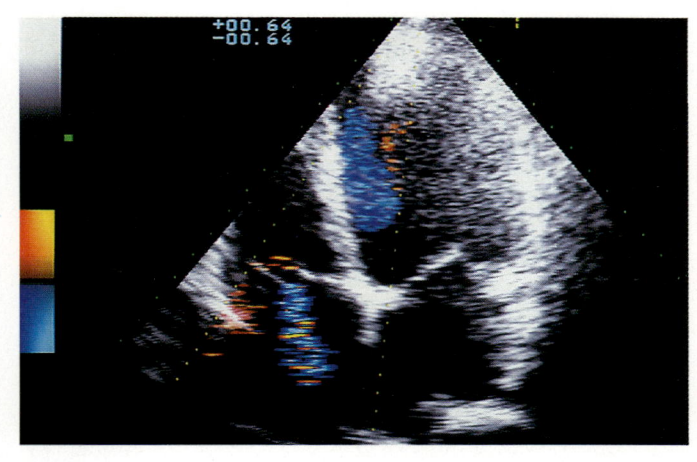

Ch. 10
Plate 12 Colour flow Doppler image of tricuspid regurgitation showing a blue jet in the right atrium in this apical four chamber view.

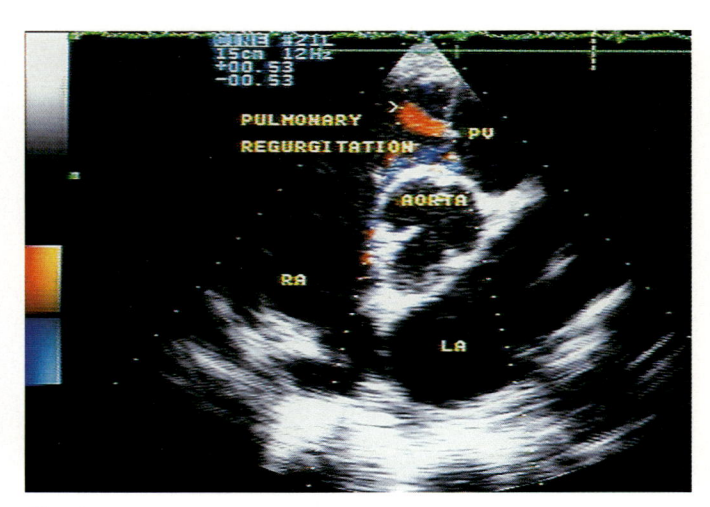

Ch. 10
Plate 15 Colour flow Doppler image of mild pulmonary regurgitation seen as a 'red flame' in this left parasternal short axis view.

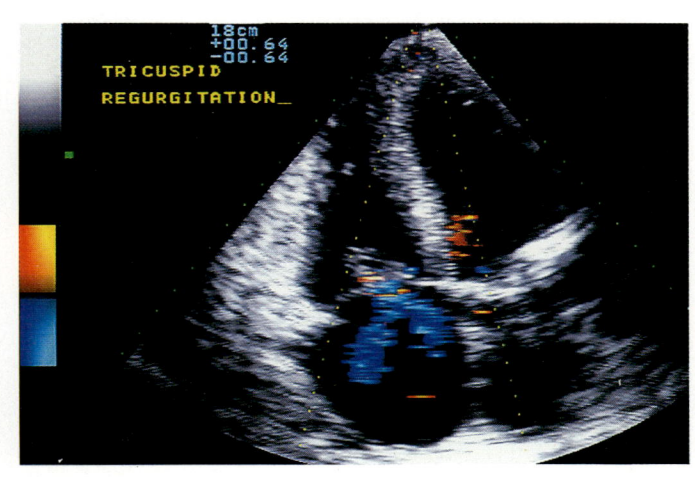

Ch. 10
Plate 13 Colour flow Doppler image of tricuspid regurgitation from the apical four chamber window. In this case the jet is in two distinct and divergent streams.

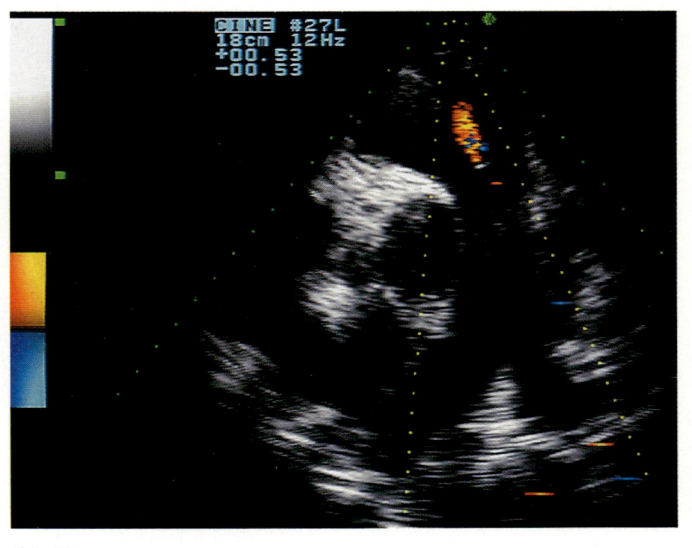

Ch. 10
Plate 16 Modified left parasternal view showing the main pulmonary artery and its bifurcation. Pulmonary regurgitation is seen as a red jet.

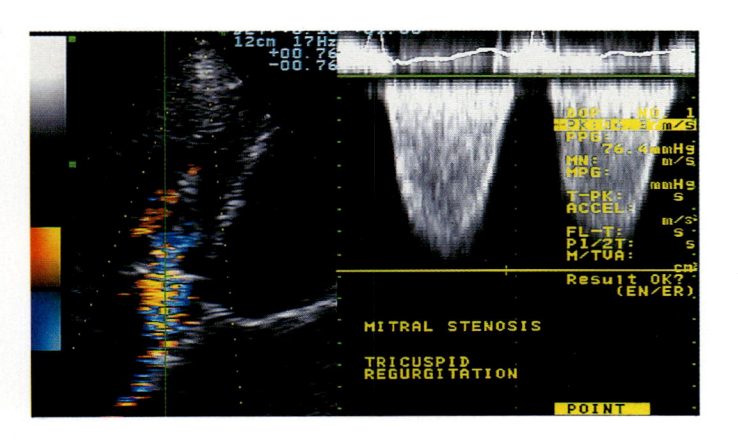

Ch. 10
Plate 14 Apical colour flow image (left) in a patient with tricuspid regurgitation secondary to mitral stenosis. The colour flow jet has been used to direct a continuous wave beam. The spectral trace (right) shows a calculated peak jet velocity of 4.3 m/s (peak pressure drop of 76.4 mmHg).

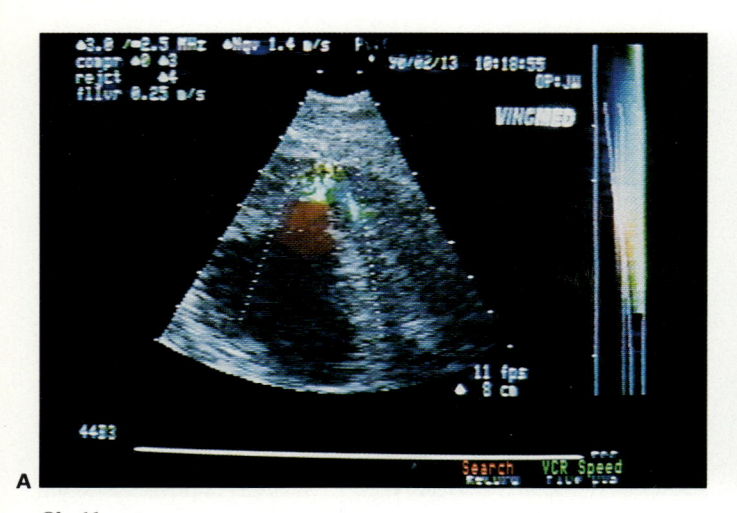

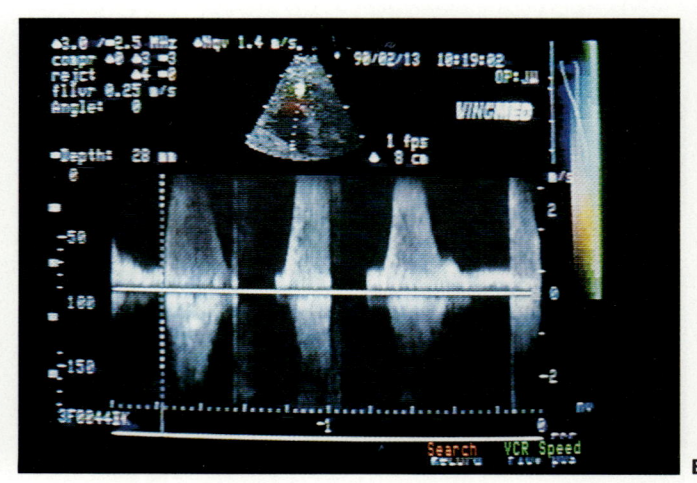

Ch. 11
Plate 1 **A: VSD colour Doppler signal from apex of right ventricle** through the distal inter-ventricular septum. **B:** Pulsed Doppler signal from apex of right ventricle in the same patient.

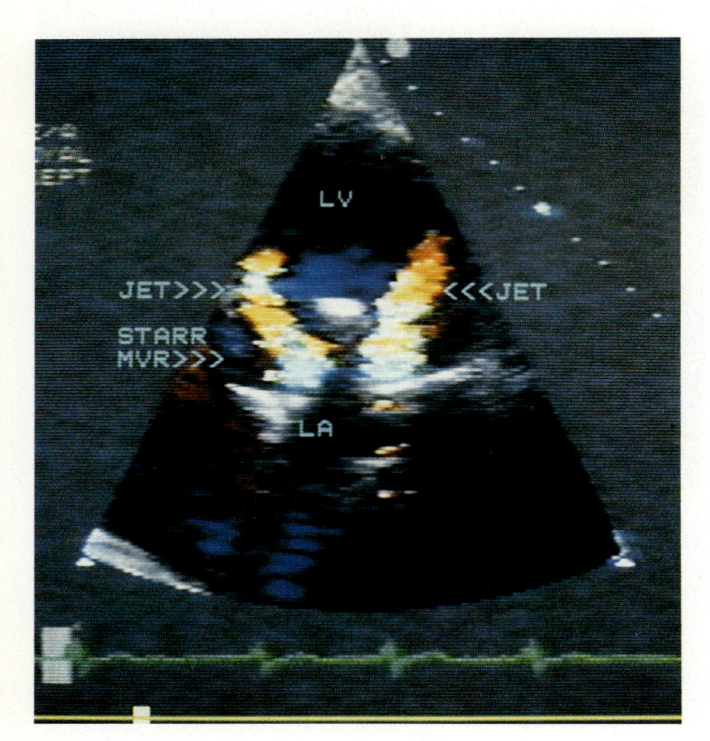

Ch. 14
Plate 1 **Doppler colour flow mapping** superimposed on the cross-sectional echocardiographic image shown in Fig. 16. This frame in early diastole demonstrates the two characteristic jets of turbulent flow at the edge of the Starr–Edwards prosthesis (MVR).

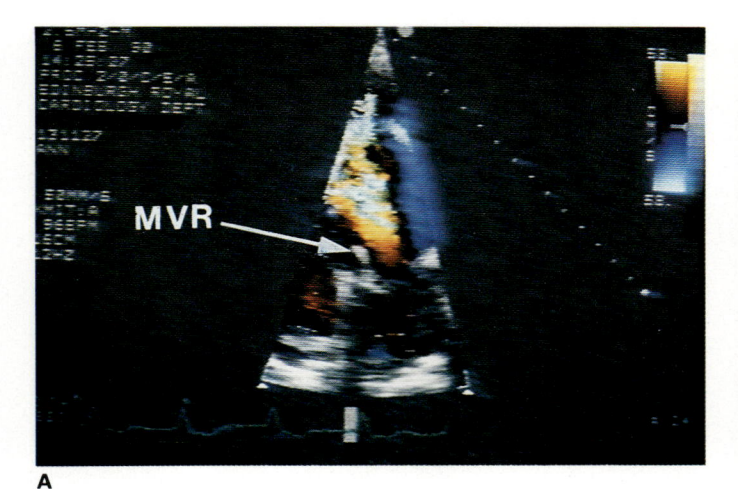

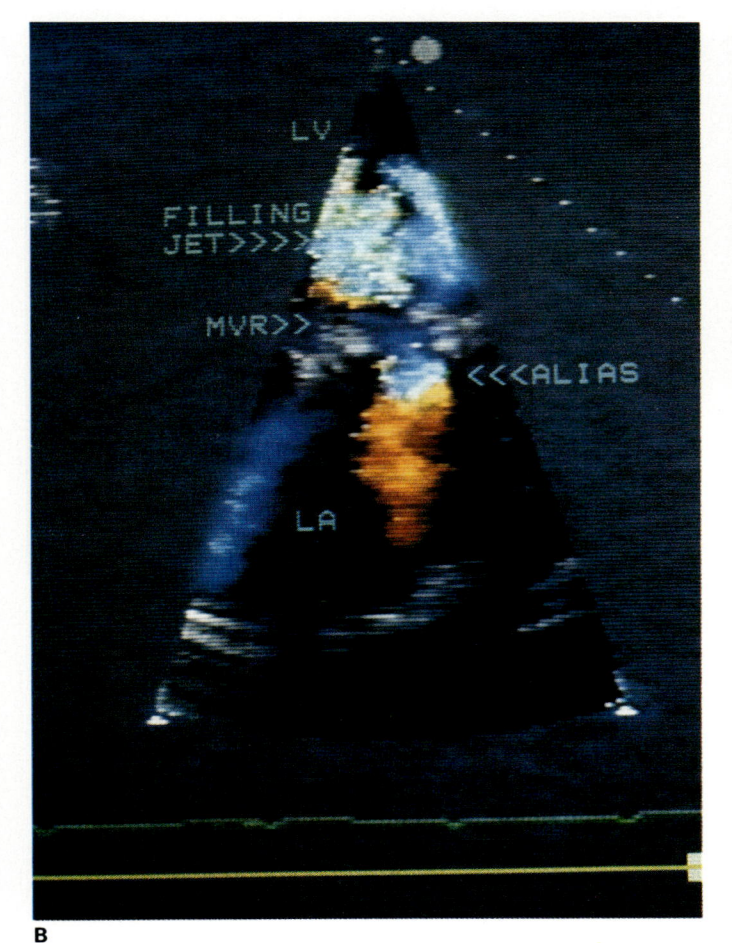

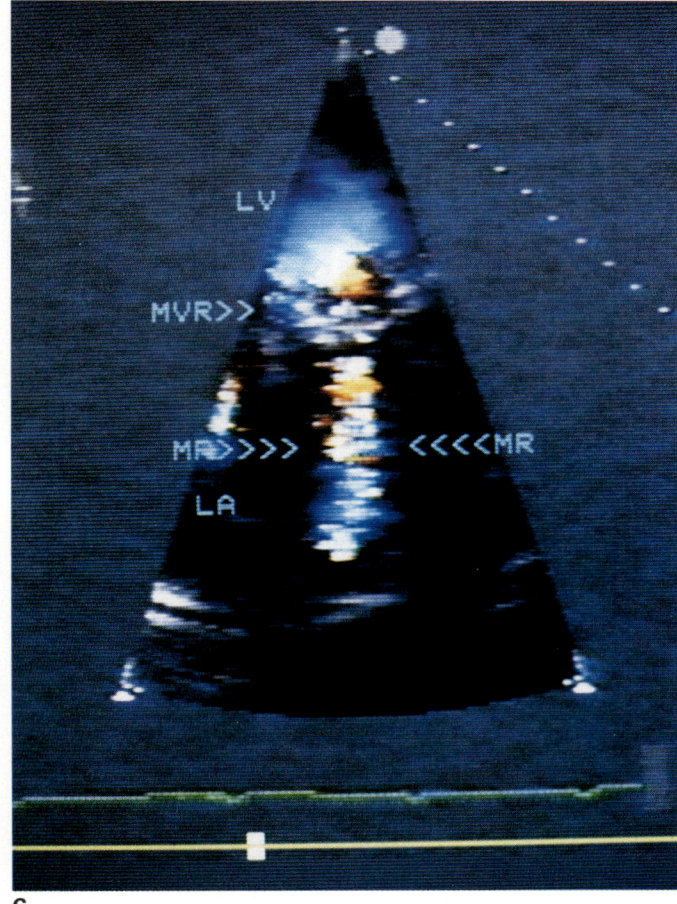

Ch. 14
Plate 2 **A: Doppler colour flow mapping** superimposed on the cross-sectional echocardiographic image shown in Fig. 17. This frame in diastole shows turbulent flow through the centre of the prosthesis (MVR) directed towards the intraventricular septum because of the angle at which the prosthesis lies. **B:** Doppler colour flow mapping from the same patient as in A showing that the valve is also relatively stenotic and the colour aliases from red to blue within the left atrium as blood accelerates from the left atrium towards the prosthesis. **C:** Doppler colour flow mapping superimposed on the cross-sectional echocardiographic image shown in Fig. 17. This frame in systole shows a turbulent mosaic of flow (jet) directed through the centre of the regurgitant prosthetic valve (MVR) in systole filling half of the left atrium.

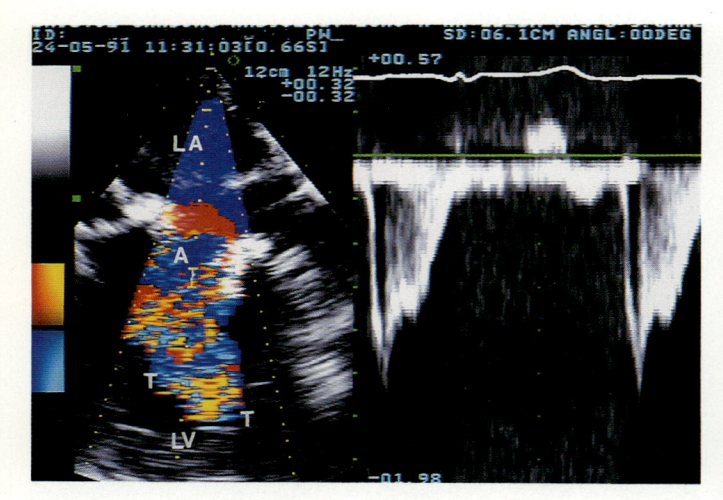

Ch. 14

Plate 3 Colour flow and pulsed Doppler examination of the same prosthetic valve shown in Fig. 21. Diastolic high velocity colour flow with central blue aliasing (A) and turbulent dissipation of the jet in the left ventricle (T) are clearly seen within the colour sector. The pulsed Doppler recording of the same flow is shown on the right, the sample volume lying in the central blue aliased flow.

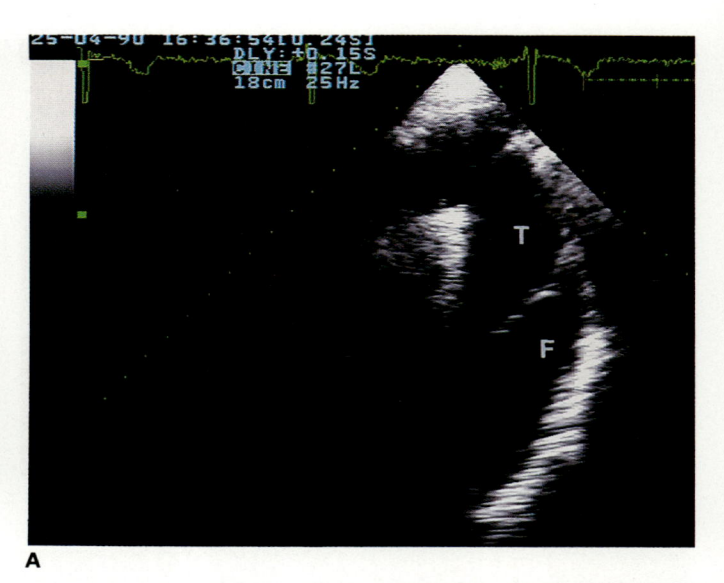

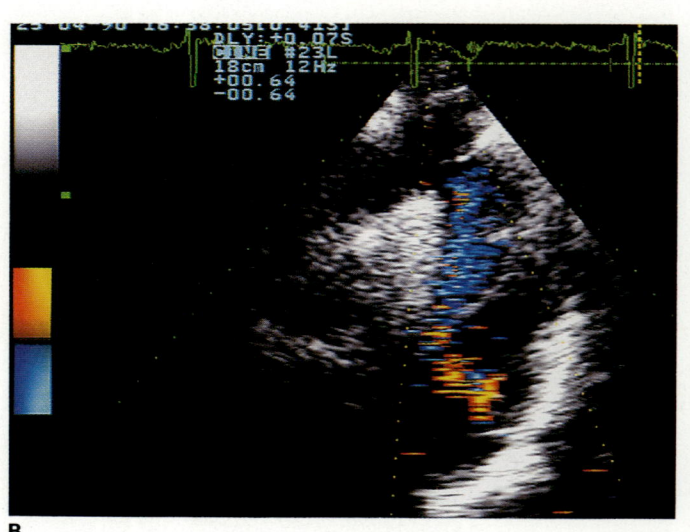

Ch. 17

Plate 1 A: Suprasternal view of the aortic arch and descending aorta showing an oblique dissection flap in a patient with type B aortic dissection. T – true lumen; F – false lumen. **B:** Colour flow image in the same section as A. The flow in the true lumen (blue, away from the transducer) is seen to alias as it passes through a tear into the false lumen.

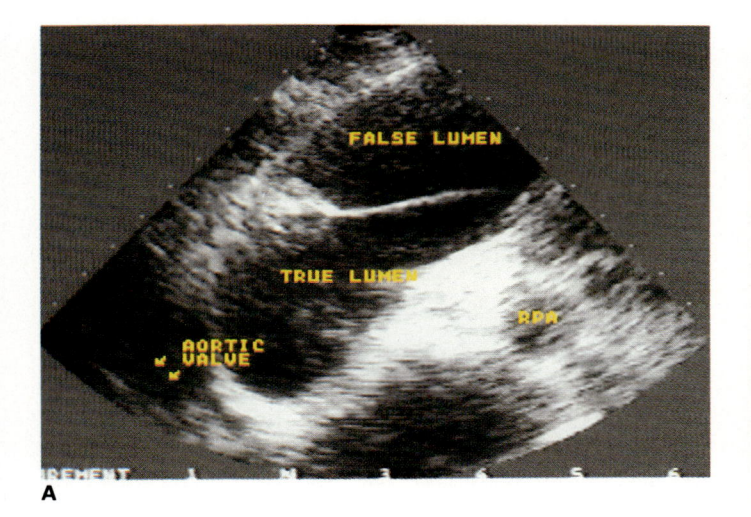

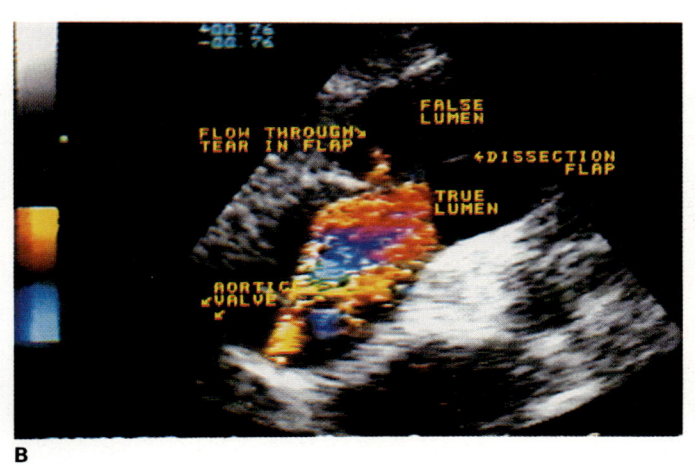

Ch. 17
Plate 2 A: Modified right parasternal view of a dissection flap in the ascending aorta. **B:** Colour flow imaging of the same section showing flow in the true lumen (with central aliasing) passing through a small tear into the false lumen.

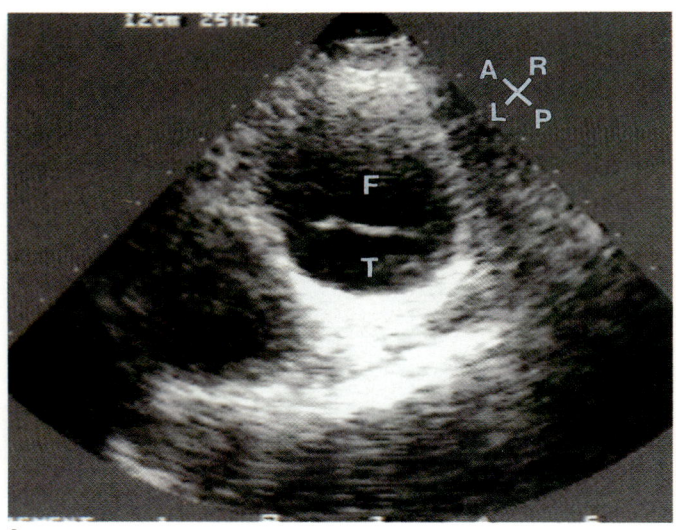

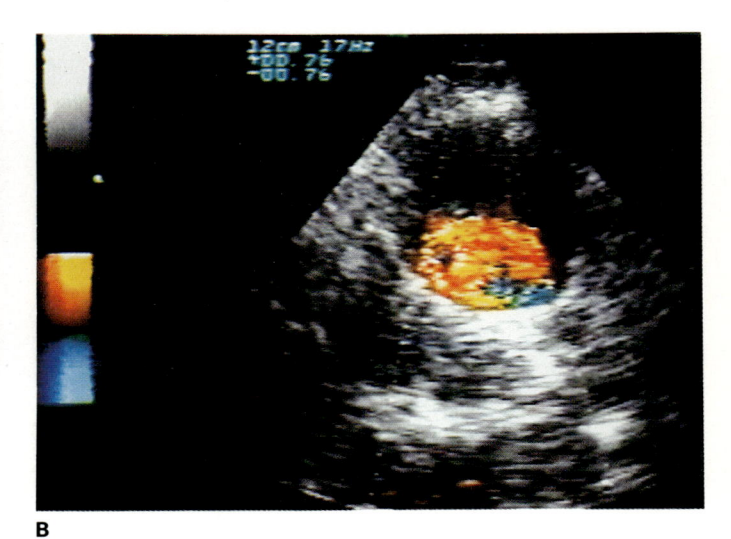

Ch. 17
Plate 3 A: Transoesophageal image of the descending aorta showing a dissection flap separating the true lumen (T) from the false lumen (F). **B:** Colour flow image of the same section as **A** showing flow in the true lumen and no detectable flow in the false lumen.

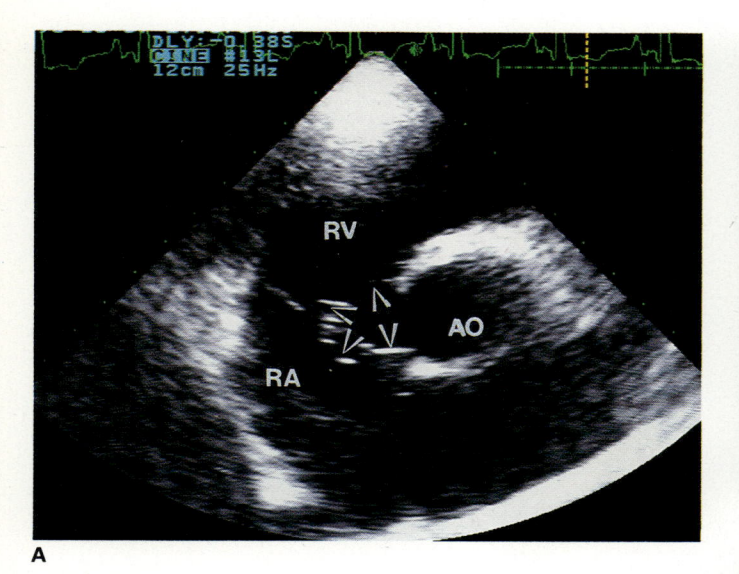

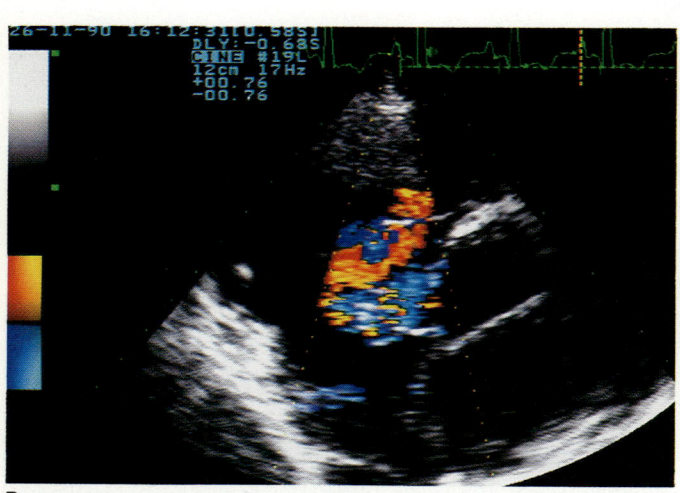

Ch. 17

Plate 4 A: **Ruptured sinus of Valsalva aneurysm** (arrowed) seen from a modified parasternal short axis view. B: Colour flow image of the same section as Figure 11A showing turbulent flow through the ruptured sinus of Valsalva aneurysm from aortic root to right ventricle.

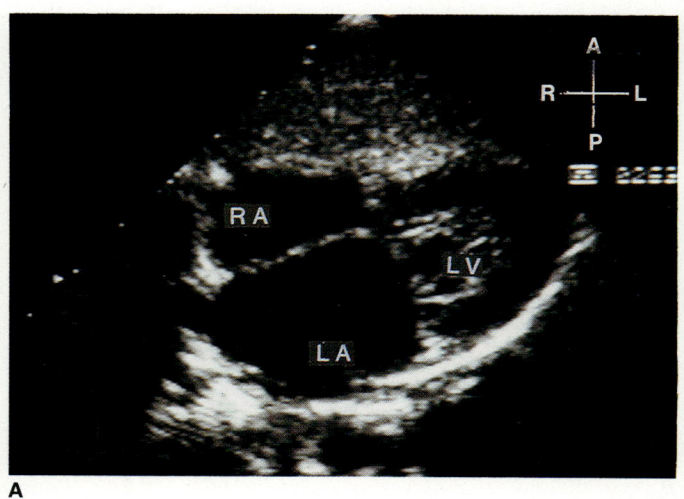

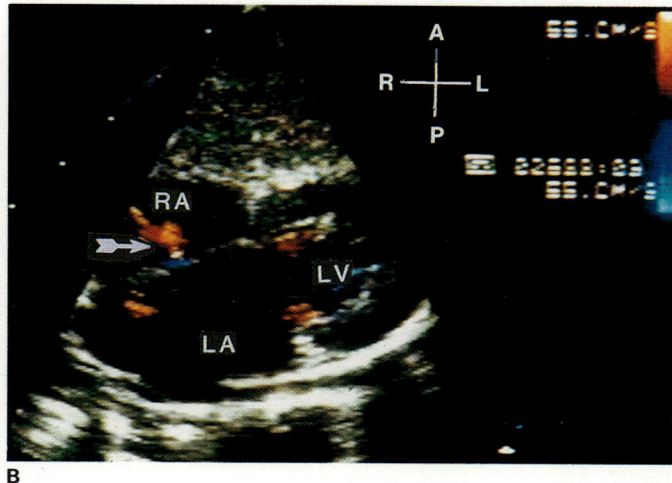

Ch. 20

Plate 1 A: **The normal neonatal atrial septum appears thin but intact on cross-sectional echocardiography.** B: However, colour flow mapping will show a small left to right shunt (arrowed) across the foramen in a high percentage of normal babies and should be regarded as a normal finding.

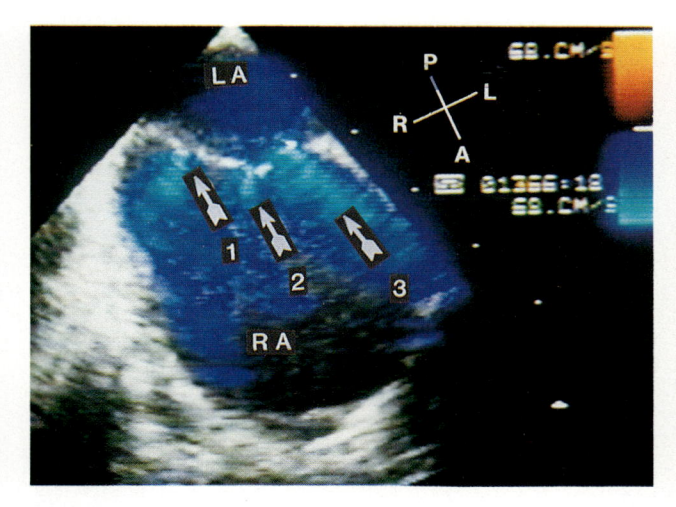

Ch. 20
Plate 2 Multiple tiny holes are present in the oval fossa. The septum appears to be intact even with transoesophageal imaging, colour flow Doppler mapping is required to demonstrate the multiple jets across the septum (arrowed).

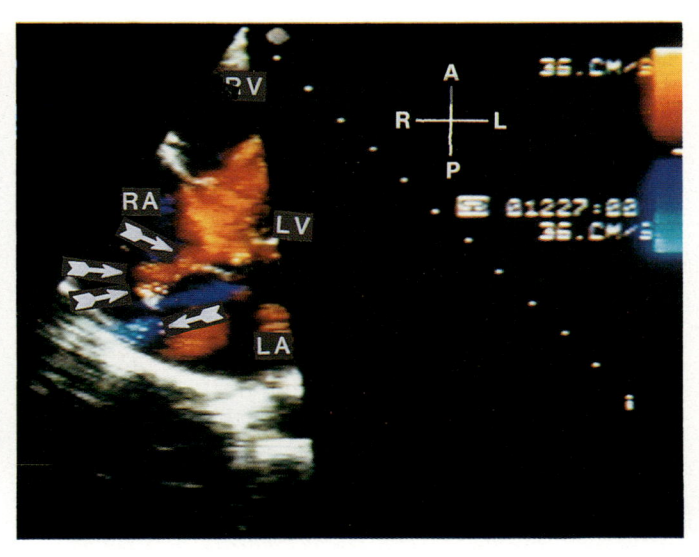

Ch. 20
Plate 3 The same case as shown in Fig. 8. Colour flow Doppler mapping clearly reveals the presence of multiple fenestrations with left to right shunting in multiple jets (arrowed).

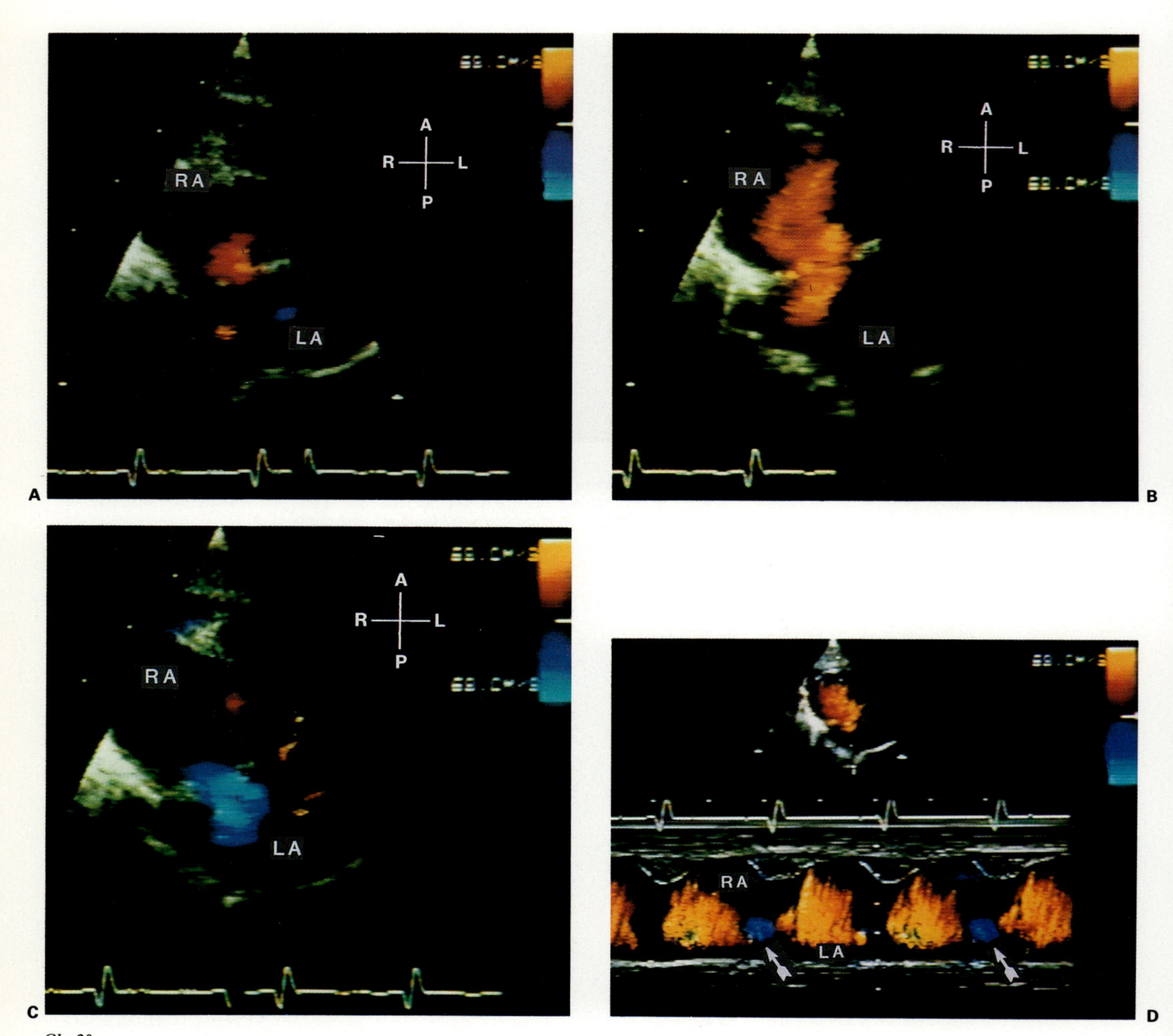

Ch. 20
Plate 4 Frame by frame analysis of colour flow Doppler mapping reveals that patterns of interatrial shunting may be complex even in the presence of a straightforward oval fossa defect, when shunting is often bidirectional but predominantly from left to right. The shunt haemodynamics vary with both the stage of the cardiac cycle and the stage of respiration. In early diastole (on the T wave of the electrocardiogram) there is usually a small left to right shunt **A**, which increases during the phases of ventricular filling **B**. **C**: At the onset of systole, however, the shunt direction in this patient can be seen to change from left to right to right to left. The timing of the changes in flow direction is best appreciated using colour flow M-mode Doppler examination **D**. Shunt reversal is shown by a change in colour of the trans septal flow from orange to blue (arrowed).

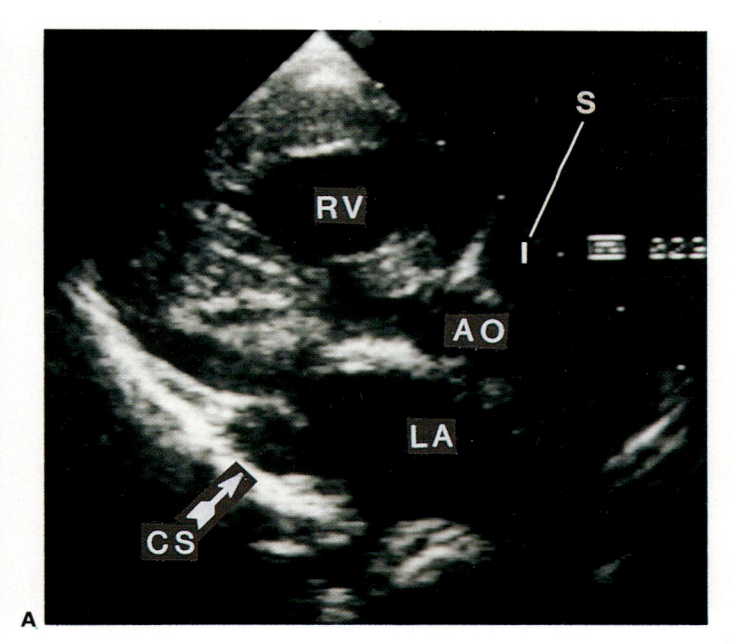

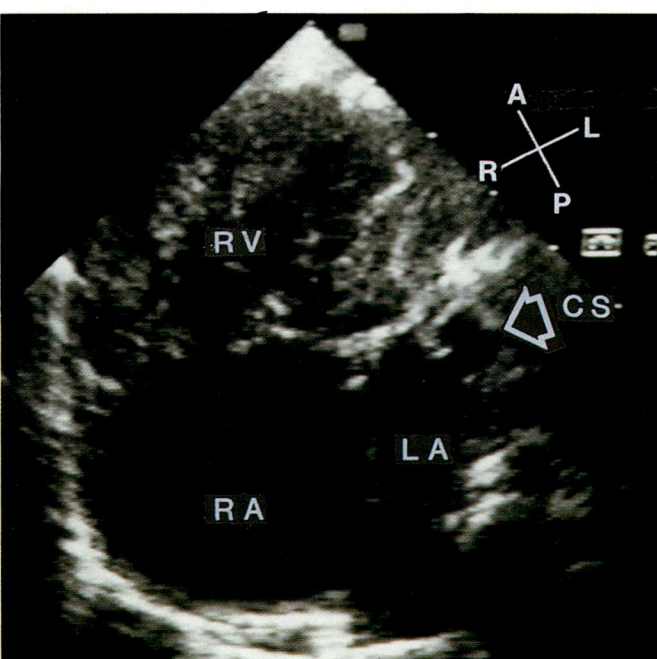

Ch. 20

Plate 5 **A: Parasternal long axis view of a coronary sinus defect.** The dilated coronary sinus (arrowed) is seen to communicate with the left atrium. **B:** Colour flow mapping shows turbulent flow (arrowed) within the coronary sinus (the patient also has mitral atresia, the coronary sinus defect being the only escape route from the left atrium). **C:** The dilated coronary sinus (arrowed) and its communication with the left atrium is also seen in an apical four chamber view. **D:** In this view colour flow mapping shows blood streaming (small arrows) from the left atrium into the coronary sinus, where the flow becomes turbulent (large arrow). There is also a jet of tricuspid regurgitation. **E:** Posterior angulation of the transducer allows visualisation of the coronary sinus draining into the right atrium (flow in blue) and thence through the tricuspid valve to the right ventricle (flow in orange).

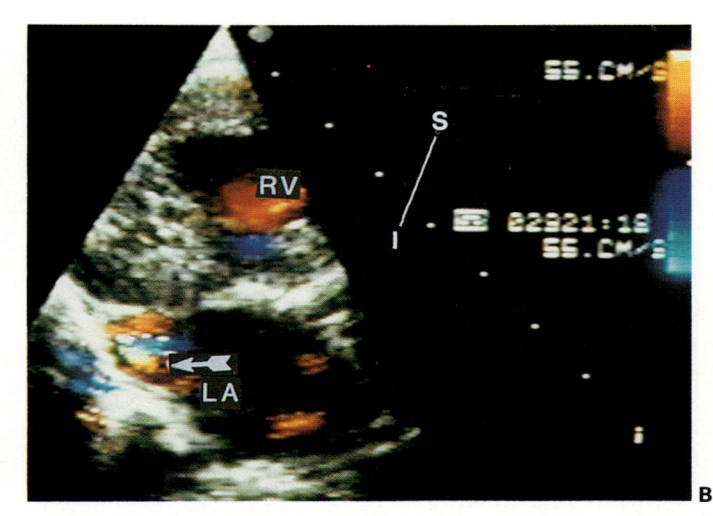

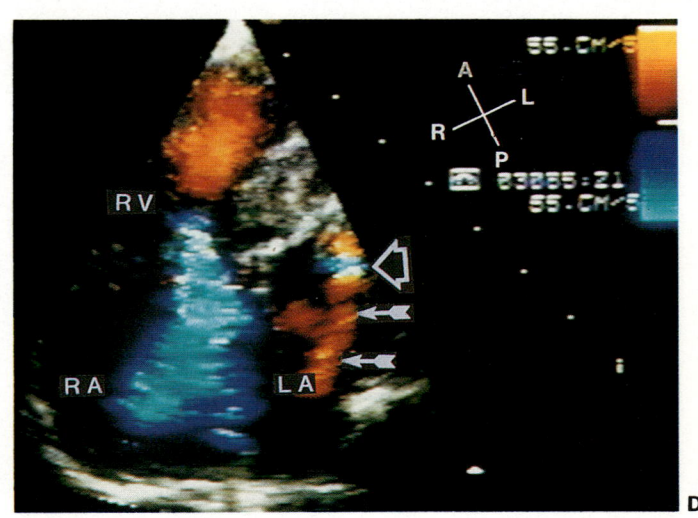

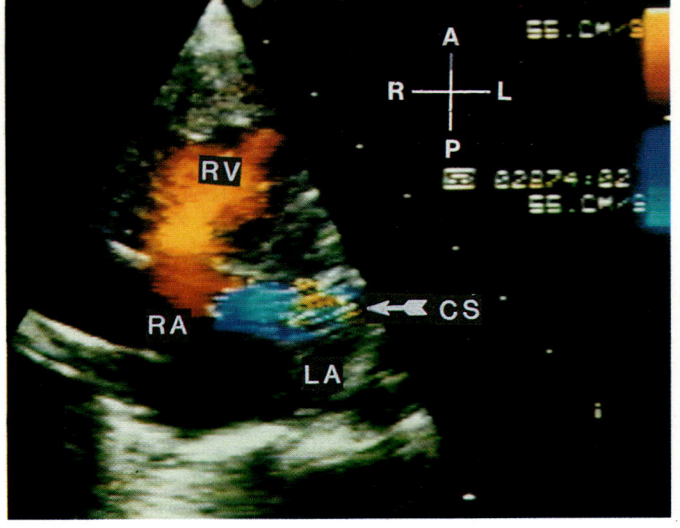

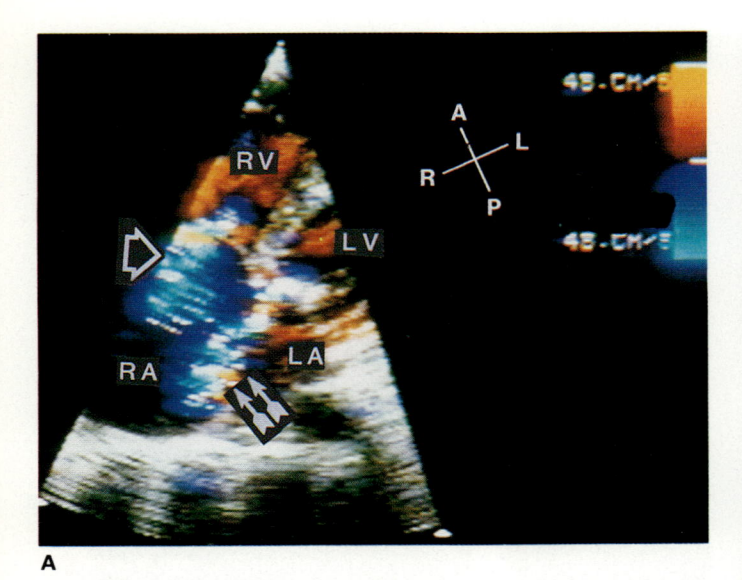

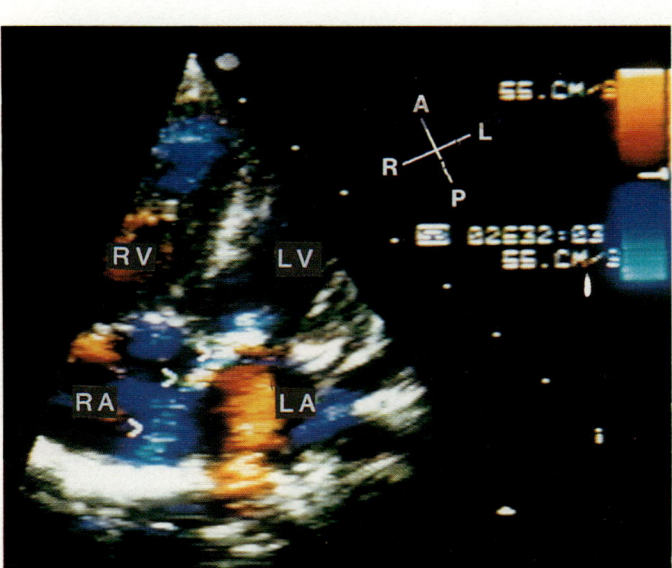

Ch. 20
Plate 6 Both left and right sided atrioventricular valve regurgitation are common with atrioventricular septal defects. **A:** In colour flow Doppler mapping, an apical view shows jets of regurgitation into both the left atrium (small arrows) and the right atrium (large arrow).
B: There is a left sided regurgitant jet which is directed across the atrial septum into the right atrium. This finding is often associated with a very large atrial shunt (effectively a left ventricular to right atrial shunt), along with particularly marked echocardiographic changes of right ventricular volume overload.

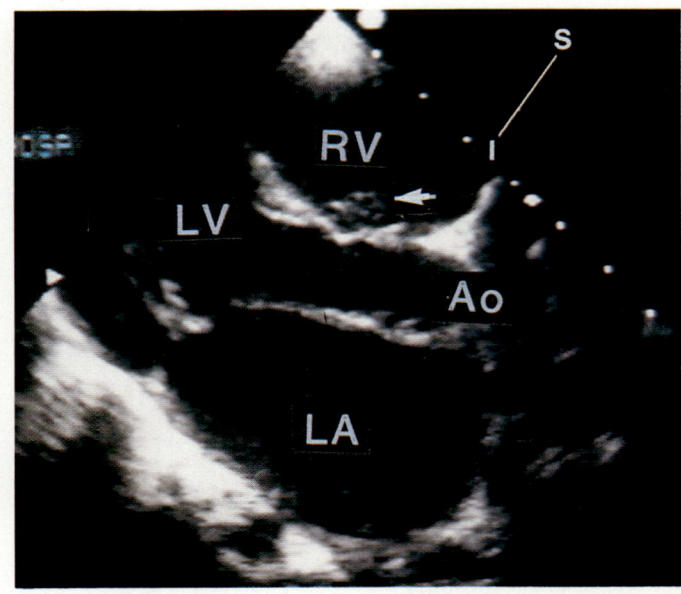

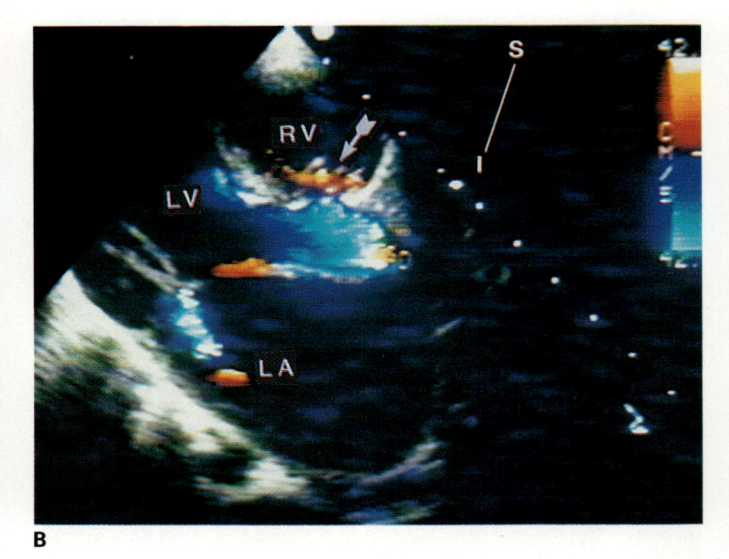

Ch. 20
Plate 7 **A:** A perimembranous defect seen in long axis left parasternal view. The defect appears to be completely closed by aneurysm formation. **B:** Colour flow Doppler mapping however shows a persistent left to right shunt across the defect (arrowed) as well as a jet of mitral regurgitation into the left atrium.

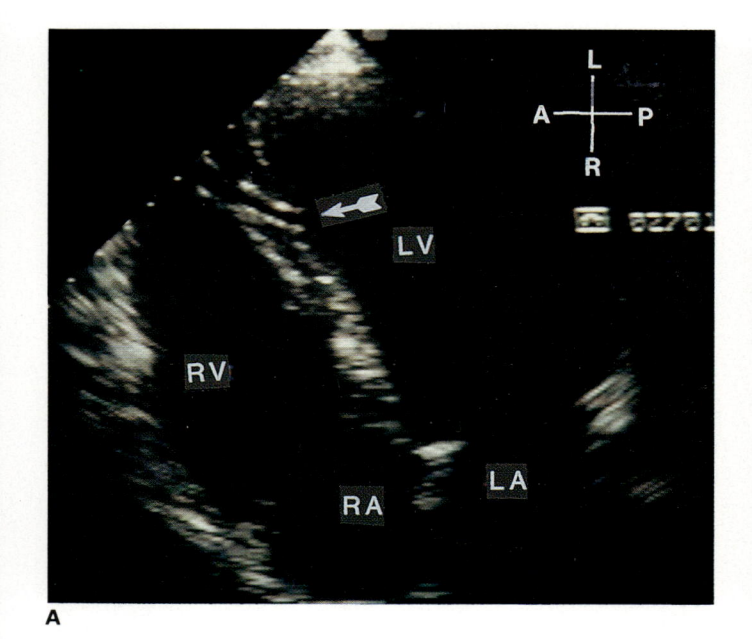

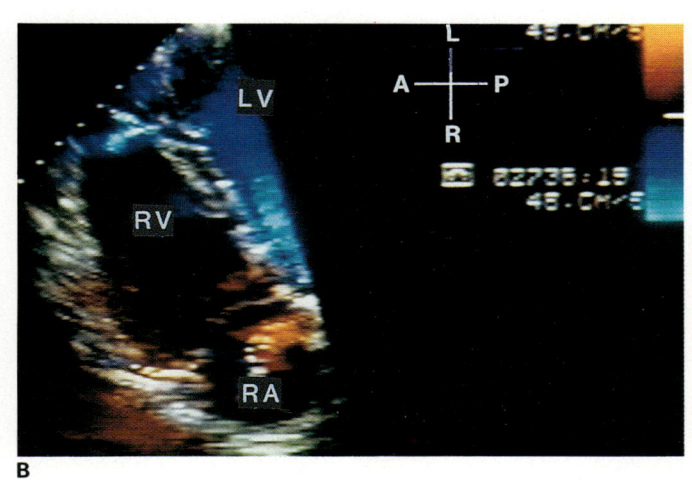

Ch. 20
Plate 8 A: An oblique muscular apical defect seen from an apical four chamber view. B: Left to right shunting across the defect is confirmed by colour flow Doppler mapping.

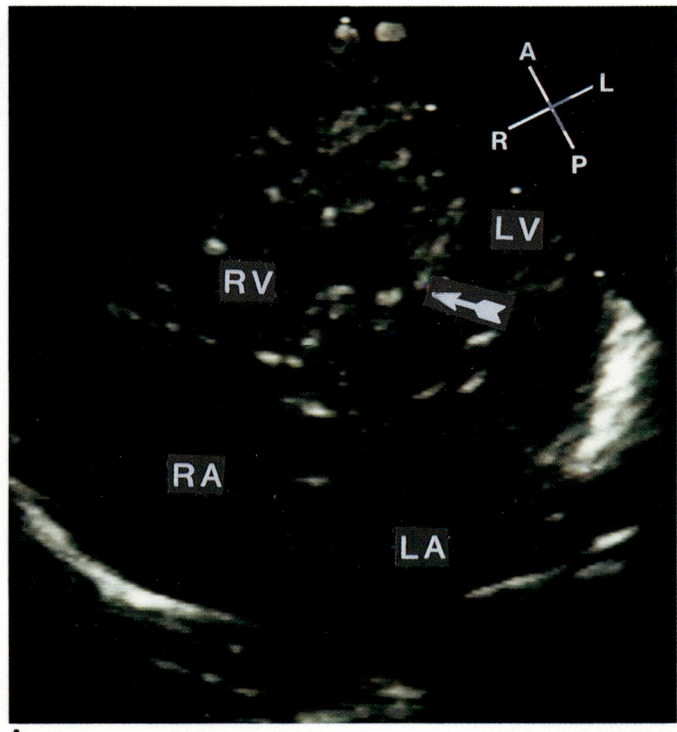

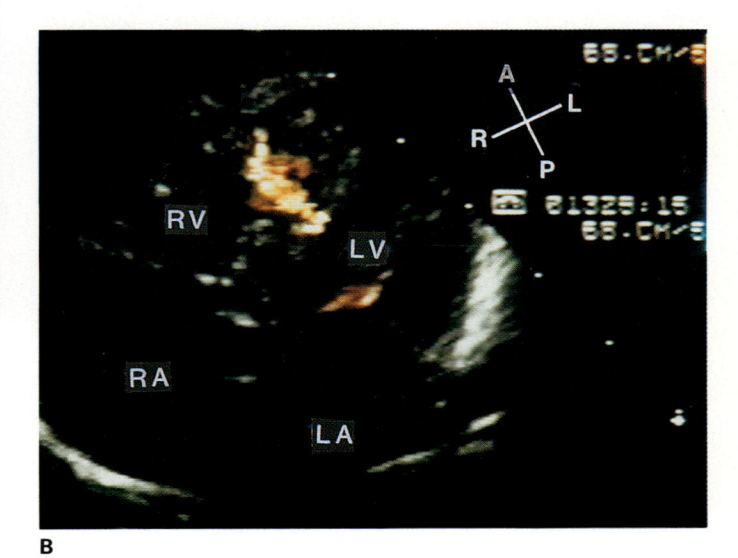

Ch. 20
Plate 9 A: A mid muscular defect. There is thinning of the ventricular septum, but an actual defect is not appreciated using imaging alone. **B:** Left to right shunting across the defect is clearly present on colour flow Doppler mapping.

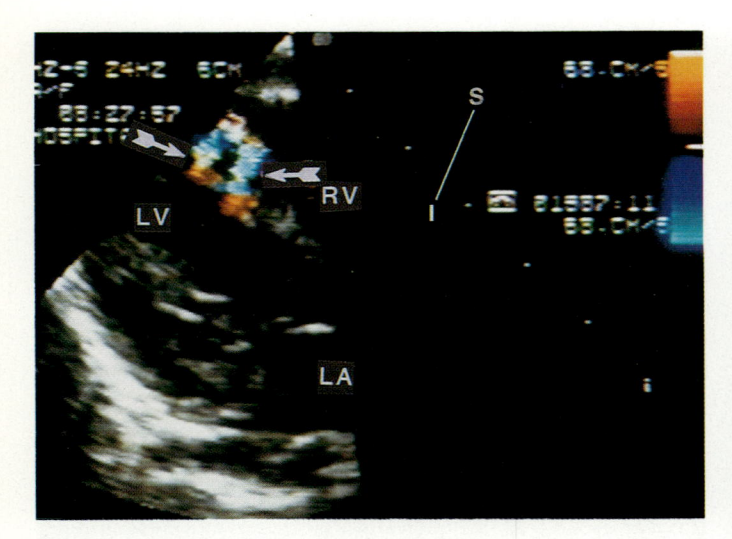

Ch. 20
Plate 10 Colour flow mapping study of multiple apical defects (arrowed) in the long axis left parasternal view.

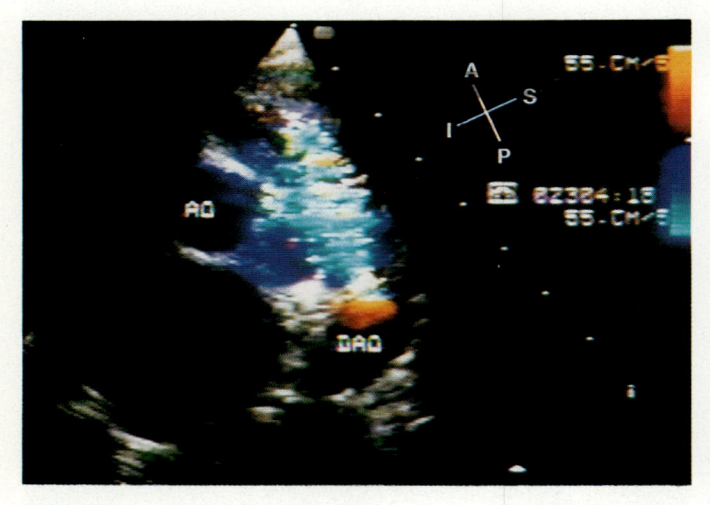

Ch. 20
Plate 11 Colour flow Doppler mapping in the left parasternal short axis view demonstrating a broad, centrally placed mosaic jet from aorta into the pulmonary artery (anatomy as in Fig. 30).

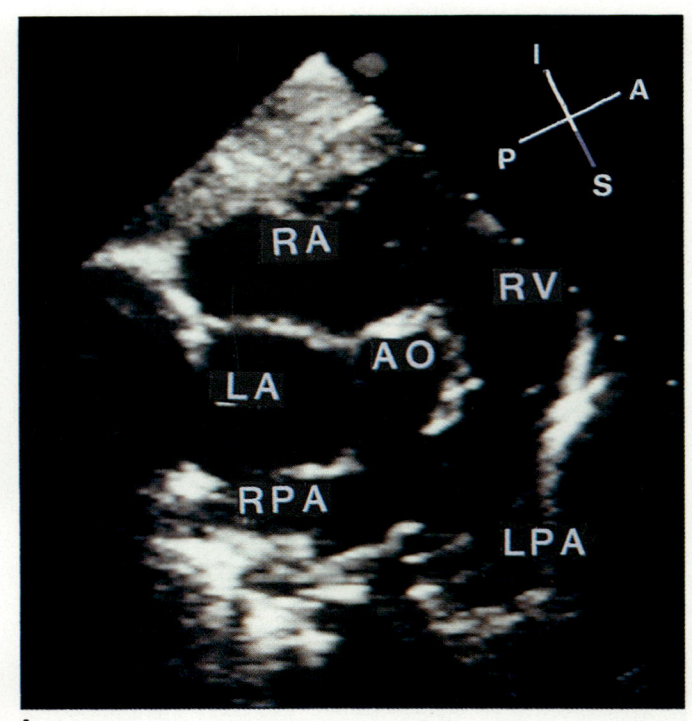

A

B

Ch. 20
Plate 12 In breathless children with aortopulmonary window the subcostal approach may prove to be useful. A: This example shows a large window between the posterior aspect of the ascending aorta and the origin of the right pulmonary artery. **B:** Colour flow Doppler mapping shows a wide, turbulent jet (arrowed) directed from the aorta into the pulmonary artery.

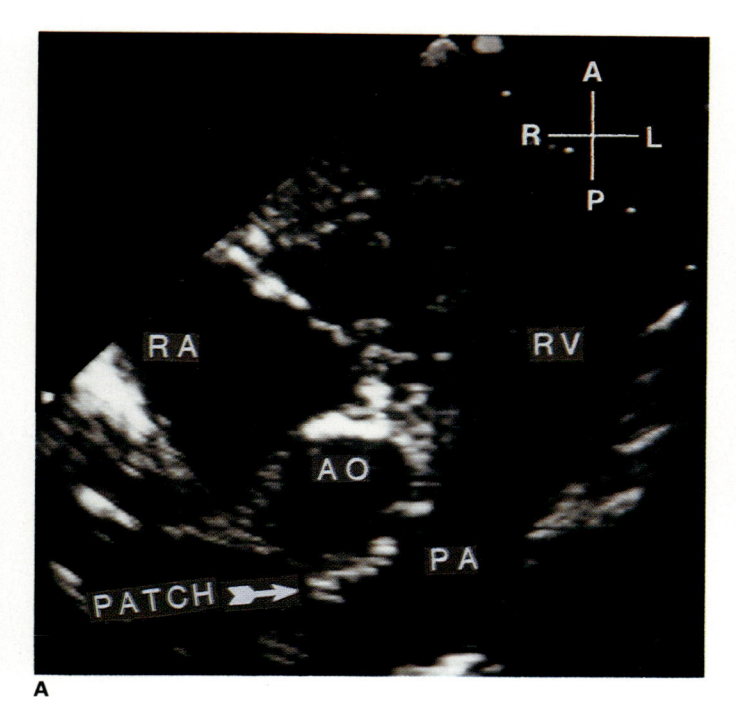

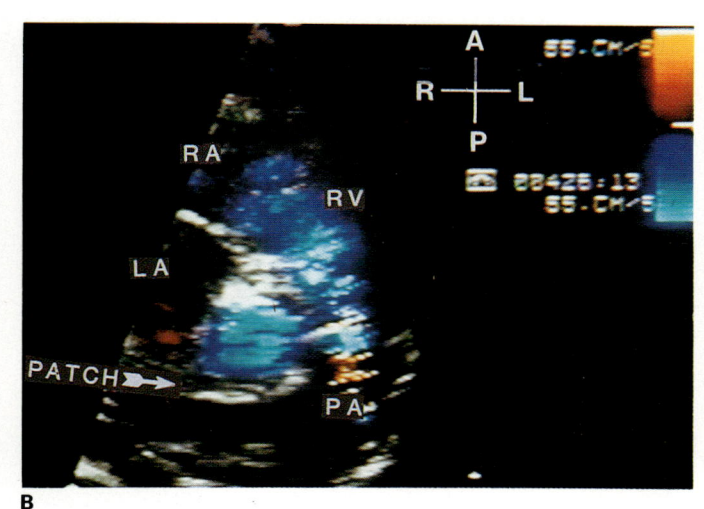

Ch. 20
Plate 13 A: After surgical repair of **aortopulmonary window** the patch closure of the defect is clearly visible on subcostal imaging.
B: Colour flow Doppler mapping shows normal flow patterns in the pulmonary artery, with no residual aortopulmonary shunt, in marked contrast to Plate 12B.

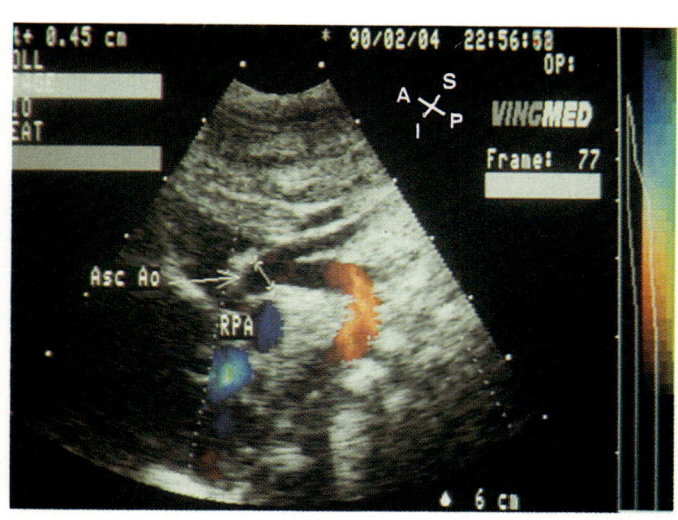

Ch. 21
Plate 1 Suprasternal view of the ascending aorta and aortic arch in hypoplastic left heart syndrome. The red/orange colour indicates retrograde flow in the arch from the descending aorta to the arch and thence to the ascending aorta.

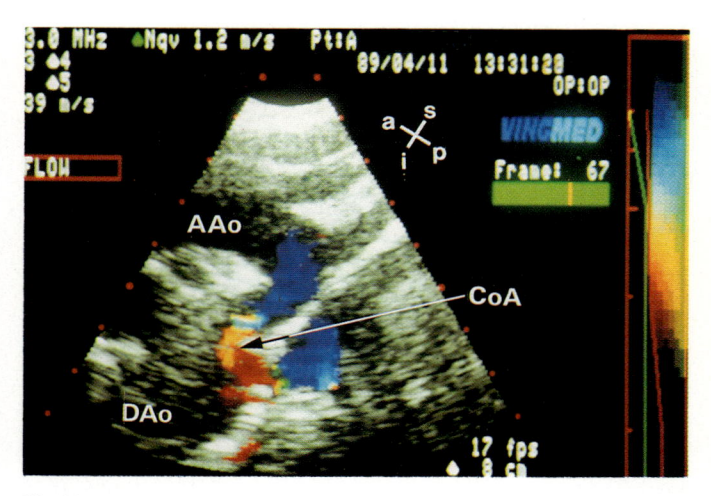

Ch. 21
Plate 2 Suprasternal view from a patient with coarctation of the aorta in whom the site of obstruction was not clearly shown with imaging. The colour signal shows acceleration towards the site of the coarctation which is outlined with the posterior aspect of the poststenotic area clearly seen outlined in red. AAo – ascending aorta; DAo – descending aorta; CoA – coarctation.

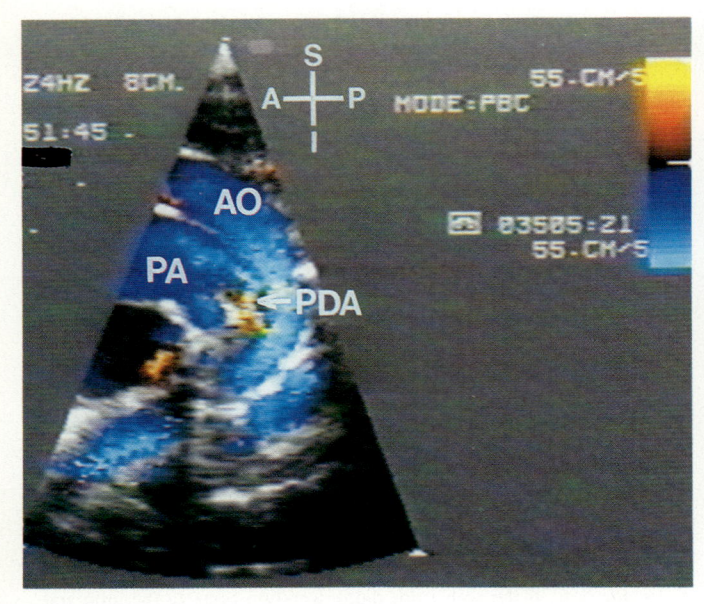

Ch. 22
Plate 1 High parasternal short axis colour flow Doppler image of the great arteries in complete transposition. The systolic (blue) flow in the aorta and pulmonary trunk can be seen with flow in the persistent arterial duct showing as an orange jet passing from descending thoracic aorta anteriorly into the pulmonary artery.

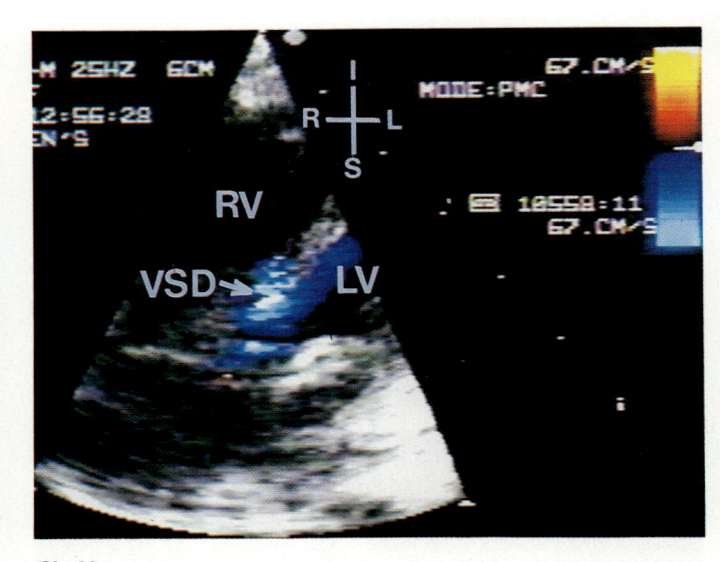

Ch. 22
Plate 3 Colour flow Doppler image in an infant with transposition and a perimembranous ventricular septal defect. Note that the flow through the defect is blue indicating right to left flow. This is the normal direction of flow in transposition where the right ventricular pressure is likely to be higher than the left.

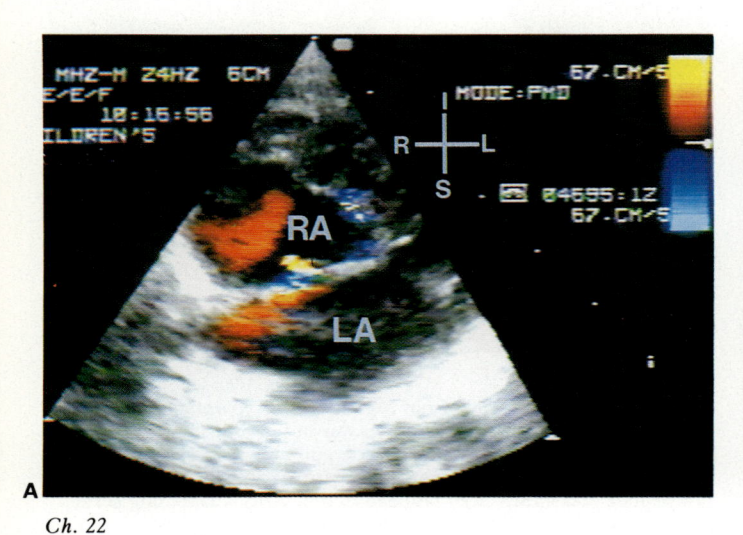

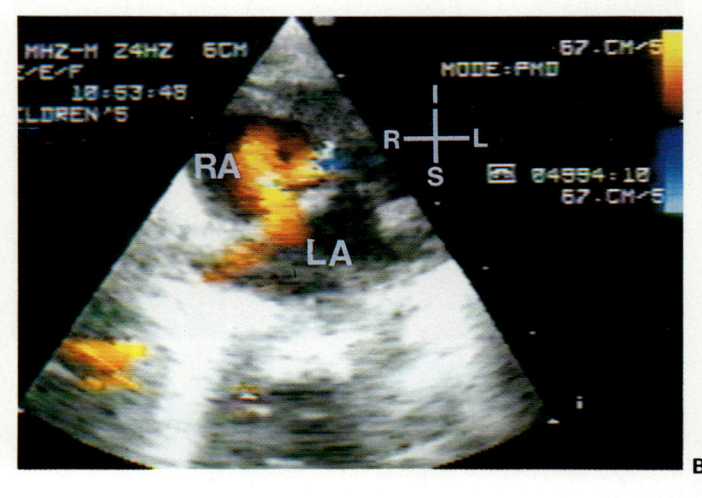

Ch. 22
Plate 2 Colour flow images before and after balloon atrial septostomy. A: Subcostal four chamber view of atrial septum showing a narrow jet of left to right flow across the foramen ovale. **B:** Similar view in same patient after balloon atrial septostomy. There is now a moderate sized atrial septal defect with low velocity (orange) left to right flow.

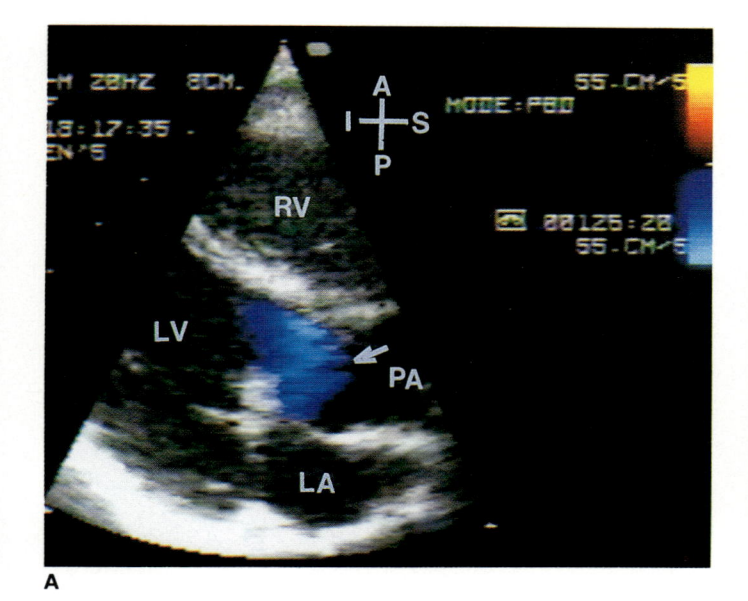

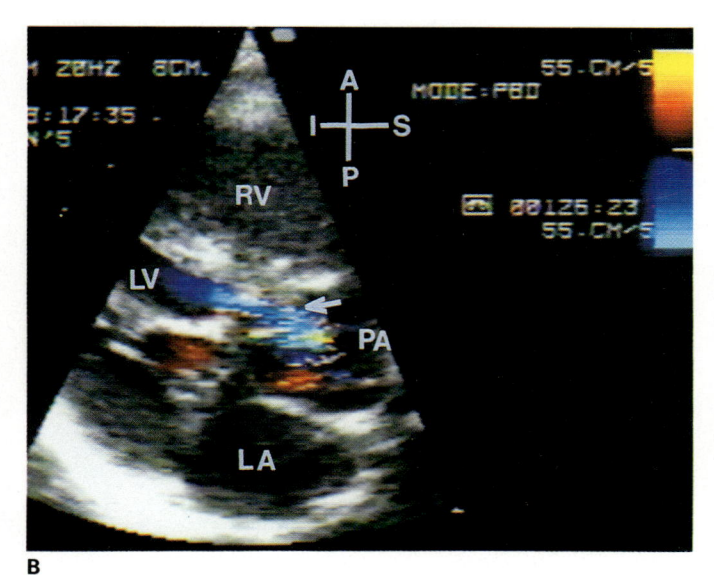

Ch. 22
Plate 4 Colour flow Doppler images showing dynamic left ventricular outflow obstruction in transposition with intact ventricular septum. A: Parasternal long axis image in early systole shows low velocity blue flow in the left ventricular outflow (arrowed). **B:** Similar view in mid systole shows that the anterior mitral valve leaflet has moved anteriorly producing obstruction to the left ventricular outflow. There is high velocity turbulent flow just distal to the mitral leaflet (arrowed).

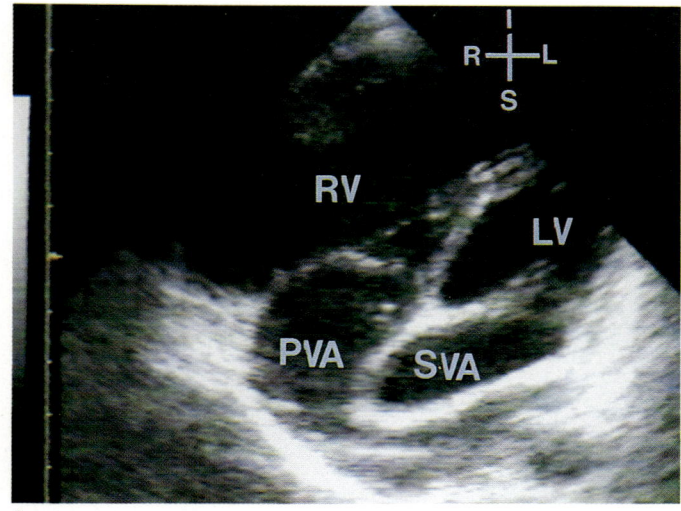

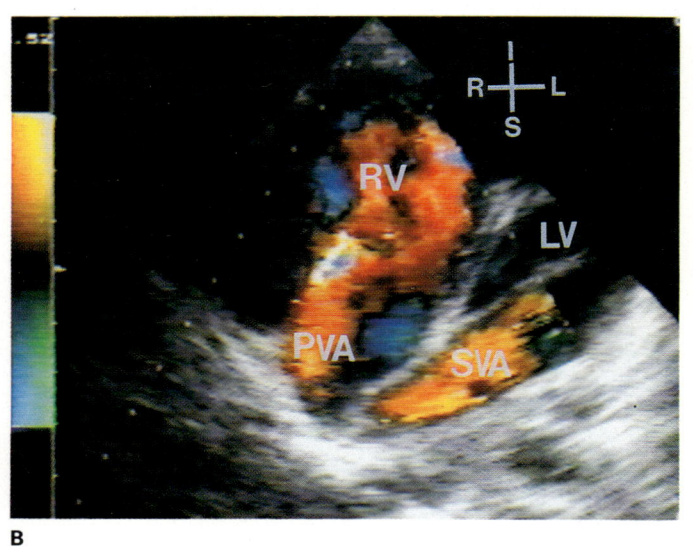

Ch. 22
Plate 5 A: Apical four chamber view after the Senning operation for complete transposition with intact ventricular septum. The pulmonary veins connect to the pulmonary venous atrium (PVA) posterior and to the right of the systemic venous atrium (SVA). **B:** Colour flow Doppler image showing low velocity, non-turbulent (orange) flow in the pulmonary and systemic venous pathways.

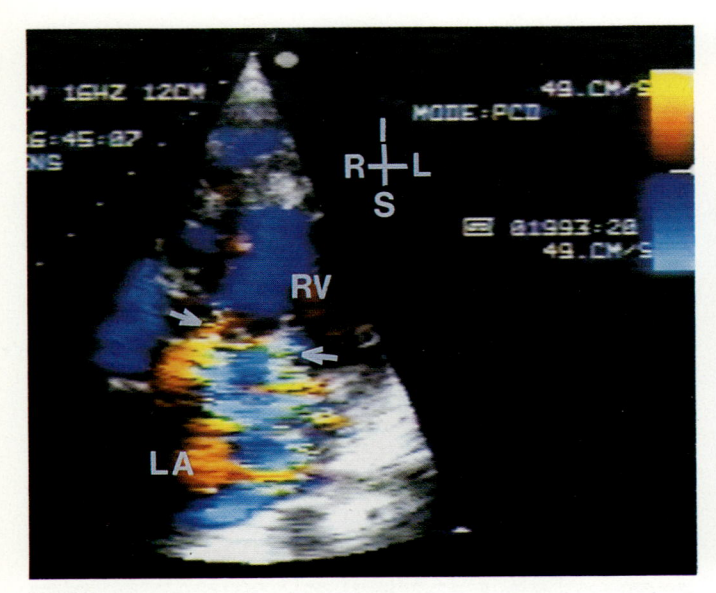

Ch. 22
Plate 6 Severe left atrioventricular valve regurgitation in congenitally corrected transposition of the great arteries. Apical view showing two separate regurgitant jets (arrowed).

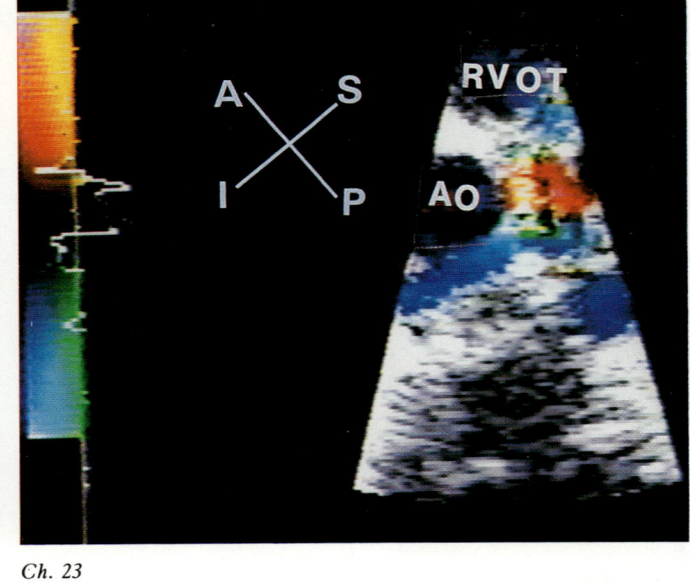

Ch. 23
Plate 2 High precordial short axis view in pulmonary atresia and ventricular septal defect demonstrating bifurcation of main pulmonary artery. Colour flow mapping documents absence of forward flow through outflow tract but flow from ductus is visualised.

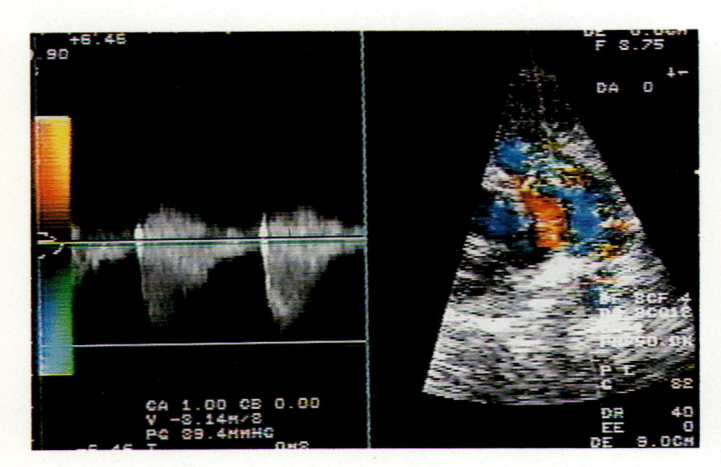

Ch. 23
Plate 1 Parasternal short axis view of pulmonary artery with colour flow mapping to guide continuous wave recording and recognition of maximal flow velocities.

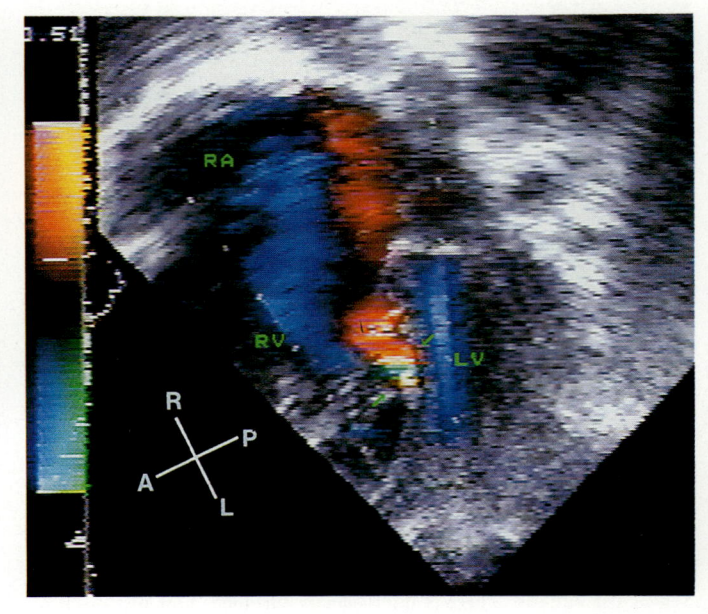

Ch. 23
Plate 3 Colour Doppler image from same patient as Fig. 21 showing direction, origin and degree of tricuspid valve regurgitation.

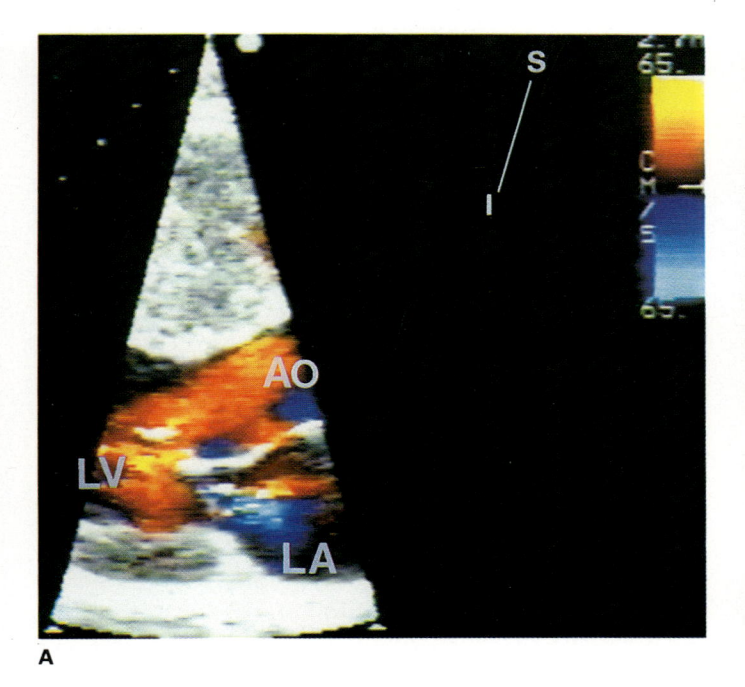

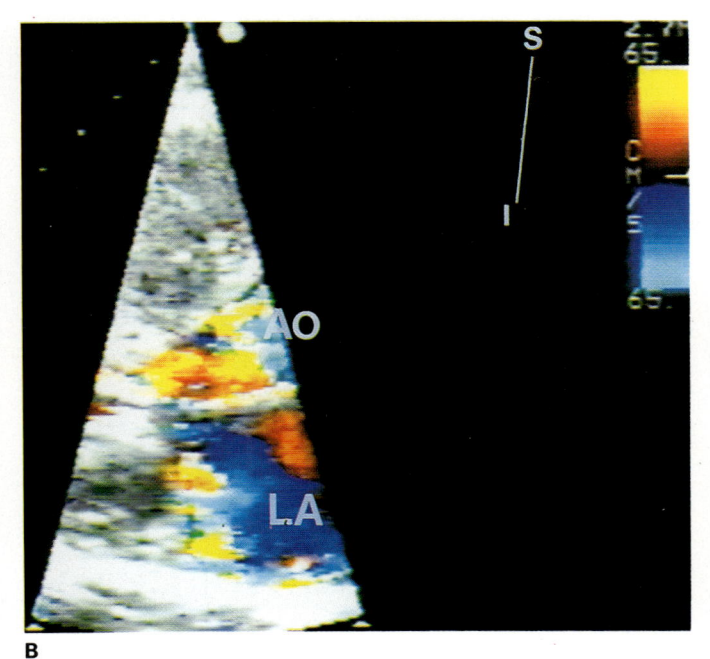

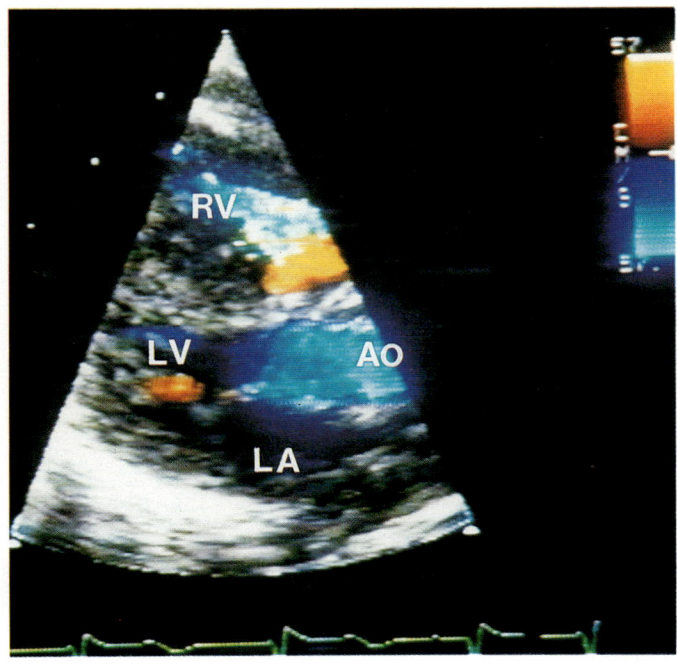

Ch. 26
Plate 2 Right ventricular outflow obstruction in an infant with hypertrophic cardiomyopathy. Parasternal long axis colour flow image with normal (blue) velocities in left ventricular outflow and high velocity aliasing flow in the right ventricular outflow.

Ch. 26
Plate 1 A: Parasternal long axis colour flow image in hypertrophic cardiomyopathy with left ventricular outflow obstruction. In early systole there is low velocity (orange) flow in the left ventricular outflow and a mitral regurgitant jet in the left atrium (blue). **B:** Later systolic frame showing high velocity aliasing flow in the left ventricular outflow due to the development of left ventricular outflow obstruction. There is also a high velocity jet in the left atrium from the mitral regurgitation.

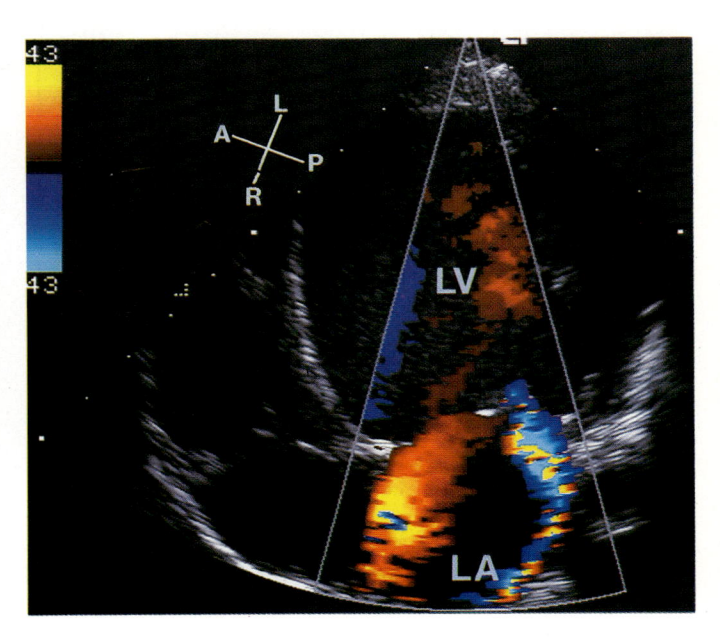

Ch. 26
Plate 3 Mitral regurgitation in dilated cardiomyopathy. Apical four chamber colour flow Doppler image. There is a high velocity turbulent jet of mitral regurgitation that hugs the lateral wall of the left atrium.

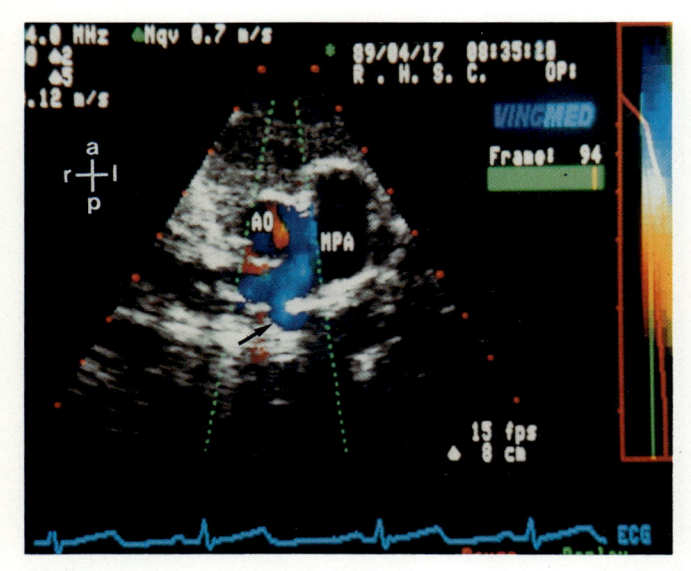

Ch. 27
Plate 1 Pulmonary artery sling. In a left parasternal short axis view the left pulmonary artery is seen to arise from the proximal right pulmonary artery (arrowed). The abnormal branching of the pulmonary artery is most easily appreciated using colour flow Doppler. (By courtesy of Dr James Gnanapragasam.)

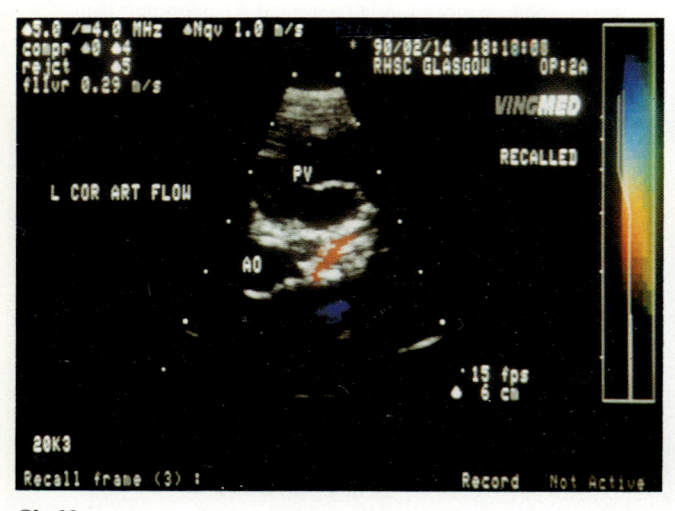

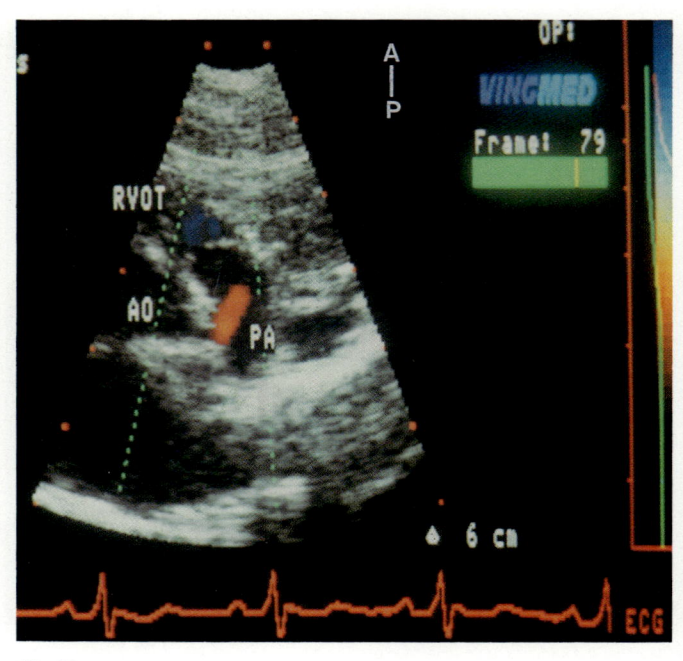

Ch. 28
Plate 2 Diastolic short axis view of the great arteries in diastole using colour flow mapping. Flow from the anomalous left coronary artery into the pulmonary artery is clearly shown in red. (RVOT – right ventricular outflow tract.)

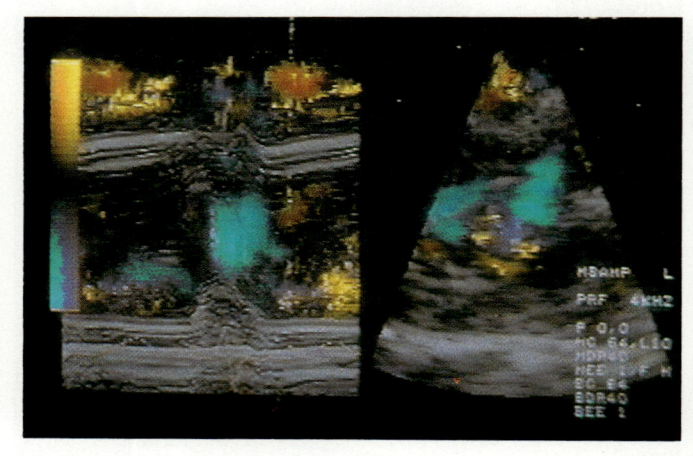

Ch. 28
Plate 1 Short axis view showing the aortic root and left coronary artery. Flow in the artery is shown in red, towards the transducer.

Ch. 30
Plate 1 Intraoperative echocardiogram obtained from the epicardial approach after bypass in a child who had undergone repair of a ventricular septal defect. On colour flow mapping in real time (right panel) turbulence was visible within the right ventricle. This was interpreted as systolic turbulence, possibly indicating a residual ventricular septal defect. The colour M-mode recording (left panel) however, demonstrates that the turbulence within the right ventricle is mostly diastolic and therefore due to turbulent inflow over the ventricular septal patch rather than to a residual defect.

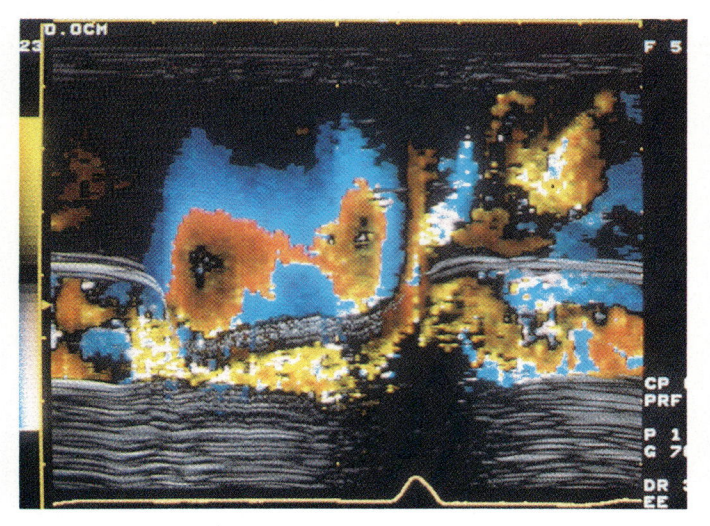

Ch. 30
Plate 2 Colour M-mode recording obtained during a trans-oesophageal study showing flow events within the left atrium (upper part of trace) and left ventricular outflow tract (lower part of trace). During diastole there is aortic regurgitation which occupied almost the whole width of the outflow tract at this level. In systole the colour M-mode confirms that there is mitral regurgitation and shows its duration and depth.

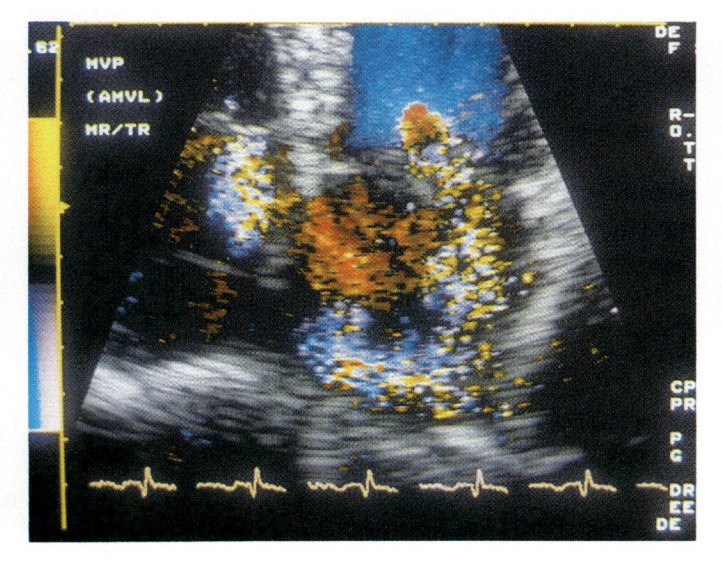

Ch. 30
Plate 3 Apical four chamber view obtained from the precordium. There is a central mitral regurgitant jet directed into the middle of the left atrium and then around the posterior wall. The convergence zone within the left ventricle (of blood accelerating into the regurgitant orifice) is clearly demonstrated. This patient also has some tricuspid regurgitation.

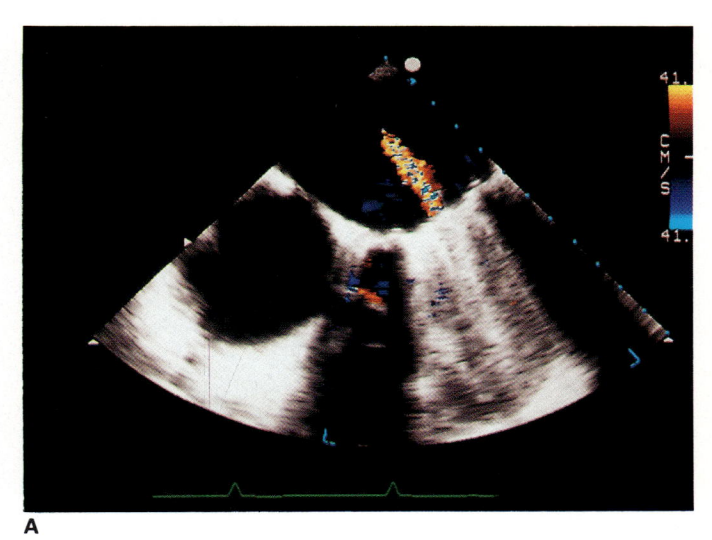

Ch. 30
Plate 4 A: Trans-oesophageal cross-sectional image and colour flow map and B: colour M-mode recording of a normally functioning Medtronic Hall tilting disc mitral prosthesis. There is a long jet of mitral regurgitation in the left atrium but it is present only at the start of systole and is therefore a normal closure jet. The colour M-mode recording also shows mild persistent regurgitation adjacent to the valve ring during the remainder of systole. This is also a normal phenomenon for this valve.

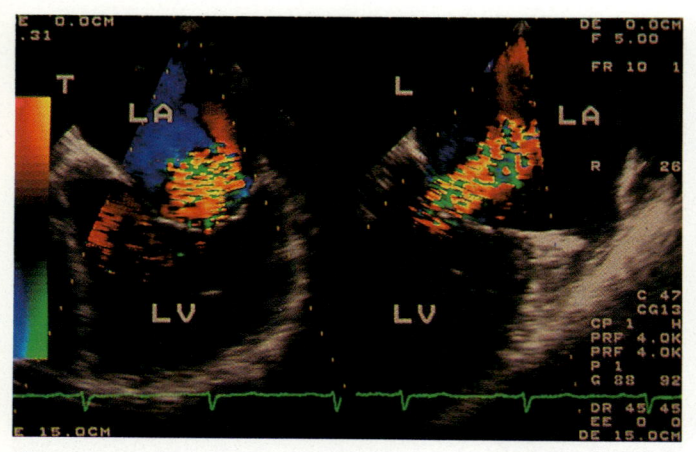

Ch. 30
Plate 5 Biplane trans-oesophageal colour flow maps of a mitral regurgitant jet. The transverse image (left panel) shows a broad jet just above the mitral valve. The longitudinal image (right panel) demonstrates that the jet is quite long but is directed superiorly within the left atrium.

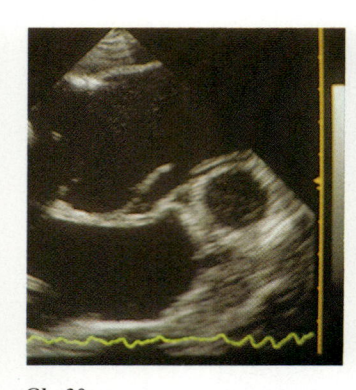

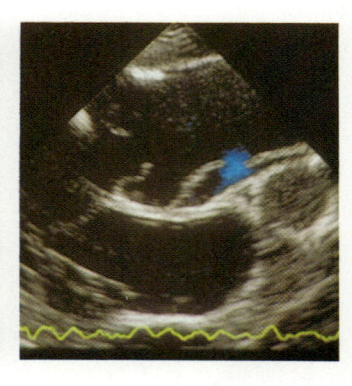

Ch. 30
Plate 7 Epivascular image and colour flow map obtained during cardiopulmonary bypass in a patient with aortic dissection. The aorta is imaged along its long axis. The cross-sectional image (left) shows the site of the intimal tear. This is confirmed on colour flow mapping (right).

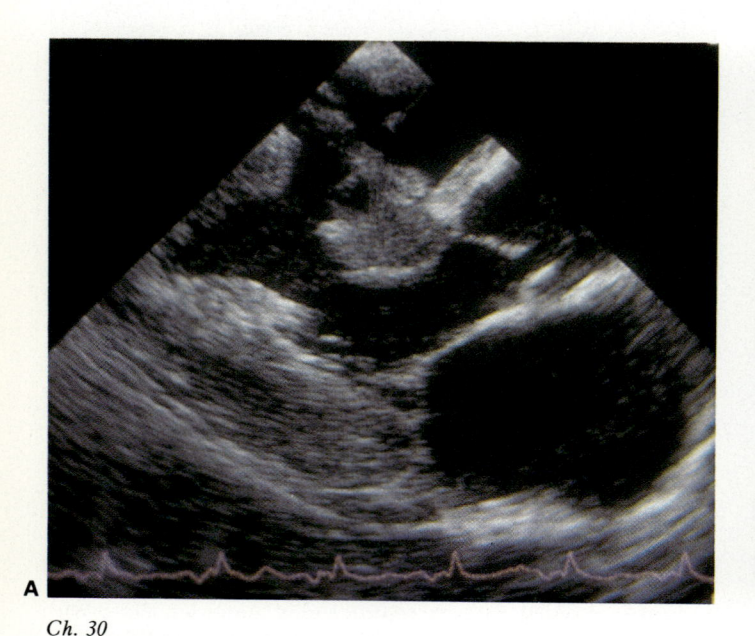

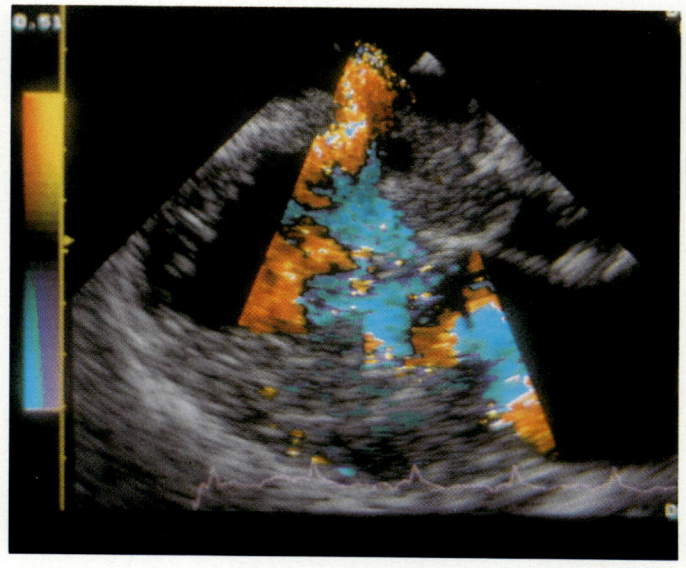

Ch. 30
Plate 6 A: Intraoperative epicardial cross-sectional image in the longitudinal axis in a patient with acute ventricular septal rupture. The margins of the defect within the mid-ventricular septum are clearly defined. There is little undermining of the adjacent edges of the septum.
B: The corresponding colour flow map confirms a left to right shunt.

… SECTION 1

Introduction to cardiac ultrasound

1

History

Origins
M-mode echocardiography
Two-dimensional scanning
Doppler methods
Duplex scanning
Doppler colour flow imaging
Intravascular and endoscopic scanning
Epilogue

Peter N. T. Wells

ORIGINS

Immediately after World War II, efforts were made to use the ultrasonic methods that had been developed for military purposes to try to solve medical diagnostic problems. These primitive systems, apparently independently invented by Firestone[1] in the USA and by Sproule[2] in the UK, used the pulse-echo principle to locate cracks for the non-destructive testing of metallic structures. A few years later, Howry and Bliss[3] in Denver and Wild and Reid[4] (the same Reid who was later to play a leading role in the development of echocardiography in Philadelphia) working in Minneapolis had constructed pulse-echo two-dimensional ultrasonic scanners for medical diagnosis. Some of the Minneapolis instruments even operated in real time. Subsequently, progress in the USA received a setback when in 1955 the Atomic Energy Commission published a report[5] stating that ultrasonic reflection techniques were unsuitable for the detection of cerebral disease, a conclusion which did not in any way exclude other areas of the body. Fortunately, the British and the Swedes were not discouraged – probably they were unaware of the American report – and the history of the disappointing research on the brain and the spectacularly successful developments in obstetrics is now well-known.

M-mode echocardiography

Whether an invention or a discovery, the credit for echocardiography belongs to Edler and Hertz, who in 1954 published the pioneering paper[6] on their work in Lund, Sweden. The first echocardiograph was an industrial A-scope flaw time-position (M-mode) recording made on continuously-moving 35 mm photographic film. One of the first recordings is shown in Figure 1. For the next decade, what was happening in Lund was watched by a few interested medical scientists with a mixture of scepticism and inactivity. Eventually, however, some – particularly Reid and Joyner[7] in Philadelphia – constructed equipment themselves and began to confirm Edler's results and to explore the potential of what is now known as M-mode echocardiography. Edler's collaborator Hertz had soon shown that the nuisance of having to wait for the film to be developed before the trace could be seen could be avoided by the use of a time-to-voltage analogue converter and an ink-jet recorder.[8] This instrument electronically gated the strong echo from an isolated structure, such as the leaflet of a valve, to produce a single-value time-varying waveform in real time on a strip chart. Although this approach was followed by others,[9] in retrospect it can be seen to have held back progress because it restricted investigations to only one strongly echogenic structure at a time. It was not until instrument manufacturers brought the fibre-optic strip-chart recorder into widespread use that the capability previously only provided by the photo-

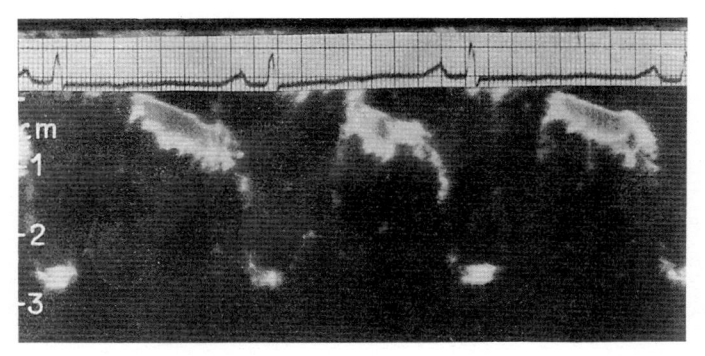

Fig. 1 One of the first recorded echocardiograms. Originally, it was thought that this characteristic pattern was that of the echo from the left atrial wall in mitral stenosis, but later it was shown to correspond to the anterior cusp of the mitral valve. (Reproduced with permission from Edler and Hertz 1954.)

graphic technique became economically available with the enormous advantage of real time operation.

Two-dimensional scanning

Quite early in the development of cardiac ultrasound, it was demonstrated by King[10] that two-dimensional images corresponding to any desired phase in the cardiac cycle could be obtained by electrocardiographic gating of the display of a conventional static contact scanner. There never was any likelihood, however, that this approach could compete with real time scanning. Already by 1967, Asberg[11] had constructed a scanner capable of operating at seven frames per second. The work of Bom[12] and his colleagues on the linear array real time scanner, despite the technical limitation imposed by the rectangular scan format, led to the realisation in 1972 that there was much of clinical value to be observed. By 1974, Griffith and Henry[13] were using the fast mechanical real time sector scanner shown in Figure 2. The earlier invention by Somer[14] in 1968 of the phased array sector scanner had to await the work of Thurstone and von Ramm[15] for its potential in echocardiography to be appreciated. Taken together, these developments laid the foundations of two-dimensional real time cardiac ultrasound and the growth in interest in the subject that has continued undiminished since the mid-1970s.

Doppler methods

The Japanese were the first to demonstrate the Doppler shift in the frequency of ultrasound backscattered by moving cardiac structures; the phenomenon was described in English in 1957 by Satomura.[16] The use of backscattered ultrasound to detect fetal heart movements was demonstrated in 1964 by Callaghan[17] and there can now hardly be an obstetrician in the industrialised countries who does not regularly use this method. It was Lube[18] in the USSR,

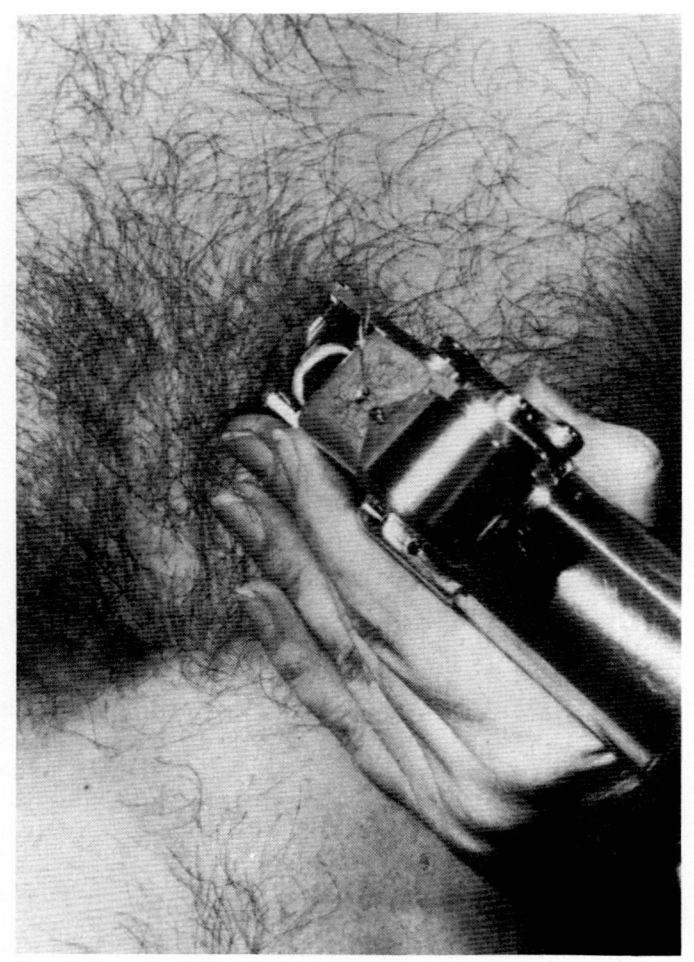

Fig. 2 A prototype real time mechanical sector scanner for echocardiography. (Reproduced with permission from Griffith and Henry 1974.)

however, who was the first to follow up Satomura's work, 10 years after the original publication. Although for a short time there was interest in simultaneous display of Doppler signals with M-mode recordings, as described by Edler and Lindstrom,[19] this has never become popular. If a timing reference is needed for cardiac Doppler signal interpretation, nowadays the electrocardiogram (ECG) is used or, as described later, the Doppler information is superimposed in colour on the M-mode display or on the real time two-dimensional display.

When Kaneko[20] showed in 1961 that blood flow itself could be detected by the Doppler effect, the idea was immediately taken up with enthusiasm by many investigators. Initially what followed was concerned with clinical applications in the study of blood flow in the peripheral and extracerebral vessels. By 1974, however, Kalmanson[21] was demonstrating that abnormalities particularly of the right heart can be easily diagnosed by studying the shape of the velocity-time Doppler flow waveforms detected trans-

cutaneously, for example, in the jugular vein. As early as 1969, Baker,[22] Peronneau[23] and Wells[24] had independently demonstrated the feasibility of range-gated pulsed Doppler operation and, by 1974, Peronneau[25] had constructed a pulsed Doppler system capable of measuring the flow velocity profile in the exposed thoracic aorta in the dog. Light[26] was making good progress in his systematic study of time-velocity waveforms in the aorta using the suprasternal notch approach and a continuous wave Doppler system with a rudimentary but ingenious real time frequency spectrum analyser. Two methods of measuring cardiac output and related aspects of cardiac function are direct descendants of Light's work. The traditional method, which is subject to errors due to non-uniform insonation and inaccuracies in estimating angles and dimensions, is now in competition with Evans'[27] attenuation-compensated blood flow volume ratemeter which simultaneously employs wide and narrow beams of ultrasound and which, in theory, avoids these difficulties.

Duplex scanning

The term 'duplex' is used somewhat imprecisely to describe scanners designed to provide both two-dimensional images and Doppler signals. The early system described by Phillips[28] in 1980, shown in Figure 3, used a mechanical real-time sector scanner and an offset pulsed Doppler transducer. Most of the subsequent development has been by commercial instrument manufacturers. At present, the most popular arrangements use either a mechanical scanner which can be stopped with the transducer directing the ultrasonic beam through the region chosen for Doppler study, or a phased array transducer. The mechanical sys-

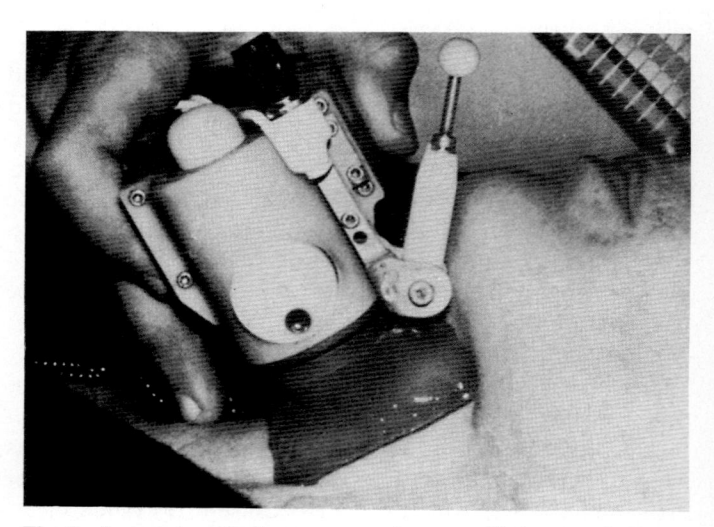

Fig. 3 A prototype duplex scanner using an oscillating transducer for real time imaging and an independently adjustable offset transducer for Doppler signal acquisition. This particular device was constructed primarily for the study of superficial vessels. (Reproduced with permission from Phillips et al 1980.)

tems do not allow simultaneous imaging and Doppler signal acquisition but the 'agile' beam of an array avoids this limitation. For duplex echocardiography, the phased array system is usually the more convenient.

Doppler colour flow imaging

The first demonstration of the feasibility of combining pulse-echo images with two-dimensional Doppler information was published by Eyers[29] in 1981. The system produced complete picture frames at the rate of four per second. It was not until Kasai[30] published his important paper in 1985 that the feasibility of carrying out the process in real time was generally appreciated. Again, most of the development work has been in commercial laboratories and so the details of the signal processing schemes adopted in modern instruments are proprietary. In general, however, either autocorrelation or multigate detection is used.

Intravascular and endoscopic scanning

The clinical use of intracardiac ultrasonic probes was first described in English by Kimoto[31] in 1964. Using ECG-gating, both two-dimensional B-scan and C-scan images were made, the latter being particularly useful for visualising atrial septal defects. Subsequent interest was slow to develop. Recently, however, intravascular devices have been constructed in several laboratories[32] and some are now commercially available.

Imaging the heart from the oesophagus using a scanner mounted on an endoscope originated in Japan, Hisanga's[33] first easily accessible publication in English having appeared in 1977 (Fig. 4). Advanced commercially-made devices now have duplex and colour Doppler capabilities.

Epilogue

Throughout its history, the development of echocardiography has been led by technological innovation. In parallel with improvements in instrumentation, analytical techniques have evolved: a good example is Holen's[34] 1977

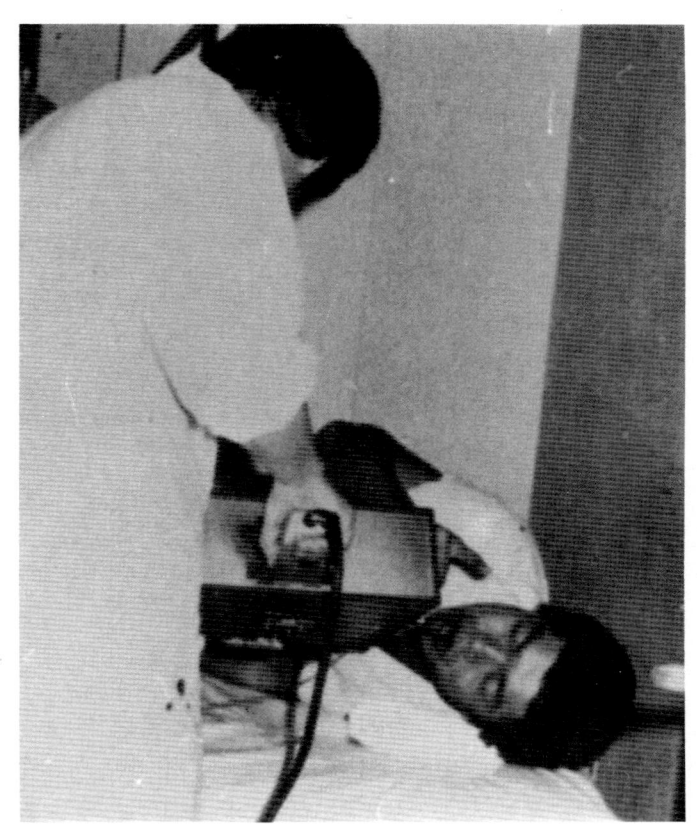

Fig. 4 An early ultrasonic endoscope being used for transoesophageal scanning of the heart. (Reproduced with permission from Hisanga and Hisanga 1977.)

method of the pressure drop estimation across an orifice from the measurement of the jet flow velocity. Another discovery of potentially great significance was that of Gramiak,[35] who demonstrated in 1969 that the echogenicity of blood can be enhanced by microbubble contrast agents. The scope and clinical value of ultrasonic techniques in cardiology can confidently be expected to continue to develop for as long as such new ideas continue to come to fruition.

REFERENCES

1. Firestone F A. The supersonic reflectoscope, an instrument for inspecting the interior of the solid parts by means of sound waves. J Acoust Soc Am 1946; 17: 287–291
2. Desch C H, Sproule D O, Dawson W J. The detection of cracks in steel by means of supersonic waves. J Iron Steel Inst Lond 1946; 153: 319–352
3. Howry D H, Bliss W R. Ultrasonic visualisation of soft tissue structures in the body. J Lab Clin Med 1952; 40: 579–592
4. Wild J J, Reid J M. Further pilot echographic studies of the histologic structure of tumors of the living intact human breast. Am J Pathol 1952; 28: 839–861
5. United States Atomic Energy Commission. Studies in methods in instruments to improve the localisation of radioactive materials in the body with special reference to the diagnosis of brain tumors and the use of ultrasonic techniques. Report AECV-3012. Minneapolis: University of Minnesota Press. 1955
6. Edler I, Hertz C H. The use of the ultrasonic reflectoscope for the continuous recording of the movements of heart walls. K Fysiogr Sallsk Lund Forh 1954; 24: 40–58
7. Reid J M, Joyner C R. The use of ultrasound to record the motion of heart structure. In: Kelly E. ed. Ultrasonic energy. Urbana: University of Illinois Press. 1964: p 278–293
8. Edler I. Ultrasound cardiography. Acta Med Scand 1961; 170; Suppl 370
9. Wells P N T, Ross F G M. A time-to-voltage analogue converter for ultrasonic cardiology. Ultrasonics 1969; 7: 171–176
10. King D L. Cardiac ultrasonography. A stop-action technique for imaging intra-cardiac anatomy. Radiology 1972; 103: 387–392

11. Asberg A. Ultrasonic cinematography of the living heart. Ultrasonics 1967; 5: 113–117
12. Bom N. New concepts in echocardiography. Leiden: Stenfert Kroese. 1972
13. Griffith J M, Henry W L. A sector scanner for real time two dimensional echocardiography. Circulation 1974; 49: 1147–1152
14. Somer J C. Electronic sector scanning for ultrasonic diagnosis. Ultrasonics 1968; 6: 153–159
15. Thurstone F L, von Ramm O T. A new ultrasound imaging technique employing two-dimensional electronic beam steering. In: Green PS. ed. Acoustical holography. Vol 5. New York: Plenum Press. 1974: p 149–159
16. Satomura S. Ultrasonic Doppler method for the inspection of cardiac function. J Acoust Soc Am 1957; 29: 1181–1185
17. Callagan D A, Rowland T C, Goldman D E. Ultrasonic Doppler observation of the fetal heart. Obstet Gynecol 1964; 23: 637
18. Lube V M, Savonof Y D, Yakiemenkov L I. Ultrasonic detection of the motions of cardiac valves and muscle. Sov Phys Acoust 1967; 13: 59–65
19. Edler I, Lindstrom K. Ultrasonic Doppler techniques used in the heart. In: Bock J, Ossoinig K. eds. Ultrasonographia medica. Vol III. Vienna: Verlag Wiener Med Akad. 1971: p 455–461
20. Kaneko Z, Kotani H, Komuta K, Satomura S. Studies on peripheral circulation by ultrasonic blood-rheograph. Jpn Circ J 1961; 25: 203–213
21. Kalmanson D, Veyrat C, Derai C, Savier Ch, Bernier J, Chiche P. Diagnostic applications of the CW directional Doppler technique in cardiology. In: de Vlieger M, White D N, McCready V R. eds. Ultrasonics in medicine. Amsterdam: Excerpta Medica. 1974: p 278–281
22. Baker D W. Pulsed ultrasonic Doppler blood flow sensing. IEEE Trans Sonics Ultrason 1970; 17: 170–185
23. Peronneau P A, Hinglais J R, Pellet M M, Leger F. Velocimetre sanguin par effet Doppler a emission ultra-sonore pulsee. Onde Elect 1970; 50: 369–384
24. Wells P N T. A range-gated ultrasonic Doppler system. Med Biol Eng 1969; 7: 641–652
25. Peronneau P A, Beynon A, Bournat J-P, Xhaard M, Hinglais J. Instantaneous bi-dimensional blood velocity profiles in the major vessels by a pulsed ultrasonic Doppler velocimeter. In: de Vlieger M, White D N, McCready V R. eds. Ultrasonics in medicine. Amsterdam: Excerpta Medica. 1974: p 259–266
26. Light L H. Initial evaluation of transcutaneous aortovelography. In: Reneman R S. ed. Cardiovascular applications of ultrasound. Amsterdam: North-Holland. 1974: p 325–360
27. Evans J M, Skidmore R, Luckman N P, Wells P N T. A new approach to the non-invasive measurement of cardiac output using an annular array Doppler technique. Ultrasound Med Biol 1989; 15: 169–178
28. Phillips D J, Powers J E, Eyer M K, et al. Detection of peripheral vascular disease using the duplex scanner III. Ultrasound Med Biol 1980; 6: 205–218
29. Eyers M K, Brandestini M, Phillips D J, Baker D W. Color digital echo/Doppler image presentation. Ultrasound Med Biol 1981; 7: 21–31
30. Kasai C, Namekawa K, Koyano A, Omoto R. Real time two-dimensional blood flow imaging using an autocorrelation technique. IEEE Trans Sonics Ultrason 1985; 32: 460–463
31. Kimoto S, Omoto R, Tsunemoto M, Moroi T, Atsumi K, Uchida R. Ultrasonic tomography of the liver and detection of heart atrial septal defect with the aid of ultrasonic intravenous probe. Ultrasonics 1964; 2: 82–86
32. Bom N, Roelandt J. eds. Intravascular ultrasound. Dordrecht: Kluwer Academic Publishers. 1989
33. Hisanga K, Hisanga A. A new real time sector scanning system of ultra-wide angle and real time recording of entire adult cardiac images. In: White D, Lyons E A. eds. Ultrasonics in medicine. Vol 4. New York: Plenum Press. 1978: p 391–402
34. Holen J, Aaslid R, Landmark K, Simonsen S, Ostrem T. Determination of effective orifice area in mitral stenosis from non-invasive Doppler data and mitral flow rate. Acta Med Scand 1977; 201: 83–88
35. Gramiak R, Shah P M, Kramer D H. Ultrasound cardiography: contrast studies in anatomy and function. Radiology 1969; 92: 939–948

2

Physics and principles

Introduction to ultrasound
Waves
Amplitude
Frequency
Wavelength
Properties of sound
Speed
Power
Intensity
Beam shapes
The pulse echo technique
Pulses
Echoes
   Specular reflection
   Non-specular reflection
Range measurement
Attenuation

The A-mode display
Sampling
The M-mode display
Real-time imaging
Combining real-time with M-mode
The Doppler effect
The influence of angle
Flow patterns
   Laminar flow
   Turbulent flow
Doppler equipment
Continuous wave Doppler
Pulsed Doppler
Display of Doppler information
Aliasing
   Nyquist frequency
   Extended pulse repetition frequency

Colour flow mapping
Doppler method (autocorrelation)
Moving target indicator
Velocity coding
Power coding
Low velocity detection
Variance
Influence of angle
Aliasing and colour flow
Image resolution
Spatial
Temporal
Contrast
Artefacts
Reverberation
Refraction
Shadowing
Enhancement
Beam width effects

Michael Halliwell

INTRODUCTION TO ULTRASOUND

Ultrasound is a mechanical form of energy. It is precisely the same as audible sound in its physical properties but, because man is unable to hear it, as its pitch is too high, it becomes ultrasound. Sound has a pitch of up to about 20 000 vibrations or cycles per second. Vibrations of ultrasound extend beyond this to over 1000 million per second; medical applications use the range from 2 to 20 million cycles per second.

Sound and ultrasound both rely on the presence of some physical medium in which to travel. For medical applications only the soft tissues of the body need be considered, since ultrasound travels very poorly in gas and bone.

Mechanical waves are fluctuations in pressure and are supported by the mechanical properties of materials. In any discussion of these properties it is useful to have a simple model of the material. Consider the tissues of the body as a lattice of balls separated and supported by a network of springs (Fig. 1).

Pressure fluctuations can be produced by vibrating surfaces, such as those of a recently struck bell. The surface moves backwards and forwards alternately rarefying and compressing the surrounding medium. Those alterations in particle density are seen as alterations in local pressure. If the individual particles (balls) of the medium are considered, the only motion they undergo is a vibration around their rest positions. It is by passing that vibration on to their neighbours (through the springs) that the *pressure* fluctuation is transmitted though the medium. There is no net movement of particles through the medium but there is movement of energy.

The unit of pressure is the pascal with an approximate relationship that 1 MPa (1 million pascals) is equivalent to ten times the normal atmospheric pressure. Ultrasound machines produce peak pressures of about 1 or 2 MPa.

Waves

Ultrasound is most easily understood in terms of a wave, a cyclical fluctuation of pressure travelling though a medium. All pressure waves, no matter what their actual shape, can be constructed by adding together a number of waves of different characteristics but all of an identical *shape*, the sinusoidal shape. Consequently every discussion of ultrasound includes a section on sine waves, simple, mathematically at least, and not too far from reality. Sinusoidal waves are characterised by their amplitude and their frequency (or periodicity), (Fig. 2).

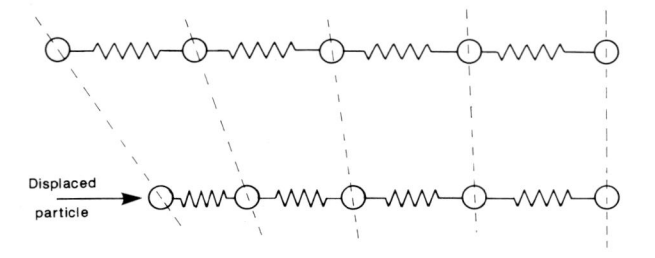

Fig. 1 **The balls on springs tissue model.** The displacement of one ball takes time to affect the others. The stiffer the springs and the lighter the balls the faster the disturbance travels.

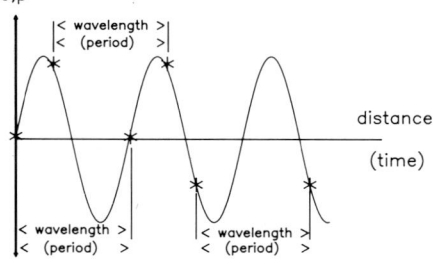

Fig. 2 **A sinusoidal wave.** This particular shape describes many of the changes associated with an ultrasound wave. The displacement of particles from their rest positions, the velocity of the particles, and the pressure in the medium can all be displayed on the vertical axis.

Amplitude

The amplitude is the range from the minimum to the maximum value of the pressure associated with the wave. In diagnostic ultrasound terms the greater the pressure amplitude the greater the power of the beam (see *Power*).

Frequency

The frequency of a sound wave is the rate at which it cycles through the pressure fluctuations. From Figure 2 it can be seen that the interval between any adjacent identical parts of the pressure cycle is constant. This interval is called the period of the wave, T. The frequency, f, of the wave is the number of cycles which would occur in 1 s. It is determined by the equation:

$$f = 1/T$$

where T is in seconds and f is in cycles per second or hertz (Hz). The frequency of the wave is the most useful descriptor in practice. Its significance is that it tells the operator what depth of penetration to expect and what clarity of image will be obtained. For diagnostic purposes frequencies in the range 2 to 20 MHz are most often used (2 000 000 to 20 000 000 cycles per second). These values correspond to penetrations of 20 and 2 cm and resolutions of about 1 and 0.1 mm respectively. In echocardiography the range of usable frequencies is from 2 to 7.5 MHz.

The higher the frequency the lower the penetration but the better the image clarity.

Wavelength

The wavelength λ of the sound wave is the distance between adjacent identical parts of the wave (see Fig. 2). The wave is a travelling wave and it moves through the medium with the speed c m/s. The distance which one cycle occupies in space is equal to the distance which the wave travels in one period. Thus we have:

$$\lambda = T.c$$

With T in seconds and c in metres per second, λ is in metres. It is usual to replace T by $1/f$ in the expression leading to the relationship:

$$\lambda.f = c$$

This is a relationship between f and λ it must not be interpreted as meaning 'the speed depends on the product of frequency and wavelength' because the speed of sound in a particular medium is essentially constant.

A 2 MHz wave in soft tissue has a wavelength of about 0.77 mm, and at 10 MHz the wavelength is 0.154 mm.

The relevance of the wavelength is that it critically governs the clarity or *resolution* of the image. The best possible resolution is about two or three wavelengths but usually it is worse. Cardiac images typically resolve structures between 1 and 2 mm in size or separation.

Properties of sound

Speed

The speed with which the pressure fluctuations travel is called the speed of (ultra)sound. It is not the same as the speed with which the balls vibrate about their rest positions. The speed of sound through a medium is constant for that medium, and for the soft tissues of the body it is about 1540 m/s.

Ultrasound speed depends on the stiffness and density of the medium; the stiffer the medium (the stronger the springs between the balls) the shorter the distance that the transmitting ball must move to exert a suitable force on the next in line and so the sooner that force will be transmitted; the more dense the medium (the heavier the balls) the greater the force required to overcome inertia and so the longer the time required. Generally more rigid media have higher speeds of sound while denser media have lower speeds.

In practice both properties change from substance to substance, so that it is not always easy to determine what the change in the speed of sound will be. For example the speed of sound in air is about 300 m/s. In steel the density is greater so one might expect a lower velocity but the increase in stiffness outweighs the increase in density and the speed of sound turns out to be about 6000 m/s.

The reason that the speed of sound in the soft tissues of the body is practically constant is that there is little dif-

Table 1 Velocity of sound in different media

Medium	Velocity of sound (m/s)
Air	330
Fat	1450
Water	1480
Kidney	1561
Blood	1570
Muscle	1585
Lens of eye	1620
Bone	3500
Average soft tissue	1540

ference in the relative densities and stiffnesses of these media. The table of speeds (Table 1) shows that fat has the lowest value while the lens of the eye has the highest. The difference between these extreme values is only about 10% and for most practical purposes the differences in sound speed are only significant in that very fat or very muscular individuals tend to yield relatively poor images because of distortions of the beam due to refraction.

Power

The power of an ultrasound beam is a measure of the energy associated with the beam. Energy is the capacity for doing work, so a more powerful beam is capable of causing a greater rate of heating at a particular site. The unit of power is the watt (or joule per second). If the amplitude of the pressure fluctuation of the wave were to double, the power associated with the wave would quadruple.

Intensity

The intensity of a sound wave is the density of energy associated with the wave. It is found by measuring the total power in the beam over a specified area and then dividing that value by the size of the area. If the power measured over an area A square metres is P watts then the intensity is:

$$P/A \text{ watts per square metre.}$$

The intensity is an easily understood concept but there are a variety of different specific definitions which are useful in quantifying different aspects of the possible effects of the beam (Fig. 3).

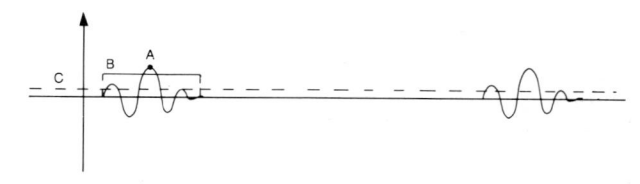

Fig. 3 A pressure against time plot for two consecutive ultrasound pulses illustrating the values of pressure used to calculate: A, peak intensity; B, mean intensity of the pulse; C, mean overall intensity.

The average intensity measured over the whole area of the beam and averaged over the whole time interval that the transducer is energised is called the spatial average, time average intensity (Isata) and relates well to the heating capacity of a beam. A statement on safety from the American Institute of Ultrasound in Medicine concludes that Isata intensities of less than 100 mW per square centimetre have not been shown to be harmful. Other definitions of intensity are used but are beyond the clinical scope of this chapter.

Intensity is not so easily related to other possible biological effects and for fundamental research into the bioeffectiveness of ultrasound more basic measures of the pressure wave, such as the peak positive and peak negative values of pressure are often used.

For an operator the significance of intensity is that reducing the transmitted intensity of sound into the patient has the effect of reducing the brightness or amplitude of all the echoes in the image.

Beam shapes

Ultrasound energy emerges from the face of the transducer in a well-organised way. From the point of view of image clarity and precision it would be most satisfactory if the beam could be made to be extremely thin throughout its length. Unfortunately the physical characteristics of the pressure wave means that the simple expedient of using a small diameter transmitter results in a very widely divergent beam, and the use of a large source reduces the spread of the beam but leaves us with a fat beam (Fig. 4). The best compromise is reached by focusing. A variety of techniques is available: a fixed mechanical lens produces a single focal region; a variable electronic 'lens' can produce a single focal region for each transmitted pulse but a variety of foci for the returning echoes.

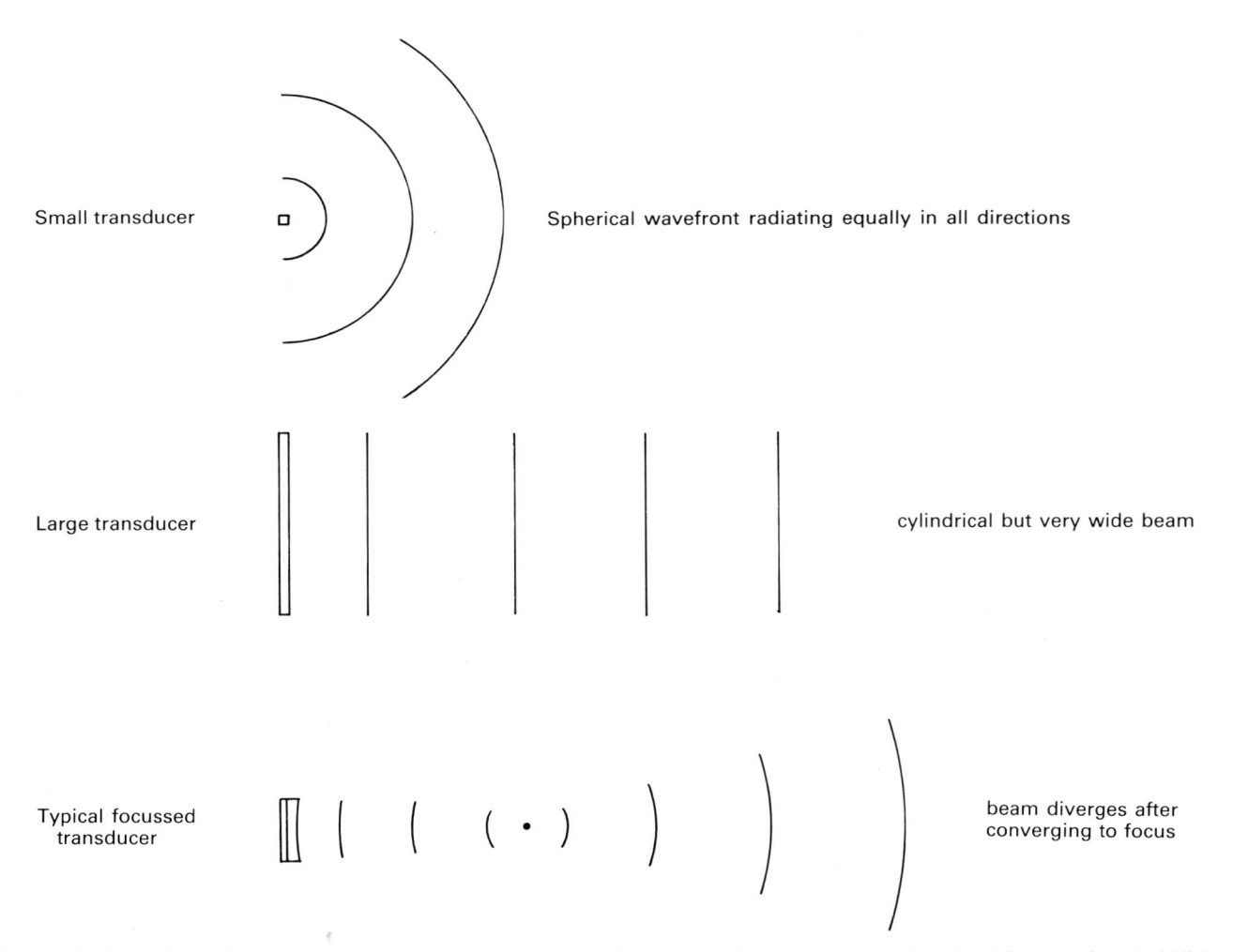

Fig. 4 **The beam shapes** from a tiny transducer with a spherical wavefront (top); a large transducer with a plate (flat) wavefront (middle), and a focused transducer with a curved wavefront (bottom).

The pulse echo technique

There are many examples in both the human and animal kingdoms where details concerning the range, trajectory and constitution of objects are determined using variations of the pulse-echo technique. The principle is that a burst or pulse of energy is transmitted toward an object and the way in which that energy is reflected at the object is analysed by observing the 'echo' returned to the source. The transmitter can be a radar antenna or a bat's larynx, the receiver of echoes can be the same device as the transmitter or a more specialised one (the ear of the bat, for example). Analysing the echo is the heart of the matter and here man and animals part company, animals using biological computers that have evolved over millions of years and are situated snugly between their ears, whilst man relies on a mixture of electrical circuits and computing techniques developed since 1940.

Pulses

Two kinds of ultrasound pulse are used for diagnostic purposes: short pulses for imaging and long pulses for Doppler purposes. Both are generated by the electrical excitation of an element which has the property of altering its dimensions under the influence of an electric field (i.e. a piezoelectric element or transducer).

Short pulses, produced by shock exciting the transducer with a voltage spike, are typically about 3–6 cycles long. They are used in imaging because they provide the best image clarity or resolution.

Long pulses, typically up to 30 or 40 cycles in length, require excitation of the transducer by a sinusoidal voltage of similar length but allow good Doppler resolution. Physically these pulses are 30–40 mm long.

Echoes

The echo is the key to all diagnostic information. It is produced whenever a travelling ultrasound wave encounters a region where the acoustic properties change, that is where the stiffness or density alter. In soft tissues these regions occur at organ boundaries, at tissue discontinuities and at cellular boundaries. Echoes are produced from areas in which acoustic changes occur on a scale greater than approximately one wavelength.

In the balls-on-springs model, acoustic property changes correspond to changes in the spring stiffness and/or the ball mass. At such places the energy travelling toward the new ball/spring system is not completely transferred from the previous ball/spring system resulting in a reflected wave of energy.

There are two kinds of reflection of importance in echocardiography: specular reflection (mirror-like from large interfaces); and non-specular reflection (scattering in all directions from tiny targets).

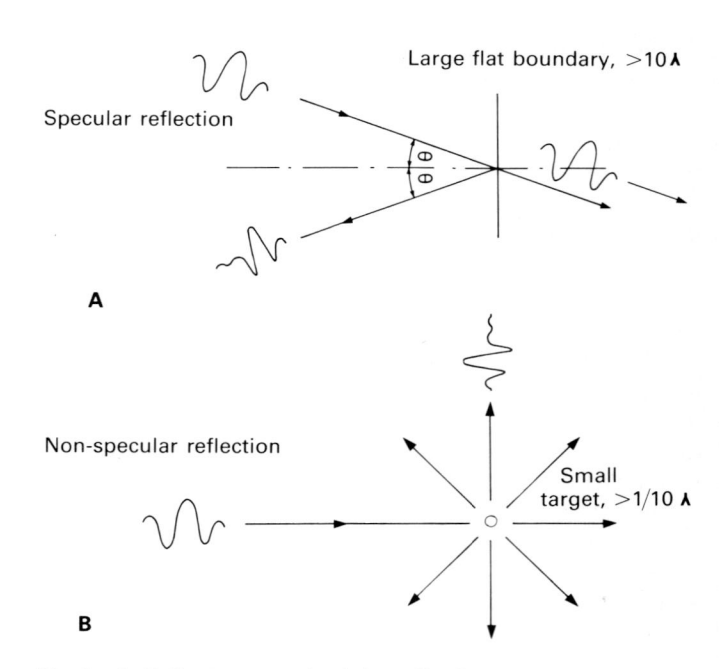

Fig. 5 A: Reflection: specular (mirror-like from large flat targets). **B:** Non-specular reflection (scatter from small targets).

Specular reflection Specular reflection gives rise to large echoes which are best picked up by the transducer when the interface is perpendicular to the beam (Fig. 5). At other orientations the echo size is less than maximum. This phenomenon means that echo size alone cannot generally be used to characterise the target. The boundary size is normally over ten times the size of the ultrasonic wavelength.

Non-specular reflection Non-specular reflection causes the low-level echoes often thought to describe the texture of the organ's parenchyma. The appearance of these low level scattered echoes depends much more on the characteristics of the pulse packet and the width of the beam. This is because the 'echo' seen at the transducer arises from the combination of a multitude of small reflected wavelets from the cellular scatterers which occupy the volume of the ultrasound pulse packet. In some circumstances the combination is a net constructive one in which case an 'echo' approximately the size of the pulse packet is seen; in other arrangements of the randomly oriented scatterers the net result is a cancellation of the reflected wavelets leading to a 'null-echo'. This pattern of 'echoes' and 'null echoes' is called *speckle*. The main problem with speckle is that it produces a false texture for the homogenous, parenchymal areas of organs. The texture depends on the physical size of the pulse packet, and scanning the same region with a different transducer produces a different pattern. In echocardiology the effect of speckle is relatively small because the movement of cardiac muscle results in an averaging out of the worst features of the phenomenon. Non-specular reflection usually occurs with a target size of one-tenth or less of the ultrasonic wavelength.

Range measurement

The time of arrival of the echo (the total time t elapsed between transmission and reception of the pulse-echo pair) is the fundamental clue for diagnostic ultrasound. The speed of ultrasound in soft tissues is assumed to have a constant value and therefore multiplying the time of arrival by this speed yields the go–return distance to the target (Fig. 6).

go–return distance = go–return time × speed
however, target distance = ½ go–return distance,
so, target distance = ½ t × c

The range of the target (half the go–return distance) is the basic information which all pulse-echo systems derive. From it can be calculated the speed of heart valves and the total excursion of the leaflets. In conjunction with the knowledge of the direction of the beam, it is used to produce anatomical images.

Attenuation

An important feature of any system which relies on the pulse-echo technique is that the echo size from identical targets is not the same for targets at different ranges. As the range is increased the echo size is reduced. This is due to the weakening or attenuation of the beam as it travels through the medium. The weakening comes about partially because some of the energy in the beam is scattered out of the beam and divergence of the beam reduces the intensity, but mainly because large fractions are converted into heat in the medium. The practical significance of this is that displayed signals from similar targets appear progressively weaker as the ranges of the targets increase. Electronic compensation for this effect is necessary to produce balanced ultrasonic images.

Attenuation is an exponential reduction in intensity. In practical terms this means that at 3 MHz the intensity is reduced to half its original value after travelling 10 mm, a further reduction of a half occurs after the next 10 mm and a further one after the next 10 mm (the intensity is now $\frac{1}{8}$ of the original value). This is an 'inverse square law' phenomenon with the intensity being halved over each new 'half value' distance (Fig. 7).

Once the pulse is launched into the tissues, nothing can change the way it loses energy but the effects of attenuation can be compensated for electronically. It is arranged that the amplification applied to the electrical signals from the transducer is doubled over each period of time corresponding to the echoes returning from each successive 'half value distance'. The signals produced by echoes from progressively deeper and deeper structures are amplified by progressively greater and greater amounts.

The increase in gain (or amplification) with time is called variously Depth Gain Compensation (DGC), Time Gain Compensation (TGC) and Swept Gain (SG). Adjusting the compensation factors to match the tissues and frequency being used is often referred to as 'balancing' because the effect is to produce displays in which the average echo height or brightness is constant with depth.

The limit of range over which compensation can be

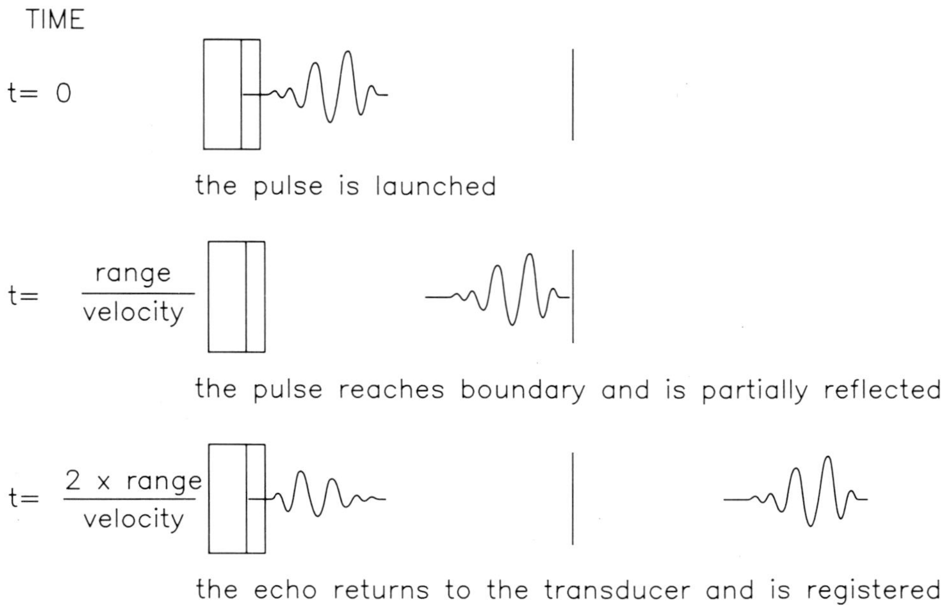

Fig. 6 The pulse echo phenomenon. Top, the pulse is launched; middle, the pulse reaches the target and is partially reflected; bottom, the echo reaches and registers at the transducer.

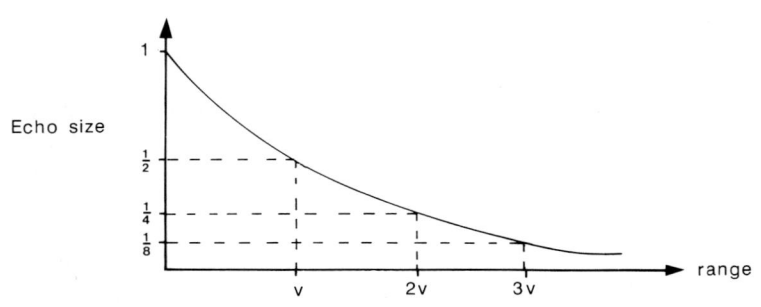

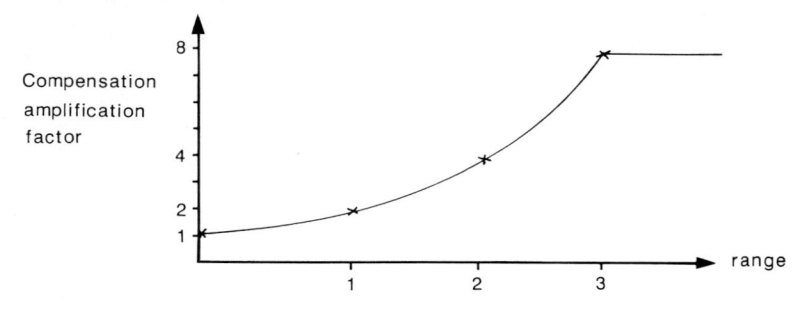

Fig. 7 **Attenuation of echo size with range** (top); The increase of the receiver amplification with time required to compensate for the attenuation (bottom).

achieved is governed by the depth from which the echo size is so small that the signal produced by it at the transducer is at the same level as the electrical noise in the amplifiers. In practice the range limit (the 'penetration depth') is reduced as the frequency is increased. At 3 MHz the typical penetration is about 150 mm; at 10 MHz it is 40 mm.

The A-mode display

The A-mode display is the most straightforward display of returning echo information. A horizontal line on a display screen travels from left to right and is vertically displaced by signals corresponding to the returning echoes.

Thus the distance of a signal from the left hand side of the display is directly related to the time of arrival of that echo (Fig. 8). This is also related to the distance of the structure from the transducer (assuming a constant speed of sound).

The size or amplitude of the signal is related to the amplitude of the corresponding echo but not usually in a linear way. The 'fine texture' echoes resulting from speckle at a cellular level of scattering are very much smaller than the echoes from organ boundaries, often by a factor of a thousand or so. Consequently for both of these kinds of echo to be visible on the same line, where the largest discernible difference in height is about 100 to 1, the small

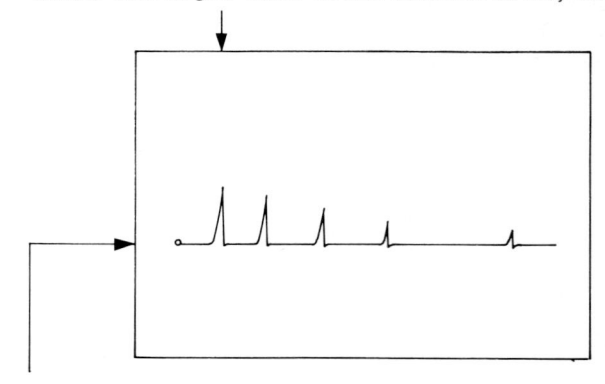

Fig. 8 The A-scan display. The time of arrival of echoes is displayed horizontally and their size vertically.

echoes are amplified to a greater extent than the larger ones. This is called non-linear or logarithmic amplification. An additional problem with the amplitude of signals on the display is that they do not reflect the nature of the boundary producing the echo.

Sampling

After the pulse is launched, echoes begin to return to the

transducer. For a 3 MHz pulse the last useful echoes return after about 200 μs (if the deepest structure is 150 mm away). To produce a visible display of the echoes the information must be constantly updated or refreshed.

A suitable speed of refreshing the display is about 20 times a second as this is just above the persistence threshold for the eye and would produce a flicker-free display. This rate however turns out to be too low for the majority of ultrasound techniques because of the limitations introduced by sampling. Each pulse effectively samples the targets in its path. If these targets are stationary then the slowest sampling rate will satisfactorily describe their non-existent motion. If however, as is usual, there is target movement then the sampling rate must be so high that negligible movement occurs in the interval between samples. If there is any 'missed' movement then the reconstructed description of the targets' motion will be erroneous.

The upper limit of sampling rate (or pulse repetition frequency) is governed by the problem of ambiguity. The echoes from the deepest structures take a finite time to return, depending on the depth and the speed of sound. In the example here the time is 200 μm. The relevance of this is that no further pulses can be launched until echoes from the deepest structures have been received. Here there must be an interval of at least 200 μm between pulses; the maximum rate of transmission of pulses is $1/200 \times 10^6 = 5000$ per second. For most body movements sampling at 5000 times per second is sufficient to produce a reasonably accurate picture. There are, however, circumstances, particularly in Doppler techniques, where increased sampling rates are needed.

The prime use of this kind of display is for purposes requiring accurate measurement of distances, for example corneal thickness for ophthalmic surgery or skin thickness in dermatology. In cardiology the A-scan must be further processed before it can be practically used.

The M-mode display

The M-mode display is a much more useful display for cardiological diagnosis. Here the timebase line no longer has signals deflecting its amplitude; now they produce bright dots along its length. The brightness is related to the echo strength but as in the A-mode scheme, not in a linear fashion. This means that as wide a range of echo sizes as possible can be accommodated on the display. The timebase line with its bright echo dots is made to move slowly in a direction perpendicular to its own direction (Fig. 9). This motion causes stationary targets to trace out a series of parallel lines across the screen. However moving targets draw lines which are a graphical representation of their movements plotted against time. The trace is a plot of distance (calculated from the ultrasonic time of arrival) against time (using the built-in slow sweep timebase). From this display a wealth of detail concerning the activity of cardiac structures is obtained. It is one of the most important display modalities for echocardiography. Usually it is combined with cross-sectional imaging for additional accuracy.

Real-time imaging (or cross-sectional imaging)

The basic pulse-echo technique provides information about

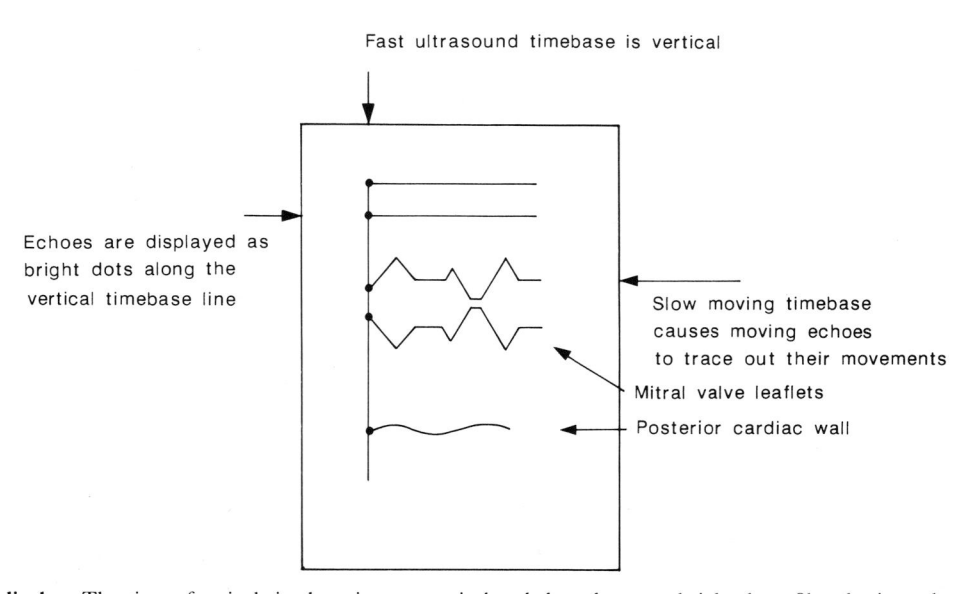

Fig. 9 The M-mode display. The time of arrival timebase is now vertical and the echoes are bright dots. Slow horizontal sweeping of the whole line graphs out moving 'dots'.

target range. Before this can be used to construct a two-dimensional image of the spatial relationships of the targets, information about the direction of the target is needed. This information is gained using a second fundamental assumption about the propagation of ultrasound: ultrasound travels in a straight line in the direction in which it was launched. (The first assumption was that the speed of sound is constant.) Consequently, by describing this direction to the equipment electronically, it is possible to display the timebase line in the direction in which the beam is launched and is assumed to be travelling.

Devices which produce two-dimensional images arrange for the timebase line direction always to follow the beam direction and physically constrain the beam to be swept in one plane. The plane of the display screen then maps the plane of the ultrasound beam. Targets within the scanned plane are drawn as bright dots on the screen in the appropriate anatomical relationships.

It is important to appreciate that the beam is not infinitely thin so that as it is swept through the tissues it interrogates a volume of tissue. The thickness of this volume in the direction perpendicular to the scan plane is termed the slice thickness. The fact that the slice may well be more than 10 mm thick, especially at large ranges from the transducer, means that artefactual echoes may well interfere with the clarity of the image.

Typically the ultrasound beam is rapidly moved either mechanically or electronically so that it describes a fan-shaped sector scan within the scan plane (Fig. 10).

Mechanical scanners incorporate transducers in rotating wheels or attached to rocking assemblies to sweep the beam through the sector. Electronic movement is achieved using an array of small transducer elements mounted side by side. Exciting the elements simultaneously generates a beam perpendicular to the front face, just as a conventional single large element transducer. However if a time delay of a fraction of a microsecond is introduced between exciting each of the small elements then a beam can be produced at angles up to 45° to the face. Since the amount of steering depends only on the size of the time delay there are no physically moving parts involved. The beam is said to be 'inertialess' because a pulse launched at 45° to the face can be followed immediately by a pulse launched straight ahead. The only changes necessary are electronic and these can be performed extremely quickly. A mechanically steered beam cannot be moved swiftly enough to copy this behaviour.

Scan formats other than the sector are possible and rectangular scans are popular in obstetric applications. However, in cardiology the small 'footprint' of the sector scanner is a major advantage as scans can be performed in situations where only small windows for ultrasound transmission are available, notably the intercostal spaces.

If each complete sector movement of the beam is completed in about 1/20 of a second, then twenty complete sectors can be produced per second. Displaying these sectors as they are produced gives rise to a sector image which is a real-time display of the targets within the scanned area, and movement of the targets are displayed in the image as they happen. Real-time scanners are essential for cardiac purposes.

Combining real-time with M-mode scanning

M-mode scans are considerably easier to obtain and are often of enhanced value if they are combined with a real-time imager. The imager ensures that an optimum anatomical view of the target is found so that the M-mode trace can rapidly and accurately be determined. The easiest system to use allows both modes to operate simultaneously but sometimes it is necessary to freeze the real-time image while the M-mode trace is taken. The difference in these approaches lies in the way in which the ultrasound beam is steered through the sector. If the beam is mechanically

Mechanical transducer movement or electronic beam steering

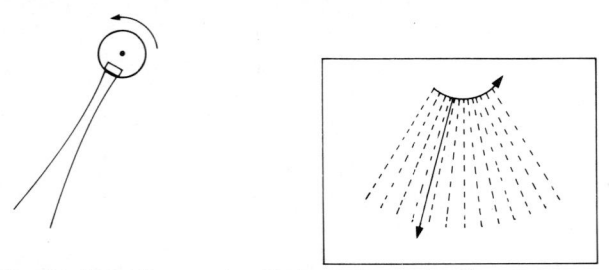

The timebase line on the display follows the direction of the ultrasound beam as the beam moves through its sector

Fig. 10 Rapid sweeping of the beam in the scan plane is achieved either by mechanical or electronic steering. The electronic method results in a beam which has no mechanical inertia and may be directed in any direction within the plane very rapidly. Such scanners (phased array scanners) allow simultaneous imaging and M-mode and pulsed Doppler operation.

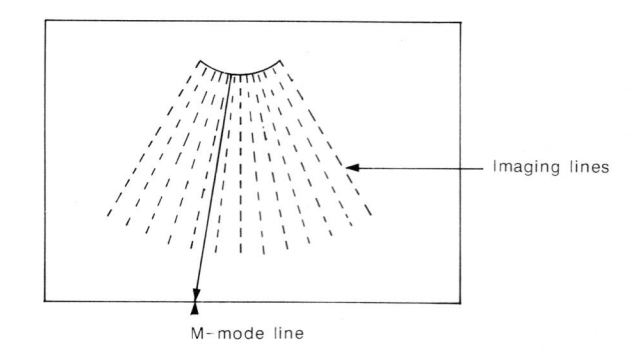

Imaging lines

M-mode line

Fig. 11 The technique of simultaneous imaging and M-mode operation. The transmitted pulses are allocated alternate functions: every other pulse is used in the imaging process and progressively swept through the scan plane while the remainder (the in-between ones) are sent along the same direction to produce the M-mode display. If the rate of pulse production is 5000 per second then the image and the M-mode are produced each with a PRF of 2500.

steered then the transducer must be halted and pointed in the M-mode direction while the M-mode recording is made. If the beam is electronically steered then its direction can be altered from pulse to pulse. The beam is said to be agile and the function of the scanner can be switched between imaging and M-mode very rapidly. Often the stream of pulses are used alternately for each function so that to the operator it appears that both are being performed simultaneously (Fig. 11). Each technique relies on sampling and if both imaging and M-mode are operating together then they have to share the available pulse repetition rate. If the image is frozen the M-mode display can make use of the maximum possible sampling rate.

The Doppler effect

Ultrasound Doppler technology has revolutionised echocardiography. It extends the measurement of cardiac activity to incorporate the investigation of blood flow velocity.

The frequency of a sound wave can be recognised by the rate at which pressure peaks reach the observer. If the observer moves towards the source of sound then more pressure peaks are encountered every second than if the observer is stationary, so the frequency is observed to increase. Similarly if the observer moves away from the source each subsequent peak has further to travel, the rate of arrival is reduced and the observed frequency falls (Fig. 12).

Ultrasound reflected from moving targets undergoes the same effect and has its frequency shifted by an amount proportional to the velocity of the target. The Doppler equation:

$$f_1 - f_0 = \Delta f = \frac{2.f_0.V.\cos\theta}{c}$$

shows that the *change* in frequency, Δf (the difference between the transmitted frequency, f_0, and the received frequency f), depends on constant factors to do with the transmitted frequency, f_0, and the sound speed, c, and is proportional to the component of target velocity in the direction of the beam, $V.\cos\theta$.

Influence of angle

The angle between the beam and the direction of movement of the target has a major effect on the Doppler shift. The more nearly the beam and velocity direction coincide, the larger the value of Doppler shift. If the beam and velocity are perpendicular then the Doppler shift is zero. The component of velocity along the beam direction is found by multiplying the target velocity by the cosine of the angle between the two directions (Fig. 13).

Flow patterns

Although Doppler signals arise from every moving target the most useful ones in cardiology come from flowing blood. Under normal conditions blood cells travel at a variety of velocities, with those in the centre of the vessel or jet moving more rapidly than those on the periphery. Each velocity will give rise to its own Doppler shift fre-

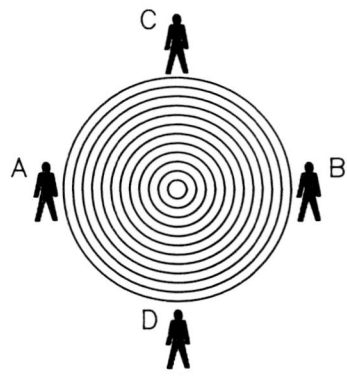

stationary source
all positions detect the same frequency

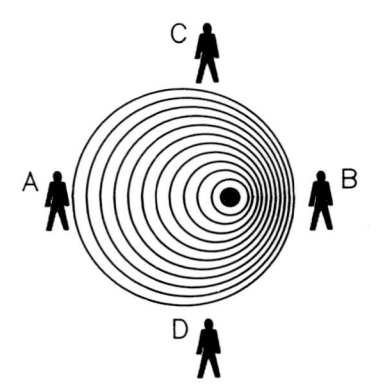

source moving towards B
lower frequency at A
higher frequency at B
unchanged frequency at C,D

Fig. 12 The Doppler effect. When the source is moving towards B, the observer at A hears a reduced frequency while at B an increase is observed. At C and D no change is noticed.

$$\Delta f \propto \cos \theta$$

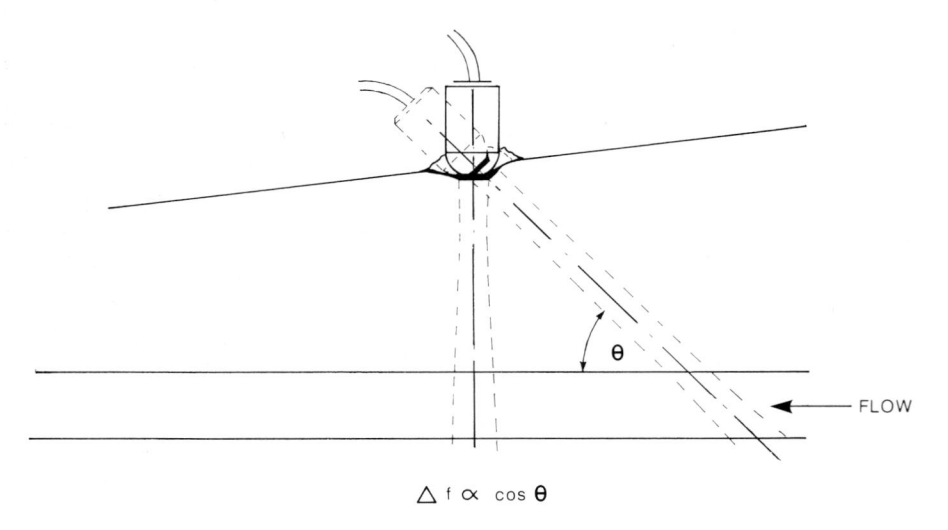

Fig. 13 **The component of velocity along the beam direction** is the product of the flow velocity and the cosine of the angle between the beam and flow directions.

quency. The total Doppler shift from 'real flow' will contain a complex spread of individual frequencies. The observed spectrum of shift frequencies then indicates the range of velocities in the flow and denotes the kind of blood cell velocity profile present.

Laminar flow Laminar flow exists when all the directions of flow velocity are the same. This is often found in normal blood vessels (especially the low pressure ones) and in large area low velocity jets. There are two usual forms of laminar flow.

Parabolic flow. If the flow is non-pulsatile and of relatively low average velocity (for example in the portal vein) then the flow is likely to be parabolic; lines whose length represents the velocity of the blood corpuscles will lie on a parabolic curve (Fig. 14).

Plug flow. Where the fluid is subjected to high fluctuating forces (for example in the ascending aorta) then the flow is likely to be plug, and all the corpuscles will have the same velocity (Fig. 14).

For parabolic flow the average velocity is equal to half the maximum velocity, for plug flow the average velocity and the maximum velocity are identical. The real-life velocity profile under laminar flow conditions will have a characteristic somewhere between parabolic flow at one extreme and plug flow at the other. Laminar Doppler audio signals are very smooth sounding and will have either a wide frequency spread if parabolic flow predominates, or a narrow spread if the flow is more plug-like.

Turbulent flow Turbulent flow is characterised by velocity directions being relatively haphazard. Often this arises in the presence of stenoses in small vessels or where high pressure drops exist across cardiac defects (Fig. 14).

The velocity profile across the flow is impossible to categorise and the relationship between maximum and average velocity is unclear. The Doppler signals are recognised by having a very coarse sound and a chaotic pattern on the spectral display due to the multidirectional and multivelocity components of the flow.

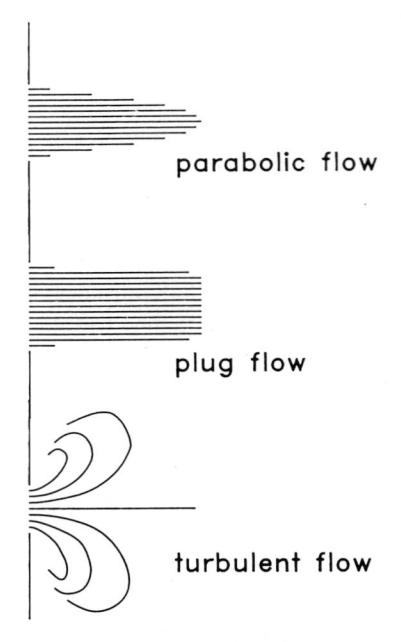

Fig. 14 **Flow patterns**: laminar (parabolic and plug) (top); turbulent (bottom).

Doppler equipment

Continuous wave Doppler

The continuous wave Doppler device is the simplest technical implementation of the effect. A two-transducer probe yielding the range at which the Doppler signal is being generated and if several moving targets exist in the path of the beam all the Doppler shifts will be summed in the final output. Range information and separation of overlying targets can be achieved by using the pulse-echo technique. Pulsed Doppler techniques are in principle no different to the A-mode but now the returning echoes are gated so that only those from a specified range are processed. The echo signal from this range is compared with the reference transmitted signal and any Doppler shift is identified as a phase difference signal. Each transmitted pulse effectively samples the Doppler shift which would have been produced if a continuous beam were used. The samples of Doppler shift are reconstructed to produce the output signal. As with M-mode systems, pulsed Doppler devices are most often used in combination with real-time imaging machines (Fig. 15B).

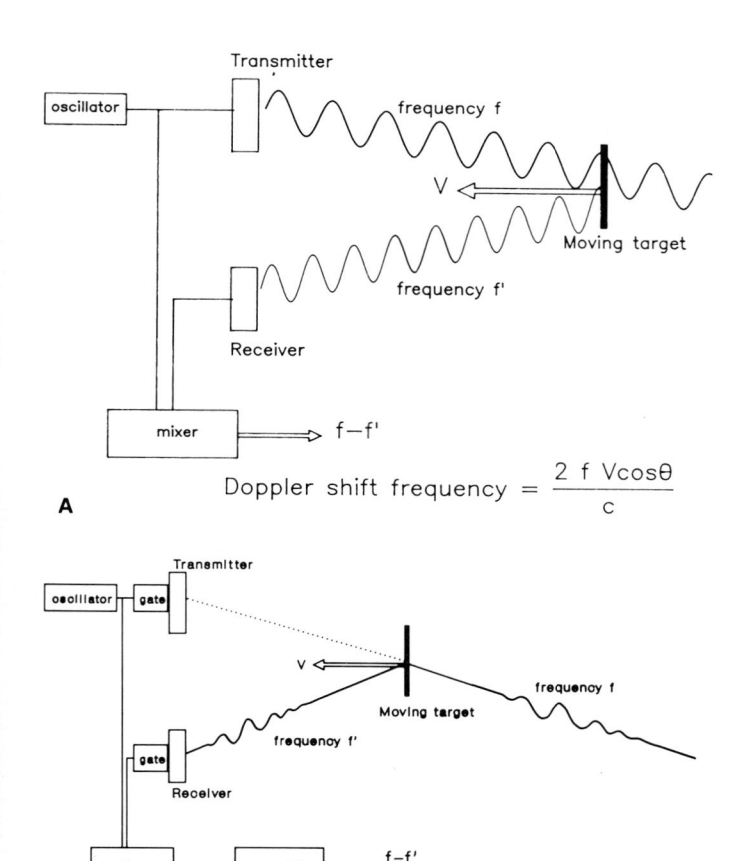

Fig. 15 A: The continuous wave Doppler device. B: The pulsed Doppler device.

is used; one transducer continually generates a beam of ultrasound whilst the second adjacent transducer continually receives the backscattered echoes. The received signals are compared with the transmitted signal and the difference signal is extracted (Fig. 15A). The difference frequency is normally in the audible range and in basic machines this signal is often fed directly to a loudspeaker where the movements can be 'heard'.

The fact that audible sounds are generated can lead to the impression that the device is no more than an 'electronic stethoscope'. It is important to realise that the 'noises' are to do with the velocity of targets and not with any audible bruit or murmur.

The direction of flow is an important physiological feature and can be determined from the Doppler signal by taking into account whether the frequency of the returned signal is higher or lower than the transmitted frequency.

Pulsed Doppler

Continuous wave Doppler techniques are incapable of

Display of Doppler information

The Doppler frequency shifts are displayed in a variety of ways. The most straightforward is to use them as the drive signal for a loudspeaker or a pair of headphones. The operator then 'listens' to the velocity components. Although it is not possible to quantify this kind of display it is extremely useful in many situations. Even when more sophisticated analysis is available, the ability to hear the Doppler signal allows the experienced operator to optimise the position of the beam and gate (for pulsed Doppler systems).

A spectrum analyser must be used for a detailed analysis of all the frequency shifts present in the Doppler waveform, and hence an indication of the kind of flow profile present. The most popular kind uses a technique termed 'Fast Fourier Analysis'. Fourier was the first mathematician to work out the details behind the construction of any waveshape from a series of sine waves of different frequencies and amplitudes. The fast Fourier transform takes any waveshape and calculates the required series of sine waves needed to construct it. Each sine wave, by definition, has only one frequency so the resultant series, when plotted against time, display the complete range of velocity components in the Doppler signal. The amplitude of each frequency component is related to the number of scatterers moving at that speed, hence the relative brightnesses in the display give an appreciation of the kind of velocity profile under investigation (Fig. 16).

Aliasing

In any sampling system an insufficient rate of sampling will produce results that are unreliable. Consider the sinusoidal Doppler signal produced by a continuous wave device observing a single target having constant velocity (Fig. 17). If this target is sampled at a rate of 5000 samples per

22 CARDIAC ULTRASOUND

Fig. 16 Doppler display.

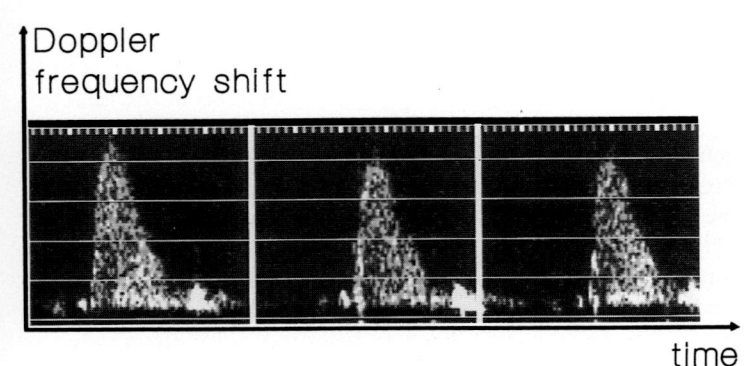

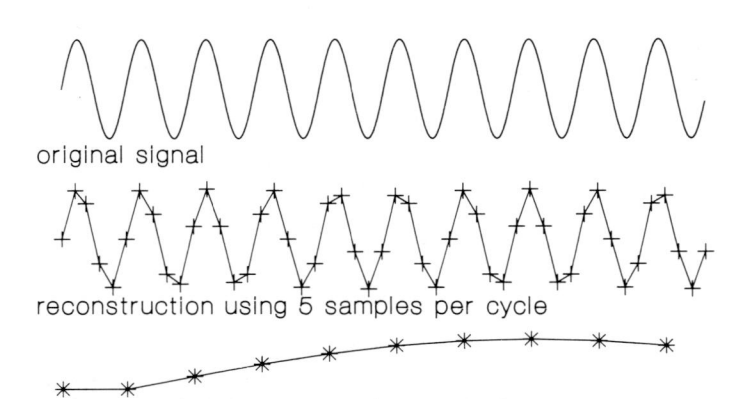

Fig. 17 If the sampling rate is too low a misleading signal is reconstructed. Sampling must be at least twice per cycle to give a recognisable reconstruction.

second then the reconstructed waveform is very close to the original. If however the sampling rate is 1000 per second then the reconstructed signal is very poor and woefully misleading. The effect of having too low a sampling rate is called aliasing. (Often the sampling rate is referred to as the sampling frequency but this nomenclature is avoided here because of the possible confusion between sampling rates and the Doppler shift frequencies being sampled.)

Nyquist frequency The minimum sampling rate for a sinusoidal wave which will enable accurate reconstruction is twice the frequency of the wave. A 2500 Hz wave needs to be sampled at 5000 samples per second. The sampling rate is set by constraints on the ambiguity of returning echoes. The maximum Doppler shift frequency which can be sampled, without aliasing, is the Nyquist frequency and this is equal to half the repetition rate. If the repetition rate is 25 000 pulses per second the Nyquist frequency is 12 500 Hz.

Aliasing is a major problem for Doppler echocardiography and a number of solutions are available. One perfectly feasible method is simply to reduce the carrier frequency by changing to a lower frequency transducer. The lower carrier frequency reduces the Doppler shift frequency and may make it fall below the Nyquist limit.

Extended pulse repetition frequency High pulse repetition frequency options make use of the fact that for Doppler purposes range ambiguity may not be a problem. By transmitting twice as many pulses per second as usual the Nyquist frequency is doubled and only a small penalty appears in the form of an extra Doppler sensitive spot along the timebase line. Pulse repetition rates can be quadrupled in some equipment. In this case three extra sensitive spots are generated. This is important if these additional spots lie in regions of important flow. This flow will be displayed along with signals from the intended region of interrogation.

Colour flow mapping

Colour flow mapping is a logical extension of the combined pulsed Doppler and two-dimensional devices. The display produced is a conventional, two-dimensional, grey scale, real-time, pulse-echo image with regions of movement overlaid in colour (Plate 1). Often the movement is that of blood and the colours describe both the direction (red towards and blue away, for example) and speed of flow (the brighter the colour the higher the speed of flow).

Doppler method (autocorrelation)

The easiest way to understand how this display may be generated is to consider that every series of returning

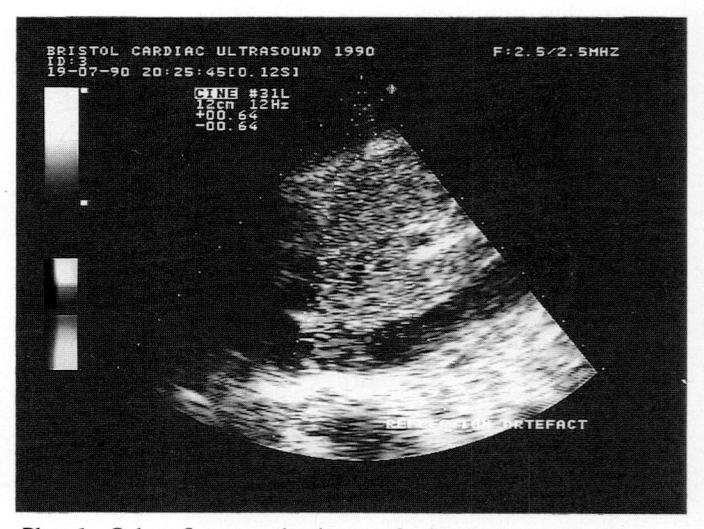

Plate 1 Colour flow mapping image of a hepatic vein draining to the inferior vena cava. Note the artefactual flow image produced by mirror-like reflection of the beam in the posterior wall of the inferior vena cava. This figure is reproduced in colour in the colour plate section at the front of this volume.

echoes is passed to a large number of electronic gates, each feeding an individual pulsed Doppler circuit. The output from each circuit is then assessed for Doppler shift. The shifts are assigned colours according to magnitude (velocity component) and direction. The colours are displayed on the image as coloured dots (or pixels), in place of the usual range gate blip shown for a single channel device. A hundred channels would allow a hundred possible coloured dots. As the ultrasound beam sweeps through the scan plane the coloured dots illuminate those regions where Doppler shifts occur. If each line of Doppler information is obtained rapidly then a real-time map of tissue or blood movement is produced (Fig. 18).

Moving target indicator

A technique by which movement can be colour coded onto the display without estimating the frequency shift of returning echoes uses direct calculation of the velocity of a cluster of blood cells. The echo patterns produced by the cluster are tracked from pulse to pulse so that the distance travelled, in the inter-pulse period, can be determined (Fig. 19).

This approach is fundamentally different to the pulsed Doppler one and does not suffer the same problems of aliasing. It is still a measure of the velocity component and dependent on the angle of attack. It too requires relatively long dwell times to estimate low velocities.

Velocity coding

The usual information coded onto the flow map is the average velocity and direction of flow. As flow velocities increase the colours become brighter with highest velocities often being represented as white. The precise colours used are often chosen by the operator.

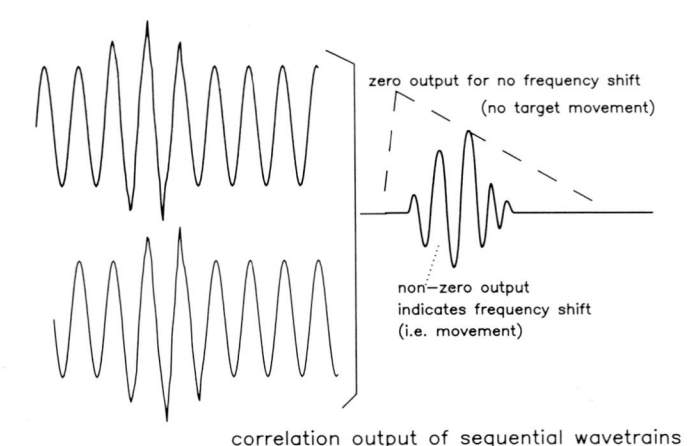

Fig. 18 Autocorrelation method for colour flow mapping.

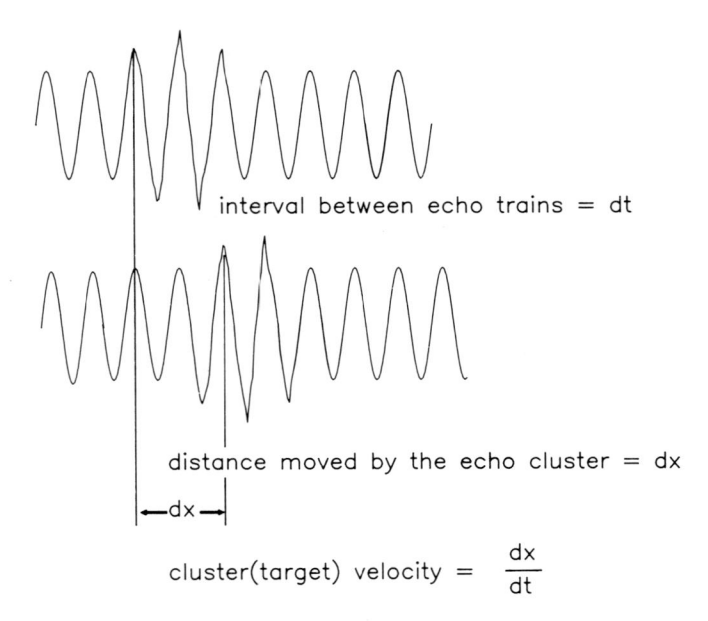

Fig. 19 Moving a cluster (direct velocity) method for colour flow mapping.

Power coding

The power option codes the backscattered energy into colour. It is chosen when the velocity of flow is too low to be estimated accurately. The backscattered energy (the power) depends on the quantity of scatterers present; consequently a useful idea of the volume and direction of flow can be obtained even if the velocity components are not measurable.

Low velocity detection

The problem of determining low flow velocities is one of being able to dwell along one line of sight for a sufficient length of time for a measurable Doppler shift or cluster movement to occur. Machines usually send ensembles of ten or 15 pulses along each colour flow timebase line direction so that the dwell time is about 2 ms. Increase of this observation time would require a reduction in the colour flow frame rate.

Variance

An additional feature often included in the coding is the variance of the Doppler signal. This is a measure of the spread of the velocities in the signal and is taken as an indicator of degree of turbulence in the flow. Laminar flow will have a smoothly changing spectral content. The presence of turbulence changes the nature of the spectrum and is obviously an important clinical feature.

Influence of angle

It is important to realise that the main feature of 'velocity coded' colour flow images is the Doppler frequency shift or cluster velocity. This feature depends on the velocity component *in the direction of the ultrasound beam*. A regurgitant jet flowing directly toward the transducer will look much more spectacular than flow through a interventricular defect if that flow is perpendicular to the beam. If 'power coding' is used this effect is less important although it is still worth noting that machines are inherently less sensitive to low flow velocities because of the dwell time difficulties referred to above and because filters are used to remove some low frequency ('wall and tissue thump') signals.

Aliasing and colour flow

The constraints of time are especially severe in the operation of a device which is producing a real-time image with simultaneous colour flow mapping and single channel pulsed Doppler output. This can lead to the use of relatively low pulse repetition rates for each modality. Aliasing then becomes a significant feature of the image. As far as colour flow mapping is concerned aliasing appears as a sudden change from one extreme colour to the extreme opposite direction colour. If there is true flow reversal then the two colours are separated by a thin black region representing flow of such low velocity that no Doppler shift is detected and no colour can be assigned. In analysing an image for the presence of aliasing it is essential to consider what flow characteristics are likely to be occurring in that clinical situation from a commonsense point of view.

Image resolution

Resolution is a term used to mean the clarity and fidelity of the image. The definition of clarity involves the minimum spatial separation of point targets which can just be distinguished on the display. The fidelity is the precision with which target velocity can be determined (temporal resolution) and with which regions of slightly different echo level can be detected (contrast resolution).

Spatial

Resolution in space is the ability of an imaging device to detect two closely spaced objects. This ability is often 'measured' by suspending two typical targets in a suitable background medium and altering their separation, measuring it just before the discrete images fuse on the screen.

Spatial resolution is often in the order of several millimetres depending on whether measured along the beam axis (axial or range resolution) or across it (lateral or azimuthal resolution). Range resolution is constant with range whereas lateral resolution improves from the transducer face to the focal zone and then worsens in the distal parts of the beam (Fig. 20).

In cardiac applications the most significant practical problem is poor lateral resolution at extreme range.

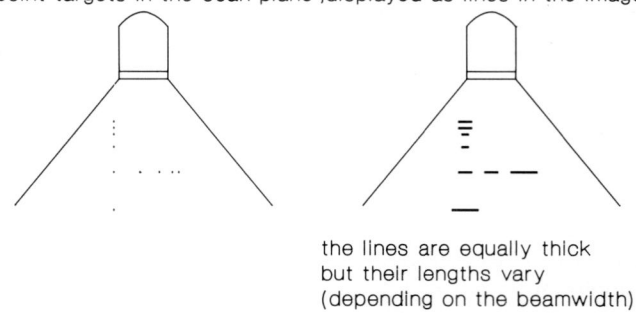

Fig. 20 Spatial resolution. Point targets in the scan plane are displayed as lines because of the physical dimensions of the ultrasound pulse.

Temporal

Temporal resolution is the precision of measurement of moving targets on the M-mode display. It has to do with the sampling rate and for all cardiac measurements is not a significant restriction.

Contrast

Contrast resolution is the ability to resolve regions of the image which differ from their surroundings only by reason of their echogenicity. If a system can detect small differences in echogenicity it is said to have good contrast resolution.

Contrast resolution is not a feature of much concern for the majority of echocardiography imaging, since most images deal with structures of fairly well defined morphology surrounded by blood. Contrast resolution becomes of more value in situations such as the detection of metastatic deposits in the liver.

Artefacts

In any ultrasound image the artefacts are almost as important as the 'real' echoes. Artefacts are appearances on the image which do not correspond to targets at that anatomical site.

Reverberation

Reverberation is the most common kind (Fig. 21) of artefact. The ultrasound pulse reflects from every surface where there is a significant acoustic difference. If a strong

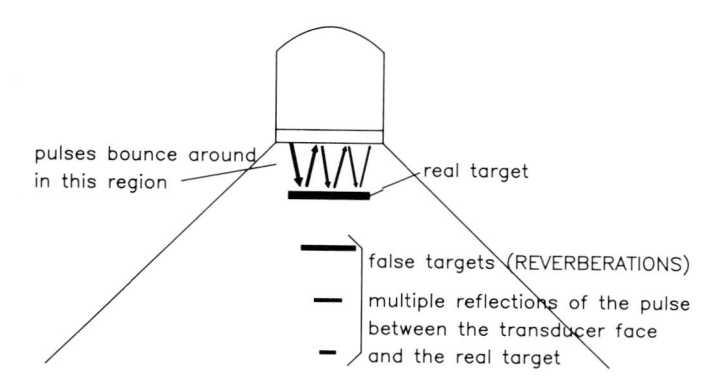

Fig. 21 Reverberation artefact caused by multiple re-reflection of the pulse between two good reflectors.

reflector is encountered close to the transducer face then the returning echo is large and the size of that part which is partially re-reflected at the transducer face back into the patient is also quite large. Meeting the same strong reflector it returns to the transducer where it is once again partially reflected back into the patient. This sequence can occur many times before the pulse is eventually attenuated into noise by the intervening tissues. Each time the reflected pulse strikes the transducer face it generates an echo signal which is registered as coming from deeper and deeper within the patient. On a real-time image the appearance of these echoes is of a gradually decreasing ladder of identically spaced echoes extending into the patient. This artefact is often seen during echocardiography.

All echoes returning to the transducer are partially reflected at its face because of the large mismatch between the transducer and the skin. One way of reducing this effect is to use matching layers of intermediate materials between them. Matching layers not only reduce reverberation artefacts but also improve the sensitivity of the transducer, enabling weaker echoes to register recognisable signals.

Refraction

Refraction is a phenomenon which occurs whenever a travelling wave passes from one medium to another with a different wave velocity (Fig. 22). It is commonly encountered in optics where it produces the 'broken stick' illusion when a straight stick is partially immersed in water. The bending of ultrasound beams certainly produces observable effects. The electronically drawn lines which map the passage of the ultrasound beam onto the display screen are straight and echoes are displayed on them as though the beam of ultrasound travelled in a straight line. Any deviation of the beam is not apparent to the machine so that echoes arising from a refracted beam are misregistered in the image.

The prime effect of refraction is to degrade the image.

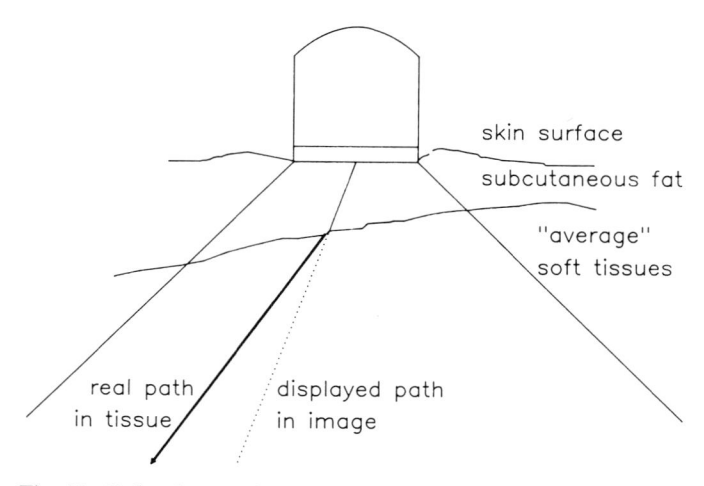

Fig. 22 Refraction artefact; the beam is deviated from its original propagation direction at the boundary between media with differing sound velocities.

If this becomes unacceptable it may be possible to scan through an alternative window to view the required site without traversing the distorting region. Alternatively the use of a larger diameter transducer, sometimes necessarily of a lower frequency, may improve image clarity by averaging more of a collection of small random deviations.

Shadowing

Shadowing in an ultrasound image is caused by the beam meeting a highly attenuating or very reflective region (Fig. 23). The echoes from the area distal to such a region are much weaker and are displayed as a relatively dark streak extending all the way from the shadowing structure to the maximum depth of the image. Often this feature is

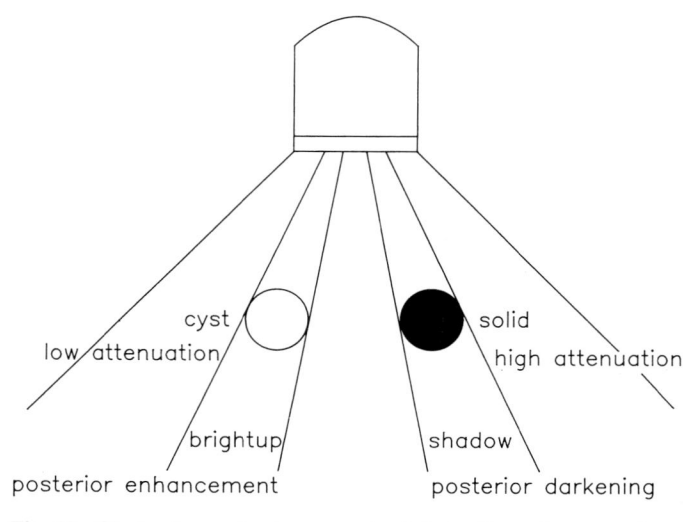

Fig. 23 Shadowing and enhancement artefacts. Strongly attenuating regions lead to posterior shadowing while posterior enhancement lies behind regions of low attenuation.

an aid to diagnosis as it yields additional information about the image; for example calcified valves and plaques can be identified more easily because of the shadowing. Where shadowing obscures the region of interest it is sometimes possible to scan from a slightly different site and avoid the worst effects of the shadow.

Enhancement

Enhancement is the inverse of shadowing and occurs when the beam interacts with an area of reduced attenuation (Fig. 23). The distal echoes are stronger than expected and on the image posterior bright streaks are displayed. These are typically seen behind cysts where again the artefact is of some diagnostic value. They do not present the problem of obscuring important detail but rather require that the overall gain or the transmitter power be reduced so that the distal echo levels are at an appropriate level.

Beam width effects

Although the display represents the beam as a very thin straight line the ultrasound beam width is considerable, even in very well focused systems. Typically the beam is the same width as the transducer face, initially reducing to about 3 or 4 mm wide over the useful depth of focus, often to a range of about 8 cm after which it diverges and can be 2 or 3 cm across at the maximum penetration depth. The effect of this shape on the image is that point targets are displayed at the full width of the beam at that range (Fig. 24). Additionally if there is a small cyst or stone located at a range where the beam width is larger than the lesion, then those parts of the beam which overlap will send echoes back to the transducer disguising any enhancement or shadowing which would otherwise be expected (Fig. 25).

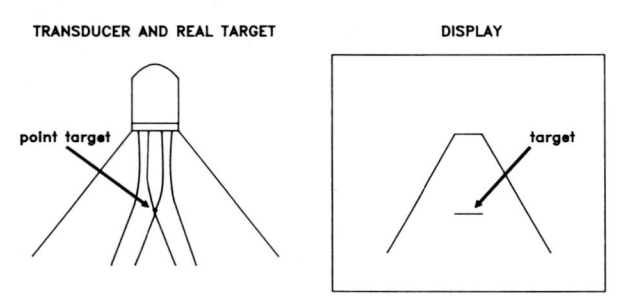

The point target is represented as a line on the display because it is picked up by several adjacent ultrasound beams. The length of the line is equal to the ultrasound beam width

Fig. 24 Beam width effect. Overestimating target widths.

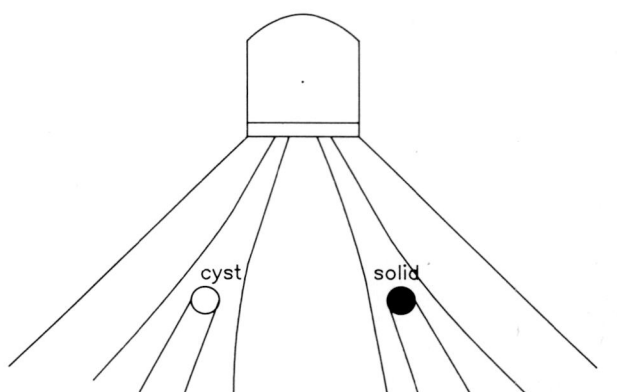

If the beam is wider than the lesion then the effects of shadowing and enhancement are diluted by echoes from the parts of the ultrasound beam that bypass the lesion.

Fig. 25 Beam width effect. Hiding cysts and stones.

BIBLIOGRAPHY

Evans J A (ed.) 1986 Physics in medical ultrasound. Institute of Physical Sciences in Medicine, York
Evans D H, McDicken W N, Skidmore R, Woodcock J P 1989 Doppler ultrasound: physics, instrumentation and clinical applications. Wiley, New York
Goldberg B B, Wells P N T (eds) 1983 Ultrasonics in clinical diagnosis. Churchill Livingstone, Edinburgh
Hill C R (ed.) 1986 Physical principles of medical ultrasonics. Ellis Horwood, Chichester

Kremkau F W 1990 Diagnostic ultrasound: physical principles and exercises, 2nd edn. Grune and Stratton, New York
McDicken W N 1991 Diagnostic ultrasonics: principles and use of instruments, 3rd edn. Wiley, New York
Shirley I M, Blackwell R J, Cusick G, Farman D J, Vicary F R 1978 A user's guide to diagnostic ultrasound. Pitman Medical, London
Wells P N T 1977 Biomedical ultrasonics. Academic Press, London

3

Equipment

Introduction
Instrument technologies
Scanhead types
Mechanical sector scanheads
   Principle of operation
   Rotating scanheads
   Oscillatory scanheads
   Practical considerations
Phased array scanheads
   Principle of operation
   Practical considerations
Phased annular array scanheads
   Principle of operation
   Practical considerations
Transoesophageal scanheads

Scanhead frequency and focus
Doppler techniques
Pulsed Doppler
High PRF Doppler
Continuous wave Doppler
Colour flow Doppler
Measurement and analysis packages
Distance and area
Volumes
Wall motion analysis
Doppler analysis
Image storage devices
Video recorders
Digital storage
Disk storage
Hard copy devices

Factors affecting instrument performance
Image aesthetics (presentation)
Imaging artefacts
Practical aspects of spectral Doppler (pulsed and continuous wave)
Practical aspects of colour flow Doppler
Future developments
Digital echocardiography
   Stress echocardiography
   Further applications of digital echocardiography
Transducer developments

Graham Thirsk

INTRODUCTION

Since their introduction, echocardiography systems have developed into sophisticated instruments capable of providing a wide range of diagnostic information. Real time, two-dimensional (2D) imaging provides valuable information about anatomical structure and has proved to be particularly useful in detecting morphological defects, for example in the evaluation of congenital heart disease and myocardial dysfunction. Systems with pulsed wave (PW) and continuous wave (CW) Doppler facilities provide additional diagnostic information about blood flow within the heart structures. Valvular stenosis, valvular regurgitation, septal defects and patent ductus arteriosus can all be detected and localised by use of Doppler techniques. Determination of pressure gradients across valves or septal defects is also possible using Doppler techniques. The recent introduction of colour flow Doppler has simplified the assessment of cardiac flow and can sometimes reduce the Doppler examination time considerably. The visual nature of colour flow often highlights small unsuspected lesions and improves the discrimination of multiple lesions.

The practical implementation of these ultrasound techniques and the success of that implementation varies enormously in individual instruments. Consequently, the prospective purchaser may be faced with a complex and difficult task when selecting the best instrument for their clinical requirements. Assessment of echocardiography system performance must be approached objectively if the true diagnostic value of the instrument is to be determined accurately. Instruments producing the most aesthetically pleasing images could be using extensive processing which may mask valuable diagnostic information. The quality of images can also be affected dramatically by the echo subject. It is generally easier to display high quality echo images from a young, thin non-smoking subject with wide intercostal spaces, than from an emphysematous obese subject with a large chest. Performance comparisons of echocardiography instruments should therefore be carried out on a side by side basis, that is, the subject should be imaged on both instruments consecutively, so that a fair assessment is made of each instrument.

Instrument technologies

All current echocardiography instruments include 2D imaging and M-mode facilities, whilst Doppler and colour Doppler facilities are either integrated into the system or available as separate options. Two-dimensional echocardiography images are most often presented in a sector format. This format provides a narrow field of view close to the scanhead with an increasing field of view as the distance from the scanhead increases. A sector format is ideal for scanning through the intercostal spaces where physical access is restricted but as much of the heart as possible must be visualised.

The ultrasound scanhead (probe) can influence greatly the performance of the echocardiography system. There are several different types of sector ultrasound probes and each type is available in a range of frequencies and focusing. Careful selection of the optimum probe type, frequency and focus for a specific clinical application is essential to obtain the best possible diagnostic performance from the instrument.

SCANHEAD TYPES

There are three major types of sector ultrasound scanhead currently used with modern cardiac ultrasound systems, namely mechanical scanheads, phased array scanheads and phased annular array scanheads.

Mechanical sector scanheads

Principle of operation

There are two types of mechanical sector scanhead, rotating or oscillatory. In both types, the scanning action is achieved by physically moving a large circular element through a predetermined arc, usually 90°. This element is physically shaped to form a concave lens producing a concentric ultrasound beam, focused at the appropriate focal point. The diameter of the element determines the effective aperture and thus influences the focal range and the sensitivity of the scanhead.

For efficient transfer of the ultrasound energy, the high impedance of the element must be matched to the much lower impedance of the skin. This impedance matching is attained by enclosing the element in a fluid whose acoustic impedance is less than that of the element but is greater than that of the skin surface. The scanhead cap also assists the impedance matching process.

Rotating scanheads

In rotating scanheads several identically matched elements are mounted on a wheel which is rotated at a constant velocity. As the element reaches the edge of the sector a microswitch is closed. This action enables electrical pulses from the ultrasound system to reach the element, and permits the received signals to return to the system. After the arc has been traversed the switch opens and the emission/reception cycle ceases. The mounting of multiple elements on the wheel allows multiple image frames to be constructed for every rotation of the wheel which optimises the frame rate and temporal resolution. In addition this type of scanhead produces very little vibration.

The maximum velocity at which the wheel can be rotated is determined by the pulse repetition frequency (PRF) which, in turn, is dictated by the depth of the structure of interest.

Oscillatory scanheads

In oscillatory scanheads, the element is swept forwards and backwards through an arc and is pulsed at the required PRF. The element and its mounting must decelerate at the end of each sweep, stop and then accelerate in the opposite direction at the beginning of the next sweep. This non-linearity of motion leads to severe distortion of the ultrasound image at the extremes of the arc. To reduce this distortion, the element is swept through a greater arc than necessary and only the linear portion of the sweep is used. This type of scanhead necessarily produces noticeable vibration when operating.

Practical considerations

Mechanical sector scanheads combine small contact area with large constant aperture and possess the ability to scan through restricted acoustic windows with high sensitivity and high resolution (Fig. 1). The single, large element design of this type of scanhead enables high frequencies to be used with increased spatial resolution.

The focal point is fixed by the size and shape of the element and so one scanhead is unable to provide ideal performance for applications requiring both superficial and deep imaging. In addition, it is not possible to provide operation in additional modes simultaneously, for example simultaneous 2D imaging and M-mode recording, since the mechanical movement of the element prevents the motion being stopped and restarted easily (see Ch. 2).

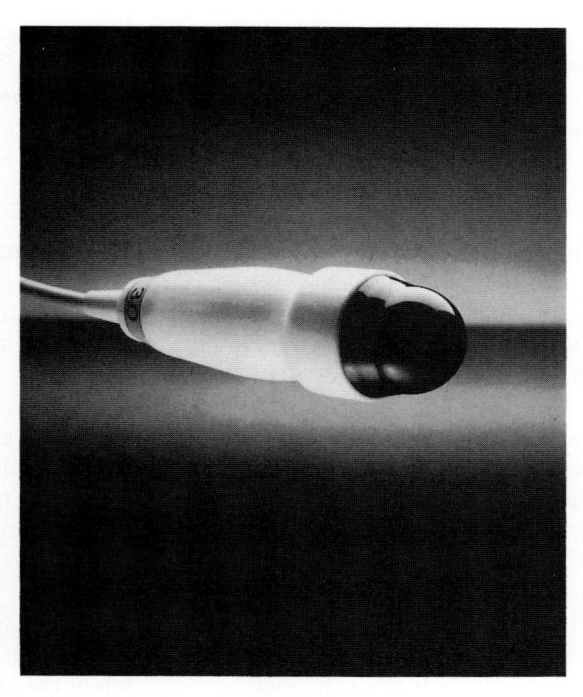

Fig. 1 Typical mechanical oscillating transducer.

Phased array scanheads
Principle of operation

Phased arrays are formed by placing a large number of electrically discrete elements side by side to form a rectangular scanhead. Individual elements are usually sub-divided into a number of smaller sub-elements in order to minimise the production of artefacts, such as grating lobes. The entire array of elements is treated as if it were one group, that is, all elements are required to produce a single ultrasound line. Each element in the array is in series with an electronically controlled delay (channel). Careful selection of the delays between each element controls both the direction and focusing of the beam. Increasing the number of elements and channels can increase focusing accuracy and the image quality, bearing in mind that the accuracy of the delays is a limiting factor in this process.

Electronic focusing can be performed only in the image plane, that is, along the array of elements. Focusing in the perpendicular plane is implemented with an acoustic lens which provides a fixed focal point. This fixed focusing in the perpendicular plane adversely affects the resolution of the scanhead.

Practical considerations

Phased array sector transducers provide good images when physical access is restricted. Electronic control of the beam direction enables the highest frame rates to be achieved and permits simultaneous operation in more than one mode, due to the agile nature of the beam. Two dimensional imaging can be achieved simultaneously with M-mode or Doppler examination. The imaging resolution of phased array sector scanheads may be less than that of a mechanical scanhead of the same frequency due to the artefacts produced as a consequence of steering the beam. Modern phased array instruments utilise several processing techniques to minimise the side lobe artefacts generated during

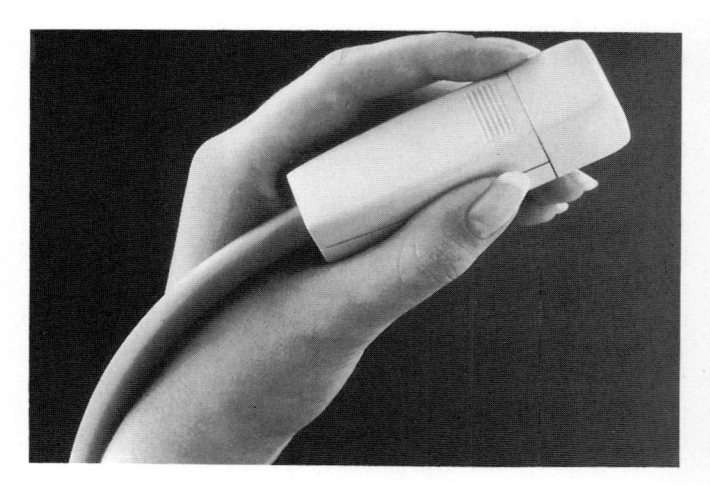

Fig. 2 Typical phased array transducer.

beam steering. Wide aperture scanheads with a large number of elements have a physically large contact area and some practical limitations may be encountered when scanning through a restricted acoustic window (Fig. 2). When scanning through narrow intercostal spaces, the effective aperture may be reduced, as the outer elements of the array are not fully able to contribute to the focusing of the beam. This reduction of aperture will affect the focusing accuracy and consequently will degrade the image quality.

Phased annular array scanheads

Principle of operation

The operation of phased annular array scanheads is similar to that of oscillatory mechanical sector scanheads but the large crystal is not single, instead being subdivided into a number of electrically discrete concentric elements or rings. Individual ring elements should be of equal surface area and should be subdivided into subelements to minimise artefact generation.

Annular phased arrays are dynamically focused in the same manner as phased array transducers but because the elements are circular rather than rectangular, the beam is focused in both the imaging and perpendicular planes simultaneously. Annular phased arrays should produce the narrowest ultrasound beam and the best lateral resolution, provided other aspects of beam formation do not degrade the performance. Increasing the number of rings improves focusing accuracy whilst increasing the surface area (aperture) improves penetration and focus at depth.

Practical considerations

The large aperture of annular array scanheads provides greater sensitivity and dynamic range, for a given frequency, than with any other type of transducer. In addition, the concentric focusing provides the best possible spatial resolution at the desired point of interest. Although annular arrays provide the best theoretical resolution, the accuracy of the focusing is restricted by the small number of elements that contribute to the process. This limitation can be minimised by very accurate control of the delays, such as that provided by digital beam forming techniques. Wide aperture annular arrays may not always produce the expected image quality because of poor physical access or the aperture restriction imposed by narrow intercostal spaces.

Transoesophageal scanheads

In some patients, it is difficult to obtain a satisfactory image through the intercostal spaces but by imaging the heart from the oesophagus using a transoesophageal (TOE) probe a significant improvement in diagnostic image quality can be achieved. This improvement results from reducing the distance from the scanhead to the heart and using a higher frequency scanhead. In addition, the echo window is not restricted by the intercostal spaces and not obstructed by the lungs.

Most TOE scanheads have phased array transducers located at the end of an endoscope, although a mechanical version is available. The TOE scanheads usually have a centre frequency of 5 MHz to optimise the resolution and depth of penetration. The active tip of the TOE is manipulated and held in contact with the oesophageal wall by means of steel control wires within the endoscope.

Early TOE probes suffered from a high number of mechanical failures. These failures were attributed to stretching of the control wires, resulting in loss of mobility of the probe tip or damage caused by the patient biting the probe. Modern probes have been designed to overcome these problems.

SCANHEAD FREQUENCY AND FOCUS

Typical probe frequencies used in echocardiography instruments are 2.25, 3.5, 5.0, 7.5 and 10.0 MHz. Increasing the probe frequency generally improves image resolution but this also decreases the sensitivity and penetration. For example, a 2.25 MHz probe can be expected to penetrate to a depth of 23 cm, whilst a 7.5 MHz probe may only penetrate to a depth of 7 cm. The lower frequencies (2.25, 3.5 MHz) are most suitable for adult and teenage patients, whilst the higher frequencies (5.0, 7.5 MHz) are most suitable for children and neonates.

The optimum frequency for Doppler performance is generally lower than that for 2D imaging since the highest possible sensitivity is required to detect the very low level scattered signals returned from blood cells. In addition, the Doppler frequency shift for a given blood velocity increases as the frequency of the probe increases and this reduces the ability to assess high velocities, especially when using pulsed wave and colour flow Doppler techniques.

When considering scanhead focus, both focal point and the focal range are important. Probes which are tightly focused have a narrow focal range so that the image will appear to be sharply in focus only over a small area, whereas probes with a wide focal range produce less sharp but more uniform images. Mechanical scanheads have a fixed focus which is determined by the shape of the element. Array scanheads may be focused electronically to provide a selectable focal point and, by dynamic focusing during reception of the echoes, extend the focal range to increase image uniformity.

Typical focal ranges are:

Short focus	2–3 cm
Medium focus	3–5 cm
Medium to long focus	5–8 cm
Long focus	8–11 cm.

DOPPLER TECHNIQUES

Most current echocardiography systems incorporate Doppler blood flow velocity measurement capability whilst colour flow Doppler capability is usually provided as an option. There are two main types of Doppler technique, pulsed wave (PW) and continuous wave (CW).

Pulsed Doppler

Pulsed Doppler systems transmit a burst of ultrasound and then receive for only a short period after a selected delay. Thus, in effect, PW systems only listen for Doppler shifts at a predetermined depth. The burst is repeated as soon as the signal is received from the desired depth. The rate at which the bursts are repeated, the pulse repetition frequency (PRF), reduces as the sample depth increases, since the burst takes longer to make the round trip to the selected depth and back.

The length of the burst and the period for which the receiver is active determine the length of the sample volume. The burst length is not usually less than three wavelengths since at least this number is needed to determine accurately the frequency of the received signal. The minimum sample volume length is usually restricted to 1.5 mm for this reason. The lateral dimensions of the sample volume are determined entirely by the width of the Doppler beam at the selected depth and may be affected by any beam focusing techniques employed.

PW systems have excellent range resolution as they only respond to motion at the selected depth. However, since the motion is sampled at a rate equal to the PRF, they are only able to determine accurately a maximum frequency shift of half the PRF. Above this maximum frequency a phenomenon known as aliasing occurs which limits seriously the maximum velocity that can be accurately determined. This maximum frequency is known as the Nyquist limit.

High PRF Doppler (HPRF)

PW Doppler systems wait until the transmitted pulse has travelled to the requisite depth and returned before activating the receive gate. The PRF is limited by the depth of the sample volume and therefore the maximum velocity that can be resolved without ambiguity is also limited. This limitation may be overcome by transmitting additional pulses whilst waiting for the return of the first pulse, thereby increasing the PRF. However, the receiver will be unable to differentiate between returning signals from each of the pulses and this introduces range ambiguity. The instrument is effectively introducing multiple sample volumes in the beam. Some instruments move automatically to HPRF if circumstances dictate and it is essential for this to be made clear to the operator by the display in order to avoid erroneous interpretations being made.

Continuous wave Doppler (CW)

Continuous wave Doppler systems continuously transmit ultrasound of a fixed known frequency from one element, or set of elements, and continuously receive ultrasound on an adjacent element, or set of elements. Motion within the beam at any depth will produce a Doppler shift in the reflected signal. Consequently, CW systems do not have any range resolution since they cannot determine where in the beam the motion occurred. They are however able to determine accurately very high flow velocities because they transmit and receive continuously. CW devices fall into two categories, single crystal devices and duplex CW. Single crystal devices have the disadvantage of being used blind, that is, no 2D image is available to assist in the optimum orientation of the beam into the flow. They display the widest dynamic range and sensitivity of all Doppler devices and the small size of the transducer simplifies the acquisition of good Doppler signals from small acoustic windows. Duplex CW systems offer the advantage of being able to use a 2D image to optimise the orientation of the Doppler beam into the flow. The larger size of these transducers often makes it more difficult to locate the optimum echo window for good Doppler signals and because the transducer aperture is now shared between transmit and receive there is a reduction in Doppler sensitivity. Peak velocities measured with this type of transducer may be underestimated by as much as 15% because of the reduced sensitivity. Some duplex CW systems use a separate CW transducer side by side with the imaging scanhead in the same housing. There is no way that the CW beam can be steered in the image with this system. Additionally, with this type of scanhead, the CW probe will not use exactly the same echo window as the imaging probe, and therefore different quality results may be obtained. Recently some manufacturers have introduced 'steerable' CW Doppler probes in which the phased array crystals produce both image and Doppler information.

Colour flow Doppler

Colour flow imaging (CFI) systems may be considered to be multigate PW Doppler systems with simultaneous 2D imaging since they acquire Doppler data from many sample volumes along each ultrasound beam. The sample volume length and resolution depend upon the digitisation rate and the depth range covered. The instantaneous mean velocity at each of these sample volumes is estimated and represented as colour overlaying the 2D image. The statistical variance of the mean velocity estimation is calculated and may also be displayed on the colour image.

The Fast Fourier Transform (FFT) method used for Doppler signal analysis takes at least 5 ms. If this method were used to analyse colour Doppler signals, it would take approximately 2 minutes to create a single colour flow image. Therefore, a different analysis method, pulse pair co-variance estimation, is used for colour flow Doppler. An auto-correlator device is used to perform the analysis.

The echo data received as a result of each pulse is digitised and stored in a memory buffer for a period equal to the time required to receive the echo data from a second pulse, which is also digitised and stored in buffer memory. Since this method is a statistical estimation, a minimum number of four pulse pairs must be transmitted to ensure a reasonably accurate estimate of the mean frequency shift. The lower the velocity to be interrogated, the more pulse pairs must be transmitted to maintain the accuracy of the estimate.

MEASUREMENT AND ANALYSIS PACKAGES

Distance and area

All echocardiography systems offer at least one pair of digital calipers for the measurement of linear distance. The actual distance is computed from the time of flight of ultrasound assuming that the average velocity of sound through tissues is a constant 1540 m/s. The speed of sound through blood is however greater than 1540 m/s and this may cause some distortion of the measurements. Multiple sets of calipers can sometimes be very useful, for example, when assessing diameter changes in a structure at different times of the cardiac cycle or in measuring the size of an irregularly sized structure.

Several methods to make perimeter measurements and calculate areas are usually provided. These methods, in order of decreasing accuracy are; continuous trace – where a continuous line is drawn around the perimeter; trace by points – where several points on the perimeter are defined and the system joins them together to reconstruct the perimeter; elliptical approximation – where an ellipse is sized in its two axes until it overlays the perimeter to be measured. The latter method is quick and easy for regular shapes such as vessels in cross-section.

Volumes

In all cases, volumes are calculated from the area or length measurements obtained directly from the M-mode or 2D image. Since only one dimension is actually measured when volumes are obtained from M-mode data the assumptions necessary to calculate such volumes must necessarily incorporate a large standard error. Various algorithms are used to calculate left ventricular volumes from M-mode recordings, all of which make different assumptions about ventricular geometry.

Several algorithms are in use for calculating volumes from 2D images. The Bullet formula assumes that the left ventricle is a truncated cone (bullet shape) and Simpson's rule uses multiple diameters in order to incorporate any irregular variation in the wall. Both of these algorithms are used to estimate global parameters of left ventricular function such as ejection fraction and end diastolic volume. Multiple views of the heart in systole and diastole are required for each method and are best obtained either by using electrocardiographically triggered image acquisition or by use of cineloop facilities. The methods are very dependent on high quality image recording and even when this is achieved assumptions about ventricular geometry are still made.

Wall motion analysis

Both qualitative and quantitative methods of wall motion analysis may be available on some instruments. The qualitative method involves scoring of the visualised regional wall motion according to a defined table of indices.

The centre line method of wall motion analysis requires the definition of a sequence of points halfway between two ventricular contours representing the endocardial surfaces in systole and diastole defined by echocardiography. Perpendiculars to this centre line at each point are then constructed. The distance between the intersections of the perpendicular with each contour is considered to be the extent of local wall motion. This method was developed because reports have shown that wall motion proceeds towards many points in the ventricle rather than a single point.

The presence of sophisticated software for volume calculations on an instrument must not lull the operators into a false sense of security about the accuracy of their results. If there is any doubt about the clarity of the imaging data being used, the calculations must not be performed.

Further discussion of the assessment of left ventricular volume is included in Chapter 5.

QUALITATIVE REGIONAL WALL

WALL MOTION TYPE LEGEND

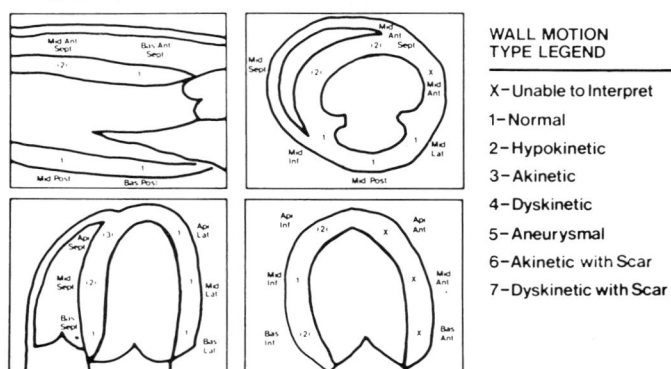

X – Unable to Interpret
1 – Normal
2 – Hypokinetic
3 – Akinetic
4 – Dyskinetic
5 – Aneurysmal
6 – Akinetic with Scar
7 – Dyskinetic with Scar

Fig. 3 Qualitative wall motion scoring method.

Doppler analysis (also Chs 6, 7 and 8)

Peak instantaneous pressure gradient can be calculated from the peak velocity, measured from the spectral display, by using a modified form of the Bernoulli equation. Most systems will calculate this value automatically if a caliper is placed at the maximum velocity point on the spectral display.

Mean pressure gradient is determined by calculating the peak pressure gradient at every point on the spectral trace during a complete cardiac cycle. It is calculated by the system after the operator has traced the outline of the spectral display throughout a single cardiac cycle, on the monitor.

Pressure half time is used to estimate functional valve area in mitral stenosis. The peak velocity is measured and the system calculates the instantaneous peak pressure gradient and the time, in ms, taken for the pressure gradient to fall to 50% of its peak value, the pressure half time. The software in many systems actually measures the slope of the curve rather than the actual pressure half time and this can give misleading results if the slope is non-linear.

Velocity time integrals (VTI) are determined by integrating the area under the spectral trace for a single cardiac cycle. The value is calculated by the system after the operator has traced the outline of the spectral display throughout one cardiac cycle. Velocity time integral values are used to estimate volume flow parameters such as cardiac output by calculating the product of mean velocity and cross-sectional area. One major source of error in such calculations is the accurate measurement of cross-sectional area. VTI may also be used in the continuity equation to estimate aortic valve area.

The sophisticated software now available on many systems will all too easily tempt the inexperienced operator to give precise quantitative reports which may be completely erroneous. Great care must be taken to perform all Doppler calculations on the highest quality signals and in an appropriate haemodynamic context.

IMAGE STORAGE DEVICES

Video recorders

There are three major types of video recorder currently used in echocardiography systems. VHS recorders use 0.25 inch tape and are small, compact and generally inexpensive. This is the standard used in domestic video recorders. Although monochrome performance is good, they are generally less able to provide the high performance required to reproduce the high dynamic range colour images obtained from modern colour flow echocardiography systems. Super VHS (S-VHS) recorders offer significant performance improvements over the standard VHS format, especially when recording colour images. In order to obtain optimum performance from these devices special high density tapes must be used which are currently more expensive than standard VHS tapes. Although standard VHS recorded tapes may be played back on S-VHS systems, the quality of playback will probably be inferior to that obtained when they are played on a standard VHS player. S-VHS tapes cannot be played on a standard VHS recorder. U-Matic recorders use wide 0.5 inch tape and provide the best possible recording quality onto cassette tape. The recorders are physically larger and more expensive than VHS recorders. U-Matic tapes are also considerably more expensive than VHS tapes.

Digital storage

Advances in computer technology have provided new methods of storing and retrieving ultrasound image data. Images may be stored either in digital memory or onto computer disks for permanent storage. Images stored in digital memory are lost if new images are acquired or power to the instrument is interrupted. The digital memory of some systems can be used to acquire a consecutive series of image frames over a short period of time. This facility may be referred to under several names, for example, cine review, cineloop or video review. All terms describe the ability to recall previous ultrasound or video frames from digital memory for review or measurement. These stored frames may also be replayed in a continuous loop at standard speed or more slowly to allow easier review of dynamic events. This has become particularly useful with the advent of colour flow Doppler imaging which presents a huge amount of data in each image.

Doppler spectral data and M-mode data, as well as 2D images, may also be stored on computer memory which simplifies the acquisition of optimum data for measurement and analysis. Some devices re-digitise the video signal and store this data in cineloop memory whilst others buffer the original ultrasound data and reformat it for display as required. Those storing the original data offer additional advantages, such as the ability to zoom (magnify) and postprocess the images.

Frame grabbers are devices that capture and digitise video frames from video tape recorders to provide a stable image that can be measured and analysed. Simple frame grabbers capture only single frames whilst the more sophisticated versions are capable of capturing a series of frames and replaying them in a loop. The digitised frame has to be recalibrated if measurements have to be taken. Some devices also record scale information on the videotape simultaneously with the image so that calibration of the frame grabbed image is not necessary before making measurements.

Disk storage

The advent of low cost, high speed microcomputers has made it possible to transfer image data from memory onto computer disks. Large capacity, hard disks provide fast storage of both single pages (frames) of video and cineloops, whilst high density floppy disks can be used to archive patient data. This digital storage of image data is considered in more detail in the section under digital echocardiography.

Hard copy devices

Chart recorders produce a continuous recording of scrolling M-mode or spectral Doppler data. Dry silver chart recorders make use of silver halide, light-sensitive paper to record the scrolling display. These recorders are very expensive and although the recordings are of excellent quality, the paper is also very expensive and does not store well. They have mostly been replaced by devices that use heat sensitive paper to record the data. The cost of thermal recorders and the paper for them, is much less than for dry silver recorders. Unfortunately the recording quality is not as good and the exposed paper has to be stored at low temperature if the image is to be retained more than a few months.

Video printers produce a single print of a still video frame rather than a continuous recording of scrolling data. Monochrome printers use similar thermal paper to that used in thermal chart recorders to record a single picture. Several qualities of printer are available which produce various image sizes and are all relatively inexpensive. These printers also incorporate a frame grabber so it is not necessary to wait for printing to be completed before continuing the examination.

Satisfactory recording of colour video images from colour flow Doppler systems requires a different technique. These printers use high gloss paper and a plastic film coated with heat sensitive dyes to record colour images. When the film is heated in a very small area, the dye sublimes onto the gloss paper to form a small colour dot or pixel. If the process is repeated for red, cyan and yellow dyes, a composite colour image is formed on the paper. The quality of the colour prints can be very good but current colour printers take approximately 90 seconds to produce a print. The integral frame grabber does allow the operator to continue whilst the print is made but additional prints cannot be made during the process time. The quality of the images is generally better than that produced on Polaroid prints.

Colour thermal printers are available in a range of qualities and prices. Some will make prints on transparency film and some will print multiple video images on a single sheet of paper.

Good quality 35 mm slides, for presentations and teaching purposes cannot be generated reliably by directly photographing a colour monitor. Instead, the image must be frame grabbed and split into the component primary colours. These components are fed to a high quality monochrome monitor and photographed through a complementary colour filter so that the correct colour is rendered onto the film. The process is fully automatic but takes some time to photograph each image. These freeze frame cameras are relatively inexpensive and can also be used to photograph images replayed from videotape.

FACTORS AFFECTING INSTRUMENT PERFORMANCE

The patient is probably the most limiting factor in the production of images of high quality. Narrow intercostal spaces, large chests, a small heart and lung dysfunction all reduce the quality of the images obtained. Conversely, patients with cardiac enlargement often provide images of exceptional clarity, since the enlarged heart is close to the surface and not obscured by the lungs.

The lungs effectively absorb ultrasound energy, so it is essential to find a position on the chest where the heart is not obscured by overlying lung. It is not unusual for a patient to have a single 'echo window' such that parasternal views are acceptable whilst apical views are poor or vice versa. The skill of the operator in positioning the patient and locating the best 'echo window' is the single most important factor in determining overall image quality.

The difference in image quality obtained by two different operators from the same patient with the same echocardiography instrument can be dramatic. It is important for the operator to be sufficiently experienced to be able to optimise the equipment control settings, gain, frame rate and so forth as well as positioning the patient and selecting the best 'echo window'. Operators that apply a firm pressure to the scanhead generally obtain better contact and improved image quality.

Whilst various processing techniques may be used to improve the aesthetic appearance of the image, the major determinant of image quality is the information content. Processing techniques may enhance the visibility of diagnostic information but they cannot add new information. Thus when evaluating a system, it is essential to distinguish true image quality, judged by information content, from apparent image quality due to software manipulation of the image.

Spatial resolution is the ability of the ultrasound system to discriminate between two or more closely spaced objects and is specified as the distance in millimetres at which two discrete objects can just be differentiated. Resolution figures specified by the manufacturer are usually determined at the focal point of the scanhead and represent the best attainable values. Resolution in the axial and lateral dimensions are commonly specified independently. Axial resolution is largely determined by the frequency of the probe but other factors such as electrical and acoustic damping and digitisation rate also have an effect. The principal parameter influencing lateral resolution is the ultrasound beam width.

Spatial resolution has a third dimension which is perpendicular to the other planes and is sometimes referred to as slice thickness. The resolution of phased array transducers in the imaging plane is superior to that in the perpendicular plane. Dynamic electronic focusing is used to reduce the beam width in the imaging plane but slice thickness is rarely specified and its effect on image quality is often overlooked.

Spatial resolution can be ascertained from the image by the ease with which relatively small objects can be observed, (for example, chordae tendinae or aortic valve leaflets). It is usually measured objectively by means of an ultrasound phantom which contains small diameter wires separated by a known distance and surrounded by a medium that has ultrasound attenuating properties that are similar to tissue.

Contrast resolution is the ability to discriminate between a low level reflector in the presence of a strong reflector and probably has more effect on the apparent clarity of ultrasound images than spatial resolution. Side lobes, which increase the effective beam width for low level reflectors, are the main determining factor of contrast resolution. Contrast resolution, in an ultrasound image, can be judged by observing small vessels, such as the coronary arteries. Instruments with good contrast resolution will show distinct walls and a black vessel lumen without spurious echoes within it.

Acoustic dynamic range is the maximum range of signal values that the system can process from the scanhead (100 dB), and is generally greater than the range that is displayed on the monitor (60 dB). The compression used to reduce the acoustic dynamic range so that it can be displayed has great influence on the image quality. The compression curves, that produce the most diagnostic images, are usually determined by experimentation. Systems with wide dynamic range provide better tissue differentiation than those with less dynamic range, provided that they also have good contrast resolution. This can be important in discriminating between thrombus formation and vegetations in cardiac structures. Differentiation of endocardium from epicardium also requires good dynamic range and contrast resolution.

Image uniformity describes how consistent the resolution remains throughout the displayed image. That is to say, tissues of the same type should have the same ultrasonic appearance, wherever they appear in the field of view. Uniformity is affected by focusing techniques, time-gain compensation, beam steering and the patient.

IMAGE AESTHETICS (PRESENTATION)

Not all echo data is of equal diagnostic value, echoes of middle range amplitude being more important in tissue differentiation than low amplitudes or high amplitudes. Consequently, faithful representation of the original ultrasound data does not always produce the most diagnostic or aesthetically pleasing images. Images reconstructed by digital scan converters can appear 'grainy' and diffraction of the ultrasound beam results in 'speckle' which tends to degrade the appearance of the images. To minimise these unwanted characteristics, the image data is processed in various ways. The 'attractiveness' of the final images is greatly affected by the processing, some of which is preset when the system is manufactured and some being user selectable.

Spatial smoothing is a commonly used form of image processing. The apparent 'graininess' in digital images is due to the emphasis of the edges of image pixels by adjacent, empty (black) pixels. These empty pixels arise from the geometric translation necessary to reconstruct a sector shaped image from the digital ultrasound data which is stored in columns. Spatial averaging of pixels can reduce the effect by filling empty pixels with a value that is calculated from adjacent pixels.

Diffraction of the ultrasound beam within the tissues results in random echoes, 'speckle', appearing in the image. In addition, random noise may also be introduced by the system electronics. This unwanted and distracting information can be removed by generating a composite image that has been constructed from a weighted average of successive images (frames), the most weight being given to the newest frame and least weight to the oldest frame. This is known as temporal smoothing. This frame averaging eliminates much of the random noise but also reduces the ability of the system to display rapid motion. Excessive temporal smoothing may remove valuable diagnostic information from images of moving structures.

The linear conversion of echo amplitude to image pixel intensity produces an image of high contrast with little tissue differentiation. Such an image has little diagnostic value so some signal processing must be used to emphasise echoes of mid-range amplitude whilst limiting echoes of high amplitude. The assignment of image pixel brightness to echo amplitude is controlled by grey scale transfer curves. Suppression or rejection of very low amplitude signals is also used to reduce the noise in the image. Grey scale processing may be performed prior to digitisation and storage, pre-processing, or afterwards, post-processing. Post-processing is the preferred method since the original data is retained in memory and only the display of the data is changed by the processing, whereas pre-processing changes the data irreversibly before storage.

IMAGING ARTEFACTS

In the assessment of instrument performance, it is important to be aware of the various ultrasonic artefacts that may occur. Grating lobes are secondary ultrasound beams generated at a large angle to the main beam. They are generated by all array transducers and are related to the frequency and inter-element spacing of the scanhead. Scanhead element spacing of less than one wavelength significantly reduces grating lobe generation. Low frequency array probes are more likely to generate significant grating lobe artefacts than higher frequency ones since the element spacing is wider. Grating lobe artefacts in the image are often visualised as double echoes from strongly reflecting objects.

Side lobes, as the name suggests, are secondary ultrasound beams occurring outside the main beam. They are produced by all types of ultrasound transducer and depend upon the frequency and active area (aperture) of the transducer. The effect of side lobes is to increase the effective beam width, so that out of plane objects are represented as being in the image plane, thereby degrading resolution.

Reverberation artefacts are caused by multiple reflections between two strongly reflecting interfaces with a low attenuation medium, such as blood, between them.

This displacement of echo information can be eliminated, in some echo instruments, by changing the frame rate of the scanhead slightly. Mechanical transducers that use fluid to transform the high impedance of the element to the low impedance of the tissues, always show near field reverberations. These artefacts are caused by multiple reflections between element and scanhead cap and appear in the image as a number of bright rings at the apex of the image.

Dense objects such as bone reflect most of the ultrasound incident upon them. Consequently, little or no ultrasound reaches deeper structures and this results in a black shadow, often sector shaped, below the reflecting object. Diagnostic ultrasound does not propagate through air because the wavelength is shorter than the distance between the molecules. Air in the lungs acts as a 'curtain' preventing ultrasound from reaching structures beyond and is often the reason for poor cardiac images.

PRACTICAL ASPECTS OF SPECTRAL DOPPLER (PULSED AND CONTINUOUS WAVE)

There are different requirements for imaging and Doppler transducers. An imaging ultrasound pulse is short and contains a band of frequencies centred about the resonant frequency of the element. Doppler beams, on the other hand, are generated by exciting the element with a sine wave of a fixed frequency, which forces the element to vibrate and emit ultrasound at that frequency. In addition, the ideal frequency for Doppler examination, including colour Doppler, is lower than that for best image resolution. The lower Doppler carrier frequency improves the sensitivity because of the lower attenuation and allows higher velocities to be detected without aliasing.

Ideally, the transducer elements should be optimised for each mode of operation. In practice, a compromise must be made between the differing requirements which adversely affect the performance of duplex transducers, especially the sensitivity. However, the development of new piezo-electric materials that have a wide frequency range (bandwidth) may lead to the development of new transducers that can perform both functions without compromise.

Signals that are back scattered from blood cells are of much lower amplitude than those reflected from anatomical structures and as a consequence, Doppler systems must have high sensitivity and good signal to noise ratio to be able to detect these signals and analyse the Doppler shift accurately. Poor sensitivity leads to underestimation of the severity of flow lesions.

The best imaging of tissue interfaces occurs when the ultrasound beam is perpendicular to the interface. For Doppler studies, however, it is important to align the ultrasound beam so that the angle of incidence is as closely aligned to the direction of blood flow as possible. This often means that different 'echo windows', from those used to obtain the best images, must be used to acquire the best Doppler signals. Ultrasound images are two-dimensional slices of a three-dimensional volume so a flow jet may not be correctly evaluated by Doppler, unless all planes of the volume are interrogated from several angles. This difference is particularly apparent when using colour flow Doppler.

The dynamic range of received Doppler signals is much greater than the electronics can process. The high amplitude, low frequency shifts, generated by the motion of anatomical structures such as heart wall, must be attenuated as much as possible using high pass filters. The cut off frequency of the filter must be carefully selected to avoid removing the signals from slow-moving blood, as in diastole, which will have an adverse effect on any volume flow calculations.

Insufficient filtering or excessive gain produces an artefact known as crosstalk, which appears in the spectral display as an exact mirror image of the true signal but at lower amplitude.

PRACTICAL ASPECTS OF COLOUR FLOW DOPPLER

Whilst aliasing impairs the clinical usefulness of pulsed wave Doppler, it can actually provide valuable diagnostic information in a colour Doppler image since it immediately highlights the highest blood flow velocities. Aliased colour is depicted as a transition from one bright colour to another bright colour, whereas reversed flow always appears as a transition from one colour through black, representing zero flow, to the opposite colour.

Each line of information in a colour Doppler image requires the transmission and reception of at least eight ultrasound pulses. As a consequence, the frame rate is much lower when performing colour Doppler than when imaging alone. The actual frame rate depends upon the depth of the image, the number of colour lines and the number of pulses used to create each line (packet size). Increasing the number of colour lines by increasing the colour sector angle, for example, will decrease the frame rate proportionately.

If the frame rate is too slow, flow jets of short duration may not be seen, since the system may not be acquiring Doppler data from that location at that time. The size of larger jets may also be underestimated for the same reasons. Many systems incorporate the use of a limited zone of colour analysis within a full sector in order to allow maintenance of a satisfactory frame rate.

Colour Doppler systems estimate the mean flow velocity by integrating the Doppler shift obtained from each of the pulses used to create a single colour line. The accuracy of the estimate depends upon the number of pulses used and the velocity being interrogated. Accurate determination of low flow velocities requires more pulses to be transmitted than for high velocities.

FUTURE DEVELOPMENTS

Digital echocardiography

Digital echocardiography is a term used to describe the digital acquisition, formatting, analysis, storage and review of ultrasound data. The technique was initially developed to reduce some of the practical difficulties encountered during the performance of a stress echocardiography examination.

Digitisation and storage of ultrasound images requires specialist computer hardware with a large amount of additional video memory, at least 2 MBytes. The resolution and format of the images, as well as the number of images that can be acquired, depends on the size of the video memory area. There is no observable loss of image quality at moderate resolution, unlike videotape storage media. The images, together with M-mode and Doppler studies if appropriate, can be stored on magnetic or optical disc for later retrieval and analysis.

Single image frames, or a sequence of images (cineloop) may be captured. The acquisition may be triggered manually or synchronised to the electrocardiogram (ECG) by triggering with the R-wave. The number of images in the cineloop and the interval between successive images determines the portion of the cardiac cycle that is recorded.

Recording eight frames at an interval of 50 ms, after triggering by the R-wave, will produce a cineloop that shows the systolic portion of the cardiac cycle. Other portions of the cardiac cycle can be observed by introducing a delay between the R-wave trigger and capture of the first image. The image loops may be replayed continuously, in slow motion, or individual image frames selected for closer examination.

The most common format used for the observation of cardiac wall motion is 'quad screen' format, where four synchronised image loops are displayed simultaneously on the screen. The four image loops display different imaging planes, parasternal long axis, parasternal short axis, apical long axis and apical four-chamber views. These four views, three of which are essentially orthogonal to each other, allow observation of the segments of the myocardium that are perfused by the main branches of the coronary arteries.

Stress echocardiography

The major application of digital echocardiography techniques at the current time is in stress echocardiography examinations, although there are additional potential applications.

Stress echocardiography aids the overall management of patients with suspected coronary artery disease and acute myocardial infarction (MI) since changes in wall motion are visible before ST segment changes are seen on the electrocardiogram (ECG) or the patient reports chest pain. Exercise ECG alone does not provide information regarding left ventricular function, and stress echo done in conjunction with routine stress ECG, increases the accuracy of stress testing. Stress echo offers real advantages over some other diagnostic techniques used to assess myocardial perfusion. It is the only technique that looks at wall thickening, it takes a relatively short time to perform the study and the results are available immediately.

Cardiac stress may be induced by exercise, pharmacological agents or by atrial pacing.

There are various approaches used in exercise stress techniques. These include use of a treadmill, an upright bicycle or a supine bicycle. The examination protocol is modified to suit the method chosen.

The treadmill method is the simplest exercise echo protocol. It requires cardiac views at rest and the same views after exercise, both sets acquired with the patient supine. The disadvantage of this protocol is that the time taken for the patient to move to the examination couch after exercise may be long enough to allow the myocardium to recover from the exercise induced hypoxia.

The upright bicycle protocol does allow the examination of the heart at peak exercise and provides a more accurate assessment of myocardial perfusion during stress, but is technically more difficult for the echocardiographer.

The supine bicycle method tries to combine the practical

advantages of the two-stage protocol with the peak exercise sensitivity of the upright bicycle. However, because the bicycle must be pedalled with the legs elevated, the patient is often unable to exercise to the maximum extent due to leg fatigue, and much of the sensitivity of the technique is lost.

The practical difficulties associated with exercise echo can be overcome to some extent by using pharmacological agents such as dipyridamole to simulate the haemodynamic effects of exercise but such agents may not produce exactly the same haemodynamic changes as physical exercise and therefore may produce false negative results.

External pacing of the heart, by means of an oesophageal pacing wire, can also be used to increase the oxygen demand of the myocardium. Despite the practical advantages of atrial pacing, the haemodynamic response is different from that produced by exercise and may lead to false positive or negative results.

Further applications of digital echocardiography

The ability to capture short, dynamic sequences of images depicting cardiac motion can reduce the examination time greatly and simplify the diagnosis. Only image sequences showing relevant clinical information need to be reviewed. The simultaneous display of synchronised, dynamic image loops, showing multiple planes, allows the motion of several cardiac wall segments to be observed and compared. This 'side by side' comparison increases the accuracy of the diagnosis of wall motion abnormalities that may occur with an acute myocardial infarction (Fig. 4). Selecting image loops that are free of respiratory artefacts also improves the quality of diagnosis.

High speed storage and retrieval of digitised, dynamic image sequences allows previous examinations to be recalled quickly and reviewed without loss of image quality. Direct 'on screen' comparison of early examinations with more recent ones, simplifies the evaluation of changes or improvements in cardiac performance after intervention or therapy. This has applications in outpatient studies, the coronary care unit and during surgical monitoring of cardiac function.

Digital echo offers an effective way of producing high quality illustrations of pathology for teaching purposes or conference presentations. Images that best depict an aspect of the pathology may be readily selected from stored dynamic image loops and high quality hard copy produced for publications or presentations. The rapid selection and recall of patient data also permits the display and review of image loops, showing dynamic cardiac events, rather than single frames.

Images that have been digitised and stored can readily be recalled for subsequent analysis at the most convenient time. No calibration is required for analysis since the original scale information is stored with the data. Many measurements can be done automatically by the computer which improves accuracy, reduces the time required to analyse the data and allows the echo instrument to be used for additional examinations.

Digitised images can be stored on magnetic media such as floppy discs and the availability of new high capacity optical storage media will make this method of data archiving even more desirable. Data is stored in a very stable, compact form and can be rapidly retrieved for review without loss of image quality.

Transducer developments

Multiplane transoesophageal echocardiography. Initially, transoesophageal (TOE) probes only offered the possibility to image the heart in a single orientation. This single plane approach does not allow some parts of the heart to be visualised. Recently, biplane TOE transducers have been introduced that have two phased array transducers aligned perpendicular to each other. In some instruments it is possible to store the images from one plane in an image loop and compare them directly with the live images obtained in the alternative plane.

The next logical development is a multiplane transducer where the phased array at the tip of the probe can be rotated mechanically to provide an infinite number of intermediate planes. Such a probe would permit the entire cardiac anatomy to be observed with extremely high image quality. In combination with modern high speed computers, multiplane transducers could provide the necessary data for the reconstruction of a three-dimensional image of the heart. This technology has not as yet reached a practical stage of development. The addition of a pacing wire to the transoesophageal probe may provide the ability to

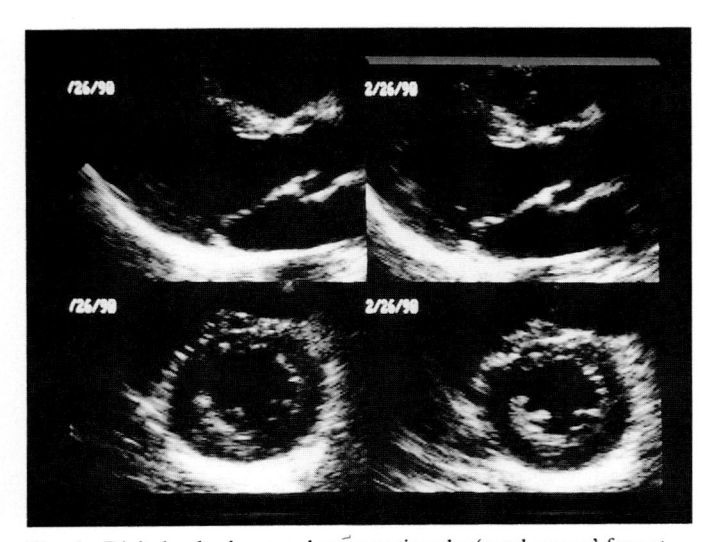

Fig. 4 Digital echo images demonstrating the 'quad screen' format and the side by side comparison of identical anatomical scan planes before (left) and after (right) stress.

perform a high quality stress echo study without the practical limitations associated with exercise echo studies.

High frequency ultrasound probes (20 MHz) mounted at the tip of an intravascular catheter have recently become available. These probes provide a 360° image of the vessel lumen and have been used to observe atherosclerotic plaque in the coronary arteries before and after percutaneous transluminal coronary angioplasty (PTCA).

Whilst their use for imaging coronary arteries is interesting, modified versions of this technique may provide other diagnostic information. For example, lower frequency transducers could be used to image the right side of the heart from the vena cava. Additionally catheter mounted Doppler transducers have been used to measure intravascular flow signals.

Intra-operative surface echocardiography utilises the excellent image quality of high frequency, short focus, transducers to achieve a flexible series of views before, during and after cardiac surgery. Whilst very high quality data are achievable, and views are more flexible than those obtained by transoesophageal studies, the technique is more disruptive to the surgeon than TOE, and it remains to be seen if this approach will become more widely utilised.

BIBLIOGRAPHY

Multi-element array transducers – K B Aerotech report 1981.
Whittingham T A. Real time ultrasonic scanning. In: Moores B M, Parker R P, Pullman B R. eds. Physical aspects of medical imaging. John Wiley: London. 1981
Goldstein A. Ultrasound devices open new diagnostic avenues. Diagnostic Imaging. September 1989
Scott Robertson W. Echocardiographic assessment of ischaemic heart disease. Advanced Technology Laboratories Publication, C-6034, 1989

Examination technique

Introduction
Environment and patient preparation
Transducer selection
Transducer positioning
Imaging and M-mode examination
Parasternal window
Apical window
Subcostal (or subxiphoid) window
Suprasternal window
Right parasternal window
Doppler examination
Mitral valve
Tricuspid valve
Aortic valve
Pulmonary valve
Vena cavae
Pulmonary veins

Control optimisation
Imaging controls
Doppler controls
   Power output
   Signal gain
   Low frequency filter
   Baseline shift
   Sweep speed
   Electrocardiogram (ECG)
   High pulse repetition frequency (high PRF)
   Sample volume size
Standard echocardiographic examination
Conclusion

Peter Wilde and Robert L. Parry

INTRODUCTION

Echocardiography is the most versatile investigative tool available for the assessment of cardiac structure and function. It has proved itself to the point where the information it provides will frequently allow surgery to be planned without the need for invasive investigations. This is especially true in paediatrics where disease of the coronary arteries is not usually a major concern. Even in adults a full haemodynamic assessment via catheter is frequently unnecessary and invasive techniques may only be needed for evaluation of the coronary arteries.

This general acceptance of the place of echocardiographic data did not come about overnight. The natural reluctance of some people to accept the echocardiographic data was only altered by the realisation that such data provided them with an accurate and reliable picture of what was happening inside the heart. Whilst this current state of affairs is all to the good it places an onus on operators to produce good quality data from a thorough and accurate examination. It is important that the limitations of the technique are recognised along with its advantages.

As technological advances allow equipment to be made more user friendly, it is all too easy for operators to think themselves competent simply because they are able to obtain reasonable quality images or traces. Whilst the ability to obtain high quality echocardiographic recordings is the most important factor in determining how useful an examination will be, it is not the only requirement. An understanding of normal and abnormal appearances is required, as is a thorough understanding of cardiac physiology and patterns of blood flow in both normal and diseased hearts. It is essential for the operator to understand and utilise the physical principles employed by the equipment. This subjective aspect of the technique is an area in which a high degree of restraint and judgement is necessary so that minor variations in anatomy, physiology and technique are not to be labelled as pathological findings or vice versa.

The American College of Cardiologists has recently published the findings of a task force established to provide guidelines for training in echocardiography (see reading list below). Such guidelines are important in maintaining the high standards which will ensure that the momentum gained by echocardiography is not lost.

No matter how great the operator's theoretical knowledge of echocardiography, the highest possible quality of cardiac imaging and recording of other data is a pre-requisite for a successful examination. If adequate cardiac images and blood flow velocity data are not recorded at the time of the examination there is little one can do to rectify the situation later.

To this end it is necessary to consider those factors which go to make a satisfactory examination possible. These include the comfort of the patient and operator both in position and environment, the selection of transducer best suited to the particular patient being examined, the correct positioning of the transducer, the scan planes and systematic conduct of the examination and optimal use of the available equipment and its controls.

The operator should have a clear idea of the patient's history before commencing the examination. The examination should thoroughly examine all valves and chambers since it is surprising how often a murmur turns out not to originate from the clinically suspected site!

ENVIRONMENT AND PATIENT PREPARATION

The room in which the examination is conducted should be large enough to allow easy access to the equipment and examination couch as well as having a private cubicle where patients can change into an examination gown. The examination couch should be low enough for patients to lie on without undue exertion and should have a tilting head end so the patient can be positioned anywhere from supine to sitting upright. Not only should the head of the couch be adjustable but the control for this should be convenient to use.

Lighting in the room is also important, since one needs little illumination whilst scanning yet full illumination for making notes and attending to the patient before and after the examination. The best set-up is to have a central light operated by a dimmer switch with a smaller anglepoise lamp which can be used to one side for note taking. Adjustable dark blinds should be available on any external windows.

Echocardiography is surprisingly hot work both for the operator and patient as the equipment produces copious amounts of hot air. Ideally the examination room should have air conditioning, but if this is not possible the room should be well ventilated with fans provided to keep the room reasonably comfortable.

A comprehensive record of all examinations should be made and a system must be devised to facilitate reference to a particular examination at a later date. Details such as patient name, hospital number, referring clinician and suspected diagnosis should be recorded in a log book. The majority of examinations are recorded on video tape and the number of the tape and recording details should be entered in the log. Diagnoses are frequently coded so that if required a computer search can be initiated to provide information on a particular condition for research purposes.

Patients should strip to the waist and are commonly provided with a gown which opens down the front. The patient is positioned for the examination in a semirecumbent position at about 45° and is rotated towards the left side. The patient's left hand is placed behind their head to open up the left sided rib spaces in order to provide better access for the transducer. Normally patients are scanned from the right side, the operators using the right hand to hold the transducer, but this is by no means a requirement. There is no reason why the examination should not proceed from the patients' left side using the operators' left hand. Indeed this position has the advantage that the patient is facing the operator and the equipment which may provide psychological reassurance. In our own department the former arrangement is used but a secondary monitor on the patient's left has proved to be reassuring even if the patient does not understand the images seen. Most operators prefer to be seated comfortably during the examination. It is important to discuss the examination with the patient before starting, to enable any fears to be allayed.

Electrodes should be placed so that an electrocardiogram can be recorded simultaneously with the echocardiographic data. The precise positioning of the electrodes is not critical since they are used for their timing rather than the actual electrocardiographic morphology. It is usual however to have a right and left arm lead and a trunk lead. Whilst more lateral placement of the electrodes allows a better recording, limb leads are more prone to muscle tremor and are more likely to become detached, especially as the patient is moved around during the course of the examination. Disposable self adhesive electrodes are commonly used and these are positioned on the front of the patient's right and left shoulders and a third electrode is positioned over the right lower ribs. In these positions the trace remains fairly stable and is not unduly affected by patient movement. As long as the P-wave and QRS complex can be readily identified, the trace is usually considered adequate for timing purposes. The alternative approach of using clips on the wrists and ankle is acceptable and cheaper but is probably less convenient.

TRANSDUCER SELECTION

The choice of transducer for a particular examination will be governed to a large extent by the body habitus of the patient. Ideally the highest frequency transducer possible should be used to provide the best resolution of intracardiac structures. However since higher transducer frequencies have poorer tissue penetration, the frequency one can use is limited by the depth and quality of the structures one wishes to image. In practice this means the larger the patient the lower the transducer frequency and the lower the resolution of the images produced. A person of average build would normally be examined with a 3 or 3.5 MHz transducer whilst heavier patients may require a 2 or 2.5 MHz transducer to produce adequate penetration. In young adults and children, penetration is not usually a problem and a 5 MHz transducer may be used which produces excellent resolution. Neonates may frequently be examined successfully using a 7.5 MHz imaging transducer. It is important to be flexible in transducer selection. Some large patients are surprisingly good subjects for examination and many patients, small as well as large, are difficult to image.

Nowadays most imaging transducers will have built in Doppler facilities. It should be remembered that the Doppler crystal often emits at the same frequency as the imaging transducer. High quality Doppler recordings necessitate higher power levels than imaging records and so the transducer which provides the best imaging resolution does not necessarily provide the best Doppler signals and a lower frequency transducer will be more efficient. Several manufacturers now offer a combined transducer in which the frequency of the Doppler signal is less than that of the imaging transducer.

Since an air interface causes marked ultrasound reflection, a transmitting substance is needed between the patient and the transducer. Usually a proprietary water soluble gel is used. It is important that this is viscous enough to allow the transducer head to be angled slightly off the chest wall and still provide adequate contact. If the gel is not viscous enough, it simply runs away down the patient's chest. If possible, the gel bottle is kept warm to reduce unpleasant shocks as cold gel is dropped onto the patient's skin.

The size of the transducer face (or 'footprint') is important. A small transducer will fit more snugly into rib interspaces or awkward sites such as the suprasternal notch or subxiphoid notch. Smaller transducers, particularly if of the phased array type, give poorer image quality, so once again a compromise must be made for any particular circumstance. Some transducer faces are rectangular, fitting snugly between ribs in one orientation but lying awkwardly across ribs when rotated through 90°. This latter problem is eliminated by transducers with a circular 'footprint' which are usually of the mechanical type. In general lower frequency transducers are larger than higher frequency transducers. All transducers have a palpable orientation or reference mark (a notch or bump) which corresponds with a mark on one side of the sector on the screen. This facilitates correct plane orientation and some operators advocate a scanning technique with a fingertip always resting on the orientation mark.

TRANSDUCER POSITIONING

Correct positioning of the patient is imperative if the best images are to be obtained. It is customary to have the patient inclined at about 45° and rotated towards their left side. This utilises the effect of gravity to bring the heart nearer the chest wall and hence nearer the transducer. Areas where the heart is not covered by lung or bone allow access to the ultrasound beam and are termed 'windows'. There are three main windows from where it is usually possible to conduct an examination of the heart. These are

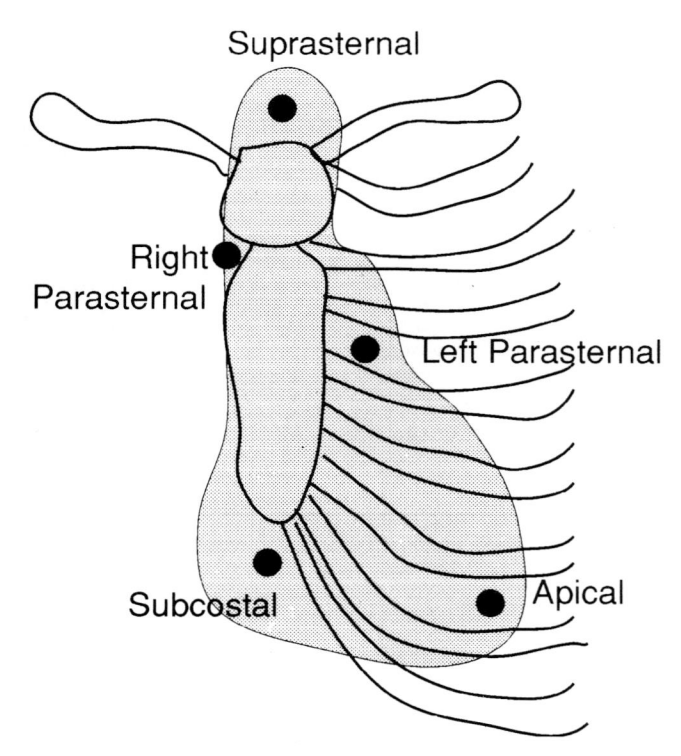

Fig. 1 Diagram illustrating anatomical sites of commonly used echocardiographic windows.

the parasternal, apical and subcostal windows (Fig. 1). (If unprefixed these terms refer to the left side. The less commonly employed right parasternal or right apical are prefixed accordingly.) There are many intermediate window positions lying between these main sites.

The parasternal window occupies the area to the left of the sternum where there is no lung overlying the heart. The apical region is where the cardiac apex contacts the chest wall and therefore usually corresponds to the region of the palpable apex beat. The subcostal or xiphisternal window uses the left lobe of the liver as a window to the heart.

The suprasternal window is a fourth site (Fig. 1), more usually used for study of the aorta and great arteries.

There are standard views which should be sought from each of these windows. The heart is imaged in planes by cross-sectional imaging and three of these planes, lying orthogonally, are used to assess the anatomy of the heart. These planes are defined by internal cardiac landmarks rather than by external body reference points and accordingly may be in significantly different positions in different patients, according to their build and their cardiac morphology. These three planes are the long axis, the short axis and the four chamber plane (Fig. 2). Such standard views allow rapid detection and assessment of any abnormality.

The reproducibility of echocardiography depends upon the operator obtaining standard views of the heart which

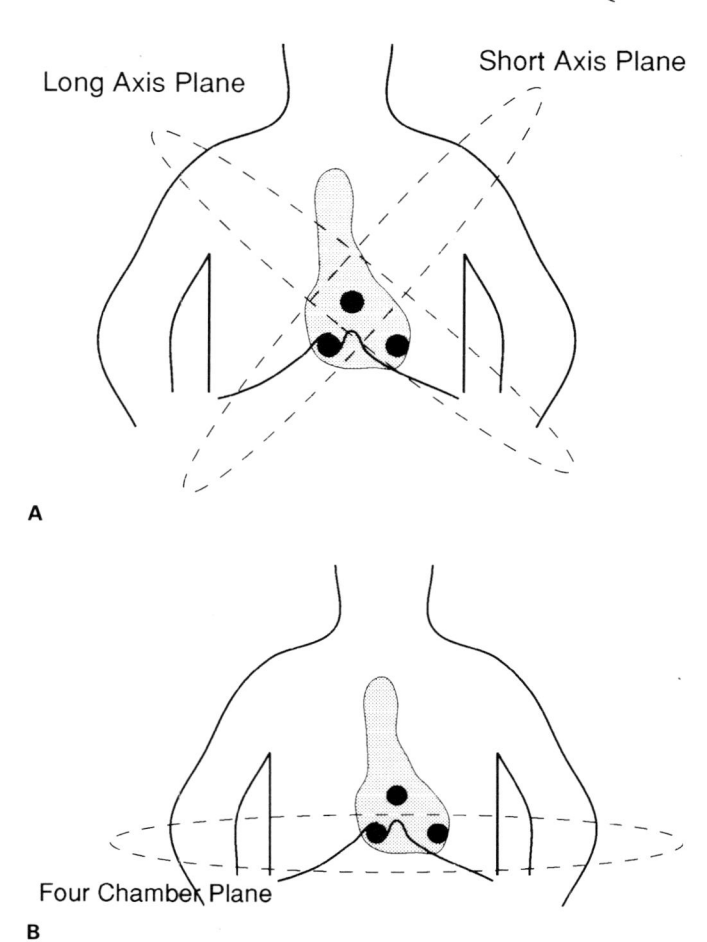

Fig. 2 **A:** Diagram showing the approximate orientation of the long axis and short axis planes. The parasternal, apical and subcostal windows are shown. Note that the long axis plane can only be achieved from the parasternal and apical windows whilst the short axis plane can only be achieved from the parasternal and subcostal windows. **B:** Diagram showing the approximate orientation of the four chamber plane. Note that the plane can only be achieved from the apical or subcostal window.

soon become easily recognisable and allow recognition of any deviations from normality. To attain these views a large degree of flexibility is required and the examination must be tailored to meet each patient's situation. Exact positions for scanning and exact angles at which to scan cannot therefore be given. The heart is more vertical in ectomorphic individuals than it is in endomorphs where it lies more horizontally. The heart also varies in its degree of rotation within the chest, especially if there is lung disease or abnormal cardiac chamber sizes. These variations must be considered when the standard views are attempted. In thin people with little tissue overlying the heart, the transducer may be rested lightly on the chest wall whilst in those more generously covered, quite firm pressure may be required to compress and displace tissue and allow approximation of the transducer to the structures to be imaged. One should remember however that having a transducer scraped painfully over ones ribs is not a pleasant sensation and excessive pressure is likely to be counterproductive.

The echocardiographic examination will be considered in two parts, namely imaging by two dimensional (or cross-sectional) and M-mode examination and then Doppler assessment of flow. The two will then be combined to outline how a practical examination would proceed.

IMAGING AND M-MODE EXAMINATION

Parasternal window

The parasternal views are obtained from the 2nd, 3rd or 4th rib interspaces to the left of the sternum. The patient should be semi-recumbent on their left side with their left arm stretched behind their head to help access between the ribs. The exact position for optimum scanning varies from patient to patient and it is probably best to start at the sternum and move out along each rib space until the best window is found. In most patients a high interspace is more likely to allow good imaging of the desirable scan planes. It is essential for the patient to be comfortable and relaxed in the selected position because a tense patient is much harder to examine.

The parasternal long axis view will be obtained with the reference or orientation point of the transducer (indicating the plane of the ultrasound beam) pointing to the patient's right shoulder. This view cuts the mitral valve and the aortic root and passes through the long axis of the left ventricle (Fig. 3). It does not normally depict the true apex of the left ventricle which lies beyond the limit of the sector. A 'false apex' can be seen if the ultrasound imaging plane cuts the medial or lateral wall of the ventricle as the valve plane is imaged, so adjustment by rotation is essential to avoid this.

The region of the apex lies on the left of the screen with the base of the heart to the right. In this position the most anterior structure is the outflow tract of the right ventricle. The interventricular septum is seen behind this, separating it from the left ventricle. The aorta is seen to arise from the left ventricle, its posterior wall being continuous with the anterior leaflet of the mitral valve. The left atrium lies behind the aorta, emptying into the left ventricle through the two leaflets of the mitral valve.

The mitral valve can be seen to move with a typical motion. The valve opens fully in early diastole due to passive ventricular filling, the ventricular diastolic pressure being lower than the left atrial pressure. The two leaflets then drift to a half-open position in mid-diastole before separating again with atrial systole. The typical M shaped movement of the anterior leaflet is seen when the M-mode beam is used to interrogate the valve (Fig. 4). The posterior leaflet, smaller and often less prominent, mirrors

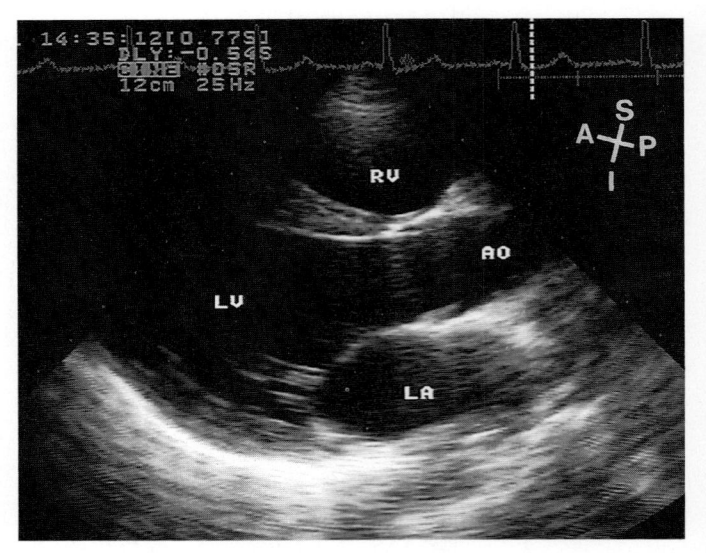

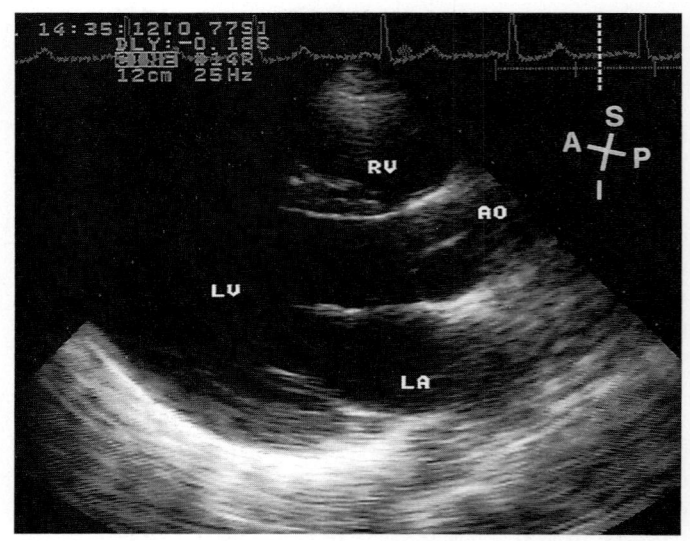

Fig. 3 Parasternal long axis view. A: In systole. The aortic valve is open and the mitral valve is closed. **B:** In diastole. The aortic valve is closed and the mitral valve is open.

the motion of the anterior leaflet, producing a W-shaped trace of smaller amplitude.

The aortic valve only appears to have two leaflets when seen from this view (Fig. 5). The left coronary cusp is not visualised as it moves to and fro, in and out of the plane of the ultrasound beam. The two visible cusps, the right and the non-coronary, can be seen clearly.

The whole of the aortic root is seen to move anteriorly in systole and posteriorly in diastole on the M-mode trace. This produces an undulating movement to the root within which can be seen the two cusps. In systole the two cusps

EXAMINATION TECHNIQUE 47

are open, producing a box-like trace before closing to form a single line in diastole.

A record of the contractility of the septum and posterior wall of the left ventricle can be gained from an M-mode trace through the left ventricle in this position (Fig. 6). This can be used to assess quantitatively the ventricular function. Most machines have a facility for calculating the ejection fraction from systolic and diastolic chamber dimensions. It is essential to ensure that the M-mode trace crosses the ventricle at 90° to the long axis of the ventricle, the latter defined as a line from the apex to the insertion of the anterior mitral leaflet on the posterior aortic root. Oblique alignment must be avoided for these measurements to be accurate and reproducible. One must also avoid crossing a papillary muscle with the M-mode beam since this will give the spurious impression of a thickened posterior wall with a reduced cavity size. The beam must be just distal to the tips of the mitral leaflets. The right ventricle can also be measured from this M-mode trace, and thicknesses of both the interventricular septum and posterior wall can be assessed.

Anterior and inferior angulation from the left parasternal window whilst keeping the sector orientated in the long axis plane will demonstrate a long axis view of the right sided cardiac chambers (Fig. 7)

M-mode traces are used for measurements of chamber size and valve diameters since its pulse repetition frequency is around 1000 Hz compared to 20–30 Hz for cross-sectional imaging. This allows better interface definition.

The next standard view, the parasternal short axis, is obtained from the same parasternal window. The transducer is rotated clockwise so that the reference mark points to the patient's left shoulder, the plane of ultrasound scan cutting at 90° to the long axis of the left ventricle.

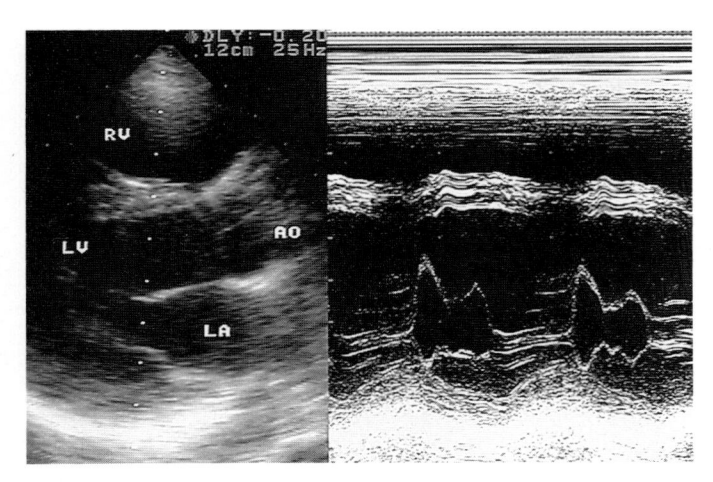

Fig. 4 Parasternal long axis view (left) with the M-mode cursor (dotted line) across the tips of the mitral valve leaflets. The M-mode trace (right) shows the typical normal opposing movements of the anterior and posterior mitral valve leaflets.

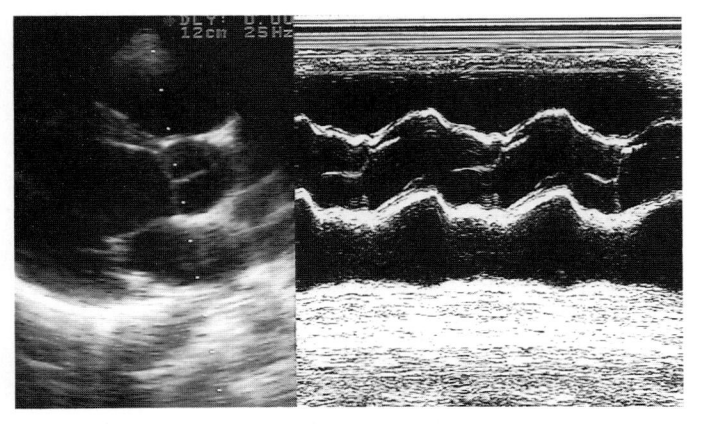

Fig. 5 Parasternal long axis view (left) with the M-mode cursor (dotted line) across the aortic valve leaflets. The M-mode trace (right) shows the typical box shaped opening of the leaflets within the aortic walls which move anteriorly in systole.

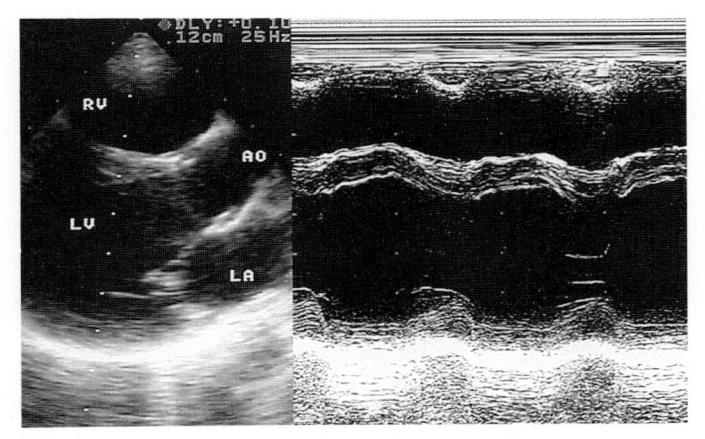

Fig. 6 Parasternal long axis view (left) with the M-mode cursor (dotted line) across the short axis of the left ventricle. The M-mode trace (right) shows the normal decrease in diameter of both ventricles during systole as well as thickening of the right ventricular free wall, the interventricular septum and the left ventricular free wall during systole.

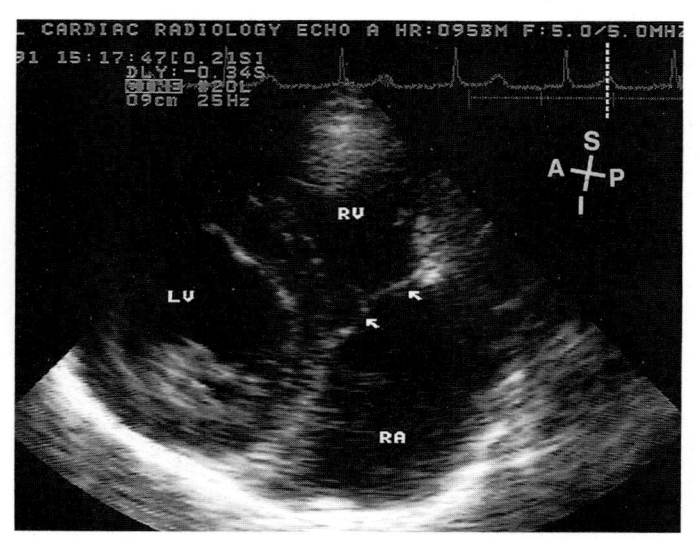

Fig. 7 Left parasternal long axis view of the right sided cardiac chambers. The view is achieved by angulating anteriorly and inferiorly from Fig. 3. The tricuspid valve is arrowed.

48 CARDIAC ULTRASOUND

One can obtain short axis cross-sectional images through the aortic root (Fig. 8A and B), the mitral valve (Fig. 9), and the left ventricle (Fig. 10A and B) depending on how much the transducer is tilted towards or away from the base of the heart.

The most basal of these views shows the tricuspid valve, the right ventricular outflow tract and the pulmonary valve wrapped around the aortic valve and root. The three aortic leaflets close as a Y-shape during diastole and the main pulmonary artery is seen with the pulmonary valve leaflets lying centrally. In systole the three leaflets of the aortic valve open to produce a circular appearance in the aortic root and as structures move anteriorly the bifurcation of the main pulmonary artery may be seen. The pulmonary leaflet closure line is lost.

If the transducer is angled slightly to the apex the mitral valve is crossed. In diastole the valve opens and there is an elliptical orifice formed by the two valve leaflets. In mid-diastole the valve half closes and then opens more fully again. In systole the two leaflets close in a single curved line.

Further angling to the apex demonstrates the two papillary muscles (antero-lateral and postero-medial) and the left ventricular cavity. A parasternal short axis M-mode trace obtained just below the level of the mitral valve is an alternative site for left ventricular recording if the long axis view was inadequate. Some operators prefer this approach for left ventricular M-mode recording.

Slight clockwise rotation of the transducer, often with the patient rotated further to their left side, will bring the main pulmonary artery and its bifurcation into view (Fig. 11). This view is relatively easy to achieve in children but is harder to achieve in many adults and may be impossible in those with emphysema or chest deformities.

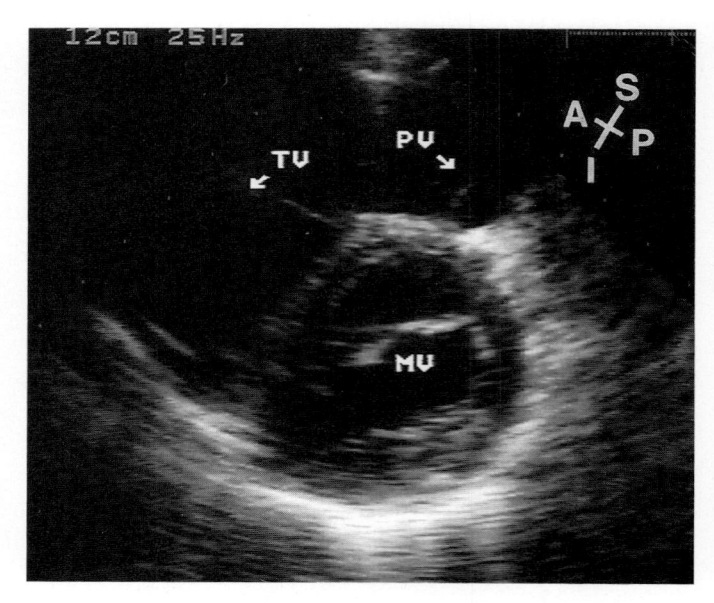

Fig. 9 Left parasternal short axis view at the level of the mitral valve orifice.

Moving of the transducer to a more inferior left parasternal window, whilst maintaining its orientation in the short axis plane, will often allow good visualisation of the tricuspid valve (Fig. 12).

Apical window

If the apex beat is palpated and the transducer reference mark directed posteriorly below the patient's left shoulder the apical four chamber view will be obtained. An upward tilt to the transducer is often required to achieve the best

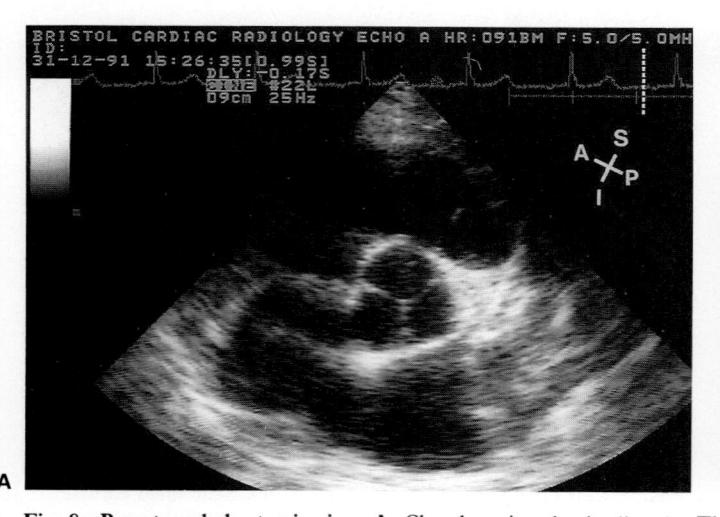

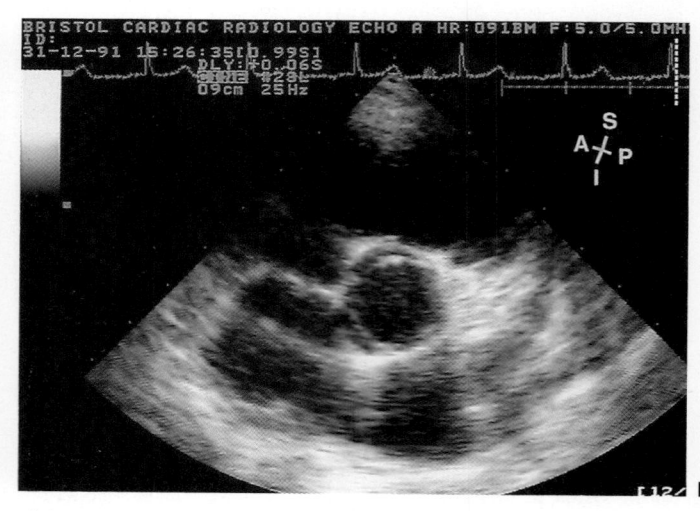

Fig. 8 Parasternal short axis view. A: Closed aortic valve in diastole. The right ventricular outflow tract and pulmonary valve (upper right) and the tricuspid valve (left) can be seen. B: The same view as in A but with the aortic leaflets open in systole.

EXAMINATION TECHNIQUE 49

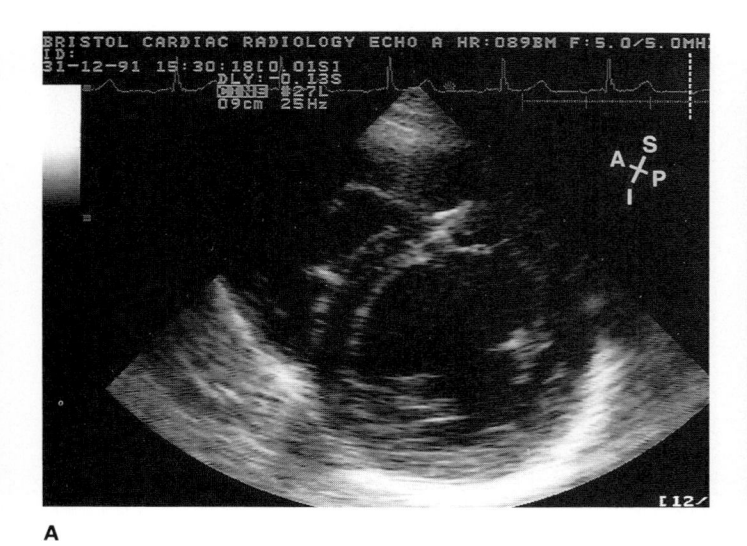

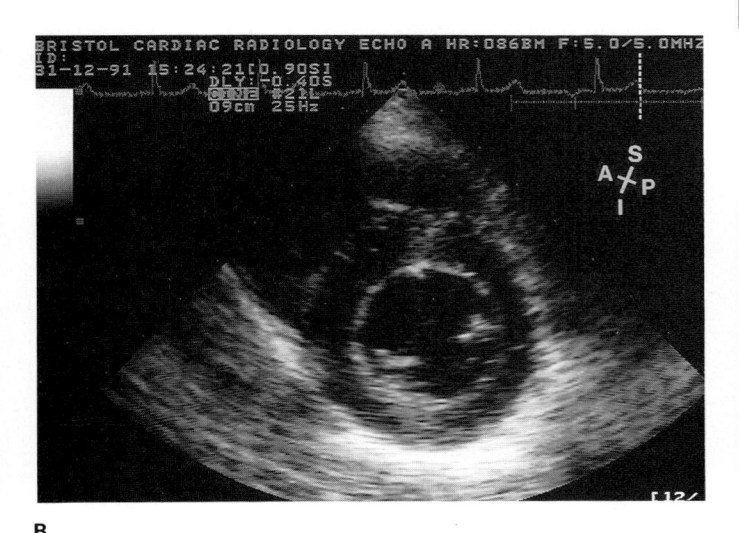

Fig. 10 Left parasternal short axis view at the level of the papillary muscles in the left ventricle. A: The image is taken in diastole. **B:** Systolic frame of the same cardiac cycle shown in A. Note enhancement of the endocardial echo pattern.

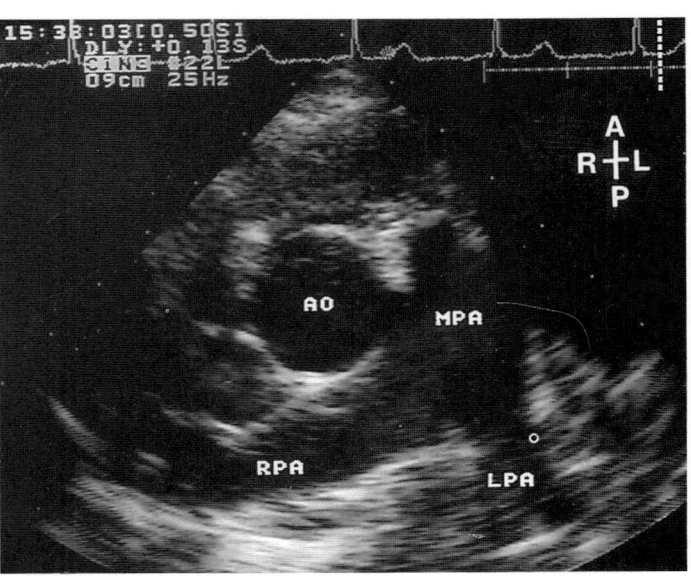

Fig. 11 Modified left parasternal short axis view. It shows the aortic root, main pulmonary artery and pulmonary bifurcation LPA – left pulmonary artery, RPA – right pulmonary artery.

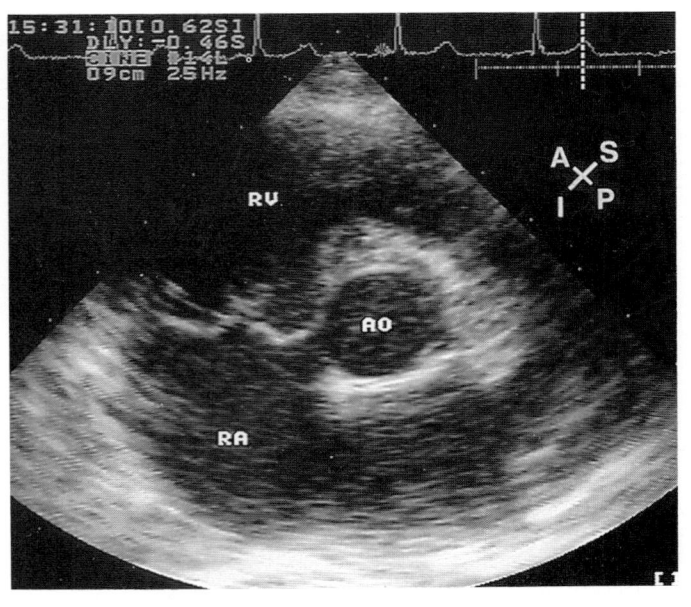

Fig. 12 Low left parasternal short axis view. It shows the closed tricuspid valve lying between right atrium and ventricle.

alignment. By common convention the structures nearest the transducer are displayed at the top of the screen. The direction of the reference mark is to the right of the screen. The heart thus appears as though with its apex uppermost and the left ventricle on the right of the screen.

The apical four chamber view displays both atria and both ventricles together with the mitral and tricuspid valves (Fig. 13). The left ventricular lateral wall together with the inflow and muscular interventricular septum can both be assessed. The interatrial septum and interventricular septum are usually both well seen although there may be some dropout of the interatrial septum and the membraneous portion of the interventricular septum as both these structures lie parallel to the ultrasound beam.

Left and right pulmonary veins are usually visible posterior to the left atrium (Fig. 14).

A slight variation is the so-called apical 'five chamber' view. To obtain this view the transducer is angled slightly anteriorly and superiorly so that the left ventricular outflow tract can be seen leading into the aorta with the aortic valve leaflets moving within it (Fig. 15). The mitral valve partially moves out of the image plane during this manoeuvre.

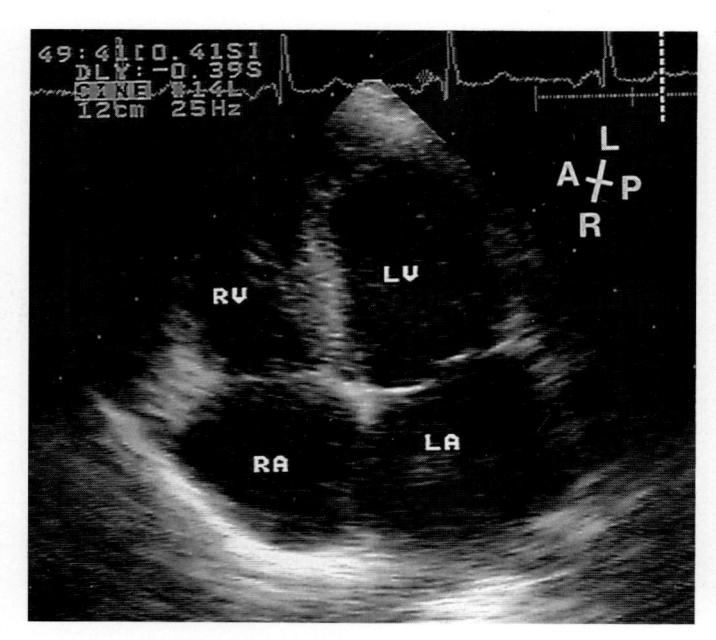

Fig. 13 Apical four chamber view. The tricuspid valve (between right atrium and right ventricle) lies closer to the cardiac apex than the mitral valve (between left atrium and ventricle).

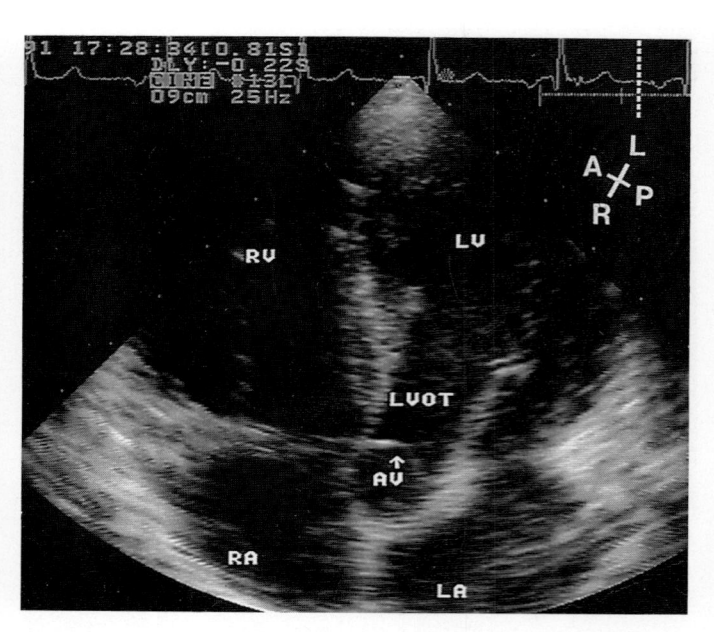

Fig. 15 Upward angulation from the apical four chamber view shows the left ventricular outflow tract (LVOT) and the lowermost leaflet of the aortic valve, the non-coronary leaflet. This is the so-called 'five chamber' view.

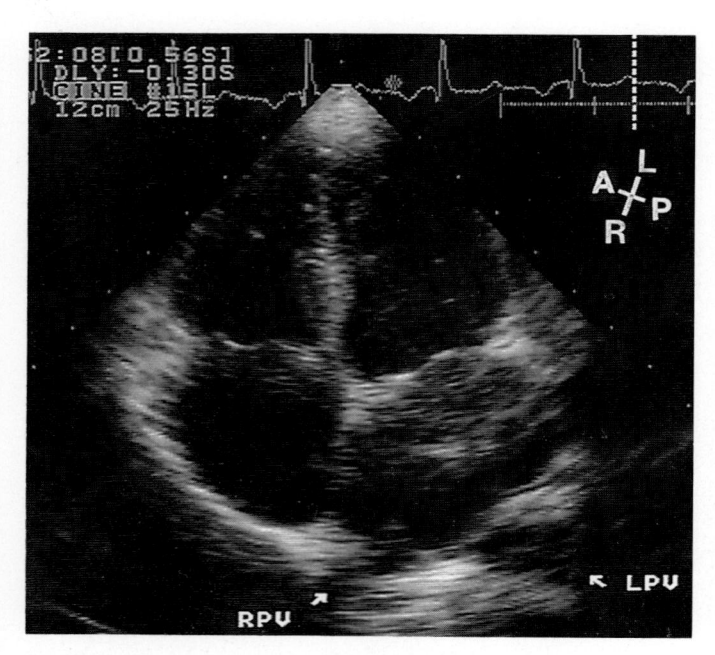

Fig. 14 Apical four chamber view showing left and right pulmonary veins (LPV, RPV). Artefactual signal occupies part of the left atrium.

If, whilst still scanning from the apex, the transducer is rotated anticlockwise through 90° so that its reference mark points anteriorly and superiorly the apical two chamber view or long axis view is seen. This is a good view for assessing the anterior and inferior walls of the left ventricle as the ultrasound scan crosses only the left sided chambers. The whole of the left ventricular wall muscle can be examined utilising the parasternal long and short axis views and the apical four chamber and long axis views.

If views from the parasternal and apical windows have been inadequate or if further information is sought then other windows may be tried.

Subcostal (or subxiphoid) window

This window may be useful in those people with hyperinflated lungs which make precordial imaging difficult. It is also very useful in young people and children. The subcostal window utilises the liver to transmit ultrasound through the diaphragm to the heart. Assessment of the abdominal vascular situs is carried out from this position. The patient should lie flat with the knees slightly drawn up to relax the abdominal muscles. The transducer is positioned below the xiphisternum with the reference mark of the transducer pointing to the patient's left side. This will give a transverse upper abdominal view showing the liver and inferior vena cava on the right side and the descending aorta on the left side (Fig. 16). These vessels can also be imaged longitudinally from this position (Fig. 17A and B) but it must be noted that in most echocardiographic laboratories the display is a left to right reversal of the usual longitudinal radiology scan of the upper abdomen.

Upward angulation and slight clockwise rotation from the transverse upper abdominal scan will give the subcostal four chamber view (Fig. 18) which is anatomically similar to the apical four chamber view but in a different orientation. The view may be more advantageous for displaying the interatrial septum which now lies more perpendicular

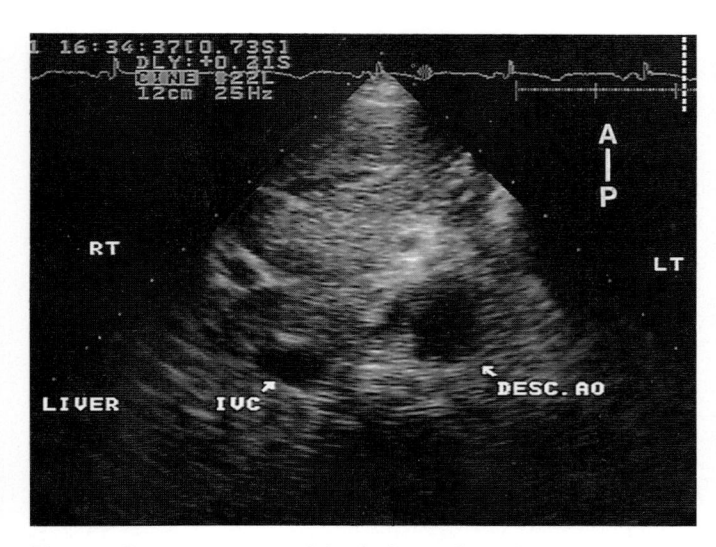

Fig. 16 Transverse upper abdominal scan from the subcostal window showing the inferior vena cava (IVC) on the right side and the descending aorta (DESC.AO) on the left.

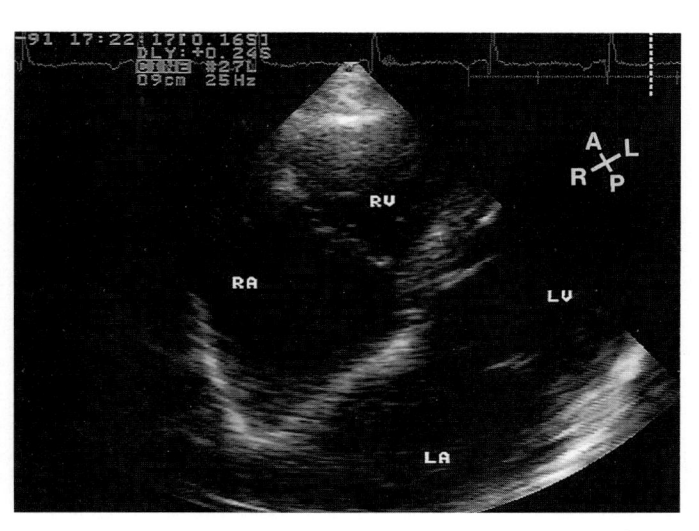

Fig. 18 Subcostal four chamber view. The inter-atrial septum is well shown.

to the ultrasound beam. This is the view of choice to exclude an atrial septal defect. Once again structures closest to the transducer are usually displayed at the top of the screen. The base of the heart is shown to the left of the screen with the apex pointing upwards to the right of the display. The quality of images from this position is very variable. Further upward angulation from the subcostal four chamber view will demonstrate the aortic valve (Fig. 19).

Short axis views similar to parasternal views can be obtained from the subcostal window by rotating the transducer anticlockwise so the reference mark is directed towards the patient's left shoulder (Fig. 20). In most children and in some adults with hyperinflated lungs, ex-cellent quality images of the pulmonary valve and main pulmonary artery can be obtained from this position.

Suprasternal window

Optimal imaging from the suprasternal notch is obtained with the patient lying almost flat and the neck gently extended over a pillow. It is usually helpful to tilt the patient's chin to the right. This window allows visualisation and assessment of the aortic arch, the ascending and descending thoracic aorta as well as the patient's branchiocephalic, left common carotid and left subclavian arteries (Fig. 21). It is a particularly useful view in children in whom coarctation

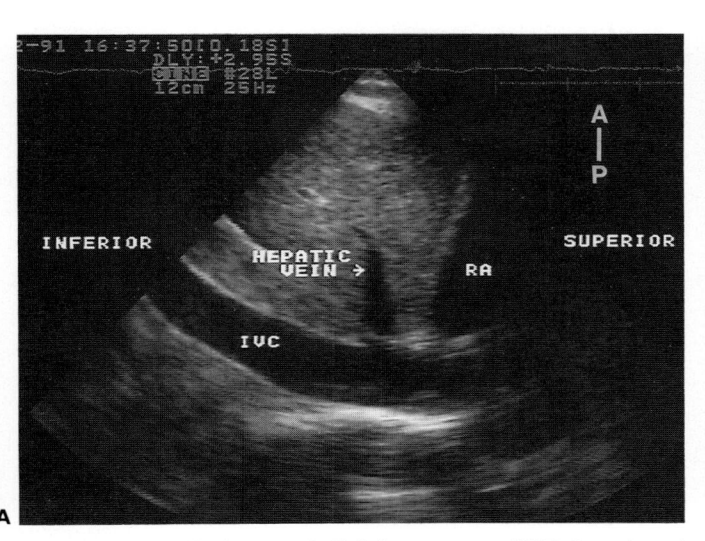

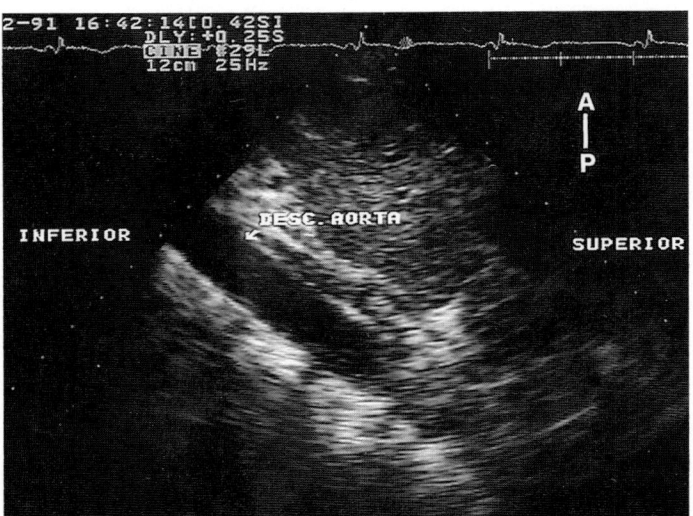

Fig. 17 Longitudinal scans. **A:** Inferior vena cava (IVC) from the subcostal window. **B:** Descending aorta from the subcostal window.

52 CARDIAC ULTRASOUND

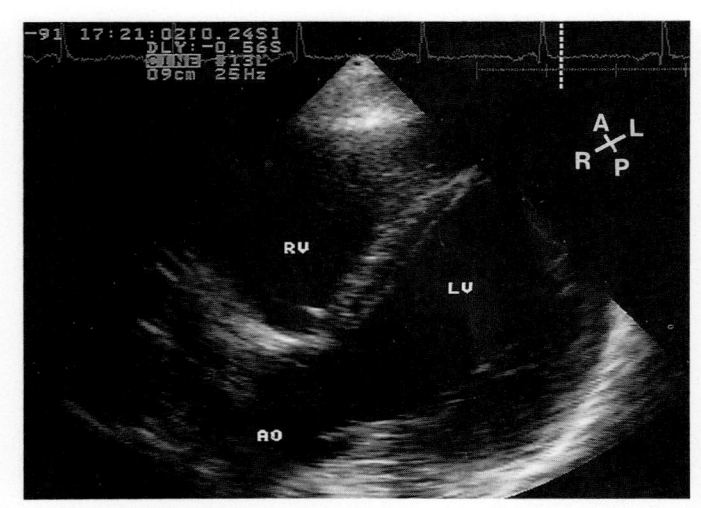

Fig. 19 Superior angulation from Fig. 18 to show the left ventricular outflow into the aorta.

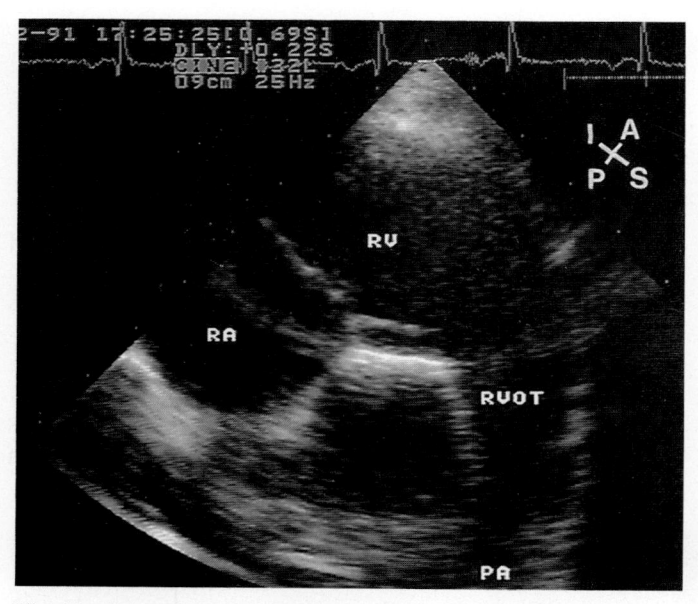

Fig. 20 Subcostal short axis view showing the right sided cardiac chambers wrapping around the left ventricular outflow tract (RVOT – right ventricular outflow tract).

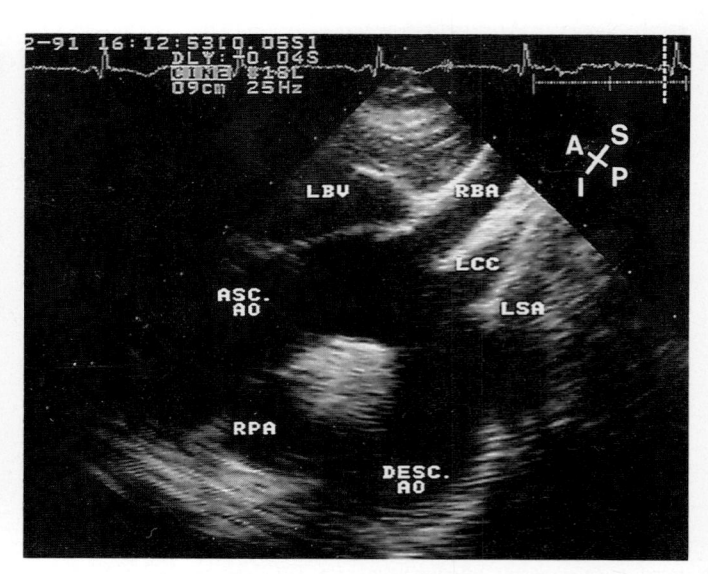

Fig. 21 Suprasternal view of the aortic arch showing its major branches (RBA – right brachiocephalic artery, LCC – left common carotid artery, LSA – left subclavian artery) and the left brachiocephalic vein (LBV). The right pulmonary artery (RPA) is seen posterior to the ascending aorta.

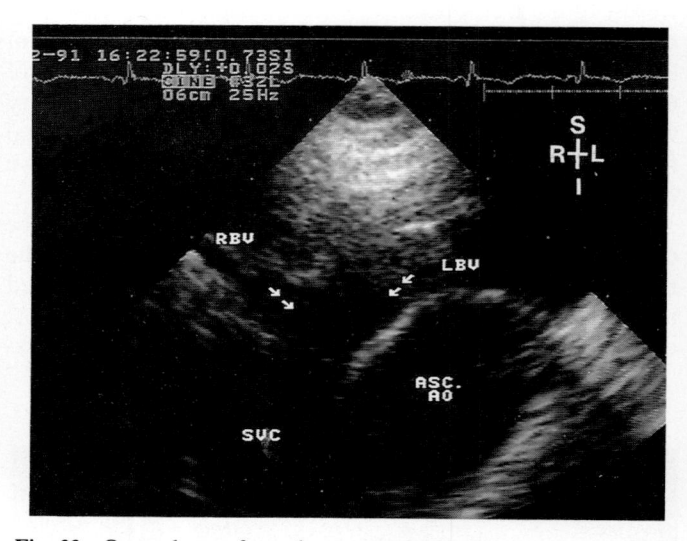

Fig. 22 Coronal scan from the suprasternal window. The left and right brachiocephalic veins (LBV, RBV) are seen draining to the superior vena cava.

is suspected or where turbulence from a patent ductus arteriosus is sought. In adults the window is primarily used for Doppler assessment of aortic flow. In some adults very poor images will be obtained from this position.

The transducer should be placed behind the sternum with the reference mark pointing posteriorly and to the left. The ascending aorta is displayed to the left of the screen with the three major branches visible and the descending aorta to the right of the screen. The right pulmonary artery will be seen in the arch of the aorta having come from the main pulmonary artery bifurcation just to the left of the plane of the aortic arch. If the transducer is now rotated anticlockwise (90° to the left) the aorta is cut in cross-section and the venous confluence to the right of the ascending aorta can be imaged (Fig. 22). In a few cases, usually children, imaging of some cardiac structures can be obtained from the suprasternal notch.

Right parasternal window

The 2nd, 3rd or 4th rib spaces to the right of the sternum can be used to give access to the ascending aorta for assessment of the jet of aortic stenosis but this is usually a poor imaging window in adults unless the heart is displaced to the right or the ascending aorta is dilated. It is worth using this view in the assessment of any case with a large ascending aorta, in which case the patient should be rotated to their right to improve ultrasonic access.

DOPPLER EXAMINATION

Although the same echocardiographic windows are used for Doppler examination as for imaging, it should be remembered that whilst the optimum angle of incidence between the ultrasound beam and tissue interfaces for imaging is 90°, one needs to be as nearly as possible parallel to the direction of blood flow for optimal Doppler examination. Thus a view such as the parasternal long axis view, whilst providing excellent visualisation of the mitral valve, is a poor position from which to interrogate mitral flow, particularly in the normal patient. Having said this, one needs to be aware in which direction blood is flowing relative to the transducer because colour flow mapping will often demonstrate flow at large angles to the interrogating beam (Plates 1A, B and C). Doppler examination is usually incorporated in an imaging probe to help placement of the Doppler beam but as the jet being sought may not be parallel to the plane of the image, this should serve only as a guide to Doppler studies.

Whenever Doppler studies are performed, the spectral display should be clean, a well-defined envelope should be obtained and the audio signal should be as nearly as possible a pure tone. Careful adjustments in transducer position and equipment controls are necessary to achieve this.

Flow through cardiac valves and the great vessels will now be considered. In this context the anatomical positions of the cardiac valves related to the precordium must be considered.

The pulmonary valve lies to the left of the midline at the level of the third sternocostal joint. The aortic valve is positioned more medially and slightly posterior to this at the level of the fourth left sternocostal joint. The mitral valve is continuous with the aortic valve but is slightly inferior to it in the fourth intercostal space at the sternal border. The tricuspid valve lies retrosternally in the midline at the level of the 6th or 7th sternocostal joints.

Mitral valve

The mitral valve is best interrogated from the apical four chamber view with the pulsed wave Doppler sample volume positioned just into the left ventricle, immediately distal to the tips of the mitral valve leaflets (Fig. 23A and B). The pulsed spectral trace is analogous to the M-mode pattern, the 'E' wave of passive ventricular filling dying away in mid-diastole before the second peak or 'A' wave

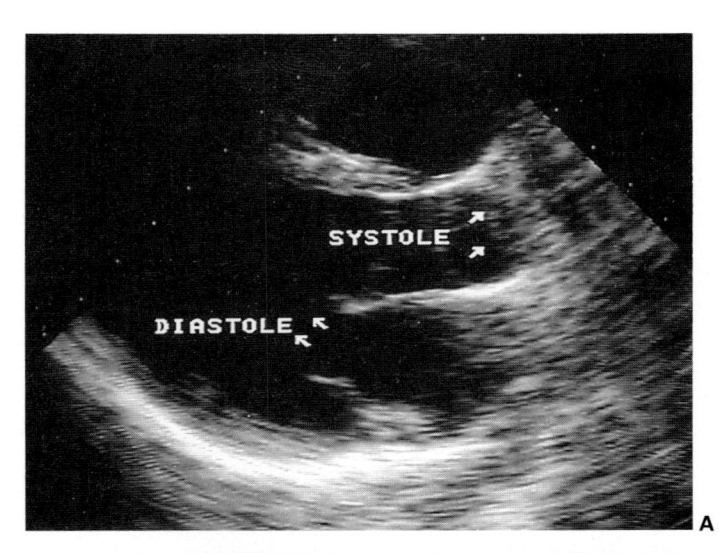

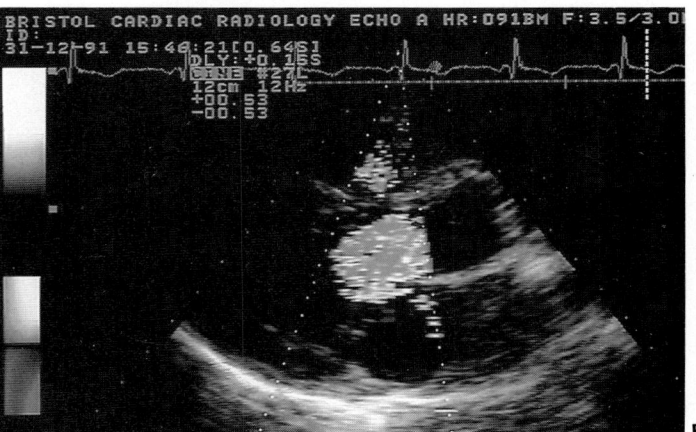

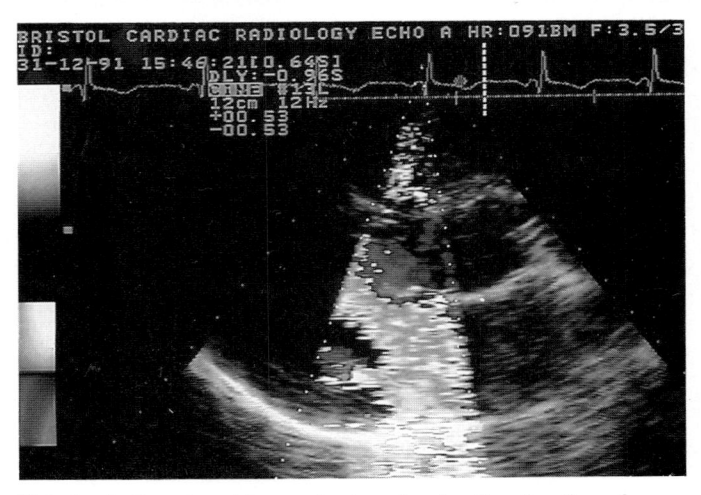

Plate 1 **A: Parasternal long axis view showing the direction of mitral inflow and of outflow towards the aortic valve.** The precise direction of flow will vary from examination to examination. **B:** Colour flow mapping of the same study as Plate 1A taken in systole and showing flow towards the aortic valve in red as it is slightly towards the transducer. Note that the colour map is only shown over a limited sector. **C:** Diastolic frame taken from the same study as Plates 1A and B showing mitral inflow in red as it is slightly towards the transducer. This figure is reproduced in colour in the colour plate section at the front of this volume.

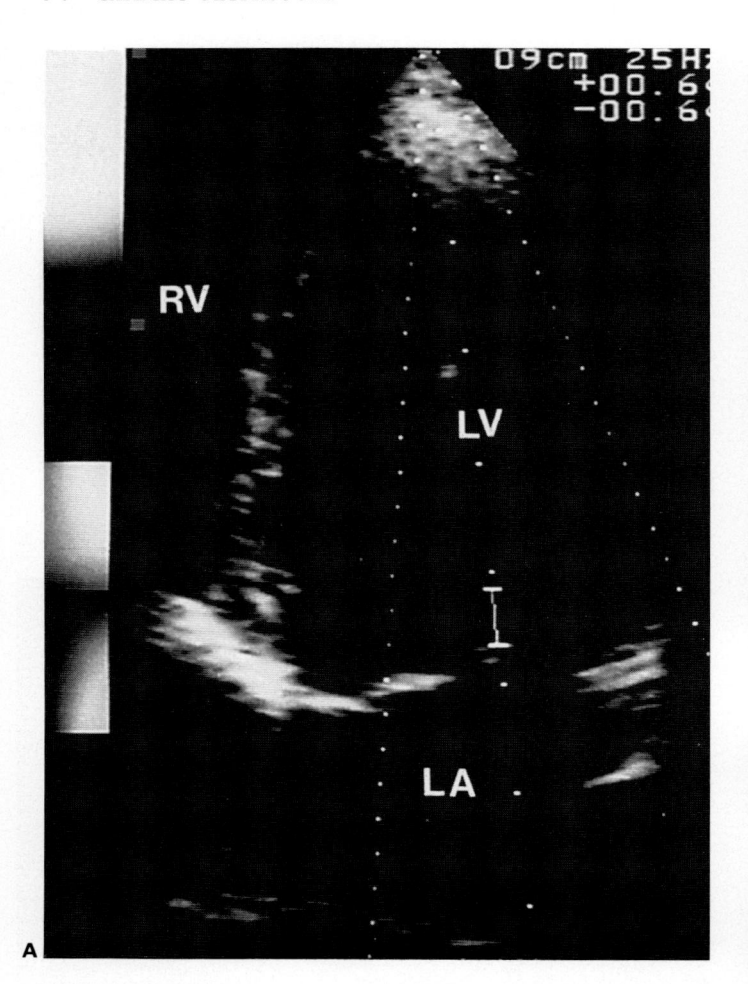

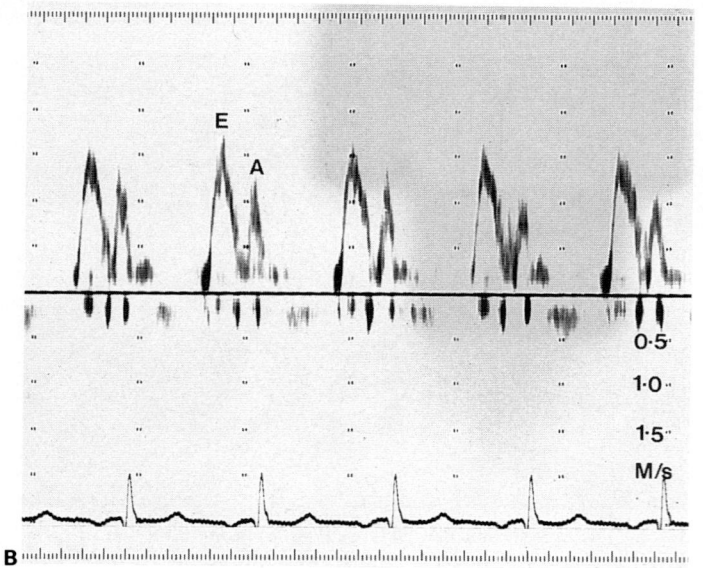

Fig. 23 Apical four chamber view. **A:** Pulsed Doppler sample volume lying in the mitral orifice. **B:** Pulsed Doppler trace taken from A. The well defined biphasic diastolic flow is clearly seen with the initial phase (the E wave) being of higher velocity than the second or atrial phase (the A wave). The well defined line of the trace shows that the flow is organised as it passes through the valve. Velocity calibration is 0.5 m/s.

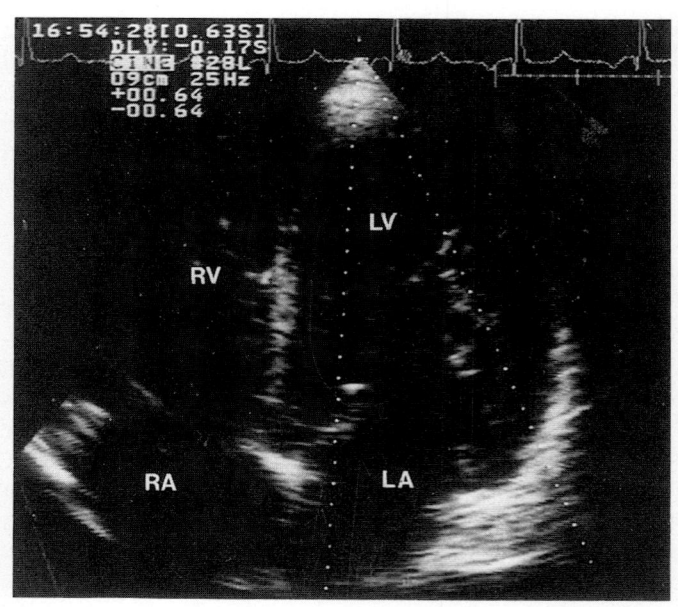

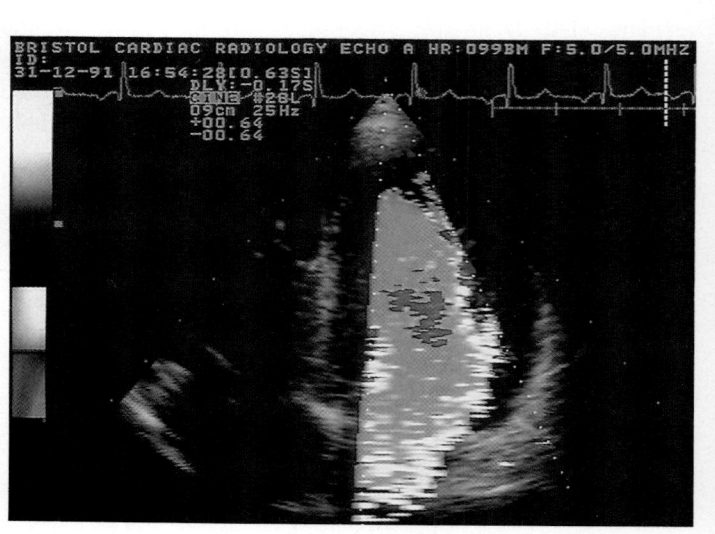

Plate 2 A: Apical four chamber view showing the mitral valve open in diastole. **B:** Colour flow image corresponding to Plate 2A showing mitral inflow towards the transducer in red. The central part of the flow shows aliasing (blue). This figure is reproduced in colour in the colour plate section at the front of this volume.

of atrial systole occurs. In normal flow the E wave has a higher velocity than the A wave. It can be useful to employ valve clicks to position correctly the pulsed wave sample volume. A click at the end of the diastolic spectral trace is due to valve closure and indicates the sample is too far into the left atrium. A click at the start of the diastolic spectral trace indicates valve opening and that the sample volume is correctly positioned distal to the valve orifice. These differences reflect the normal movement of the mitral valve away from the transducer during diastole.

The normal transmitral flow will have a clear envelope on pulsed wave Doppler traces indicating laminar (or organised) flow across the mitral valve. Colour flow imaging from the apex will demonstrate mitral inflow very clearly (Plates 2A and B).

A similar position is also used to assess the presence or absence of mitral regurgitation but the sample volume must be a little more deeply placed in the left atrium. If colour flow Doppler interrogation is available, a regurgitant jet and its extent will rapidly be identifiable in systole. If colour flow mapping is not available, the left atrium should be interrogated at several levels to determine the extent of the regurgitation into the left atrium. Semiquantitative assessment of regurgitation in this way corresponds approximately with the grades of severity assessed at left ventriculography.

Normal mitral flow velocities are usually adequately recorded by pulsed wave Doppler and continuous wave Doppler recordings are not required. If there is an increase in velocity through the mitral orifice as for example in mitral stenosis either high pulse repetition frequency pulsed wave Doppler or continuous wave Doppler techniques must be considered. Continuous wave Doppler traces show the same overall envelope shape as pulsed wave traces, but show spectral broadening because data from the turbulent areas of flow proximal and distal to the valve are included. In these instances the clean outline of the normal pulsed wave envelope becomes infilled with lower velocity flow data.

Continuous wave transducers can be separate non-imaging devices ('stand-alone CW'), they can be mounted integrally in the probe having a side-by-side arrangement or, more recently, the phased array probe can be used to produce 'steerable CW' within the sector scan. In the latter two cases the accompanying imaging data is helpful in aligning the continuous wave interrogation line but this is at the expense of a more bulky transducer. The simple 'stand-alone' or 'pencil' probe is easier to place in small windows and generally produces the best quality results but the lack of imaging makes it a more difficult technique to master.

Tricuspid valve

The apical four chamber view is usually the view from which the tricuspid valve is interrogated. Flow patterns are similar to those of the mitral valve although the velocities are lower and there is a greater degree of spectral broadening (Fig. 24A and B). Again pulsed wave Doppler will adequately record normal flow velocities. In many normal people it is possible to detect a systolic jet of tricuspid regurgitation. If the jet is of low intensity and has a velocity not exceeding 2.5 m/s it should be regarded as physiologi-

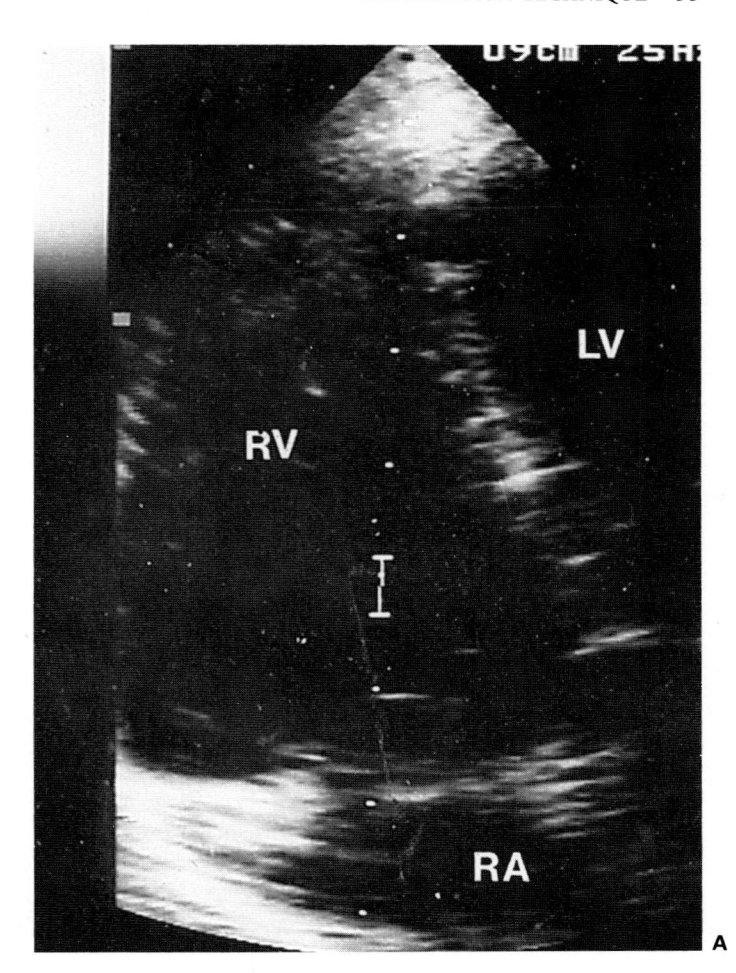

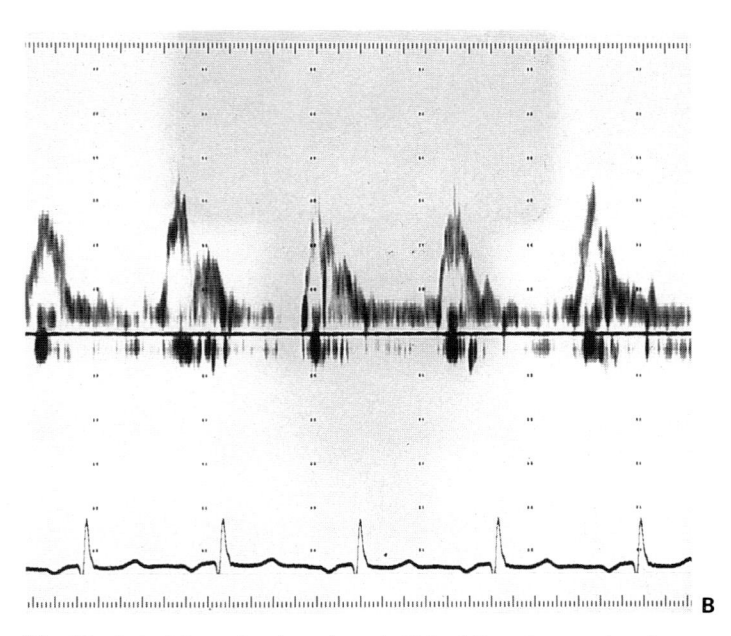

Fig. 24 Apical four chamber view. A: Pulsed Doppler sample volume lying in the tricuspid orifice. **B:** Pulsed Doppler trace taken from A. The tricuspid flow is of slightly lower velocity than the mitral flow (Fig. 23B) and is less well organised (spectral broadening). The settings of the machine are the same as for Fig. 23B.

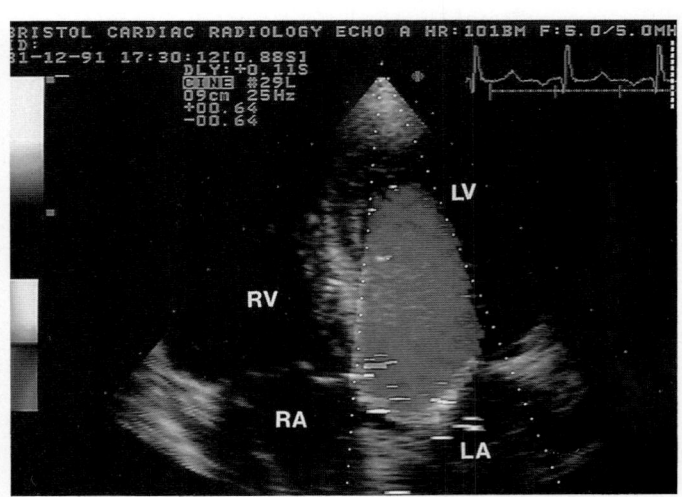

Plate 4 Apical four chamber view angled upwards towards the left ventricular outflow tract. Colour flow mapping shows flow away from the transducer in blue. This figure is reproduced in colour in the colour plate section at the front of this volume.

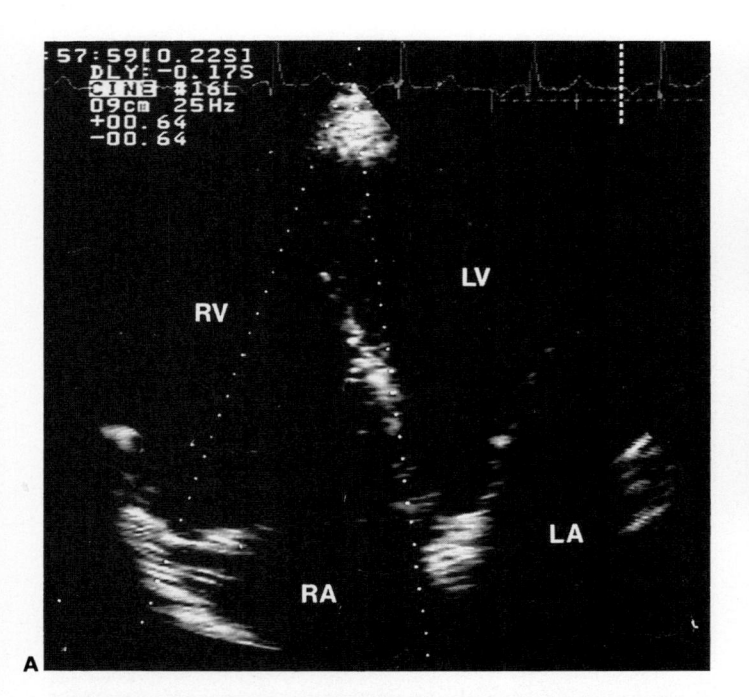

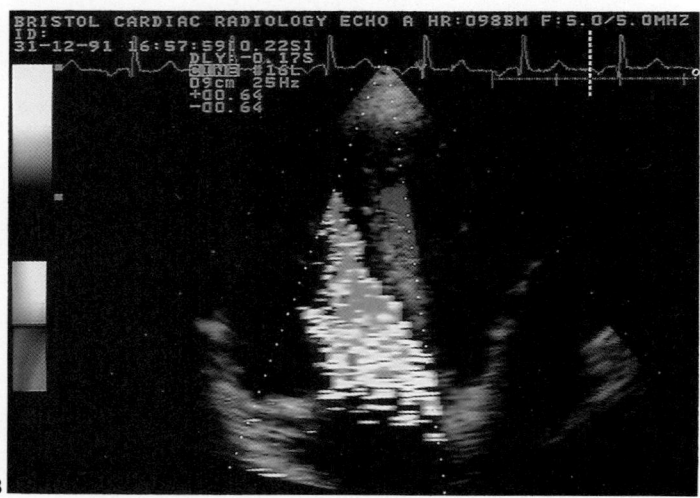

Plate 3 A: Apical view of the tricuspid valve taken from the same study as Plate 2A. B: Colour flow image corresponding to Plate 3A showing diastolic tricuspid inflow in red but there is no aliasing present as the velocity is lower than that of mitral inflow. This figure is reproduced in colour in the colour plate section at the front of this volume.

cal. Colour flow mapping will also show tricuspid flow clearly (Plates 3A and B). A modified low left parasternal window is also useful for examination of the tricuspid valve.

Aortic valve

The aortic valve is best assessed initially from the apical window using a superiorly tilted apical four chamber view (the apical 'five chamber' view) or an apical long axis view. It is important, if using a pulsed Doppler sample volume, to distinguish between a position in the left ventricular outflow tract and one in the aortic root distal to the valve. The apical four chamber view shows the left ventricular outflow satisfactorily (Plate 4) but the apical long axis view is superior in its ability to show flow right through the aortic valve (Plate 5A) and is also the best view for distinguishing mitral from aortic flow (Plate 5B). Even in normal patients there is a small but significant increase in velocity across the aortic valve (Fig. 25A and B). Normal flow is characterised by a rapid initiated acceleration to an early peak velocity of around 1 m/s to 1.5 m/s. Pulsed wave recordings show this to be plug flow with a clean envelope of narrow spectral width. However, if there is any suggestion of valve stenosis the velocity quickly increases so that continuous wave Doppler will be required to determine the peak velocity of flow. If aortic stenosis is detected then the aorta should be interrogated from a range of other windows since an eccentric jet may produce its maximum velocity in differing directions. It may be helpful to use a 'stand alone' continuous wave probe from the subcostal, right parasternal and suprasternal windows since this will have a smaller footprint and be easier to manipulate. The probe should be directed towards the upper left sternal edge from the subcostal region, towards the apex of the heart from the right parasternal window, and downwards anteriorly and slightly left of centre from the suprasternal notch.

The suprasternal window is used to demonstrate flow in the ascending and descending aorta (Fig. 26A and B; Plates 6A and B). If coarctation is being considered it is important that the increased flow velocity is shown and continuous wave studies may be needed. Flow may normally approach 2 m/s in the descending aorta. It is important to distinguish between arterial and venous flow when scanning from the suprasternal window (Plate 7). The ascending aortic flow

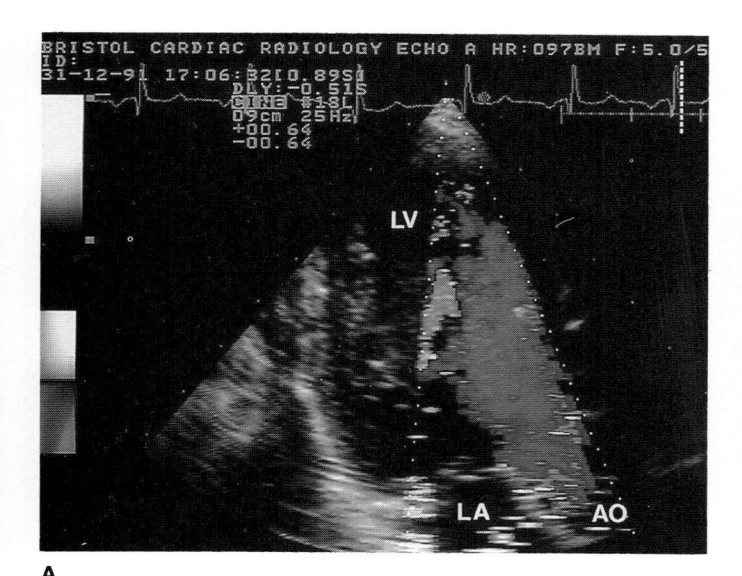

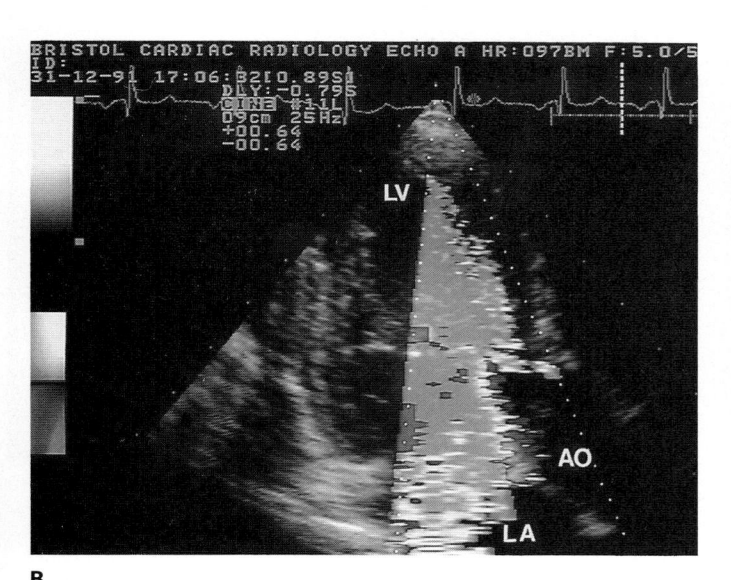

Plate 5 A: Apical long axis view with the colour sector placed over the left ventricular outflow tract. Systolic flow through the aortic valve is shown in blue (compare with Fig. 25). B: Apical long axis view showing diastolic mitral inflow in red. This figure is reproduced in colour in the colour plate section at the front of this volume.

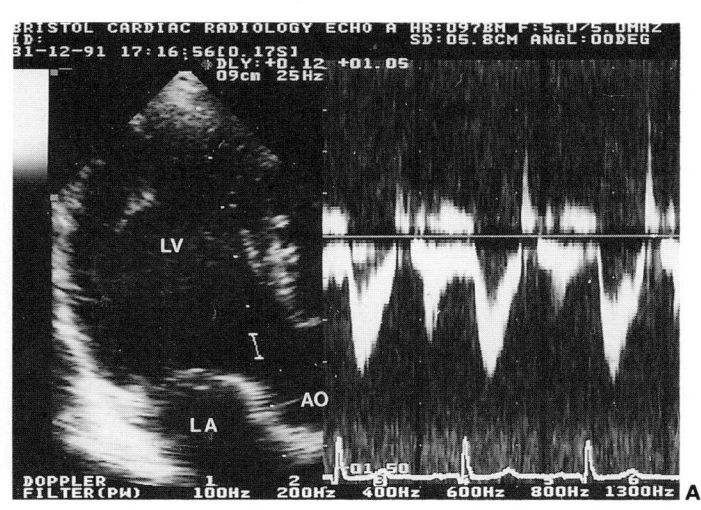

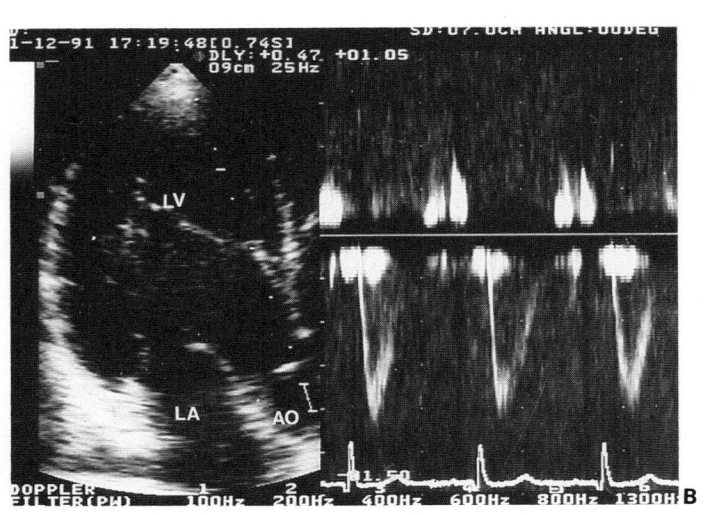

Fig. 25 A: Apical long axis view (left) showing a pulsed Doppler sample volume lying in the left ventricular outflow tract. The resulting trace (right) shows flow towards the aortic valve (away from the transducer). B: The same examination as A. The sample volume has been moved deeper, past the aortic valve and into the aortic root. The resulting trace shows slight acceleration as the blood passes through the normal aortic valve.

has a clean systolic envelope above the zero flow baseline on pulsed Doppler examination (Fig. 27A) whilst superior vena caval flow has marked spectral broadening below the zero flow line and is of lower velocity (Fig. 27B).

Aortic regurgitation is best demonstrated using spectral or colour flow mapping from the apical views but analysis of the descending aortic flow may show a reversal of velocity in diastole due to regurgitation of blood into the left ventricle.

Occasionally there may be confusion as to whether a systolic jet is due to aortic stenosis or mitral regurgitation. This is a situation in which the relationship of the jets to valve clicks may be helpful. The two valve clicks detected at the end of systole are due to aortic closure followed by mitral valve opening. If the detected jet ends with the first click it is due to aortic flow. Mitral regurgitation will overlay the first click and end only with the second click as the mitral valve opens. Conversely the two clicks at the beginning of systole are due to mitral valve closure followed by aortic valve opening (Fig. 28).

Pulmonary valve

The parasternal short axis view through the base of the heart displays the pulmonary valve. Colour flow mapping

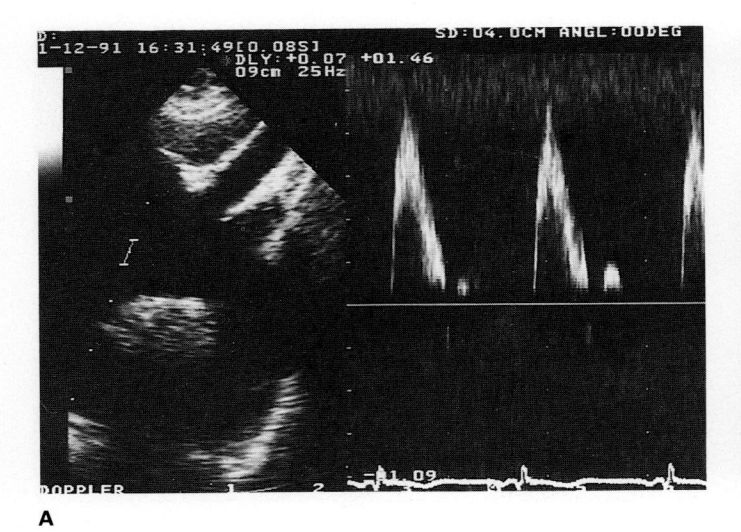

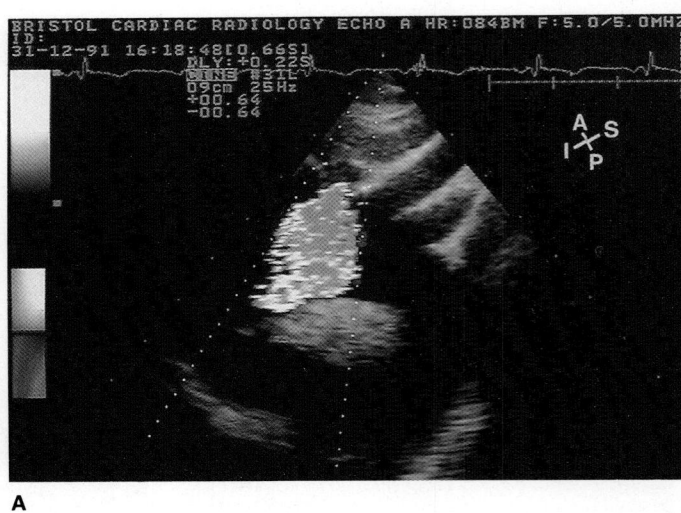

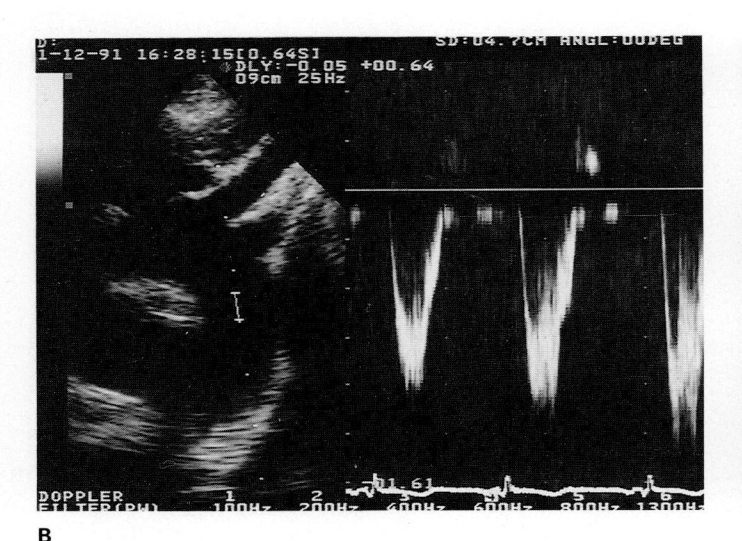

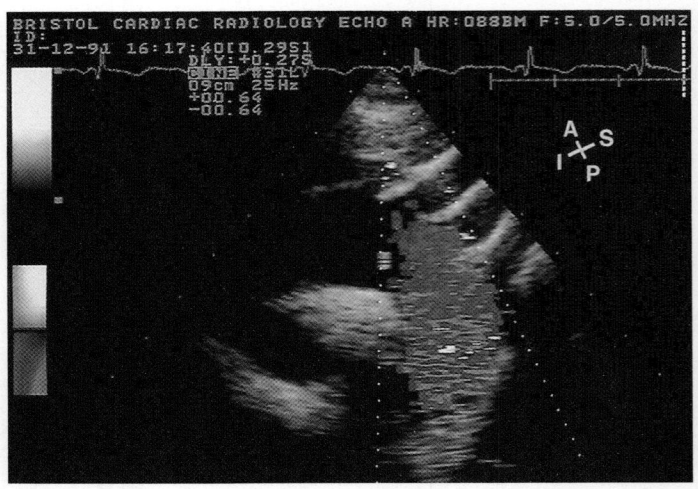

Fig. 26 A: Suprasternal image of the aortic arch with the pulsed Doppler sample volume in the ascending aorta (left). The resulting trace (right) shows aortic flow above the baseline towards the transducer. **B:** The sample volume has been moved to the descending aorta and the flow is now away from the transducer.

Plate 6 A: Suprasternal view of the aortic arch. The colour sector has been placed over the ascending aorta and shows the flow towards the transducer in red. **B:** Similar view to Plate 6A with the colour sector placed over the descending aorta, showing the flow away from the transducer in blue. This figure is reproduced in colour in the colour plate section at the front of this volume.

shows flow in the main pulmonary artery away from the transducer (Plate 8). The leaflets can be seen to lie closed in diastole and the pulsed Doppler sample can be positioned in the main pulmonary artery (Fig. 29A and B). Normal flow is laminar with a peak velocity of approximately 1.0 m/s. As with the tricuspid valve, there may be physiological regurgitation (Plate 9 and Fig. 30). Its velocity should not exceed 1.5 m/s. It may be necessary, particularly in adult patients, to position the subject well round to the left, sometimes even in a left lateral position, in order to produce an adequate echo window to the pulmonary artery. Flow in the pulmonary artery can sometimes be shown from the subcostal window in suitable subjects (Plate 10).

Vena cavae

Flow in the superior vena cava is best seen from the suprasternal notch and good alignment can usually be achieved. The inferior vena cava and hepatic veins can be assessed subcostally but the hepatic veins are better aligned than the inferior vena cava, flow in the latter vessel often being difficult to record.

EXAMINATION TECHNIQUE 59

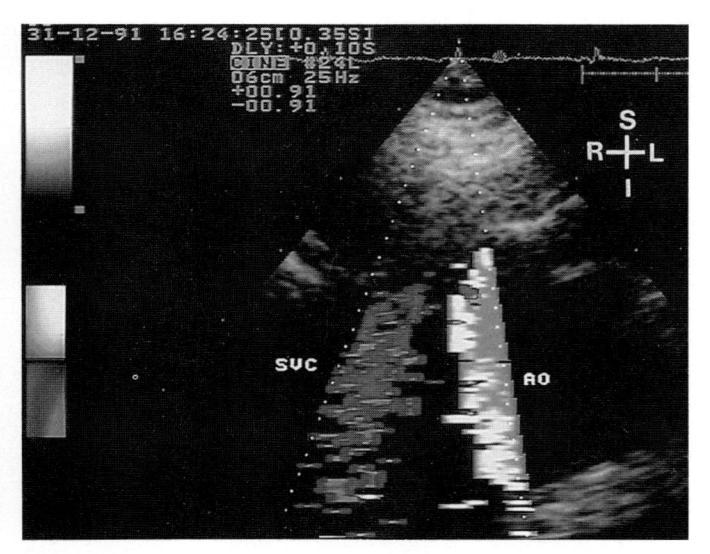

Plate 7 Coronal suprasternal view in the same orientation as Fig. 22 showing flow in the superior vena cava away from the transducer in blue and flow in the ascending aorta towards the transducer in red. This figure is reproduced in colour in the colour plate section at the front of this volume.

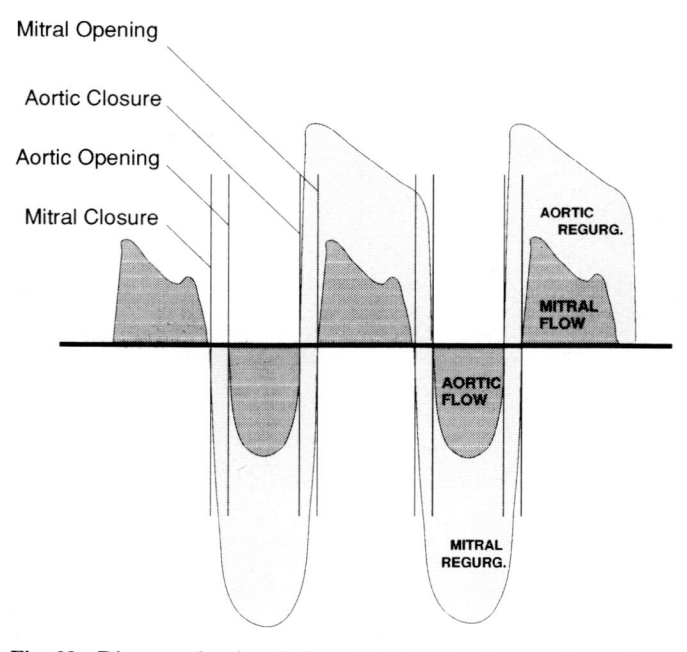

Fig. 28 Diagram showing timing of left sided valve opening and closure in relation to the normal valve flow and regurgitation through the same valves.

Pulmonary veins

Flow is difficult to assess precordially due to their depth behind the left atrium but is achievable with careful technique in a proportion of patients. The pulmonary veins can however be well demonstrated by transoesophageal echocardiography.

CONTROL OPTIMISATION

Imaging controls

These are relatively straightforward and their principles have been covered in Chapter 3 on instrumentation.

Familiarity with the various controls of the machine is

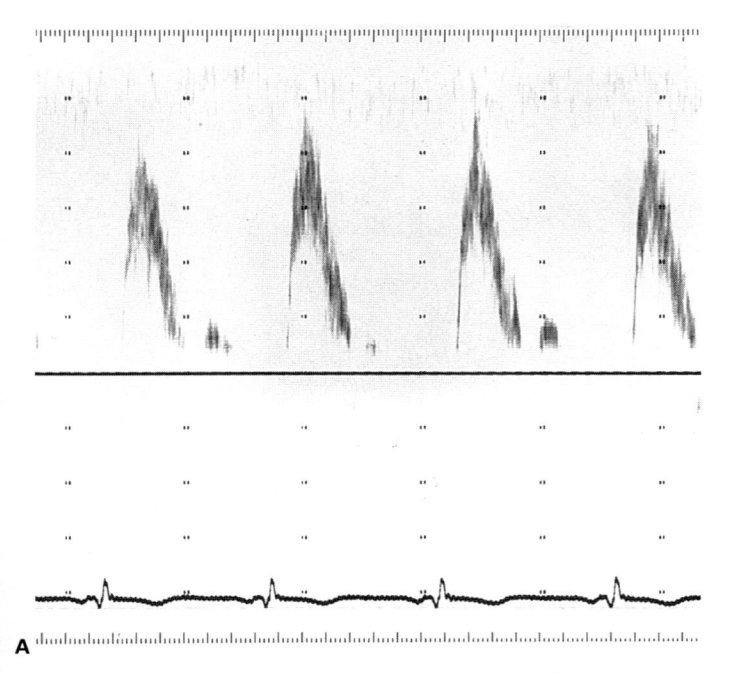

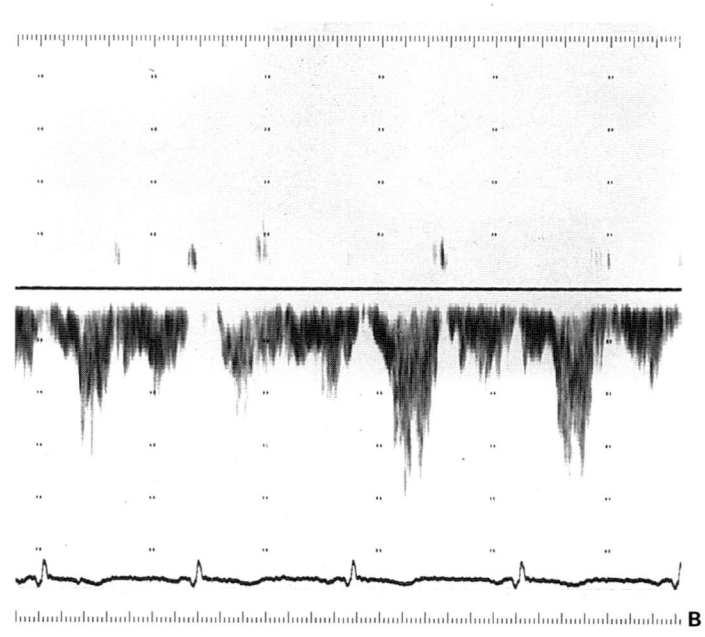

Fig. 27 Suprasternal pulsed Doppler recordings. A: The ascending aorta (taken from a coronal approach as in Fig. 22). B: Flow in the superior vena cava taken from the same window as A. The flow is of lower velocity and is continuous and more turbulent than arterial flow.

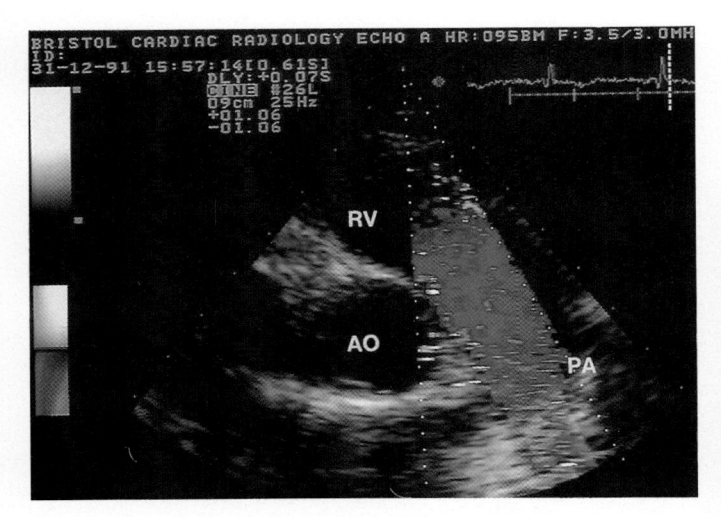

Plate 8 Left parasternal short axis view showing flow in the right ventricular outflow tract and pulmonary artery. Flow away from the transducer is shown in blue (compare with Fig. 29). This figure is reproduced in colour in the colour plate section at the front of this volume.

important before the examination commences. If these are incorrectly set, it will not be possible to produce satisfactory results. The two most important controls to regulate are the power and the gain. The power mode will control the overall intensity of the recorded image. It is good practice to use the lowest power level which is consistent with a good quality examination. In general the easiest way to judge a satisfactory power setting is to adjust the overall gain control to its mid-position and then adjust the power until an adequate image is obtained. If this is done on a fairly typically sized patient then use of the overall gain should provide enough flexibility to make frequent alterations of the power setting unnecessary. In normal operation it is important to have the overall gain suited to the patient being examined and the transducer in use. Too much overall gain will amplify noise and produce a distracting speckle across the image whilst too low a gain setting risks missing important detail. Ideally the blood-filled chambers should just contain a minimal level of signal. In some machines M-mode and sector scan gain can be adjusted separately. Depth gain compensation should be set to ensure adequate imaging according to the circumstances, but it is important to avoid using this control in conflict with the overall gain. It is unhelpful to have the depth gain control (usually a set of sliding knobs) all at maximum if the overall gain is set too low and vice versa. If good penetration is achieved with low gain settings this is a sign that a higher frequency transducer could be used.

The depth gain compensation should then be adjusted to ensure that echoes returning from various depths in the patient all have the same intensity on the display. Without this control, echoes from deep structures would be swamped by echoes from closer structures. Machines

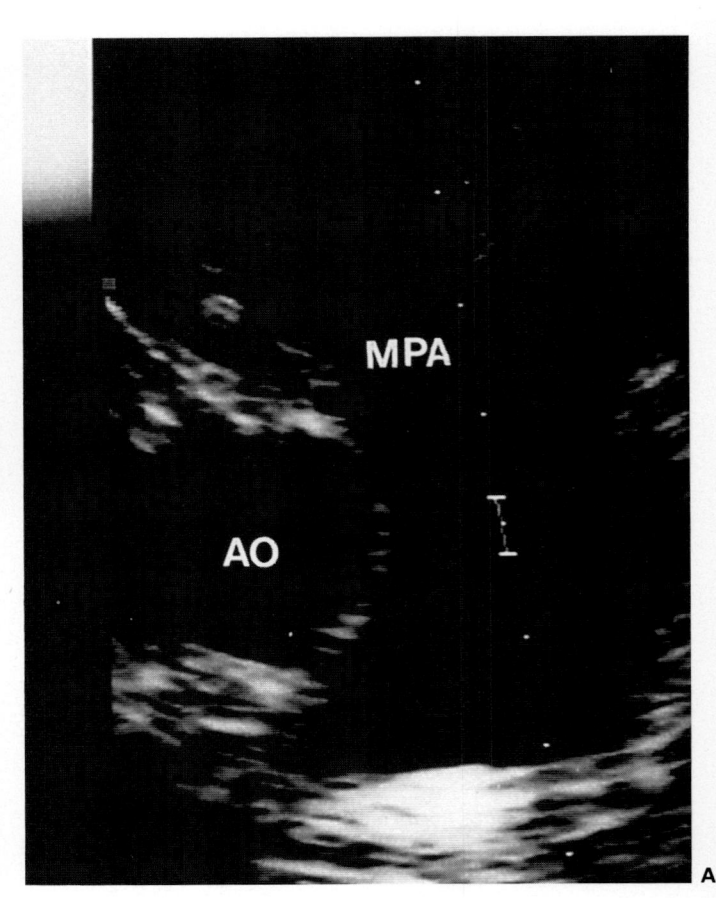

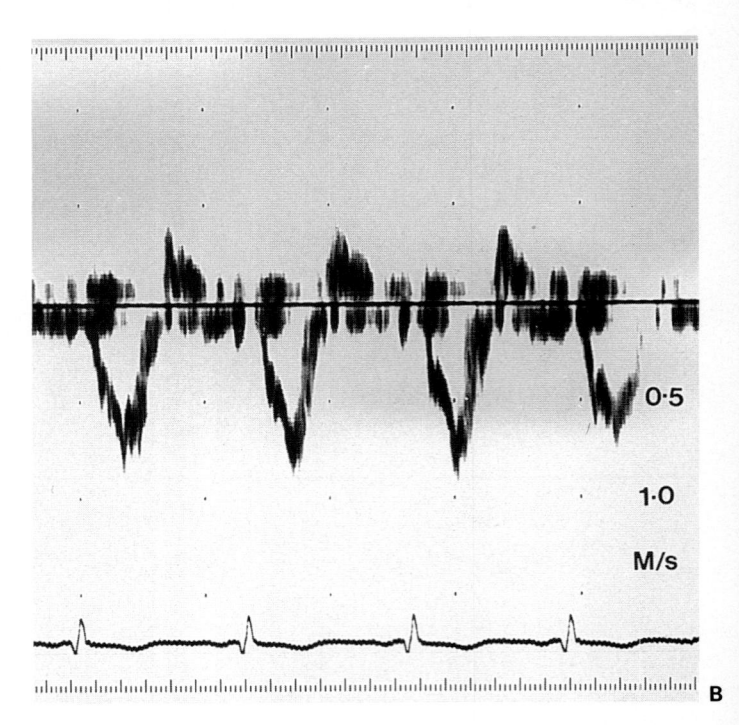

Fig. 29 A: Left parasternal view of the main pulmonary artery with a centrally positioned pulsed Doppler sample volume. B: Spectral trace from A showing normal well-organised pulmonary artery flow away from the transducer in systole. Velocity calibration is 0.5 m/s.

EXAMINATION TECHNIQUE 61

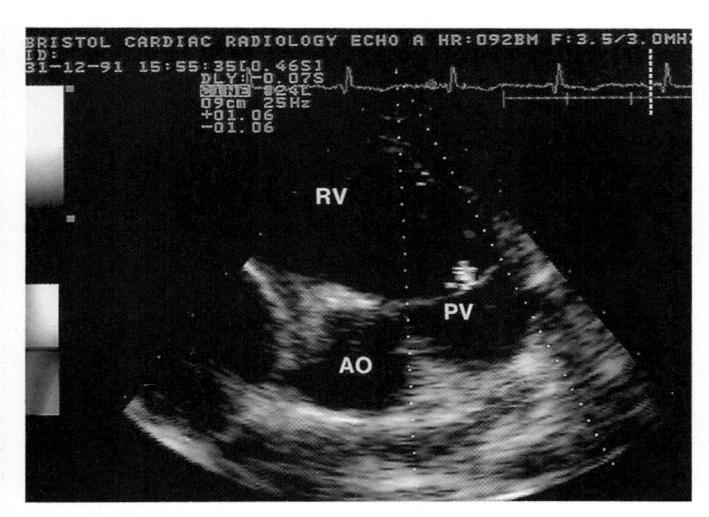

Plate 9 Diastolic frame from the same examination as Plate 8. A small orange jet of physiological pulmonary regurgitation is seen just proximal to the pulmonary valve. This figure is reproduced in colour in the colour plate section at the front of this volume.

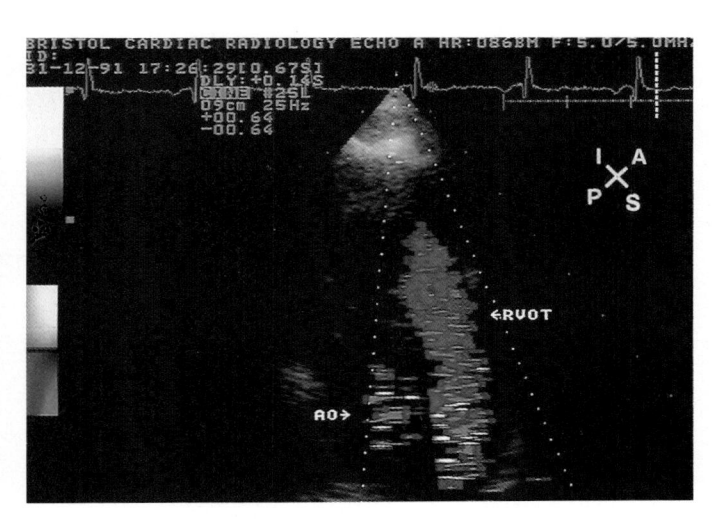

Plate 10 Subcostal short axis view taken in systole showing systolic flow (in blue) in both the aortic root and the right ventricular outflow tract (compare Fig. 20). This figure is reproduced in colour in the colour plate section at the front of this volume.

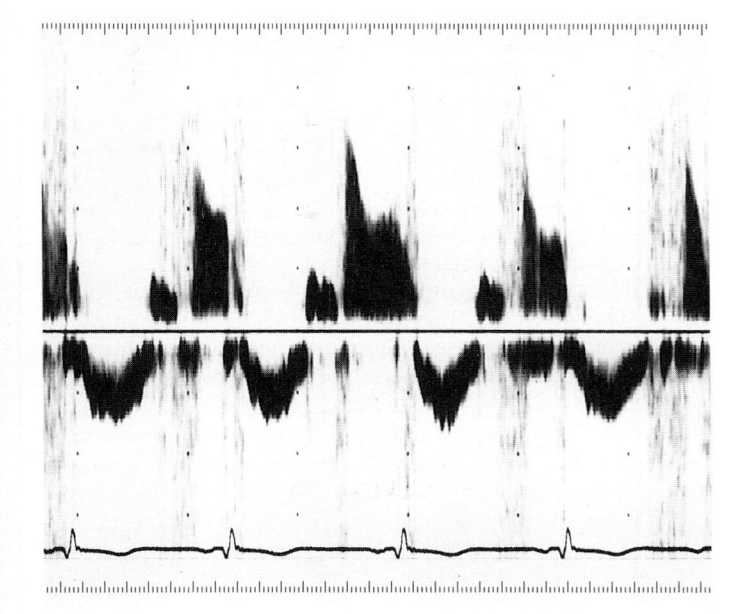

Fig. 30 Spectral trace taken from the left parasternal position with the sample volume placed just proximal to the pulmonary valve. Normal (physiological) pulmonary regurgitation is seen as a diastolic signal towards the transducer (above the baseline). Normal flow in the right ventricular outflow tract is seen in systole (below the baseline).

commonly have a bank of sliders to adjust to produce a satisfactory image but some systems offer near gain, slope and far gain controls which have a similar effect but are generally less flexible in adjustment. The image produced should be altered until structures from all depths appear uniformly bright on the display. If larger or smaller patients are imaged it will be necessary to alter this time gain compensation.

The overall depth setting of the sector scan or M-mode trace must ensure that important deep structures are not inadvertently excluded from the study (e.g. a posterior pericardial effusion).

Doppler controls

Understanding and adjustment of controls becomes even more important during a Doppler examination because the Doppler signals are amplified and electronically adjusted to an even greater degree than those used for image production. Considerable experience and patience is needed to perform a thorough Doppler examination, especially in subjects with limited access because of poor echo windows.

Again, the same details of patient positioning should be followed. The comfort of the operator should not be neglected. Arm, wrist and hand fatigue can quickly set in when the operators hand is trying to 'lock on' to a suitable signal.

Power output

As with imaging, the power output for the Doppler system should be adequate to produce good signal production. As present no harm has been documented from the use of diagnostic ultrasound but it seems unwise to use more power than is necessary.

Signal gain

Most Doppler systems have automatic gain control capabilities as well as an operator adjustable control. If a clear good quality trace is detected the automatic gain con-

STANDARD ECHOCARDIOGRAPHIC EXAMINATION

The outline below is a suggested approach to a full routine adult cardiac examination (Table 1 shows normal cardiac dimensions). Clearly it is not mandatory to adhere to this particular approach but it has proved useful in clinical practice. It is essential to modify such a protocol in the light of different equipment, patients and operators.

1. Obtain the best parasternal long axis view. Take time to do this as it is the key to much of the examination. Don't do M-mode, Doppler or colour flow examinations before you achieve this. Once you have it, record 10–20 s on video.

2. Record optimal M-mode traces of the left ventricle, aortic valve and mitral valve. Record on video but only on thermal paper when tracing is excellent. Continuous strip chart recording of the M-mode trace (rather than a single frozen digitised frame) gives the highest fidelity recording but is probably best reserved for special cases as it results in considerable paper usage.

3. Whilst in this plane, examine the subaortic and submitral areas for regurgitation using colour flow mapping. Set the gain control correctly. Careful adjustment of the scan plane is required to ensure no small jets are missed. Record normal or abnormal findings on video.

4. Turn the transducer to the parasternal short axis view. Record two-dimensional images of the left ventricle, mitral valve and aortic valve on video. Check for mitral regurgitation into the left atrium using colour flow mapping when imaging at the level of the aortic valve. Also check for tricuspid regurgitation, pulmonary valve regurgitation and abnormal colour flow patterns in the pulmonary artery (i.e. patent ductus or pulmonary valve stenosis). Position a pulsed Doppler sample volume just after the pulmonary valve and determine the pulmonary artery acceleration time. Record all findings on video.

5. Move to the apical position and obtain the best apical four chamber view. Record 10–20 s on video. Check with pulsed Doppler for stenosis of the mitral and tricuspid valves. Colour flow mapping may be used as an aid to locate the area of maximum trans-valvular velocity. Assess the mitral and tricuspid valves for regurgitation using colour flow mapping. If any significant tricuspid regurgitation is found, quantitate the degree of pulmonary hypertension by measuring the velocity of the tricuspid regurgitation using continuous wave Doppler examination. Record all findings on video, and record Doppler traces of the mitral valve and any continuous wave Doppler traces of the tricuspid regurgitation on thermal paper.

6. Elevate the four chamber plane superiorly to obtain the aortic root ('five chamber') view. Assess the aortic valve and left ventricular outflow tract using two dimensional imaging, colour flow mapping, pulsed Doppler and continuous wave Doppler. Record findings on video and any abnormal Doppler findings on thermal paper.

7. Rotate to the apical long axis view. Reassess the aortic valve and outflow tract. The apical long axis is the view of choice to carry out left ventricular contractility assessment utilising the area length calculation (only if images are of sufficiently high quality). Record the findings on video making thermal prints of optimal images.

8. If considered appropriate, move to the subcostal position. This may not always be necessary, depending on the quality of the above recordings and/or the patients clinical diagnosis (e.g. it will be necessary if a ventricular septal defect or an atrial septal defect is suspected).

9. Use the suprasternal view to image the aortic arch in cases of aortic regurgitation and assess flow in the descending aorta using pulsed Doppler. Use this position with other cases of suspected aortic pathology.

10. When assessing aortic stenosis using continuous wave Doppler, apical, sternal notch, right parasternal and subcostal approaches must all be used for accurate quantitation.

11. At this stage a full qualitative assessment should have been achieved. Quantitation, if required, should be attempted thoroughly or not at all – a 'quick look' at an aortic or tricuspid jet will lead to erroneous results.

Notes

Frozen two-dimensional images on paper are often poor, it is often best to avoid them and use video.

Thermal paper is expensive, do not record rubbish.

When recording on video, remember those who have to view the scan later. Record enough but not too much.

trol has no problem in selecting a suitable gain level. If, however, a signal which is weak in relation to the background noise is to be analysed some velocity information may be lost if the automatic gain is relied upon. In these circumstances the manual control must be adjusted to detect all the information in the weak signal. If the manual gain control is set too high for the power level selected, the phenomenon of cross talk will occur. This causes mirror-like artifacts on the opposite side of the Doppler baseline. Not only may these distort the main trace they may also be mistaken for separate flow. If cross talk occurs, both the overall Doppler power and/or the gain should be reduced.

Low frequency filter

Any moving structure within the line of the Doppler beam will produce a frequency shift and hence be detectable on the Doppler trace. Structures such as cardiac valves and the myocardial walls themselves, although slowly moving, produce high intensity signals that may interfere with normal recording of blood flow velocity. Machines have a low frequency Doppler filter to allow removal of these low velocity recordings. The low frequency is also removed from the audio signal and the removal of the thumps and bumps allows the blood flow to be heard more easily. Some degree of filtering is always required usually in the range 200 to 400 Hz but sometimes 800 Hz or even 1600 Hz is required in some recordings. It should be realised that some low velocity blood flow information will necessarily be lost by this filtering but this is not usually clinically relevant. Too high a filter setting will start to reduce useful flow information and must be avoided by keeping the filter setting at the lowest value commensurate with good flow signals.

Baseline shift

The baseline that indicates zero shift or no flow is usually positioned in the centre of the display. Conventionally, flow towards the transducer is recorded above the baseline whilst flow away is recorded below the baseline. If velocity is such that it cannot all be represented on one side of the baseline this can be shifted so that the full waveform can be displayed in one channel. This can mask aliasing to a certain extent when using pulsed wave recording and apparently allows twice the velocity to be recorded. This is often a helpful display but it should be remembered that flow in the opposite direction will now be displayed in the same part of the trace.

Sweep speed

A useful point is the use of increased sweep speed (on the screen or on paper) to allow more accurate evaluation of flow curves. Whilst the normal speed of 50 mm/s is usually adequate the speed can be increased to allow easier analysis, particularly if the heart rate is high.

Electrocardiogram (ECG)

The simultaneous electrocardiogram recording allows timing of flows or movement of structures on images. The ECG should always be set properly with a stable baseline, reasonable gain and should be positioned on the screen in a position where it does not obscure important data.

High pulse repetition frequency (high PRF)

Pulsed wave systems will alias once the Nyquist limit (half pulse repetition frequency) is exceeded. This limit will depend on the depth at which the blood flow is sampled

Table 1 Normal dimensions by M-mode echocardiography (from St. John Sutton et al. Circulation 1980; 62 (Suppl III): 100)

		cm		cm
Right ventricle	End diastole	2.1 ± 0.4	Left atrial dimension (maximum)	3.3 ± 0.5
	End systole	1.8 ± 0.4	Aortic root diameter	2.9 ± 0.4
Left ventricle	End diastole	4.8 ± 0.4	Left ventricle	
	End systole	3.0 ± 0.4	LV Dilatation – Approximate working guidelines (P. Wilde)	
Interventricular septal thickness	End diastole	0.9 ± 0.2	Mild ESD 4.0–4.5 EDD 5.5–6.0	
	End systole	1.3 ± 0.2	Moderate ESD 4.5–5.0 EDD 6.0–6.5	
			Severe ESD > 5.0 EDD >6.5	
Left ventricular posterior wall thickness	End diastole	0.8 ± 0.1		
	End systole	1.3 ± 0.2		

EDD – end diastolic diameter
ESD – end systolic diameter
The base of the left ventricle can function normally whilst the apex is dilated or impaired. Under these circumstances the M-mode study can give misleading information about the overall state of the left ventricle.

and the velocity of the blood flow. The greater the depth the longer it takes for each pulse to travel to the required depth and return to the transducer. As the sample volume is placed appropriately (usually guided by the two dimensional image) many machines automatically adjust the pulse repetition frequency to the maximum available for that depth. If aliasing occurs, either changing to continuous wave sample or the use of high PRF pulsed Doppler may allow successful velocity measurements.

In high PRF pulsed Doppler examination a second, third or fourth pulse is emitted before the first pulse is received back by the transducer. The additional pulse positions are indicated on the Doppler line indicator on the two dimensional image as extra sample volumes. It is usually possible to position the extra pulse in an area of low flow where it will add little to the spectral display. The main sample remains positioned in the jet and this increased PRF raises the Nyquist limit and allows increased velocity of flow to be recorded. It is important not to be misled in situations where a shallower sample volume picks up another flow pattern which swamps the original signal from the site of intent. This technique falls half way between pulsed and continuous wave in its ability to localise blood flow but the limitations of its velocity range mean it must be used with caution.

Sample volume size

The sample volume size of the pulsed wave systems can be altered from about 1 mm in length up to about 15 mm. The length is controlled by altering the receive time of the returning pulses. This may be usefully employed when searching for small flows in a relatively large chamber. Obviously in this situation the use of colour flow Doppler mapping can save time by alerting one to the presence of high or turbulent flow. It should be remembered that although the actual sample volume appears narrow when displayed on the screen it is in fact as wide as the ultrasound beam itself.

CONCLUSION

It should be stated finally that a high quality audit and review system is essential for the maintenance of standards in any echocardiographic department. Clinical feedback, the results of other investigations, joint meetings and consultations should all be used to monitor the accuracy of any results. Operators should view each others work frequently in order to maintain a consistent approach to reporting.

RECOMMENDED READING

1 Hatle L, Angelsen B. Doppler ultrasound in cardiology: physical principles and clinical applications, 2nd edition. New York: Lea and Febiger. 1985.
2 Fiegenbaum H. Echocardiography, 4th edition. New York: Lea and Febiger. 1986.
3 Houston A B, Simpson I A. Cardiac Doppler ultrasound – a clinical perspective. Wright 1988.
4 St. John Sutton M, Oldershaw P. Textbook of adult and pediatric echocardiography and Doppler. Oxford: Blackwell Scientific. Publications. 1989.
5 Wilde P. Doppler echocardiography – an illustrated clinical guide. Edinburgh: Churchill Livingstone. 1989.
6 Jawad I A. A practical guide to echocardiography and cardiac Doppler ultrasound. New York: Little, Brown. 1990.
7 ACP/ACC/AHA Task Force on Clinical Privileges in Cardiology. Clinical competence in adult echocardiography. J Am Coll Cardiol 1990; 15 (7): 1465–1468

5

Left ventricular function

Introduction
Ventricular shape, size and function
Left ventricular wall thickness and mass
Left ventricular stress indices
Systolic function
Diastolic function
Effects of age
Right ventricular/left ventricular relationship
Exercise and left ventricular function
Summary

Jamie Weir

INTRODUCTION

Left ventricular function is a rather nebulous concept and the term has come to have various meanings. There are many parameters to ventricular function, some of which are measurable by echocardiography, whilst others need different techniques. The combined use of M-mode, cross-sectional and Doppler ultrasound does allow a considerable 'attack' on many aspects of ventricular function and can be used as a basis for assessing the heart's physiology and more importantly, its pathophysiology.

The action of a ventricle can be broken down to include anatomical measurements which can be linked to other monitoring techniques to obtain physiological data. The anatomical measurements include diameters, areas and volumes of cavities at different phases of the cardiac cycle together with wall thicknesses (Figs 1 and 2). Physiological measurements include velocity recordings, the electrocardiogram (ECG), pressure monitoring and phonocardiography. Combination of many parameters will allow a global picture of function to be produced. Derivation of cardiac output, systolic and diastolic function, contractility and compliance can be assessed and this adds to the understanding of the heart as a pump, albeit a complicated one. The effects of afterload and preload, heart rate and rhythm, drugs, age and fitness level all produce variables which need to be known before categorising a particular ventricle's performance. Preload is the force which distends the ventricle in diastole while afterload is the complex force distributed in the ventricular wall during systole.

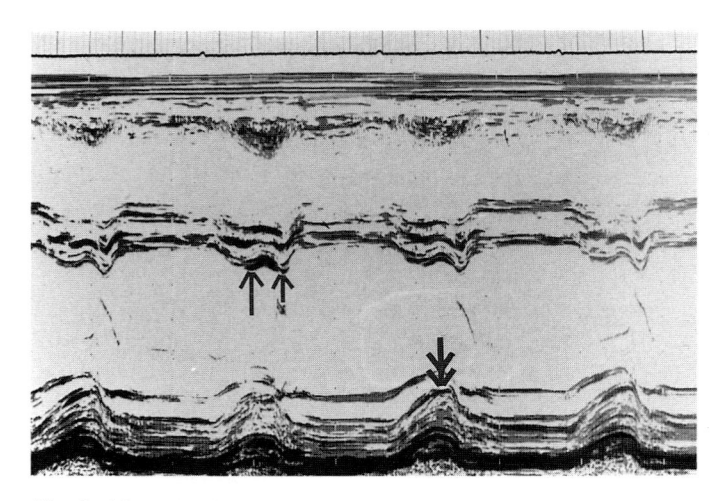

Fig. 2 Normal left parasternal M-mode echocardiogram. Note the normal double posterior wall movement (arrows) of the inter-ventricular septum at the end of systole which makes it more appropriate to use the posterior wall movements to delineate the end of ventricular systole (double arrow).

VENTRICULAR SHAPE, SIZE AND FUNCTION

The shape of a normal left ventricle can be described in simple terms as a truncated ellipsoid, one apex being cut off to simulate the base of the left ventricle. The basic concept of this shape is that the long axis is approximately twice the distance of the short axis and the volume can be calculated as

$$\frac{\pi r^3}{3}$$

where r is the short axis diameter (i.e. the volume is approximately the cube of the radius). This shape is maintained throughout the cardiac cycle allowing end systolic and end diastolic volumes to be measured, together with stroke volume. Although this may be a simplified assessment of the left ventricular shape, it does closely correlate to other methods of cavity measurement such as biplane cine-angiocardiography. Many modified versions of the left ventricular cavity geometry have been suggested with appropriate changes to the volume calculation formula depending on the model used.[1-5] Mercier[6] analysed eight algorithms of left ventricular volume calculations and found the best correlation with biplane cine-angiography to be that of an ellipsoid model using the short axis at the level of the papillary muscles and the apical four chamber view for the long axis and cavity shape contours.

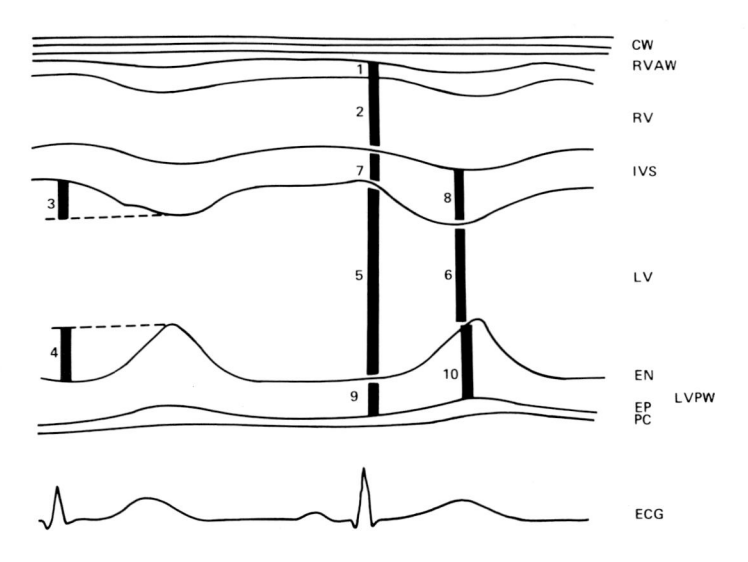

Fig. 1 Typical adult values of left ventricular indices taken from a left parasternal M-mode echocardiogram at the level of the chordae tendinae. 1. Right ventricular anterior wall thickness <6 mm; 2. Right ventricular internal dimension <30 mm; 3. Amplitude of septum 4–8 mm; 4. Amplitude of posterior left ventricular wall 8–14 mm; 5. Left ventricular end diastolic dimension 39–56 mm; 6. Left ventricular end systolic dimension Variable; 7. Septal thickness in end diastole 6–12 mm; 8. Septal thickness in end systole +30% of No. 7; 9. End diastolic LVPW thickness 6–12 mm; 10. End systolic LVPW thickness +30% of No. 9. CW = chest wall; RVAW = right ventricular anterior wall; RV = right ventricular cavity; IVS = interventricular septum; LV = left ventricular cavity; EN = endocardium; LVPW = left ventricular posterior wall; EP = epicardium; PC = pericardium; ECG = electrocardiogram.

The concepts of 'ejection fraction (EF)' and 'stroke volume (SV)' are volume dependent whereas non-volume dependent parameters include circumferential fibre shortening (Vcf) and fractional shortening (FS). The ejection fraction is the percentage of blood ejected during systole and is calculated as follows:

$$\text{EF in \%} = \frac{\text{EDV} - \text{ESV}}{\text{EDV}} \times 100$$

where EDV is the end diastolic volume and ESV is the end systolic volume. The EF in normals is approximately 70%. The SV is a measure of the volume of blood ejected each systole and is therefore given as:

$$\text{SV} = \text{EDV} - \text{ESV in ml.}$$

Cardiac output (CO) is derived from the stroke volume (SV) times the heart rate (HR) as:

$$\text{CO} = \text{SV} \times \text{HR in ml/min.}$$

As both ejection fraction and the stroke volume are volume dependent, the concept of a 'normal' ejection fraction does not hold for dilated ventricles. To take an example, a stroke volume of 70 ml may be produced by a markedly dilated ventricle with an ejection fraction of only 20%, yet the resting cardiac output will be normal at 5 litres/min if the heart rate is 70/min. In other words there is a normal cardiac output despite a very low ejection fraction.

Mean circumferential fibre shorting (mean Vcf) is calculated as:

$$\text{Mean Vcf} = \frac{\text{EDD} - \text{ESD}}{\text{EDV} \times \text{LVET}} \text{ circumferences per second}$$

where EDD = end diastolic diameter, ESD = end systolic diameter, LVET = left ventricular ejection time. As LVET is dependent on the heart rate (and age) the mean Vcf varies in normal subjects. Peak Vcf or peak normalised rate of decrease in left ventricular dimension, has also been used as an index of left ventricular performance.

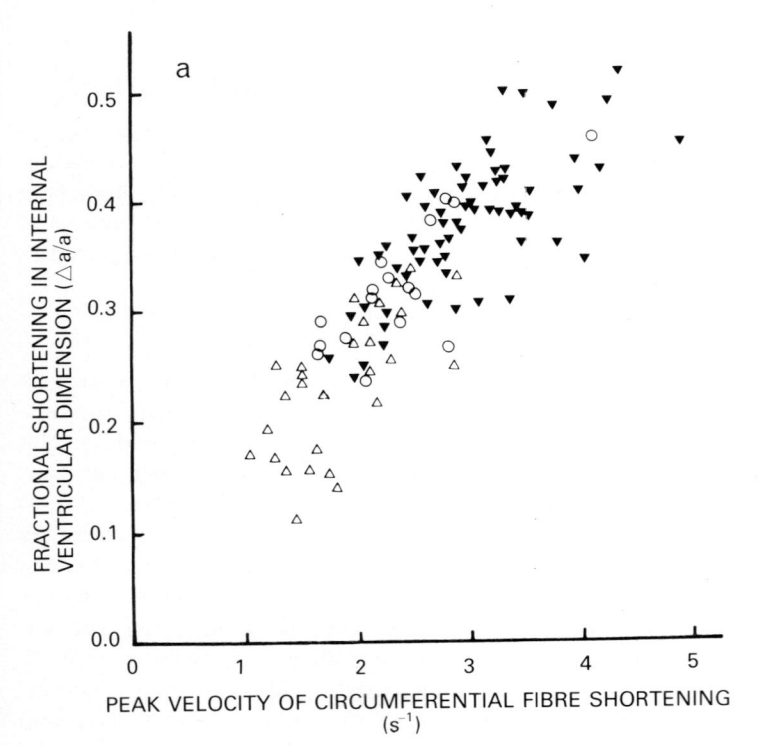

Fig. 3 Peak Vcf against FS. ▼ – normal subjects; ○ – IHD with normal left ventricular angiograms; △ – IHD with dyskinetic areas on angiography. (Vcf – mean circumferential fibre shortening, FS – Fractional shortening, IHD – ischaemic heart disease.)

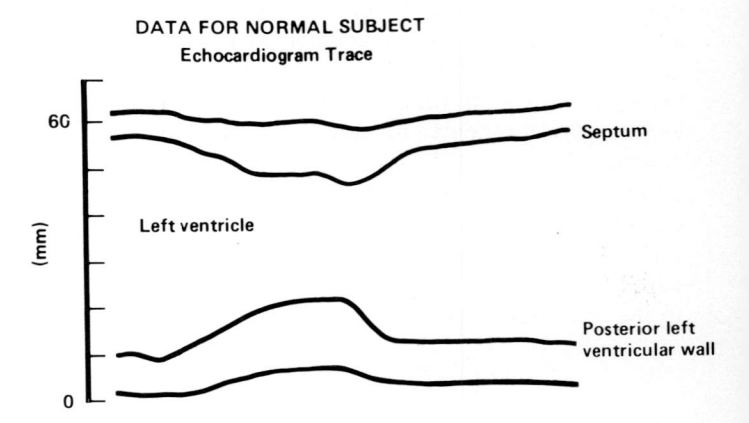

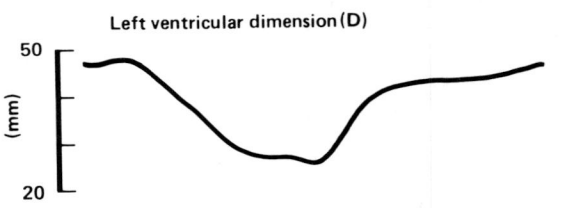

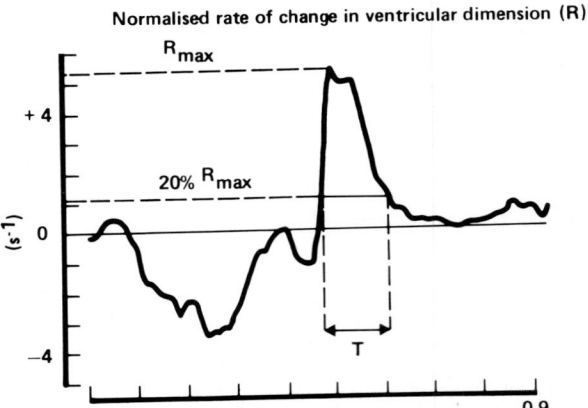

Fig. 4 Digitised trace of the inter-ventricular septum and the posterior left ventricular wall. The change in left ventricular dimension is calculated together with the normalised rate of change. R max gives the maximum normalised rate of change and 20% R max has been found to give the most accurate computing of the length of the early diastolic filling phase.

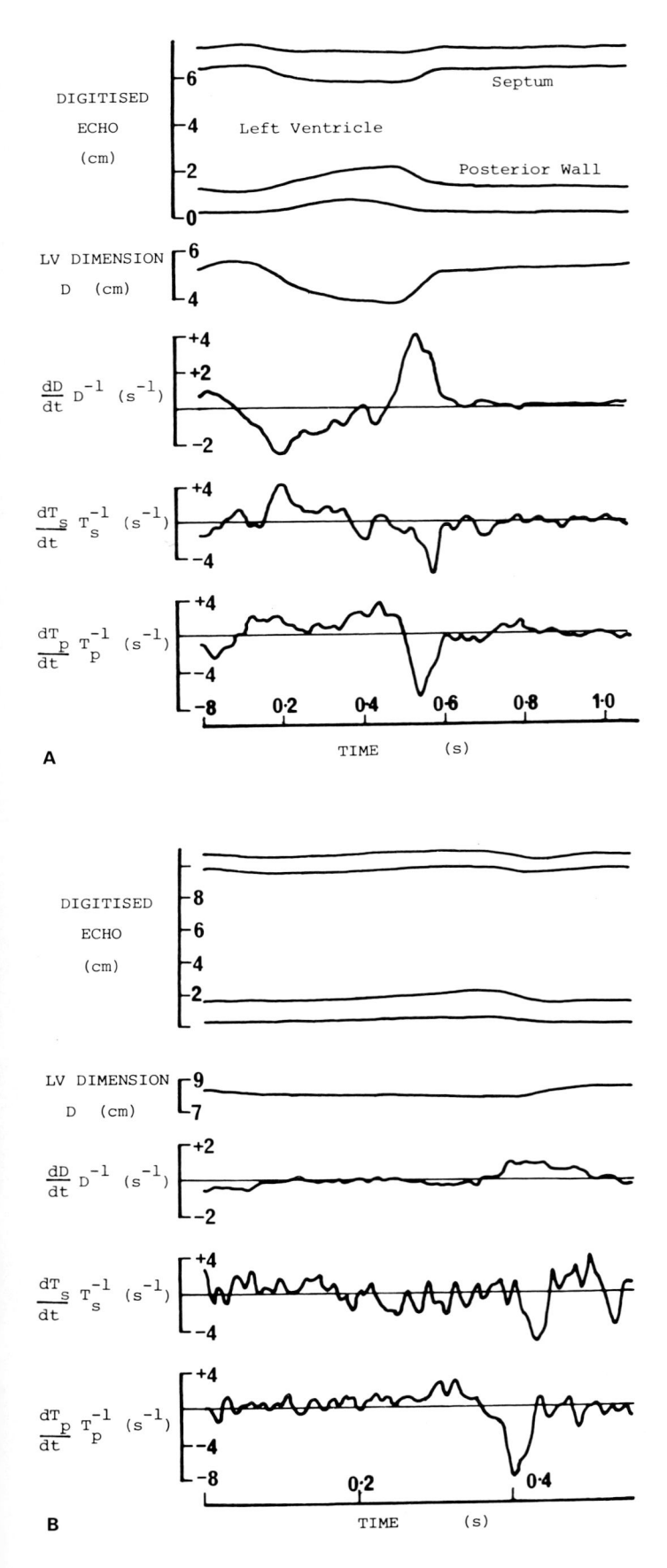

Fractional shortening (FS) is a percentage figure calculated from:

$$FS = \frac{EDD - ESD}{EDD}$$

and as LVET is omitted, FS is not dependent on the heart rate. FS is an accurate measurement only in normal ventricles with a correct septal movement and normal regional left ventricular wall contraction. If paradoxical septal movement or regional areas of dyskinesia occur, FS becomes invalid and essentially meaningless. Figure 3 demonstrates the results of FS and peak Vcf in normal subjects and in a group with ischaemic heart disease (IHD). The patients with IHD and normal ventricular contraction on angiography are within the normal range whereas those with dyskinesia have an overall reduction in FS and peak Vcf.

Digitisation of the movements of the inter-ventricular septum and the posterior left ventricular wall on the M-mode scan allows an analysis of the changes in left ventricular dimension. On a digitised plot, the normalised rate of change in ventricular dimension can be derived which indicates systolic inward wall movement and diastolic outward wall movement (Fig. 4). The differences in normalised rates of change of wall thickness and dimension in a normal ventricle and a severely dyskinetic dilated ischaemic left ventricle are demonstrated in Figure 5. The parameters described above are at their most accurate when used as serial measurements in the same patient. D'Cruz et al[7] used the distance from the inter-ventricular septum to the mitral E point in order to differentiate normal from abnormal ejection fractions. If there is a distance greater than 10 mm, the ejection fraction is probably abnormal. False positives may occur if there is an oblique or angled transducer position and inaccurate recordings may result. It is not a measurement that has found universal acceptance.

Fig. 5 A: Digitisation of a normal left ventricle. B: Digitisation of a severely ischaemic poorly functioning left ventricle.

$$\frac{dD}{dt} \; D^{-1} \, (s^{-1})$$

is the normalised rate of change in ventricular dimension.

$$\frac{dT_s}{dt} \; T_s^{-1} \, (s^{-1})$$

is the normalised rate of change in septal thickness.

$$\frac{dT_p}{dt} \; T_p^{-1} \, (s^{-1})$$

is the normalised rate of change in posterior wall thickness. Note the dilated end systolic and end diastolic dimensions, the reduced rate of change in dimension and the abnormal wall thickness rates of change in B.

LEFT VENTRICULAR WALL THICKNESS AND MASS

Before the advent of cross-sectional echocardiography, all measurements were taken 'blind' with M-mode studies. If any structure was obliquely imaged, false thicknesses and cavity dimensions were recorded. Now that M-mode recordings can be taken directly off cross-sectional images, sampling errors are reduced. The electrocardiographic criteria of left ventricular hypertrophy are poor[8] even though articles by Short and Weir[9,10] showed certain T wave changes were more reliably associated with increased left ventricular muscle mass than conventional ECG voltage criteria. Echocardiography is more accurate in determining left ventricular muscle mass than any other non-invasive technique, with the possible exception of magnetic resonance imaging. Devereux[11] used a modified formula (Penn Convention) to ascertain left ventricular mass, and his results compared favourably to anatomical studies. The formula used is:

$$LV\ mass = 1.04\ (LVID + PWT + IVST)^3 - (LVID)^3 - 13.6\ g$$

where LVID is left ventricular internal dimension, PWT posterior wall thickness, IVST inter-ventricular septal thickness. This formula produces a high correlation with anatomical studies in ventricles which are uniform in normality or hypertrophy, but results deteriorate once muscle asymmetry, infarction, aneurysm formation or right ventricular volume overload occur. Weiss et al[12] developed a technique of three-dimensional ventricular reconstruction and claimed a high degree of accuracy in measuring left ventricular mass irrespective of the shape or condition of the ventricle.

It is most valuable to correlate LV mass with body surface area as a means of determining whether hypertrophy (and hence increase in muscle mass) is present in any particular individual. Devereux[13] gives figures of left ventricular (M-mode calculated) mass index of 134 g/M^2 for men and 110 g/M^2 for women as being the upper limits of normality. Figures for children and adolescents are quoted by Daniels et al.[14] Left ventricular mass increases with age and variations in the formulae for the calculation of left ventricular mass based on M-mode echocardiographic recordings are given by Gardin et al.[15] Serial calculations of left ventricular mass by echocardiography in individual patients are more accurate in determining the development of left ventricular hypertrophy than ECG recordings or wall thickness measurement alone.

LEFT VENTRICULAR STRESS INDICES

The mechanical performance of the heart is a complex function of the contractile behaviour of individual muscle fibres and the overall geometry of the ventricles. Myocardial performance can be evaluated in terms of wall thickening and the extent and velocity of fibre shortening in relation to ventricular wall stress (Figs 6 and 7). Stress is calculated by the formula:

$$Stress = \frac{pressure \times radius}{wall\ thickness}$$

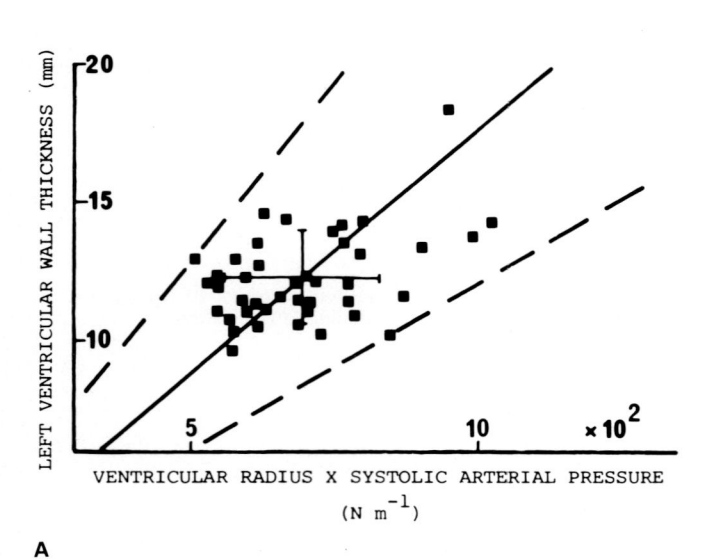

Fig. 6 Wall stress index (ventricular radius × systolic arterial pressure). **A:** Against left ventricular wall thickness in normal subjects with mean and standard deviations. **B:** Against velocity of circumferential fibre shortening in the same normal subject group.

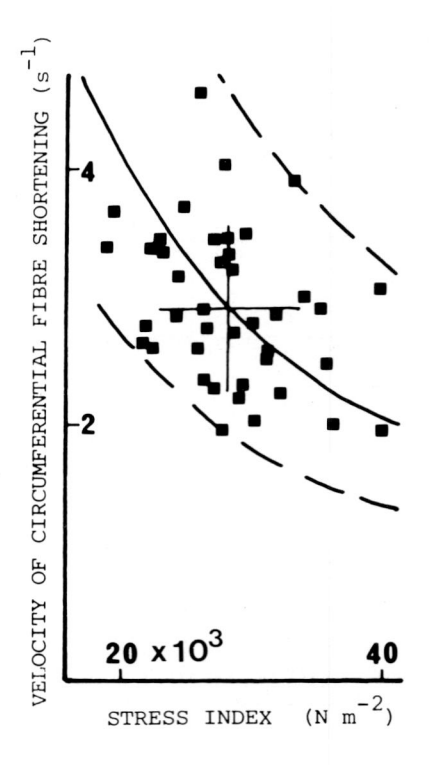

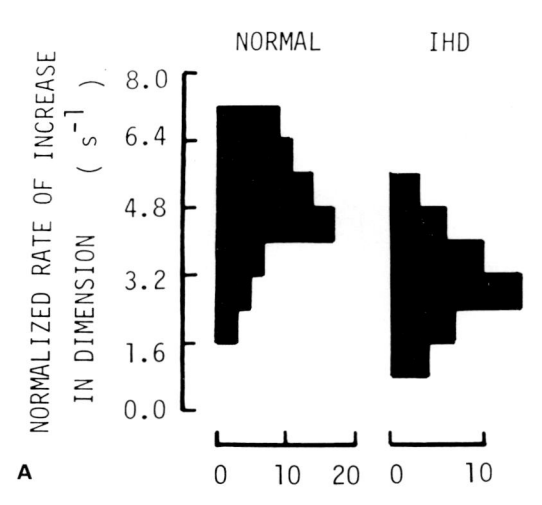

Fig. 7 A: Comparison of normalised rates of increase in dimension in a group of normal subjects and in patients with ischaemic heart disease (IHD). Blocks indicate numbers of patients. B: Comparison of wall stress in the same groups as Fig. 7A.

This stress is made up of three components. Meridional stress acts in the direction of the long axis, circumferential stress acts in a direction perpendicular to the long axis and there is a small radial stress component due to myocardial tissue pressure. The largest component is the circumferential wall stress. There are also three components of elemental power with the largest and most important component being the instantaneous circumferential elemental power which is equal to the product of circumferential wall stress and velocity of circumferential fibre shortening.

There are numerous formulae for the calculations of stress and power, most assuming that the left ventricle is an ellipsoid shape.[16–18] Once a ventricle becomes abnormal in shape for any reason, then changes have to be made to the calculations for stress and power in order to avoid misinterpretation. Correlation of left ventricular end systolic wall stress (ESS) with the mean Vcf has been measured against changes in heart rate, preload and afterload.[19] The ESS – mean Vcf relationship has been shown to be independent of any change in heart rate and afterload, but may depend on preload. The stress relationships in the normal and abnormal ventricle are shown in Figure 8. Appropriate hypertrophy occurs when an increase in mass to volume ratio parallels an increased pressure load. Inappropriate hypertrophy occurs when the left ventricular mass is out of proportion to volume and inadequate hypertrophy results from excessive dilatation of the ventricle without mass increase. A chronic pressure or volume overload in the left ventricle will give rise to an increased wall stress unless hypertrophy develops to compensate for the increased load.[20–21]

Any increase in wall stress will give rise to a reduction in the velocity of fibre shortening through the force-velocity relationship equation.[22,23] The results of M-mode echocardiography have been compared to those from cross-sectional images and differences are apparent. Meridional and circumferential stress in dilated, almost spherical, cardiomyopathic ventricles had a ratio larger than normal indicating that effective afterload would be overestimated if meridional stress alone was used in the calculation.[24] Nakano et al[25] have suggested that regional myocardial work is a more precise indicator of function than simple shortening fraction. They defined that regional work of the ventricle normalised to a unit volume of myocardium (RWM) is related to the mean wall stress and the logarithm of reciprocal of wall thickness. The functional state of different regions of the myocardium can be calculated and this is of particular use in assessing function of the left ventricle after myocardial infarction.

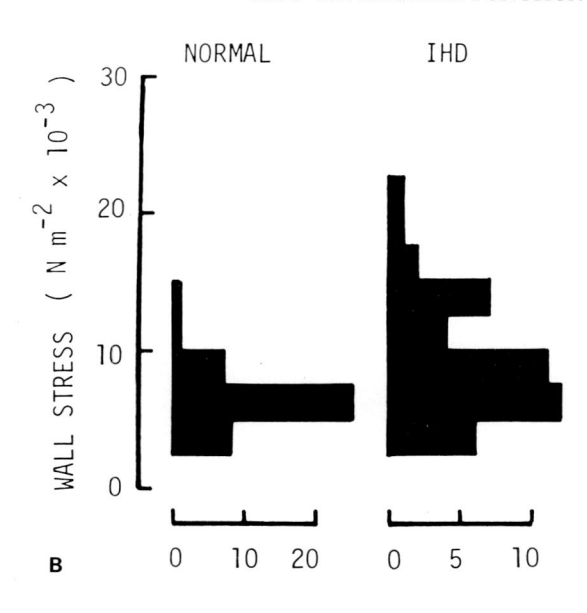

SYSTOLIC FUNCTION

At the onset of systole, the pre-ejection phase occurs when

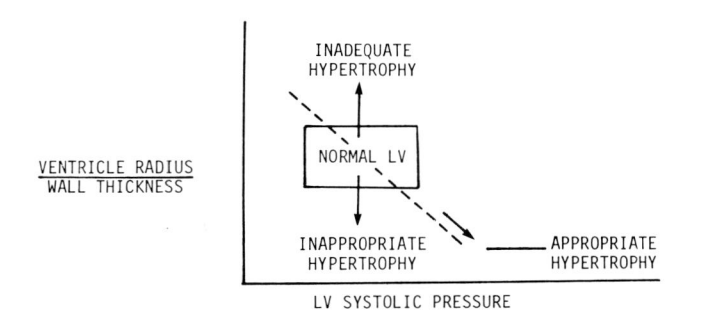

Fig. 8 Relationship of hypertrophy to pressure.

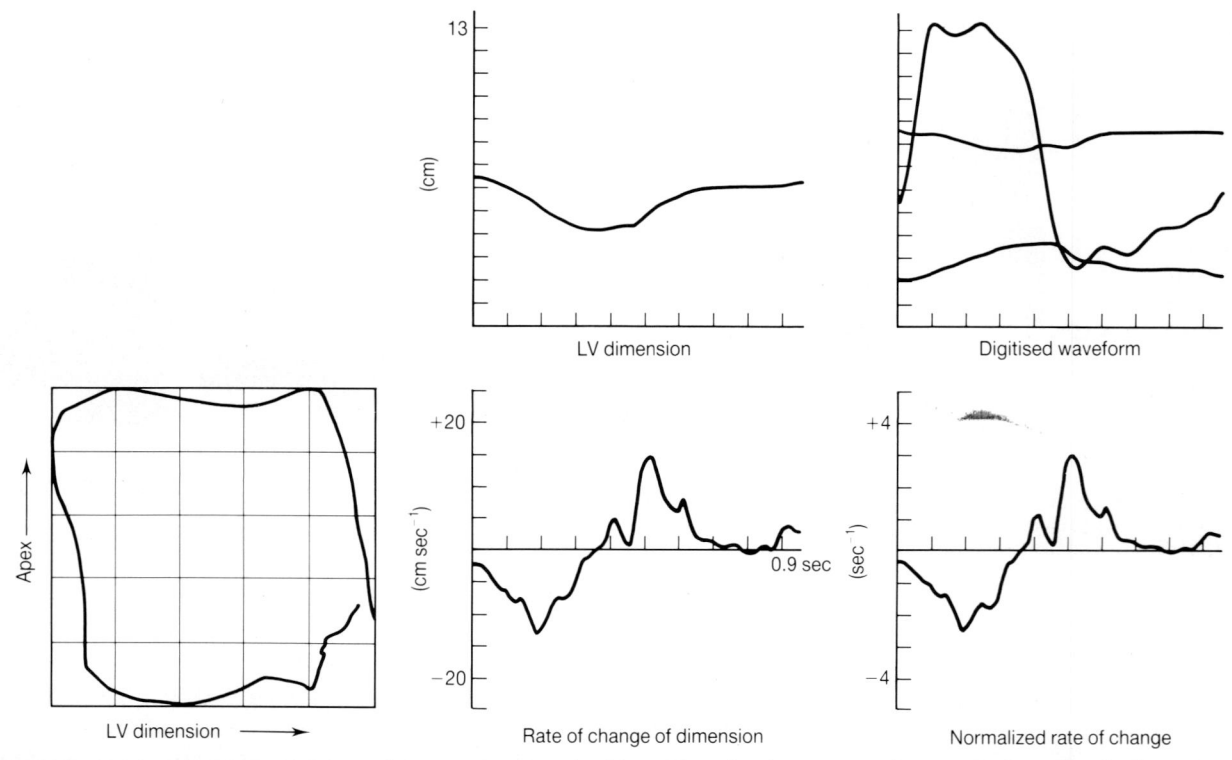

Fig. 9 Digitised apex cardiogram and echocardiogram of a normal subject. Note the almost square loop, normal systolic ejection rate and the length of the early rapid diastolic filling phase.

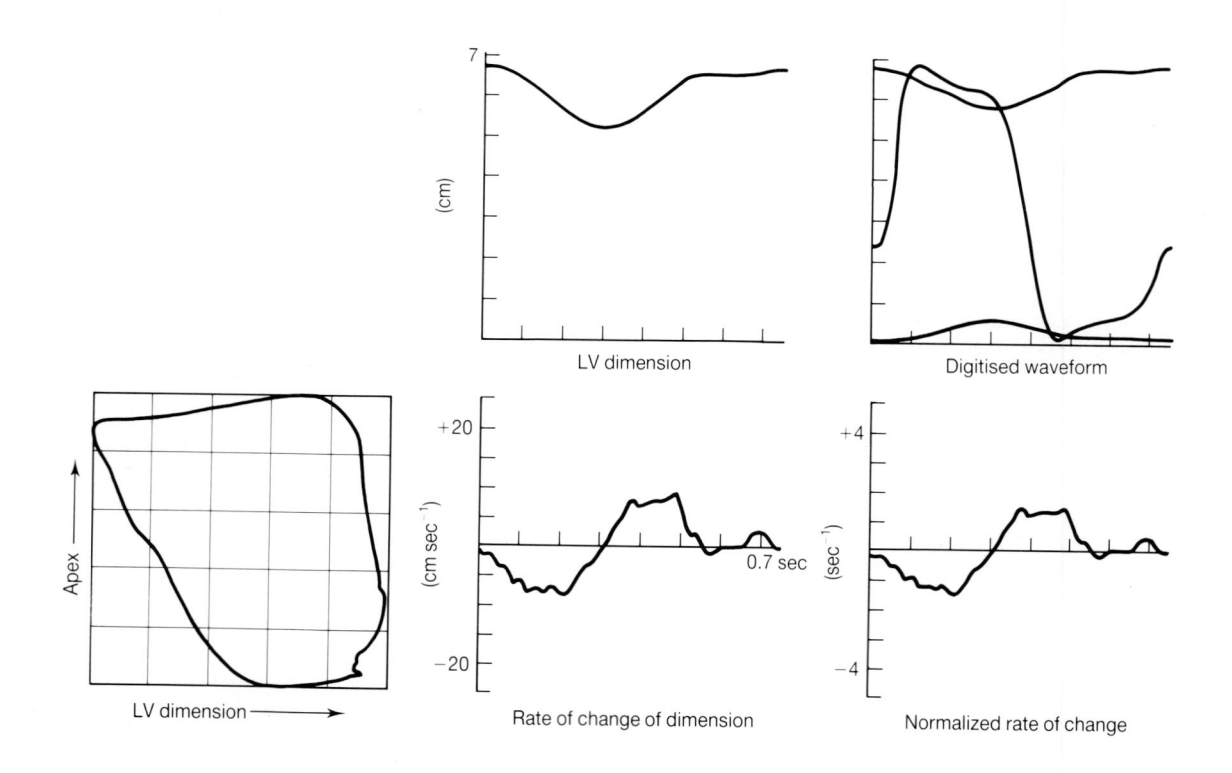

Fig. 10 Digitised apex cardiogram and echocardiogram of a patient with ischaemic heart disease and no evidence of mitral regurgitation.
Note the increased 'dimension' change occurring during isovolumic relaxation indicating abnormal response and shape change of the ultrasonically interrogated myocardium. There is also a reduced systolic rate of change of dimension, a prolonged early diastolic filling phase and a reduced rate of change in diastolic dimension increase. Systolic and diastolic functions are both impaired.

the pressure in the ventricle rises, causing the mitral valve to close and the aortic valve to open. The time from mitral valve closure to aortic valve opening is known as the isovolumic contraction phase and is prolonged in conditions such as systemic hypertension and aortic stenosis. It is a period when both aortic and mitral valves are closed and minimal shape change normally occurs to the left ventricle. Significant shape changes may be seen in some pathological states, for example in patients with mitral regurgitation and ischaemic heart disease where areas of ventricular muscle abnormality such as aneurysm formation are present. Mean and peak rates of circumferential fibre shortening can be used to determine systolic function with the peak rate of ejection occurring at the opening of the aortic valve. The rise in ventricular pressure during the isovolumic contraction phase can be monitored by a pressure transducer in the left ventricular cavity or qualitatively demonstrated by the upstroke of an apex cardiogram.[26,27] There is good correlation of timing between both the upstroke and the downstroke of the apex cardiogram and the pressure changes occurring in the left ventricle during the isovolumic phases of the cardiac cycle. By plotting ventricular dimension changes against the apex cardiogram, a loop can be produced which may be significantly altered in disease states (Figs 9 and 10).[28-30] The apex cardiogram/left ventricular dimension loop is formed from a short axis M-mode echocardiogram at the level of the chordae tendinae with simultaneous recording of the apex cardiogram. The traces are digitised and plotted allowing the various stages of the cardiac cycle to be analysed in greater detail (Fig. 11). Point 'C' of the apex cardiogram marks the beginning of the upstroke of isovolumic contraction which ends at the 'E' point. It has been shown that the 'E' point occurs approximately 40 m/s before the onset of the ejection phase. During the ejection phase, the left ventricular dimension falls to its minimum level and the 'knee' occurs at the onset of the isovolumic relaxation phase. The 'O' point is the nadir of the apex cardiogram but does not coincide with mitral valve opening. This occurs at a variable point before the 'O' point. For analytical purposes, it is better to use an 80% decrease drop in the apex cardiogram signal rather than relying on the 'O' point. The 80% level is better in differentiating normal from abnormal ventricles.

It is often assumed that wall stress and circumferential fibre shortening are relatively constant around the short axis of the left ventricle but experimental evidence suggests there may be considerable variation in normal ventricles depending on where the measurements are made. The pattern tends to be biphasic and circumferential fibre shortening may vary by a factor of two (Fig. 12).

Abnormal systolic function depends on several processes, the main ones being regional myocardial contraction abnormality, dilatation and abnormal architecture of the ventricular cavity and reduction in the peak rate of wall movement. The addition of Doppler information is of great benefit when considering global systolic left ventricular function and parameters including stroke volume and cardiac output can be assessed using this extra information. Cardiac output is the product of stroke volume and heart rate. The stroke volume can be calculated from the following formula:

$$\text{Stroke Volume} = \text{SVI} \times \text{AoCSA}$$

where SVI is the systolic velocity integral calculated from the area encompassed under the curve of the Doppler signal of aortic peak flow velocity and AoCSA is the aortic root cross-sectional area measured either on M-mode or cross-sectional imaging.[31-33] It is also possible to use the mitral valve orifice area to determine cardiac output but it is difficult to measure and has a relatively high observer error rate (see Ch. 8). Peak aortic blood flow velocity and acceleration rates are good measures of global left ventricular function and they are related to end diastolic volume, drugs, heart rate, aortic valve opening time, age and other variables affecting the myocardium.[34] The flow

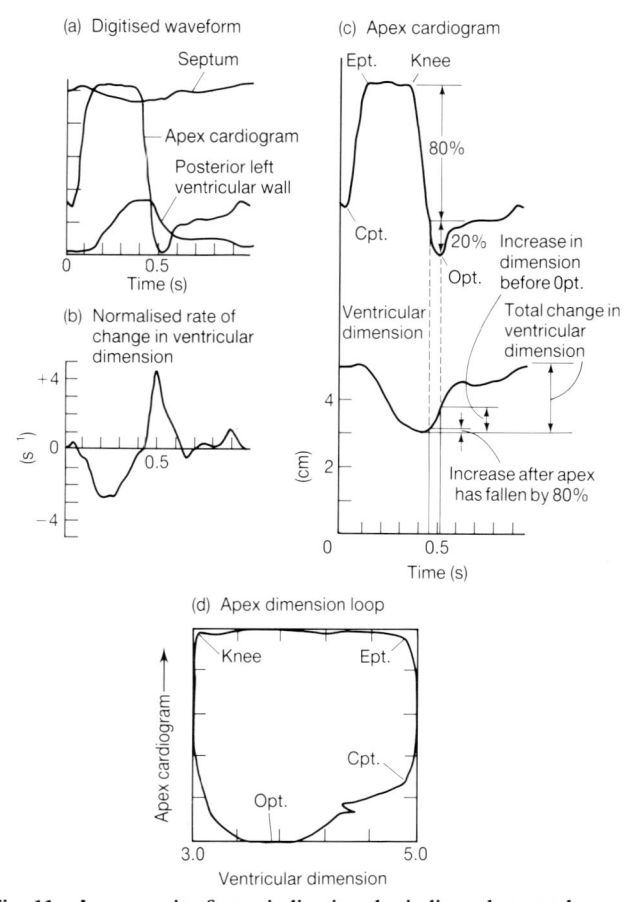

Fig. 11 A composite figure indicating the indices that can be derived from digitisation of the apex cardiogram and the echocardiogram. A: Digitised waveform. B: Ventricular dimension changes. C: Apex cardiogram. D: Apex dimension loop.

74 CARDIAC ULTRASOUND

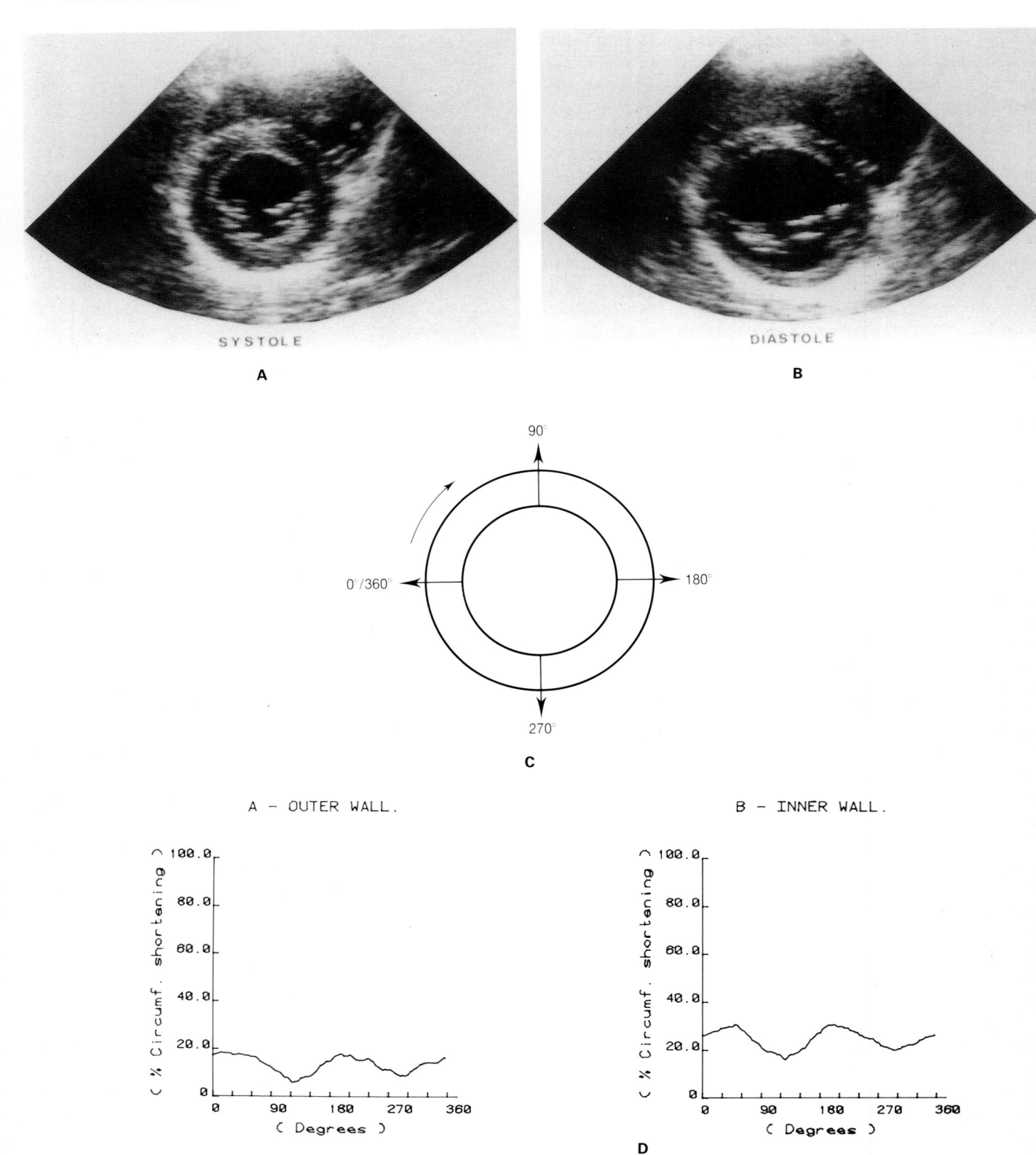

Fig. 12 **A** and **B: End systolic and diastolic short axis views of a normal left ventricle. C:** The diagrammatic representation of the walls of the left ventricle in a short axis plane, with degrees indicating the reference point for measurement of inner and outer wall movement. **D:** The circumferential fibre shortening of both the inner and outer walls of the left ventricle taken at different degree points on the circle. A biphasic pattern is seen indicating variation in circumferential fibre shortening across the ventricle. The peaks and troughs are in the same compass point positions for most normal ventricles. There is some evidence to suggest a change in the degree position if ventricular dilatation is present.

through the aortic valve during systole may fall off towards the end and can even stop prior to aortic valve closure in patients who have severe left heart disease. The left ventricular ejection time (LVET) may therefore appear longer on M-mode echocardiography at the aortic root level than on Doppler flow studies across the valve itself, a point to be taken into consideration whenever the LVET is used in calculations.

In practice, regional systolic left ventricular function is best assessed using multiple cross-sectional images of the left ventricle and analysing the movement of the myocardium in the various sections. Analyses can either be computer based or be carried out by direct visualisation.[35-37]

DIASTOLIC FUNCTION

More research has been carried out into the diastolic function of the left ventricle than the systolic function. This reflects the importance of the relationship between the behaviour of the left ventricle and its diastolic function patterns. The isovolumic relaxation phase heralds the onset of diastole. At the end of ventricular systole, the aortic valve closes and the pressure falls within the left ventricular cavity during the isovolumic phase. The mitral valve opens once the left ventricular pressure has fallen below that in the left atrium. If there is a significant volume increase during this phase then aortic regurgitation is present. The time from aortic valve closure to mitral valve opening may be extended in numerous heart conditions including that of ischaemic heart disease. The downstroke of the apex cardiogram reflects this pressure fall and when taken in conjunction with M-mode recordings can be analysed for normality. The minimum left ventricular diastolic pressure is often reached after mitral valve opening during the early rapid filling phase and this suggests, together with other evidence, that there is an active relaxation process occurring in the myocardium. The early rapid filling phase of the left ventricle occurs immediately after mitral valve opening[38] and lasts in normal subjects about 100 to 200 msec. It is relatively unchanged by heart rate and, in tachycardia induced states such as vigorous exercise, is the most important part of left ventricular filling. In mid-diastole, the volume and pressure increase simultaneously and slowly. It is this part of the cycle that is maximally altered and decreased by an increase in heart rate, to such an extent that it may completely disappear. Late diastolic filling due to atrial contraction accounts for approximately 10% of the volume entering the left ventricle during diastole. Doppler evidence of blood flow correlates closely with left ventricular volume changes and mirrors movement of the mitral valve leaflets shown on M-mode recordings.

Diastolic compliance refers to the pressure/volume relationship (dp/dV) of the ventricle, known as 'stiffness' or 'elasticity'. The compliance falls as the diastolic filling pressure rises, and the dp/dV relationship is not linear. Abnormal patterns of left ventricular diastolic filling have been found in numerous conditions such as ischaemic heart disease and hypertrophic cardiomyopathy. The abnormalities include delayed mitral opening, reduced velocity of early rapid filling, prolonged early filling, increased velocity and volume flow during atrial contraction and conversely reduced atrial filling due to high left ventricular end diastolic pressure. There is Doppler evidence[39] that peak early diastolic pressure is independent of left ventricular size. The Doppler 'E' wave of early diastolic filling and the 'A' wave of atrial contraction have been analysed in normal subjects and the E/A ratio has been shown to decline with age but has little variation with other physiological variables.[40] There is also day to day variability in certain Doppler indices, mainly affecting those concerned with events in late diastole.[41] Little variation occurs in early filling but there are substantial differences in atrial diastolic flow velocity and in the E/A ratio within individuals. There has been considerable interest over the years in the possibility of non-invasively determining absolute pressures, in particular left ventricular end diastolic pressure (LVEDP) from these flow patterns. A prominent 'B' point on the A-C slope of the atrial downstroke of the M-mode echocardiogram was initially thought to be indicative of a raised LVEDP but it is not accurate. If there is mitral valve closure at or before the 'P' wave of the electrocardiogram (ECG) then, by inference, LVEDP must be significantly raised. Severe acute aortic regurgitation is the only significant cause of mitral valve closure before the 'P' wave of the ECG. Minor closure abnormalities are of less predictable value in assessing end diastolic pressure changes. Doppler evidence has suggested that LVEDP can be measured with some accuracy but Ettles et al[42] found no correlation between Doppler trans-mitral flow velocity and pressure measurements at catheterisation. Small changes in LVEDP may have significant clinical effects on the patient and there is still no reproducible non-invasive method of accurately estimating LVEDP.

EFFECTS OF AGE

The percentage of early diastolic filling decreases with age and there is a reciprocal increase in isovolumic relaxation time.[43] Stroke volume and peak left ventricular ejection velocity are unaltered. This suggests that there is a tendency towards later diastolic filling with increasing age. This may play an important and significant role in the development of left ventricular failure when an elderly person suffers atrial fibrillation and associated tachycardia. Spirito and Maron[44] showed an increasing atrial flow velocity with age together with changes in five out of six of the Doppler echocardiographic diastolic function indices.

RIGHT VENTRICULAR/LEFT VENTRICULAR RELATIONSHIP

There is an inter-dependence between the right and left ventricles in diastole. In inspiration, there are changes in the left ventricular filling pattern involving a decrease in peak early diastolic filling velocity and a decrease in the E/A ratio.[45] Atrial emptying is unaltered. in the right ventricle, both the E and A waves of early filling and late atrial filling are enhanced due to the increased venous return. The changes in the left side on inspiration are more complicated, the changes only occurring in some of the Doppler indices.

EXERCISE AND LEFT VENTRICULAR FUNCTION

The function of the heart in subjects undergoing physical training to a high level of fitness has been studied by a number of authors.[46-51] Endurance trained international-class marathon runners[49] increase their left ventricular end diastolic dimension on exercise together with increasing their meridional wall stress. Comparing endurance trained athletes with body builders,[50] Urhausen and Kindermann found that there were significant differences in the left ventricular mass/volume ratio. The body building programme leads to increased body dimensions and a proportionate increase in left ventricular thickness, while endurance athletes increase their end diastolic volume without significant change in their left ventricular mass. It is also suggested[47] that endurance athletes increase their work by reducing their end systolic volume as opposed to untrained subjects who achieve the same work rate by increasing their end diastolic volume alone. Fisher et al[51] compared four groups of athletes with controls and again confirmed that increase in left ventricular wall thickness in strength athletes occurs without an increase in cavity dimension and that left ventricular mass was related to the increase in lean body weight. Endurance athletes, however, increased their end diastolic dimensions.

The response of the ventricle therefore depends on the type of training undertaken. Strength training with a large increase in body muscle mass may lead to marked left ventricular hypertrophy on echocardiography, an important factor when assessing the normality or otherwise of an individual's ventricle. Similarly, a 'dilated' ventricle in an endurance athlete may also be 'normal'.

SUMMARY

A wide range of data concerning all aspects of systolic and diastolic function is available using combinations of M-mode, cross-sectional and Doppler echocardiograms. Each laboratory must develop its own protocols and calculate normal parameters in order to be able to compare and contrast different groups of patients as well as monitor serial investigations in the same patient. Each operator must also know his or her error variability and have a high degree of reproducibility for the examination.

What function tests should be performed? This largely depends on equipment available together with the expertise of the operator, the amount of time available for the investigation and the clinical requirements. The more information acquired, providing it is accurate, the better will be the understanding of a particular ventricle's function and this will lead to better patient care. It is essential, however, to avoid making important clinical judgements based on apparently precise quantitative measurements which are not of satisfactory quality or accuracy.

REFERENCES

1 Teichholz L E, Kreulen T, Herman M V, Gorlin R. Problems in echocardiographic volume determinations: echocardiographic–angiographic correlations in the presence or absence of asynergy. Am J Cardiol 1976; 37: 7
2 Bennett D H, Rowlands D J. Test of reliability of echocardiographic estimation of left ventricular dimensions and volumes. Br Heart J 1976; 38: 1133
3 Linhart J W, Mintz G S, Segal B L, Kawai N, Kotler M N. Left ventricular volume measurement by echocardiography: fact or fiction? Am J Cardiol 1975; 36: 114
4 Gibson D G, Brown D J. Continuous assessment of left ventricular shape in man. Br Heart J 1975; 37: 904
5 Fortum N J, Hood W P, Sherman M E, Craige E. Determination of left ventricular volumes by ultrasound. Circulation 1971; 44: 575
6 Mercier J C, Disessa T G, Jarmakani J M, et al. Two dimensional echocardiographic assessment of left ventricular volumes and ejection fraction in children. Circulation 1982; 65: 962–969
7 D'Cruz I A, Laimalani G G, Sambasivan V, Cohen H C, Glick G. The superiority of mitral E point-ventricular septum separation to other echocardiographic indicators of left ventricular performance. Clin Cardiol 1979; 2: 140
8 Sokolow M, Lyon T P. The ventricular complex in left ventricular hypertrophy as obtained by unipolar precordial and limb leads. Am Heart J 1949; 37: 161–186
9 Short D, Weir J. Significance of asymmetrically inverted T wave. Br Heart J 1983; 49: 564–567
10 Short D, Weir J. Positive T wave overshoot as a sign of ventricular enlargement. Br Heart J 1984; 51: 288–291
11 Devereux R B, Reichek N. Echocardiographic determination of left ventricular mass in man. Anatomic validation of the method. Circulation 1977; 55: 613–620
12 Weiss J L, McGaughey M, Guier W H. Geometric considerations in determination of left ventricular mass by two-dimensional echocardiography. Hypertension 1987; 8: 1185–1189
13 Devereux R B, Casale P N, Kligfield P, et al. Performance of primary and derived M-mode echocardiographic measurements for detection of left ventricular hypertrophy in necropsied subjects and in patients with systemic hypertension, mitral regurgitation and dilated cardiomyopathy. Am J Cardiol 1986; 57: 1388–1393
14 Daniels S R, Meyer R A, Liang Y C, Bove K E. Echocardiographically determined left ventricular mass index in normal children, adolescents and young adults. J Am Coll Cordial 1988; 12: 703–708
15 Gardin J M, Savage D D, Ware J H, Henry W L. Effects of age,

sex, and body surface area on echocardiographic left ventricular wall mass in normal subjects. Hypertension 1987; 9: 1136–1139
16 Sandler H, Dodge H T. Left ventricular tension and stress in man. Circ Res 1963; 13: 91–104
17 Falsetti H L, Mates R E, Grant C, Green D G, Bunnell I L. Left ventricular wall stress calculated from one plane cineangiography – an approach to force-velocity in man. Circ Res 1970; 16: 71–83
18 McHale P A, Greenfield J C Jnr. Evaluation of several geometric models for estimation of left ventricular circumferential wall stress. Circ Res 1973; 33: 303–312
19 Watanabe K, Kishida K, Haneda N, Horino N, Nishio T, Mori C. Effect of heart rate on the end systolic wall stress – mean ventricular contraction in man. Am J Cardiol 1976; 38: 322–331 18: 451–456
20 Grossman W, Jones D, McLaurin L P. Wall stress and patterns of hypertrophy in the human left ventricle. J Clin Inv 1975; 56: 56–64
21 Gaasch W H. Left ventricular radius to wall thickness ratio. Am J Cardiol 1980; 43: 1189–1194
22 Gould K L, Kennedy J W, Frimer M, Pollack G H, Dodge H T. Analysis of wall dynamics and directional components of left ventricular contraction in man. Am J Cardiol 1976; 38: 322–331
23 Quinones M A, Gaasch W H, Cole J S, Alexander J K. Echocardiographic determination of left ventricular stress-velocity relations in man with reference to the effects of loading and contractility. Circulation 1975; 51: 689–700
24 Douglas P S, Reichek N, Plappert T, Muhammad A, St. John-Sutton M G. Comparison of echocardiographic methods for assessment of left ventricular shortening and wall stress. J Am Coll Cardiol 1987; 9: 945–951
25 Nakano K, Sugawara M, Kato T, et al. Regional work of the human left ventricle calculated by wall stress and the natural logarithm of reciprocal of wall thickness. J Am Coll Cardiol 1988; 12: 1442–1448
26 Gibson D G, Brown D J. Assessment of left ventricular systolic function in man from simultaneous echocardiographic and pressure measurements. Br Heart J 1976; 38: 8–17
27 Venco A, Gibson D G, Brown D J. Relationship between apex cardiogram and change in left ventricular pressure and dimension. Br Heart J 1977; 39: 117–125
28 Martin C J, Weir J, Gemmell H G. Assessment of left ventricular function by synchronous echocardiography and apex cardiography. Br J Radiol 1982; 55: 342–351
29 Martin C J, Weir J, Ng K H. Use of computer analysis of echocardiograms for assessment of left ventricular function. Clin Phys Physiol Meas 1983; 4: 381–394
30 Doran J K, Traill T A, Brown D J, Gibson D G. Detection of abnormal left ventricular wall movement during isovolumic contraction and early relaxation. Br Heart J 1978; 40: 367–371
31 Magnin P A, Steward J A, Myers S, VonRamm O, Kisslo J A. Combined Doppler and phased-array echocardiographic estimation of cardiac output. Circulation 1981; 63: 388
32 Steingart R M, Meller J, Barovick J, Patterson R, Herman M V, Teichholz L E. Pulsed Doppler echocardiographic measurement of beat-to-beat changes in stroke volume in dogs. Circulation 1980; 62: 542
33 Gardin J M, Dabestani A, Matin K, Allfie A, Russell D, Henry W L. Reproducibility of Doppler aortic blood flow measurements: studies on intraobserver, interobserver and day-to-day variability in normal subjects. Am J Cardiol 1984; 54: 1092

34 Merino A, Alegria E, Castello R, Martinez-Caro D. Influence of age on left ventricular contractility. Am J Cardiol 1988; 62: 1103–1108
35 Haendchen R V, Wyatt H L, Maurer G, et al. Quantitation of regional cardiac function by two-dimensional echocardiography. I. Patterns of contraction in the normal left ventricle. Circulation 1983; 67: 1234
36 Guyer D E, Foale R A, Gillam L D, Wilkins G T, Guerrero J L, Weyman A E. An echocardiographic technique for quantifying and displaying the extent of regional left ventricular dyssynergy. J Am Coll Cardiol 1986; 8: 830
37 Edwards W D, Tajik A J, Seward J B. Standardized nomenclature and anatomic basis for regional tomographic analysis of the heart. Mayo Clin Proc 1981; 56: 479
38 Prewitt T, Gibson D G, Brown D J, Sutton G. The 'rapid filling wave' of the apex cardiogram. Its relationships to echocardiographic and cine angiographic measurements of ventricular filling. Br Heart J 1973; 37: 1256–1262
39 Takenaka K, Dabestani A, Waffarn F, Gardin J M, Henry W L. Effect of left ventricular size on early diastolic left ventricular filling in neonates and in adults. Am J Cardiol 1987; 59: 138–141
40 Van-Dam I, Fast J, de Boo T, et al. Normal diastolic filling patterns of the left ventricle. Eur Heart J 1980; 9: 165–171
41 Spirito P, Maron B J, Verter I, Marrill J S. Reproducibility of Doppler echocardiographic measurements of left ventricular diastolic function. Eur Heart J 1988; 9: 879–886
42 Ettles D F, Davies J, Williams G J. Can left ventricular end diastolic pressure be estimated non-invasively? Int J Cardiol 1988; 20: 239–245
43 Myreng Y, Nitter-Hauge S. Age-dependency on left ventricular filling dynamics and relaxation as assessed by pulsed Doppler echocardiography. Clin Physiol 1989; 9: 99–106
44 Spirito P, Maron B J. Influence of aging on Doppler echocardiographic indices of left ventricular diastolic function. Br Heart J 1988; 59: 672–679
45 Riggs T W, Snider A R. Respirating influence on right and left ventricular diastolic function in normal children. Am J Cardiol 1989; 63: 858–861
46 Adams T D, Yanowitz F G, Fisher A G, Ridges J D, Lovell K, Pryor T A. Non invasive evaluation of exercise training in college-age men. Circulation 1981; 64: 958
47 Bar-Shlomo B Z, Druck M N, Morch J E, et al. Left ventricular function in trained and untrained healthy subjects. Circulation 1982; 65: 484
48 Giunta A, Maione S, Biagina R, del-Rosso-P, Sifola C, Tuccillo B. Echo Doppler evaluation of diastolic filling in differently induced left ventricular hypertrophy. Cor Vasa 1989; 31: 195–202
49 Fagard R, Van-der-Broeke C, Amery A. Left ventricular dynamics during exercise in elite marathon runners. J Am Coll Cardiol 1989; 14: 112–118
50 Urhausen A, Kindermann W. One and two dimensional echocardiography in body builders and endurance trained subjects. Int J Sports Med 1989; 10: 139–144
51 Fisher A G, Adams T D, Yanowitz F B, Ridges J D, Orsmond G, Nelson A G. Non invasive evaluation of world class athletes engaged in different modes of training. Am J Cardiol 1989; 63: 337–341

Doppler quantitation – pressure drop estimation

Introduction
Pressure gradients
Theory of gradient estimation by Doppler ultrasound
Extended Bernoulli equation
Discrete obstructions
Confined jets
Free jets
Modified Bernoulli equation
Application of Doppler ultrasound techniques
Practical aspects of quantitation

Quantitative Doppler techniques in the clinical setting
Aortic stenosis
Mitral stenosis
Tricuspid and pulmonary stenosis
Non-discrete, tunnel and multiple obstructions
Problems and pitfalls of pressure gradient estimation
Quantitative colour Doppler flow mapping
Basic principles of colour quantitation
Clinical applications of colour flow quantitation
Conclusions

Iain A. Simpson

INTRODUCTION

There are many areas of cardiology where Doppler ultrasound has been able to provide valuable *qualitative* information by detecting the presence of abnormal flow patterns and localising their site. However, Doppler techniques can also be *quantitative* and in certain situations they can provide new clinical information. Serial investigations can be performed, if necessary, which obviate the need for more invasive investigations. The publications of Holen[1] and Hatle[2] have been instrumental in the birth of quantitative cardiac Doppler techniques and have led to the established and widespread use of the basic principles initially described for the noninvasive quantitation of mitral stenosis using continuous wave Doppler ultrasound.

Estimation of pressure gradients by spectral Doppler ultrasound is now well established in mitral and aortic stenosis and this forms an important clinical diagnostic tool in adult cardiology. In infants and children Doppler ultrasound can accurately estimate left and right ventricular outflow tract gradients. Quantitative information from colour Doppler flow mapping is less well established but considerable research is currently being directed at quantitating the vast amount of flow information available from this exciting technology and it is likely that this will enhance the quantitative capabilities of cardiac Doppler ultrasound.

PRESSURE GRADIENTS

The term 'gradient' is widely used to mean 'pressure drop' although the latter term is, strictly speaking, more precise. In practice the two terms are used interchangeably.

The measurement of pressure gradients at cardiac catheterisation is well established as one of the most important techniques for quantitating the severity of valve lesions in clinical cardiological practice and it is widely accepted that this information is essential for making judgements about patient management. The use of Doppler ultrasound in estimating pressure gradients across stenosed cardiac valves has been the single most important factor in establishing the role of quantitative Doppler ultrasound in clinical cardiology. It is essential in the application of quantitative Doppler techniques that both the operator and the recipient of the report have a clear understanding of the principles of gradient estimation. Both parties must also have a grasp of the problems and pitfalls associated with Doppler ultrasound examination, particularly with respect to potential underestimation or overestimation of pressure gradients and the relationship of gradients estimated by Doppler ultrasound to those obtained by more conventional invasive means.

Theory of gradient estimation by Doppler ultrasound

Doppler ultrasound cannot be used to measure pressure or pressure gradients directly but it can be used to measure blood flow velocity very accurately and from this measurement pressure gradient can be derived since velocity and pressure drop are closely interrelated.

To understand the relationship between pressure drop and velocity it is necessary to be aware of two important concepts.

1. As fluid passes through an obstruction it accelerates to a higher velocity so that the flow velocity is greater within an obstruction than proximal to it. If, for example, one compresses the end of a garden hose, the water will come out of the end at a higher velocity. If we imagine a tube with a fluid flowing through it at a constant flow rate (Fig. 1A), then the volume of fluid leaving the end of the tube will be identical to the volume of fluid entering the tube. Since the flow rate will be the same at both ends of the tube, and fluid such as blood is incompressible, then the flow rate must be the same at any cross section along the length of the tube. Flow rate in ml/s or cm^3/s is the product of the tube cross sectional area (cm^2) and the velocity of flow at that point within the tube (cm/s). If part of the tube is narrowed (Fig. 1B) then the velocity of flow at the narrowing must increase in proportion to the cross sectional area decrease, in order to maintain the same flow rate. Therefore the product of area and velocity within the tube will be constant at any point, providing the flow is within a closed system. This is known as the *continuity principle*.

Flow rate = 10ml/s   Flow rate = 10ml/s

A

Flow rate = 10ml/s   Flow rate = 10ml/s

1   2

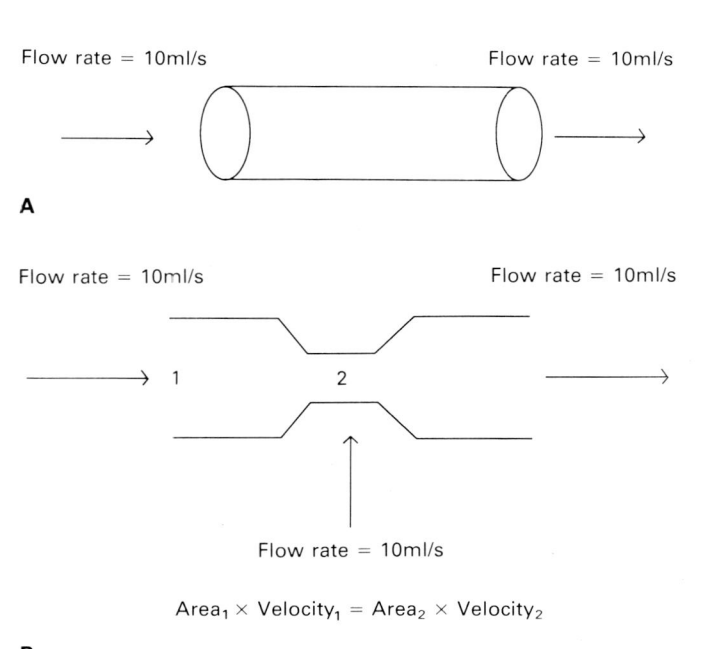

Flow rate = 10ml/s

$Area_1 \times Velocity_1 = Area_2 \times Velocity_2$

B

Fig. 1 A: Diagram of tube flow at constant velocity. The rate of flow entering the tube is identical to that leaving the tube. **B:** Diagram of tube flow at constant flow rate with a narrowed segment in the body of the tube. Since flow rate entering and leaving the tube are identical then flow rate must be the same within the narrowed segment. Flow rate is a function of area multiplied by velocity and hence as the tube area lessens the velocity must increase proportionally.

2. The relationship between pressure drop and velocity was recognised by Bernoulli[3] and is given by the Bernoulli equation:

$$p_1 - p_2 = \tfrac{1}{2} \rho (v_2^2 - v_1^2)$$

where p_1 is the pressure proximal to an obstruction, p_2 is the pressure within the obstruction and v_1 and v_2 are the velocities of blood flow at points 1 and 2, ρ is the mass density of blood. The left hand side of the equation represents the change in pressure or potential energy of the fluid from position 1 to position 2 and the right hand side of the equation represents the associated change in kinetic energy of the fluid.

Aortic valve stenosis can be used as an example of a simple and common obstruction within the cardiovascular system. The high pressure generated within the left ventricle during systole is a source of potential energy. This energy is used to accelerate blood to a high velocity through the narrowed aortic valve. This increased velocity allows cardiac output through the narrowed orifice to be maintained, representing a change from potential energy to kinetic energy as a result of the convective acceleration of blood through the aortic valve. As kinetic energy is increased through an increase in velocity, then potential energy must be lost and so pressure will fall. A difference in pressure, or pressure drop, will then exist between the left ventricle and the region within or immediately distal to the obstructive aortic valve. The larger the pressure drop across the aortic valve, then the greater will be the transfer of potential energy to kinetic energy and hence the higher the velocity that will be achieved at the site of maximal obstruction within the aortic valve. As the pressure falls the velocity increases and consequently the increase in velocity generated by the obstruction can be used to estimate the pressure drop across the obstruction.

This is the basis for estimation of pressure gradients by measurement of blood flow velocity using Doppler ultrasound.

Extended Bernoulli equation

In using the relationship of velocity and pressure drop to make quantitative determinations from Doppler derived velocity information it is important to understand the potential for other energy losses to dissipate some of the available potential energy which would otherwise be converted to velocity. Most of these are displayed in the extended Bernoulli equation:

$$p_1 - p_2 = \underbrace{\tfrac{1}{2} \rho (v_2^2 - v_1^2)}_{\text{convective acceleration}} + \underbrace{R(\vec{v})}_{\text{viscous friction}} + \underbrace{\rho \int_1^2 \frac{d\vec{v}}{dt} d\vec{s}}_{\text{flow acceleration}}$$

where p_1 is the proximal pressure, p_2 is the pressure within the obstruction, v_1 is the proximal velocity, v_2 is the velocity within the obstruction, ρ is the mass density of the fluid, $\frac{d\vec{v}}{dt} d\vec{s}$ is the energy loss due to flow acceleration and $R(\vec{v})$ is the energy loss due to viscous friction.

The first part of this equation deals with the convective acceleration of blood from a particular velocity at one point within the heart to a higher velocity at the site of obstruction. This is the conversion of potential energy to kinetic energy as described above. The second part of the equation deals with energy losses due to viscous friction. These relate to shear forces that exist at the boundary layer between blood flow and the vessel wall. If we use Doppler ultrasound to measure blood flow velocity in the centre of a vessel or chamber (i.e. away from the boundary layer) it may be reasonable to assume that dissipation of this energy will be small and negligible in comparison to the conversion of potential to kinetic energy. It may be possible to ignore this energy loss in clinical practice, but, it should still be remembered that changes in blood viscosity may have a significant effect on the quantitative estimation of obstructive lesions. The third and final part of the extended Bernoulli equation relates to energy used to accelerate blood from a low velocity at the onset of systolic contraction to a high velocity during peak systole. This form of acceleration is quite different from the convective acceleration described above in that it is a change in velocity over time, the so-called temporal or local acceleration, rather than convective acceleration which is a change in velocity as a function of distance. If we imagine any single point within the heart, this will experience local or temporal acceleration as the velocity of blood at this point alters throughout the cardiac cycle. Local or temporal acceleration is therefore a function of pulsatile flow.

In contrast, in the constant flow example described above, the velocity at any single point in the tube will not alter with time, even in the presence of an obstruction. Velocity may be quite different at different points within the tube if there is an obstruction present (see continuity principle above) so there is convective acceleration present but no temporal acceleration. This situation applies in the heart, where at any moment within the cardiac cycle there may be a difference between the velocity in the body of the left ventricle and that within the flow stream at the site of a stenotic aortic valve.

The energy loss due to temporal rather than convective acceleration is most important at the beginning and towards the end of systole. The maximum velocity through an obstruction such as aortic stenosis occurs at peak systole at a time when temporal acceleration is minimal and again it may be reasonable to regard these forces as negligible in comparison to the convective forces and allow us to ignore them for clinical purposes. Thus the first part of the Bernoulli equation is of most clinical importance in the determination of pressure drop from velocity in an obstruction.

Discrete obstructions

The principles described above are generally valid for discrete and single obstructive lesions. Discrete obstructions are common in the heart, both in obstructive lesions such as valvular stenoses and also in regurgitant valvular lesions which in hydrodynamic terms function as very severe obstructions. The general principles governing the pressure/velocity relationships described above are most easily extrapolated to these lesions. Difficulties can arise when these simple principles are applied to a more complex flow situation such as a non-discrete or tunnel-like obstruction or to serial obstructions that may occur in the ventricular outflow tracts.

Discrete obstructions have several distinct flow regions where Doppler techniques can be applied and from where quantitative information can be derived. An obstructive or regurgitant lesion within the heart will produce a jet of high velocity blood flow whose hydrodynamic characteristics will be determined by its surrounding environment. In hydrodynamic terms jets are either confined by their surroundings or they are free jets.[4] Spectral Doppler ultrasound can provide quantitative information about jet velocity and colour Doppler flow mapping can characterise the spatial velocity characteristics of jets.

Confined jets

Aortic and pulmonary valve stenosis are examples of discrete obstructions where confined or bounded jets are found. There are at least three important flow regions related to these obstructions (Fig. 2). Proximal to the obstruction the flow begins to accelerate as it approaches the obstruction. This is because the functional flow area becomes progressively smaller as it approaches the orifice. In order to maintain flow rate, the smaller flow area must contain flow of a high velocity and so flow must accelerate towards the orifice. This increase in kinetic energy is at the expense of potential energy (or pressure) and as flow accelerates then the measured pressure decreases, i.e. a pressure gradient or pressure drop develops. This flow proximal to a discrete orifice is not very susceptible to the development of turbulence and thus Doppler ultrasound techniques are likely to provide accurate velocity information in this region.

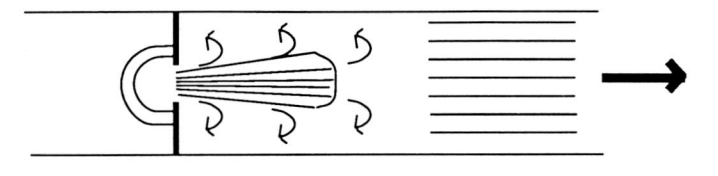

Flow reaches its maximum velocity within the obstruction itself or, more correctly, at its narrowest flow point, the so-called vena contracta of the orifice. At this point the transfer of potential energy to kinetic energy is at its greatest and therefore this is the point where the maximum pressure drop occurs. The position of the vena contracta may not necessarily be at the orifice itself, particularly for a discrete obstruction where the flow continues to contract for a small distance past the narrowest anatomical orifice. The vena contracta is therefore defined as the position of the narrowest flow diameter rather than the narrowest anatomical diameter and for discrete obstructions the area of the vena contracta is usually slightly less than the area of the orifice (see Fig. 2). The extent to which the flow area contracts beyond that of the orifice is dependent to a large extent on the characteristics of the orifice and the viscosity of blood and is defined as the coefficient of orifice contraction, which is the ratio of the flow area of the vena contracta divided by the flow area of the orifice. The ratio can range from 0.6 to 1.0, depending on the nature of the orifice.[5] It is important to realise that the peak velocity measured by Doppler techniques will reflect the functional flow area at the vena contracta rather than the anatomical orifice area and the variable position of the vena contracta has important implications for the comparison of quantitative information derived by Doppler techniques with similar information obtained by other means such as cardiac catheterisation.

Downstream of the vena contracta the jet begins to expand and vortices are formed at the edges of the jet (see Fig. 2). As the jet expands it slows down by entraining surrounding fluid. This flow region tends to be highly turbulent because of the deceleration and the viscous forces encountered. The flow relaminarises and reattaches to the boundaries of the confining chamber at a variable distance downstream which is dependent on multiple factors. As the jet flow slows down distal to the vena contracta, the pressure is recovered. In other words, kinetic energy is converted back to potential energy as the reverse of the process proximal to the obstruction. This is a very important concept because it means that the pressure measured downstream from the vena contracta of the orifice may well be higher than the pressure measured at the vena contracta. This 'pressure recovery' is never complete because of the significant energy losses associated with viscous friction and flow turbulence distal to the obstruction. It is important to recognise that as a result of pressure recovery the pressure measured at one point distal to the orifice may well be different from that measured at another position. This can influence the comparison of pressure gradients across a stenotic valve since Doppler ultrasound will reflect the velocity at the vena contracta and may estimate a

Fig. 2 Diagram of a confined jet through a narrowed orifice. Proximal to the orifice there is a zone of flow acceleration to the position of narrowest flow diameter (vena contracta). The downstream jet expands and becomes turbulent. Flow then relaminarises and reattaches to the walls of the confined receiving chamber.

pressure gradient higher than that obtained by cardiac catheterisation where the distal pressure may be measured further downstream.

Free jets

Free jets occur through orifices where the intrusion of the jet into the receiving chamber is unaffected by the boundaries of the receiving chamber. It is therefore the conditions downstream of the orifice that separate confined jets from free jets. This situation arises when the diameter of the receiving chamber is considerably larger than the diameter of the jet. Examples of free jets occurring within the heart would be mitral and tricuspid regurgitation where the regurgitant orifice is invariably small in comparison to the diameter of the left or right atrium.

As with the confined jets described above, free jets have a zone of flow convergence proximal to the orifice as flow accelerates towards the vena contracta of the orifice. It is in the flow region distal to the orifice that free jets differ (Fig. 3A). Since free jets are by definition unaffected by the boundaries of the receiving chamber, there is no zone of reattachment as occurs with confined jets. These jets conform to the principle of momentum conservation. In essence this means that throughout the intrusion of the jet into the receiving chamber the product of mass and velocity (momentum) remains constant. As the jet intrudes into the receiving chamber it increases its mass by entraining flow from the receiving chamber. Mass increases as the jet intrudes further into the receiving chamber and velocity decreases. Thus, the composition of a free jet is not entirely the result of flow traversing the orifice. Jets of mitral and tricuspid regurgitation will be composed not only of regurgitant flow but also of entrained flow from the atrium. This has important implications when we try to make quantitative measurements of regurgitant flow from jets imaged by colour Doppler flow mapping as it will not be possible to separate true regurgitant flow from entrained flow. The hydrodynamic characteristics of free jets, whether they are laminar or turbulent jets, is determined by the relationship of inertial and viscous forces given by the empirical Reynolds number.[6] Laminar flow is characterised by Reynolds numbers below 2000 and turbulent flow by Reynolds numbers greater than 3000 with the intermediate range encompassing transitional flow. Mitral regurgitant jets, for example, often have Reynolds numbers in the region of 10 000 and clearly fall well into the turbulent range. Turbulent free jets characteristically have a laminar central core with a zone of surrounding turbulence (Fig. 3B).

In the clinical situation it is rare to find such idealised jet flows and the effects of pulsatile flow, chamber compliance, interaction of multiple jets, interaction with chamber walls and so forth, must be taken into consider-

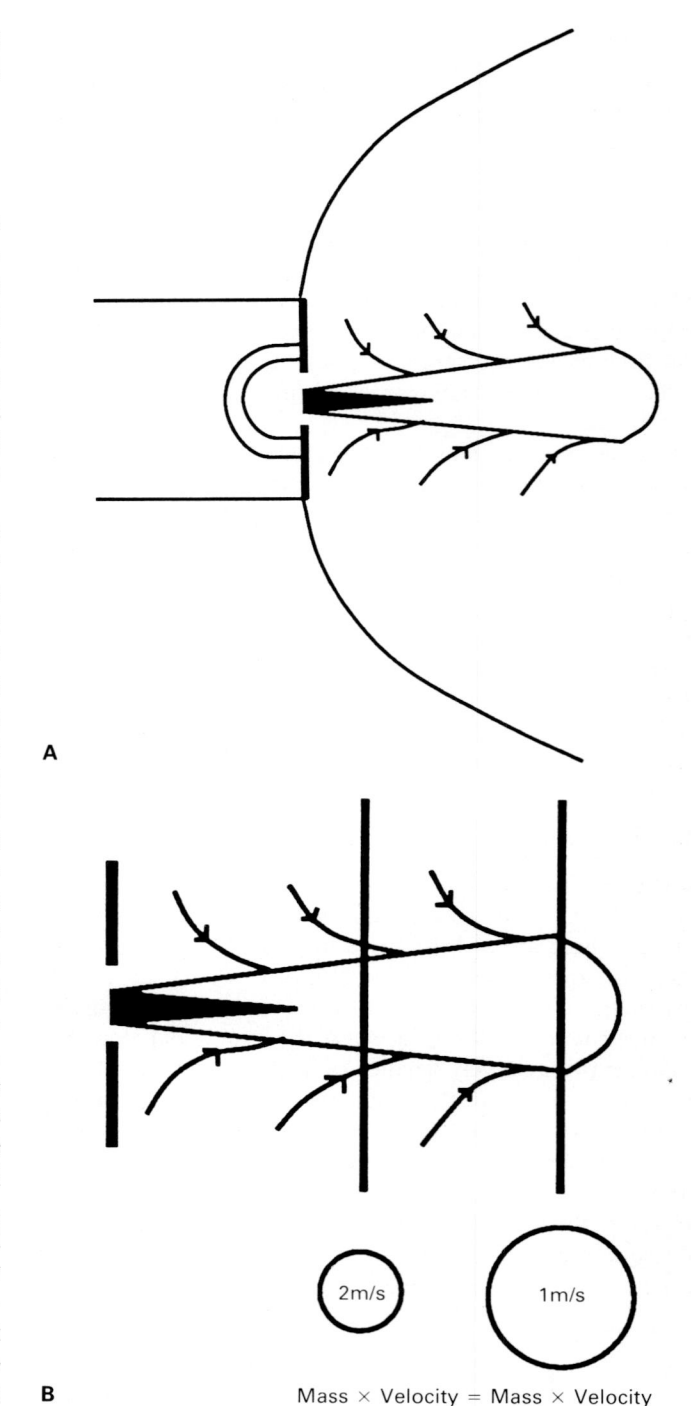

Fig. 3 A: Diagram of a free jet. As with the confined jet there is a zone of proximal flow acceleration towards the vena contracta. The jet flow within the receiving chamber expands and becomes turbulent but does not relaminarise or reattach as it is unaffected by the distant boundaries of the receiving chamber. **B: Diagram of a turbulent free jet** through a restrictive orifice demonstrating the central zone of laminar flow surrounded by a zone of turbulence. These jets conform to the laws of momentum conservation such that the product of mass and velocity remains essentially constant. As the jet slows down within the receiving chamber it entrains surrounding flow into the jet, conserving momentum by increasing mass.

ation when quantitative determinations are to be attempted. Nevertheless, understanding the basic principles of jet formation and structure allows a more rational approach to the quantitative application of Doppler techniques in the clinical setting.

Modified Bernoulli equation

The practical difficulties of applying the extended Bernoulli equation to clinical practice are considerable. As described above, the forces associated with flow acceleration early in systole are small and are not relevant to peak systole. They can largely be ignored in the estimation of peak pressure drop. Similarly viscous friction occurs mainly at the boundary layer between blood flow and the vessel or chamber wall rather than more centrally where Doppler velocity information is usually obtained. These energy losses are usually small and it does not seem unreasonable to ignore these forces for clinical purposes. This leaves us with a direct relationship between pressure drop and the convective acceleration, or velocity change, from one point to another as:

$$p_1 - p_2 = \tfrac{1}{2} \rho (v_2^2 - v_1^2)$$

If the mass density of blood (ρ) is included and the appropriate correction made to convert to mmHg, $1/2\,\rho$ becomes approximately 4 (more correctly 3.98). If the velocity proximal to an obstruction (v_1) is 1 m/s or less as is commonly the case within the heart, then v_1^2 becomes negligible (that is 1 or less) and as such can, for practical purposes, be ignored. The modified Bernoulli equation then becomes:

$$p_1 - p_2 = 4\, v_{max}^2$$

This modified Bernoulli formula, first described in this form by Hatle et al[2] has been the single most important factor in establishing the role of Doppler ultrasound for providing quantitative estimates of pressure gradients and the severity of obstructive lesions in the heart and great vessels. The pressure drop across an obstruction such as aortic or mitral stenosis can be estimated simply by using this simple equation once the peak flow velocity across the obstruction is measured. Ignoring the proximal velocity factor is valid when this velocity is 1 m/s or less but it should be remembered that the velocity proximal to an obstruction may be significantly greater in certain clinical situations, particularly where severe valve regurgitation coexists, and errors in the Doppler estimation of pressure gradients may occur if this is not taken into account. The problems and pitfalls of the modified Bernoulli equation and the potential for either overestimation or underestimation of pressure gradients will be discussed in more detail below.

APPLICATION OF DOPPLER ULTRASOUND TECHNIQUES

Current technology allows the combination of Doppler ultrasound examination and cross-sectional echocardiographic imaging (duplex systems) in addition to simple 'stand alone' Doppler systems. The availability of both these options is essential for accurate quantitation of pressure drops and gradients from Doppler ultrasound. Cross-sectional imaging combined with Doppler ultrasound allows appreciation of structural and functional associations and insights into the origin of Doppler signals. 'Stand alone' Doppler systems, usually employing continuous wave technology, provide the highest quality Doppler information as they are not compromised by integration with the somewhat different technical requirements for imaging and they are invariably smaller than larger imaging transducers and can therefore provide Doppler information from inaccessible areas of the precordium.

Pulsed wave spectral Doppler ultrasound is the best method to use for velocity quantitation where the velocities to be measured lie within the range of the pulsed system. Single sample pulsed wave Doppler can produce high resolution velocity information especially when combined with the structural information obtained by simultaneous cross-sectional imaging. Once the flow velocity causes the frequency shift to exceed the Nyquist limit of the pulsed Doppler system, aliasing occurs and ambiguity of velocity direction occurs (Fig. 4). This means that the high velocities associated with flow through obstructive and regurgitant lesions (up to 6 m/s) cannot be resolved by pulsed Doppler techniques and as such they have limited value for quantitation except within the normal heart where velocities rarely cause the Nyquist velocity limit to be exceeded.

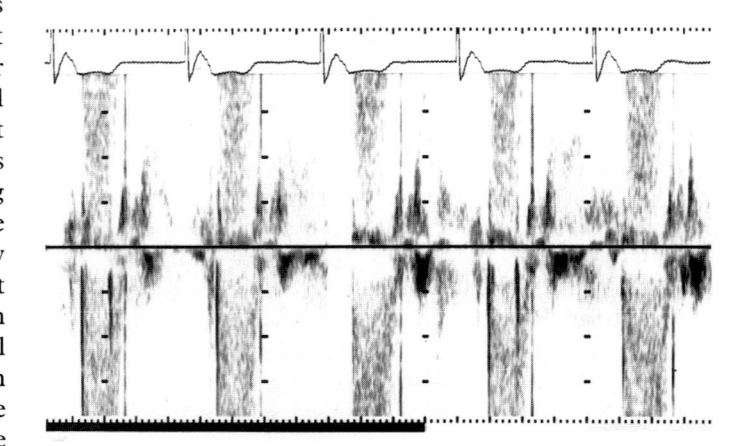

Fig. 4 Spectral Doppler recording of tricuspid regurgitation demonstrating the phenomenon of aliasing. Velocities directed away from the transducer are displayed below the zero velocity line but as the Nyquist velocity limit is exceeded then velocity information is cut off and displayed in the opposite velocity channel.

High pulsed repetition frequency (HPRF) Doppler examination can resolve much higher velocity values than single sample pulsed Doppler techniques but they introduce range ambiguity and the exact origin of the Doppler signal may not be apparent. In comparison, continuous wave Doppler examination allows no range resolution at all but essentially has no limitation in the velocity it can resolve. The latter is the most useful technique for the quantitation of pressure gradients in cardiology though HPRF Doppler examination can be valuable in situations where determination of the exact site of origin of the highest velocity signal is unclear, as in serial outflow tract obstructions.

Colour Doppler flow mapping is also emerging as having quantitative applications either in its own right or as a useful method of guiding the positioning of the continuous wave Doppler line of sight. It should be remembered that all these techniques are complementary and several may be useful in providing the most accurate quantitative information in a particular clinical setting. Nevertheless, for the practical purposes of estimation of pressure gradients continuous wave Doppler examination will generally be required to measure accurately the high velocities associated with the majority of important intracardiac lesions.

Practical aspects of quantitation

In order to estimate pressure gradients accurately using the modified Bernoulli equation it is critical that the maximum velocity occurring through an obstruction is correctly measured by Doppler ultrasound. Any underestimation of the true velocity value could result in a substantial underestimation of pressure gradient because Doppler ultrasound does not measure velocity directly, but rather the frequency shift of the transmitted ultrasound frequency, which in turn is dependent on the angle of incidence between the direction of flow and the ultrasound beam. If the ultrasound beam is not in the direct line of blood flow (parallel to flow) then the true velocity value will be underestimated. If this angle is small (less than 20°) then the resultant underestimation of velocity will also be small, but above 20° velocity underestimation becomes important. An angle of 20° will produce a 6% underestimation of velocity but an angle of 40° will give a 24% underestimation. Since it is the square of the velocity which is related to pressure gradient, any velocity underestimation will be magnified further when the modified Bernoulli equation is used to estimate pressure gradient. If Doppler ultrasound is to be used for the quantitative assessment of pressure gradients in clinical practice then it is essential that velocity estimates are obtained with the ultrasound beam as close as possible to the direction of blood flow at the vena contracta of the orifice.

It is quite common for operators to use two-dimensional imaging to line up the Doppler ultrasound beam with the assumed direction of blood flow in order to minimise the angle of incidence with the ultrasound beam. In the normal heart this is probably valid, since the direction of blood flow generally conforms to the patterns predicted by the surrounding anatomy. This is not so in diseased situations where distorted anatomy makes the direction of jet flow quite unpredictable. The clinical situations where quantitative Doppler information is particularly important, such as aortic and mitral valve disease, are almost always associated with distorted valve anatomy, and it is not possible to assume that the jet direction can be predicted from the anatomical appearance.

The single most important factor in ensuring that Doppler information is obtained as parallel to jet flow as possible, is the performance of the Doppler interrogation from as many precordial imaging sites as is practically possible. This is particularly so for aortic valve stenosis where the jet direction is extremely variable and in this situation Doppler examination from as many as five or six different positions may be necessary to ensure that the maximum velocity signal has been obtained.

Colour Doppler flow mapping allows a spatial appreciation of flow velocities in relation to surrounding structural detail and this information can be utilised when attempting to predict jet direction for the purposes of accurate velocity estimation. Guiding the direction of a continuous wave Doppler beam using colour Doppler flow mapping can be extremely valuable, particularly where the origin of the jet, as well as its direction, is unpredictable. This is common in congenital heart disease where, for example, the site of a small ventricular septal defect may be identified by colour Doppler flow mapping and the continuous wave Doppler beam can be appropriately directed. Similarly the origin of a regurgitant jet and its direction within the receiving chamber can often be visualised by colour Doppler flow mapping and this can be used to direct the continuous wave Doppler beam (Plate 1). The direction of regurgitant jets in particular can be extremely variable and on occasions it can be very difficult and time-consuming to obtain a satisfactory signal on continuous wave Doppler examination without using colour Doppler flow mapping to predict the direction of the jet.

If the direction of a high velocity jet through an obstructive or regurgitant orifice can be identified by colour Doppler flow mapping it is theoretically possible to use this information to correct for the angle between the ultrasound beam and the jet direction using the Doppler equation, rather than attempting to align the ultrasound beam with the jet. In clinical practice, however, angle correction results in a considerable overestimation of the true velocity value and hence a large overestimation of the pressure gradient. The reason for this overestimation has been elegantly demonstrated in a study by Yoganathan et al.[7]

This in-vitro experiment used streak photography to illustrate the nature of jets occurring through stenotic

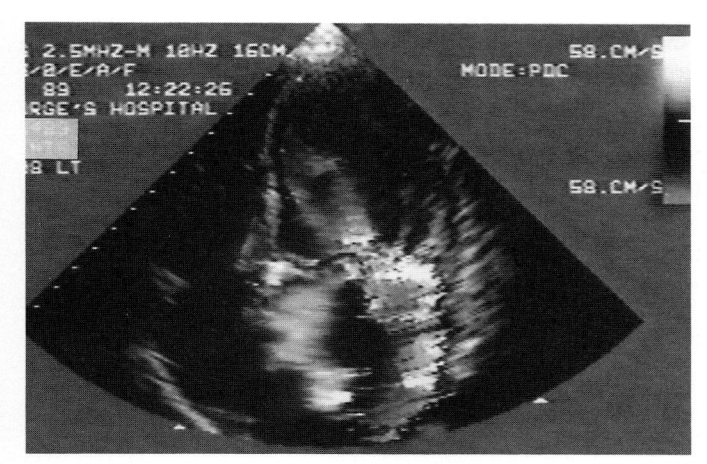

Plate 1 Colour Doppler flow map image of mitral regurgitation showing that the jet is directed posteriorly within the left atrium rather than centrally. This information can be used to aid alignment of the continuous wave Doppler beam. This figure is reproduced in colour in the colour plate section at the front of this volume.

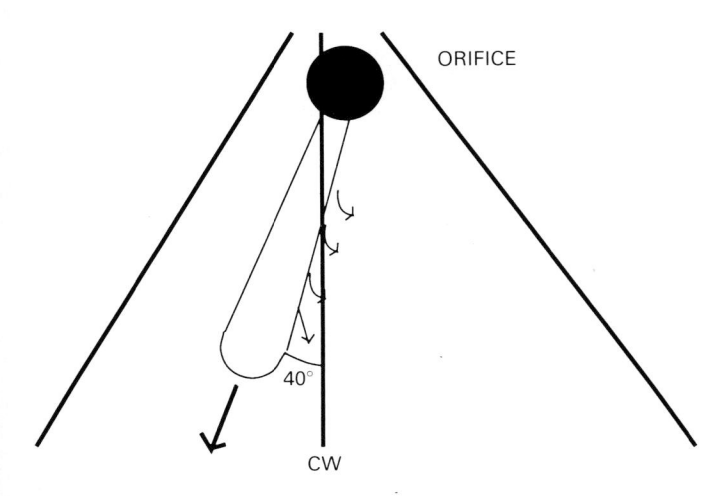

Fig. 5 Diagram demonstrating that if a continuous wave Doppler beam is aligned at a 40° angle to a jet it will pick up signals from side lobe vectors spraying from the main jet direction and it will be in direct line with some of the side lobes. If angle correction factors for 40° are applied to the measured velocity this will result in significant overestimation of the true jet velocity.

orifices and laser Doppler anemometry to measure true velocity values at different individual points within the core of the jet. These velocities were measured in the direct line of flow and at several known angles to flow which were subsequently angle corrected. It was apparent that as the jet comes through the orifice it generates a spray effect with side-lobe vectors occurring at directions oblique to the main jet direction (see Fig. 5). These oblique side-lobe jets are at a slightly lower velocity than the true maximum velocity at the vena contracta but they can be parallel to a continuous wave ultrasound beam which is positioned at a significant angle to the main jet direction. The resultant

velocity on continuous wave Doppler at, for example, an angle of 40° may only be slightly lower than the true maximum velocity because of the parallel side lobe vectors. Colour Doppler flow mapping would rightly suggest that the main jet direction was 40° to the angle of the continuous wave Doppler beam but because of the resolution of the system and the angle effects, it would be unable to identify the oblique vectors. Angle correction of the continuous wave Doppler velocity of 40° would result in a calculated velocity that was considerably higher than the true maximum velocity value. All high velocity jets occurring in the heart in disease situations will spray to some extent and as such any angle correction of these jets will be inappropriate. In order to obtain a true maximum velocity value from Doppler ultrasound it is essential that all efforts are directed at aligning the ultrasound beam as closely as possible with the high velocity jet and under no circumstances should angle correction be performed using colour flow directed continuous wave Doppler techniques.

QUANTITATIVE DOPPLER TECHNIQUES IN THE CLINICAL SETTING

Since the original descriptions of the use of Doppler ultrasound to predict the severity of mitral stenosis[1,2] there has been an explosion of its quantitative use so that it is now a well established and clinically valuable technique in both adult and paediatric cardiology. The basic principles of application of the Bernoulli equation for the quantitative estimation of pressure gradients is essentially the same for all valve lesions but the practical application can vary considerably. The main 'gold-standard' for the clinical measurement of pressure gradients has been cardiac catheterisation and it is the results of measurements from this procedure that are familiar to most clinicians.

Pressure gradients estimated by Doppler ultrasound are not necessarily directly comparable for several reasons. Firstly, there is a slight time delay due to viscous effects[8] between the development of a pressure gradient and the resultant flow velocity. However, this delay is very small (about 10–20 ms) and is of little relevance for clinical purposes even when estimates of mean valve gradients are made.

Pressure gradients across stenotic valves are dependent on both the valve orifice area and the flow through the valve. Since cardiac output can vary, it is well recognised that pressure gradients can also vary at different times and under different physiological circumstances. It is not always appropriate to compare a pressure gradient estimated by Doppler ultrasound at an outpatient clinic with one measured invasively on a different occasion. In addition, many institutions use routine sedation for cardiac catheterisation and this can also decrease pressure gradients. In contrast, unsedated patients may be very anxious during the catheterisation procedure and this can cause a rise in the pressure gradient to higher levels than estimated by Doppler ultrasound prior to catheterisation.

Even when Doppler derived pressure gradients are compared to simultaneously measured invasive gradients, other differences can be apparent. Pressure gradients (or pressure drop) across stenotic aortic and pulmonary valves are usually measured by withdrawal of the catheter across the stenotic valve. This withdrawal technique compares the peak pressure in the proximal chamber (left ventricle for aortic stenosis) with the peak pressure in the distal chamber (aorta for aortic stenosis) as a 'peak-to-peak' pressure gradient. Since these peak values may occur, and often do, at significantly different times within the cardiac cycle, this 'measured' gradient is one which does not actually exist during cardiac ejection and it is thus not a physiological gradient. Doppler ultrasound however, is measuring the peak velocity and hence the peak pressure gradient occurring at one instant in the cardiac cycle, the so-called 'peak instantaneous pressure gradient'. The peak-to-peak pressure gradient and the peak instantaneous pressure gradient are therefore quite different measurements and there may be a considerable and clinically important difference between these two measurements, although the peak-to-peak value cannot be higher than the peak instantaneous gradient (Fig. 6).

The maximum velocity and hence the maximum pressure gradient occurs at the vena contracta of the orifice and Doppler examination of pressure gradients will reflect this value. The distal pressure measurement obtained at cardiac catheterisation is often at some distance downstream from the vena contracta. Some degree of pressure recovery will occur in this distal region as the expanding jet slows down beyond the narrow orifice. A cardiac catheter positioned distally may measure a higher pressure than that occurring at the vena contracta itself, causing underestimation of the true maximum pressure gradient across the obstruction. This pressure recovery is minimal for discrete obstructive lesions and it rarely affects the clinical assessment of valve gradients, but the effects of pressure recovery can be significant in serial outflow tract obstructions as discussed below.

Comparison of pressure gradients obtained by Doppler techniques with those obtained at cardiac catheterisation should be done with full knowledge of the physiological circumstances during which the measurements were obtained and the exact methodology used for each technique if clinically useful results are to be achieved.

Aortic stenosis

Aortic valve gradient

Doppler techniques have proved to be particularly valuable for the quantitative assessment of aortic valve stenosis. Peak valve gradient is a very useful measurement of the severity of aortic valve stenosis and estimation of this can be performed easily by applying the modified Bernoulli equation to the measured maximum velocity through the stenotic valve. This was first described by Hatle et al[9] who found an excellent correlation between pressure gradients estimated by Doppler ultrasound and those measured at cardiac catheterisation. The accuracy of pressure gradient estimates in aortic stenosis by Doppler ultrasound have since been confirmed by other workers[10-15] and it is now well established as a valuable part of the non-invasive clinical evaluation of these patients.

An example of a continuous wave Doppler velocity recording from a patient with a normal aortic valve and one with significant aortic stenosis is shown in Figure 7. Several differences are apparent. Firstly, the maximum velocity is considerably higher in the patient with aortic stenosis, reflecting the significant pressure gradient across the aortic valve. The peak velocity in this case is 4 m/s, giving a calculated peak instantaneous pressure drop of 64 mmHg. The peak velocity occurs quite early in systole across the normal aortic valve, but, in the patient with significant aortic stenosis it occurs later, in mid systole, producing a more parabolic shape to the velocity recording. This is due to the characteristically slower rise of the aortic pressure curve in severe aortic stenosis. This pattern is in itself semi-quantitative and one should always consider the presence of severe aortic stenosis when a parabolic velocity profile is obtained, even if the maximum velocity is less than expected. Severe aortic stenosis in the presence of poor left ventricular function will produce this appearance and the shape of the velocity curve can be important in distinguishing this from the contrasting situation of mild

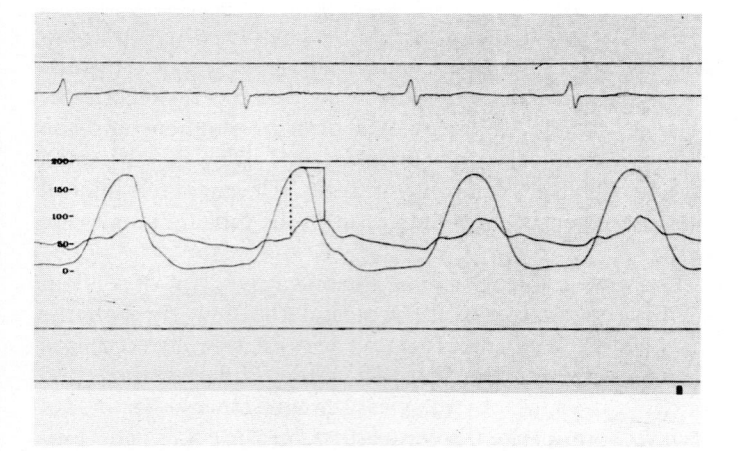

Fig. 6 Pressure tracing obtained simultaneously from the left ventricle and aorta at cardiac catheterisation in a patient with aortic stenosis. The peak-to-peak pressure gradient measured from the two peak pressures at different times in the cardiac cycle is significantly less than the peak instantaneous gradient measured at one point in time.

aortic stenosis and good left ventricular function. These observations are particularly important where echocardiographic imaging of left ventricular function is suboptimal.

The high velocity component of the signal from aortic stenosis can be of quite low amplitude or signal strength. Since small changes in velocity can make considerable differences to estimated pressures, particularly at the higher velocities, accurate determination of the true maximum velocity is of paramount importance. Gain settings should always be adjusted to demonstrate the maximum velocity value but should not be so excessive as to cause random noise which may be mistaken for a high velocity flow signal. Estimates of pressure gradient across the aortic valve should only be made where a spectral Doppler signal with a distinct spectral envelope or outline can be obtained (Fig. 8). The quality of the Doppler signal can also be judged from the audio signal where a clean, high pitched noise should be heard. If such a signal is heard but no high velocity signal is seen on the spectrum analyser, then the gain setting may be too low. If a high velocity signal is apparent on the spectral analyser but only a low pitched signal is heard then the gain setting may be too high.

Continuous wave Doppler recordings can contain low velocity signals which may be of high signal amplitude and these can mask the low intensity high velocity signals, so it is important that the high pass filter is set correctly to exclude these low velocity signals. Only when the highest quality spectral signals are obtained should an estimate of valve gradient be made.

Even when a 'clean' spectral envelope is obtained, it is important to ensure that the Doppler ultrasound beam is as close as possible to the direct line of blood flow through the stenotic aortic valve. In order to do this, signals of aortic flow should be obtained from multiple precordial positions including the cardiac apex, suprasternal notch, right parasternal position, supraclavicular and even subcostal positions. In most cases, the best signal with the highest recordable velocity will be obtained from the apical position but the direction of blood flow through the aortic valve is unpredictable and all positions should be used routinely in order to detect the maximum frequency shift. It is not possible to use two-dimensional imaging to predict the best precordial position and colour Doppler flow mapping is rarely of value in this respect as jets through stenotic aortic valves tend to spray almost immediately and the direction of the high velocity jet is often not apparent. In addition, acoustic shadowing from a calcified aortic valve can mask the flow information of colour Doppler flow mapping. Although the maximum velocity of aortic stenosis can be recorded in almost all individuals[13,15] this may require considerable time and effort, combining duplex and stand alone continuous wave Doppler systems from multiple precordial positions, in order to exclude significant aortic stenosis.

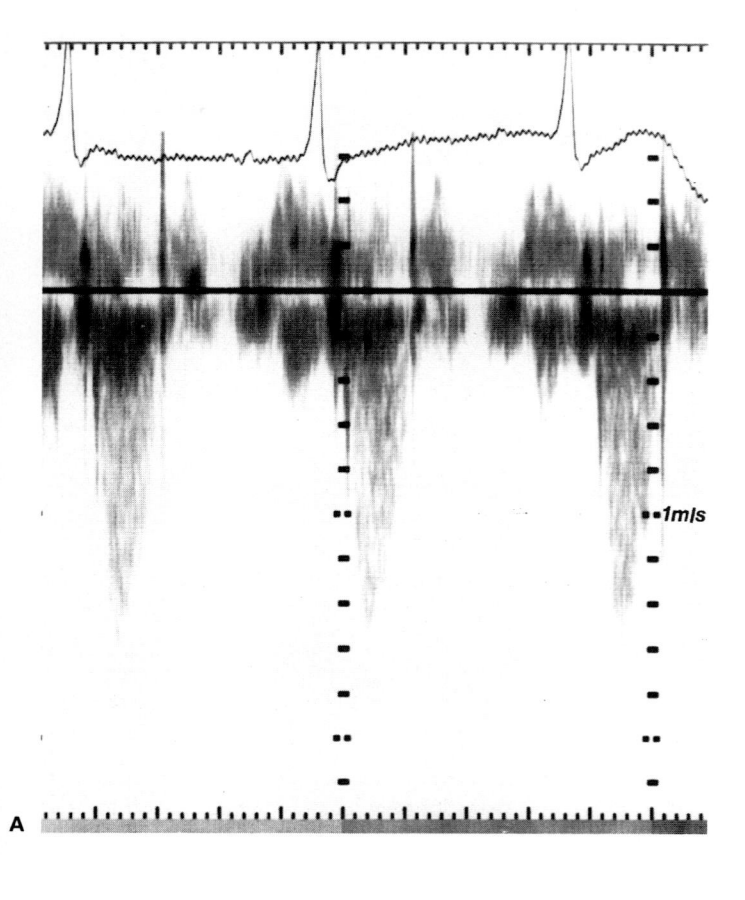

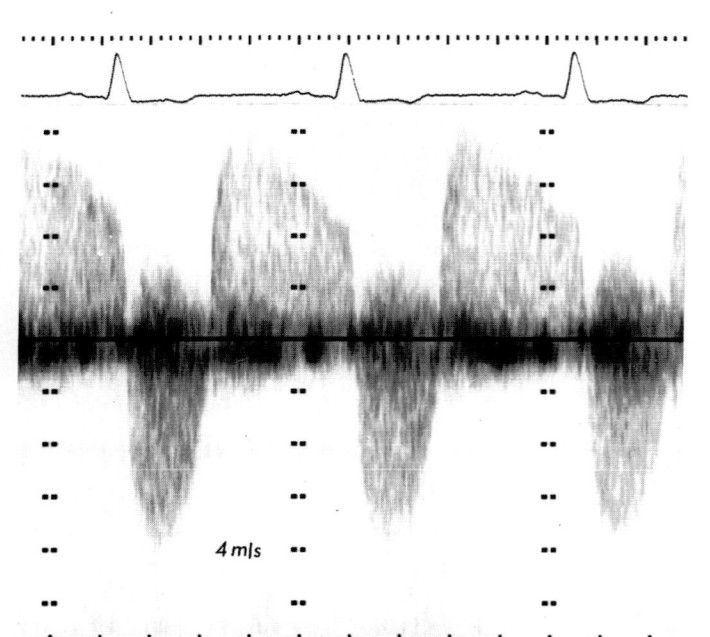

Fig. 7 A: Spectral Doppler recording of a normal aortic valve from the apex. The peak velocity is 1.4 m/s. **B:** In a patient with significant aortic valve disease the peak velocity is 4 m/s with an estimated gradient of 64 mmHg using the modified Bernoulli equation. There is also diastolic flow towards the transducer indicating aortic regurgitation.

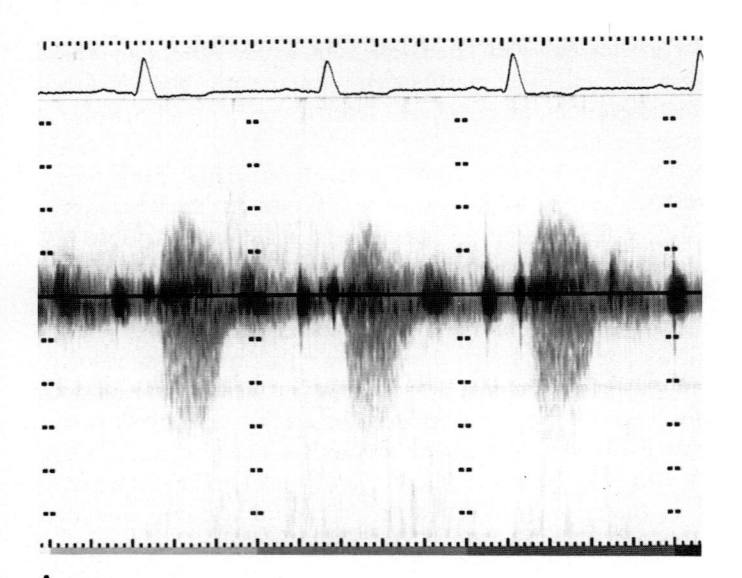

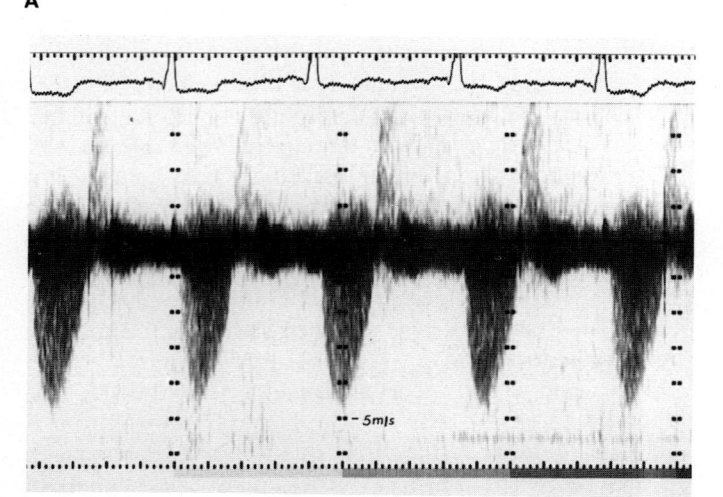

Fig. 8 A: Spectral continuous wave Doppler in a patient with aortic stenosis. Although the peak velocity is greater than 3 m/s the maximum velocity is not well defined and this signal is not suitable for accurate quantitative measurements. **B:** The continuous wave Doppler signal from this patient has a well demarcated spectral envelope with a maximum velocity of 5 m/s indicating a peak instantaneous pressure gradient of 100 mmHg.

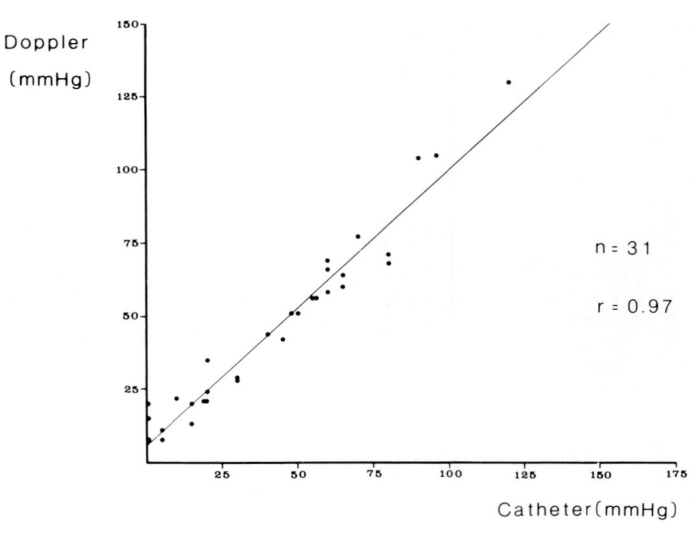

Fig. 9 Correlation graph comparing Doppler derived pressure gradients using the modified Bernoulli equation with those measured at cardiac catheterisation in patients with aortic stenosis. There is an excellent correlation between the two techniques with only small errors which are acceptable for clinical purposes. (Reproduced from Simpson et al, Br Heart J 1985; 53: 636–639.)

When continuous wave Doppler ultrasound is used to estimate the transaortic pressure gradient in patients with aortic stenosis, the estimated pressure gradient compares well with measurements obtained at cardiac catheterisation.[13-15] The relationship between gradients obtained by Doppler ultrasound and those obtained at cardiac catheterisation is illustrated in Figure 9. Currie et al[14] have demonstrated in the clinical setting the differences that exist between the peak instantaneous valve gradient as measured by Doppler ultrasound and peak-to-peak measurements obtained at cardiac catheterisation. They have also demonstrated that when true instantaneous pressure gradients are measured at cardiac catheterisation using two separate catheters, then pressure gradients estimated by continuous wave Doppler very closely reflect the gradients measured invasively. Therefore, in clinical studies, it is clear that Doppler ultrasound can accurately predict the pressure gradients across stenotic aortic valves providing attention is paid to the above precautions.

It is also clear from published studies that sedation during cardiac catheterisation can make considerable differences to the pressure gradient across a stenotic aortic valve. Doppler derived gradients obtained at a different time may give quite different results. This raises the question of the significance of Doppler derived gradients obtained at times other than during cardiac catheterisation. Rather than causing confusion between valve gradients obtained at different times or under different physiological conditions, Doppler ultrasound now allows us to observe the effects of different physiological conditions and it may be possible to use this information to improve the assessment of these patients and predict the appropriate timing of surgical intervention.

Pressure gradients will vary in an individual patient as a result of changing cardiac output, yet the functional area of the aortic valve remains essentially unchanged in the short term. If Doppler ultrasound could provide information about aortic valve orifice area rather than just valve gradient, it would circumvent the problems of estimating valve gradient under different physiological conditions.

Aortic valve area

The obvious attraction of using aortic valve area as opposed to aortic gradient is that it eliminates the problems associated with overestimation and underestimation of gradients particularly in the situation where there is coexistent aortic valve regurgitation. In addition, patients with poor left ventricular function may have critical aortic stenosis but are unable to generate a large gradient. Despite a low transvalve gradient, the severity of aortic stenosis will be reflected by a very small aortic valve area. Two methods have been described for the estimation of aortic valve area by Doppler ultrasound and it has become clear that in many cases this provides significantly better information about the severity of aortic stenosis and its progression over months or years than gradient estimation alone.[16]

Firstly it is possible to estimate aortic valve area by application of the Gorlin formula[17,18] which is also used to estimate aortic valve area from invasive measurements. This formula relates the calculated flow across the valve, the systolic ejection period and the mean aortic valve gradient to the estimated valve area as follows:

Aortic valve area = cardiac output/44.5 SEP × MTG

where SEP is the systolic ejection period and MTG is mean transvalve pressure gradient. Cardiac output is calculated from the left ventricular outflow tract diameter on cross-sectional imaging and the left ventricular outflow tract velocity. Systolic ejection period is calculated as the time between onset and cessation of aortic flow on continuous wave Doppler examination. Mean transaortic pressure gradient is calculated from the continuous wave Doppler signal using the modified Bernoulli equation.

Aortic valve area can also be calculated using the continuity principle.[19,20] Since the product of area and velocity at one position in the flow stream will be identical to the product of area and velocity at a different position, this principle can be used to estimate aortic valve area such that:

Area (LVOT) × velocity (LVOT) = area (Ao) × velocity (Ao)
LVOT = left ventricular outflow tract; Ao = aortic valve orifice.

The area of the left ventricular outflow tract (LVOT) can be estimated from cross-sectional imaging using the LVOT diameter from the parasternal long axis view and the velocity of the left ventricular outflow tract can be measured by pulsed Doppler echocardiography from the cardiac apex. The velocity through the aortic valve can, as we know, be measured using the continuous wave Doppler technique and therefore estimation of aortic valve area becomes:

$$\text{Ao valve area} = \frac{\text{area (LVOT)} \times \text{velocity (LVOT)}}{\text{velocity (Ao)}}$$

It is important to note that the continuity principle defines the velocity in question as an average velocity across the cross-sectional area of the 'tube'. The left ventricular outflow tract is subject to an 'inlet effect' which allows us to assume that the velocity profile across the left ventricular outflow tract is fairly flat and that the velocity measured by pulsed Doppler at one position is representative of the average velocity across the whole of the outflow tract. An inlet effect occurs in any situation where flow is moving from a large diameter structure such as the left ventricle to a smaller diameter structure such as the aortic valve. Within this inlet portion, the velocity profile should be quite flat and the velocity is therefore similar across the entire cross-section of the outflow tract. In aortic stenosis, the velocity profile at the vena contracta of the orifice should also be flat and as the continuous wave Doppler beam will probably encompass all of the stenotic jet diameter, this velocity recording will also be representative of the velocity profile through the stenosed aortic valve. These assumptions seem to be valid for clinical purposes since excellent correlations of aortic valve area estimated by Doppler techniques with those obtained by invasive measurement have been reported. Skjaerpe et al[20] reported a correlation coefficient of 0.89, and also made the important point that the velocity in the left ventricular outflow tract should not be measured too close to the aortic valve as acceleration of flow occurs towards the stenotic orifice. If the velocity is measured within 2 cm of the valve, then an unrepresentative high velocity may be obtained. Colour Doppler flow mapping can accurately identify the area of spatial flow acceleration proximal to the aortic valve and this may be useful for ensuring that the velocity is recorded from the appropriate position.

Mitral stenosis

Quantitative assessment of the severity of mitral stenosis can be made from the spectral Doppler recording as illustrated in Figure 10. Characteristically, mitral stenosis will cause an increase in the diastolic flow velocity. As with aortic valve stenosis, the peak velocity across the mitral valve during diastole can be converted to a peak pressure gradient using the modified Bernoulli equation. Estimation of the peak mitral pressure drop is, however, of little value in the clinical assessment of these patients as the relatively low pressure drop in comparison to aortic stenosis can be markedly altered by changes in cardiac output or by the presence of significant mitral regurgitation. The end diastolic pressure drop is often measured at cardiac catheterisation and this can easily be derived from the maximum velocity recording at end diastole by application of the modified Bernoulli equation. Even in severe mitral stenosis, however, the end diastolic pressure gradient may fall to zero following a long diastolic time period and it is for this reason that the mean pressure gradient has more traditionally been measured at cardiac catheterisation.

Estimating mean mitral valve gradient from the maximum velocity recording on spectral Doppler ultrasound is achieved by applying the Bernoulli equation throughout diastole at each point of the maximum velocity curve and then averaging the multiple pressure gradients obtained.

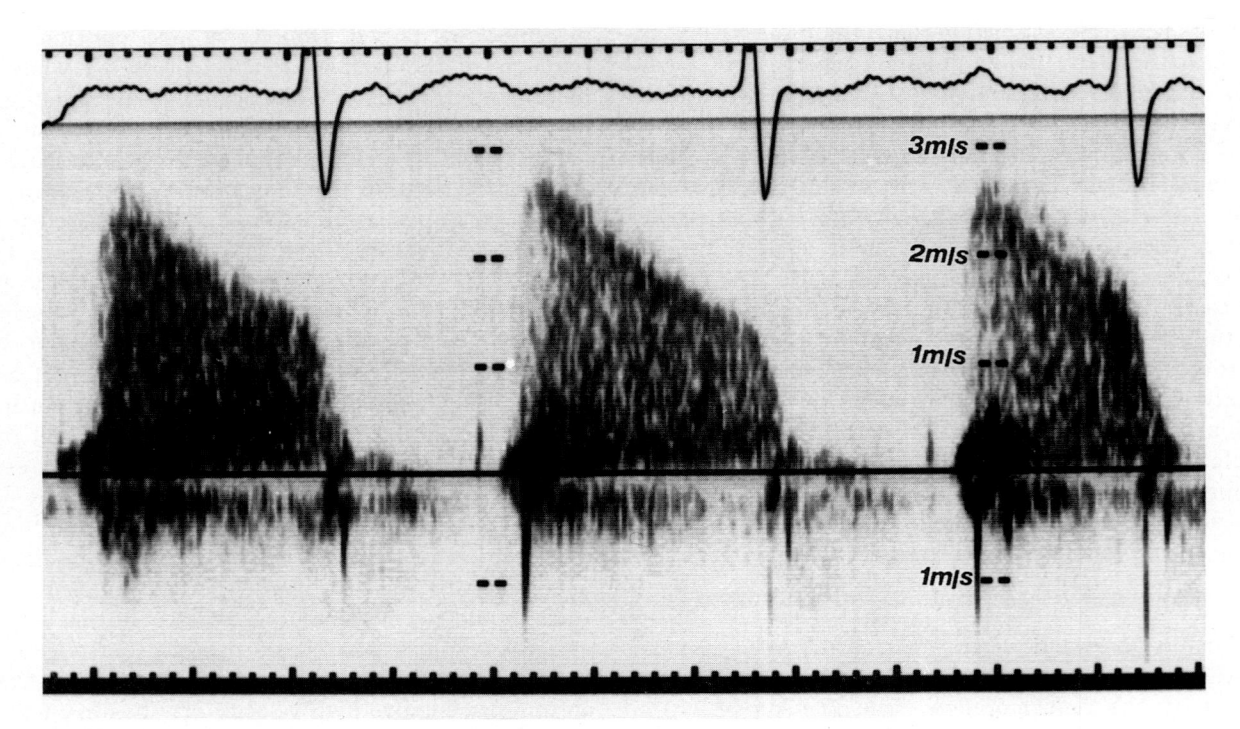

Fig. 10 Continuous wave Doppler recording of mitral stenosis. This is characterised by an increase in velocity throughout diastole. Not only is the initial peak velocity increased but there is a slower rate of velocity decrease from this initial peak.

This is a very cumbersome process to do by hand but fortunately most modern ultrasound equipment will perform this automatically when the maximum velocity envelope is traced on the screen. Excellent correlation between the mean diastolic pressure drop across the mitral valve estimated using Doppler ultrasound and that obtained at cardiac catheterisation has been reported.[2] Mean diastolic pressure gradient, however, is still dependent on such factors as cardiac output, diastolic time period and the presence of mitral regurgitation and this value may not always accurately reflect the true anatomical severity of mitral stenosis. This is true not only for mean valve gradients estimated by Doppler ultrasound but also those measured at cardiac catheterisation. The most consistently accurate way to determine the severity of mitral stenosis is to assess the mitral valve area by measuring the mitral pressure half-time.

Mitral pressure half-time

Mitral stenosis causes not only an increase in the initial diastolic flow velocity but it also affects the rate of decrease of this velocity during diastole. Mitral pressure half-time is a measurement of the rate of decrease of the mitral flow velocity from its initial peak flow and it is, to a large extent, directly related to the mitral valve area. The more severe the mitral stenosis, the slower the rate of velocity decrease during diastole and hence the longer the mitral pressure half-time. The pressure half-time in milliseconds is the time taken for the initial peak pressure drop to fall to a value equivalent to half its original level (Fig. 11). Note that this is not the same as the time taken to reach half the peak velocity value because the relationship between velocity and pressure gradient described in the Bernoulli equation is not linear but squared. The peak velocity in early diastole should first be converted to a pressure drop using the modified Bernoulli equation. Half this value is then used to back calculate the appropriate velocity value. The time difference between the peak velocity value and the calculated velocity representing half the initial pressure drop is the mitral pressure half-time.

In practice the calculation of mitral pressure half-time can be simplified. The maximum velocity relates to maximum pressure drop as $4 V_{max}^2$ and hence pressure half-time is the time for the velocity to decrease to $\frac{1}{2} 4 V_{max}^2$. This velocity is not V_{max}^2 but $V_{max}/\sqrt{2}$. Hence the velocity equivalent to half the initial pressure drop is $V_{max}/1.4$. Mitral pressure half-time can be estimated quickly by measuring the maximum velocity, dividing this by 1.4 and measuring the time difference in milliseconds (ms) between the two values on the maximum velocity curve. The normal value for mitral pressure half-time across a non-stenotic valve is less than 80 ms. Mild mitral stenosis is present when the pressure half-time is between 100–150 ms and severe mitral stenosis exists when the pressure half-time exceeds 220 ms.

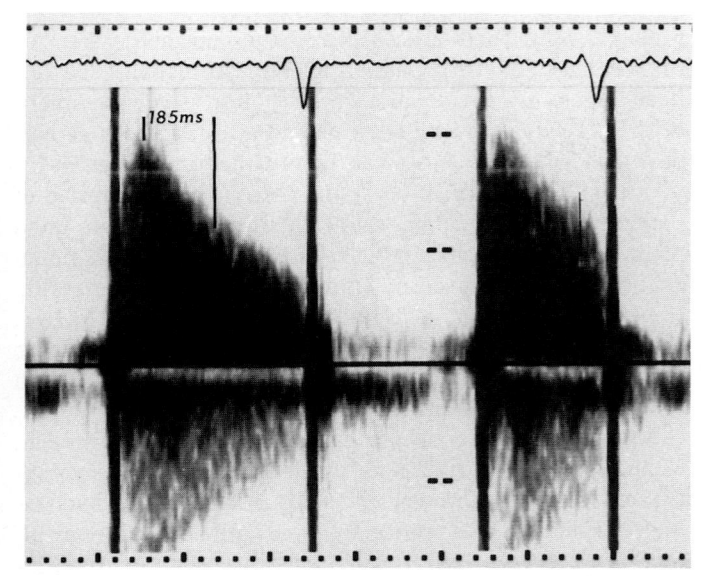

Fig. 11 Continuous wave Doppler recording from a patient with moderate mitral stenosis. The mitral pressure half-time of 185 ms is the time taken for the initial peak velocity to decrease to a value equivalent to half the initial peak pressure drop.

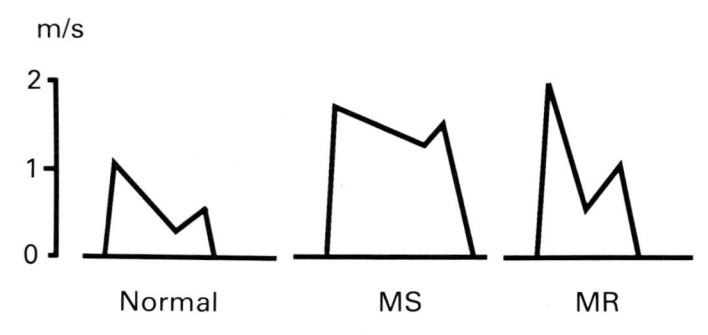

Fig. 12 Schematic representation of the flow velocity across normal, stenotic and regurgitant mitral valves. Mitral stenosis results in an increased peak velocity and a prolonged pressure half-time whereas mitral regurgitation causes an increase in the peak diastolic velocity but the pressure half-time remains normal.

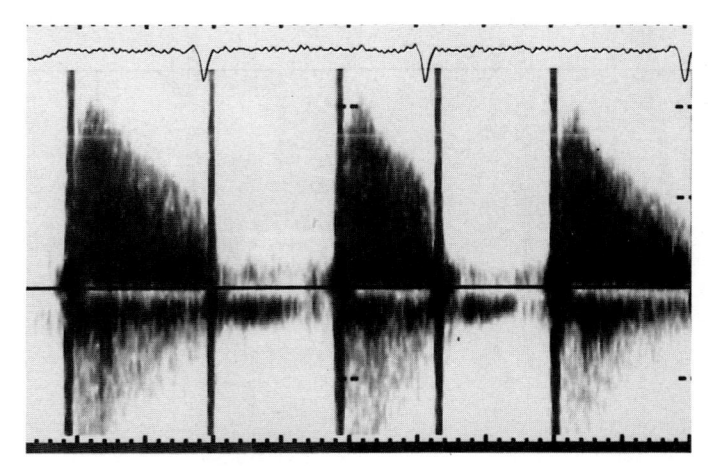

Fig. 13 High amplitude signals of mitral valve opening as illustrated should not be confused with the peak velocity signal or significant errors in the estimation of mitral pressure half-time may result.

Since mitral pressure half-time is related to the anatomical severity of mitral stenosis it is relatively unaffected by alteration in cardiac output or by the presence of mitral regurgitation. Figure 12 demonstrates the pattern of mitral diastolic flow velocity in normals, mitral stenosis and mitral regurgitation. Although the presence of significant mitral regurgitation will increase the peak mitral diastolic flow velocity, the rate of decrease of velocity is relatively unaffected and hence, the mitral pressure half-time remains within the normal range. This is despite the fact that the mean pressure gradient across the valve will have increased. Hatle and co-workers[21] have demonstrated that mitral pressure half-time provides an accurate estimation of the severity of mitral stenosis when compared to invasive estimation of mitral valve area. They have suggested that mitral valve area in square centimetres can be estimated by dividing 220 by the mitral pressure half-time. The figure of 220 is an empirical value chosen as a result of the comparative information gained from the invasive investigation of a group of patients with mitral stenosis. A mitral pressure half-time of 220 ms correlates with a mitral valve area of 1 cm^2. Pressure half-times of greater than 220 ms will therefore predict a functional mitral valve area less than 1 cm^2.

Accurate estimation of the mitral pressure half-time is dependent on a number of factors, not least of which is accurate identification of the peak mitral flow velocity. It is usually quite easy to align the Doppler beam with the direction of mitral inflow from the cardiac apex and concerns about underestimating the true velocity as a result of a significant angle of incidence are rarely justified. This is not so when attempting to obtain the maximum velocity across a prosthetic valve where the direction of blood flow may be significantly influenced by the type of prosthesis and its direction of insertion. Here, colour Doppler flow mapping may be of considerable value in aligning the spectral Doppler beam with the direction of valve flow.

High amplitude signals resulting from mitral valve opening may in some cases cause masking of the initial peak velocity recording. Such errors in identifying the true maximum velocity may cause significant underestimation of the mitral pressure half-time if the high amplitude, high frequency signal of valve leaflet motion is taken as the maximum velocity signal of mitral inflow (Fig. 13). With experience it is usually easy to separate visually the two signals.

Accurate estimation of mitral pressure half-time depends on the assumption that the mitral flow velocity signal decreases in a linear fashion but it is not uncommon for mitral velocities to decrease exponentially (Fig. 14). Measurement in the early part of the diastole will result in a

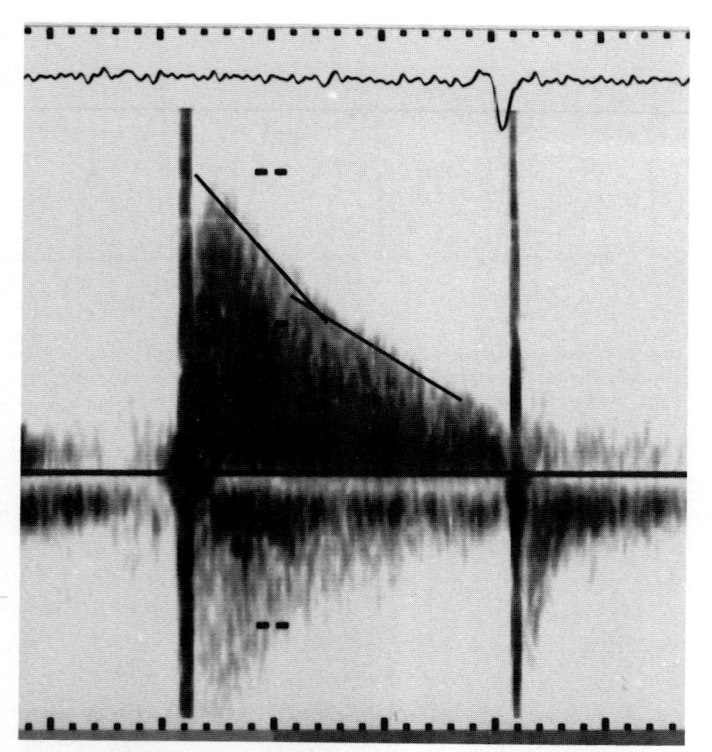

Fig. 14 Mitral flow velocity curve demonstrating an exponential decrease throughout diastole. If the initial slope early in diastole is used for estimation of mitral pressure half-time this will result in a significantly shorter half-time in comparison to the rate of velocity decrease in late diastole.

shorter pressure half-time than that obtained if the slope occurring later in diastole was used. In cases of doubt the method described above for determining the actual half-time should be adhered to although some authors claim that measurement over a longer period of time is more accurate.

Many patients with mitral valve stenosis will be in atrial fibrillation and therefore there will be no 'a' wave on the mitral flow velocity recording. Estimation of mitral pressure half-time in these patients is quite easy. In patients who remain in sinus rhythm, the mitral flow velocity may not have fallen to a value reflecting half the initial pressure drop before the onset of the 'a' wave velocities, particularly if the heart rate is quite rapid. In these patients it is necessary to extrapolate the slope of decreasing diastolic velocity in order to obtain a measurement of mitral pressure half-time. One can imagine that in these patients the onset of atrial fibrillation will cause loss of the 'a' wave velocities and hence the mean diastolic pressure gradient across the mitral valve will decrease as a result. However, the estimation of functional valve area from the mitral pressure half-time should remain unchanged.

Estimates of mitral pressure half-time do, to a large extent, reflect the functional area of the mitral valve and this measurement can be affected by changes in heart rate, preload, ventricular afterload and the contractile state of the ventricle. Nevertheless, mitral pressure half-time has been shown to provide an accurate noninvasive assessment of the severity of mitral stenosis and as satisfactory signals of mitral inflow velocities can be obtained in almost all individuals, it can easily be applied to the vast majority of patients. It is certainly more consistently accurate than planimetry of the mitral valve area using cross-sectional echocardiographic imaging, and the measurement can often be obtained using a dedicated, stand-alone Doppler transducer in patients who are poor echocardiographic subjects. The method is subject to less variability than other available techniques.

Mitral pressure half-time estimation is also of value in excluding mitral valve stenosis in patients who have increased diastolic flow velocities for other reasons such as high cardiac output states or significant mitral regurgitation. In native mitral valve regurgitation, or regurgitation through a tissue mitral valve prosthesis[22] a peak mitral diastolic flow greater than 2 m/s in the presence of a normal mitral pressure half-time is highly suggestive of significant mitral regurgitation.

Tricuspid and pulmonary stenosis

The principles applied to the mitral valve are also applicable to the tricuspid valve although, to date, very little information is available to verify this.[23] This is mainly due to the fact that tricuspid valve stenosis is a relatively rare finding. For prosthetic tricuspid valves, the general principles applied to the mitral valve also hold true though the accepted values for normal tricuspid gradients and half-time measurements for tricuspid valve replacements are slightly different.[24] The peak diastolic inflow velocity for normally functioning tricuspid valve replacements ranges from 0.6–1.6 m/s with pressure half-times from 38–197 ms.[24] The use of pressure half-time estimates for the quantitative assessment of tricuspid prosthetic valve obstruction appears to be valid, in that 5 reported patients with significant tricuspid prosthetic obstruction had pressure half-times ranging from 237–570 ms.

Pure valvar pulmonary stenosis will behave in an identical manner to aortic valve stenosis and pressure gradients estimated by Doppler ultrasound across the pulmonary valve using the Bernoulli equation will be an accurate reflection of similar pressure gradients measured invasively. Clinical studies using Doppler derived pressure gradients have demonstrated that this technique does provide accurate quantitative data about the severity of pulmonary valve stenosis.[25,26]

Non-discrete, tunnel and multiple obstructions

Quantitative estimation of the severity of discrete obstructive lesions by Doppler ultrasound is relatively straightforward. Non-discrete, tunnel-like obstructions or multiple obstruction conform to different haemodynamic principles which have considerable bearing on their quantitation using Doppler techniques. Multi-level obstructions are most common in paediatric cardiology where both left and right ventricular outflow tract obstruction may have subvalve, valve and supravalve components. Tunnel-like obstructions occur with subvalve muscular obstruction such as infundibular pulmonary stenosis, in coarctation of the aorta and with muscular ventricular septal defects. These lesions are potentially quantifiable using Doppler techniques and the spatial velocity information now available using colour Doppler flow mapping combined with the high resolution velocity information of spectral Doppler ultrasound allows quantitation of such complex lesions to a degree not previously possible even with conventional catheter investigation.

Right ventricular outflow tract obstruction

The general principles applied to serial right ventricular outflow tract obstruction are also relevant to similar obstructions occurring across the left ventricular outflow tract. Teirstein et al described the application of the Bernoulli equation across irregular, dual, and tunnel-like obstructions[27] and demonstrated that Doppler ultrasound accurately predicted the pressure gradient across tunnels with cross-sectional areas as small as 0.25 cm^2. In the case of tunnel lengths greater than 3 cm or tunnel cross-sectional areas below 0.25 cm^2, however, Doppler derived pressure gradients significantly underestimated the manometer derived pressure gradients.

In a clinical study of infundibular pulmonary stenosis[28] accurate estimation of the measured pressure drop across the obstruction has been obtained using continuous wave Doppler ultrasound and application of the modified Bernoulli equation. In this study a variation of 20 mmHg between the Doppler derived pressure gradient and that measured by catheterisation was not uncommon although this was not usually considered to be of any clinical significance in individual patients. Nevertheless it does suggest that the pressure/flow relationships across tunnel-like obstructions in the clinical situation may be quite complex. Yoganathan et al[29] have elegantly demonstrated that Doppler ultrasound can significantly 'overestimate' the measured pressure drop across tunnel-like obstructions both in vitro and in vivo. Figure 15 shows a tunnel-like obstruction in series with a non-stenotic valve, a situation seen with infundibular pulmonary stenosis. The maximum pressure drop in this outflow tract obstruction occurs across the tunnel and the pressure gradient across the tunnel plus valve is less than across the tunnel alone. This paradox is explained by flow expansion distal to the tunnel, with decrease in flow velocity and partial pressure recovery. This pressure recovery continues up to and

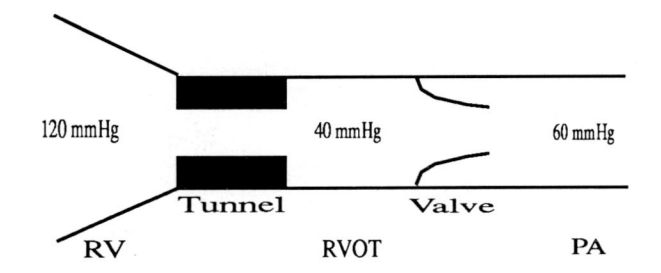

Fig. 15 Diagram of serial subvalve tunnel, and an unobstructed valve in right ventricular outflow tract obstruction. The measured pressure difference across the tunnel obstruction is greater than that across the total because of a degree of pressure recovery distal to the valve.

beyond the level of the valve such that distal to the valve the measured pressure will actually be higher than between the tunnel and valve. Pressure recovery will be incomplete because of energy losses due to turbulence and viscous friction and so the pressure proximal to the tunnel obstruction will still be higher than that distal to the valve. In other words, there will still be a significant pressure gradient across the total obstruction. Continuous wave Doppler ultrasound has no depth resolution and will measure the maximum velocity wherever it occurs and will thus allow estimation of the maximum pressure gradient, in this example the one across the tunnel. Cardiac catheterisation will frequently be used to measure the pressure proximal to the tunnel within the right ventricle and distal to the valve in a region where significant pressure recovery may already have occurred. This pressure gradient will therefore be lower than that predicted by continuous wave Doppler examination.

Continuous wave Doppler ultrasound does not overestimate the maximum pressure gradient in tunnel-like obstructions, but invasive catheter pressure measurements may significantly underestimate the true maximum pressure gradient. In some cases this underestimation may be as much as 40%.[29] Cardiac catheterisation may miss important physiological information in serial obstruction unless extreme care is taken with measurements and apparent overestimation of pressure gradient by Doppler ultrasound in this situation should never be discounted as erroneous. Since continuous wave Doppler examination has no depth resolution, the exact origin of the maximum velocity signal may not be apparent but the character of flow is different at the two sites with maximum infundibular obstruction characteristically occurring towards the end of systole and valvar obstruction occurring in mid systole. Thus, despite the lack of depth resolution with continuous wave techniques it may still be possible to separate the relative components of the serial obstruction. Figure 16 illustrates a continuous wave Doppler signal where the valve obstruction is seen as a parabolic velocity profile but the more significant infundibular obstruction is

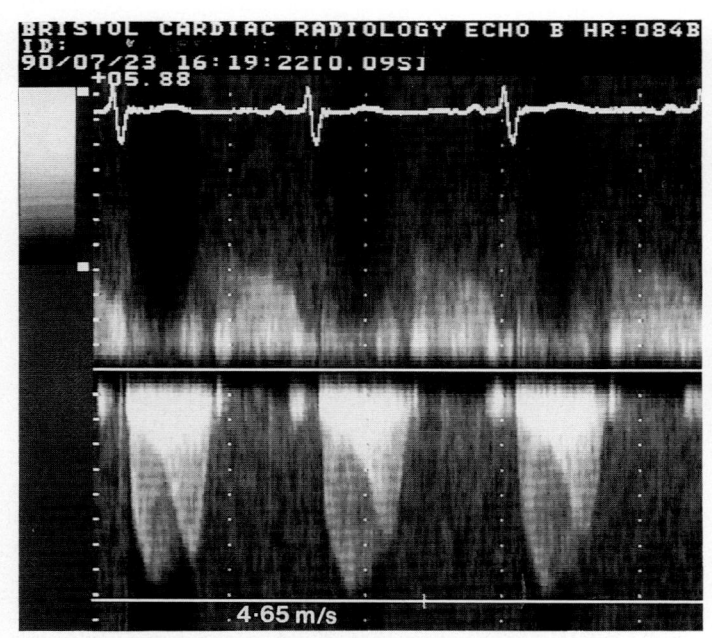

Fig. 16 Continuous wave Doppler signal of serial obstruction. A parabolic flow velocity profile of valvular obstruction is combined with a flow velocity profile maximum in late systole associated with dynamic subvalve muscular obstruction. (Dr P Wilde.)

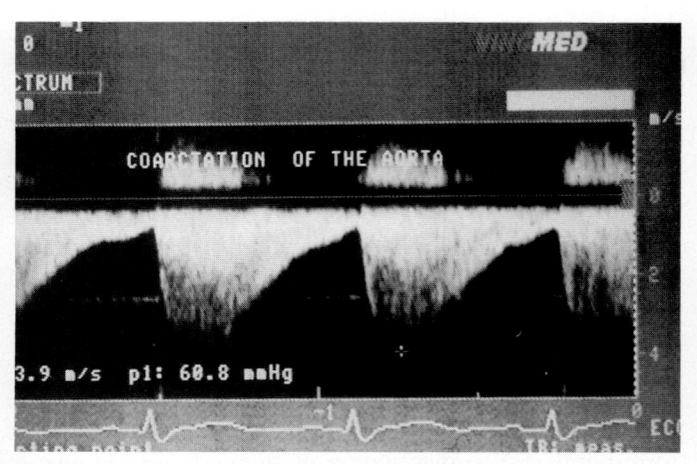

Fig. 17 Continuous wave Doppler recording of coarctation of the aorta from the suprasternal notch. High flow velocities away from the transducer are recorded in the descending aorta with a peak systolic gradient over 60 mmHg. Note that flow velocities >1 m/s persist throughout diastole.

seen as a superimposed flow velocity signal with its peak in late systole. The relative contribution of valve and subvalve obstruction can easily be distinguished.

If the site of obstruction is not readily apparent from the shape of the velocity signal then high pulse repetition frequency (HPRF) Doppler may be helpful. Colour Doppler flow mapping can now provide spatial information and may also have a valuable quantitative role to play in serial obstruction in its own right.

Coarctation of the aorta

Doppler techniques can be used to provide quantitative information about the severity of coarctation of the aorta. This lesion is often a tunnel-like obstruction and therefore concerns about the application of the Bernoulli equation are also relevant to this lesion. Continuous wave Doppler signals of coarctation are usually obtained from the suprasternal notch or occasionally from the upper sternal borders. The pattern of velocities on the spectral Doppler display can be quite characteristic (Fig. 17). There is a high velocity systolic signal with a gradual decrease in velocity throughout diastole such that high velocities are often seen throughout diastole, with an end diastolic velocity greater than 1 m/s being quite common. The pattern of diastolic velocities in coarctation of the aorta can, however, be quite variable, and to a large extent this reflects the development of collateral flow around the site of coarctation.[30] The peak velocity obtained from continuous wave Doppler examination will reflect the peak systolic pressure gradient across the coarctation but actual results suggest that this relationship is less accurate in this clinical setting than might be anticipated[30] and is certainly worse than the correlation between Doppler and invasive measurements in discrete valve obstruction. This may be due, in part, to the nature of the tunnel-like obstruction. Other workers have suggested that the relationship is considerably improved when the velocity proximal to the coarctation is taken into account.[31]

Coarctation of the aorta presents additional problems in terms of quantitation. Even if the pressure difference across the coarctation can be accurately estimated by Doppler techniques, this pressure difference will be highly dependent on the presence and extent of collateral vessels and may not reflect the true anatomical severity of the coarctation. Although a high pressure gradient will determine the presence of a significant coarctation, at least in older infants and children, the absence of a high velocity may not exclude the presence of severe coarctation because of extensive collateralisation.

In the neonatal period, confusion may arise between severe coarctation and aortic arch interruption if there is right to left shunting through a restrictive ductus arteriosus.[30] Flow through a restrictive ductus arteriosus may produce a high velocity signal away from the transducer which can be misinterpreted as a coarctation, particularly if stand-alone (non-imaging) continuous wave Doppler examination is used to obtain a satisfactory signal from the suprasternal notch.

Colour Doppler flow mapping can be extremely useful for defining the origin of high velocity flow signals in this situation. Colour flow mapping may also be useful for quantitation in coarctation of the aorta,[32] by using the colour flow diameter at the coarctation site and also by applying digital computer analysis to the flow velocity zone proximal to the coarctation.

PROBLEMS AND PITFALLS OF PRESSURE GRADIENT ESTIMATION

It is worthwhile summarising some of the potential causes of underestimation or overestimation of pressure gradients by Doppler ultrasound as knowledge of these is of paramount importance for the practical applications of quantitative Doppler techniques.

Underestimation of the true pressure gradient across a stenotic valve can occur for a variety of reasons (see Table 1). The simplest reason is that the Doppler ultrasound beam fails to interrogate the high velocity jet at the site of the stenosis. This happens commonly if the ultrasound examination is difficult and precordial views are limited or if the jet is eccentric. It is more likely to occur in severe stenosis where the high velocity jet will flow through an

Table 1 Causes of gradient underestimation by Doppler ultrasound

Jet not interrogated
Significant angle of incidence
Severe obstruction resulting in significant viscous energy losses
Comparative measurements obtained under different physiological conditions

orifice with a small cross-sectional area and the Doppler beam is aiming for a small target. If the ultrasound beam is positioned beside the jet rather than within the body of the jet then underestimation of velocity will occur. If there is a significant angle of incidence between the ultrasound beam and the direction of jet flow then the maximum velocity, and hence the pressure gradient, will be underestimated. Energy losses due to viscous friction are usually significant only through extremely small orifices or through long tunnel-like orifices but in these cases the measured maximum velocity may be an underestimation of the true maximum pressure drop. Apparent underestimation can also occur if Doppler ultrasound measurements are compared with inappropriate catheter derived measurements.

Overestimation of pressure gradient is also an important consideration in the quantitative application of Doppler ultrasound (Table 2). As mentioned above, apparent overestimation may occur with serial obstructions where the maximum pressure gradient and hence the maximum velocity occurs between the two obstructions. Invasive pressure measurements across the total obstruction at cardiac catheterisation will therefore not reflect the true maximum pressure drop occurring between the obstructions. Similarly, if there is a significant recovery of pressure distal to a tunnel-like obstruction, then cardiac catheterisation may underestimate the true maximum pressure drop if the distal pressure is measured at some distance from the obstruction.

Table 2 Causes of gradient overestimation by Doppler ultrasound

Serial obstruction
Invasive measurements obtained downstream after significant pressure recovery
Peak-to-peak versus peak instantaneous pressure measurements
Effects of sedation or other physiological variables during invasive pressure measurement
Ignoring significant velocity proximal to obstruction

In patients with aortic stenosis, peak-to-peak withdrawal gradients are often measured at cardiac catheterisation yet Doppler ultrasound will measure the peak instantaneous maximum gradient which can result in apparent overestimation of pressure gradient by the continuous wave Doppler technique. Doppler derived pressure gradients and those obtained on different occasions. The Doppler derived gradient obtained at an outpatient visit may be considerably higher than one obtained at cardiac catheterisation under sedation.

Finally, the use of the most simplified Bernoulli equation of $4 V^2$ ignores the velocity of flow proximal to an obstruction. If this flow is significantly elevated because of an increased cardiac output or the pressure of significant valve regurgitation then the maximum velocity obtained distal to the obstruction will overestimate the true pressure gradient. When applying the Bernoulli equation, the velocity of flow proximal to an obstruction should always be checked and if this is elevated above 1 m/s it should be included in the Bernoulli equation to obtain an accurate estimation of pressure gradient.

When all these factors are taken into account and Doppler ultrasound is performed with knowledge of these associated problems and pitfalls then accurate quantitative and clinically valuable measurements can be achieved non-invasively in the vast majority of patients providing care is taken to obtain the highest quality Doppler information.

QUANTITATIVE COLOUR DOPPLER FLOW MAPPING

Since the introduction of colour Doppler flow mapping it has rapidly become established as a valuable qualitative imaging technique. It can also enhance the quantitative aspects of spectral Doppler studies by aiding alignment of the continuous wave Doppler ultrasound beam with the direction of jet flow. Quantitative aspects of Doppler ultrasound examination, however, are no longer confined to spectral Doppler as there is considerable potential for quantitation of the vast amount of spatial flow velocity information inherent in colour flow map images.

In its simplest form quantitative colour flow mapping can be performed by measuring the diameter of colour flow jets or their spatial distribution. Colour flow diameter can provide additional quantitative information in patients with a ventricular septal defect[33] or coarctation of the aorta.[34]

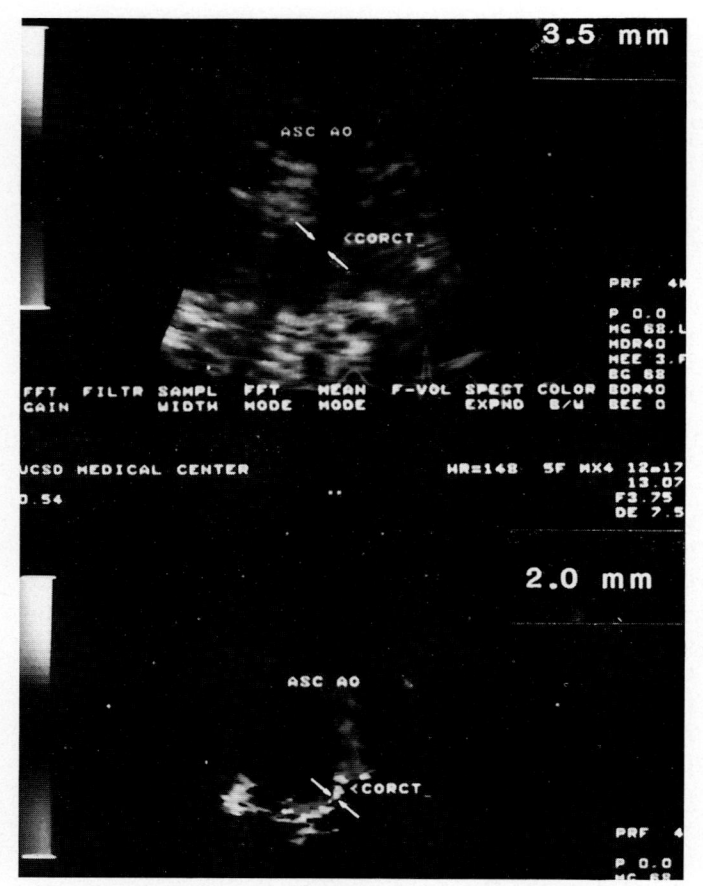

Plate 2 Two dimensional echo image (top) and colour Doppler flow map image (bottom) from a patient with coarctation of the aorta. The colour flow diameter was identical to that measured on magnetic resonance imaging and at surgery but two-dimensional imaging alone significantly underestimated the anatomical severity of the lesion. (Reproduced from Simpson et al. Circulation 1988; 77: 736–744, by permission of the American Heart Association.) This figure is reproduced in colour in the colour plate section at the front of this volume.

In these cases it probably provides more accurate information about the anatomical size of the defect than two-dimensional imaging alone (Plate 2).

Spectral Doppler techniques already provide accurate quantitation of stenotic lesions and so it is in the quantitative assessment of valve regurgitation that colour Doppler flow mapping probably has its greatest potential. With the introduction of colour Doppler flow mapping, the spatial distribution of regurgitant jets was seen as an obvious way to quantitate valve regurgitation yet the initial enthusiasm for this was somewhat tempered by disappointing results demonstrating that colour Doppler flow mapping was at best semi-quantitative.[35-37] Quantitation of regurgitation from the spatial distribution of regurgitant jets was improved by looking at orthogonal imaging planes[38] or by looking at changes in mitral regurgitation rather than absolute volume.[39] Accurate quantitation of the volume of regurgitation is not possible by simply measuring the spatial distribution of colour jets and this has prompted investigation of the display characteristics of colour Doppler flow mapping. The size of regurgitant jets imaged by colour Doppler flow mapping can be greatly affected by varying haemodynamic conditions as well as a number of instrumentation factors and this has led to an improved understanding of colour Doppler flow mapping, forming a basis for quantitation of these images.

Basic principles of colour quantitation

The major advantage of colour Doppler flow mapping over conventional spectral Doppler is its ability to provide spatial flow velocity information. Velocities can be identified in relation to structural detail and also in relation to adjacent velocity information. Colour Doppler flow mapping utilises the technique of autocorrelation rather than the more time consuming Fourier transform spectral analysis to estimate flow velocity information within a colour flow pixel. Because the image can contain several thousand pixels there is not enough time available to perform spectral analysis whilst maintaining real-time imaging. Autocorrelation does allow spatial flow velocity information to be displayed in real-time but this involves a loss of accuracy in velocity determination. Colour Doppler flow mapping is still a form of pulsed Doppler technique and is therefore subject to the physical limitations imposed on any pulsed wave Doppler examination. The maximum velocity that can be resolved by colour Doppler flow mapping prior to the onset of aliasing is determined by the transducer frequency and the pulse repetition frequency.

Typically, there may be 32 colour assignments for flow velocities towards the transducer which are displayed as increasing colour intensities of red and 32 colour assignments for flow velocities away from the transducer, displayed as increasing colour intensities of blue. These colour intensities and the maximum or Nyquist velocity limit will be displayed as a colour calibration bar on colour flow map images (Plate 3). The number of possible velocity answers up to the Nyquist velocity limit is thus limited and therefore the velocity resolution of colour Doppler flow mapping is not as good as single sample spectral pulsed Doppler. Nevertheless the velocity difference between colour assignments may be as small as 1 or 2 cm/s which is unlikely to be significant for clinical purposes. It is thus possible to obtain velocity information for individual colour pixels by utilising the information provided on the colour calibration bar. Some systems introduce a third colour, green, to designate areas of turbulent or other complex flow.

Quantitative velocity determination from colour Doppler flow map images can be performed by digital computer analysis of the colour flow map images, decoding the colour image into its red, blue and green components. The colour intensitites can be calibrated against the colour bar to

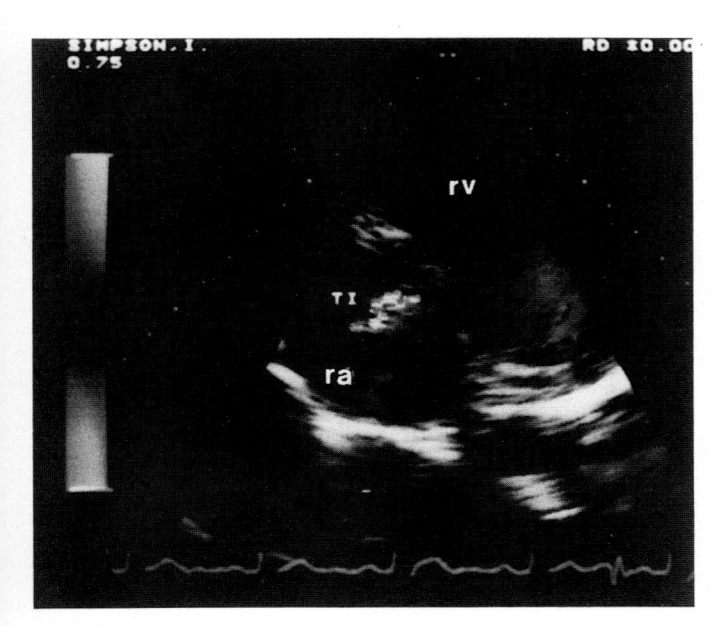

DOPPLER QUANTITATION — PRESSURE DROP ESTIMATION 99

Plate 3 Colour Doppler flow map image of the author's own physiological tricuspid regurgitation. Note the colour calibration bar at the left of the image with a Nyquist velocity limit for both red (towards) and blue (away) flow of 0.75 m/s (displayed above the colour bar). This figure is reproduced in colour in the colour plate section at the front of this volume.

designate an actual velocity to each colour pixel. This can be performed throughout the entire colour flow map image to provide a digital velocity map rather than a colour display (Fig. 18). The individual colour components of each pixel can be decoded and calibrated against the on-screen colour calibration bar. This provides digital maps for the red, blue and green pixel components for the same spatial distribution as the colour flow image (Fig. 19). The numerical values are absolute numbers of colour intensity and relate to velocity values dependent on the maximum or Nyquist velocity limit. That is, the same colour intensity may relate to a different velocity value for a different Nyquist velocity. This altered Nyquist velocity limit will be displayed on the colour calibration bar for each pulse repetition frequency or transducer frequency and this is used for appropriate calibration.

Accurate velocity estimation can be achieved up to the maximum Nyquist velocity limit using this method but beyond this, as the maximum velocity is exceeded, aliasing will occur. When colour Doppler flow aliasing occurs because the Nyquist limit is exceeded the highest red value changes to the highest value of blue or vice versa (Plate 4). Higher velocities will be displayed as decreasing intensities of colour which finally increase again in intensities of the original colour. Therefore a particular colour intensity of red may represent a non-aliased velocity value or a higher velocity multiple resulting from one or more aliases above the Nyquist velocity limit. Aliasing is a significant problem with single sample spectral pulsed Doppler as it limits the maximum velocity that can be measured. Aliasing with colour Doppler flow mapping can be advantageous, however, as its presence is a rapid visual indication of the presence of abnormal flow. It also allows quantitative information about the spatial changes of velocity within the heart to be obtained more easily by combining the pattern of aliasing with the rational sequence of colour changes resulting from increasing velocity values.

With single sample spectral pulsed Doppler, the number of aliases is usually impossible to determine and the true velocity value of an individual pixel of high velocity flow is unknown. Since colour Doppler flow mapping displays the spatial pattern of aliasing, and therefore the change in velocity over a portion of the colour Doppler flow map image, the potential exists to determine the extent of aliasing. In other words, it may be possible to 'unwrap' colour aliasing by looking at the sequence of colour changes occurring from one point in the image to another. As flow accelerates towards a stenotic orifice it will change from a low velocity value proximal to the stenosis to a high velocity value at the vena contracta of the orifice. This so-called convective or spatial acceleration will occur progressively towards the stenosis and the colour Doppler flow map should therefore demonstrate the rational sequence of colour change that relates to this increasing

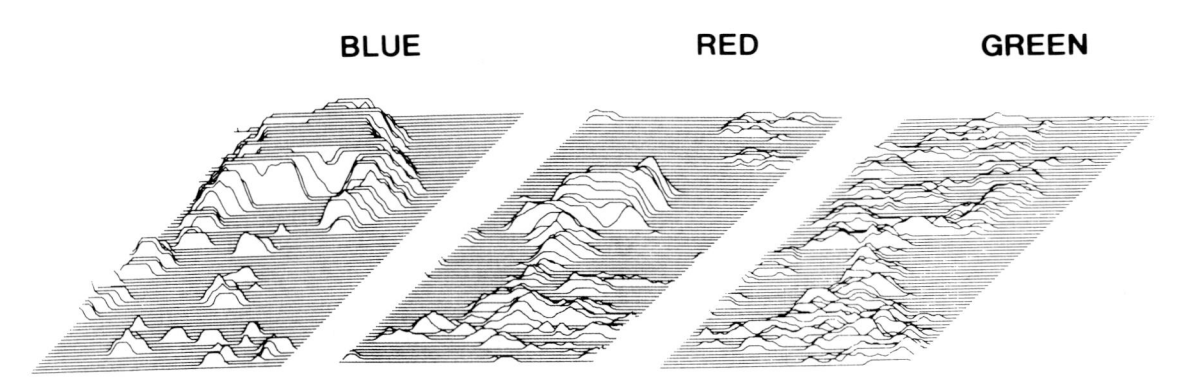

BLUE   **RED**   **GREEN**

Fig. 18 Digital velocity map displayed as a pseudo three dimensional map for the blue, red and green components of the colour image shown in Plate 6. The height of the 'mountain peaks' corresponds to the individual colour intensities.

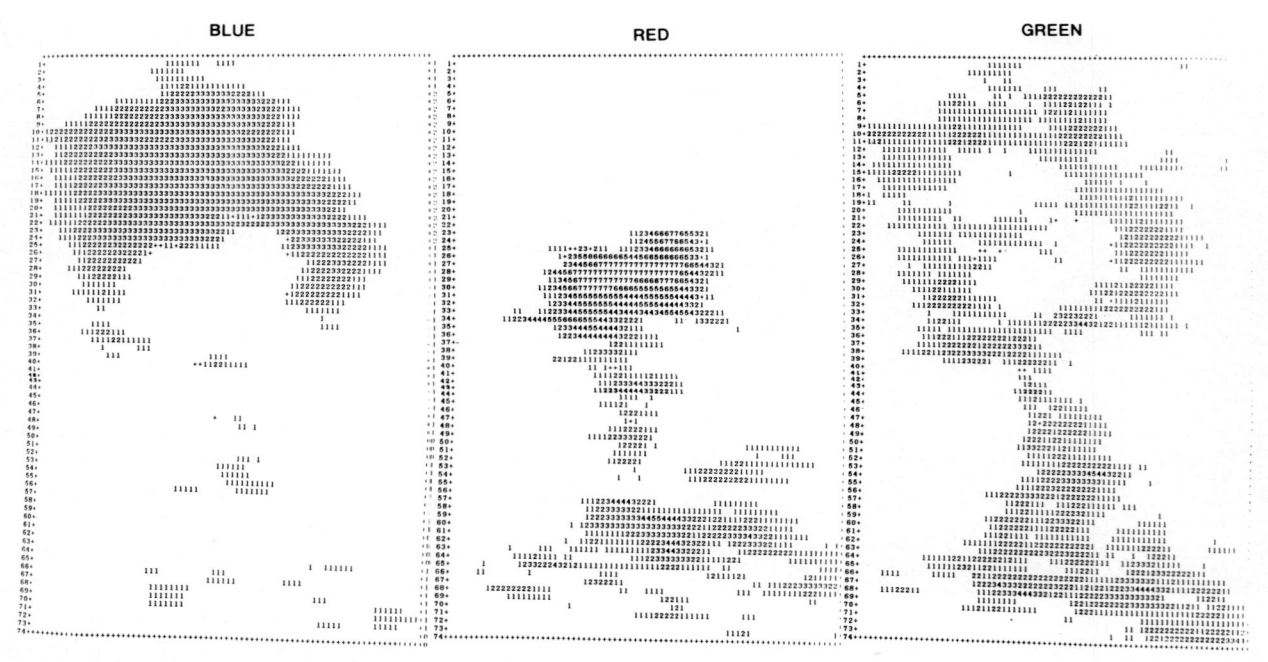

Fig. 19 Numerical velocity map identical to that in Fig. 18 but displaying digital information for each pixel rather than a height above the baseline. The digital information can then be used to provide quantitative spatial velocity information for a portion of the colour display or for the entire spatial distribution of the jet.

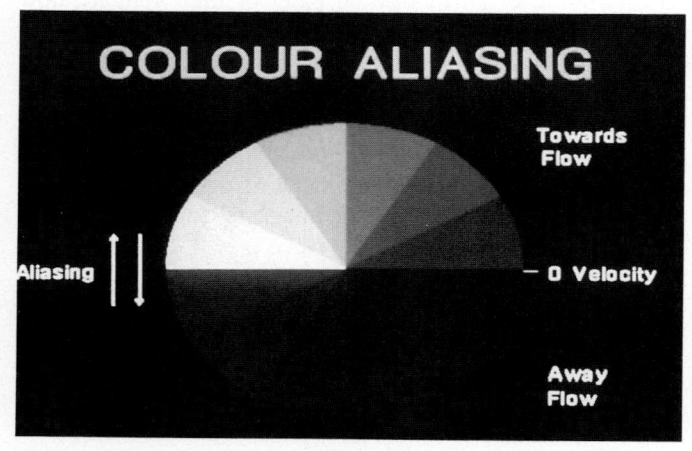

Plate 4 Diagram to illustrate the effect of colour aliasing. As flow velocities away from the transducer (display as increasing colour intensities of blue) exceed the Nyquist velocity limit an alias to the highest red value will occur producing apparent directionally opposite colour encoding. Similarly flow towards the transducer which exceeds the maximum velocity limit will alias from increasing colours of red to the highest blue value with further velocity increases towards the transducer being displayed as decreasing colours of blue eventually aliasing again back to increasing colours of red. This figure is reproduced in colour in the colour plate section at the front of this volume.

velocity. Plate 5 demonstrates the flow acceleration that occurs proximal to an obstruction imaged by colour flow mapping. Since it is known that flow is towards the transducer in this example, the initial low velocity flow will be seen as increasing intensities of red. As flow continues to accelerate towards the orifice (and towards the transducer) an alias to the highest blue value will occur, with continuing acceleration identified as decreasing blue values. Even closer to the orifice the increasing velocity values will be seen as a further alias back to the lowest value of red and so on, up to the maximum velocity occurring at the vena contracta of the orifice. It is only possible to determine the increases in velocity from the rational sequence of colour changes because we can visualise velocity values all the way up to the orifice. The colour pixels to be decoded into their digital red, blue and green components using digital computer analysis and actual velocity values for each individual colour pixel can be obtained. Quantitative determinations can be made not only of individual velocities but also of the change in velocity or acceleration over a portion of the colour flow map image, the so-called spatial flow acceleration.

With the velocity-variance colour flow map algorithms that are currently available in most colour flow systems, green is added to the primary velocity colours of red and blue, as a function of the range or variation of velocities occurring within the colour pixel (Plate 6). This statistical variation in velocity or 'variance' does to some extent reflect the presence of turbulent flow although there are many other factors that can affect the display of variance. Quantitative analysis of colour flow map images can provide information about the spatial distribution of this variance and, as with the red and blue velocity information,

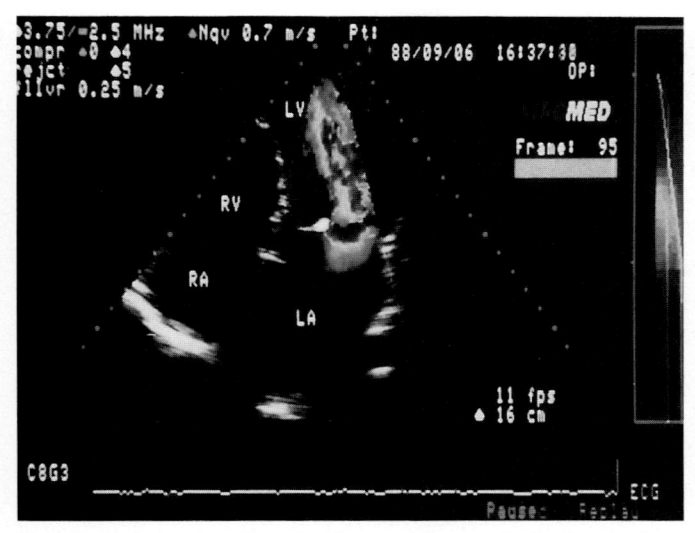

Plate 5 **Apical colour Doppler flow map image of mitral stenosis imaged using a velocity-variance colour flow map algorithm.** Green is added to one side of the colour calibration bar such that high velocity, turbulent flow has green added to the red and blue velocity assignment. Distal to the mitral stenosis within the left ventricle, there is a considerable display of green rapidly identifying the presence and spatial distribution of abnormal flow. The region of acceleration towards the stenotic valve is clearly seen in the left atrium. This figure is reproduced in colour in the colour plate section at the front of this volume.

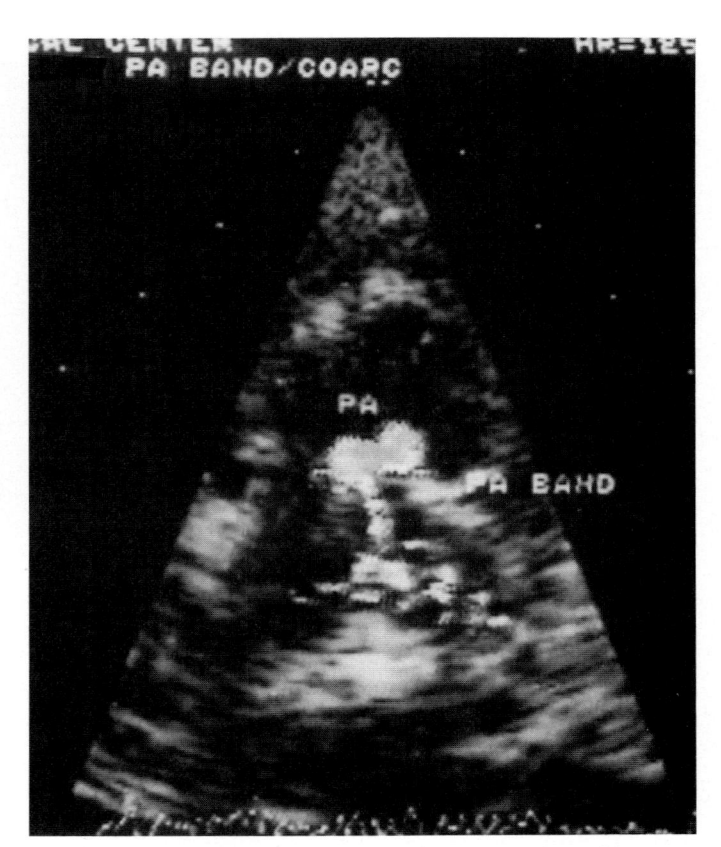

Plate 6 **Colour Doppler flow map image from a patient with a pulmonary artery band.** As flow accelerates away from the transducer towards the band in the main pulmonary artery, this spatial acceleration is identified by a rational sequence of colour changes. Increasing colours of blue alias to the highest red value with decreasing values of red nearer the orifice indicating continued spatial acceleration. Distal to the obstruction a multi-colour mosaic pattern with high green values indicates the presence of high velocity, turbulent flow. This figure is reproduced in colour in the colour plate section at the front of this volume.

it can be assigned a numerical value which relates to the intensity of green within the colour pixel. It may prove possible to provide quantitative information about the turbulence caused by a particular lesion as well as identifying its distribution. With increasingly sophisticated technology and image analysis quantitative aspects of variance displays may eventually provide valuable and clinically useful information but this is not yet available.

Clinical applications of colour flow quantitation

Serial obstruction

Quantitation of colour flow map images is currently most valuable in complex flow situations such as serial outflow tract obstruction. It is also useful in lesions such as mitral regurgitation where current methods of quantitation have proved disappointing. Quantitative aspects of colour Doppler flow mapping are still rapidly expanding. In serial outflow tract obstruction, quantitative colour Doppler flow mapping yields some interesting results.[40] Firstly, the zone of proximal flow acceleration within the outflow tract can be identified easily (see Plate 5) and in-vitro investigation has demonstrated that the length of the zone of proximal flow acceleration is dependent on the pressure gradient across the obstruction. In addition the rate of spatial flow acceleration in cm/s^{-2} can be calculated from the digital velocity maps described above. The maximum rate of spatial flow acceleration proximal to a subvalve obstruction is, to a large extent, related to the anatomical severity of obstruction. Potentially, colour Doppler flow mapping may be able to determine the relative severity of subvalve obstruction and provide quantitative information even in situations where adequate continuous wave Doppler signals cannot be obtained.

Valve regurgitation

Quantitation of aortic regurgitation is fraught with difficulty. Colour Doppler flow mapping has taught us that the jet of aortic regurgitation invariably mixes with mitral inflow and separation of the spatial distribution of flow resulting purely from aortic regurgitation becomes impossible. As a result, the majority of work related to quantitative colour Doppler flow mapping has concentrated on mitral valve regurgitation. It quickly became apparent that the spatial distribution of mitral regurgitant jets imaged by colour Doppler flow mapping did not provide accurate quantitation and subsequent research work was directed towards investigating the haemodynamic determinants of colour jets, using more sophisticated analysis techniques in an attempt to extract important quantitative information. The spatial distribution of regurgitant jets on colour flow mapping is highly dependent on flow rate rather than the volume of regurgitation[41,42] and under pulsatile flow conditions, the velocity or driving pressure regurgitation is the single most important factor in determining spatial jet distribution. Indeed, using the conventional velocity-variance colour flow algorithms, colour encoding of regurgitant jets is almost independent of volume[42] down to the small, critical volume necessary for any colour encoding.

Digital computer analysis of colour flow map images allows estimation of jet kinetic energy[42,43] and momentum analysis of colour jets[44] and in vitro optical visualisation studies have enhanced our understanding of factors influencing the structure of these jets.[45] However, accurate clinical quantitation of mitral regurgitant volume remains elusive. The development of newer colour flow map algorithms such as the power mode which encode colour not only on the basis of velocity but also, to a large extent, on the amplitude of the Doppler signal, may hold some promise for quantitation of volume flow.[42] At present colour Doppler flow mapping of mitral regurgitation remains a semi-quantitative technique[46] but clinically useful quantitative information from colour Doppler flow mapping seems increasingly likely as our understanding of both colour flow mapping and the characteristics of regurgitant jets continues to improve.

It should be said that there is no simple 'gold standard' for measuring valve regurgitation volumes. Cardiac angiography is the standard taken by most clinicians but this technique, in spite of its invasive nature, is at best only semi-quantitative and at worse is misleading.

CONCLUSIONS

Quantitative Doppler techniques have provided the basis for the acceptance of Doppler ultrasound and promoted its routine use in clinical cardiology. The ability to predict the severity of an obstruction noninvasively using the modified Bernoulli equation has allowed accurate serial quantitation of mitral and aortic stenosis in adults, right ventricular outflow tract obstruction in children, and can provide a method for predicting pulmonary artery systolic pressure. The application of quantitative Doppler techniques has also made us reassess the accuracy of traditional 'gold standard' measurements such as cardiac catheterisation and has led to a widespread understanding of the physiological basis of jet formation within the heart and its relation to pressure gradients. Continuous wave Doppler ultrasound is firmly established as a valuable quantitative technique in adult and paediatric cardiology and now colour Doppler flow mapping with its spatially accurate flow velocity information, has added a new dimension to quantitative Doppler ultrasound. Ever advancing technology combined with an improved basic understanding of the hydrodynamics of cardiac flow, will continue to enhance our abilities to provide valuable quantitative information about the haemodynamic effects of cardiac pathology using a combination of spectral Doppler ultrasound and colour Doppler flow mapping.

REFERENCES

1 Holen J, Aaslid R, Landmaker K, Simonsen S. Determination of pressure gradient in mitral stenosis with a non-invasive ultrasound Doppler technique. Acta Med Scand 1976; 199: 455–460
2 Hatle L, Brubakk A, Tromsdal A, Angelsen B. Non-invasive assessment of pressure drop in mitral stenosis by Doppler ultrasound. Br Heart J 1978; 40: 131–140
3 Bernoulli D. Hydrodynamics. Translated from Latih (1968). Dover Publications, New York
4 Yoganathan A P, Cape E G, Sung H W, Williams F P, Jimoh A. Review of hydrodynamic principles for the cardiologist: applications to the study of blood flow and jets by imaging techniques. J Am Coll Cardiol 1988; 12: 1344–1353
5 Shames I H. Mechanics of fluids. 2nd Ed. McGraw-Hill, New York, 1982; 192
6 Caro C G, Pedley T J, Schroter R C, Seed W A. The Mechanics of the Circulation. Oxford University Press, Oxford 1978; 54–56
7 Yoganathan A P, Recusani F, Valdes-Cruz L M, Sung H W, Sahn D J. Oblique flow vectors from dispersing jets produce the velocity overestimation on angle-corrected continuous wave Doppler studies: in vitro laser Doppler investigations. Circulation 1987; 76, Suppl IV: IV-355 (Abstract)
8 Hatle L, Angelsen B. Doppler ultrasound in cardiology: physical principles and clinical applications. Lea and Febiger, Philadelphia, 1985, pp 126–128
9 Hatle L, Angelsen B A, Tramsdal A. Non-invasive assessment of aortic stenosis by Doppler ultrasound. Br Heart J 1980; 43: 284–292
10 Lima C O, Sahn D J, Valdes-Cruz L M, Allen H D, Goldberg S J, Grenadier E, Vargas Barron J. Prediction of the severity of left ventricular outflow tract obstruction by quantitative two-dimensional echocardiographic Doppler studies. Circulation 1983; 68: 348–354
11 Stamm B R, Martin R P. Quantification of pressure gradients across stenotic valves by Doppler ultrasound. J Am Coll Cardiol 1984; 2: 707–718
12 Berger M, Berdoff R L, Gallerstein P E, Goldberg E. Evaluation of aortic stenosis by continuous wave Doppler ultrasound. J Am Coll Cardiol 1984; 3: 150–156
13 Simpson I A, Houston A B, Sheldon C D, Hutton I, Lawrie T D V. Clinical value of Doppler echocardiography in adults with aortic stenosis. Br Heart J 1985; 53: 636–639
14 Currie P J, Seward J B, Reeder G S et al. Continuous wave Doppler echocardiographic assessment of severity of calcific aortic stenosis: a simultaneous Doppler-catheter correlative study in 100 adult patients. Circulation 1985; 71: 1162–1169
15 Hegrenaes L, Hatle L. Aortic stenosis in adults: non-invasive estimation of pressure differences by continuous wave Doppler echocardiography. Br Heart J 1985; 54: 396–604

16 Otto C M, Pearlman A S, Gardner C L. Hemodynamic progression of aortic stenosis in adults assessed by Doppler echocardiography. J Am Coll Cardiol 1989; 13: 545–550
17 Ohlsson J, Wranne B. Noninvasive assessment of valve area in patients with aortic stenosis. J Am Coll Cardiol 1986; 7: 501–508
18 Teirstein P, Yeager M, Yock P G, Popp R L. Doppler echocardiographic measurement of aortic valve area in aortic stenosis: a noninvasive application of the Gorlin formula. J Am Coll Cardiol 1986; 8: 1059–1065
19 Otto C M, Pearlman A S, Comess K A, Reamer R P, Janko C L, Huntsman L L. Determination of the stenotic aortic valve area in adults using Doppler echocardiography. J Am Coll Cardiol 1986; 7: 509–517
20 Skjaerpe T, Hegrenaes L, Hatle L. Noninvasive estimation of valve area in patients with aortic stenosis by Doppler ultrasound and two-dimensional echocardiography. Circulation 1985; 72: 810–818
21 Hatle L, Angelsen B, Tromsdal A. Noninvasive assessment of atrioventricular pressure half-time by Doppler ultrasound. Circulation 1979; 60: 1096–1104
22 Simpson I A, Reece I J, Houston A B, Hutton I, Wheatley D J, Cobbe S M. Noninvasive assessment by Doppler ultrasound of 155 patients with bioprosthetic valves: a comparison of the Wessex porcine, low profile Ionescu Shiley and Hancock pericardial bioprostheses. Br Heart J 1986; 56: 83–88
23 Hatle L, Angelsen B. Doppler ultrasound in cardiology: physical principles and clinical applications. Lea and Febiger, Philadelphia, 1985; pp 151–153
24 Pye M, Weerasana N, Bain W H, Hutton I, Cobbe S M. Doppler echocardiographic characteristics of normal and dysfunctioning prosthetic valves in the tricuspid and mitral position. Br Heart J 1990; 63: 41–44
25 Lima C O, Sahn D J, Valdes-Cruz L M et al. Non invasive prediction of transvalvular pressure gradients in patients with pulmonary stenosis by quantitative two-dimensional echocardiographic Doppler studies. Circulation 1983; 67: 866–871
26 Houston A B, Sheldon C D, Simpson I A, Doig W B, Coleman E N. The severity of pulmonary valve and artery obstruction in children estimated by Doppler ultrasound. Eur Heart J 1985; 6: 786–790
27 Teirstein P S, Yock P G, Popp R L. The accuracy of Doppler ultrasound measurement of pressure gradients across irregular, dual, and tunnel-like obstructions to blood flow. Circulation 1985; 72: 577–584
28 Houston A B, Simpson I A, Sheldon C D, Doig W B, Coleman E N. Doppler ultrasound in the estimation of the severity of pulmonary infundibular stenosis in infants and children. Br Heart J 1986; 55: 381–384
29 Yoganathan A P, Valdez-Cruz L M, Schmidt-Dohna J, Jimoh A, Berry C, Tamura T, Sahn D J. Continuous-wave Doppler velocities and gradients across fixed tunnel obstructions: studies in vitro and in vivo. Circulation 1987; 76: 657–666
30 Houston A B, Simpson I A, Pollock J C S,. Jamieson M P G, Doig W B, Coleman E N. Doppler ultrasound in the assessment of severity of coarctation of the aorta and interruption of the aortic arch. Br Heart J 1987; 57: 38–43
31 Marx G R, Allen H D. Accuracy and pitfalls of Doppler evaluation of the pressure gradient in aortic coarctation. J Am Coll Cardiol 1986; 7: 1379–1385
32 Simpson I A, Sahn D J, Valdes-Cruz L M, Chung K J, Sherman F S, Swensson R E. Color Doppler flow mapping in patients with coarctation of the aorta: new observations and improved evaluation with color flow diameter and proximal acceleration as predictors of severity. Circulation 1988; 77: 736–744
33 Hornberger L K, Sahn D J, Krabill K A et al. Elucidation of the natural history of ventricular septal defects by serial Doppler color flow mapping studies. J Am Coll Cardiol 1989; 13: 1111–1118
34 Simpson I A, Sahn D J, Valdes-Cruz L M, Chung K J, Sherman F S, Swensson R E. Color Doppler flow mapping in patients with coarctation of the aorta: new observations and improved evaluation with color flow diameter and proximal acceleration as predictors of severity. Circulation 1988; 77: 736–744
35 Omoto R, Yokote Y, Takamoto S et al. The development of real-time two-dimensional Doppler echocardiography and its clinical significance in acquired valvular diseases, with specific reference to valvular regurgitation. Jpn Heart J 1984; 25: 325–340
36 Miyatake K, Okamoto M, Konoshita N et al. Clinical applications of a new type of real-time two-dimensional flow imaging system. Am J Cardiol 1984; 54: 857–868
37 Miyatake K, Izumi S, Okamoto M et al. Semi-quantitative grading of severity of mitral regurgitation by real-time two-dimensional Doppler flow imaging technique. J Am Coll Cardiol 1986; 7: 82–88
38 Helmcke F, Nanda N C, Hsuing M C et al. Color Doppler assessment of mitral regurgitation with orthogonal planes. Circulation 1987; 75: 175–183
39 Otsuji Y, Tei C, Kisanuki A, Natsugoe K, Kawazoe Y. Color Doppler echocardiographic assessment of the change in the mitral regurgitant volume. Am Heart J 1987; 114: 349–354
40 Simpson I A, Valdes-Cruz L M, Yoganathan A P, Sung H W, Jimoh A, Sahn D J. Spatial velocity distribution and acceleration in serial subvalve tunnel and valvular obstructions: an in-vitro study using Doppler color flow mapping. J Am Coll Cardiol 1989; 13: 241–248
41 Davidoff R, Wilkins G T, Thomas J D, Achorn D M, Weyman A E. Regurgitant volumes by color flow overestimate injected volumes in an in-vitro model (abst). J Am Coll Cardiol 1987; 9: 110A
42 Simpson I A, Valdes-Cruz L M, Sahn D J, Murillo A, Tamura T, Chung K J. Doppler color flow mapping of simulated in-vitro regurgitant jets: evaluation of the effects of orifice size and hemodynamic variables. J Am Coll Cardiol 1989; 13: 1195–1207
43 Bolger A F, Eigler N L, Pfaff J M, Reser K J, Maurer G. Computer analysis of Doppler color flow mapping images for quantitative assessment of in vitro fluid jets. J Am Coll Cardiol 1988; 12: 450–457
44 Thomas J D, Liu C M, Flachskampf F A, O'Shea J P, Davidoff R, Weyman A E. Quantification of jet flow by momentum analysis: an in vitro color Doppler flow study. Circulation 1990; 81: 247–259
45 Krabill K A, Sung H W, Tamura T, Chung K, Yoganathan A P, Sahn D J. Factors influencing the structure and shape of stenotic and regurgitant jets: an in vitro investigation using Doppler color flow mapping and optical flow visualisation. J Am Coll Cardiol 1989; 13: 1672–1681
46 Spain M G, Smith M D, Grayburn P A, Harlament E A, DeMaria A N. Quantitative assessment of mitral regurgitation by Doppler color flow imaging: angiographic and hemodynamic correlations. J Am Coll Cardiol 1989; 15: 585–590

Doppler quantitation – pulmonary artery pressure

Tricuspid regurgitation method
Measurement of the velocity of
tricuspid regurgitation
Calculation of right ventricle to right
atrium pressure gradient
Clinical estimation of right atrial
pressure
Alternative solutions for assessing right
atrial pressure
Lack of detectable tricuspid regurgitation
Pulmonary regurgitation method
Pulmonary forward flow method
**Right ventricular isovolumic relaxation
time method**
Conclusions

Thierry Touche

Pulmonary hypertension is observed in a wide spectrum of cardiac and pulmonary disease, and pulmonary artery pressure measurement is an important element in the assessment of cardiac and pulmonary function. Several Doppler methods for non-invasive pulmonary pressure measurement have been described during the last decade. Each method has its own limitations in terms of feasibility and/or accuracy. Mastering the various methods enables the echocardiographer to assess the pulmonary artery pressure in the vast majority of patients and to check the consistency of results provided by two or more of the different methods.

Four main methods have been reported. The tricuspid regurgitation method calculates the systolic pulmonary artery pressure, the pulmonary regurgitation method calculates the diastolic pulmonary artery pressure, the pulmonary forward flow method evaluates the mean pulmonary artery pressure and the right ventricular isovolumic relaxation time method evaluates the systolic pulmonary pressure. The normal pulmonary pressures are presented in Figure 1.

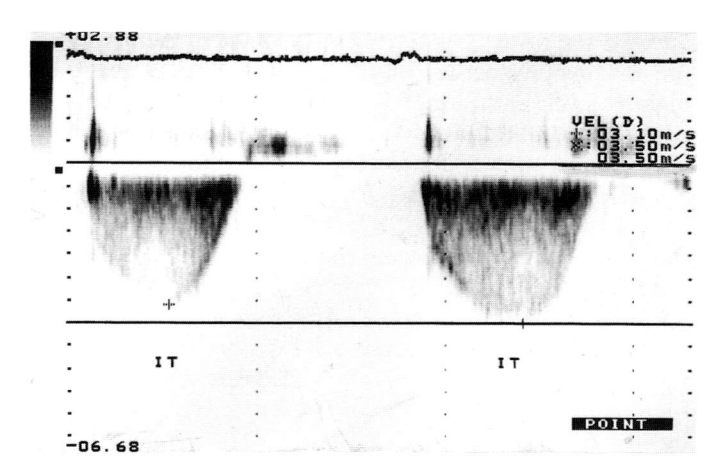

Fig. 2 **Apical continuous wave recording** of a jet of tricuspid regurgitation. The peak velocity is estimated at 3.5 m/s.

regurgitation signals are detected by the Doppler technique in a high proportion of patients with a suspicion of increased pulmonary artery pressure or an enlarged right heart as judged by clinical examination, chest X-ray or cross-sectional echocardiography.[2] Tricuspid regurgitation is also detected in a substantial percentage of normal subjects.[3]

Measurement of the velocity of tricuspid regurgitation

The examination[2] is performed using cross-sectional, continuous wave (CW) and colour flow Doppler echocardiography. The patient is positioned in the left lateral recumbent position and cross-sectional images are used to delineate the tricuspid valve from parasternal, mid-precordial, apical and/or subcostal windows (Fig. 3). Continuous wave Doppler examination is then used to seek a tricuspid regurgitant jet from these windows. The position

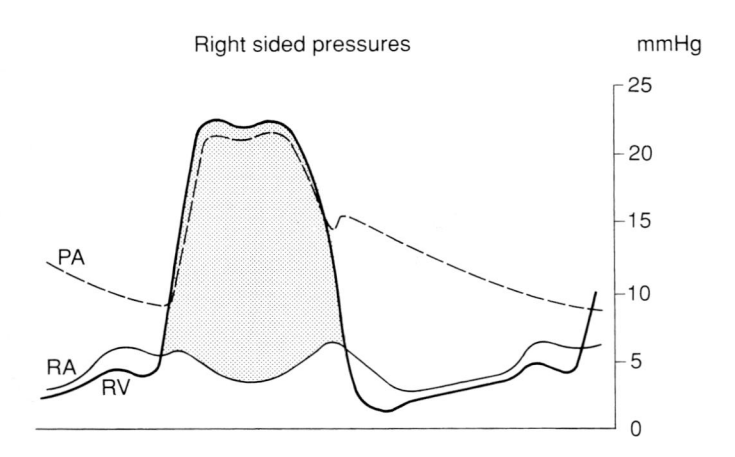

Fig. 1 Diagram of normal right heart pressures.

TRICUSPID REGURGITATION METHOD

If tricuspid regurgitation is present (Fig. 2) the pressure gradient between the right ventricle and the right atrium during systole can be estimated by measuring the maximal velocity of the regurgitant jet and applying the Bernoulli equation.[1] It has been demonstrated that right ventricular systolic pressure can be estimated reliably by addition of this pressure gradient to the right atrial pressure estimated by clinical examination.[2] If there is no significant pressure gradient across the pulmonary valve or right ventricular outflow tract, right ventricular systolic pressure is equivalent to pulmonary artery systolic pressure. Tricuspid

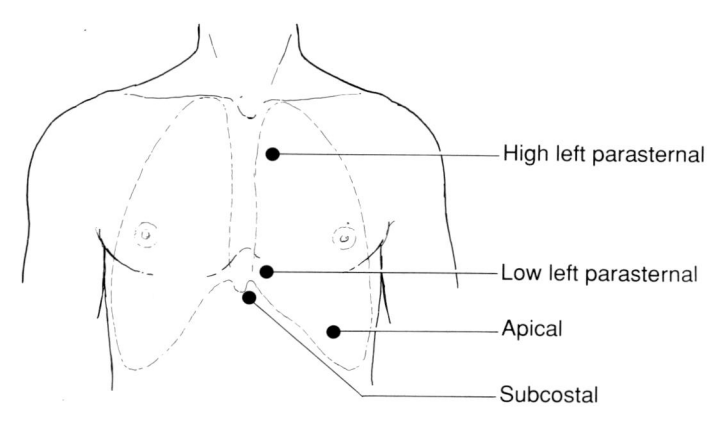

Fig. 3 Diagram showing possible precordial sites for recording tricuspid regurgitation.

selected for pressure gradient calculation is the one where the maximal velocities of the spectral display reach the highest level, indicating that the best possible alignment with flow has been obtained. A characteristic high-pitched audio signal and a dense representation of the maximal velocities of the spectral display are additional clues to an adequate alignment. Combined CW and imaging transducers shorten the time required to select the optimal position. Colour-coded Doppler mapping enables the operator to superimpose the CW beam on the axis of the colour-coded jet. The combination of both techniques on the same probe, however, often leads to compromises in the quality of each technique. If Doppler curves provided by combined probes are suboptimal, it is mandatory to switch to the small non-imaging transducer since it has both increased manoeuvrability and higher signal-to-noise ratio. When important variations of peak velocities are observed from cycle to cycle, especially in atrial fibrillation, one should average several beats. Ideally, a sequence of consecutive beats of adequate signal quality should be used.

Calculation of right ventricle to right atrium pressure gradient

The final value for the peak velocity of tricuspid regurgitation is squared and multiplied by four according to the simplified Bernoulli equation, giving the right ventricle-to-right atrium pressure gradient in mmHg. This pressure gradient correlates remarkably well with the invasive pressure gradient ($r = 0.97$), without significant underestimation or overestimation and with a small standard error (7 mmHg), according to one of the first studies.[2]

Clinical estimation of right atrial pressure

Pulmonary artery pressure determination necessitates the addition of an adequate value for right atrial pressure. Right atrial pressure or jugular pressure can be estimated clinically.[4] It is equal to the height difference between the highest level of dilatation and pulsatility of internal jugular veins and the estimated level of the centre of the right atrium (Fig. 4).

Patients are examined in a semi-sitting position at 45° elevation of the thorax and head, under adequate lighting conditions for the right side of the neck. Pulsations of the right internal jugular vein are transmitted to the sternocleidomastoid muscle and can be differentiated from arterial pulsations by simultaneous palpation of the left carotid artery. When venous pulsations are not clear, higher or lower angles of elevation of the thorax should be tried in high and low jugular venous pressures respectively. Height of jugular pulsations are measured in cm above the sternal angle. The centre of right atrium can be estimated

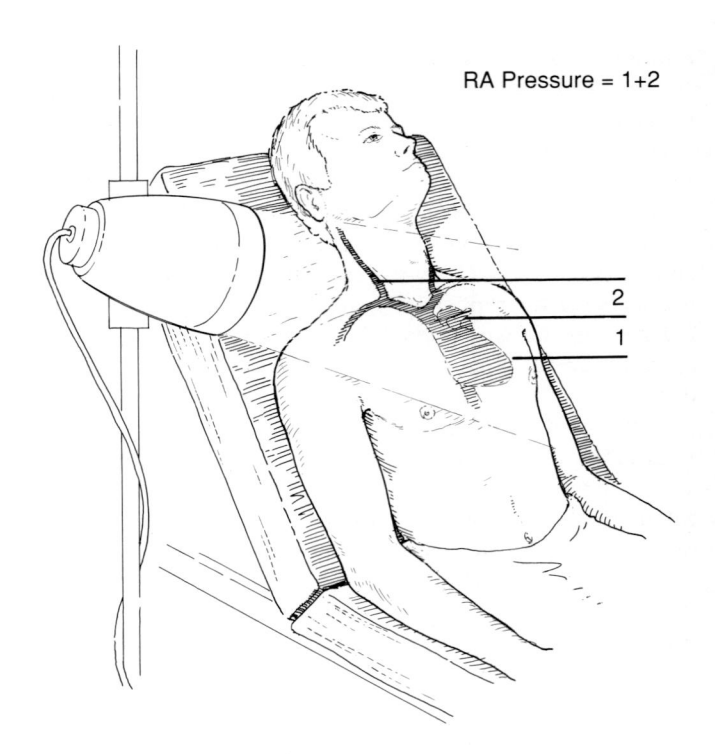

Fig. 4 Diagram illustrating the clinical method of estimating jugular venous pressure.

to be 5 cm under the sternal angle whatever the patient's size and the degree of elevation of the thorax.[4] In our personal experience one can also measure the height difference between the sternal angle and a cross-sectional imaging probe maintained in a horizontal position and located so as to visualise the right atrium. Mercury is 13 times more dense than blood at normal body temperature. Thus, the total height difference in cm divided by 1.3 gives the right atrial pressure in mmHg. The correlation between clinical and invasive right atrial pressure has been reported[2] with this method to be relatively low ($r = 0.80$). In the same study, however, the standard error of the estimate (SEE) was small (2 mmHg) due to the relatively low range of variation of mean right atrial pressure (1 to 24 mmHg) encountered in the population with cardiac diseases. In this same study there was an important underestimation of several high right atrial pressures by the clinical method. It is unclear whether or not this can be related to the decision of the authors not to take into account prominent 'V' waves in the clinical estimation of jugular venous pressure. The clinical estimation of right atrial pressure was concluded to be a significant but unavoidable source of error in pulmonary artery pressure measurement.

The overall correlation of this Doppler technique and invasive absolute pulmonary artery pressures was excellent ($r = 0.93$) with a reasonably small SEE (8 mmHg) and without significant underestimation or overestimation.

Alternative solutions for assessing right atrial pressure

More recent studies have challenged the usefulness of the clinical estimation of right atrial pressure. It has been proposed that regression equations deriving right ventricular systolic pressure solely from Doppler gradients[5,6] can be used. Alternatively, a fixed value for right atrial pressure (10 or 14 mmHg) can be taken.[5,7] In a comparative study[5] these two methods and the jugular venous pressure method correlated identically with invasive pressures (r = 0.89 to 0.90) but the regression equation method was reported to provide a more accurate result, with a negligible mean underestimation (1 mmHg). This study used two different regression equations: systolic pressure = 20 + 1.1 × Doppler gradient when right atrial pressure was over 15 mmHg and systolic pressure = 14 + Doppler gradient when right atrial pressure was below or equal to 15 mmHg. In the latter case the equation corresponds to the addition of a fixed 4 mmHg value for right atrial pressure. Thus, clinical estimation of jugular venous pressure was still necessary with this method, in order to select one of the two equations.

Another study[7] proposes the use of the same regression equation for all patients: systolic pressure = 1.23 × Doppler gradient. Such an equation implies that the higher the pulmonary artery pressure, the higher the right atrial pressure. This may be untrue in certain clinical situations. Severe right heart failure (high right atrial pressure) can occur without important pulmonary hypertension, as in constrictive pericarditis, right ventricular myocardial infarction and severe tricuspid regurgitation. Conversely severe pulmonary hypertension can be observed without any degree of right heart failure (with a normal right atrial pressure), as in the long-standing pulmonary hypertension of congenital heart disease which is well-compensated because of important right ventricular hypertrophy.

Regression equations and/or fixed values for right atrial pressure compensate not only for right atrial pressure but also for underestimation of the right ventricle-to-right atrium gradient. This is apparent when fixed values of 10 mmHg or even 14 mmHg are used in normal subjects, the normal values for right atrial pressure being 5 mmHg ± 3 mmHg.[8] The risk of suboptimal alignment may have been higher in some studies that were simultaneous to catheterisation because of a limited access to thoracic windows and limited possibilities for modifying the patient's position.

The level of right atrial pressure depends on the population that is studied. In a recent personal unpublished series of 18 patients with chronic respiratory disease and adequate tricuspid regurgitation signals, a high correlation between simultaneous invasive and Doppler pressure gradients was observed (r = 0.92, standard error = 5.4 mmHg). Only four patients had signs of right heart failure. The best estimation of pulmonary artery pressure was obtained using 15 mmHg for the right atrial pressure value in these four cases, and 5 mmHg in all the other cases.

An echocardiographic estimation of right atrial pressure has been proposed recently.[9] The method is referred to as 'sonospirometry' and it is used to study the respiratory variations in the diameter of the terminal segment of the inferior vena cava using cross-sectional imaging. The inferior vena cava fails to collapse during inspiration with increased right atrial pressure. Patients perform increasing graded sustained inspirations from 2.5 to 20 mmHg, measured on a manometer. The right atrial pressure is estimated as the inspiratory pressure required to decrease the inferior vena cava diameter to 85% or more of the difference between maximal and minimal diameters. The study suggests that useful information can also be obtained without the procedure of quantified graded inspiratory pressures. A review of the presented graphs suggests that a minimum vena cava diameter of less than 8 mm and a percent decrease on inspiration of more than 50% of the maximum diameter are almost always associated with a right atrial pressure below 10 mmHg. Conversely, a percent diameter reduction of less than 50% indicates that the right atrial pressure is over 10 mmHg. According to the same group of investigators the right atrial pressure can be approximated to 5 mmHg in the former case and to 15 mmHg in the latter case.[10] Another reason for using a 5 mmHg value in normal subjects is that the upper limit of peak tricuspid velocities in normal subjects is 2.5 m/s (slightly higher velocities can be obtained in elderly normal subjects). A peak velocity of 2.5 m/s with a 5 mmHg right atrial pressure gives a 30 mmHg systolic pulmonary artery pressure, which corresponds to the upper limit of invasive normal values.[8]

Lack of detectable tricuspid regurgitation

An obvious limitation of the method is the requirement for a detectable jet of tricuspid regurgitation. Although such a jet is frequently found in normal subjects and almost constantly found in patients with severe pulmonary hypertension and/or dilated right hearts, the tricuspid regurgitant jets can be impossible to record in certain populations of patients. A 50% failure rate has been reported in patients with severe chronic obstructive disease when pulmonary hypertension is sought at an early stage.[11] The same failure rate was observed in our personal experience with a similar population of patients. The success rate for recording the jet adequately in such patients could be increased up to 91% by the use of contrast injection to enhance the Doppler signal.[12] Obviously the drawback of such contrast studies is the necessity for a venous injection. Very high transvalvular

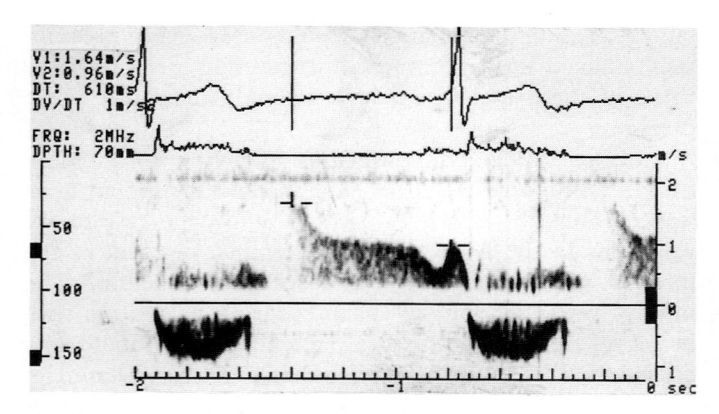

Fig. 5 Physiological pulmonary regurgitation recorded from the parasternal position. The signal is most intense in late diastole possibly due to decreasing coaptation of pulmonary valve leaflets during diastole.

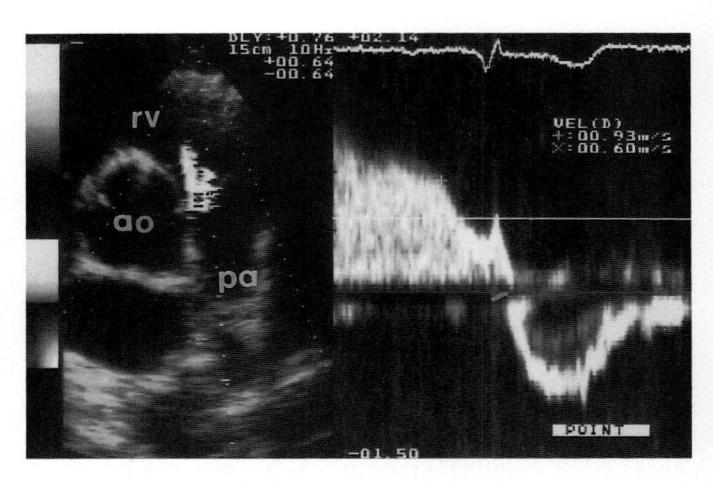

Plate 1 Colour flow Doppler illustration of pulmonary regurgitation (left) with an accompanying pulsed Doppler recording from the left parasternal position. This figure is reproduced in colour in the colour plate section at the front of this volume.

pressure gradients are generally associated with the presence of tricuspid regurgitation, probably because of annular dilatation and/or modification of the geometry and function of right ventricular walls and papillary muscles, but valvular coaptation may be tighter at moderately elevated pressure gradients than at low transvalvular pressure gradients. This is suggested by the spectral display of the signal of many cases of 'physiological' pulmonary regurgitation which are intense in end diastole and extremely weak in early diastole (Fig. 5).

Although the tricuspid regurgitation method has become the leading method for pulmonary artery pressure measurement, its lack of feasibility in certain patients justifies the need for alternative methods.

PULMONARY REGURGITATION METHOD

The end diastolic pressure gradient between pulmonary artery and right ventricle can be measured applying the Bernoulli equation to the end diastolic velocity of pulmonary regurgitation.[12] As in the case of the tricuspid orifice, regurgitant signals can be recorded in the pulmonary orifice in the majority of patients with important pulmonary hypertension and in a high proportion of normal subjects.[12] Similar correlation coefficients with invasive measurements have been obtained with and without correction for incident angle, respectively $r = 0.97$ and $r = 0.94$, and the standard error was the same (3 mmHg), Angle correlation provided the best correlation agreement between the two measurements (Doppler gradient = $0.91 \times$ catheterisation gradient), being performed assuming that regurgitant jets were perpendicular to the plane of the pulmonary valve, because colour coded Doppler location (Plate 1) was not available at the time of the study. Addition of a catheterisation determined right atrial pressure provided a Doppler end diastolic pulmonary artery pressure that correlated closely with the invasive measurement, without important underestimation ($r = 0.96$, standard error = 4 mmHg, Doppler pressure = $0.93 \times$ catheterisation pressure). The errors that are introduced when evaluating the right atrial pressure clinically are more significant with the pulmonary regurgitation method than with the tricuspid regurgitation method because right atrial pressure is much higher when compared to diastolic pulmonary artery pressure than when compared to systolic pulmonary artery pressure. Normal values of end diastolic pulmonary regurgitation velocities are up to 1.3 m/s, corresponding to an end diastolic pressure of 12 mmHg with a 5 mmHg right atrial pressure.

The same authors[12] have noted that the early diastolic pulmonary artery-to-right ventricle pressure gradient correlates well ($r = 0.92$) with the mean pulmonary artery pressure. The correlation coefficient is the same with angle correction ($r = 0.92$) and there is only a minor underestimation by Doppler examination (Doppler gradient = $0.91 \times$ mean pulmonary pressure − 3). This slight underestimation is probably related to the right atrial pressure which was low in this study (more than 10 mmHg in only 3/31 patients). Thus the addition of an estimated right atrial pressure can also be used in this situation and if added to the early diastolic pressure gradient it is likely to provide a valuable estimation of the mean pulmonary artery pressure. Normal values for early diastolic pulmonary regurgitation velocities are up to 1.9 m/s, corresponding to normal mean pulmonary artery pressures up to 20 mmHg.

PULMONARY FORWARD FLOW METHOD

In patients without pulmonary hypertension the pattern of systolic forward flow in the right ventricular outflow tract and main pulmonary artery exhibits a dome-like contour

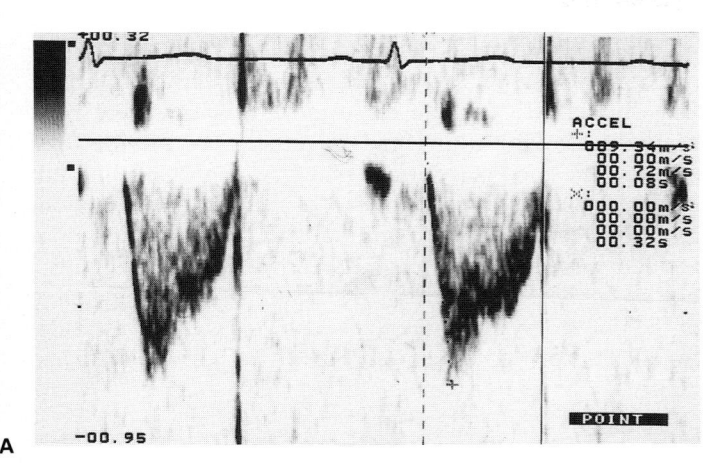

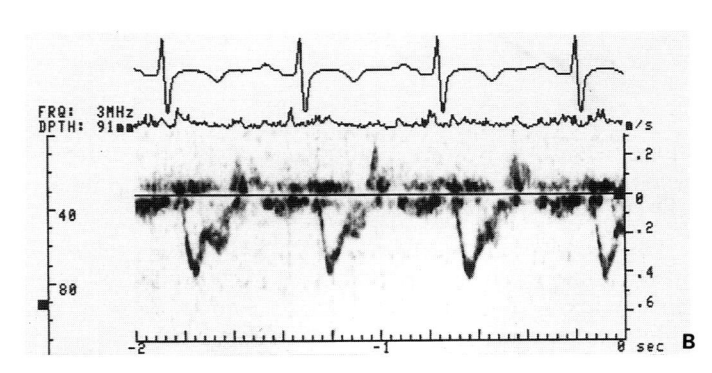

Fig. 6 **Patterns of pulmonary artery flow in pulmonary hypertension. A:** Early peak velocity with a consequent increase in rate of acceleration and a shorter AT/ET ratio (AT, acceleration time; ET, ejection time). **B:** Notching of the pulmonary flow trace due to premature reflection of the pressure wave front on the periphery of the pulmonary arterial tree.

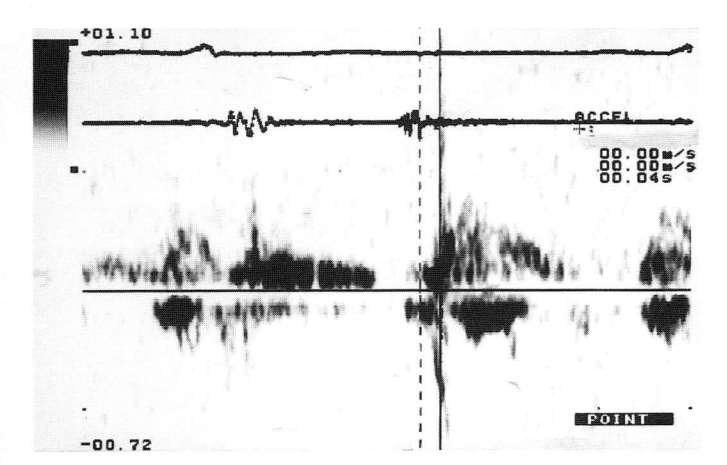

Fig. 7 **Measurement of the right ventricular isovolumic relaxation time** using a phonocardiogram (top) and a tricuspid flow trace (bottom).

in systole, with peak velocity occurring in mid-systole.[13] In patients with pulmonary hypertension, two other patterns are observed[13] (Fig. 6). The first resembles a triangle, with a rapid acceleration and a peak velocity that is earlier than in normals. The second consists of an early peak followed by a rapid deceleration, in turn followed by a secondary slow rise (notching). These patterns are related to premature reflections of the pressure wave front on the periphery of the pulmonary arterial tree which interrupts the forward flow. These premature reflections are related not only to pulmonary hypertension but to the associated modifications of the physical properties of the pulmonary arterial tree. They are also related to the magnitude of the stroke volume that is ejected into the pulmonary tree. Furthermore eddy currents are present around the pulmonary valve within a dilated main pulmonary artery. It has therefore been recommended that when using pulsed Doppler examination the forward flow should be sampled just below the pulmonary cusps in the right ventricular outflow tract rather than within the pulmonary artery.[13] Two indices are reported to correlate with directly measured mean pulmonary artery pressure, acceleration time (AT) and the ratio of acceleration time to ejection time (AT/ET) (Fig. 6). Correlation coefficients from 0.75 to 0.88 have reported for AT[13-17] and between 0.71 and 0.90[13-17] AT/ET. Logarithmic correlations were described by Kitabatake and co-authors[13] and linear relations have been described by Dabestani and co-authors.[15] Dabestani and co-authors have used pulmonary artery sampling which was found to be less reproducible than right ventricular outflow sampling. However, they found regression equations that were reasonably concordant with those reported by Kitabatake et al. The equations can be used over a wider range of AT and AT/ET values but they necessitate the use of more complex formulas.

RIGHT VENTRICULAR ISOVOLUMIC RELAXATION TIME METHOD

The interval between closure of the pulmonary valve and opening of the tricuspid valve, or right isovolumic relaxation time (RIRT) is governed by the rate of pressure drop in the right ventricle between these two events and the absolute pressure difference between the systolic pressure of right ventricle and the pulmonary artery, except in right heart failure and/or severe tricuspid regurgitation. This approach was used nearly 30 years ago to develop a phonomecanographic method for evaluation of the systolic pulmonary artery pressure[19] which was assumed to be linearly related to RIRT and to heart rate. A table was constructed on the basis of preliminary observations and its accuracy was verified on 120 patients. Examination of this table indicates that it can be conveniently summarised by the following formula:

$$SPAP = RIRT + HR - 108.5\ (+/-\ 2.5)$$

where SPAP is systolic pulmonary artery pressure in mmHg, RIRT is right isovolumic relaxation time in ms, and HR is heart rate in beats per minute.

These results were applied by Hatle and co-authors using Doppler ultrasound to record the timing of valve movements.[20] Since the two valves cannot be recorded simultaneously by Doppler examination, the timing of pulmonary valve closure was noted on a simultaneous phonocardiogram, and the phonocardiogram was used to measure the RIRT on the Doppler tricuspid record (Fig. 7). Another approach records the intervals between Q or R waves of the electrocardiogram and the separately recorded two valve movements and calculates the difference between these two intervals. The two intervals should be measured at the same time in the respiratory cycle, or in a short, quiet end-expiratory breath-holding state. Hatle and co-authors found a correlation coefficient of 0.89 applying Burstin's table to their Doppler data. Sources of error are right heart failure and important tricuspid regurgitation, which should both be ruled out by clinical examination and by the rest of the ultrasound data. One should also exclude those patients with severe right heart disease whose tricuspid valve only opens with atrial systole. The good correlations that were reported using this method should not mask the fact that the two assumptions made by Burstin are both questionable. These assumptions include a linear decrease of RIRT with heart rate and a rate of fall of right ventricular pressure that is independent of height of systolic pressure and of right ventricular function. Normal values for RIRT are between 20 and 65 ms.[19]

CONCLUSIONS

The tricuspid regurgitation method has become the most popular and probably the most accurate method for estimation of pulmonary artery pressure but the method is not feasible in all patients. Even when it is feasible, the result may indicate a pulmonary artery pressure around the upper limit of normal values resulting in the need to employ other comparative measurements to differentiate normal from abnormal results. The variety of available methods is fortunate, since they may provide a check on one another.[18]

REFERENCES

1. Skjaerpe T, Hatle L. Diagnosis and assessment of tricuspid regurgitation with Doppler ultrasound. In Risterborgh H, Ed: Echocardiography. The Hague: Martinus Nijhoff, 1981, p 299
2. Yock P G, Popp R L. Noninvasive estimation of right ventricular systolic pressure by Doppler ultrasound in patients with tricuspid regurgitation. Circulation 1984: 70: 657–662
3. Yock P G, Naasz C, Schnittger I, Popp R L. Doppler tricuspid and pulmonic regurgitation in normals: is it real? Circulation 1984; 70: Supp II: II-40 (abstract)
4. Braunwald E, editor: Heart disease, Philadelphia: W B Saunders, 1988, p 19
5. Currie P J, Seward J B, Chan K L et al. Continuous wave Doppler determination of right ventricular pressure: a simultaneous Doppler-catheterisations study in 127 patients. J Am Coll Cardiol 1985; 6: 750–756
6. Berger M, Haimowitz A, Van Tosh A, Berdoff R L, Goldberg E. Quantitative assessment of pulmonary hypertension in patients with tricuspid regurgitation using continuous wave Doppler ultrasound. J Am Coll Cardiol 1987; 6: 359–365
7. Chan K L, Currie P J, Seward J B, Hagler D J, Mair D D, Tajik A J. Comparison of three Doppler ultrasound methods in the prediction of pulmonary artery pressure. J Am Coll Cardiol 1987; 9: 549–554
8. Grossman W. Cardiac catheterisation and angiography. Second edition. Philadelphia, Lea and Febiger, 1980, p 415
9. Simonson J S, Schiller N B. Sonospirometry: a new method for noninvasive estimation of mean right atrial pressure based on two-dimensional echographic measurement of the inferior vena cava during measured inspiration. J Am Coll Cardiol 1988; 11: 557–564
10. Himelman R B, Stulbarg M, Kircher B et al. Non invasive evaluation of pulmonary artery pressure during exercise by saline-enhanced Doppler echocardiography in chronic pulmonary disease. Circulation 1989: 79: 863–871
11. Himelman R B, Struve S N, Brown J K, Namnum P, Schiller N B. Improved recognition of cor pulmonale in patients with severe chronic obstructive pulmonary disease. Am J Med 1988; 84: 891–898
12. Masuyama T, Kodama K, Kitabatake A, Sato H, Nanto S, Inoue M. Continuous wave Doppler echocardiographic detection of pulmonary regurgitation and its application to noninvasive estimation of pulmonary artery pressure. Circulation 1986; 74: 484–492
13. Kitabatake A, Inoue M, Asao M et al. Noninvasive evaluation of pulmonary hypertension by a pulsed Doppler technique. Circulation 1983; 68: 302–309
14. Kosturakis D, Goldberg S J, Allen H D, Leober C. Doppler echocardiographic prediction of pulmonary arterial hypertension in congenital heart disease. Am J Cardiol 1984; 53: 1110–1115
15. Dabestani A, Mahan G, Gardin J M, Takenaka K, Burn C, Allfie A, Henry W L. Evaluation of pulmonary artery pressure and resistance by pulsed Doppler echocardiography. Am J Cardiol 1987; 59: 662–668
16. Isobe M, Yazaki Y, Takaku F et al. Prediction of pulmonary arterial pressure in adults by pulsed Doppler echocardiography. Am J Cardiol 1986; 57: 316–321
17. Martin-Duran R, Larman M, Trugeda A et al. Comparison of Doppler-determined elevated pulmonary arterial pressure with pressure measured at cardiac catheterisation. Am J Cardiol 1986; 57: 859–863
18. Stevenson J G. Comparison of several noninvasive methods for estimation of pulmonary artery pressure. J Am Soc Echo 1989; 2: 157–171
19. Burstin L. Determination of pressure in the pulmonary artery by external graphic recordings. Br Heart J 1967; 29: 396
20. Hatle L, Angelsen B A J, Tromsdal A. Non-invasive estimation of pulmonary artery systolic pressure with Doppler ultrasound. Br Heart J 1981; 45: 157–165

8

Doppler quantitation – volume flow estimation

Aortic flow
Theoretical basis
Diameter measurement
Velocity measurement
Aortic orifice: volumetric flow calculation
Mitral flow
Measurement at the annulus level
Measurement at the tip of the mitral leaflets
Pulmonary flow
Tricuspid flow
Cardiac output
Valvular stenosis
Valvular regurgitation
Cardiac shunts
Conclusions

Thierry Touche

One of the first reported applications of Doppler techniques was the recording of blood velocities in ascending aorta and aortic arch from the suprasternal notch.[1-5] These early studies emphasised the potential value of Doppler techniques for the follow-up of variations in blood velocity, stroke volume and cardiac output.[2,4,5] The combination of echographic measurement of dimensions and Doppler measurement of blood velocities opened the way to the calculation of absolute values of cardiac output in various sampling sites. Ascending aorta and aortic arch,[6-14] aortic valve and left ventricular outflow tract,[14-20] mitral valve,[16,21-26] pulmonary artery and pulmonary valve,[7,14] and tricuspid valve[27] have been proposed for these calculations. Validation and standardisation of measurement methods have been considerably more difficult for volumetric flow than for other quantitative Doppler measurements such as pressure gradients and pulmonary pressures. Some of the difficulties were technical, a considerable variety of equipment being used for measurements in the aorta and aortic orifice. Probes were either non-imaging[1-5,10-15,17,18,20] or combined cross-sectional echocardiography and Doppler examination.[6-9,14,16,19] Doppler emissions were pulsed,[3,5-9,13,14,16] continuous[1,2,4,10-12] or both, with recording techniques being switched between the two modes on the same probe.[15] Processing of the Doppler signal was provided by either zero-crossing counters and other velocity estimators[1-6,10-13,15] or real-time spectral analysis.[7-9,14,16-20] Aortic diameters were measured using two-dimensional,[6-9,14-17,20] M-mode,[13,18,19] or A-mode[10-12] methods of distance calculation. Most of the currently available echocardiographic systems offer all or almost all of these technical capabilities, facilitating the optimal choice of modality for each particular measurement.

The difficulties that have been encountered more recently are methodological. It has been necessary to define the exact level where measurements of dimension and velocity had to be made for each sampling site. The main problem has been the selection of such sites where it was reasonable to assume a flat velocity profile across the lumen.[15] In this situation the velocities that are recorded by Doppler examination in a limited part of the lumen are representative for the velocities present in the whole lumen. This requirement led to a decreasing interest in ascending aortic measurements[6-14] and to an increasing use of the aortic orifice and the left ventricular outflow tract[15-20] in the assessment of aortic flow.

At present volumetric flow measurements have reached a level of accuracy that permits their use in clinical echocardiography, at least in specialised hands. Further development of the clinical use of these measurements is justified by their multiple fields of application in the assessment of cardiac diseases. Cardiac output measurement is central to the assessment of cardiac function, since it measures the ability of the heart to deliver a sufficient amount of blood to meet the demands of the body. Doppler examination can be used to assess the changes in stroke volume and cardiac output in varying physiological circumstances,[28-30] for example with exercise,[31,32] pharmacologic interventions,[33] or with various types of pacing.[34,35] Measurement of stroke volume at different sites provides a method for checking the internal correlation of echo-Doppler measurements[36-38] and can be used as a control of the validity of M-mode[39] or cross-sectional measurements of left ventricular stroke volume and ejection fraction. Pressure gradients through valvular stenosis should be interpreted taking into account volumetric flow through the stenotic valve. This is the basis for the calculation of valvular areas.[40-44] In valvular insufficiency regurgitant fractions may be evaluated[45-49] by a comparison between the increased forward flow in the regurgitant valve and the normal or decreased forward flow through another sampling site. In the case of cardiac shunts, the ratio of pulmonary flow to systemic flow can be evaluated.[50-53]

AORTIC FLOW

Theoretical basis

In the aortic orifice or aortic lumen at a given level along the vessel (Fig. 1), instantaneous volumetric flow $q(t)$ in cm^3/s or ml/s is the product of instantaneous cross-sectional

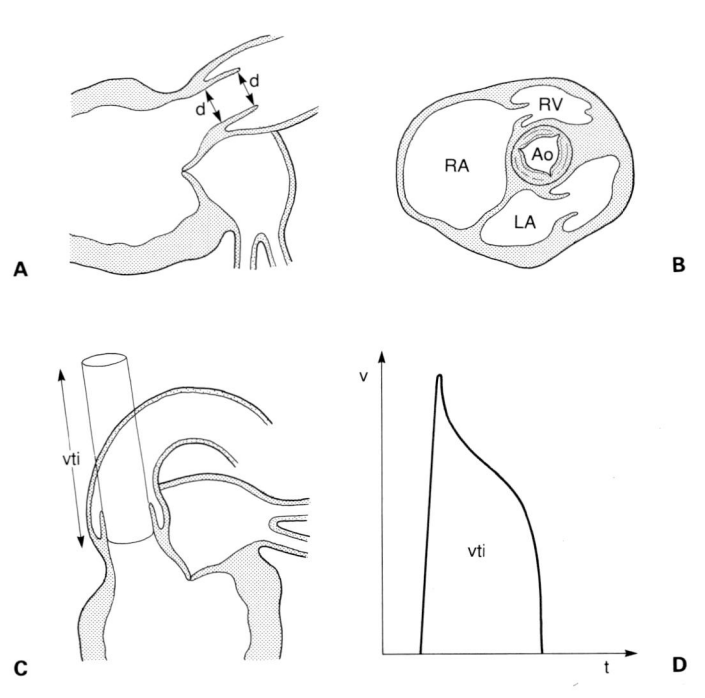

Fig. 1 Diagrams showing aspects of cardiac output calculation from the aortic orifice. **A:** Parasternal long axis view; d is the annulus and leaflet tip diameter. **B:** Parasternal short axis view; Ao is the aortic orifice area. **C:** Diagram illustrating stroke distance calculated at the aortic orifice; vti is the velocity time integral. **D:** Trace from the aortic orifice showing the velocity (v) plotted against time (t). The velocity time integral (vti) is the area under the curve.

area $a(t)$ in cm² and instantaneous blood velocity $v(t)$ in cm/s:

$$q(t) = a(t) \times v(t) \qquad (1)$$

The t in the parentheses indicate that the variables are a function of time. In the case of the aorta and particularly the aortic annulus it is generally accepted that the variations in the aortic cross-sectional area with time can be neglected. This can be verified by M-mode recording or cross-sectional frame-by-frame study of aortic diameter. Thus in the above equation the factor $a(t)$ can be replaced by a constant value a:

$$q(t) = a \times v(t) \qquad (2)$$

The aortic section a is circular in the great majority of patients. This can be verified on a cross-sectional short axis view (Fig. 1) of the aortic annulus of the aortic root. Thus a can be calculated from the aortic diameter d in cm:

$$a = (\pi/4) \times d^2 \qquad (3)$$

Equations 1, 2 and 3 give:

$$q(t) = (\pi/4) \times d^2 \times v(t) \qquad (4)$$

Integration of both parts of equation 4 throughout one systole gives:

$$SV = (\pi/4) \times d^2 \times vti \qquad (5)$$

where integration of $q(t)$ during one systole is the stroke volume SV in cm³ or ml, and integration of $v(t)$ is the systolic velocity-time integral vti in cm. The latter is calculated by planimetry of the area under the velocity curve during ejection (Fig. 1). On the velocity recording the x axis is time in seconds and the y axis is velocity in cm/s. Thus the dimension of the planimetered area is cm/s × s = cm. Thus, vti is also called stroke distance or systolic traverse distance. It is the theoretical distance that the stroke volume would occupy in the aorta if the aorta itself were a perfectly cylindrical conduit, without branches, which had a constant diameter equal to the diameter of the sampling site in the aortic valve orifice (Fig. 1). The fact that vti is a distance can be illustrated by the analogy of the blood velocity curve with the velocity curve of a vehicle throughout a trip. In the later case the x axis is time in hours and the y axis is velocity in km/h or mph. The area surface under the curve is the length of the trip in km or miles.

The stroke volume given by equation 5 should be calculated from several cycles and averaged or alternatively one representative systole can be selected for calculation. Then cardiac output (CO) in ml/min is the product of stroke volume and heart rate (HR):

$$CO = SV \times HR \qquad (6)$$

The instantaneous velocity $v(t)$ in equations 1, 2 and 4 is the spatial average velocity, or the mean of all the velocities that are present across the aortic lumen at instant t. Doppler techniques do not, however, provide uniform insonation of the lumen, blood velocities being recorded from a limited part of the cross-sectional area. The Doppler velocities can only be extrapolated to the whole section in sites where the velocity profile can be assumed to be flat.

Ihlen et al[15] first reported that in adult patients (mean age 53 in their study) a considerable overestimation of cardiac output was observed when maximal recordable velocity in the proximal aortic root was used together with the aortic diameter measured at the sino-tubular junction, i.e. the junction of the sinuses of Valsalva with the tubular part of the ascending aorta (Fig. 2A). In adult patients whose ascending aortic diameter is markedly larger than the diameter of the aortic annulus, there is a central high velocity core issuing from the aortic orifice which remains at some distance from the walls of the ascending aorta. Multiplying the velocity of this central core by the cross-sectional area of the whole lumen causes severe overestimation of stroke volume, whereas substituting the dimension of the aortic orifice in the same calculation provides more accurate results.[15] These results contradicted previous studies which reported adequate results when using the diameter of the ascending aorta.[7,9,10–12] Good results using the diameter of the ascending aorta can be explained as far as children, young adults or experimental animals were studied,[7,9] because in these cases the variation in aortic diameter between annulus and ascending aorta is small (Fig. 2B). In children the results obtained

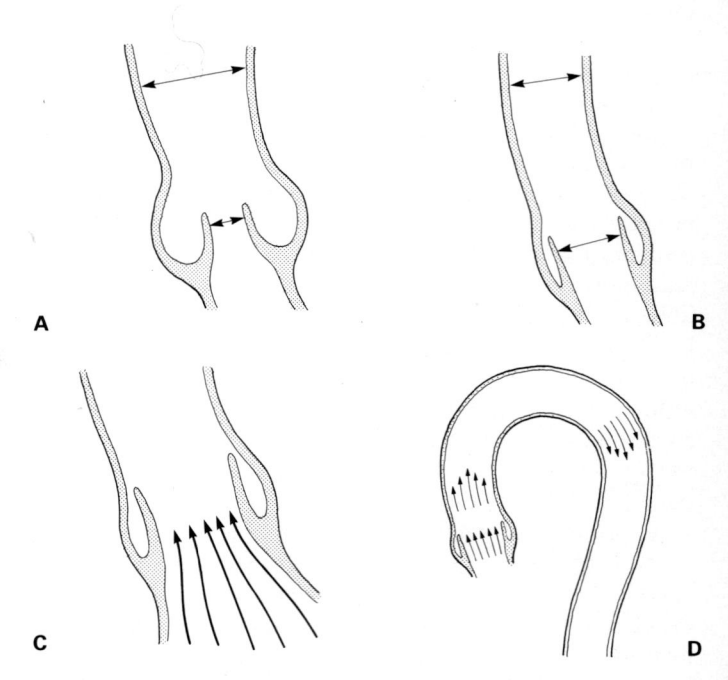

Fig. 2 Diagrams showing aortic flow patterns. **A**: A typical adult aorta in which the ascending aorta is wider than the aortic annulus. **B**: A typical child's aorta in which the annulus and ascending aorta are similar in diameter. **C**: Convergent flow in the left ventricular outflow tract. **D**: Changing velocity profiles in the aorta.

using the diameter of aortic orifice are still better than with the diameter of the ascending aorta, but only slightly.[19] Studies reporting good results with the diameter of the ascending aorta in adults[10-12] are more difficult to explain. In these studies, some underestimation of maximal aortic velocities because of suboptimal sampling may have compensated for the overestimation of flow area.

Although few data about velocity profiles in the upper left ventricular outflow tract and aortic orifice are available (Fig. 2C), theoretical and practical data suggest that the assumption of a flat velocity profile in this site is justified. Theoretically, the velocity profile is flat in the inlet orifice of a conduit. In the aortic orifice, both convective acceleration of flow into the orifice and acceleration of flow with time in early systole tend to flatten the velocity profile. In practice, when pulsed Doppler sampling is being performed immediately under or above the aortic valve (from apex or suprasternal notch) and small changes in probe orientation are made, it is not possible to create significant variations in the amplitude or shape of the velocity curve. This contrasts with the variations that can be created when sampling further from the valve in the lower left ventricular outflow tract or in the ascending aorta.

Discussion of velocity profiles further down the aorta (aortic arch)[54] is of less practical interest for cardiac output measurements because of the proven validity of volumetric flow measurements in the aortic orifice and because of the irregularities of velocity profiles that appear even at a short distance from the orifice. The region of curvature between horizontal and descending segments of the arch, however, is a superb site for sampling aortic velocities, because of a relatively small sampling depth and a close to zero intercept angle[2] (Fig. 2D). In early studies the velocity curve in this site has been proposed for the follow-up of changes in cardiac output,[2] or as a substitute to the curve of the ascending aorta for cardiac output calculation.[8,9,14] In experimental animals the velocity curve in the aortic arch has been reported to be similar in shape and amplitude to that recorded in the ascending aorta.[9] In patients with cardiac and/or aortic disease, however, the unpredictable variations of velocity amplitudes and velocity profiles along the aortic arch seem to preclude the use of distal aortic velocity sampling for cardiac output calculation.

Diameter measurement

Measurement of aortic orifice dimension can be performed at the level of the aortic annulus, in the upper left ventricular outflow tract or at the tips of the aortic valve leaflets. Our recommendation is to begin the procedure of cardiac output measurement by a detailed cross-sectional examination of these structures, in order to identify a short cylindrical segment of the aortic conduit where both dimension and velocity can be confidently measured. A long axis view of the aortic orifice is obtained in early systole (since maximal instantaneous flow occurs in this period), adjusting the sector orientation in order to maximise both the annulus diameter and the distance between the tips of aortic leaflets (Fig. 3). Figure 4 summarises various appearances that can be found when using this view. The view provides a guide as to whether or not volumetric flow can be measured in any particular situation. In many patients the diameter of the upper left ventricular outflow tract, the aortic annulus and the maximal leaflet separation are similar. These three structures form the cylinder used for measurement (Fig. 4A). In such

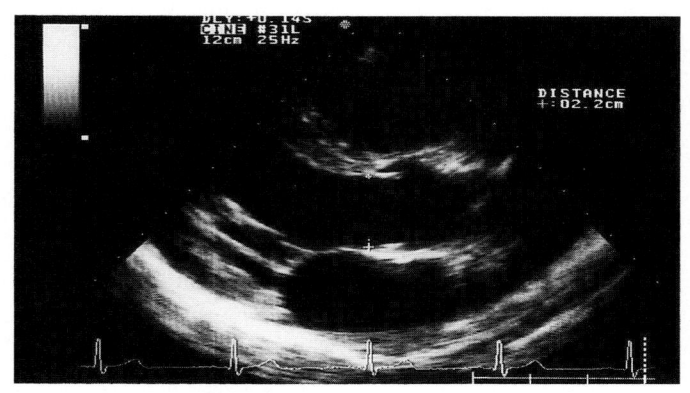

Fig. 3 **Measurement of the aortic annulus** from the parasternal long axis view.

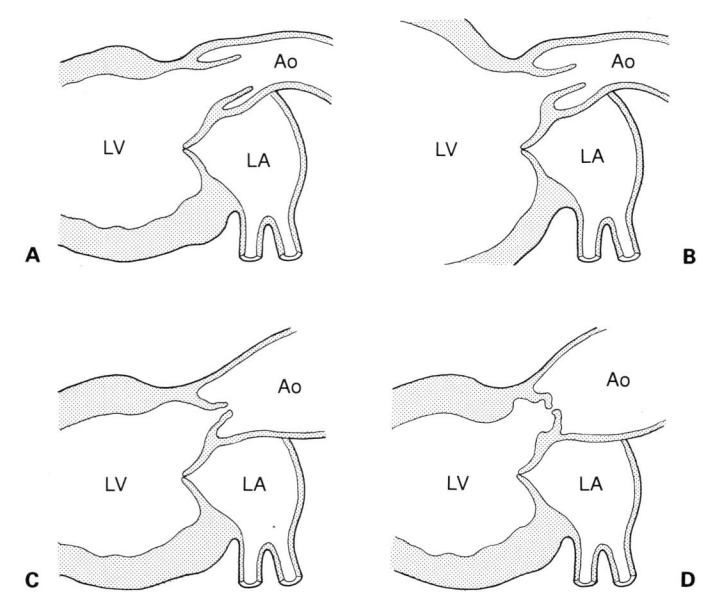

Fig. 4 **Diagrams showing different anatomical patterns in left ventricular outflow. A:** Uniform outflow tract and valve annulus in a normal young person. **B:** Funnel-shaped left ventricular outflow tract in a patient with a dilated left ventricle. **C:** Thickened and irregular aortic leaflets above a normal outflow tract. **D:** Thickened and irregular left ventricular outflow and aortic valve leaflets.

patients pulsed Doppler velocity sampling is possible either immediately above, within, or immediately under the valve. Velocity recording as described below is performed from the apex and/or from the suprasternal notch. The incidence providing the best alignment with flow giving the highest velocity peak is used for cardiac output calculation. In patients with enlarged left ventricles, the left ventricular outflow tract is dilated and funnel shaped. A cylindrical segment may still be identifiable but only at the level of aortic leaflets (Fig. 4B). In these cases velocity measurement can still be attempted from both suprasternal notch and apex. In another group of patients, cross-sectional examination of the aortic orifice demonstrates that the opening of aortic leaflets in early systole is incomplete, whether or not this corresponds to significant aortic stenosis. In some of these patients (Fig. 4C) a short cylindrical conduit can still be imaged at the level of the left ventricular outflow tract. Velocity sampling can still be performed but this is only possible under the valve from the apical approach. In other patients there are both abnormalities of the aortic valve leaflets and the left ventricular outflow tract, such as the association of calcified aortic stenosis and subaortic septal thickening or important calcification in the root of the anterior mitral leaflet. In these patients attempts to measure aortic volumetric flow should probably be avoided.

It should be noted that aortic leaflet opening can be incomplete (leaflet separation measuring less than the annulus diameter) even in the lack of structural abnormalities of the aortic valve, as seen in patients with a low cardiac output or those with dilatation of the ascending aorta. In some patients the leaflet opening may be full in early systole at the time of peak flow but becomes reduced in mid or late systole. Sometimes there is a change in the shape of the orifice formed by the tips of the leaflets, which becomes triangular and thus cannot be calculated from a single diameter measurement. In fact the geometry of this type of orifice is more complex than that of a simple triangle since it is not localised to a single plane (Fig. 5). In this latter situation the measurement at the tip of the leaflets should be avoided.

In order to reduce inaccuracy in dimension measurements, the cross-sectional technique should be used with maximal enlargement of the image, with a high frequency probe whenever possible, and with a gain setting just sufficient for adequate definition of the structures to be measured. We use the trailing edge–leading edge measurement method. The leading edge–leading edge method which was devised for early echo instruments with low axial resolution artificially adds the thickness of the endocardium of the proximal wall to the lumen dimension.

Some technical variants can be used for the measurement of aortic orifice dimension. M-mode recording under cross-sectional guidance permits further improvement in resolution for axial distance measurement. Colour Doppler

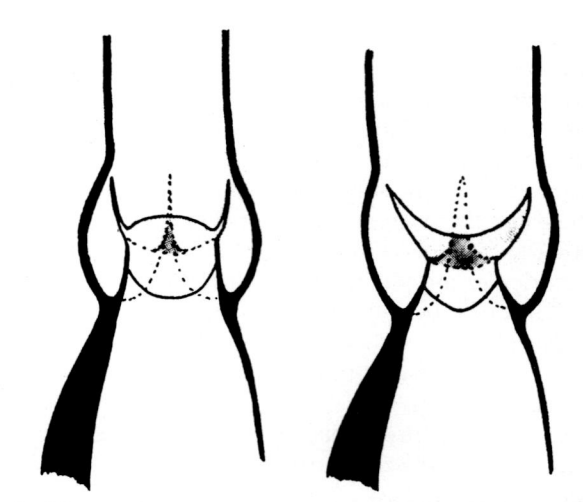

Fig. 5 **Diagram showing the three dimensional nature** of the aortic valve leaflets.

flow mapping is interesting since it shows the diameter of the column of blood flow itself. The angle of incidence of the beam of ultrasound should not be perpendicular to the left ventricular outflow tract and aortic root for optimal colour Doppler imaging to be achieved. High parasternal, low parasternal and apical views should all be tried. Apical views offer the opportunity to measure two orthogonal sub-aortic diameters, on the 4 chamber view with aorta (the so-called 5 chamber view) and on the long axis (2 chamber) view.

Velocity measurement

Blood velocity within or close to the aortic orifice can be recorded by pulsed wave (PW) Doppler examination under cross-sectional guidance, PW Doppler examination under continuous wave (CW) Doppler guidance, or CW Doppler examination alone. PW Doppler examination combined with cross-sectional imaging is the technique of choice for sampling the aortic orifice and the upper left ventricular outflow tract from the apex. In contrast, sampling the aortic orifice from the suprasternal notch requires a small, easy to handle probe. Only non-imaging probes can be inserted sufficiently deeply into the suprasternal notch and angled toward the aortic root to obtain consistently good results. Non-imaging probes are usually used in the CW mode. In this case the highest velocities of the CW spectrum are assumed to come from the narrowest portion of the blood path, i.e. the aortic orifice. Many non-imaging probes also permit PW emission under CW guidance. The switch to PW mode improves the quality of the spectral tracing. Location of the sample volume with respect to the aortic leaflets can be determined using the Doppler clicks of valvular movement. The aortic orifice moves down towards the cardiac apex during systole. Thus, when the fixed sample volume is immediately above the orifice, it only records the aortic opening click at the beginning of the systolic flow curve. When the sample volume is within the orifice it records both the opening and closing clicks. In this position leaflet vibrations are frequently recorded between the two clicks. With the sample volume immediately under the leaflets, only the closing click is recorded (Fig. 6).

Aortic orifice: volumetric flow calculation

Stroke volume is calculated using equation 5. The calculation is made automatically by current machines after the manual tracing of the velocity envelope (Fig 7). Tracings should be performed on one representative cycle, or on several consecutive cycles. The cardiac output is obtained by equation 6.

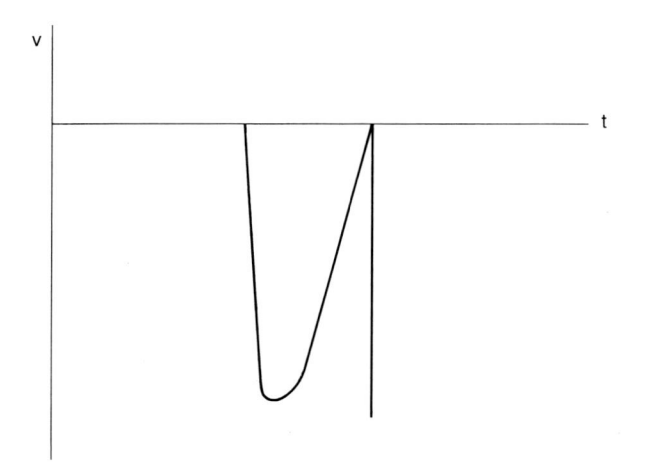

Fig. 6 Diagram showing an apical pulsed wave Doppler recording with the sample volume just below the leaflets in systole. Only the closing click is recorded.

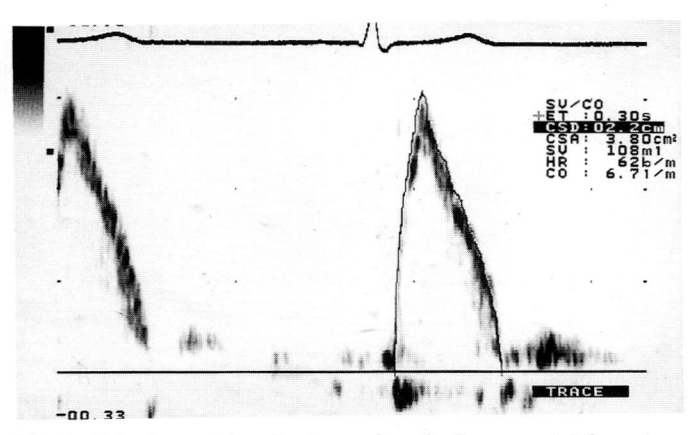

Fig. 7 Pulsed wave Doppler trace of aortic flow recorded from the suprasternal position. The outline of the second curve has been traced on the computer.

MITRAL FLOW

The open mitral orifice can be assumed to be a conduit (Fig. 8) whose inlet and outlet are the mitral annulus and the tips of mitral leaflets respectively. Both sites have been proposed for volumetric flow calculation. Whatever the selected sampling site, the dimension and the velocities should be measured at the same level.

Measurement at the annulus level

Mitral annulus area is assumed to be constant throughout diastole. The annulus diameter from the apical four chamber view is used to calculate the annulus area ($\pi d^2/4$).[16,25] If the orthogonal diameters are measured the annulus area is calculated as the surface of an ellipse ($\pi d_1 d_2/4$).[26] Volume flow measurement at the mitral annulus level can be performed with the same theoretical basis and practical techniques as the measurement at the aortic annulus level which is described above.

Only a few studies[16,25,26] have reported the measurement of volumetric flow at mitral annulus level and there are significant methodological differences between these studies which include variations in the sites of diameter measurement and velocity sampling. This contrasts with measurement at the tip of mitral leaflets, which has been validated by more numerous and more concordant studies.[21-24,31,45,47,52]

Measurement of mitral annulus diameter from the apex is performed at a greater depth than the measurement of aortic annulus diameter from the parasternal window, which may result in poorer resolution. In addition, the ultrasound beam is parallel to the mitral conduit whereas it is perpendicular to the aortic conduit and so the accuracy of mitral annulus measurement depends upon lateral imaging resolution which is inferior to axial resolution. If only one diameter is measured an erroneous value so obtained will be squared in the formula for flow calculation. Finally, distance between the mitral annulus and the apex varies constantly throughout diastole, whilst the sample volume is locate at a fixed depth. Thus the sample volume can be located in the left atrium in early diastole and can be pos-

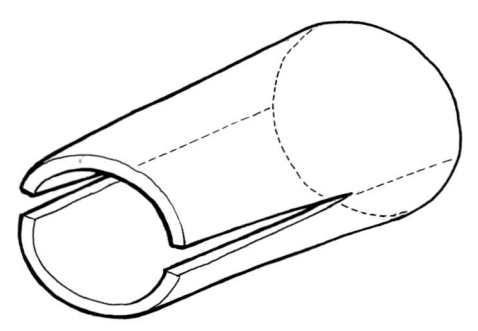

Fig. 8 Diagrammatic representation of the three dimensional nature of the two mitral leaflets.

120 CARDIAC ULTRASOUND

itioned between the mitral leaflets in late diastole (Fig. 9). Since the annulus region of the mitral conduit is funnel-shaped the likelihood of measuring a correct diameter at precisely the same level as the Doppler sampling volume is questionable.

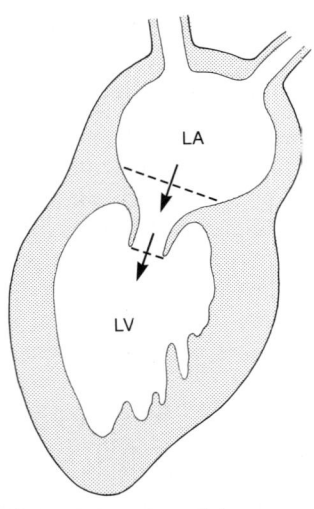

Fig. 9 **Diagrammatic representation of the narrowing diameter** from left atrium to mitral valve orifice.

Measurement at the tip of the mitral leaflets

The orifice delineated by the tip of the mitral leaflets has constant area variations throughout diastole. Two solutions have been proposed in order to take these variations into account. Both methods use the same four basic recordings (Fig. 10): (1) parasternal short-axis image of the mitral leaflets at the time of maximal leaflet opening (either the E wave or the A wave) which is easily obtained using the cinememory available on present machines; (2) M-mode recording of the mitral leaflets guided by the cross-sectional short axis view, with the M-mode cursor adjusted across the middle of the mitral leaflets; (3) apical four chamber view with positioning of the pulsed Doppler sample volume at the tip of the leaflets; (4) pulsed Doppler recording at the corresponding sampling depth with the sample volume position adjusted in order to maximise mitral velocities. The first method[21,23,29,45,47,52] is to measure the maximal mitral area on the cross-sectional short axis view and to calculate a ratio of mean-to-maximal valve separation from the M-mode recording. In the initial report using this method[21] planimetry of the valve orifice image was done through the middle of the leaflet thickness (this gives area values that are intermediate between those of the leading edge–trailing edge method and the trailing edge–leading

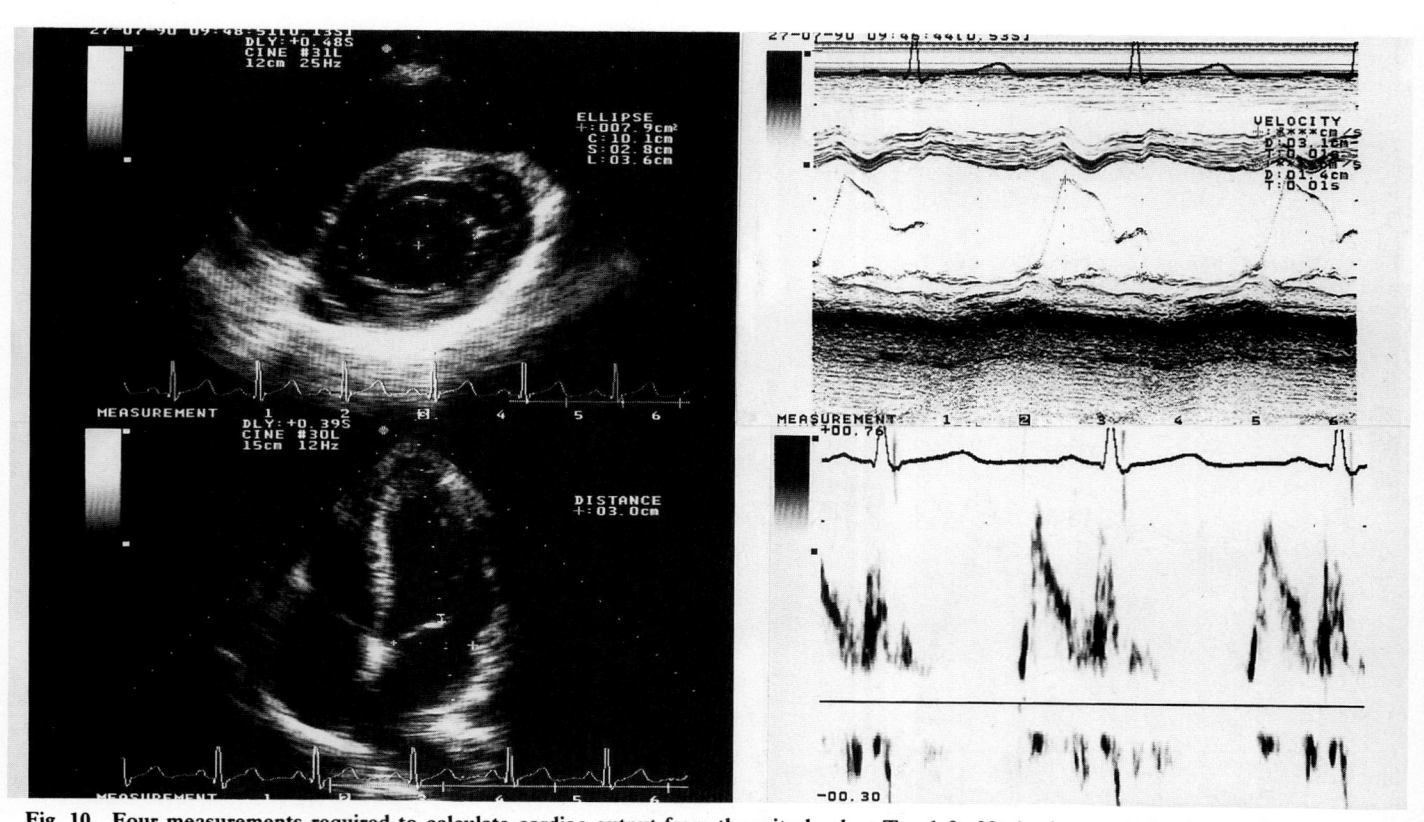

Fig. 10 **Four measurements required to calculate cardiac output from the mitral valve. Top left:** Maximal cross-sectional area of opening measured from a parasternal short axis view. **Top right:** M-mode trace of mitral leaflet separation. **Bottom left:** Mitral annulus diameter measured from an apical four chamber view. **Bottom right:** Pulsed Doppler record of mitral flow.

edge method). The mean leaflet separation was calculated by averaging the values obtained by manual measurement of leaflet separation on vertical lines traced at successive 50 ms intervals. Mean leaflet separation can be determined more conveniently by planimetry of the M-mode area between the leaflets and division by the duration of diastolic mitral opening.[23] Planimetry of M-mode tracings is not normally available on echo systems but can be performed if the machine permits the off-line analysis of video records. The M-mode record is reanalysed as if it were a cross-sectional image, with y axis calibration in cm and x axis calibration in arbitrary units. Mean leaflet separation is obtained by dividing the planimetered area by the diastolic mitral opening period measured in the arbitrary units.

Finally, a mean diastolic mitral valve orifice area corrected for diastolic variations is calculated as the product of the cross-sectional maximal area and the M-mode ratio of mean-to-maximal leaflet separation. This single value (a) of mitral valve area is used to calculate instantaneous flow. Stroke volume and cardiac output:

$$q(t) = a \times v(t) \qquad (2)$$

After integration throughout one diastole:

$$MIV = a \times vti \qquad (7)$$

And finally:

$$CO = MIV \times HR \qquad (8)$$

In equations 7 and 8, MIV is the mitral inflow volume during one diastole in cm^3.

The second method for calculation of flow at the tip of the mitral leaflets is the instantaneous flow integration method.[22,24] This method takes into account the fact that instantaneous flow is the product of instantaneous velocity times instantaneous orifice area:

$$q(t) = a(t) \times v(t) \qquad (1)$$

The mitral orifice is approximated to an ellipse with a constant long axis l measured on cross-sectional images, and a variable short axis d, the mitral leaflet separation sampled by the M-mode record. The mitral area is:

$$a(t) = (\pi/4) \times d(t) \times l \qquad (9)$$

and instantaneous flow is:

$$q(t) = (\pi/4) \times d(t) \times l \times v(t) \qquad (10)$$

It was found difficult to measure l on the cross-sectional short axis view, since the contour of the mitral leaflets was frequently poorly defined in the vicinity of mitral commissures in adult patients with normal mitral valves.[24] Thus, l was measured at the level of the annulus on the 4 chamber view, assuming that the long axis of the outlet orifice of the mitral canal was identical to the long axis of the inlet orifice. In patients with abnormal mitral valves this may not be the case and l should be derived from the maximal cross-sectional short axis view, either through direct measurement or through calculation.

Integration of the product of leaflet separation and blood velocities throughout diastole (equation 10) necessitates a specific computer programme[24] based on Simpson's rule of integration. This programme is similar to the programme used for the calculation of ventricular volumes from biplane angiography or echocardiographic images. It necessitates the matching of M-mode and Doppler tracings of exactly the same diastolic duration.[24] Correlation with thermodilution was significantly better with this method than with a method using a mean leaflet separation throughout diastole.[24]

A simplified method for instantaneous flow integration is depicted in Figure 11. The E wave and the A wave are computed separately. The Doppler curve is traced completely for each wave and on the M-mode recording only the maximal leaflet separation is measured. The method uses the assumption that the leaflet separation before and after the peak is directly proportional to flow velocity, i.e. that the ratio of separation to velocity (d/v) is constant and

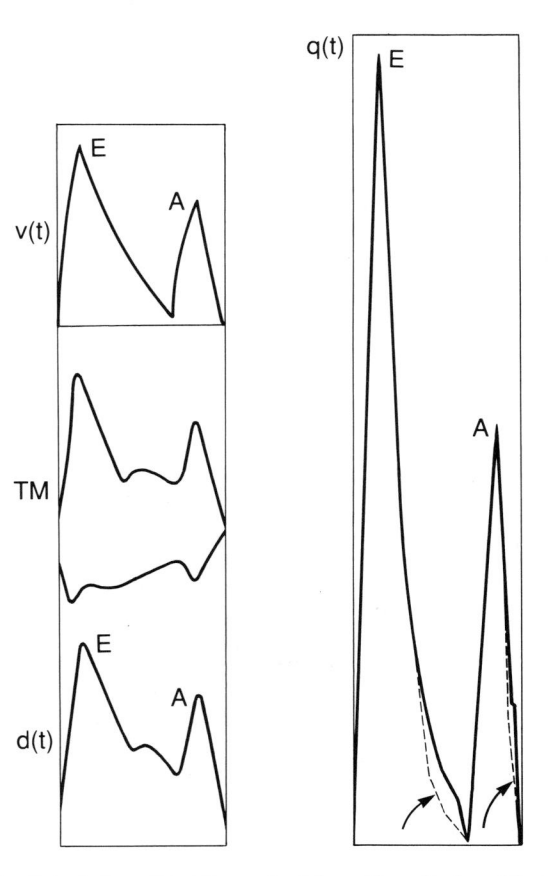

Fig. 11 Calculation of cardiac output from the mitral position. On the left are v(t) (the Doppler curve with its E and A waves), TM (the M-mode trace), and d(t) (the changing leaflet separation with time). On the right is the composite calculation of flow q(t).

equal to the ratio measured at the time of peak flow (d_{max}/v_{max}). Thus:

$$d(t) = v(t) \times (d_{max}/v_{max}) \qquad (11)$$

and:

$$q(t) = v(t)^2 \times (\pi/4) \times 1 \times (d_{max}/v_{max}) \qquad (12)$$

This approximation is inaccurate in mid-diastole but instantaneous flow is minimal during this period. The interest of this simplified formula is that its integration during the E wave and the A wave can be done on present echocardiographic equipment. Integration of $v(t)^2$ can be derived from the programme for calculation of the mean pressure gradient of stenosis (G), which integrates instantaneous gradient G(t) equal to $4 \times v(t)^2$ according to the simplified Bernoulli equation.

PULMONARY FLOW

The basis for pulmonary flow measurement is similar to the basis for aortic flow measurement. As for aorta, diameter measurement was performed above the valve in initial studies[7,50,51] and at the level of the annulus or upper ventricular outflow tract in more recent publications.[14,29,41,48] The anterior part of the pulmonary annulus is located at a very shallow depth and is best defined with a high frequency cross-sectional imaging probe (Fig. 12). Optimal images of the pulmonary orifice in early or mid systole are obtained from a high parasternal position with the patient in a marked left lateral recumbent position. The best Doppler alignment with pulmonary flow is obtained from a low parasternal position or from a subcostal position.

TRICUSPID FLOW

Absolute measurement of tricuspid flow has been validated by only one study.[27] The valve diameter was measured at the level of the annulus and the velocity was measured at the tip of the leaflets. This is valid because of the three-leaflet geometry of the valve which allows complete opening of the leaflets as for aortic and pulmonary valves. Another study reported good correlation between flows measured in the aortic, pulmonary and tricuspid valves, but there were discrepancies with flow measured at the tip of mitral leaflets.[36] Validation of the measurement of tricuspid flow would probably benefit from further studies and from better knowledge of tricuspid annulus geometry and of respiratory variations in tricuspid flow.

CARDIAC OUTPUT

Measurement of cardiac output is one of the main parameters in the assessment of cardiac function. In our experience one can obtain normal values similar to those obtained by invasive techniques, 2.6 to 4.2 l/min/m^2 for cardiac index and 30 to 65 ml/m^2 for stroke volume index.[55] Cardiac output decreases with age and we use normal values calculated with both body surface area and age. The cardiac index decreases from 2.7–4.8 l/min/m^2 at 20 years of age, to 2.3–3.5 l/min/m^2 at 80 years of age, and stroke volume decreases from 35–65 ml/m^2 at 20 years of age to 26–48 ml/m^2 at 80 years of age. A considerable advantage of noninvasive techniques is the possibility of studying a large series of normal subjects and these normal values will certainly be more precisely defined in the future.

Cardiac Doppler examination has the unique capability of following up changes in stroke volume and cardiac output. It is the only technique to assess beat-to-beat chambers in stroke volume. The majority of causes of error in Doppler cardiac output determination are related to the measurement of dimensions and to the possibility of significantly large incident angles. These aspects are of no consequence when one studies variations of flow in a single individual while using the same window of access and the same sampling depth. Changes in stroke volume and cardiac output have been studied in animals under fluid infusion, exsanguination or drug infusion[4,5] or when controlling cardiac output with a roller pump.[29] In patients changes have been induced by dobutamine infusion,[28] upright exercise,[30,31] supine exercise,[30,31,32] vasodilators[33] and various pacing modalities.[34,35] Flow augmentation at the aortic annulus is associated with an increase in the velocity-time integral.[29,31] Changes in aortic cross-sectional area were only observed with major variations of cardiac output in the experimental animal.[29] In contrast, increase in flow rate measured at the tip of the mitral leaflets is predominantly due to an increase in diastolic mitral valve area.[29,31]

In the absence of shunts and significant valvular regurgitation, the measurement of volumetric flow at different sampling sites[14,16,29,36,37,38] should yield similar results,

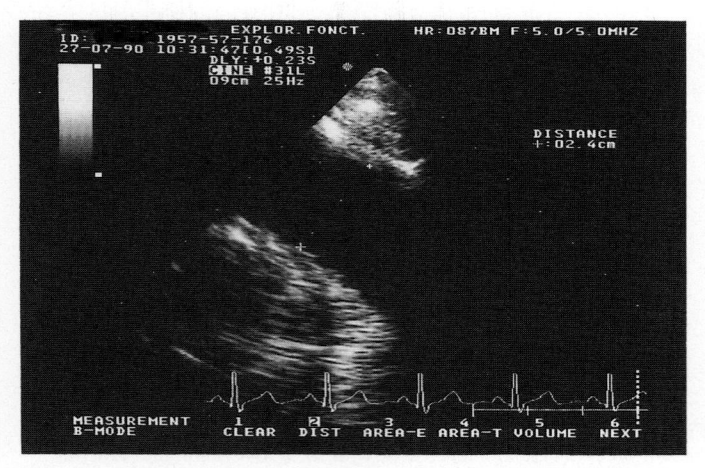

Fig. 12 Measurement of the pulmonary valve annulus from the parasternal position.

thus permitting an internal control of the Doppler measurements which reduces the risk of error. Left ventricular measurements should be included in this comprehensive view of the overall consistency of echocardiographic measurements. In the absence of segmental abnormalities of left ventricular geometry and kinetics, end-diastolic and end-systolic volumes can be evaluated from M-mode diameters (Fig. 13), using the Teichholz formula which uses a left ventricular short axis–long axis relationship derived from angiographic data. This method was the only one to provide a reasonable assessment of stroke volume and cardiac output,[39] before the advent of Doppler techniques, provided patients with segmental abnormalities were discarded from calculation. The cross-sectional examination permits the selection of patients adequate for such an M-mode measurement of stroke volume. We use the model of the 'maximal sphere' that can be inscribed in the left ventricle (Fig. 14). Left ventricular volumes can be derived from M-mode diameters provided that this imaginary sphere (a) can be inscribed between the left ventricular walls, (b) has a diameter recorded by the M-mode beam in both end-diastole and end-systole, and (c) has an area contraction that can be considered representative of the overall kinetics of the left ventricle. The systematic use of both parasternal and subcostal views permits a control of the validity of M-mode measurements of the left ventricle (Fig. 13). Present equipment permits an instantaneous display of ventricular volumes, ejection fraction and cardiac output.

Doppler measurement of stroke volume can be helpful for the calculation of ejection fraction in some cases. In patients with segmental wall motion abnormalities but with conservation of the ellipsoidal geometry of the left ventricle in end-diastole, the ratio of Doppler derived stroke volume to image derived end-diastolic volume can probably be used to evaluate the ejection fraction.

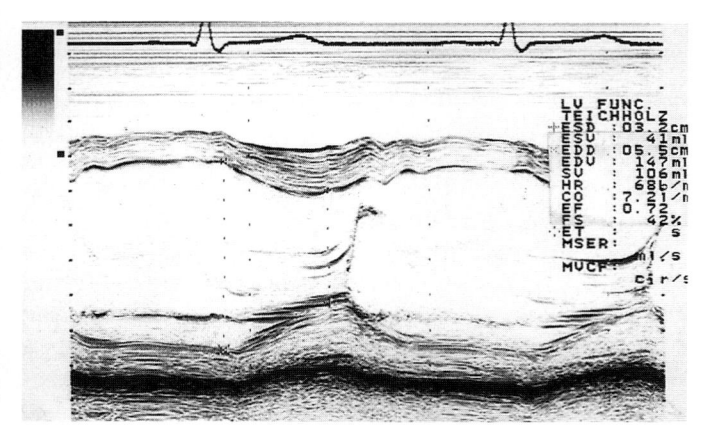

Fig. 13 M-mode trace of left ventricular dimensions.

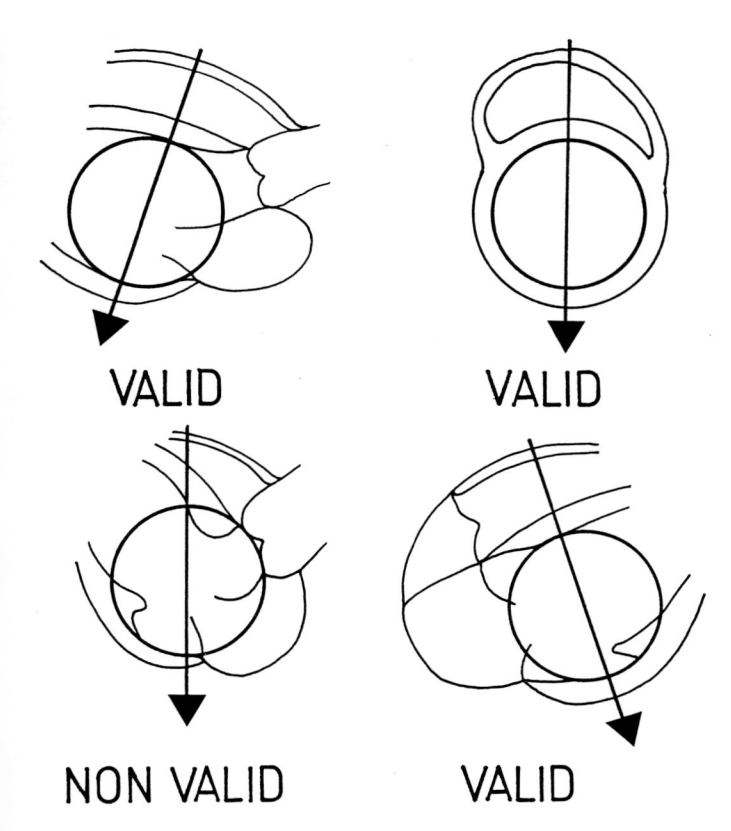

Fig. 14 Diagram showing valid and non-valid left ventricular measurements using the maximal sphere method.

VALVULAR STENOSIS

The measurement of the pressure gradient is an important element in the assessment of valvular stenosis since it indicates the haemodynamic consequence of the stenosis under the conditions of the examination. However, transvalvular velocities and pressure gradients must be interpreted in the context of the volumetric flow through the stenotic valve. This is the purpose of area calculations and the basis for those area calculations is the continuity equation. This equation indicates that volumetric flow is the same at the stenotic valve and at another sampling site in the same conduit. In the case of aortic stenosis the other sampling site can be the upper left ventricular outflow tract.[40] Maximal instantaneous volumetric flow (q) is the same in the outflow tract (site 1) and in the stenotic aortic valve (site 2). In both sites q is equal to peak velocity (v) times surface area (a):

$$q_1 = v_1 \cdot a_1 = q_2 = v_2 \cdot a_2 \qquad (13)$$

Thus:

$$a_2 = v_1 \cdot a_1/v_2 \qquad (14)$$

Similarly, integration of instantaneous volumetric flow over one systole (equal to stroke volume SV) is the same in the outflow tract (site 1) and in the stenotic aortic valve (site

2), and in both sites SV is equal to the velocity time-integral (vti) times surface area (a):

$$SV_1 = vti_1 \cdot a_1 = SV_2 = vti_2 \cdot a_2 \quad (15)$$

Thus:

$$a_2 = vti_1 \cdot a_1/vti_2 = SV/vti_2 \quad (16)$$

The area values that are obtained by equations 14 and 16 are very close to each other,[40,41] but equation 14 is preferred because it is quicker to calculate. The additional time required by equation 16 however, only corresponds to the time taken for tracing of the envelopes of the two velocity curves, which only needs a few seconds on present machines. Equation 16 has the considerable importance of indicating clearly the value of stroke volume and cardiac output that leads to the final area value. Thus one can assess its consistency with the clinical status of the patient (body surface area, age, possible clinical symptoms of low cardiac output) and with cardiac output values obtained in other sites, including the left ventricle. The principle of the continuity equation in the form of equation 16 can be applied to the calculation of valve area in mitral stenosis and mitral prostheses, and to the measurement of stroke volume either in the aortic orifice (in the absence of mitral regurgitation and of aortic regurgitation) or in the pulmonary orifice (in the absence of mitral regurgitation).[42–44]

One should note both similarities and differences between the continuity equation and the Gorlin equation.[55] The latter uses pressure gradients to calculate flow velocities which cannot be measured directly using conventional catheterisation techniques. The continuity equation can be written in the following equivalent forms:

$$a = SV/vti \quad (16)$$

and:

$$a = (CO/HR) / (v \times DFP \text{ or } SEP) \quad (17)$$

This second form can be compared to the Gorlin equation:

$$a = (CO/HR) / (44.3 \times C \times \sqrt{G} \times DFP \text{ or } SEP) \quad (18)$$

In equations 17 and 18, a = orifice area in cm^2, CO = cardiac output in ml/min, HR = heart rate in beats/min, v = mean velocity within the stenotic valve in cm/s, DFP = diastolic filling period in s, SEP = systolic ejection period in s, G = mean pressure gradient in mmHg, and C = empiric constant. C has been set at 0.85 for mitral stenosis (by comparison to anatomical specimens) and to 1 for other orifices. C is the product of C_c (contraction coefficient expressing that the effective orifice is smaller than the anatomical orifice) and a conversion factor correcting for expression of G in mmHg instead of a height of a blood column in cm. This conversion factor is equal to $\sqrt{1.36/1.06} = 1.132$.

Comparing equations 17 and 18 and neglecting the contraction phenomenon ($C_c = 1$ and $C = 1 \times 1.132$), one can verify that the term v in equation 17 corresponds to the term $44.3 \times C \times \sqrt{G}$ in equation 18, since:

$$v = 44.3 \times 1.132 \times \sqrt{G} = 50\sqrt{G} \quad (19)$$

is equivalent to:

$$G = 4v^2 \quad (20)$$

which is the simplified Bernoulli equation used in Doppler methods with v expressed in m/s instead of cm/s.

Thus, the Gorlin equation differs from the continuity equation by the use of C_c leading to the calculation of an anatomical area, greater than the haemodynamic (physiological or effective) area calculated by the continuity equation. Another difference is the use of the term $\sqrt{G}$ in the Gorlin equation instead of the more accurate term G.[42,43] With the term $\sqrt{G}$ the Gorlin equation tends to overestimate v and thus to underestimate the area, especially in the peaked gradient and velocity curves that are observed in moderate stenosis and in the non-obstructive prosthesis.[42] These two differences between continuity and Gorlin equations should be kept in mind when comparing invasive and non-invasive assessment of valvular stenosis and prosthetic valves.

VALVULAR REGURGITATION

Volumetric flow measurements contribute to the quantitation of valvular regurgitation. In our experience of invasive results in adult patients with moderately severe (regurgitant fractions 40% to 60%, grade 3/4) and severe (regurgitant fractions 60 to 80%, grade 4/4) aortic or mitral regurgitation, values obtained for left ventricular output are almost always between 7 and 20 l/min, and values for effective cardiac output are almost always between 2.5 and 6 l/min. With M-mode and/or cross-sectional echo cardiography the increase in left ventricular output can be appreciated taking into account end-diastolic and end-systolic dimensions of the left ventricle and heart rate. In severe mitral regurgitation the echo-Doppler examination demonstrates the discrepancy between signs of increased left ventricular output (or increased mitral inflow) and signs of normal or decreased aortic outflow. The difference between the total left ventricular output (or mitral inflow) and the aortic flow is equal to the regurgitant flow and the ratio of regurgitant flow to total ventricular output (or mitral inflow) is the regurgitant fraction.[45–47] The accuracy of the estimation of regurgitant flow is limited by the cumulative errors from the measurement of each of the two flows that are used for the calculation. In the future, progress in the spatial resolution of colour-coded Doppler systems may provide a direct measurement of the regurgitant flow. Theoretically regurgitant flow is equal to the product of the velocity-time integral of the regurgitant jet (which can be measured using continuous wave Doppler examination) and the cross-sectional area of the root of the jet. The width of the root of regurgitant jets is already proposed as an important clue in the assessment of the severity of regurgitation.

In aortic regurgitation it has been suggested that regurgitant fraction can be calculated by comparing systolic aortic flow and systolic pulmonary flow.[48] Another possibility is the comparison of forward and backward flow in the aortic arch in the bend between the horizontal and descending segments.[49] Regurgitant fraction can only be calculated in patients with a high systolic flow pattern in the arch (peak systolic velocity of over 1/s and ejection time over 0.24 s). In other patients the normal early diastolic backward flow that is present in the aortic isthmus has too great a relative magnitude and leads to overestimations of the regurgitant fraction.[49]

CARDIAC SHUNTS

Volumetric flow measurements in two different sites permits the calculation of pulmonary to systemic flow ratios.[50-53] In atrial septal defects systemic flow should be measured in the aortic orifice and pulmonary flow in the pulmonary orifice. In patent ductus arteriosus, systemic flow should be measured in the pulmonary orifice and pulmonary flow in the aortic orifice. Aortic and pulmonary orifices are preferred to ascending aorta and main pulmonary artery as explained above. In addition, flow in the main pulmonary artery is disturbed in patients with patent ductus arteriosus and laminar flow can only be expected beneath the valve. In ventricular septal defect the systemic flow is measured in the aortic orifice. Systolic flow in the right ventricular outflow tract and pulmonary orifice is frequently disturbed, due to the propagation of the shunt jet. In these cases pulmonary flow should be measured in the mitral valve.[52,53]

CONCLUSIONS

The concept of volumetric flow underlies the assessment of many cardiac diseases. In daily practice the echocardiographer can frequently be satisfied with the observation of indirect signs of increased or decreased flow in cardiac valves and ventricular cavities. A severe valvular stenosis can be excluded in the presence of a low pressure gradient associated with lack of signs of a low cardiac output (normal M-mode left ventricular diameters and kinetics, normal velocities in the left ventricular outflow tract). In the presence of M-mode measurements indicating an increase in left ventricular output aortic regurgitation or mitral regurgitation are likely to be severe and a ventricular septal defect is probably associated with an important left-to-right shunt. In the presence of cross-sectional and M-mode signs of increased right ventricular output (the association of enlarged right ventricle and paradoxical motion of the ventricular septum), tricuspid regurgitation is probably severe, and an atrial septal defect can be anticipated to cause an important left-to-right shunt. Truly quantitative assessment of volumetric flow in various cardiac sites can provide a substantial improvement in the study of heart disease by ultrasound, but it would be naive to expect clinically relevant results without spending adequate time to gather accurately and compute the data that are required for these detailed calculations.[37]

REFERENCES

1 Huntsman L L, Gams E, Johnson C C, Fairbanks E. Transcutaneous determination of aortic blood flow velocities in man. Am Heart J 1975; 89: 605–612
2 Sequeira R F, Light L H, Cross G, Raftery E B. Transcutaneous aortovelography: a quantitative evaluation. Br Heart J 1976; 38: 443–450
3 Angelsen B A J, Brubakk A O. Transcutaneous measurement of blood flow velocity in the human aorta. Cardiovasc Research 1976; 10: 368–379
4 Colocousis J S, Huntsman L L, Curreri P W. Estimation of stroke volume changes by ultrasonic doppler. Circulation 1977; 56: 914–917
5 Steingart R M, Meller J, Barovick J, Patterson R, Herman M V, Teichholz L E. Pulsed Doppler echocardiographic measurement of beat-to-beat changes in stroke volume in dogs. Circulation 1980; 62: 542–548
6 Magnin P A, Stewart J, Myers S, Von Ramm O, Kisslo J A. Combined Doppler and phased-array echocardiographic estimation of cardiac output. Circulation 1981; 63: 388–392
7 Goldberg S J, Sahn D J, Allen H D, Valdes-Cruz L M, Hoenecke H, Carnahan Y. Evaluation of pulmonary and systemic blood flow by 2-dimensional Doppler echocardiography using fast Fourier transform spectral analysis. Am J Cardiol 1982; 50: 1394–1400
8 Touche T, Vervin P, Curien N, Merillon J P, Gourgon R. Cardiac output measurement in adult patients with combined pulsed Doppler and two dimensional echocardiography. Circulation 1982; 66: II-121 (abstract).
9 Fisher D C, Sahn D J, Friedman M J, Larson D, Valdes-Cruz L M, Horowitz S, Goldberg S J, Allen H D. The effect of variations on pulsed Doppler sampling site on calculation of cardiac output: an experimental study in open-chest dogs. Circulation 1983; 67: 370–376
10 Huntsman L L, Stewart D K, Barnes S R, Franklin S B, Colocousis J S, Hessel E A. Non-invasive Doppler determination of cardiac output in man: clinical validation. Circulation 1983; 67: 593–602
11 Chandraratna P A, Nanna M, MacKay C, Nimalasuriya A, Swinney R, Elkayam U, Rahimtoola S H. Determination of cardiac output by transcutaneous continuous-wave ultrasonic Doppler computer. Am J Cardiol 1984; 53: 234–237
12 Nishimura R A, Callahan M J, Schaff H V, Ilstrup D M, Miler F A, Tajik A J. Noninvasive measurement of cardiac output by continuous-wave Doppler echocardiography: initial experience and review of the literature. Mayo Clin Proc 1984; 59: 484–489
13 Loeppky J A, Hoekenga D E, Greene E R, Luft U C. Comparison of noninvasive pulsed Doppler and Fick measurements of stroke volume in cardiac patients. Am Heart J 1984; 107: 339–346
14 Labowitz A J, Buckingham T A, Habermehl K, Nelson J, Kennedy H L, Williams G A. The effects of sampling site on the

two dimensional echo doppler determination of cardiac output. Am Heart J 1985; 109: 327–332
15 Ihlen H, Amlie J P, Dale J, Forfang K, Nitter-Hauge S, Otterstad J E, Simonsen S, Myhre E. Determination of cardiac output by Doppler echocardiography. Br Heart J 1984; 51: 54–60
16 Lewis J F, Kuo L C, Nelson J G, Limacher M C, Quinones M A. Pulsed Doppler echocardiographic determination of stroke volume and cardiac output: clinical validation of two new methods using the apical window. Circulation 1984; 70: 425–431
17 Rein A J J T, Hsieh K S, Elixson M, Colan S D, Lang P, Sanders S P, Castaneda A R. Cardiac output estimates in the pediatric intensive care unit using a continuous-wave Doppler computer: validation and limitations of the technique. Am Heart J 1986; 112: 97–103
18 Bouchard A, Blumlein S, Schiller N B, Schlitt S, Byrd III B J, Ports T, Chatterjee K. Measurement of left ventricular stroke volume using continuous wave Doppler echocardiography of the ascending aorta and M-mode echocardography of the aortic valve. J Am Coll Cardiol 1987; 9: 75–83
19 Sholler G F, Whight C M, Celermajer J M. Pulsed Doppler echocardiographic assessment, including use of aortic leaflet separation, of cardiac output in children with structural heart disease. Am J Cardiol 1986; 57: 1195–1197
20 Touche T. Mesure Doppler des debits intracardiaques. Coeur 1987; 18: 113–119
21 Fisher D C, Sahn D J, Friedman M J, Larson D, Valdes-Cruz L M, Horowitz S, Goldberg S J, Allen H D. The mitral valve orifice method for non-invasive two-dimensional echo-Doppler determinations of cardiac output. Circulation 1983; 67: 872–877
22 Touche T, de Zuttere D, Nitenberg A, Prasquier R, Gourgon R. Echo-Doppler quantitation of transmitral flow: a new method tested in adult patients (abstract). J Am Coll Cardiol 1985; 5: 425
23 Zhang Y, Nitter-Hauge S, Ihlen H, Myhre E. Doppler echocardiographic measurements of cardiac output using the mitral orifice method. Br Heart J 1985; 53: 130–136
24 De Zuttere D, Touche T, Saumon G, Nitenberg A, Prasquier R. Doppler echocardiographic measurement of mitral flow volume: validation of a new method in adult patients. J Am Coll Cardiol 1988; 11: 343–350
25 Valdes-Cruz L M, Horowitz S, Sahn D J, Mesel E, Fisher D C, Larson D, Scagnelli S. A simplified mitral valve method for cross-sectional echo Doppler cardiac output. Circulation 1983; 62: III-230 (abstract).
26 Goldberg S J, Dickinson D F, Wilson N. Evaluation of an elliptical area technique for calculating mitral blood flow by Doppler echocardiography. Br Heart J 1985; 54: 68–75
27 Meijboom E J, Horowitz S, Valdes-Cruz L M, Sahn D J, Larson D F, Oliveira Lima C. A Doppler echocardiographic method for calculating volume flow across the tricuspid valve: correlative laboratory and clinical studies. Circulation 1985; 71: 551–556
28 Ihlen H, Myhre E, Amlie J P, Forfang K, Larsen S. Changes in left ventricular stroke volume measured by Doppler echocardiography. Br Heart J 1985; 54: 378–383
29 Steart W J, Jiang L, Mich R, Pandian N, Guererro J L, Weyman A E. Variable effects of changes in flow rate through the aortic, pulmonary and mitral valves on valve area and flow velocity: impact on quantitative Doppler flow calculations. J Am Coll Cardiol 1985; 6: 653–662
30 Loeppky J A, Greene E R, Hoekenga D E, Caprihan A, Luft U C. Beat-by-beat stroke volume assessment by pulsed Doppler in upright and supine exercise. J Appl Physiol 1981; 50: 1173–1182
31 Rassi A, Crawford M H, Richards K L, Miller J F. Differing mechanisms of exercise flow augmentation at the mitral and aortic valves. Circulation 1988; 77: 543–551
32 Christie J, Sheldahl L M, Tristani F E, Sagar K B, Ptacin M J, Wann S. Determination of stroke volume and cardiac output during exercise: comparison of two-dimensional and Doppler echocardiography, Fick oximetry and thermodilution. Circulation 1987; 76: 539–547
33 Elkayam U, Gardin J M, Berkley R, Hughes C A, Henry W L. The use of Doppler flow velocity measurement to assess the hemodynamic response to vasodilators in patients with heart failure. Circulation 1983; 67: 377–383

34 Schuster A H, Nanda N C. Doppler echocardiography and cardiac pacing. Pace 1982; 5: 607–612
35 Labowitz A J, Williams G A, Redd R M, Kennedy H K. Non invasive assessment of pacemaker hemodynamics by Doppler echocardiography: importance of left atrial size. J Am Coll Cardiol 1985; 6: 196–200
36 Loeber C P, Goldberg S J, Allen H D. Doppler echocardiographic comparison of flows distal to the four cardiac valves. J Am Coll Cardiol 1984; 4: 268–272
37 Sahn D J. Determination of cardiac output by echocardiographic Doppler methods. Relative accuracy of various sites for measurement. J Am Coll Cardiol 1985; 6: 663–664
38 Touche T, Dutoit C, Tcheng P, Bonnet N, de Zutere D. Debits aortique, mitral et ventriculaire gauche en echo-Doppler: degre de concordance des mesures. Arch Mal Coeur 1989; 82: 635 (abstract 35).
39 Kronik G, Slany J, Mosslacher H. Comparative value of eight M-mode echocardiographic formulas for determining left ventricular stroke volume. A correlative study with thermodilution and left ventricular single plane cineangiography. Circulation 1979; 60: 1308–1316
40 Skjaerpe T, Hegrenaes L, Hatle L. Non invasive estimation of valve area in patients with aortic stenosis by Doppler ultrasound and two-dimensional echocardiography. Circulation 1985; 72: 810–818
41 Zoghbi W A, Farmer K L, Soto J G, Nelson J G, Quinones M A. Accurate noninvasive quantification of stenotic aortic valve area by Doppler echocardiography. Circulation 1986; 73: 452–459
42 Holen J, Nitter-Hauge S. Evaluation of obstructive characteristics of mitral disc valve implants with ultrasound Doppler techniques. Acta Med Scand 1977; 201: 429–434
43 Wilkins G T, Gillam L D, Kritzer G L, Levine R A, Palacios I F, Weyman A E. Validation of continuous-wave Doppler echocardiographic measurements of mitral and tricuspid prosthetic valve gradients: a simultaneous Doppler-catheter study. Circulation 1986; 74: 786–795
44 Nakatani S, Masuyama T, Kodama K, Kitabatake A, Fujii K, Kamada T. Value and limitations of Doppler echocardiography in the quantification of stenotic mitral valve area: comparison of the pressure half-time and the continuity equation methods. Circulation 1988; 77: 78–85
45 Ascah K J, Steart W J, Jiang L, Guerrero J L, Newell J B, Gillam L D, Weyman A E. A Doppler-two-dimensional echocardiographic method for quantification of mitral regurgitation. Circulation 1985; 72: 377–383
46 Blumlein S, Bouchard A, Schiller N B, Dae M, Byrd III B F, Ports T, Botvinick E. Quantification of mitral regurgitation by Doppler echocardiography. Circulation 1986; 74: 306–314
47 Zhang Y, Ihlen H, Myhre E, Levorstad K, Nitter-Hauge S. Measurement of mitral regurgitation by Doppler echocardiography. Br Heart J 1985; 54: 384–391
48 Kitabatake A, Ito H, Inoue M et al. A new approach to noninvasive evaluation of aortic regurgitant fraction by two-dimensional Doppler echocardiography. Circulation 1985; 72: 523–529
49 Touche T, Prasquier R, Nitenberg A, De Zuttere D, Gourgon R. Assessment and follow-up of patients with aortic regurgitation by an updated Doppler echocardiographic measurement of the aortic regurgitant fraction in the aortic arch. Circulation 1985; 72: 819–824
50 Sanders S P, Yeager S, Williams R G. Measurement of systemic and pulmonary blood flow and QP/QS ratio using Doppler and two-dimensional echocardiography. Am J Cardiol 1983; 51: 952–956
51 Valdes-Cruz L M, Horowitz S, Mesel E, Sahn D J, Fisher D J, Larson D. A pulsed Doppler echocardiographic method for calculating pulmonary and systemic blood flow in atrial level shunts: validation studies in animals and initial human experience. Circulation 1984; 69: 80–86
52 Valdes-Cruz L M, Horowitz S, Mesel E, Sahn D J, Fisher D C, Larson D, Goldberg S J, Allen H D. A pulsed Doppler echocardiographic method for calculation of pulmonary and systemic flow: accuracy in a canine model with ventricular septal defect. Circulation 1983; 68: 597–602

53 Vargas Barron J, Sahn D J, Valdes-Cruz L M, Oliveira Lima C, Goldberg S J, Grenadier E, Allen H D. Clinical utility of two-dimensional Doppler echocardiographic techniques for estimating pulmonary to systemic blood flow ratios in children with left to right shunting, atrial septal defect, ventricular septal defect or patent ductus arteriosus. J Am Coll Cardiol 1984; 3: 169–178

54 Shultz D L. Pressure and flow in large arteries. In: Bergel D H, ed. Cardiovascular fluid dynamics. London, Academic Press, 1972, p 287–314

55 Grossman W. Cardiac catheterisation and angiography. Second edition. Philadelphia, Lea and Febiger, 1980

Transoesophageal examination

Introduction
Historical background
Equipment
Technique
Transoesophageal cross-sectional echocardiographic anatomy
Indications for outpatient and emergency transoesophageal echocardiography
Infective endocarditis
Aortic pathology
Intracardiac masses
Coronary artery disease
Congenital heart disease
Valvular heart disease
Transoesophageal echocardiography during interventional procedures
Intra-operative and intensive care applications
Biplane transoesophageal echocardiography
Conclusion

Duncan F. Ettles

INTRODUCTION

All echocardiographic techniques are limited by the behaviour of transmitted ultrasound in the tissues through which it passes. Attenuation of ultrasound due to interposed air, muscle and lung tissue leads to suboptimal imaging of cardiac structures in a significant proportion of adult patients using the precordial approach. Diagnostic M-mode and cross-sectional echocardiography are operator dependent and interpretation of findings is subjective. The ability of an echocardiographic study to answer a specific clinical question within acceptable limits of confidence is therefore influenced by a number of variables. While few exact data concerning the incidence of technically inadequate or non-diagnostic precordial echocardiograms are available, a figure of between 10% and 20% is often quoted for routine diagnostic examinations in adults.[1]

Such practical difficulties first prompted investigation into the possibility of ultrasonic imaging of the heart from the oesophagus more than a decade ago.[2] Transoesophageal echocardiography allows imaging of the heart and great vessels that is virtually interference free by virtue of the close proximity of the transducer to the heart. High quality diagnostic images with excellent signal to noise ratio can be obtained irrespective of chest wall configuration or pulmonary disease and evaluation of certain regions of the heart and great vessels rarely visualised by the precordial approach is possible. The rapid developments in technique and equipment which have followed the introduction of transoesophageal echocardiography have already made it the investigation of choice for the investigation of some patients with particular cardiovascular disorders. Transoesophageal echocardiography can be performed easily in anaesthetised patients without disturbing the surgical procedure and its use in intra-operative monitoring of ventricular function in cardiac and other high risk patients is increasing.

HISTORICAL BACKGROUND

The first application of ultrasound to study cardiac function using an intra-oesophageal transducer was reported by Side and Gosling in 1971, who used a simple system for aortic Doppler flow velocimetry.[3] Transoesophageal imaging of the heart and great vessels became possible in 1976 when Frazin developed an oesophageal transducer for use in patients in whom precordial echocardiography gave inadequate results.[2] A single crystal M-mode transducer was attached to a thin coaxial cable and could be swallowed by the patient after topical oropharyngeal anaesthesia. In spite of the lack of steerability of the transducer and the restricted number of views obtained, the introduction of this system represented an important advance in diagnostic cardiac ultrasound.

Experimental two-dimensional endoscopic imaging in animals using a linear array transducer mounted on a conventional gastroscope was reported by DiMagno in 1980.[4] Later that year, real time transoesophageal cross-sectional imaging of the heart and great vessels became feasible in humans with the introduction of a high speed rotating mechanical sector scanner by Hisanga.[5] The variable frequency transducer was mounted on a flexible rotating shaft within an elastic oil filled bag to maintain contact with the oesophageal wall for adequate acoustic coupling. Although the transducer was 'non-steerable', a series of wide sector horizontal cross-sectional images could be obtained as the transducer was advanced and withdrawn within the oesophagus. The superior near field resolution of mechanical transducers and the technical problems of maintaining acceptable endoscope diameter in a phased array system, favoured the development of mechanical transducers but a clinical evaluation of a 3.5 MHz miniature transoesophageal phased array transducer was achieved by Schluter 2 years later.[6] Mounted on a conventional gastroscope, the transducer could be deflected within the oesophageal lumen to maintain contact with the oesophageal wall and by manipulation in two orthogonal planes, provided multiple cross-sectional views. The increased line density of the phased array system yielded better anatomical resolution than the mechanical scanner and the absence of transducer vibration was claimed to improve patient comfort.

Higher frequency phased array transducers have further improved tissue resolution and since 1987 combined transoesophageal imaging and Doppler colour flow mapping has been possible.[7] Smaller endoscopes for paediatric use and endoscopic transducers with the capability of scanning in horizontal and vertical planes are now available.

The evolution of transoesophageal echocardiography has, until recently, been subject to differing philosophies in Europe and the United States. While in America transoesophageal imaging was largely developed by anaesthetists as a tool for intra-operative cardiac monitoring, the greater emphasis in Europe has been towards diagnostic applications of the technique as a result of the extensive work of Hanrath, Schlutter and colleagues. More widespread recognition of the potential value of transoesophageal echocardiography to surgeons, anaesthetists and physicians is reflected by a rapid increase in the literature documenting its many uses.

EQUIPMENT

A commercially available cardiac endoscopic transducer is shown in Figure 1. This instrument incorporates a 5 MHz miniature phased array transducer end-mounted on a conventional 100 cm gastroscope with orientation of the transducer elements to produce a horizontal sector scan at right angles to the long axis of the gastroscope shaft. The transoesophageal transducer is capable of M-mode

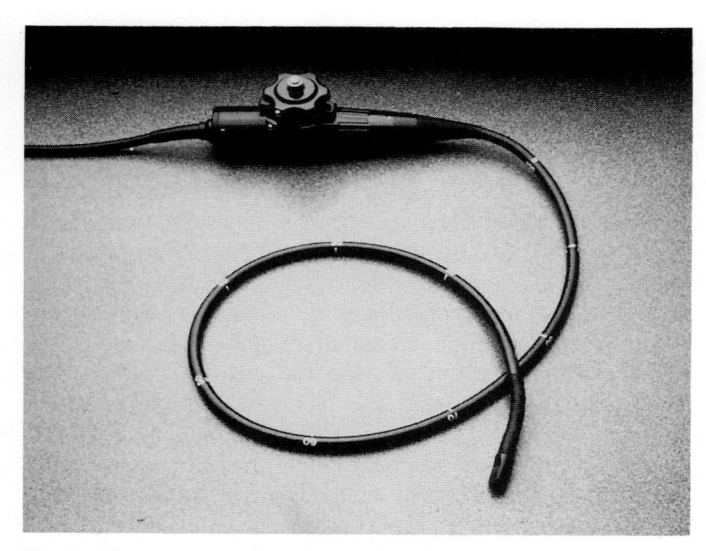

Fig. 1 The transoesophageal transducer is mounted on a flexible gastroscope.

and cross-sectional imaging, spectral pulsed Doppler and colour flow mapping. There is no fibre-optic channel and so the instrument must be introduced without direct vision. Deflection controls at the proximal end of the gastroscope allow combined anteroposterior and lateral motion of the transducer through arcs of approximately 180° and 140° respectively.

To eliminate the theoretical danger of thermal damage to the oesophageal mucosa most instruments incorporate a thermocouple in the tip of the endoscope which automatically switches off electrical power to the transducer if its surface temperature exceeds pre-defined limits. Electrical safety must be ensured by careful inspection of the endoscopic transducer before and after each examination and by frequent electrical testing.

Attention to correct cleaning and disinfection procedure of the transoesophageal transducer is required to prevent possible exposure of medical personnel and patients to pathogenic microorganisms. Additional protection from contamination of the endoscope may be achieved by the use of a disposable sheath which covers the transducer and endoscope shaft in patients examined under general anaesthesia and which does not affect image quality. The echocardiographic equipment to which the transoesophageal transducer is connected may require minor electronic modification.

TECHNIQUE

Physician training

Transoesophageal echocardiography should only be performed by medical personnel competent in upper GI endoscopy. This experience is best obtained by a period of attachment to an endoscopy unit under the supervision of a gastroenterologist. Additional familiarity with transoesophageal echocardiographic views and technique can be gained by initially performing studies in patients undergoing general anaesthesia before attempting studies in awake or sedated patients. The lack of serious reported serious complications of transoesophageal echocardiography to date reflects adequate operator training and competence rather than the intrinsic safety of endoscopy.

Interpretation

Initial unfamiliarity with transoesophageal echocardiographic appearances may lead to difficulties in interpretation of findings. Visualisation of left ventricular bands and the pectinate muscles of the left atrium is common and should not lead to erroneous diagnoses of intracardiac pathology. The operator should be aware of the possibility of ultrasound artefact in the ascending thoracic aorta and in close relation to the course of the left coronary artery.[8,9] Caution is required in the interpretation of transoesophageal colour flow Doppler studies, for instance the increased sensitivity of transoesophageal colour flow mapping making the detection of even minor degrees of mitral regurgitation possible.[10] The use of the technique in the quantification of regurgitation remains to be established.

Intra-operative and intensive care examination

Introduction of the endoscopic transducer in the unconscious patient rarely poses a problem and is conveniently performed shortly after endotracheal intubation and insertion of monitoring lines. A sterile sheath containing ultrasound coupling medium may be used to cover the endoscope. The use of a laryngoscope facilitates passage of the endoscope into the oesophagus and minimises the possibility of pharyngeal trauma or damage to the delicate transducer. The deflection controls are always placed in the unlocked or 'freewheeling' position when advancing or withdrawing the transducer. Once in place, the endoscope is conveniently supported by a clamp at the head of the operating table and the echocardiographer should ensure that the transducer connector cable is kept clear of anaesthetic and pressure monitoring equipment. Preliminary cross-sectional, M-mode and Doppler recordings are then made, if required, for later reference. During cardiac surgery the transducer should be disconnected during any period of hypothermic cardiac arrest although it may be left in situ within the oesophagus.

Introduction of the endoscope in the intensive care unit is performed in a similar manner. Most patients are examined in a supine or semi-recumbent position because of the limitations imposed by mechanical ventilation and monitoring equipment. In the semi-conscious intubated patient 10% lignocaine spray is administered to produce topical pharyngeal anaesthesia before the endoscope is introduced. If the patient experiences any more than minor difficulty in swallowing the transducer, is agitated or in discomfort, then a small dose of a short-acting benzodiazepine is given intravenously unless contra-indicated.

Outpatient examination

Patient preparation

An informed and relaxed patient is better able to cooperate with any form of ultrasound examination and this is particularly true of transoesophageal echocardiography. In most instances the patient will have already attended for preliminary diagnostic precordial echocardiography and an explanation of the need for supplementary transoesophageal echocardiography should therefore be given, although not in a way that might provoke undue anxiety or alarm. The patient is asked to fast overnight before attending for the examination and written consent is taken before the procedure. It is the responsibility of the endoscopist to ensure that the procedure is indicated and clinically justified in view of the small but significant risks of oesophageal instrumentation. The operator should ensure that there is no history of swallowing difficulties and the condition of the teeth is checked. It is helpful if rapport can be established between patient and operator and staff should be sensitive to the anxieties and fears which many patients have of such procedures.

Topical anaesthesia

Topical hypopharyngeal anaesthesia is given in all cases using a 10% lignocaine spray (Xylocaine) or equivalent. Careful attention to achieving adequate anaesthesia greatly reduces the difficulty of the procedure and improves patient comfort.

Sedation

Successful endoscopic cardiac ultrasound can be performed in the majority of patients using topical pharyngeal anaesthesia alone. The use of intravenous sedation is reserved for those patients who are unable to swallow the instrument because of anxiety and in other selected groups of patients such as those with suspected aortic dissection. Whilst transoesophageal echocardiography is well-tolerated by the majority of patients, it is also unpleasant for many and there is nothing to be gained from persistent attempts to pass the endoscope in awake patients who are clearly intolerant of it. The chief advantage of performing the examination without sedation is that the patient is free to leave the department soon after the procedure. In all cases the patient should be advised not to eat or drink until the effects of the topical anaesthesia have worn off. During transoesophageal echocardiography in the unsedated patient, the operator and ancillary staff should refrain from inappropriate discussion or comment on the echocardiographic findings which might be overheard by the patient.

Where sedation is required, a small intravenous dose of midazolam hydrochloride is administered (Hypnovel, 2.5 to 5 mg). This produces a rapid onset of short-lived sedation and antegrade amnesia. The risks of intravenous sedation have been minimised by the availability of the specific benzodiazepine antagonist flumazenil. Use of intravenous sedation increases the time spent by each patient in the endoscopy room and calls for the presence of appropriately trained nursing staff and full resuscitation facilities. However, these factors result in little added inconvenience in a well-organised department.

Antibiotic prophylaxis

There are no established recommendations for antibiotic prophylaxis before transoesophageal echocardiography.

Endoscopic technique

With the patient in the left lateral decubitus position, the oesophageal transducer is introduced through the mouth and into the oesophagus using standard technique. Sterile ultrasound or lignocaine jelly is used to lubricate the transducer and a mouthguard is inserted to prevent the patient inadvertently biting the endoscope. The transducer is initially advanced 25 cm to 30 cm from the teeth. Minor gagging is not uncommon until the endoscope has been advanced beyond the tracheal carina, but the instrument should never be advanced against resistance which most commonly occurs if the endoscope has not been introduced in the mid-line. This is simply corrected by withdrawing and redirecting the endoscope centrally.

Once the endoscope is in place and it has been ensured that the patient is in no discomfort, the transducer is gently rotated anticlockwise until the aortic valve comes clearly into view. The aortic valve acts as a convenient landmark from which a systematic examination of the heart and great vessels may be commenced. Care is taken to avoid any more than the minimum transducer deflection needed within the oesophagus to obtain the necessary views, although almost 90° anterior angulation is needed when the endoscope is passed to the fundus of the stomach for adequate short-axis views of the right and left ventricles. Most views can be obtained by a combination of small changes in anteroposterior angulation of the transducer and axial rotation of the shaft of the endoscope. For examination of the aortic arch and descending thoracic aorta, the endoscope is rotated further anticlockwise to face posteriorly.

Instrumentation time is kept to a minimum with most studies not exceeding 10 minutes duration.

Contra-indications

Transoesophageal echocardiography is contra-indicated in patients with a history of previous oesophageal stricture or oesophageal surgery and in patients who have previously undergone radiotherapy for breast or lung neoplasms. It should not be performed in the presence of uncontrolled hypertension. Where there is any suspicion of oesophageal pathology the examination must be deferred until this has been evaluated and a gastro-enterological opinion sought if necessary.

Complications

The potential hazards of oesophageal instrumentation include oesophageal trauma and ulceration, oesophageal perforation, and electrical shock but none of these has been reported. Acute asthma, transient atrioventricular block and rare episodes of non-sustained ventricular tachycardia have been reported in awake patients undergoing endoscopic ultrasound, but the overall complication rate is less than 1% even in patients with severe heart disease.[11,12] There is an isolated report of recurrent laryngeal nerve palsy following transoesophageal echocardiography in a sedated neurosurgical patient following intra-operative use of a prototype transducer.[13] A small proportion of patients complain of minor throat discomfort after endoscopy which quickly resolves.

There is a reported failure rate of approximately 3% in awake patients who are unable to tolerate the procedure.[11] A small rise in blood pressure is usual during the procedure and continuous monitoring of the electrocardiogram and blood pressure throughout the procedure is recommended.[12,14]

TRANSOESOPHAGEAL CROSS-SECTIONAL ECHOCARDIOGRAPHIC ANATOMY

By convention left sided cardiac structures are displayed on the right side of the monitor screen with posterior structures at the top of the screen.[15,16] Nomenclature has been proposed to allow standardisation of transoesophageal cross-sectional echocardiographic views,[15,16] but it should be emphasised that in many circumstances multiple and often non-standard views are required for adequate transoesophageal echocardiographic evaluation of cardiac pathology. The following section describes the more commonly used transoesophageal cross-sectional echocardiographic views. The reader should refer to the line drawing in Figure 2 in conjunction with each cross-sectional view. Distances given between transducer and teeth are approximate.

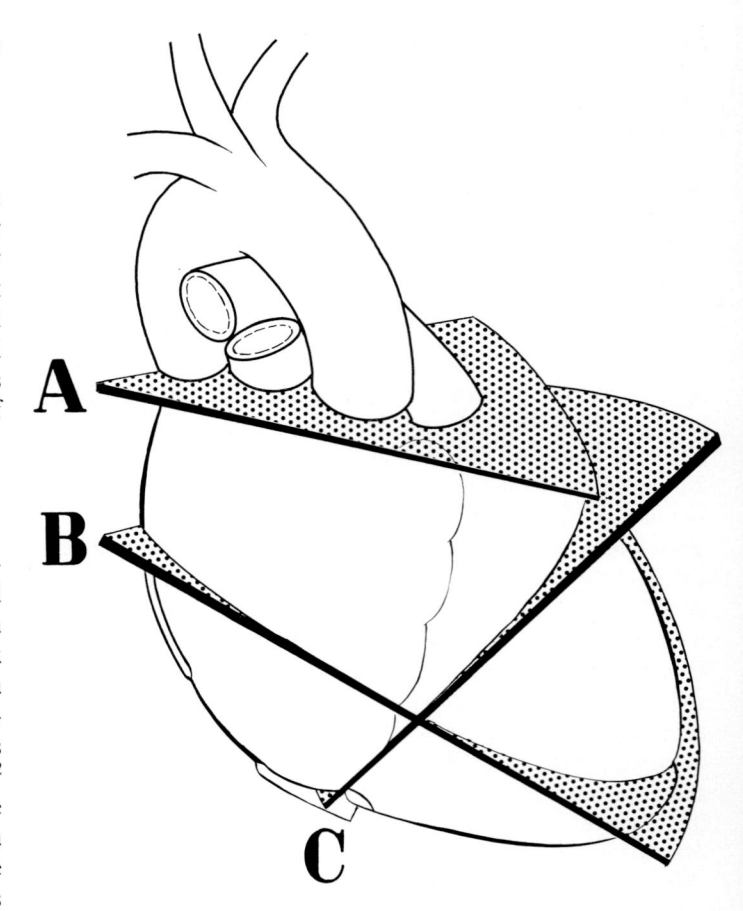

Fig. 2 Basic imaging planes used in transoesophageal echocardiography. **A:** Basal short axis view. **B:** Four chamber view. **C:** Ventricular short axis view. For corresponding echocardiographic sections refer to Figures 3A, 4A and 5.

Basal short axis view (Figs 2 and 3A)

With the endoscope advanced to between 25 and 30 cm and facing anteriorly, the aortic valve occupies the centre of the scan sector and its leaflets can be identified clearly. The superior part of the left atrial cavity lies behind the aortic valve with the right ventricular outflow tract in the left anterolateral position and the superior vena caval–right atrial junction in the right anterolateral position. Rotation of the endoscope anticlockwise at this level brings the left atrial appendage into view as shown in Figure 3B. Clockwise rotation of the transducer produces a bi-atrial view which is of particular value for the detection and assessment of patent foramen ovale. Slight withdrawal of the transducer allows visualisation of the superior vena cava, aorta and pulmonary arteries. The pulmonary artery can be followed from the pulmonary valve to its bifurcation and the major portion of the right pulmonary artery is also seen. Minor rotation and angulation of the transducer just above the level of the aortic valve brings the coronary arteries into view.

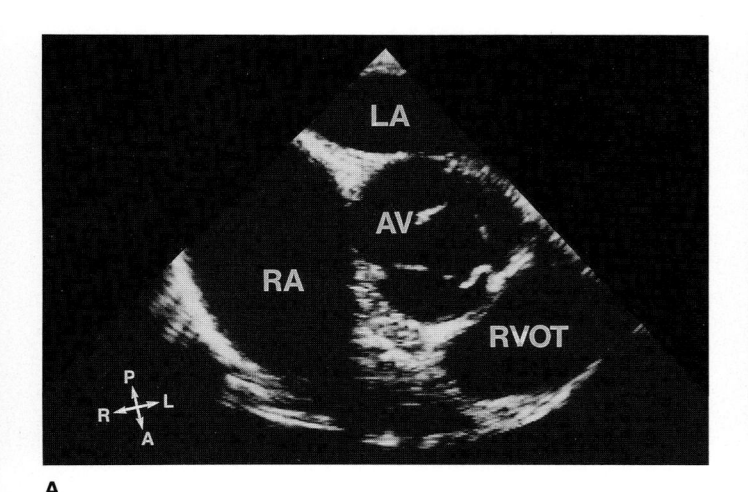

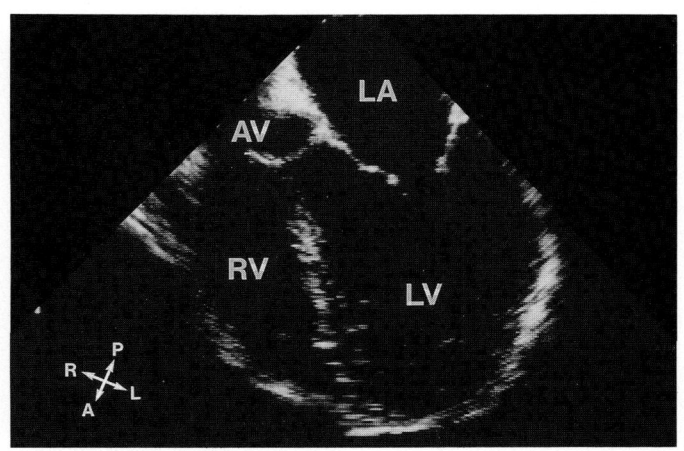

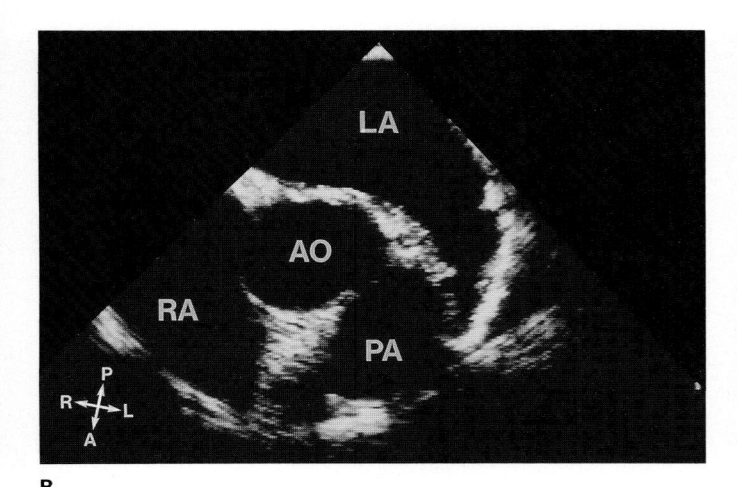

Fig. 3 A: Basal short axis view. The transducer has been positioned in mid-oesophagus allowing clear visualisation of aortic valve (AV), atria and right ventricular outflow tract (RVOT). **B:** Slight rotation and angulation of the transducer has been used at the same level to bring the left atrial appendage into view.

Fig. 4 A: Four chamber view. Angulation of the transducer anteriorly allows better visualisation of the aortic valve (AV) and left ventricular outflow tract, while slight posterior deflection provides optimum views of the mitral valve. **B:** Rotation of the transducer at this level is used to inspect the right heart although only limited views are obtained in the absence of right heart enlargement.

Four chamber view (Figs 2 and 4A)

By further advancement of the transducer to approximately 30 cm, longitudinal views of the mitral valve, left atrial cavity, left ventricle and aortic outflow tract are obtained. A variable portion of the right ventricle and right atrium are seen. Angulation of the transducer upwards brings the aortic valve and outflow tract more clearly into view while straightening or slight posterior angulation of the transducer brings the mitral valve into view. Doppler colour flow mapping of mitral regurgitation is best performed in this latter position. A true long axis view of the aortic valve cannot be obtained but the tangential section of the aortic valve and outflow tract is suitable for the detection of aortic regurgitation.

In a small proportion of normal subjects, rotation of the endoscope clockwise allows a two chamber view of the right heart to be obtained as shown in Figure 4B. Where the right heart is enlarged as part of the disease process, much larger portions of the right atrium and ventricle are accessible.

Ventricular short axis view (Figs 2 and 5)

A short axis view of the right and left ventricles is obtained by advancing the tip of the endoscope to the fundus of the stomach and angling the transducer anteriorly. The origins of the papillary muscles are often visualised and occasionally a true short axis view of the mitral valve is obtained. The ventricular short axis view is used for intraoperative monitoring of left ventricular function.

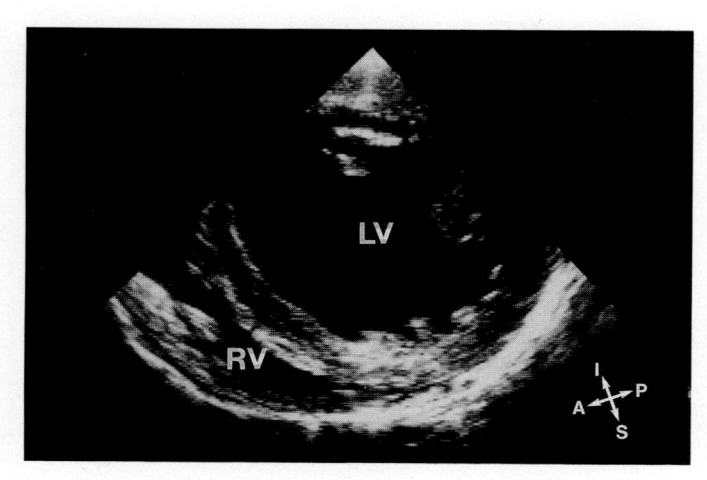

Fig. 5 Ventricular short axis view obtained with the transducer tip located in the gastric fundus or terminal oesophagus. This view is of particular value intra-operatively for monitoring left ventricular size and contractility.

Thoracic aorta

Transoesophageal echocardiography allows the greater portion of the thoracic aorta to be imaged from the level of the aortic root to the diaphragm. The aortic valve and aortic root are visualised with the transducer facing anteriorly and approximately 60° anticlockwise rotation of the endoscope allows the aortic arch and descending aorta to be examined. The upper portion of the ascending aorta and proximal part of the arch are less consistently visualised due to interposition of the left main bronchus. When the ascending aorta is dilated this region is usually well-visualised.

Limitations of views

The difficulties in imaging the upper ascending aorta have already been discussed. While multiple long-axis sections of the left ventricle can be obtained, a true long-axis view corresponding to the conventional precordial image is unobtainable using horizontal scanning transducers. The apices of both ventricles are rarely visualised and except in the presence of right heart pathology, only limited views of the right atrium and ventricle are obtained. The introduction of endoscopic transducers which allow imaging in more than one orthogonal plane is beginning to increase the number of cross-sectional views obtained and will overcome some of these important limitations.

INDICATIONS FOR OUTPATIENT AND EMERGENCY TRANSOESOPHAGEAL ECHOCARDIOGRAPHY

Infective endocarditis

The definitive diagnosis of infective endocarditis is based upon clinical features and isolation of the causative microorganism from the bloodstream,[17] but echocardiography has an important role in the identification of vegetations and detection of complications. The diagnosis of endocarditis may rely solely on echocardiographic findings when blood cultures are negative.[18] The sensitivity of combined precordial M-mode and cross-sectional echocardiography for the detection of valvular vegetations is between 60% and 80%,[19,20] but confident echocardiographic exclusion of infective vegetations can pose considerable difficulties especially in poor imaging subjects with concomitant lung disease or obesity. Further difficulties are encountered in the presence of prosthetic valves where multiple echoes from the valve itself can easily mask the presence of vegetations.

Comparison between precordial and transoesophageal echocardiography in proven native and prosthetic valve endocarditis demonstrates the increased sensitivity of transoesophageal echocardiography for the detection of vegetations.[21,22] The advantages of the oesophageal approach are due to superior image resolution which is of particular value in the detection of small vegetations. Figure 6 shows the transoesophageal echocardiographic appearances in a patient presenting with digital gangrene and confusion in whom blood cultures were negative and precordial echocardiography failed to demonstrate vegetations conclusively. The value of transoesophageal echocardiography in the investigation of patients with

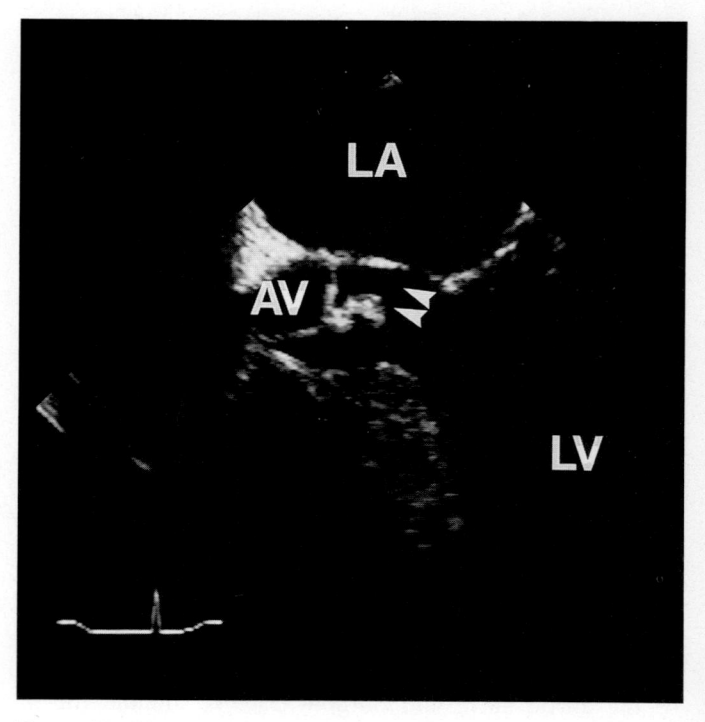

Fig. 6 Modified four chamber view. A large vegetation is clearly visible (arrowed) on the ventricular surface of the aortic valve (AV). Precordial echocardiography had previously failed to reveal a cause for this patient's confusion and digital gangrene.

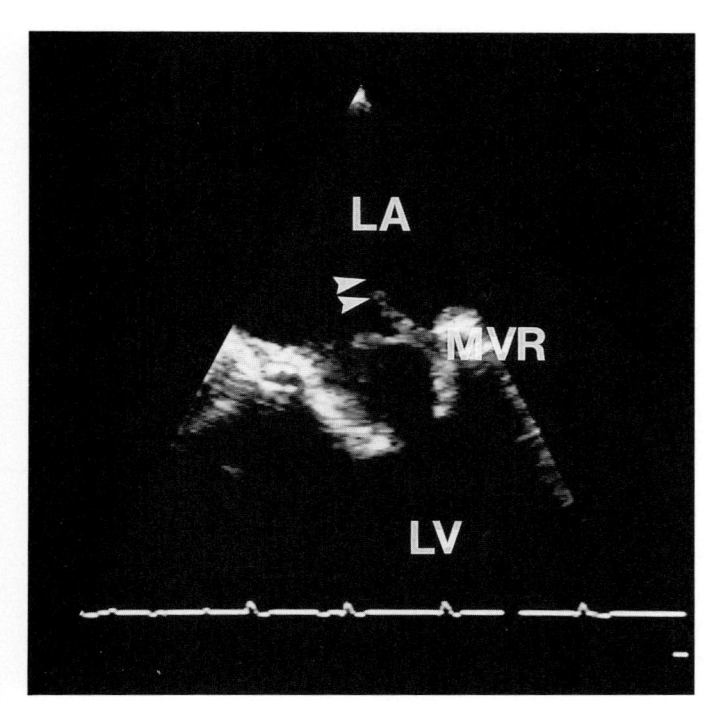

Fig. 7 Long axis scan (modified four chamber view) showing a vegetation (arrowed) attached to the sewing ring of a Carpentier–Edwards xenograft (MVR). The orientation of the transducer to the mitral orifice overcomes the problems of artefact and acoustic masking often encountered using the transthoracic approach.

suspected prosthetic valve endocarditis is illustrated in Figure 7 which shows a large vegetation attached to the valve sewing ring which went undetected using precordial cross-sectional imaging.

Further use of transoesophageal echocardiography in this condition will provide useful insights into the natural history of infective endocarditis and the effects of antibiotic therapy on vegetation size and morphology. What effects the earlier detection of vegetations and subsequent therapeutic intervention will have on the morbidity and mortality of infective endocarditis remains uncertain.

Complications of infective endocarditis such as paravalvular abscess and prosthetic valve dehiscence are readily detected using the transoesophageal approach.[21,23,24] The addition of Doppler colour flow mapping provides important haemodynamic information that is of particular value in the evaluation of mitral prosthetic dysfunction. The site and extent of paraprosthetic regurgitation can be determined quickly without the need for potentially hazardous angiographic studies. Periodic follow up examinations will detect any further deterioration.

The precise role of transoesophageal echocardiography in the diagnosis and management of endocarditis has yet to be established. Preliminary studies suggest that where a high index of clinical suspicion exists, haematological and bacteriological evidence is inconclusive and conventional echocardiography is unhelpful, then transoesophageal echocardiography should be undertaken, especially in the presence of prosthetic valves. The increased sensitivity of transoesophageal cross-sectional echocardiography for the detection of vegetations underscores the importance of critical evaluation of precordial examinations.

Aortic pathology

The close apposition between oesophagus and thoracic aorta provides a unique ultrasonic window for the study of aortic pathology. The thoracic aorta can be studied in its entirety except for the upper segment of the ascending aorta where the trachea and left main bronchus intervene. Detailed studies of aortic aneurysm and acute and chronic aortic dissection are therefore possible.[8,25]

Correct management of acute thoracic aortic dissection hinges on accurate assessment of the site of intimal disruption and the extent and haemodynamic effects of dissection.[26,27] Perhaps the most exciting potential application of transoesophageal echocardiography is in the diagnosis and management of this often fatal condition.

Transoesophageal cross-sectional echocardiography has high sensitivity and specificity for the detection of acute thoracic aortic dissection and visualisation of the intimal tear is possible in approximately half of cases.[28–30] While reliable diagnosis of type I and III dissection is possible, false negative and false positive results have been reported in cases of type II dissection.[8,28] False positive diagnosis of type II aortic dissection relates to aortic wall motion artefact in the upper ascending aorta. Further improvement in diagnostic accuracy may be possible using combined imaging and colour flow Doppler to detect the site of intimal tear and differentiate true and false aortic lumina.[30,31] Plate 1A and B shows imaging alone and combined imaging with colour flow Doppler in the same patient with acute type I aortic dissection. Absence of laminar flow in the false lumen at this level is confirmed by the Doppler findings.

The results of a European Co-operative Study into the value of echocardiography in thoracic aortic dissection demonstrate that combined transthoracic and transoesophageal cross-sectional echocardiography offers superior sensitivity and specificity ($> 90\%$) to both angiography and computed tomography in the diagnosis of aortic dissection. Transoesophageal echocardiography has proved to be a reliable bedside technique for the assessment of suspected dissection. Endoscopy can be performed in the intensive care unit or anaesthetic room and a confident diagnosis made within minutes of hospital admission, in some cases allowing the patient to proceed to operation without further investigation.[8,28,30] Careful control of the blood pressure is mandatory during transoesophageal echocardiography in patients with suspected dissection and intravenous sedation is advised. The avoidance of lengthy and potentially hazardous angiographic examinations in this high risk group with significant early mortality (2%

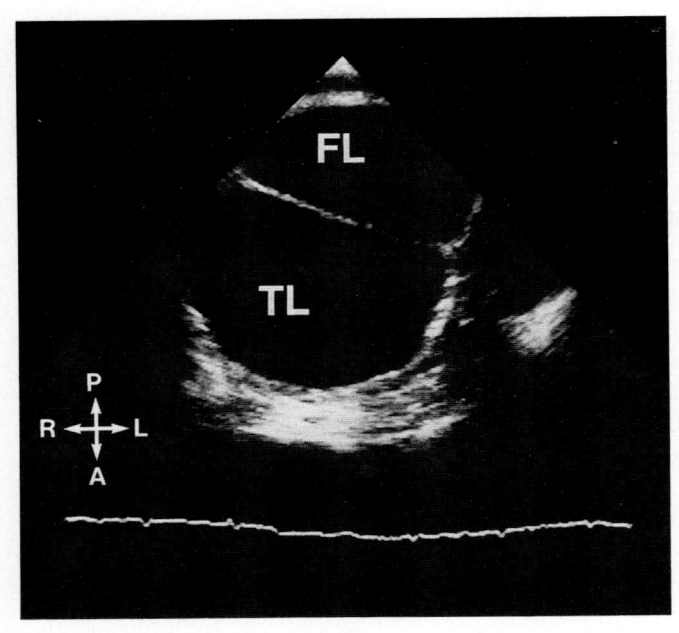

Early and accurate diagnosis of the type and extent of aortic dissection by transoesophageal echocardiography should in turn lead to improvement in patient care and a reduction in early associated mortality. In the follow up of thoracic aortic dissection, serial transoesophageal echocardiography allows documentation of persistence or thrombosis of the false lumen and recognition of complications for which surgery may be indicated.[32]

Intracardiac masses

Transoesophageal cross-sectional echocardiography allows clear imaging of the greater portion of the left atrial cavity and appendage, while more limited views of the right atrium are obtained. The left ventricle may be examined in at least two planes but only limited views of the right ventricular cavity are obtained in the non-dilated heart. The apices of both ventricles cannot be adequately examined in most patients. The potential of transoesophageal echocardiography in the investigation of intracardiac space occupying lesions is perhaps best illustrated in the assessment of atrial pathology.

Atrial myxoma

Precordial cross-sectional echocardiography plays an important role in the pre-operative diagnosis and long-term follow up of atrial myxomata.[33,34] Characterisation of atrial masses may however be difficult and even sizeable tumours can go undetected.[35] Figure 8 shows the transoesophageal echocardiographic appearances of a solitary atrial myxoma. This illustration emphasises the value of transoesophageal echocardiography to the surgeon in determining the anatomical relationships of the tumour prior to operation and thus helping to plan the surgical approach. Evaluation of the remaining cardiac chambers may be undertaken also

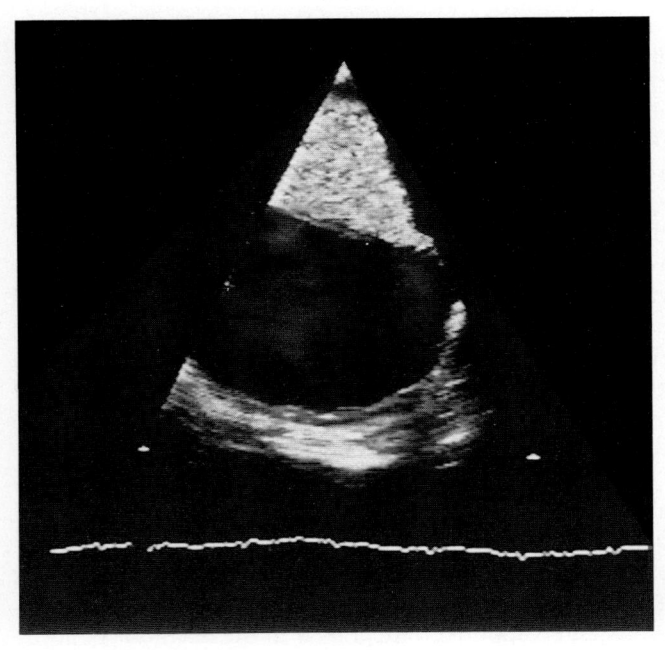

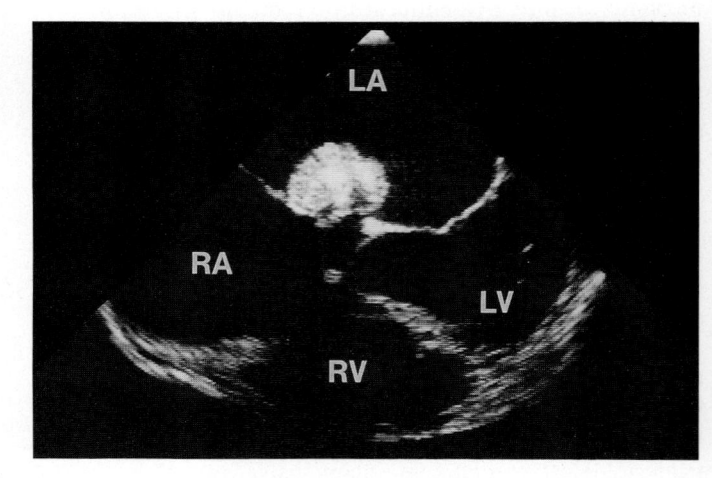

Plate 1 **A:** True (TL) and false lumina (FL) are clearly identified in the ascending aorta in this case of Type I dissection. The transducer is directed anteriorly. **B:** Colour flow mapping shows a normal pattern of flow within the true lumen while a jet of turbulent flow is demonstrated in the false lumen. This figure is reproduced in colour in the colour plate section at the front of this volume.

per hour)[32] is a major advantage provided by transoesophageal echocardiography. The most important limitation of the technique is failure to visualise the brachiocephalic vessels for which supplementary angiography or other imaging techniques may be required.

Fig. 8 Four chamber view. Pre-operative transoesophageal echocardiography was used to determine the size and anatomical relationship of this solitary atrial myxoma.

to exclude additional tumours within the limitations of the cross-sectional views obtained. Superior image resolution allows recognition of tissue characteristics that cannot be appreciated by precordial imaging. Small fluid-filled cysts and flecks of calcification are typically seen within myxomata using the transoesophageal approach.[36] The practical value of this technique is well illustrated in a case report by Ezekowitz et al., where platelet scintigraphy led to the erroneous diagnosis of atrial thrombus in the presence of an atrial mass that was subsequently shown to be a myxoma by transoesophageal echocardiography.[37]

Transoesophageal echocardiography offers clear advantages over precordial imaging in the diagnosis and pre-operative assessment of atrial myxomata,[38] but may have an equally important role in post-surgical follow up. Early detection of new or recurrent tumours may be especially useful in younger patients presenting with multiple lesions where recurrence can follow a more aggressive course.

Intracardiac thrombus

The left atrial appendage is infrequently and inconsistently imaged using the precordial approach, but can be visualised in the majority of patients transoesophageally.[16] For this reason, the common clinical problem of excluding an intracardiac source of emboli in patients with neurological signs and symptoms may be best approached using transoesophageal cross-sectional echocardiography.

In patients with atrial fibrillation and mitral valve disease spontaneous contrast within the left atrium and appendage

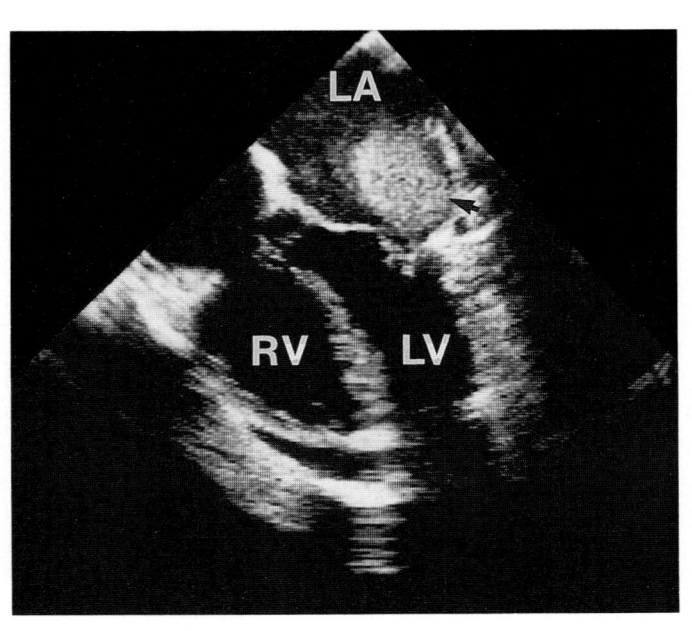

Fig. 10 Four chamber view. Acute thrombus formation within the left atrium in the presence of severe mitral stenosis. The patient presented in a low cardiac output state and transoesophageal echocardiography was performed in the intensive care unit during assisted ventilation. Spontaneous formation of thrombosis occurred over a period of several minutes.

is a frequent transoesophageal echocardiographic finding. The precise temporal relationship of this phenomenon to thrombus formation is unclear but it reflects the presence of turbulent and relatively slow moving blood within the atrium. Figure 9 shows an example of spontaneous contrast within the left atrial appendage of a patient with functional mitral regurgitation secondary to ischaemic papillary muscle dysfunction. The 'shifting sands' pattern of echoes is clearly visible. A more dramatic example of this phenomenon is seen in Figure 10 where acute thrombus formation is demonstrated in a patient with severe mitral stenosis.

100% specificity and sensitivity for transoesophageal echocardiographic detection of left atrial appendage thrombus has been reported in one study of a small number of patients with advanced mitral valve disease.[39] However, single plane endoscopic transducers fail to visualise all portions of the atrium and further research to establish the incidence of both false positive and false negative findings in the investigation of suspected atrial thrombi is needed. Figure 11 shows atrial thrombus in a patient presenting with transient loss of vision who had undergone mitral valve replacement 3 years previously. The patient was not taking anticoagulant therapy.

In the investigation of unexplained systemic embolic episodes when precordial echocardiography fails to detect intracardiac thrombus, the incidence of left atrial appendage thrombus detected by transoesophageal echocardiography may be as high as 50%.[40] This finding has

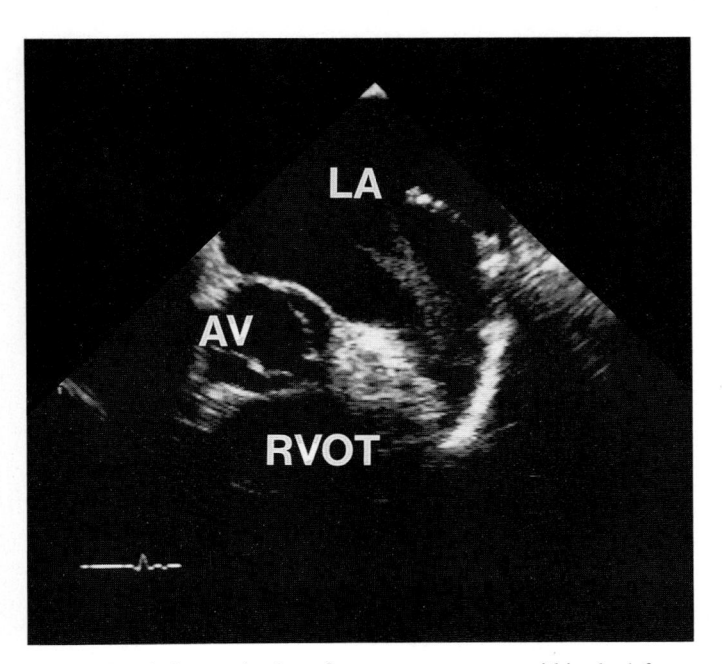

Fig. 9 Basal short axis view. Spontaneous contrast within the left atrial appendage due to mild mitral regurgitation after myocardial infarction (AV – aortic valve, RVOT – right ventricular outflow tract).

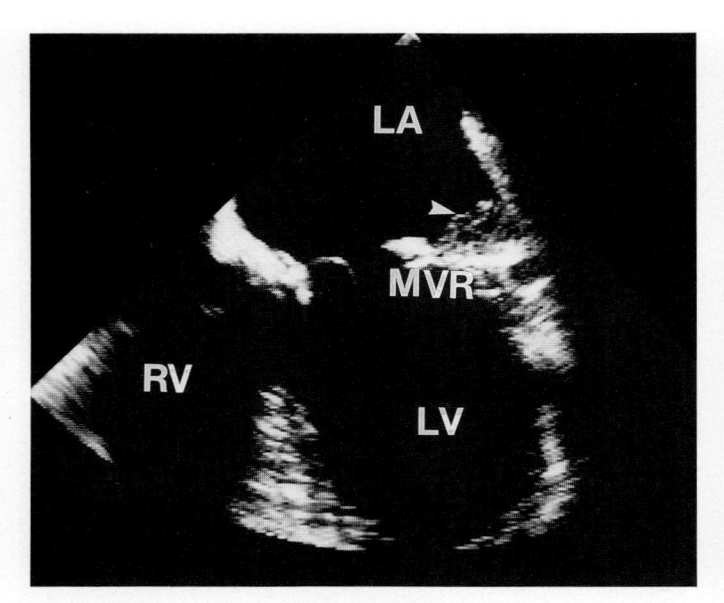

Fig. 11 Four chamber view showing atrial thrombus (arrowhead) and mitral xenograft (MVR).

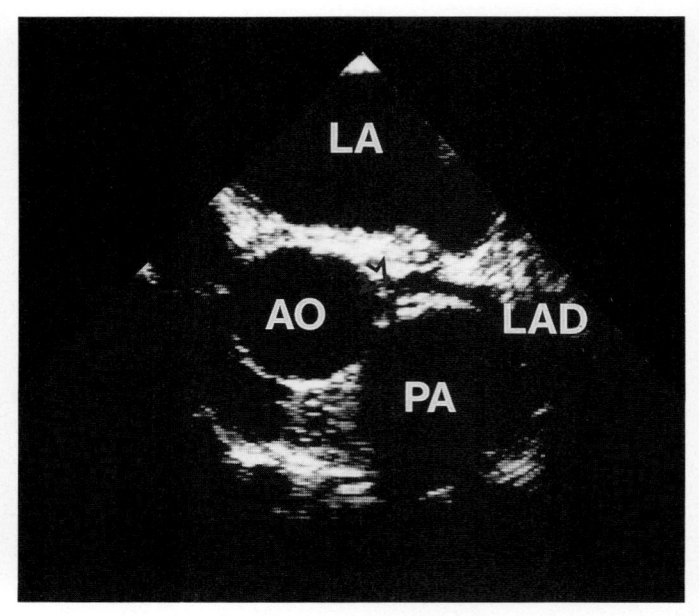

Fig. 12 Basal short axis view. Visualisation of the left main coronary artery (arrowed) and its continuation as left anterior descending artery (LAD) is possible in a significant proportion of subjects.

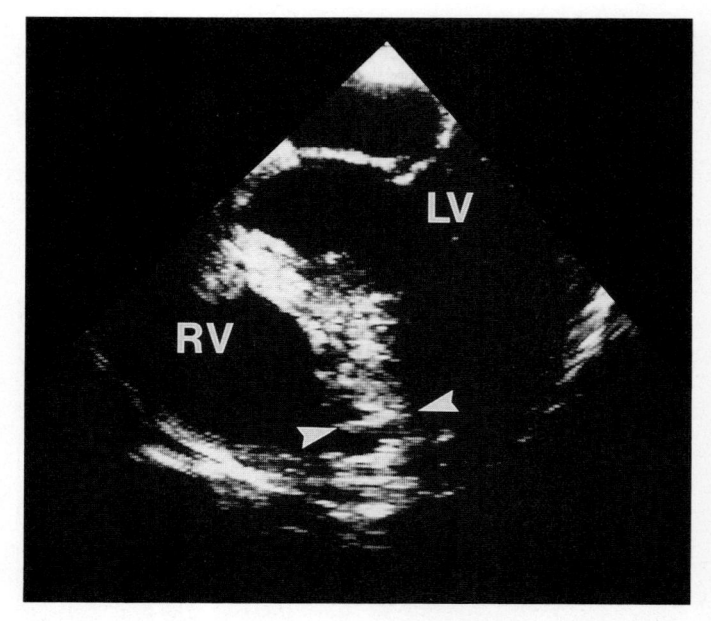

Fig. 13 Four chamber view. A small apical ventricular septal defect (between arrowheads) is demonstrated following acute occlusion of the right coronary artery. Note the thickened appearance of the remainder of the septum due to peri-infarctional oedema. Successful closure of the defect was possible.

important implications for cardiologists and neurologists in the investigation and management of patients with and without valvular disease who present with unexplained neurological symptoms.

Transoesophageal cross-sectional echocardiography has been used successfully for the localisation of thrombus within the pulmonary artery following pulmonary embolism.[41] In selected patients, it may therefore be possible to assess the need for emergency thrombectomy or thrombolytic therapy without the need for cardiac catheterisation and pulmonary angiography. Clear visualisation of the fossa ovalis is possible using transoesophageal echocardiography and Doppler colour flow mapping may reveal even minor degrees of inter-atrial shunting.[42] Dramatic presentation of impending paradoxical embolism correctly identified by endoscopic ultrasound and prevented by emergency surgery has been reported.[43]

Coronary artery disease

Reliable ultrasonic imaging of the coronary arteries would have many important clinical applications, but despite advances in transducer performance and digital image processing,[44] precordial echocardiography remains of limited value in the assessment of coronary artery disease.[45,46] Visualisation of the left main coronary artery and proximal circumflex arteries is possible in a high proportion of patients undergoing transoesophageal echocardiography. The left anterior descending artery is less frequently seen and limited views of the right coronary artery are obtained in a minority of patients. Figure 12 shows the proximal branches of the left coronary system in a patient with normal coronary arteries.

Transoesophageal cross-sectional echocardiography has been shown to be a reliable screening investigation for the detection of atherosclerotic lesions in the proximal circumflex and left main coronary arteries,[9] but with a tendency for overestimation of the severity of stenotic lesions. Doppler colour flow mapping can be used to delineate diastolic flow within the coronary arteries but its application to the detection and quantification of coronary stenosis is unexplored. The right coronary artery is seen in a minority of patients only and evaluation of proximal atheromatous disease seems less hopeful. Therefore, while transoesophageal imaging of the left main and circumflex arteries may prove useful as a screening procedure during routine examinations by alerting the clinician to possible underlying coronary atheroma, its role is limited and cannot be regarded as an alternative to conventional angiographic techniques.

In the management of patients with acute myocardial infarction, transoesophageal echocardiography can be used for the diagnosis of acute ventricular septal rupture and papillary muscle dysfunction in patients whose precordial echocardiograms are unhelpful.[47] Figure 13 shows a small post-infarction ventricular septal defect in a patient who suffered acute inferior myocardial infarction 3 days previously.

Transoesophageal cross-sectional echocardiography has proved reliable for the recognition of angiographically demonstrated dyskinetic ventricular wall motion and even transoesophageal exercise studies have been successfully performed.[48,49] As neither precordial nor transoesophageal echocardiography provides comprehensive views of all ventricular segments, the two techniques may be complementary in the non-invasive detection of ischaemic myocardial dysfunction.

Congenital heart disease

The use of transoesophageal echocardiography in congenital heart disease is currently of more use in adolescent and adult patients. Precordial imaging rarely presents a problem in the paediatric population, but the development of high resolution small diameter endoscopic probes for use in infants and small children will yield important advantages in the peri-operative assessment of surgery for complex congenital cardiac anomalies.

Conventional cross-sectional and contrast echocardiography allow reliable detection of atrial septal defects (ASD) with sensitivity approaching 90% for the common secundum type defect.[50–52] The problems of false positive diagnoses due to echo drop out are largely overcome by the use of a subcostal transducer position but in poor imaging subjects, the diagnosis can be difficult. The proximity and orientation of the endoscopic transducer to the interatrial septum make transoesophageal echocardiography a sensitive and reliable technique for the detection of ASDs and differentiation of secundum, primum and the more difficult sinus venosus defects is possible.[53–55] The technique should be regarded as complementary to, rather than a substitute for, right heart catheterisation, allowing anatomical rather than functional assessment of the atrial shunt. Combined with accurate pulsed Doppler shunt quantification and the increased anatomical information promised with biplane scanning, transoesophageal echocardiography may further reduce the need for cardiac catheterisation prior to surgery although anomalous venous drainage cannot be identified using this technique.

Figure 14 shows an example of a secundum ASD in a 34-year-old male patient in whom precordial echocardiography was technically inadequate. Coronary angiography was performed prior to surgical closure of the defect because of a strong family history of ischaemic heart disease.

Valvular heart disease

Precordial cross-sectional echocardiography is of limited value in the direct measurement of aortic valve orifice area[55] and has been replaced largely by continuous wave Doppler techniques for estimation of peak pressure drop[56,57] or valve area calculation using the continuity equation.[58] Transoesophageal echocardiographic measurement of aortic valve orifice area appears to correlate well with invasive determination of orifice area by the Gorlin equation,[59] although difficulties in obtaining appropriate cross-sectional views make it unsuitable in some patients. Where retrograde catheterisation of the aortic valve is contraindicated or unsuccessful, transoesophageal echocardiography performed in conjunction with precordial Doppler measurements may yield sufficient information on which therapeutic decisions can be based.

Transoesophageal echocardiography has been shown to be of value in the differential diagnosis of flail mitral valve

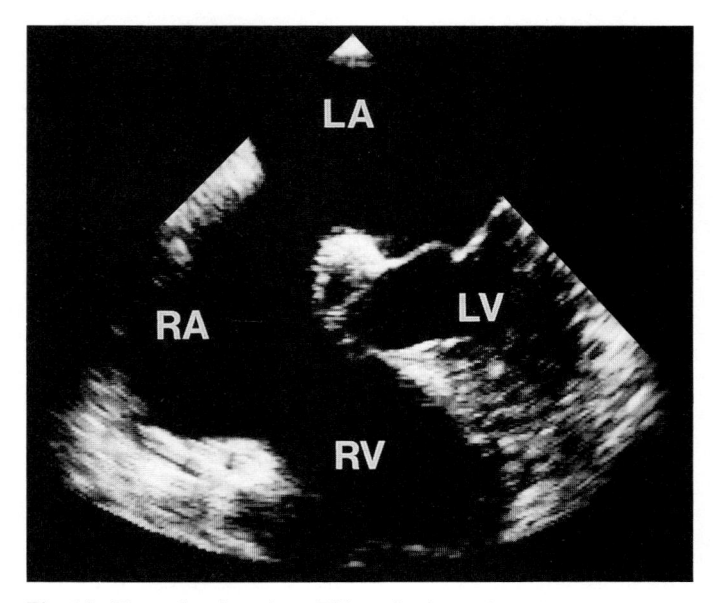

Fig. 14 **Four chamber view.** This patient's stocky build prevented a definitive diagnosis by transthoracic echocardiography. The atrial septal defect was easily visualised endoscopically.

and cor triatiatum.[60,61] Transoesophageal pulsed wave and colour encoded Doppler are sensitive for the detection of even minor degrees of mitral regurgitation although accurate quantification of the regurgitant fraction is not yet feasible.[62] Accurate measurement of left and right atrial dimensions is possible and could provide a means of evaluating atrial dynamics in various cardiac disorders and the interaction between left and right atria.[63]

Using spectral or colour encoded transoesophageal pulsed Doppler echocardiography, blood flow velocity patterns may be studied in the left atrium, thoracic aorta, pulmonary veins and through the aortic and mitral valves. The use of colour flow mapping in aortic pathology has already been discussed.

The alignment of the transducer to the mitral valve and the absence of intervening tissues makes the transoesophageal approach sensitive for the detection of native and prosthetic mitral regurgitation.[62,64] In Plates 2 and 3 transoesophageal colour Doppler studies of mitral regurgitation are shown from patients with angiographically mild and severe mitral regurgitation respectively. Further correlative studies are needed to determine whether clinically reliable quantification of mitral regurgitation according to the size, extent and colour encoding information of the regurgitant jets is possible. Conflicting evidence exists over the reliability of this technique.[64,65,66]

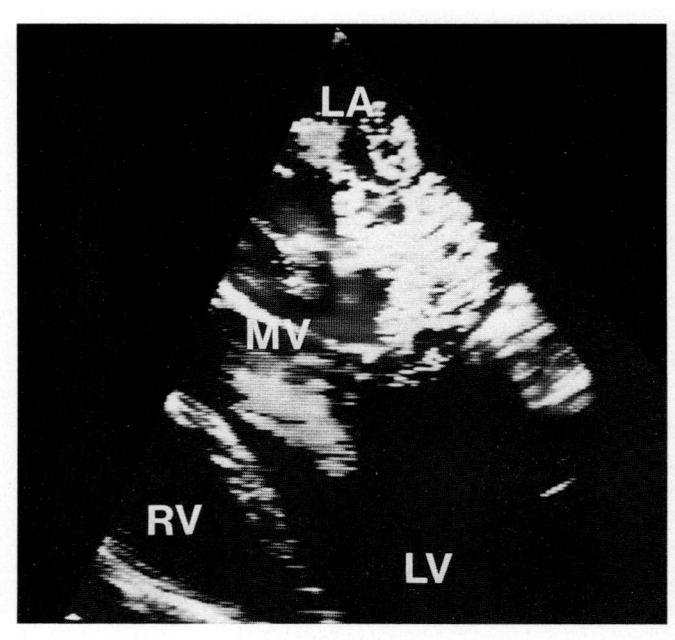

Plate 3 Four chamber view. Mitral regurgitation in the presence of mitral valve prolapse. A widely based regurgitant flow jet is seen within the atrium and angiography confirmed the severity of regurgitation. This figure is reproduced in colour in the colour plate section at the front of this volume.

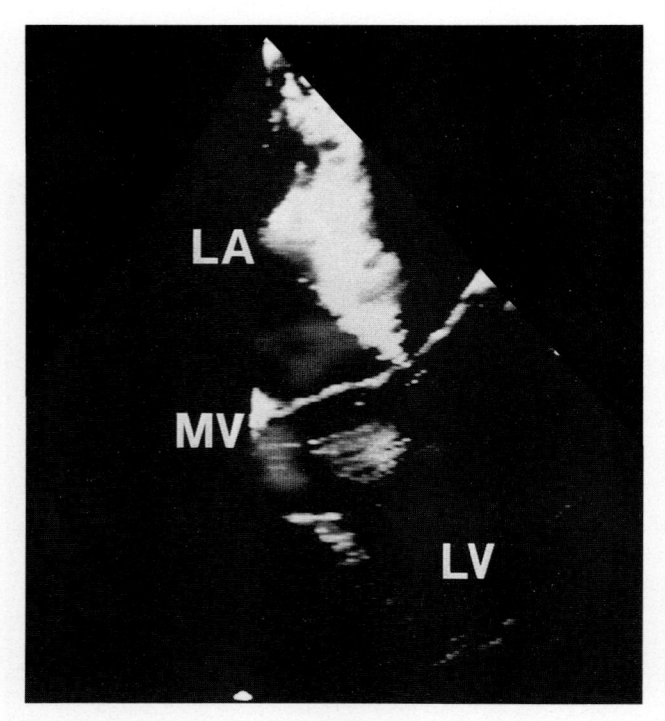

Plate 2 Four chamber view. Colour flow mapping shows a 'candle flame' jet of regurgitation in an elderly subject with angiographically mild mitral regurgitation. This figure is reproduced in colour in the colour plate section at the front of this volume.

Transoesophageal colour flow mapping has been found of particular use in the evaluation of suspected mitral prosthetic valve dysfunction where the common problem of acoustic masking, encountered in precordial Doppler echocardiographic studies of mechanical mitral valve prostheses,[67] is avoided due to the ideal orientation of the ultrasound beam to the prosthesis. It is possible to differentiate pathological from 'physiological' prosthetic mitral regurgitation according to colour flow characteristics of the regurgitant jets and the precise location and extent of paraprosthetic leaks can be determined.[65,66]

In the seriously ill patient with suspected acute prosthetic valve failure, precordial Doppler echocardiography may be limited due to respiratory distress and cardiac catheterisation may be hazardous. Combined transoesophageal cross-sectional echocardiography and colour flow Doppler allows confirmation of prosthetic dysfunction at the bedside and in some cases no further investigation is required prior to re-operation. Figure 15 shows the transoesophageal basal short axis view in a patient presenting in acute pulmonary oedema 6 weeks after aortic valve replacement in whom a short aortic diastolic murmur was audible. Precordial echocardiography showed abnormal rocking of the valve but could not confirm the presence of paraprosthetic regurgitation. Transoesophageal echocardiography revealed extensive dehiscence of the aortic valve sewing ring which was confirmed at successful reoperation.

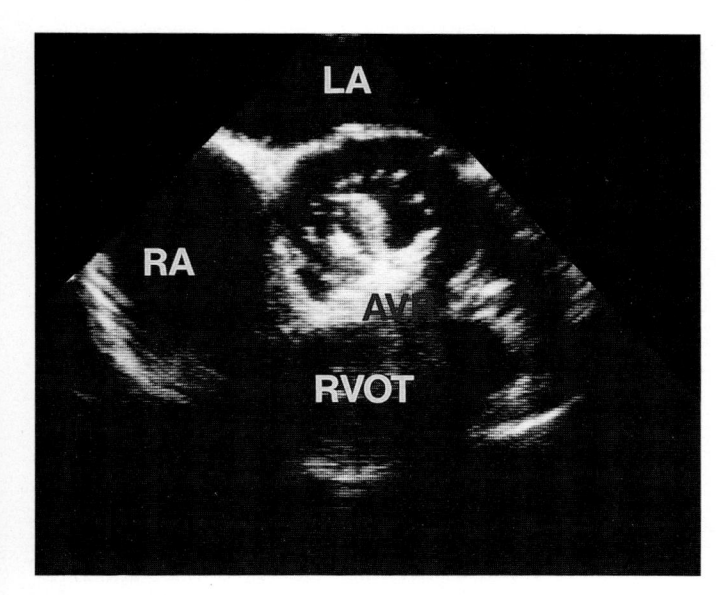

Fig. 15 Basal short axis view. Acute prosthetic aortic valve dehiscence (AVR – aortic valve prosthesis, RVOT – right ventricular outflow tract).

Pulmonary venous inflow to the left atrium can be detected by spectral and colour flow Doppler in a large proportion of cases. Transoesophageal pulsed Doppler studies of pulmonary venous return have been used to differentiate constrictive and restrictive disorders of the left ventricle[68] and the study of trans-mitral diastolic flow velocity patterns by this approach may yield further insight into diastolic behaviour of the left ventricle.

TRANSOESOPHAGEAL ECHOCARDIOGRAPHY DURING INTERVENTIONAL PROCEDURES

Successful localisation and retrieval of an intracardiac catheter embolus from the right heart using combined fluoroscopy and transoesophageal echocardiography highlights the broad range of applications of the technique.[69] A similar technique has been used to guide accurate bioptome placement in the biopsy of right atrial mass.[70] Correct siting of valvuloplasty balloons is possible and transoesophageal echocardiography has been used to monitor the immediate effects of aortic balloon valvuloplasty on ventricular function, aortic valve anatomy and regurgitation.[71] Potential advantages of such a technique include the avoidance of repeat aortograms and the prevention of complications due to incorrect balloon size. Transoesophageal monitoring of such procedures may be better performed in the anaesthetised patient.

Patient selection

The introduction of any new diagnostic technique leads to a period of optimism closely followed by one of rationalisation. Thus the eventual place of transoesophageal imaging and Doppler studies in patient management is still uncertain. Preliminary evaluation of transoesophageal echocardiography suggests that two of the major applications will be the investigation of atrial and aortic pathology. The superiority of transoesophageal echocardiography over conventional Doppler echocardiographic studies both in the detection of infective vegetations and prosthetic mitral valve dysfunction is of major clinical importance.

Increasing familiarity with transoesophageal cross-sectional echocardiography has a noticeable influence on expectations of precordial imaging and perception of image quality that may lower the threshold for recommending endoscopic cardiac ultrasound. It has been proposed that for a routine diagnostic ultrasound service approximately 10% of echocardiographic examinations may have to be performed transoesophageally,[21] but this will depend on the availability of equipment and local expertise. Unfortunately endoscopic transducers are relatively expensive and have a limited lifespan.

Outpatient transoesophageal echocardiography is a semi-invasive and, for the patient, moderately unpleasant procedure. It is complementary to other ultrasound and diagnostic imaging techniques and its use cannot be justified where an adequate diagnosis can be arrived at using conventional echocardiography. Appropriate clinical application of transoesophageal echocardiography depends on close communication between the clinician and cardiac ultrasound department.

INTRA-OPERATIVE AND INTENSIVE CARE APPLICATIONS OF TRANSOESOPHAGEAL ECHOCARDIOGRAPHY

Detection of intracardiac air

Transoesophageal echocardiography has been used to document the high incidence of intracardiac air emboli occurring during neurosurgical procedures[13] and intra-operative paradoxical venous air embolism has been observed in upright neurosurgical patients.[13,72] In coronary artery and valve replacement surgery, following termination of cardiopulmonary bypass, ejection of intracardiac air bubbles may be observed for prolonged periods in between 40% and 80% of cases.[73,74] In one series, neurological sequelae were associated with this finding in almost a quarter of cases while no documented neurological deficit occurred in the patients with no detectable intracardiac air. There is, however, conflicting evidence to suggest that despite the high incidence of observed intracardiac microbubbles, neurological deficit is a very rare event although the possibility of subclinical organ damage cannot be excluded.[73,75] Echocardiography is extremely sensitive for the detection of intracardiac air and allows visualisation of microbubbles as small as 10 μm which are often seen

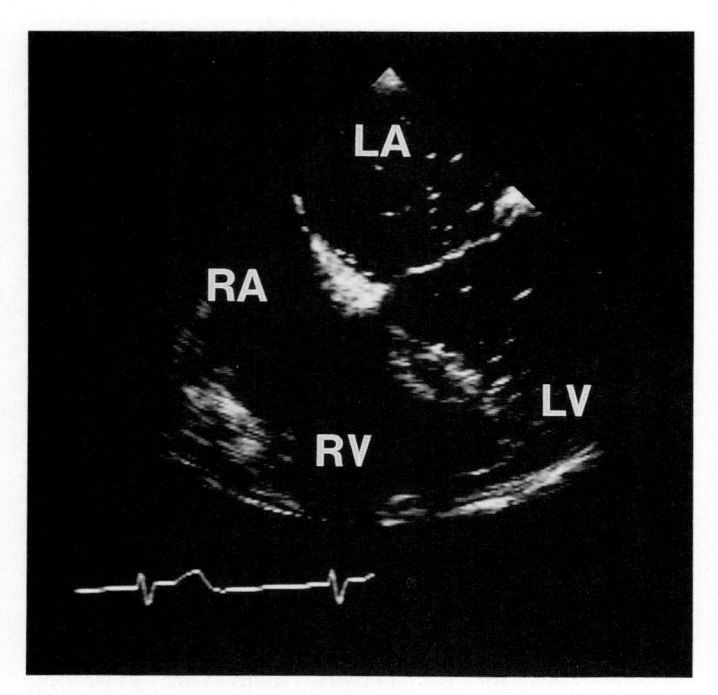

Fig. 16 Four chamber view. Microbubbles within the left heart chambers after coronary artery bypass surgery.

intra-operatively following drug or fluid administration through atrial catheters.[76] The quantity of air required to produce neurological damage in humans is unknown and it is uncertain whether transoesophageal echocardiography can differentiate these microbubbles reliably from larger and potentially more hazardous air emboli. Figure 16 demonstrates the typical appearance of microbubbles within the left atrium and ventricle in a patient undergoing aortocoronary bypass shortly after release of the aortic cross-clamp.

Post-operative hypotension and ventilated patients

Prompt and accurate assessment of the cause of hypotension in the post-operative period is vital to the management of patients after cardiac surgery. Precordial echocardiography in this group is subject to severe limitations imposed by the presence of sternotomy dressings, mediastinal air entrapment and assisted ventilation. Transoesophageal echocardiography has been used for the evaluation of intraoperative and post-operative hypotension and reliably detects the presence of cardiac tamponade and ventricular dysfunction.[77,78] In certain instances this approach may yield more information about left ventricular function and loading than pulmonary wedge pressure or invasive cardiac output measurement.[79] In patients receiving assisted ventilation with positive end expiratory pressure (PEEP), transoesophageal echocardiography has provided new insight into the mechanism by which this technique leads to a reduced cardiac output.[80,81]

Reconstructive valve surgery

Preliminary reports suggest that transoesophageal echocardiography is of potential value in the evaluation of mitral valve repair surgery.[82,83] Intra-operative transoesophageal contrast and Doppler echocardiographic studies have been used to assess the outcome of reconstructive surgery and determine the need for early valve replacement.[84] The application of transoesophageal colour flow mapping for quantitation of valve regurgitation has obvious applications for reconstructive surgery but further angiographic-transoesophageal correlative studies are required before this technique can be recommended for clinical use.

Ventricular function

By advancing the transoesophageal transducer to the fundus of the stomach, a short axis view of the left and right ventricles is obtained (Fig. 5). This view provides direct monitoring of left ventricular size and function to the anaesthetist and surgeon throughout the operation. Once the position of the transducer has been fixed, preliminary cross-sectional and M-mode recordings of left ventricular function and size can be made for reference later in the surgical procedure. To make the detection of changes in ventricular function easier, some commercially available echocardiographic equipment provides a split screen cine loop facility so that changes in global and segmental ventricular function can be more readily observed 'on-line'.

The use of transoesophageal echocardiography for intra-operative diagnosis and management of left ventricular dysfunction has been the subject of intensive research. M-mode and cross-sectional transoesophageal echocardiography have been used for intra-operative evaluation of left ventricular dimensions and function during cardiac and major vascular surgery.[85–88] The effects of altered fluid loading and anaesthetic agents on left ventricular performance have been documented[89] and there is some evidence to suggest that transoesophageal monitoring of left ventricular dimensions is more reliable than pulmonary artery wedge pressure for the assessment of left ventricular filling pressure during general anaesthesia.[90]

Transoesophageal echocardiography allows earlier detection of myocardial ischaemia and infarction than conventional electrocardiographic monitoring by the detection of left ventricular segmental wall motion abnormalities.[88,91,92,93] Appropriate therapeutic intervention to reverse ischaemia and correct fluid load may therefore be instituted at an earlier stage and not surprisingly this impressive monitoring technique has already found a place in the routine intra-operative care of high-risk patients in the United States. The effects of coronary grafting can be evaluated intra-operatively and in one study of patients undergoing coronary revascularisation, immedi-

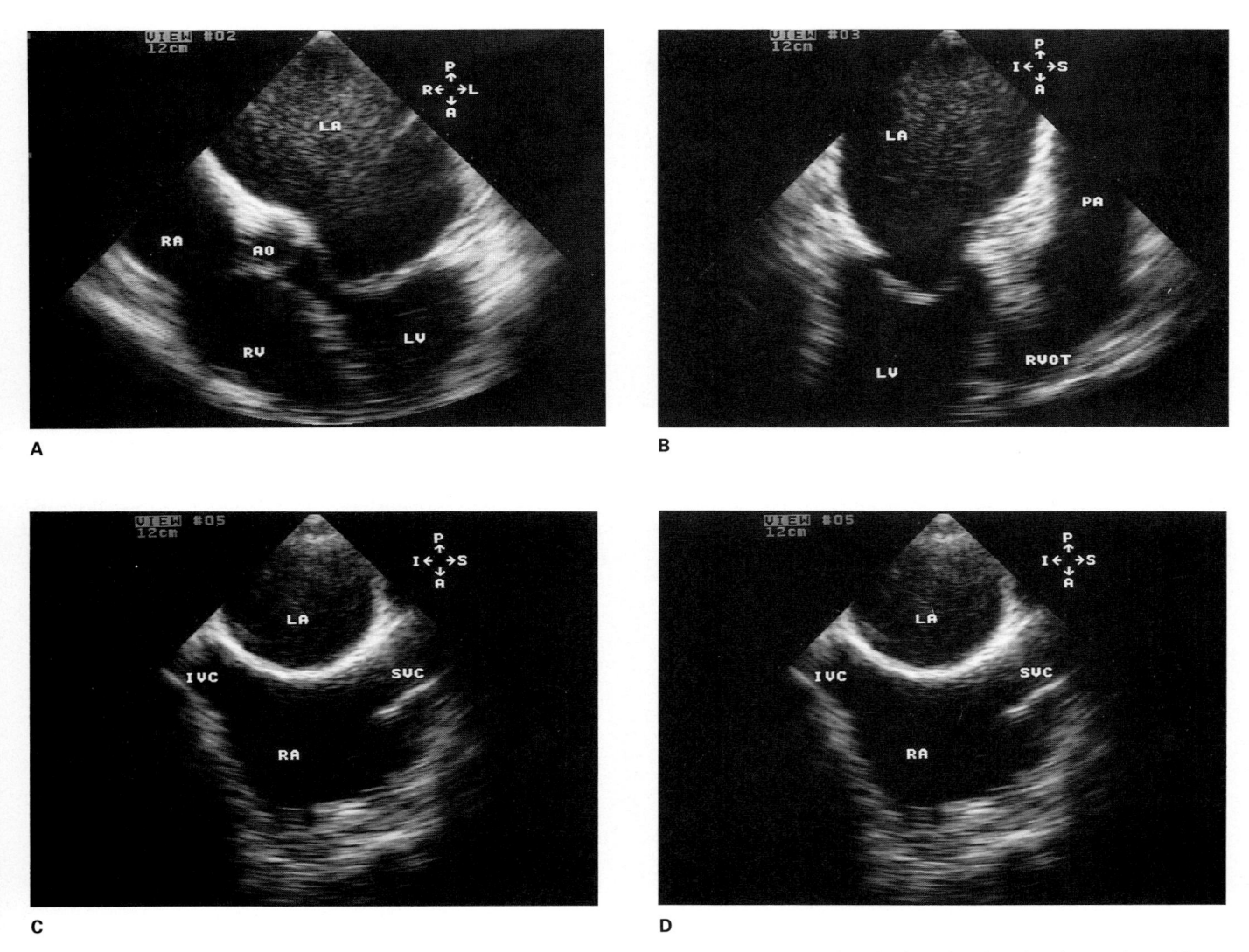

Fig. 17 Biplane transoesophageal examination. A: Transverse plane transoesophageal image showing the four chamber view in a patient with mitral stenosis. Note the spontaneous contrast in the left atrium. B: Longitudinal (sagittal) view in the same patient as (A) again showing the left atrium and left ventricle but also showing the right ventricular outflow tract (RVOT) leading to the pulmonary artery. C: Clockwise rotation of the transducer from the position shown in (A) showing the interatrial septum with the right atrium lying anterior to the left atrium. D: Longitudinal (sagittal) view from the position shown in (C) showing the superior vena cava and inferior vena cava entering the right atrium. The curvature of the interatrial septum is more pronounced in this plane.

ate improvement of segmental wall motion in previously ischaemic areas was observed.[94]

Cardiac output measurement

The first documented application of transoesophageal ultrasound was for the measurement of aortic blood flow velocity.[3] One of the most recent developments of endoscopic ultrasound has been the development of continuous wave transducers for intra-operative and intensive care measurement of cardiac output.[95,96] The transducer is mounted at an angle on the end of a thin flexible catheter and positioned to obtain the optimum Doppler flow velocity signal from the descending aorta. Impressive correlations have been achieved between non-invasive oesophageal estimates of cardiac output and direct haemodynamic measurements. The obvious advantages of this technique are the avoidance of risks associated with central venous cannulation and infection of indwelling catheters.

BIPLANE TRANSOESOPHAGEAL ECHOCARDIOGRAPHY

The limitations of single transverse plane imaging have been described. Some of these may be overcome by the

Table 1 Transoesophageal echocardiography

Outpatient and emergency applications
1. Inadequate precordial examination
2. Suspected infective endocarditis
3. Evaluation of intracardiac masses
4. Investigation of unexplained embolic events
5. Assessment of native and prosthetic valves
6. Adult congenital heart disease
7. Aortic dissection

Intraoperative and intensive care applications
1. Monitoring of left ventricular function
2. Detection of intracardiac emboli
3. Assessment of valve repair and prosthetic valve function
4. Assessment of perioperative complications
5. Cardiac output measurement
6. Mechanically ventilated patients

introduction of biplane endoscopes which incorporate a second longitudinally orientated transducer. Imaging, though not simultaneous, is thus possible in two orthogonal planes. Use of biplane systems allows improved visualisation of the pulmonary outflow tract, atrio-ventricular valves, superior vena cava and distal ascending aorta. The latter may assume particular importance in the investigation of suspected thoracic aortic dissection. Disadvantages include reduction in image quality due to a smaller number of elements in each transducer and a slightly more complicated endoscopic technique. This and further developments in transoesophageal echocardiography are also discussed in Chapter 30. Figures 17A–D show examples of biplane transoesophageal echocardiograms in a patient with mitral stenosis.

CONCLUSION

Transoesophageal echocardiography provides a safe and valuable addition to other currently available ultrasound techniques and has already found applications in a wide variety of clinical situations. In selected patients it provides information that is unobtainable even by more invasive and potentially hazardous techniques.

REFERENCES

1. Bansal R C, Tajik J, Seward J B, Offord K P. Feasibility of two-dimensional echocardiographic examination in adults. Prospective study of 200 patients. Mayo Clin Proc 1980; 55: 291
2. Frazin L, Talano J V, Stephanides L, et al. Oesophageal echocardiography. Circulation 1976; 54: 102–108
3. Side C D, Gosling R G. Non-surgical assessment of cardiac function. Nature 1971; 232: 335–336
4. DiMagno, E P, Regan P T, Wilson D A, et al. Ultrasonic endoscope. Lancet 1980; 1: 629–631
5. Hisanga K, Hisanga A, Hibi N, Nishimura K, Kambe T. High speed rotating scanner for transoesophageal cross-sectional echocardiography. Am J Cardiol 1980; 46: 837–842
6. Schluter M, Langenstein B A, Polster J, et al. Transoesophageal cross-sectional echocardiography with a phased array transducer system. Technique and initial clinical results. Br Heart J 1982; 48: 67–72
7. de Bruijn N P, Clements F M, Kisslo J A. Intraoperative transoesophageal colour flow mapping: initial experience. Anaesth Analg 1987; 66: 386–390
8. Taams M A, Gussenhoven W J, Schippers L A, et al. The value of transoesophageal echocardiography for the diagnosis of thoracic aorta pathology. Eur Heart J 1988; 9: 1308–1316
9. Taams M A, Gussenhoven E J, Cornel J H, et al. Detection of left coronary artery stenosis by transoesophageal echocardiography. Eur Heart J 1988; 9: 1162–1166
10. Schluter M, Langenstein B A, Hanrath P, Kremer P, Bleifield W. Assessment of transoesophageal pulsed Doppler echocardiography in the detection of mitral regurgitation. Circulation 1982; 66: 784–789
11. Erbel R, Borner N, Steller D et al. Detection of aortic dissection by transoesophageal echocardiography. Br Heart J 1987; 58: 45–51
12. Geibel A, Kasper W, Behroz A, Prezewolka U, Meinertz T, Just H. Risk of transoesophageal echocardiography in awake patients with cardiac diseases. Am J Cardiol 1988; 62: 337–339
13. Cucchiara R F, Nugent M, Seward J B, Messick J M. Air embolism in upright neurosurgical patients: Detection and localisation by two-dimensional transoesophageal echocardiography. Anesthesiology 1984; 60: 353–355
14. Engberding R, Hasfeld I, Chiladakis I, Dohrmann W, Grosse-Heitmeyer W, Stoll V. Transoesophageale echokardiographie: erhotes untersuchungsrisikiko durch blutdruckansteig und herzrhythmusstorungen? Herz 1988; 20: 233–236
15. Schlutter M, Hinrichs A, Thier W, et al. Transoesophageal two-dimensional echocardiography: Comparison of ultrasonic and anatomic sections. Am J Cardiol 1984; 53: 1173–1178
16. Seward J B, Khandheria B K, Oh J K, et al. Transoesophageal echocardiography: technique, anatomic correlations, implementation and clinical applications. Mayo Clin Proc 1988; 63: 649–680
17. Freedman L R. Infective endocarditis and other intravascular infections. New York: Plenum Medical. 1982
18. Rubenson D S, Tucker C R, Stinson E B, et al. The use of echocardiography in diagnosing culture negative endocarditis. Circulation 1981; 64: 641
19. Martin R P, Meltzer R S, Chia B L, Stinson E B, Rakowski H, Popp R L. Clinical utility of two-dimensional echocardiography in infective endocarditis. Am J Cardiol 1980; 46: 379
20. Hickey A J, Wolters J, Wicken DEL. Reliability and clinical relevance of detection of vegetations by echocardiography in bacterial endocarditis. Br Heart J 1981; 46: 624–628
21. Daniel W G, Schroder E, Mugge A, Lichtlen P R. Transoesophageal echocardiography in infective endocarditis. American Journal of Cardiac Imaging 1988; 2: 78–85
22. Erbel R, Rohmann S, Drexler M, et al. Improved diagnostic value of echocardiography in patients with infective endocarditis by transoesophageal approach. A prospective study. Eur Heart J 1988; 9: 43–53
23. Polak P E, Gussenhoven W J, Roelandt J R T C. Transoesophageal cross-sectional echocardiographic recognition of an aortic valve ring abscess and a subannular mycotic aneurysm. Eur Heart J 1987; 8: 1235–1239
24. Gussenhoven E J, Taams M A, Roelandt J R T C. Transoesophageal two-dimensional echocardiography: its role in solving clinical problems. J Am Coll Cardiol 1986; 8: 975–979
25. Engberding R, Bender F, Grosse-Heitmeyer W, et al. Identification of dissection or aneurysm of the descending thoracic aorta by conventional and transoesophageal two-dimensional echocardiography. Am J Cardiol 1987; 59: 717–719

26 De Bakey M E, Henly W S, Cooley D A, Morris G C, Crawford S C, Beall A C. Surgical management of dissecting aneurysms of the aorta. J Thorac Cardiovasc Surg 1965; 49: 130–149

27 Dinsmore R E, Willerson J T, Buckley M J. Dissecting aneurysm of the aorta. Radiology 1972; 105: 567–572

28 Erbel R, Daniel W, Visser C, Engberding R, Roelandt J, Rennollet H. Echocardiography in diagnosis of aortic dissection. Lancet 1989; 1: 458–460

29 Borner N, Erbel R, Braun B, et al. Diagnosis of aortic dissection by transoesophageal echocardiography. Am J Cardiol 1984; 54: 1157–1158

30 Mohr-Kahaly S, Erbel R, Borner N, et al. Kombination von Farb-Doppler und transoesophagealer echokardiographie in der notfalldiagnostik bei aortendissektionen vom typ I. Z Kardiol 1986; 75: 616–620

31 Takomoto S, Omoto R. Visualisation of thoracic dissecting aneurysm by transoesophageal Doppler colour flow mapping. Herz 1987; 12: 187–193

32 Mohr-Kahaly S, Erbel R, Rennollet H, et al. Ambulatory follow-up of aortic dissection by transoesophageal two-dimensional and colour-coded Doppler echocardiography. Circulation 1989; 80: 24–33

33 Wolfe S B, Popp R L, Feigenbaum H. Diagnosis of atrial tumours by ultrasound. Circulation 1969; 39: 615–620

34 Perry L S, King J F, Zeft H O, et al. Two dimensional echocardiography in the diagnosis of left atrial myxoma. Br Heart J 1981; 45: 667–671

35 Come P C, Riley M F, Markis J E, Malagold M. Limitations of echocardiographic techniques in the evaluation of left atrial masses. Am J Cardiol 1981; 48: 947–953

36 Thier W, Schlutter M, Krebber H, et al. Cysts in left atrial myxomas identified by transoesophageal echocardiography. Am J Cardiol 1983; 51: 1793–1795

37 Ezekowitz M D, Smith E O, Rankin R, Harrison L H, Krous H F. Left atrial mass: diagnostic value of transoesophageal two-dimensional echocardiography and indium-111 platelet scintigraphy. Am J Cardiol 1983; 51: 1563–1564

38 Obeid A I, Marvasti M, Parker F, Rosenberg J. Comparison of transthoracic and transoesophageal echocardiography in the diagnosis of left atrial myxoma. Am J Cardiol 1989; 63: 1006–1008

39 Aschenberg W, Schlutter M, Kremer P, Schroder M, Siglow V, Bleifield W. Transoesophageal two-dimensional echocardiography for the detection of left atrial appendage thrombus. J Am Coll Cardiol 1986; 7: 163–166

40 Daniel W G, Nikutta P, Schroder E, Nellessen U. Transoesophageal echocardiographic detection of left atrial appendage thrombi in patients with unexplained arterial embolism. Circulation 1986; 74: 391

41 Nixdorff U, Erbel R, Drexler M, Meyer J. Detection of thromboembolus of the right pulmonary artery by transoesophageal two-dimensional echocardiography. Am J Cardiol 1988; 61: 488–489

42 Mugge A, Daniel W G, Klopper J W, Lichtlen P R. Visualisation of patent foramen ovale by transoesophageal colour-coded Doppler echocardiography. Am J Cardiol 1989; 62: 837–838

43 Nellessen U, Daniel W G, Matheis G, Oelert H, Depping K, Lichtlen P R. Impending paradoxical embolism from atrial thrombus: correct diagnosis by transoesophageal echocardiography and prevention by surgery. J Am Coll Cardiol 1985; 5: 1002–1004

44 Ryan T J, Armstrong W F, Feigenbaum H. Prospective evaluation of the left main coronary artery using digital two-dimensional echocardiography. J Am Coll Cardiol 1988; 11: 565–571

45 Block P J, Popp R L. Detecting and excluding significant left main coronary artery narrowing by echocardiography. Am J Cardiol 1985; 55: 937–940

46 Rink L D, Feigenbaum H, Weyman A E, et al. Echocardiographic detection of left main coronary artery obstruction. Circulation 1982; 65: 719–724

47 Koenig K, Kasper W, Hofmann T, Meinertz T, Just H. Transoesophageal echocardiography for diagnosis of rupture of the ventricular septum or left ventricular papillary muscle during acute myocardial infarction. Am Heart J 1987; 59: 362

48 Matsuzaki M, Matsuda Y, Ikee Y, et al. Esophageal echocardiographic left ventricular anterolateral wall motion in normal subjects and patients with coronary artery disease. Circulation 1981; 63: 1085–1092

49 Matsumoto M, Hanrath P, Kremer P, et al. Evaluation of left ventricular performance during supine exercise by transoesophageal M-Mode vechocardiography in normal subjects. Br Heart J 1982; 48: 61–66

50 Lieppe W, Scallion R, Behar V S, Kisslo J A. Two-dimensional echocardiographic findings in atrial septal defect. Circulation 1977; 56: 447–456

51 Schapira J N, Martin R P, Fowles R E, Popp R L. Single and two-dimensional echocardiographic features of the interatrial septum in normal subjects and patients with an atrial septal defect. Am J Cardiol 1978; 43: 816–819

52 Bourdillon P D, Foale R A, Rickards A F. Identification of atrial septal defects by cross-sectional contrast echocardiography. Br Heart J 1980; 44: 401–405

53 Hanrath P, Schluter M, Langenstein B A, et al. Detection of ostium secundum atrial septal defects by transoesophageal echocardiography. Br Heart J 1983; 49: 350–358

54 Oh J K, Seward J B, Khandheria B K, Danielsen G K, Tajik A J. Visualisation of sinus venosus atrial septal defect by transoesophageal echocardiography. Journal of the American Society of Echocardiography 1988; 1: 275–277

55 De Maria A, Bommer W, Joye J, Lee G, Bouteller J, Mason D T. Value and limitations of cross-sectional echocardiography of the aortic valve in the diagnosis and quantification of valvular aortic stenosis. Circulation 1980; 62: 304–312

56 Hatle L, Anglesen B A, Tromsdal A. Non-invasive assessment of aortic stenosis by Doppler ultrasound. Br Heart J 1980; 43: 707–718

57 Currie P J, Seward J B, Reeder G S, et al. Continuous wave Doppler echocardiographic assessment of severity of calcific aortic stenosis: a simultaneous Doppler-catheter correlative study in 100 adult patients. Circulation 1985; 71: 1162–1169

58 Richards K L, Cannon S R, Miller J F, Crawford M H. Calculation of aortic valve area by Doppler echocardiography: a direct application of the continuity equation. Circulation 1986; 73: 964–969

59 Hofmann T, Kasper W, Meinertz T, Spillner G, Schlosser V, Just H. Determination of aortic valve orifice area in aortic valve stenosis by two-dimensional transoesophageal echocardiography. Am J Cardiol 1987; 59: 330–335

60 Schluter M, Kremer P, Hanrath P. Transoesophageal 2-D echocardiographic feature of flail mitral leaflet due to ruptured chordae tendinae. Am Heart J 1984; 108: 609–610

61 Schluter M, Langenstein B A, Their W, et al. Transoesophageal two-dimensional echocardiography in the diagnosis of cor triatriatum in the adult. J Am Coll Cardiol 1983; 2: 1011–1015

62 Schluter M, Langenstein B A, Hanrath P, Kremer P, Bleifield W. Assessment of transoesophageal pulsed Doppler echocardiography in the detection of mitral regurgitation. Circulation 1982; 66: 784–789

63 Toma Y, Matsuda Y, Matsuzaki M, et al. Determination of atrial size by oesphageal echocardiography. Am J Cardiol 1983; 52: 878–880

64 Sprecker D L, Adamick R, Adams D, Kisslo J. In vitro colour flow, pulse and continuous wave Doppler ultrasound masking by prosthetic valves. J Am Coll Cardiol 1987; 9: 1306–1310

65 Nellessen U, Schnittger I, Appleton C P, et al. Transoesophageal two-dimensional echocardiography and colour flow velocimetry in the evaluation of cardiac valve prostheses. Circulation 1988; 78: 848–855

66 Van der Brink R B A, Visser C A, Basart D C G, Duren D R, de Jong A P, Dunning A J. Comparison of transthoracic and transoesophageal colour Doppler imaging in patients with mechanical prostheses in the mitral valve position. Am J Cardiol 1989; 63: 1471–1474

67 Taams M A, Gussenhoven E J, Cahalan M K, et al. Transoesophageal Doppler colour flow imaging in the detection of native and Bjork-Shiley mitral valve regurgitation. J Am Coll Cardiol 1989; 13: 95–99

68 Schiavone W A, Calafiore P A, Salcedo E E. Transoesphageal Doppler echocardiographic demonstration of pulmonary venous flow velocity in restrictive cardiomyopathy and constrictive pericarditis. Am J Cardiol 1989; 63: 1286–1288
69 Neumann H P H, Hofmann T, Koester W, Billmann P, Kaufmann G W. Extraction of an intracardial catheter embolus using combined radiography and transoesophageal echocardiography. Clinical Cardiology 1988; 11: 427–429
70 Scott P J, Ettles D F, Rees M R, Williams G J. The use of combined transoesophageal echocardiographic and fluoroscopy in the biopsy of a right atrial mass. Br J Radiol 1990; 63: 222–224
71 Cryan S E, Kimball T R, Schwarz D C, Meyer P R A, Steed R D, Kaplan S. Evaluation of balloon aortic valvuloplasty with transoesophageal echocardiography. Am Heart J 1988; 115: 460–462
72 Furuya H, Okumura F. Detection of paradoxical air embolism by transoesophageal echocardiography. Anesthesiology 1984; 60: 374–377
73 Topol E J, Humphrey L S, Borkon A M, et al. Value of intraoperative left ventricular microbubbles detected by two-dimensional transoesophageal echocardiography in predicting neurologic outcome after cardiac operations. Am J Cardiol 1985; 56: 773–775
74 Oka Y, Moriwaki K M, Hong Y, et al. Detection of air emboli in the left heart by M-mode transoesophageal echocardiography following cardiopulmonary bypass. Anesthesiology 1985; 59: 1047–1051
75 Rodigas P C, Meyer F J, Haasler G B, Dubroff J M, Spotnitz H M. Intraoperative 2-D echocardiography: Ejection of microbubbles from the left ventricle after cardiac surgery. Am J Cardiol 1982; 50: 1130–1132
76 Meltzer R S, Tickner E G, Sahines T P, Popp R L. The source of ultrasound contrast effect. JCU 1980; 8: 121
77 Chan K-L. Transoesophageal echocardiography for assessing the cause of hypotension after cardiac surgery. Am J Cardiol 1988; 62: 1142–1143
78 Ettles D F, Firth N, Nair R U, Williams G J. Fatal acute left ventricular outflow obstruction due to interventricular septal haematoma – diagnosis by transoesophageal echocardiography. Eur Heart J 1989; 10: 479–481
79 Topol E J, Humphrey L S, Blanck T J J, et al. Characterisation of post cardiopulmonary bypass hypotension with intraoperative transoesophageal echocardiography. Anesthesiology 1983; 59: A2
80 Terai C, Uenishi M, Sugimoto H, Shimazu T, Yoshioka T, Sugimoto T. Transoesophageal echocardiographic dimensional analysis of four cardiac chambers during positive end-expiratory pressure. Anesthesiology 1985; 63: 640–646
81 Koolen J J, Visser C A, Wever E, et al. Transoesophageal two-dimensional echocardiographic evaluation of biventricular dimension and function during positive end-expiratory pressure ventilation after coronary artery bypass grafting. Anesthesiology 1985; 63: A191
82 Dahm M N, Iversen S, Drexler M, Oelert H. Intraoperative beurteilung der rekonstruktion von atriovenrtikularklappen mittels transoesophagealer echokardiographie. Z Kardiologie 1987; 76: 779–783
83 Drexler M, Oelert H, Dahm M, Scherhag A, Meyer J. Assessment of successful valve reconstruction by intraoperative transoesophageal echocardiography. Circulation 1986; 74: 390
84 Shiveley B, Cahalan M K, Benefiel D, Schiller N. Intraoperative assessment of mitral valve regurgitation by transoesophageal Doppler echocardiography. J Am Coll Cardiol 1986; 7: 228A
85 Matsumoto M, Oka Y, Strom J, et al. Application of transoesophageal echocardiography to continuous monitoring of left ventricular performance. Am J Cardiol 1980; 46: 95–105
86 Abel M D, Nishimura R A, Callahan M J, Rehder K, Ilstrup D M, Tajik J. Evaluation of intraoperative transoesophageal two dimensional echocardiography. Anesthesiology 1987; 66: 64–68
87 Clements F M, de Bruijn N P. Perioperative evaluation of regional wall motion by transoesophageal two-dimensional echocardiography. Anesth Analg 1987; 66: 249–261
88 Roizen M F, Alpert R A, Beaupre P N, et al. Monitoring with two-dimensional transoesophageal echocardiography: comparison of myocardial function in patients undergoing supraceliac, suprarenal-infraceliac, or infrarenal aortic occlusion. J Vasc Surg 1984; 1: 300–303
89 Beaupre P N, Cahalan M K, Kremer P F, Lurz F W, Schiller N B, Hamilton W K. Isoflurane, halothane and enflurane depress myocardial contractility in patients undergoing surgery. Anesthesiology 1983; 59: A59
90 Beaupre P N, Cahalan M K, Kremer P F, et al. Does pulmonary artery pressure adequately reflect left ventricular filling during anaesthesia and surgery? Anesthesiology 1983; 59: A3
91 Smith J S, Cahalan M K, Benefiel D J, et al. Intraoperative detection of myocardial ischaemia in high risk patients: electrocardiography versus two-dimensional transoesophageal echocardiography. Circulation 1985; 72: 1015–1021
92 Beaupre P N, Cahalan M K, Kremer P F, Lurz F W, Schiller N B, Hamilton W K. Intraoperative detection of changes in left ventricular segmental wall motion by transoesophageal two-dimensional echocardiography. Am Heart J 1984; 107: 1021–1023
93 Cahalan M K, Kremer P F, Beaupre P N, et al. Intraoperative myocardial ischaemia detected by two-dimensional transoesophageal echocardiography. Anesthesiology 1983; 59: A164
94 Topol E J, Weiss J L, Guzman P A, et al. Immediate improvement of dysfunctional myocardial segments after coronary revascularisation: detection by intraoperative transoesophageal echocardiography. J Am Coll Cardiol 1984; 4: 1123–1134
95 Freund P R, Padavich C A. A comparison of cardiac output techniques: transoesophageal Doppler versus thermodilution cardiac output during general anaesthesia in Man. Anesthesiology 1985; 63: A191
96 Kumar A, Minagoe S, Thangathurai D, et al. The continuous wave Doppler oesophageal probe: A new method for measurement of cardiac output during surgery. J Am Coll Cardiol 1986; 7: 2A

SECTION 2

Acquired heart disease

10

Valvular disease

Introduction
Mitral valve
Normal mitral valve
Mitral stenosis
Mitral regurgitation
Aortic valve
Normal aortic valve
Aortic stenosis
Aortic regurgitation

Tricuspid valve
Normal tricuspid valve
Tricuspid stenosis
Tricuspid regurgitation
Pulmonary valve
Pulmonary stenosis
Pulmonary regurgitation
Conclusion

Paula Murphy

INTRODUCTION

The diagnosis of valvular heart disease has been greatly facilitated by the introduction of echocardiography and before echocardiography was widely available the diagnosis of aortic and mitral valve disease was based mainly on clinical acumen and in severe cases where surgery was contemplated, by cardiac catheterisation.

Echocardiography nowadays includes M-mode, cross-sectional imaging and Doppler examination. M-mode echocardiography was first reported by Edler in 1956 in the same year that an ultrasonic Doppler technique was described by Satomura but it was M-mode examination which became the early mainstay of echocardiography. Doppler techniques took a back seat until the development of real time cross-sectional imaging, first with mechanical sector scanners in 1974 and later with phased array sector scanning. In 1978, Barber and his colleagues reported a further advance, namely the combination of cross-sectional imaging and Doppler facility to produce the duplex scanner. It now became possible to use pulsed Doppler techniques to measure blood flow at specific sites within the heart. The most recent development in echocardiography has been the arrival of colour flow mapping. This is a combination of cross-sectional imaging with a form of pulsed Doppler analysis across the area being imaged. In colour flow Doppler mapping the colours, usually blue and red, are coded to represent flow away from and towards the probe. This is the equivalent of a pulsed Doppler trace where flow towards the probe would be above the baseline and flow away from the probe would be beneath the baseline. The main advantage of colour flow mapping lies in increasing the speed of assessment of abnormal flow patterns, particularly if they have an eccentric or unusual course. Colour flow mapping is particularly effective in picking up turbulence and this can guide the operator to assess a jet in more detail when this flow might have been missed or might have been discovered by pulsed Doppler examination after a much longer time. Current echocardiography gives accurate analysis of haemodynamic abnormalities, in particular the pressure drop across valvular stenoses. The diagnosis of the cause of cardiac murmurs has now become considerably simplified.[1-5] The advent of the microchip has made this possible and rapid advancement of software has facilitated many calculations.

The mitral, aortic, tricuspid and pulmonary valves will be assessed in terms of:

1. Cross-sectional imaging
2. M-mode examination
3. Pulsed wave Doppler examination
4. Colour flow Doppler examination
5. Continuous wave Doppler examination

MITRAL VALVE

Normal mitral valve

The normal mitral valve is best assessed in the long axis parasternal view and in the four chamber apical view (Fig. 1). The mitral valve has two cusps, an anterior and a posterior one. These are seen to open widely in diastole and to close firmly in systole. The chordae will be seen to extend from the cusps to the papillary muscles. In the long axis parasternal view the close relationship of the anterior leaflet of the mitral valve to the posterior wall of the aortic root can be seen. The four chamber apical view complements the parasternal view and can be particularly useful in assessing the mitral valve when there is a poor parasternal window (Fig. 2). The short axis parasternal view

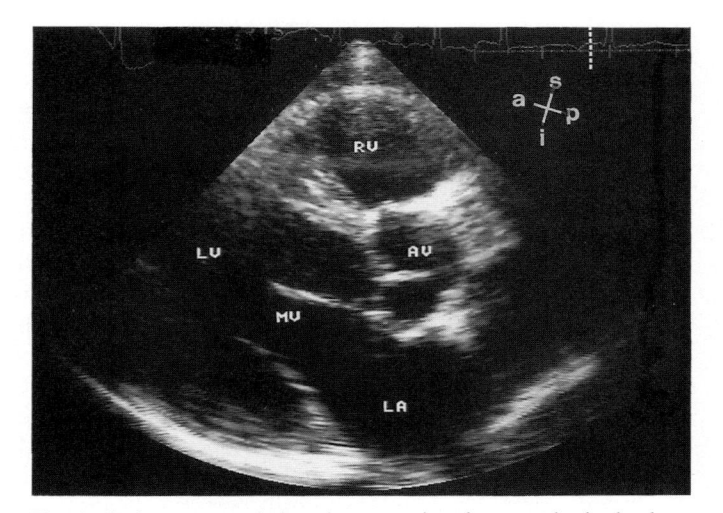

Fig. 1 **Left parasternal view** demonstrating the opened mitral valve cusps in diastole. The aortic valve cusps are closed. The close relationship of the posterior aortic root and anterior mitral valve leaflet should be noted.

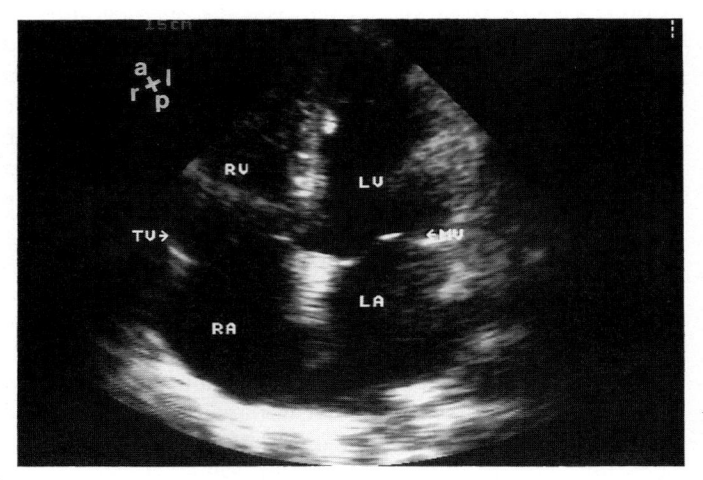

Fig. 2 **Four chamber apical view**. Note the slightly offset positioning of the mitral and tricuspid valves, i.e. the mitral valve lies a little more basally than the tricuspid valve.

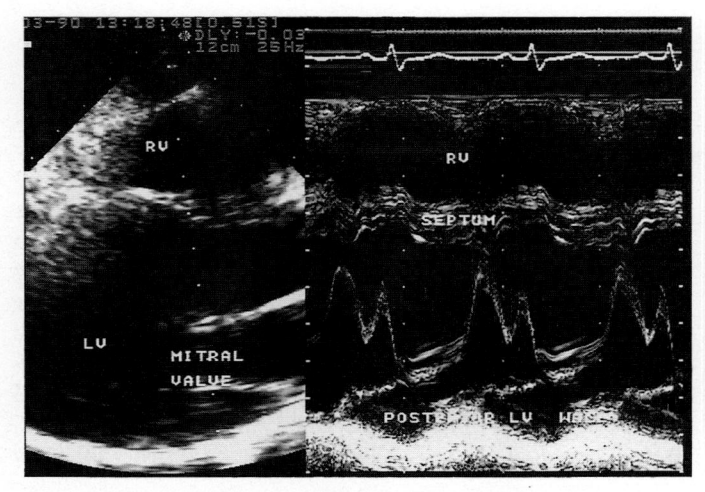

Fig. 3 M-mode tracing of **normal mitral valve** (right) with the corresponding long axis cross sectional image (left).

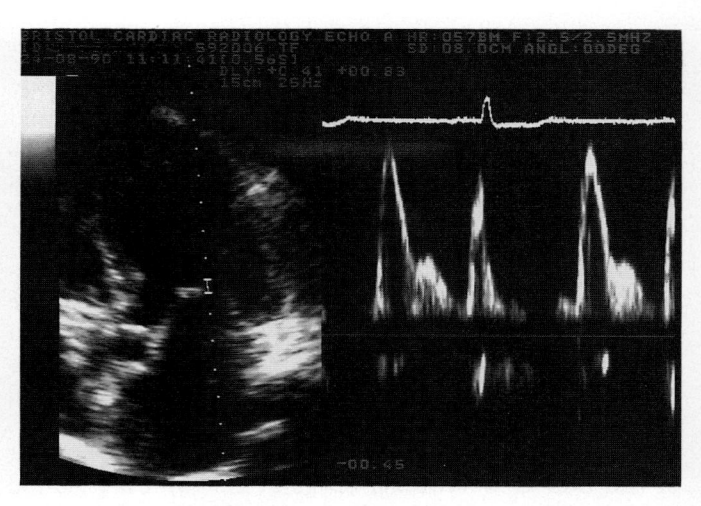

Fig. 4 Apical pulsed Doppler trace from a normal mitral valve (right) with the sample volume cursor placed between the opening anterior and posterior leaflets of the valve (left).

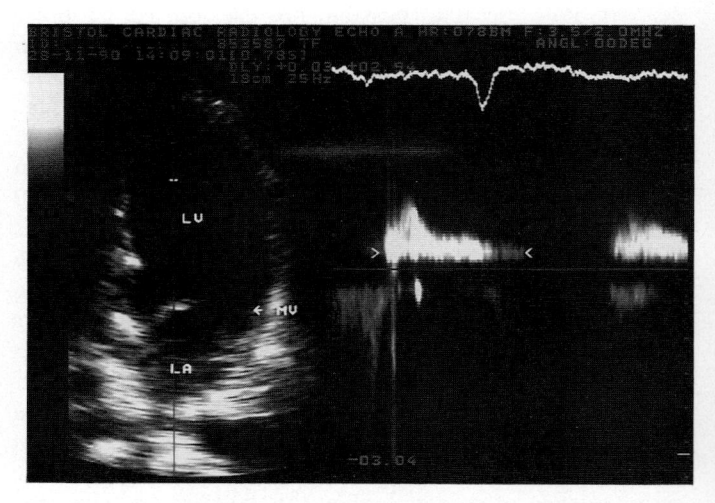

Fig. 5 Apical continuous wave Doppler trace from a normal mitral valve.

gives a transaxial view of the mitral valve cusps opening and closing and inferior angulation of the transducer in this plane towards the apex of the left ventricle will show the two papillary muscles.

M-mode examination is performed from the left parasternal long axis position. A trace against time will demonstrate the normal opening and closing of the valve when the M-mode line is placed perpendicularly through the valve leaflet tips (Fig. 3). The M-mode trace of a normal mitral valve shows rapid opening in early diastole due to passive flow which is followed by mid-diastolic closure and then atrial systole produces a final opening at the end of ventricular diastole. This produces the characteristic M-shaped trace. The anterior and posterior leaflets of a normal mitral valve oppose one another throughout ventricular systole.

Pulsed Doppler examination of the mitral valve is performed from the apical four chamber position with the sample volume being placed between the opening anterior and posterior leaflets (Fig. 4). The best results are obtained by placing the cursor as parallel to the mitral jet as possible. The pulsed Doppler trace of a normal mitral valve has an M shape with a sharp upstroke above the baseline in early diastole, with a sharp drop off throughout mid diastole followed by the late peak of atrial systole in late ventricular diastole.

Colour flow mapping of the mitral valve is again best assessed from the apical four chamber window. Most systems colour code in red and blue and flow through the normal mitral valve towards the probe can be seen as red. Flow away from the probe in this position (either normal flow through the left ventricular outflow tract or abnormal flow through the mitral valve into the left atrium in mitral regurgitation) would be coded in blue. High velocity turbulent jets of mitral regurgitation usually show a multicoloured mosaic pattern.

Continuous wave Doppler examination can be performed by either a 'stand alone' probe (non-imaging) or by a dual probe where cross-sectional imaging is possible. The cross-sectional image in continuous wave Doppler studies must be aligned with the continuous wave beam on most echocardiography machines but some equipment now includes 'steerable' continuous wave examination. The combination of imaging and continuous wave Doppler examination has the advantage over the independent probe in that there is more certainty as to the position of the continuous wave jet for the less experienced operator (Fig. 5). The advantage of the stand alone probe is that it is much smaller and can be placed in more awkward areas such as between small gaps in tightly spaced ribs. The 'stand alone' probe is usually more sensitive than the continuous wave Doppler beam produced by a phased array transducer.

Mitral stenosis[6-10]

The majority of cases of mitral stenosis are due to rheumatic heart disease, but in the older patient it is occasionally due to fibrosis of the annulus. Mitral valve annular calcification on its own is quite a common finding in patients over 60 years of age and is usually of no clinical significance and is unrelated to mitral stenosis or mitral regurgitation. Congenital mitral stenosis is an uncommon condition and must be distinguished from supra-mitral ring.

Cross-sectional imaging has replaced M-mode echocardiography as the echocardiographic method of choice to diagnose this condition. The leaflets of the mitral valve are seen to be thickened in both the long axis parasternal view (Fig. 6) and the four chamber apical view. The thickening is often most marked at the edge of the leaflets. In both these views, doming of the cusps can be seen during diastole. The leaflets are often quite markedly increased in echogenicity as well as being thickened. Only a small orifice remains between the anterior and posterior cusps in diastole. Cross-sectional imaging can also demonstrate a dilated left atrium and even without Doppler echocardiography the combination of thickened doming mitral valve leaflets and a large left atrium would establish the diagnosis of mitral stenosis (Fig. 7A). The differential diagnosis of doming of the mitral valve is stretching of the annulus due to a dilated left ventricle. This can give apparent doming of the valve, but unlike mitral stenosis the valve orifice is normal.

In the absence of mitral regurgitation, the degree of dilatation of the left atrium usually reflects the severity and duration of the mitral valve stenosis. In situations where the left atrium is not compliant and does not dilate, the increased back pressure from the stenotic mitral valve is reflected by increased pulmonary artery pressure. This can be estimated by continuous wave Doppler examination of a tricuspid regurgitant jet or by estimation of the pulmonary acceleration time in the pulmonary artery distal to the pulmonary valve. Both of these features will be dealt with under the tricuspid and pulmonary valve sections. The possibility of thrombus within the left atrium should be excluded on cross sectional imaging (Fig. 7B).

Historically, M-mode tracings of mitral stenosis were one of the first applications of echocardiography. The trace is extremely characteristic and demonstrates the loss of the normal opposite motion of the anterior and posterior leaflets due to fusion of the commissures which results in both cusps moving almost together (Fig. 8). M-mode echocardiography also demonstrates thickening of the leaflets, some of which may be due to calcification. There is loss of the abrupt downslope of valve closure in early diastole which is seen in the normal mitral valve. The slope instead is shallow and the time over which it takes the

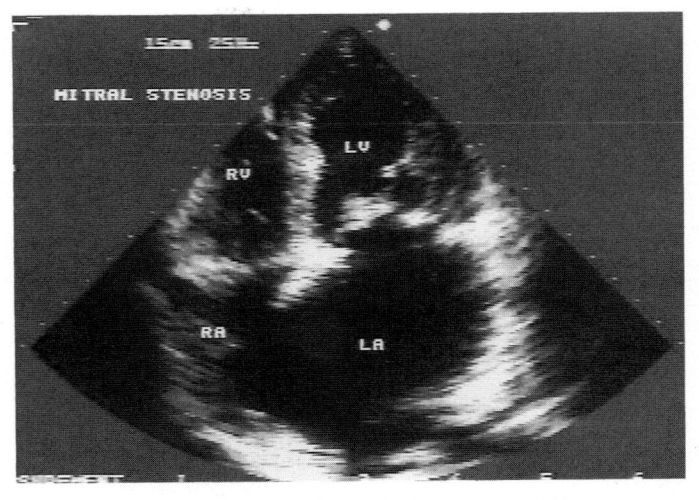

Fig. 7A: Apical four chamber view of mitral stenosis with thickening and increased echogenicity of both cusps of the valve.

Fig. 6 Long axis parasternal view showing doming of the anterior cusp of the mitral valve.

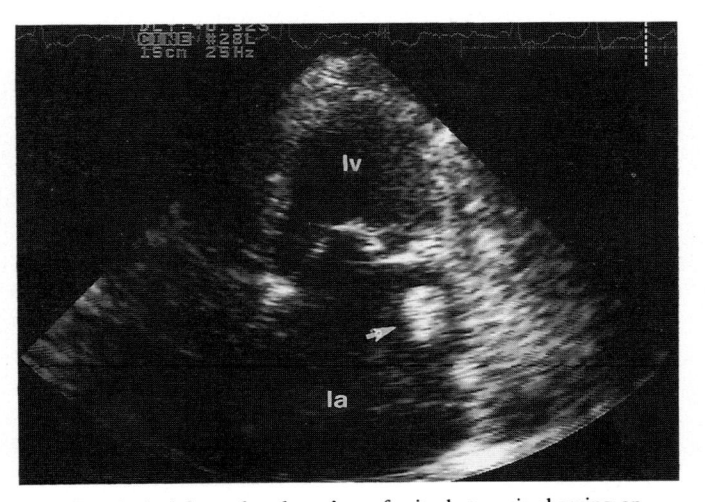

Fig. 7B: Apical four chamber view of mitral stenosis showing an echogenic thrombus (arrowed) near the posterior left atrial wall.

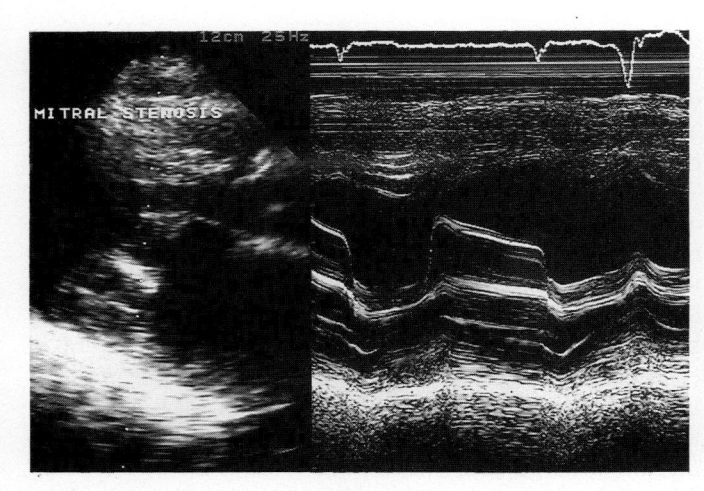

Fig. 8 M-mode tracing of mitral stenosis showing thickening of the leaflets and loss of the abrupt posterior movement of the anterior leaflet in early diastole which is seen in the normal mitral valve.

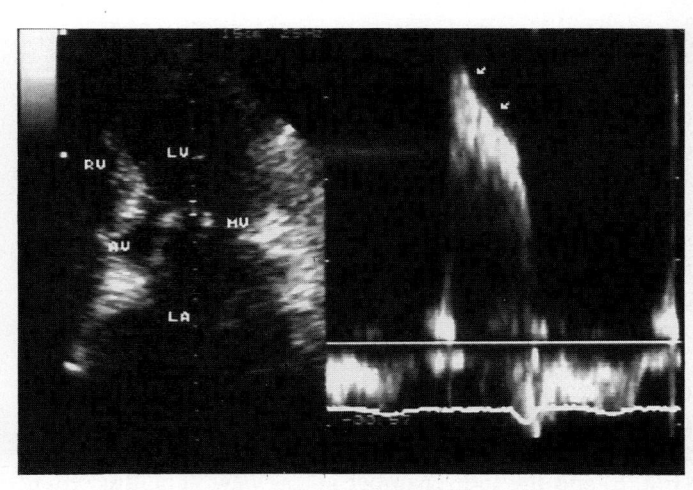

Fig. 10 Pulsed Doppler trace of a patient with mitral stenosis showing the slow decrease in high velocity in early diastole (arrowed). There is still a significant pressure drop across the valve at the end of diastole.

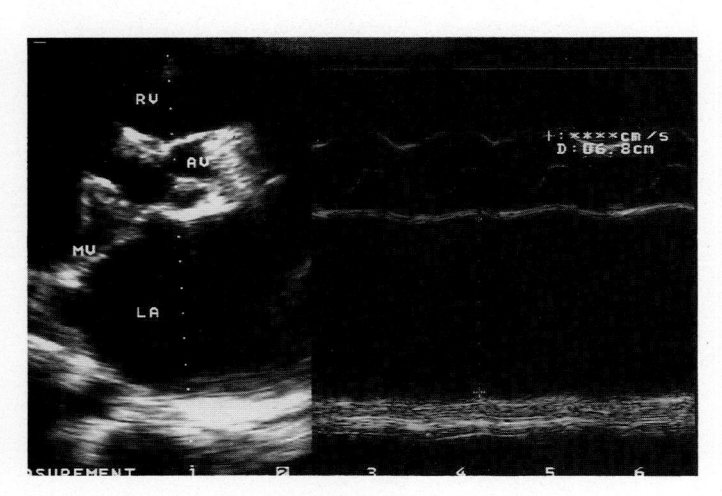

Fig. 9 M-mode tracing of a dilated left atrium in a patient with mitral stenosis. The left atrial diameter is measured at 6.8 cm.

mitral valve to close is markedly lengthened. It is also useful to perform M-mode examination of the left ventricle for function and left atrium for size (Fig. 9). M-mode echocardiography of the mitral stenotic valve can also be directed from the short axis parasternal view. The valve area can be calculated on two dimensional imaging from this view also, but this is relatively inaccurate and has, to a large extent, been negated by the use of Doppler studies to estimate the valve area.

Pulsed wave Doppler examination is performed from the four chamber apical view to allow parallel alignment of the ultrasound beam with the high velocity jet of mitral stenosis. It is vital that the sample volume is placed in the centre of the jet and this usually involves placing the cursor between the tips of the mitral valve cusps. Occasionally the jet may be eccentric and mapping has to be performed using the pulsed Doppler cursor. Colour flow mapping allows easier assessment of an eccentric jet. It is important to get a clear and pure trace both on the audio signal and on the spectral trace otherwise calculations will be inaccurate. Many patients with mitral stenosis have atrial fibrillation and this results in variable lengths of the cardiac cycle. An average cardiac cycle must be sought and it is wise to base calculations on several cardiac cycles. Atrial fibrillation also results in loss of the second or atrial peak of mitral flow.

Mitral stenosis is characterised by increased peak flow velocity through the valve orifice, the peak usually being over 2 metres per second. There is a slow decrease in this high velocity in diastole due to the slower equalisation of the pressure difference between the left ventricle and the left atrium. This means that a considerable flow velocity may still be seen in late diastole (Fig. 10).

The centre of the jet passing through this narrow orifice may still have laminar flow, but there will be turbulent flow towards its periphery and also where the jet enters the left ventricle. Flow through the valve is closely related to the pressure gradient across the valve and this can be calculated from the modified Bernouilli equation. However, as the mean pressure gradient across the valve is greatly influenced by heart rate and cardiac output, a more accurate means of quantitation of stenosis severity is required.

The pressure half time is the time taken for the initial peak pressure gradient to drop to half its value.[11] The rate of decrease in pressure gradient during diastole is much less influenced by heart rate and cardiac output than is the mean or end diastolic pressure and it has a more direct and consistent relationship with the severity of stenosis of the valve. Longer pressure half times are associated with more severe mitral stenosis. It can also be used to estimate the valve orifice area. The normal pressure half time is approximately 50-70 milliseconds. In severe cases of mitral stenosis it can exceed 250 milliseconds. Calculations are best performed on a trace with a fast sweep speed. The functional mitral valve orifice cross-sectional area can be estimated from the pressure half time. Hatle and colleagues[8] showed that there was a linear relationship between pressure half time and the orifice area of a stenotic mitral valve. A valve with an orifice of 1 cm had a pressure half time of 220 milliseconds and the relationship between the two is described in the equation:

$$\text{Functional cross sectional area} = \frac{220}{\text{Pressure half time (milliseconds)}}$$

This formula can be used to estimate the functional mitral valve orifice size. An area of under 1 cm^2 is consistent with severe mitral stenosis and 1-1.5 cm with moderate mitral stenosis. This area is quick to calculate from the mitral valve Doppler trace and involves placing a point at the beginning of diastole and a second point along the slope of the curve (Fig. 11). It is important that the calculation is performed on a trace that shows an even drop of pressure throughout diastole. If the calculation is performed on a trace with an uneven drop in pressure, the pressure half time and mitral valve orifice size will be inaccurate. This technique is particularly useful when the mitral valve is difficult to visualise on cross-sectional imaging.

The independent small continuous wave probe can be particularly helpful in this instance in assessing mitral stenosis. The small probe can be used to confirm the presence of a normal mitral valve where there is a normal mitral valve and poor echo window. The calculation of pressure half time and estimation of the mitral valve orifice area can be calculated from the continuous wave trace as well as from the pulsed Doppler wave trace. The character of the trace is different from that seen with pulsed Doppler examination. In the latter case a well-positioned sample volume will produce a well-defined laminar trace from the central jet but in the continuous wave Doppler trace, the envelope will be filled in by the multiple lower velocities recorded as the flow accelerates in the left atrium and decelerates in the left ventricle.

Colour flow Doppler examination is particularly useful if the stenotic jet is eccentric. It allows the pulsed Doppler cursor to be more accurately placed within the jet and it allows the transducer position to be adjusted in order to minimise the angle between the jet and the ultrasound beam. Colour flow mapping of a stenotic mitral valve often shows aliasing, as the maximal mean velocity which can be recorded with colour flow mapping is very limited (Plate 1). Colour flow examination itself is not useful in accurate quantitation of the severity of mitral stenosis. Colour flow examination will often show the narrow jet of flow through the stenoic valve even when the examination beam is almost perpendicular to flow (Plate 2).

Mitral regurgitation[12-15]

The causes of mitral regurgitation are much more numerous than those of mitral stenosis. Like mitral stenosis, it may be due to rheumatic heart disease and there is often a combination of both stenosis and regurgitation in this condition. In the older patient with ischaemic heart disease and in patients with dilated cardiomyopathy, it is often seen secondary to stretching of the mitral valve annulus which accompanies left ventricular dilatation. Mitral valve prolapse can be a cause of regurgitation in the younger patient with myxomatous or 'floppy' valves and in older patients with degenerative valves.

In mitral stenosis imaging can usually establish the diagnosis and Doppler echocardiography quantifies the degree of stenosis; but with mitral regurgitation the lesion is usually detected by Doppler echocardiography, with cross-sectional imaging often having little to contribute except in cases where there is major valve disruption such as severe prolapse or a flail leaflet due to ruptured chordae tendinae.

Mitral valve prolapse is best seen in the long axis parasternal view (Fig. 12). The apical four chamber view is also a good echo window (Fig. 13) for mitral valve prolapse and in some patients it allows easier visualisation of the prolapsing cusps than the long axis left parasternal view. Oblique views of the cusps can give a false impression of valve prolapse.

Infective endocarditis is another setting for mitral regurgitation and in this condition a vegetation can restrict or obstruct the valve in its efforts to close and can cause regurgitation (Fig. 14).

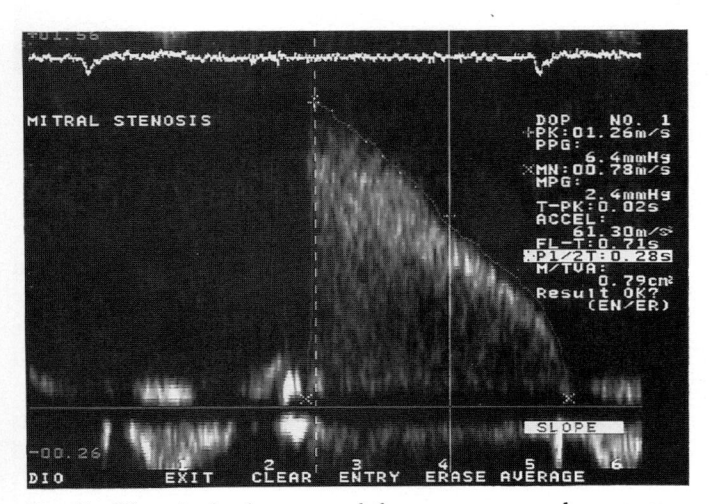

Fig. 11 The mitral valve area and the mean pressure drop across the mitral valve have been calculated from the pulsed Doppler trace. The valve area is estimated at 0.79 square centimetres, i.e. severe stenosis but the mean pressure drop is only 2.44 mmHg.

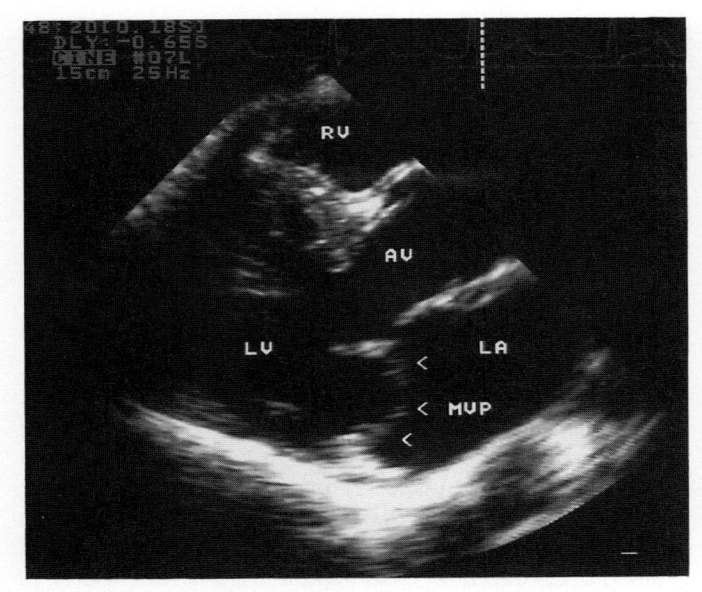

Fig. 12 Long axis left parasternal view of systolic prolapse of the posterior cusp of the mitral valve (MVP).

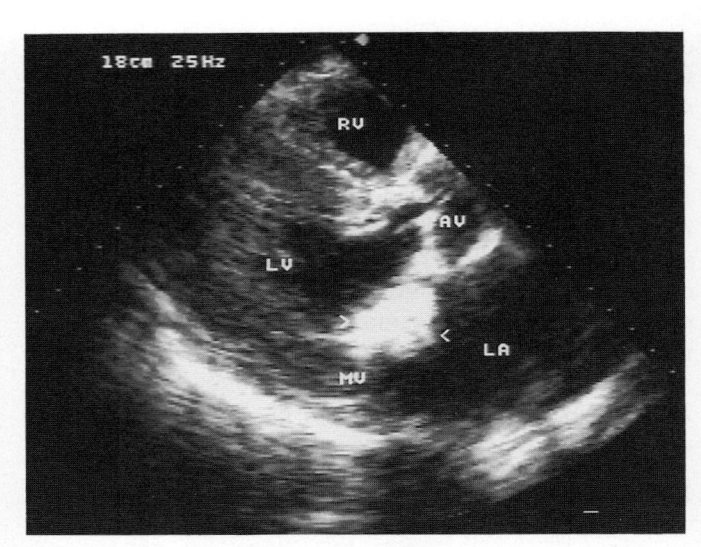

Fig. 14 Parasternal long axis view. Infective endocarditis of the mitral valve showing a large echogenic vegetation (arrowed).

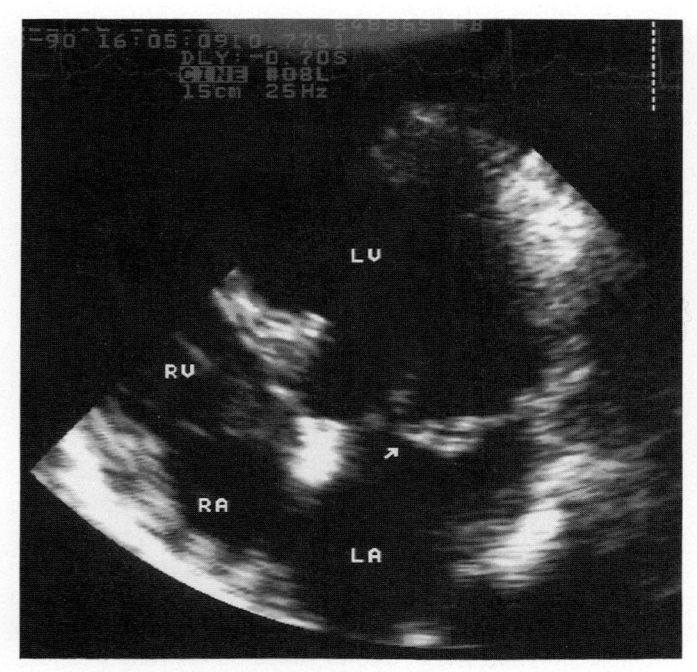

Fig. 13 Apical four chamber view showing prolapse of the posterior leaflet of the mitral valve (arrowed).

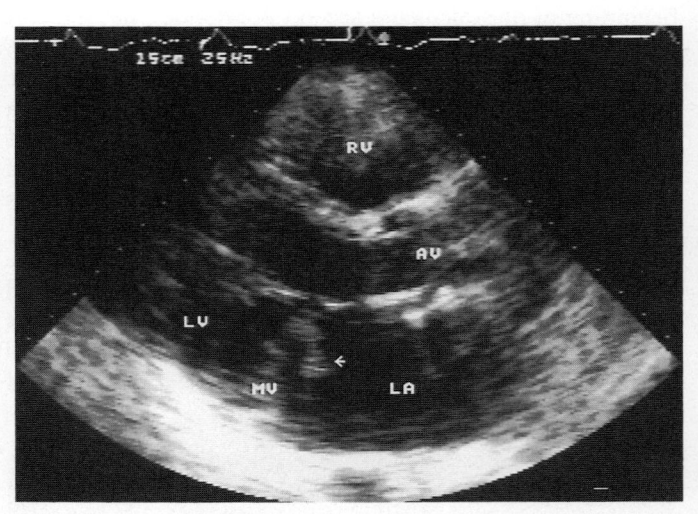

Fig. 15 Parasternal long axis view showing a flail mitral valve leaflet (arrowed).

Whereas the mitral regurgitation found secondary to left ventricular dilatation is functional and will often resolve when cardiac failure is treated and the chamber returns to normal size, ischaemic heart disease can also cause a more acute and serious form of mitral regurgitation if acute myocardial infarction causes rupture or dysfunction of a papillary muscle. This will produce a flail mitral valve cusp (Fig. 15). Cross-sectional imaging is particularly useful in myocardial infarction where the patient develops a new systolic murmur and acute heart failure which may be due to a post infarction ventricular septal defect or mitral regurgitation due to papillary muscle damage.[16]

Imaging is particularly helpful in Marfan's Syndrome as the valve cusps have a particularly floppy appearance and can suggest mitral regurgitation. The presence of particularly thickened, floppy or 'myxomatous' leaflets is associated with a greater incidence of associated complication such as systemic embolus or endocarditis.

Clues to the presence and severity of mitral regurgitation can be gained from assessment of left ventricular function. Severe regurgitation leads to a dilated and hyperdynamic ventricle but caution must be exercised in patients with damaged ventricles. These patients may still have significant regurgitation without obvious ventricular effects. Left atrial enlargement and right heart changes are very variable and depend on the aetiology of the regurgitation, its duration and the presence of any co-existing mitral stenosis.

M-mode echocardiography has little to help in the diagnosis of mitral regurgitation except in confirming on M-mode traces conditions such as mitral valve prolapse (Fig. 16), a thickened cusp in rheumatic heart disease, vegetation in infective endocarditis and the absence of complete apposition of the anterior and posterior leaflets in systole in stretching of the mitral valve annulus, secondary to left ventricular dilatation. Left ventricular function can also be assessed. Occasionally in very severe cases there will be premature closure of the aortic valve due to emptying of the left ventricle into the left atrium.

Though colour flow mapping is now the quickest and usually the most comprehensive Doppler method of assessing mitral regurgitation, for those operators who do not have colour flow Doppler equipment available (and even for those who do) pulsed Doppler mapping is still a very accurate though more time consuming method than colour flow Doppler mapping for assessing mitral regurgitation. The sample volume is placed between the valve cusps on the left atrial side in the apical four chamber position and is moved around the chamber to map the jet distribution. Mitral regurgitation can produce turbulence over a widespread area in the left atrium and the three dimensions of the chamber must be interrogated, often from more than one window. It is not always necessary to have the cursor completely aligned with the mitral regurgitant jet as the turbulence is usually multi-directional. The velocity of the mitral regurgitant jet is extremely high due to the marked difference in pressure between the left atrium and left ventricle and this results in aliasing on the pulsed Doppler trace. Pulsed Doppler sampling can be used to estimate semiquantitatively the severity of regurgitation by mapping out the regurgitant jet within the left atrium. This can be done from the left parasternal window as well as the apical window and the former may be particularly helpful where there is an eccentric jet which more commonly occurs in prolapse of one mitral cusp. In the case of prolapse of the posterior mitral valve cusp, the regurgitant jet is directed superiorly towards the posterior aspect of the root of the aorta. Anterior mitral leaflet prolapse usually leads to an inferiorly directed jet.

Regurgitation in rheumatic valvular disease is usually associated with some degree of mitral stenosis and in this case the jet is often more centrally placed between the stiff opening cusps. Determining the severity or degree of mitral regurgitation remains one of the difficult challenges for Doppler echocardiography. A small thin jet of mitral regurgitation can sometimes reach the most posterior aspect of the left atrium whereas severe longstanding mitral regurgitation may produce an intense swirling pattern in the more proximal part of a markedly dilated left atrium.

Some now believe that colour flow mapping has now become the 'gold standard' of Doppler echocardiography in assessing regurgitant jets, particularly those of mitral regurgitation. Colour flow mapping is particularly sensitive to turbulent jets and colour map turbulence is encoded by the presence of increasing intensities of green in some velocity maps. A more detailed analysis of the jet can be assessed frame by frame, either on cine loop facilities if present on the machine used or on video playback. Narrowing the width of the sector being scanned improves the quality of the colour flow map by increasing the sampling frame rate within the narrowed sector. It is wise to set the Doppler gain as high as possible without producing too much background speckling as very low velocities are not assigned any colour and on a lower setting the degree of regurgitation may therefore be underestimated.

The main advantage of colour flow Doppler examination is that it saves time by quickly demonstrating the site and direction of turbulent flow or any abnormal laminar flow jet. Pulsed or continuous wave Doppler can then be used for further detailed analysis of the jet. The apical four chamber view is usually the best echo window for assessment of the mitral regurgitant jet by colour flow mapping in rheumatic disease or in cases of a dilated annulus, the jet is usually centrally directed. The jet is blue, away from the probe into the left atrium (Plate 3). Eccentric mitral regurgitant jets can often be detected with ease on colour flow mapping (Plates 4, 5A, 5B).

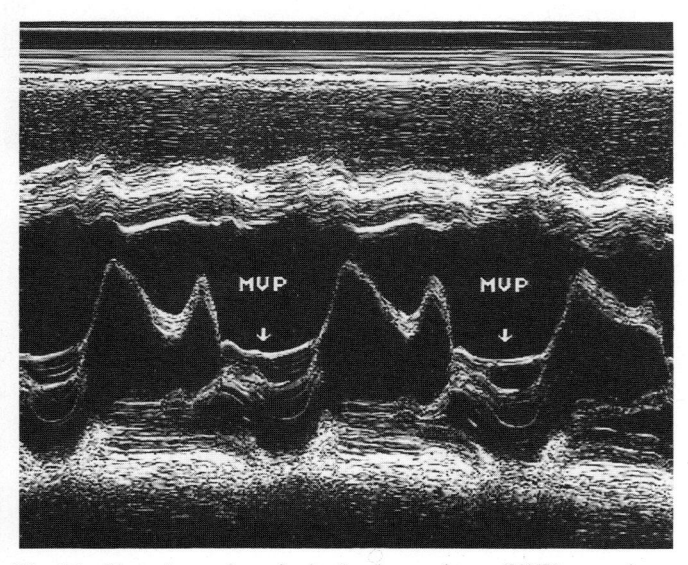

Fig. 16 M-mode tracing of mitral valve prolapse (MVP) occurring in late systole.

160 CARDIAC ULTRASOUND

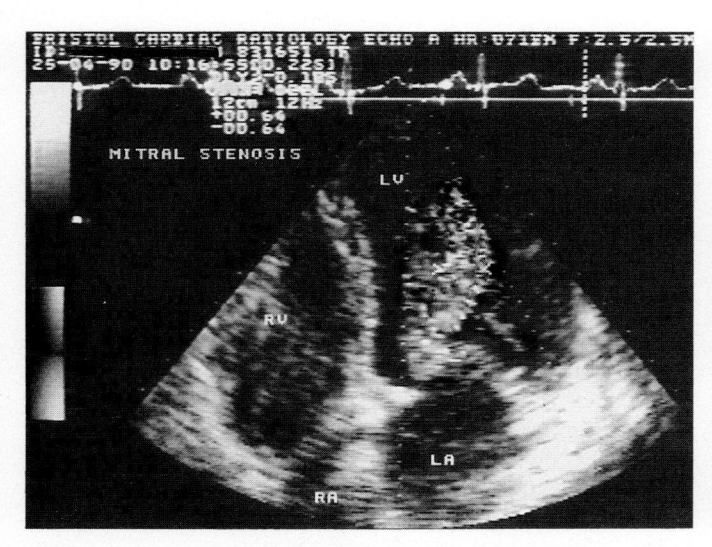

Plate 1 Colour flow Doppler image of mitral stenosis from the apex showing turbulence and aliasing as the maximum velocity which can be recorded with colour flow Doppler examination is limited. This figure is reproduced in colour in the colour plate section at the front of this volume.

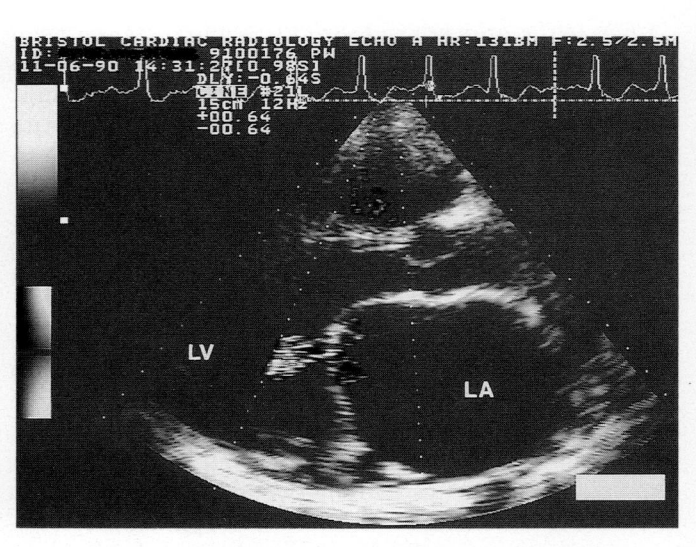

Plate 2 Parasternal long axis view in a case of mitral stenosis. Colour flow mapping shows blood flow accelerating through the narrow orifice. This figure is reproduced in colour in the colour plate section at the front of this volume.

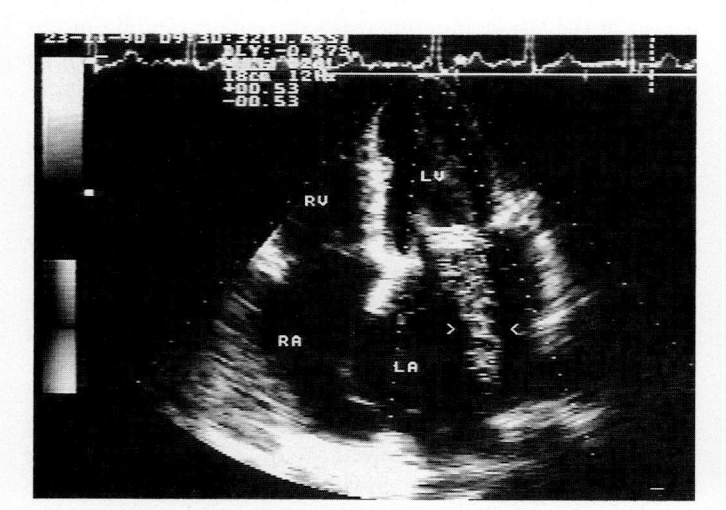

Plate 3 Apical colour flow Doppler image of mitral regurgitation showing a blue jet (arrowed) away from the probe within the left atrium. There is aliasing and a mosaic pattern within the jet. This figure is reproduced in colour in the colour plate section at the front of this volume.

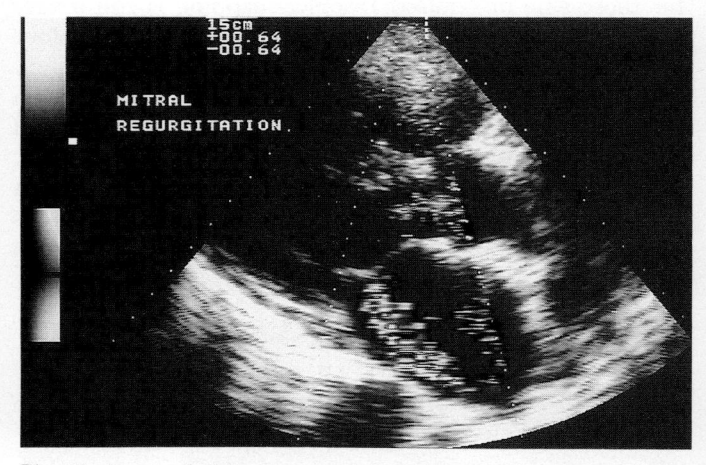

Plate 4 Long axis left parasternal view showing mitral regurgitation as a blue jet into the left atrium. There is aliasing and a mosaic pattern in the jet. This figure is reproduced in colour in the colour plate section at the front of this volume.

VALVULAR DISEASE 161

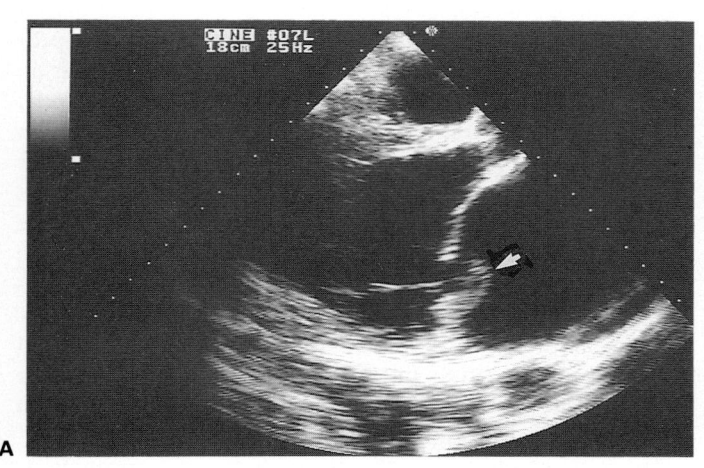

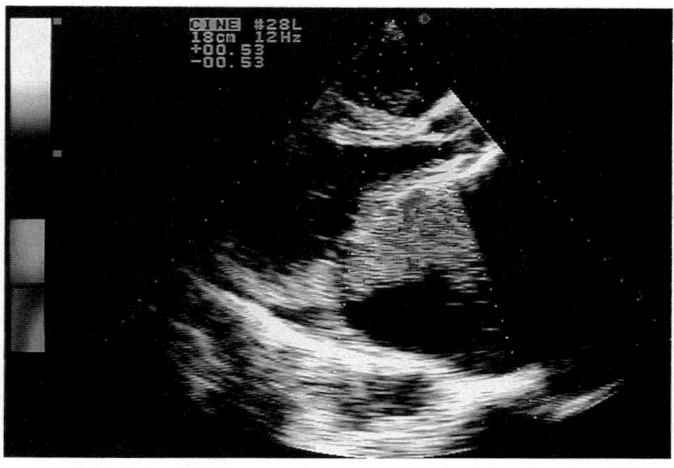

Plate 5 A: Parasternal long axis view showing prolapse of the posterior mitral leaflet arrowed. **B:** Colour flow image simultaneously with **A** showing an intense mosaic jet of mitral regurgitation directed superiorly in the left atrium. This figure is reproduced in colour in the colour plate section at the front of this volume.

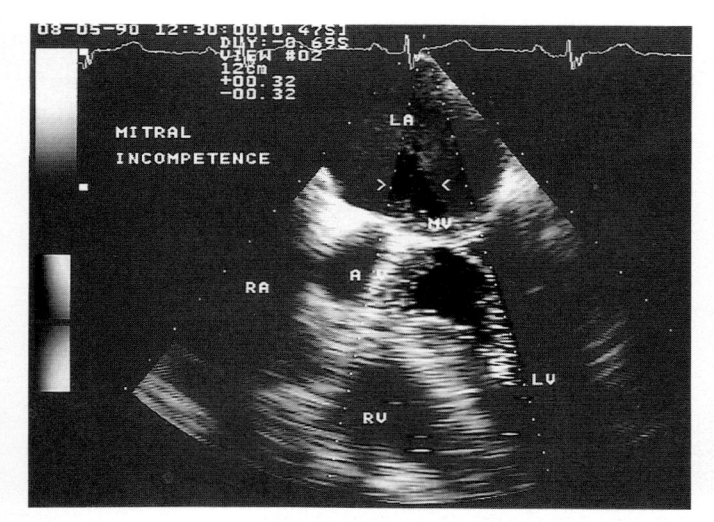

Plate 6 Trans-oesophageal colour flow echocardiogram of mitral regurgitation showing a red jet (arrowed) extending posteriorly from the mitral valve into the left atrium towards the probe in the oesophagus. There is also an intense red signal in the left ventricular outflow tract indicating normal flow towards the mitral valve. This figure is reproduced in colour in the colour plate section at the front of this volume.

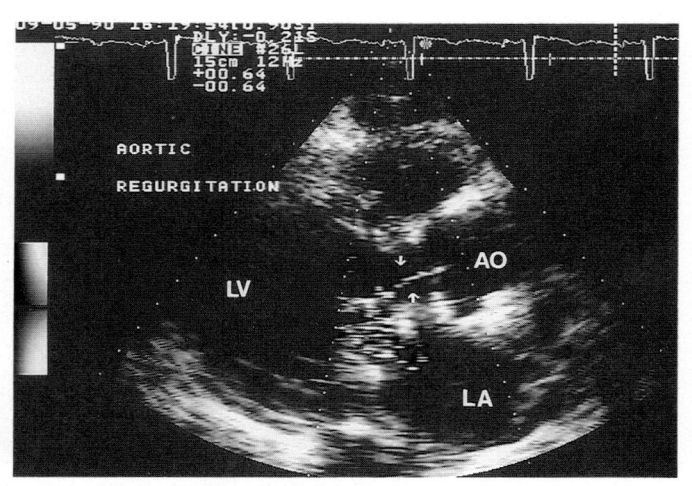

Plate 7 Parasternal long axis view with colour flow Doppler mapping showing a tiny physiological jet of aortic regurgitation (arrowed). This figure is reproduced in colour in the colour plate section at the front of this volume.

In patients with poor precordial echo windows trans-oesophageal echocardiography offers an alternative approach and with the transducer placed behind the left atrium it is in an ideal position to assess mitral regurgitation. In a four chamber view from this approach, the mitral regurgitant jet will of course be red towards the transducer in the oesophagus (Plate 6) whereas from the apical four chamber precordial view the regurgitant jet will be blue. Trivial degrees of mitral regurgitation have been observed on trans-oesophageal echocardiography of otherwise normal mitral valves. This approach is also of particular use in the presence of a heavily calcified valve or a valve prosthesis where precordial examination may not afford good access to the left atrium.

Many operators find continuous wave Doppler examination a satisfying way to prove or disprove the presence of mitral regurgitation, particularly in patients with poor echo windows. As mentioned before, the velocity of the regurgitant jet of the mitral valve often is extremely high because of the wide pressure differences between the left atrium and the ventricle (Fig. 17). Only in severe mitral regurgitation does the velocity markedly reduce due to the reduction in pressure difference between the two chambers. Duplex probes with fixed or steerable continuous wave beams are available but in both cases the mitral valve on imaging needs to be aligned with the continuous wave beam position. A continuous wave independent probe has the advantage of being smaller and can therefore be placed between the ribs more easily. This is a non-imaging procedure which in experienced hands usually provides no problem for the operator, but in less experienced hands, the two jets of mitral regurgitation and aortic stenosis can be confused. Angling the probe from one valve to the other usually establishes the valve of origin of the particular jet and an accurate study of the relationship of the jet to the opening and closing of valves can usually differentiate the two jets.

Continuous wave examination with a good quality non-imaging system is probably the most sensitive of all methods for detecting mitral regurgitation. The presence of a well-defined jet should not, therefore be taken to indicate clinically significant regurgitation.

In spite of all the available methods of examination, Doppler assessment of the severity of mitral regurgitation is still difficult and remains at best an approximate technique and at worst it can be a misleading technique.

AORTIC VALVE

Normal aortic valve

In most patients, the best window for visualising the aortic valve is the left parasternal one. The long axis view from this position will immediately tell the echocardiographer

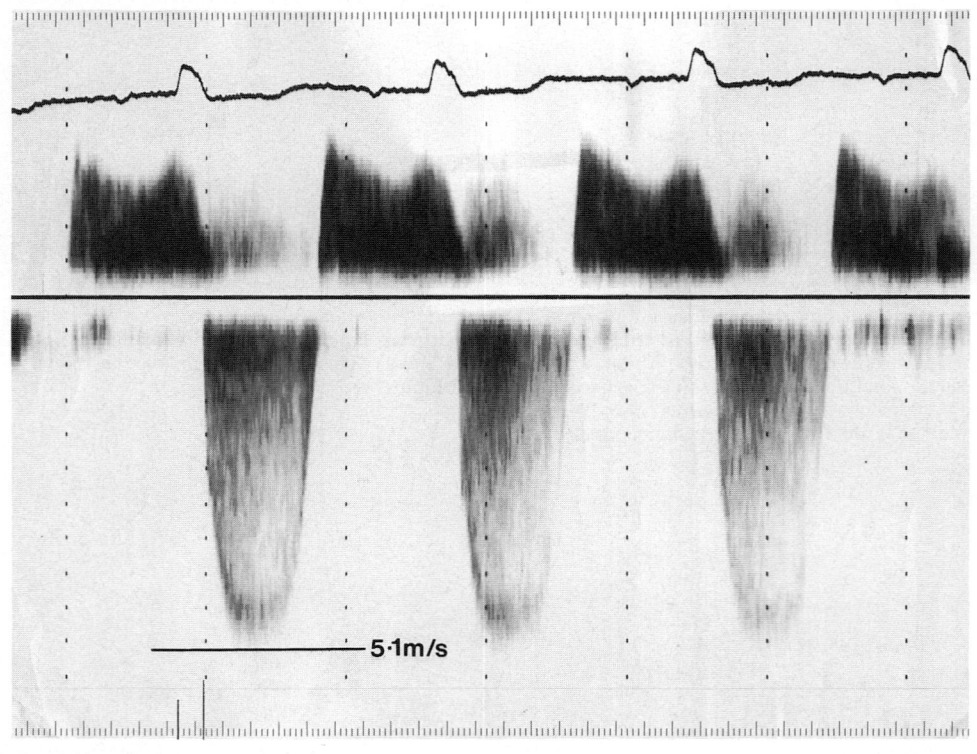

Fig. 17 **Apical continuous wave Doppler examination** of mitral stenosis and regurgitation. The peak velocity of the mitral regurgitant jet is 5.1 m/s.

whether the valve is opening normally or is restricted in movement (Fig. 18). In young patients, the valve cusps are very thin with little echogenicity but with age the cusps become more echogenic. In old age the cusps may be quite markedly echogenic without any restriction in movement.

In the left parasternal view, the relationship of the aortic valve to the proximal aortic root should be observed as well as its relationship to the mitral valve. The left parasternal short axis view gives additional information. It confirms the presence of a tricuspid or a bicuspid aortic valve and in older patients with some calcification in the aortic root wall it confirms that this calcification lies within the wall and not on a valve cusp. Echocardiographic imaging, unlike X-ray imaging, is not specific for calcification but the particularly echogenic character of calcified tissue will frequently suggest its presence.

When the normal tricuspid aortic valve closes there is a 'Y' shape within the aortic root (Fig. 19). The bicuspid valve may produce a horizontal line across the root when closed which becomes two lines in the horizontal position, both slightly bulging convexly towards the superior and inferior walls of the root respectively when the valve opens (Fig. 20). This clear cut pattern is not always seen with bicuspid valves as there is sometimes partial fusion of two commissures which gives an intermediate appearance. Exact diagnosis depends on the image quality of the individual examination. It is often helpful to place the patient well over on his or her left side to get a good view of the aortic valve from the left parasternal short axis view. The apical four chamber view is less suited to aortic valve imaging but in some patients with a poor left parasternal window, the apical long axis view may afford the best view of the aortic valve.

M-mode tracings of the aortic valve are performed from the left parasternal window usually with the heart in the

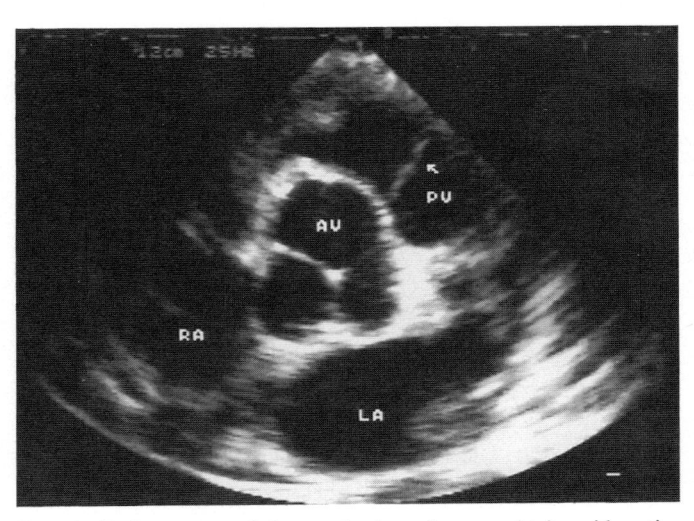

Fig. 19 Left parasternal short axis view of a normal tricuspid aortic valve, the closed cusps producing a 'Y' shape within the aortic root.

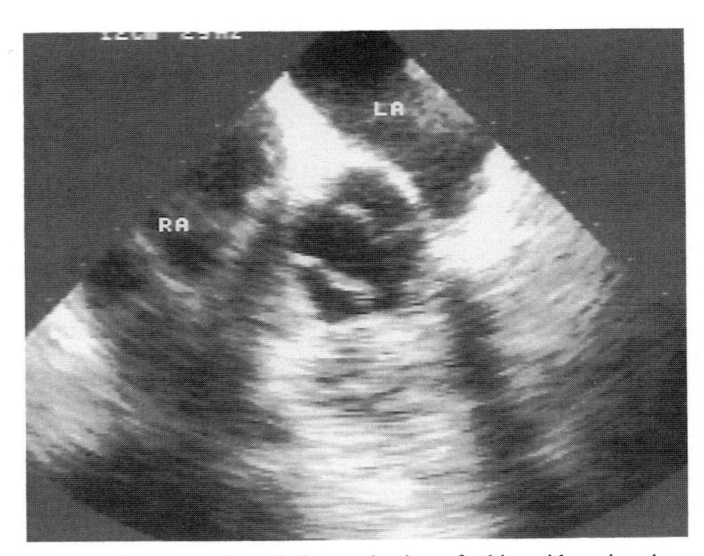

Fig. 20 Transoesophageal short axis view of a bicuspid aortic valve.

long axis position (Fig. 21) but the short axis view can also be used to produce satisfactory M-mode tracings (Fig. 22). The normal aortic valve has a box-shaped appearance of M-mode tracing, with the open box representing the divergent valve cusps in systole.

Pulsed Doppler echocardiography is optimally performed from the apical position with the cursor sampling in the left ventricular outflow tract just below the aortic valve. This demonstrates flow away from the probe towards the aortic valve (Fig. 23). This normal flow is seen in systole and because of the adjacent position of the anterior cusp of the mitral valve, mitral flow is often noted on this trace in diastole. The left parasternal window is not normally suitable for pulsed Doppler examination of the subaortic region as flow through the aortic valve in this position is perpendicular to the probe.

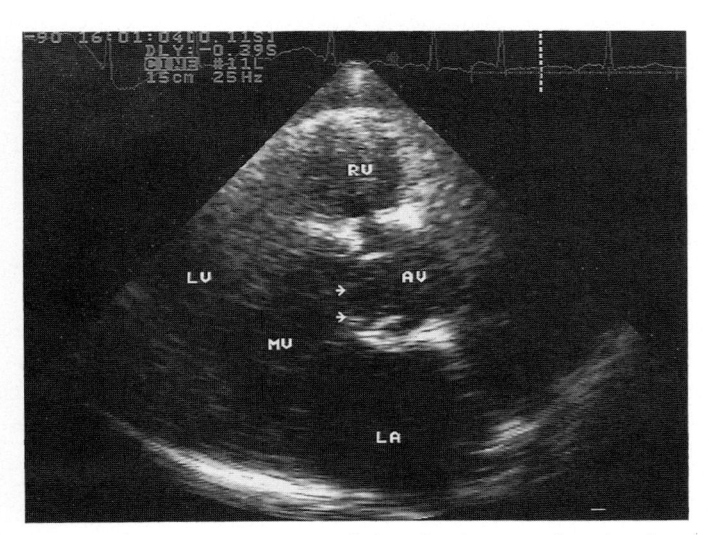

Fig. 18 Long axis left parasternal view showing normal aortic valve cusps opened in systole (arrowed).

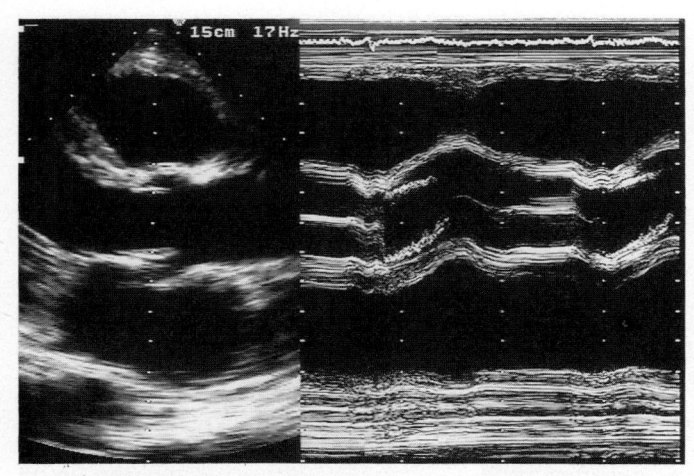

Fig. 21 M-mode tracing of a normal aortic valve (right) performed from the left parasternal window in the long axis position (left). A normal aortic valve produces a box shaped trace in systole and in diastole a single line when the valve cusps oppose one another.

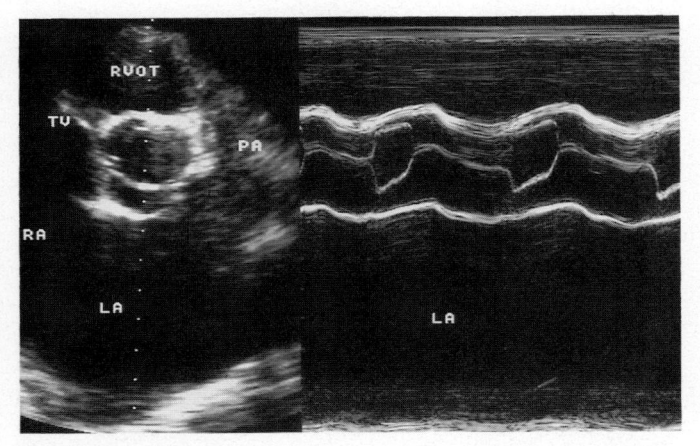

Fig. 22 Short axis view of a normal aortic valve (left) with M-mode tracing (right).

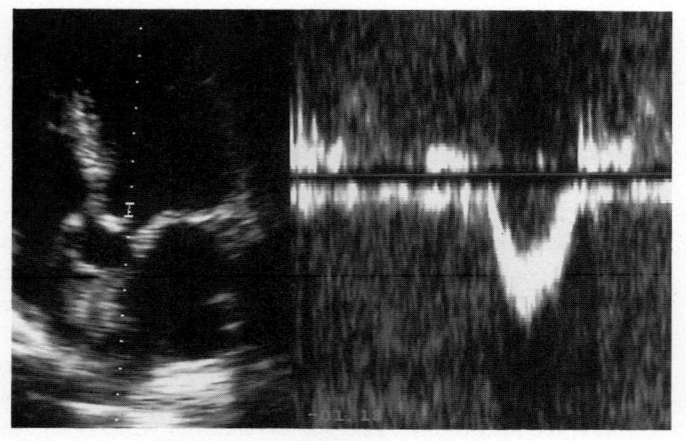

Fig. 23 Pulsed Doppler examination of a normal aortic valve (right) with the cursor placed in the left ventricular outflow tract in this apical four chamber view (left). Flow is away from the probe and therefore below the baseline.

In the normal aortic valve, colour flow Doppler has little to add to cross-sectional imaging and M-mode echocardiography which usually establish the presence of normality. In the apical four chamber position the flow through the left ventricular outflow tract and through the aortic valve is coded blue (away from the probe). In the long axis parasternal view, flow is usually coded red as the flow is commonly slightly towards the probe in this position but this can vary with slightly different cardiac and transducer orientations. In very high quality examinations a tiny jet of 'physiological' regurgitation is sometimes seen (Plate 7) but in general the detection of aortic regurgitation by colour flow mapping is an abnormal finding.

Continuous wave Doppler studies have little part to play in assessing the normal aortic valve. Peak flow velocities across the aortic valve do not normally exceed 1.5 m/s.

Aortic stenosis[17–25]

Aortic stenosis is the commonest stenotic valvular abnormality encountered by the echocardiographer today. In years gone by, rheumatic heart disease was the commonest cause of aortic stenosis, usually in conjunction with mitral stenosis but this has now been relegated to second position with degenerative aortic stenosis in older patients now becoming the main cause of this condition. There is usually an underlying bicuspid aortic valve in these patients. The third cause of aortic stenosis is congenital and this is therefore seen in the younger patient and is usually diagnosed nowadays shortly after birth. These patients often have a bicuspid valve as well.

The valve cusps in acquired aortic stenosis will appear thickened, markedly increased in echogenicity and the degree of restriction in movement will depend upon the severity of the stenosis. The left parasternal long axis and short axis (Figs 24 and 25) views will quickly establish the diagnosis. The more long-established the aortic stenosis, the more calcification is usually seen not only on the valve cusps but in the aortic root surrounding the valve. Established aortic stenosis usually gives rise to left ventricular hypertrophy and this again will be seen on cross sectional and M-mode imaging. When aortic stenosis is severe and the patient begins to go into heart failure the left ventricle will also become dilated and show impaired contractility. At this stage there is usually post-stenotic dilatation of the aortic root which is visible on two dimensional imaging. The common differential diagnosis of aortic stenosis in the adult is sub-aortic stenosis. Sub-aortic stenosis is usually due to hypertrophic cardiomyopathy with dynamic left ventricular outflow obstruction[26,27] but occasionally adults present with fixed sub-aortic stenosis.

M-mode echocardiography is extremely useful in confirming the presence of aortic stenosis. Older patients can have thickened aortic valve cusps without aortic stenosis and M-mode echocardiography discriminates between the

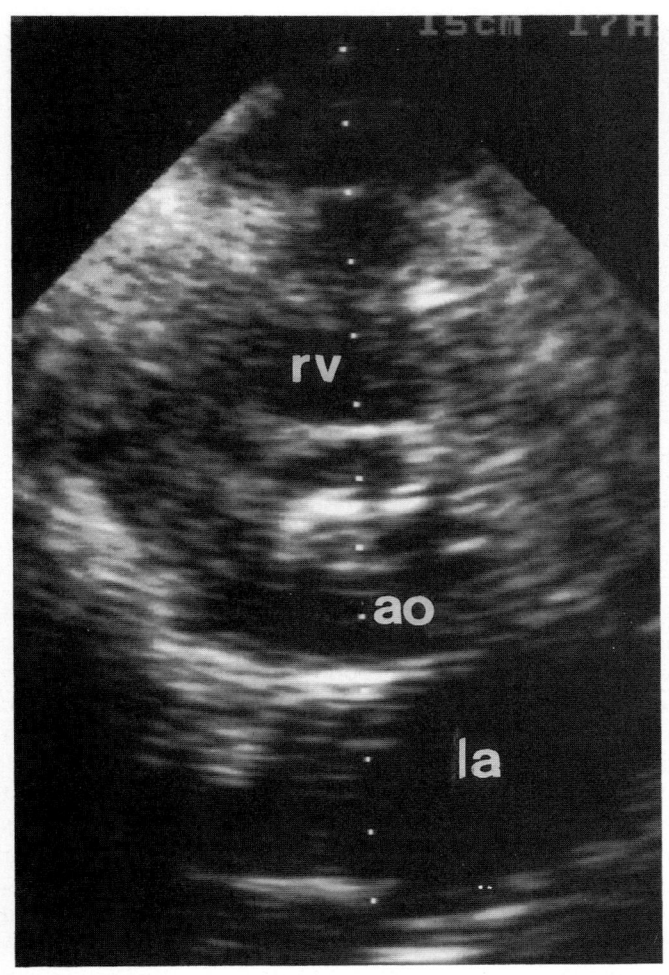

Fig. 24 Left parasternal short axis view of a stenotic aortic valve.

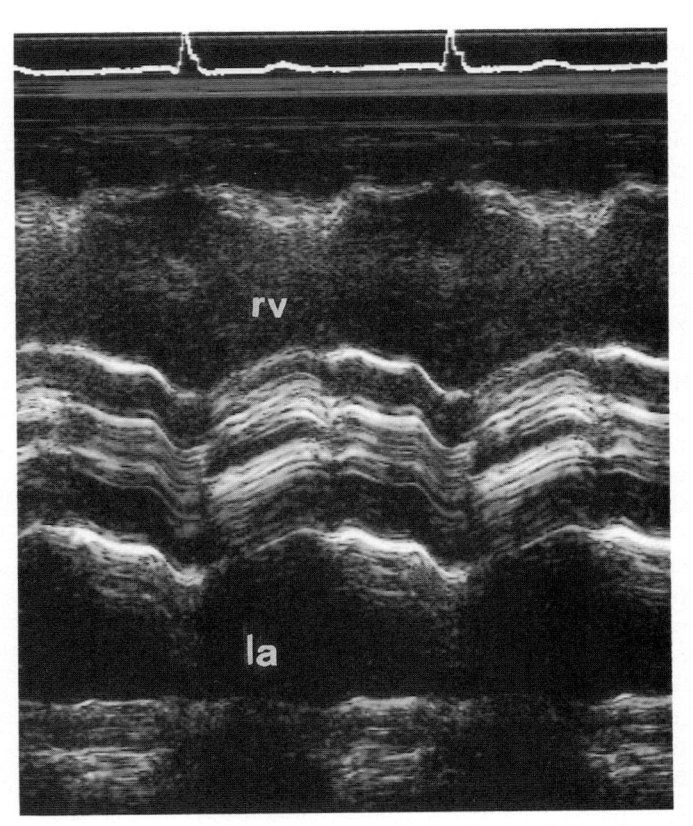

Fig. 25 M-mode trace of aortic stenosis showing restriction of cusp movement producing a compressed rather than a widely opened squared box.

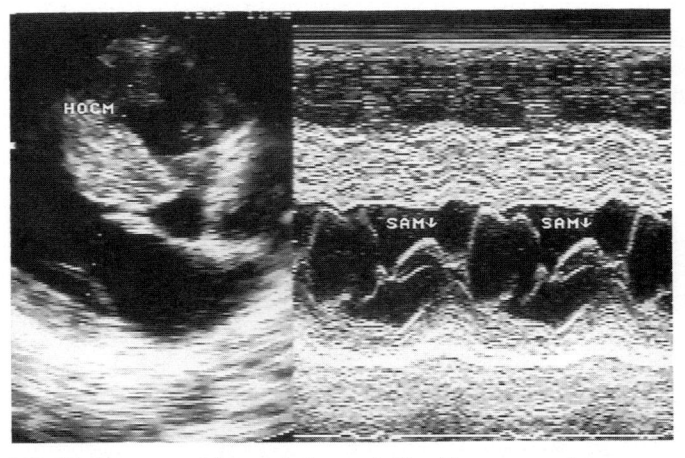

Fig. 26 Parasternal long axis image (left) with accompanying M-mode tracing of hypertrophic obstructive cardiomyopathy showing a markedly thickened septum and systolic anterior motion of the mitral valve (SAM).

ageing process of cusps and true aortic stenosis. The M-mode trace of aortic stenosis shows restriction of cusp movement and produces a compressed rather than a widely open squared box. It will be noted that the thickened aortic valve cusps produce a thicker line on the trace, but in older patients who do not have aortic stenosis the slightly thickened cusps will have a normal 'box' configuration on M-mode echocardiography. M-mode is also useful in establishing subaortic stenosis where there is hypertrophic cardiomyopathy and Figure 26 shows the classical appearance of obstruction of the left ventricular outflow tract by systolic anterior motion of the mitral valve. In some cases where there is obstruction to left ventricular outflow, there can be premature closure of the aortic valve due to cessation of systolic flow.

Pulsed wave Doppler examination is less suitable than continuous wave Doppler examination for assessing aortic stenosis. This is because the jet of aortic stenosis is of high velocity and the aortic valve lies at quite a depth from the probe which enhances the production of aliasing. Pulsed wave examination is useful, however, in assessing sub- aortic stenosis as the cursor can be used to sample areas within the left ventricular outflow tract and detect that the level of obstruction is below the valve itself.

Colour flow Doppler has little to add to the diagnosis of aortic stenosis. Turbulence is usually seen both above and below the aortic valve and aliasing can be seen in the colour flow jet.

The diagnosis of aortic stenosis on echocardiography is usually made by cross-sectional imaging and continuous wave Doppler is usually used to assess its severity. A duplex probe combining two dimensional imaging and a continuous wave transducer can be used but frequently a small non-imaging probe with only a continuous wave transducer is more suitable. The line of the continuous wave should be placed in the left ventricular outflow tract from the apex. The audio signal is extremely useful in detecting the jet and the trace of aortic stenosis will show an extremely high velocity jet below the baseline when examination is carried out from the apex (Fig. 27). This may not be the peak jet and in order to ascertain this at least three other areas should be sampled for a possible higher peak jet. The non-imaging probe should be placed in the subcostal position angling up towards the head, in the right parasternal position with the patient turned completely onto the right side and the probe placed in the second intercostal space to the right of the sternum. The final position is suprasternal with the pencil probe directed inferiorly towards the ascending aorta. The jets detected from the right parasternal and suprasternal windows will be shown as traces above the baseline (Fig. 28). The right parasternal window is a particularly useful site to detect peak jets of aortic stenosis in patients in whom the apical position is not satisfactory in detecting a jet. Obviously, if a jet with a velocity which indicates a peak instantaneous pressure drop of over 100 mmHg is detected at the apex, it is less necessary to assess the other sites, but confirmation of the jet from other positions is always useful. The modified Bernoulli formula is applied to the jet trace. The pressure gradient (or more precisely the pressure drop across the valve) measured by Doppler examination is instantaneous whereas that measured during a cardiac catheterisation by catheter 'pull-back' from left ventricle to aorta is a 'peak to peak' gradient. In the latter situation the peak aortic and peak ventricular pressures are not simultaneous. This usually results in the 'gradient' at cardiac catheterisation being a little lower than that estimated by Doppler examination. Continuous wave Doppler studies can also underestimate a pressure drop if the beam is not absolutely parallel with the jet through the valve. Underestimation of the valve stenosis, though not of the actual pressure drop is also present when there is poor left ventricular function and a reduction in the cardiac output. This will also be noted at cardiac catheterisation because it is a real event as the reduced cardiac output produces a reduction in the jet velocity and this will therefore decrease the gradient across the valve, though of course the valve will be still just as narrowed. This is where cross-sectional imaging plays a vital role as the tightly stenotic aortic valve and the dilated and poorly contracting left ventricle would be appreciated and taken into account in the reporting of what would otherwise appear to be a moderate or even mild gradient. When an aortic valve appears normal, i.e. there is no evidence of stenosis and a high velocity jet is detected from the suprasternal position this should raise the suspicion of a cause for stenosis at another level, above or below the valve. In the case of hypertrophic cardiomyopathy, the obstructed flow produces a characteristic trace with peak velocities occurring in late systole. Figure 29 shows a typical trace produced by hypertrophic obstructive cardiomyopathy.

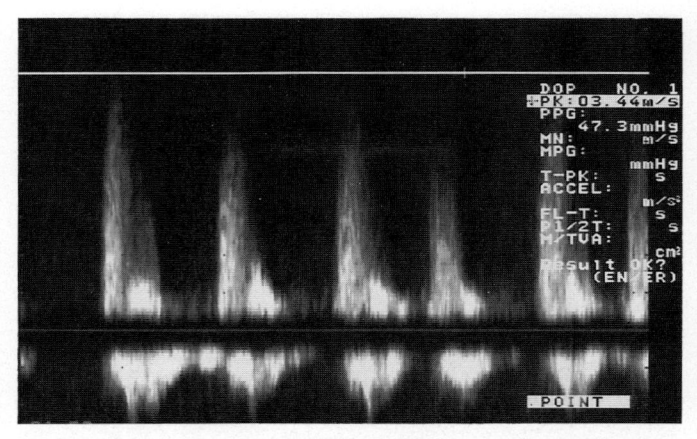

Fig. 28 Continuous wave Doppler trace of aortic stenosis taken from the right parasternal window showing the jet above the baseline as flow in this position is towards the probe. Peak velocity is 3.44 m/s.

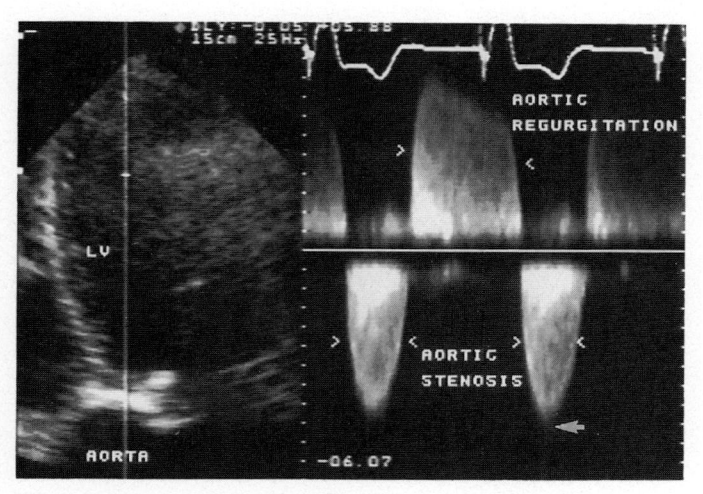

Fig. 27 Apical continuous wave Doppler trace of aortic stenosis (right). The gradient across the valve can be calculated from the velocity of the jet. In this case a velocity of 4.5 m/s gives a peak gradient of 81 mmHg. There is also accompanying aortic regurgitation. Cross-sectional image shows beam position (left).

Aortic regurgitation[28-33]

Aortic regurgitation is most often seen in the setting of both aortic stenosis and regurgitation. This is usually due

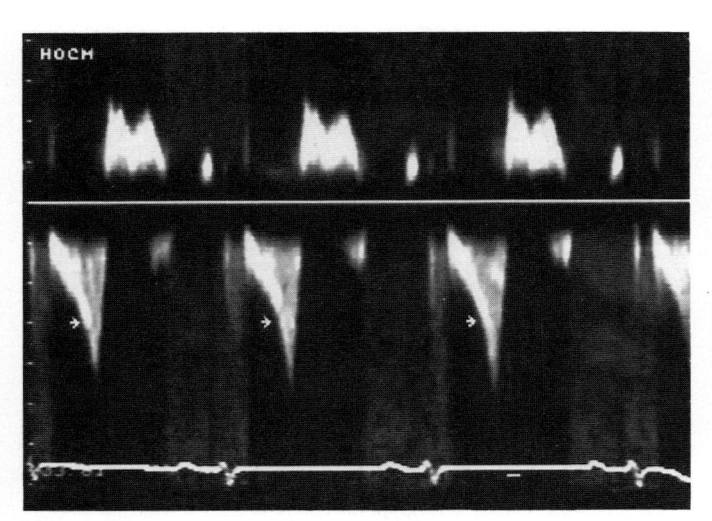

Fig. 29 Continuous wave Doppler trace from a patient with hypertrophic obstructive cardiomyopathy showing a characteristic curve which has a skewed shape produced by the increasing obstruction in the left ventricular outflow tract produced by the markedly hypertrophied septum.

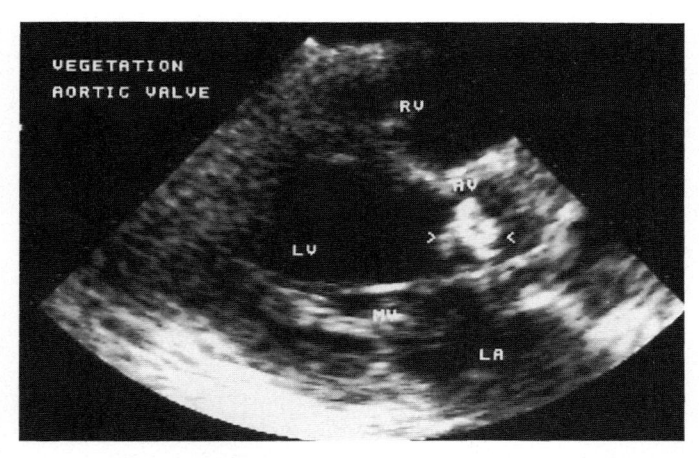

Fig. 30 A large vegetation is seen on the aortic valve in this left parasternal long axis view of a patient with infective endocarditis.

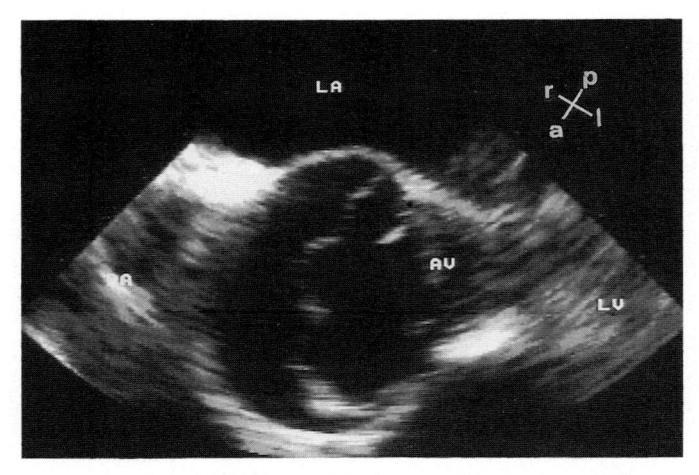

Fig. 31 An intimal flap is noted in the ascending aorta, extending to the aortic valve in this patient with aortic dissection (transoesophageal echo).

to rheumatic heart disease but it is also seen when aortic stenosis is degenerative and often the valve is bicuspid. Regurgitation can be the dominant valvular lesion and of course it can occur on its own without any stenosis. Acute aortic regurgitation is seen in infective endocarditis where a vegetation interferes with closure of the valve cusps or where a valve cusp itself becomes flail or perforated. Aortic dissection is also the setting for acute aortic regurgitation, and Marfan's syndrome and ankylosing spondylitis have an increased incidence of aortic regurgitation. Aortic regurgitation in a child or teenager is usually associated with a bicuspid aortic valve.

Aortic regurgitation is usually diagnosed by Doppler examination rather than by cross-sectional echocardiography. However, the causes of aortic regurgitation such as a vegetation or aortic root abscess occurring in infective endocarditis (Fig. 30) can often be imaged. A flail cusp, commonly with an infective cause, can usually be seen on cross-sectional imaging. These findings may not always be very apparent on a static hard copy image but in real time they can easily be appreciated. When the intimal flap of dissection of the ascending thoracic aorta extends as far as the aortic valve, aortic regurgitation will occur and echocardiography is extremely helpful in confirming or ruling out this diagnosis (Fig. 31) in the patient who presents with acute and severe chest pain and a new murmur of aortic regurgitation. Patients with Marfan's syndrome often develop aneurysmal dilatation of the aortic root and in particular of the sinuses of Valsalva. Floppy valve cusps involving both the aortic and mitral valves are features of Marfan's syndrome and even without an aneurysm of the aortic root, some minor degree of aortic regurgitation is often noted in these patients. With more severe forms of aortic root regurgitation the aortic valve may be replaced and if there is an aneurysm of the aortic root, this may also be grafted. Aortic regurgitation produces volume overload of the left ventricle and with time the ventricle dilates. Volume overload of this chamber initially produces more vigorous contractions of the ventricular walls in an effort to offload this volume, but when decompensation sets in, sometimes after many years, the ventricle fails and is then quite markedly dilated and poorly contracting. There is often associated left ventricular hypertrophy or increase in left ventricular muscle mass.

M-mode tracings have little to add to the diagnosis of aortic regurgitation other than the demonstration of fine vibrations which sometimes occur on the anterior leaflet of the mitral valve when the regurgitant aortic jet strikes the cusp.[34] When a combination of colour flow and M-mode

168 CARDIAC ULTRASOUND

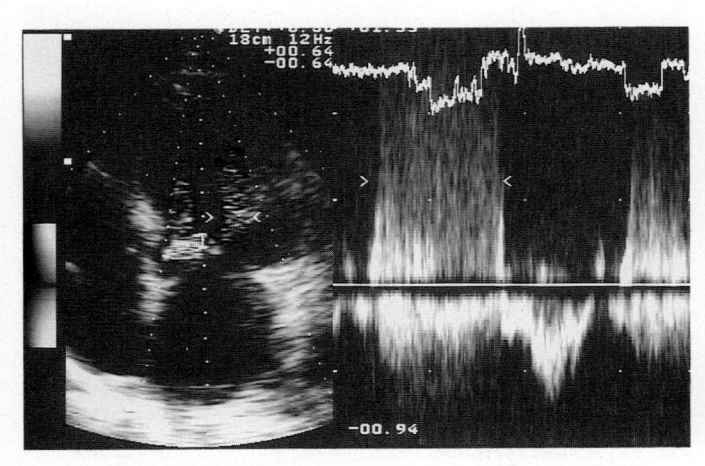

Plate 8 Pulsed Doppler trace of aortic regurgitation (right) with accompanying colour flow image (left). The cursor is placed in the left ventricular outflow tract and mapping of the regurgitant jet can be performed by tracing the cursor back into the left ventricle. This figure is reproduced in colour in the colour plate section at the front of this volume.

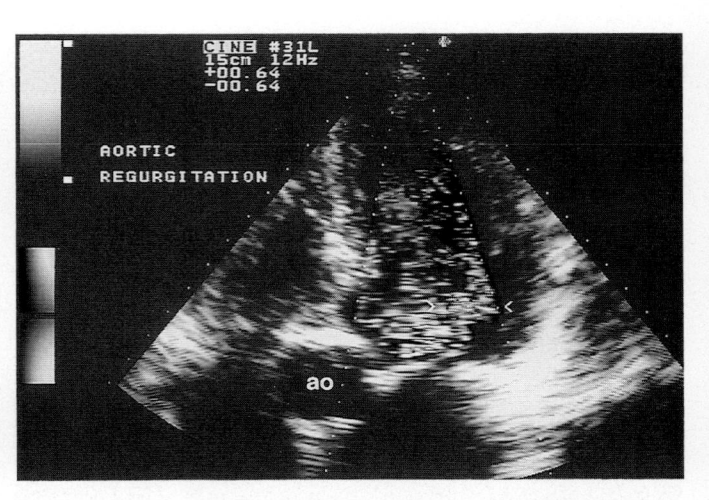

Plate 9 Apical colour flow Doppler image of aortic regurgitation. In this apical four chamber view the regurgitant jet is red towards the probe but shows aliasing and a mosaic pattern. This figure is reproduced in colour in the colour plate section at the front of this volume.

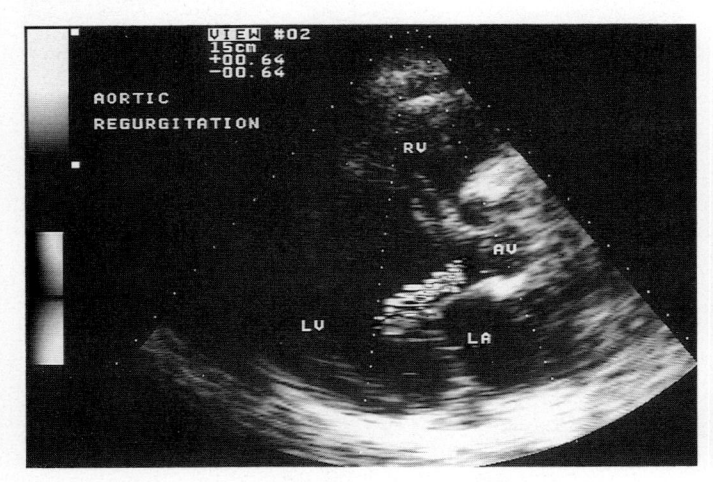

Plate 10 Left parasternal long axis view showing aortic regurgitation as an aliasing blue jet directed towards the anterior mitral leaflet. This figure is reproduced in colour in the colour plate section at the front of this volume.

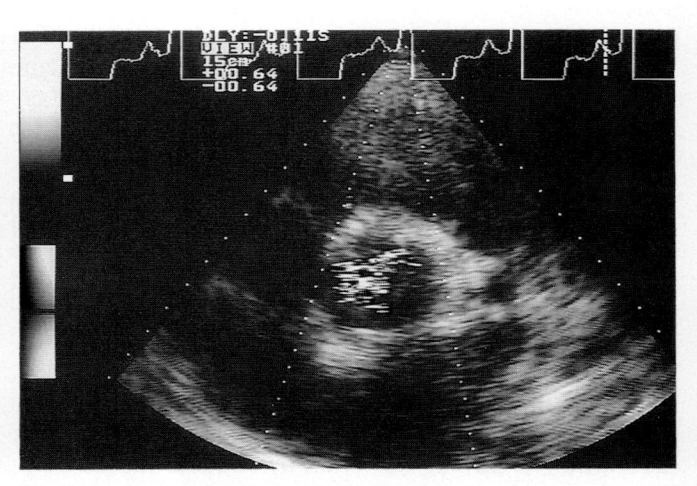

Plate 11 Parasternal short axis colour flow image showing a moderately large jet of aortic regurgitation in the left ventricular outflow tract. This figure is reproduced in colour in the colour plate section at the front of this volume.

examination is used to assess the aortic valve, the regurgitant jet can be seen to pass through the valve when the cusps are closed in diastole. M-mode traces of left ventricular dimensions are also helpful in following patients on a long term basis as serial measurements can help in assessing the severity of aortic regurgitation and the response of the left ventricle to volume overload. There is no universally agreed criterion for deciding the correct time for surgical intervention but an end systolic left ventricular diameter of over 5 cm is often taken as an important upper limit of acceptable dilatation.

Pulsed wave Doppler examination of aortic regurgitation is best performed from the apical four chamber view with the sample volume of the pulsed Doppler placed in the left ventricular outflow tract just below the aortic valve. Pulsed Doppler traces of aortic regurgitation often show aliasing (see Plate 8). Mapping of the jet to assess its severity can be done by moving the sample volume back into the left ventricle and tracing the course of the jet. Care needs to be taken to look for an eccentric jet, particularly along the septum or posterior wall of the left ventricle. There is often controversy and debate about the ability of pulsed Doppler to assess the degree of severity of aortic regurgitation. As colour flow Doppler examination can trace jets much more easily than pulsed Doppler mapping, the role of the latter has diminished.

Pulsed Doppler techniques are still extremely useful when the sample volume is placed from the suprasternal position into the descending thoracic aorta and the degree of diastolic reverse flow is noted. Flow will be away from the probe below the baseline with only minor degrees of reverse flow being seen in a patient without aortic regurgitation (Fig. 32) but in those with significant aortic regurgitation the degree of reverse flow detected can almost equal that of the amount of flow away from the probe and down the aorta (see Fig. 33).

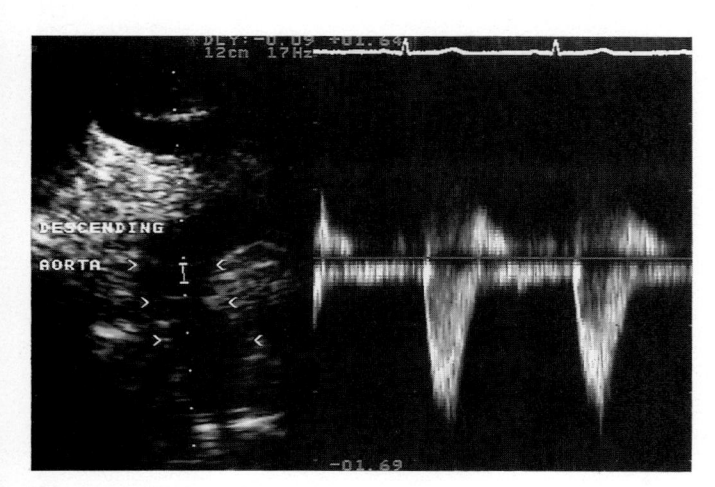

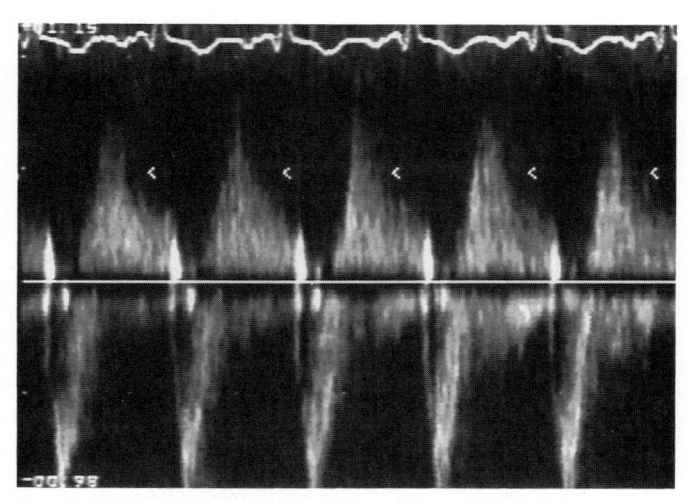

Fig. 33 Severe aortic regurgitation producing significant backflow in a pulsed Doppler trace from the descending thoracic aorta. The transducer has been positioned in the suprasternal position (compare Fig. 32).

Fig. 32 Pulsed Doppler sample volume is placed in the descending aorta (left) showing normal aortic flow with no significant aortic regurgitation (right). A small amount of backflow seen above the baseline in early diastole is normal.

The advent of colour flow Doppler examination has greatly eased both the detection and quantitation of aortic regurgitation. In some ways, colour flow studies can be too sensitive and it is observed that many patients have trivial amounts of aortic regurgitation which must be considered clinically insignificant and are only seen because of the high sensitivity of the technique. In the apical four chamber view, aortic regurgitation will be seen as a red jet with aliasing or a mosaic pattern coming towards the left ventricular apex and the probe (Plate 9). The jet of aortic regurgitation can often be seen in the long axis left parasternal view, particularly if the jet hits the anterior leaflet of the mitral valve (Plate 10). The size of the jet can be seen in the short axis view as it passes down the left ventricular outflow tract (Plate 11).

Assessing the degree of aortic regurgitation can be more difficult. Very mild or severe aortic regurgitation can often be easy to establish. It is the assessment of moderate degrees of aortic regurgitation that can be more difficult. The experience of the operator helps in this regard and also the serial examination of patients helps the operator to assess when there is a change in the degree of aortic regurgitation. The peak velocity in a jet of aortic regurgitation is usually high due to the high pressure differential between the aorta and the left ventricle in diastole. There is a characteristic envelope shape to the trace of aortic regurgitation produced by continuous wave Doppler examination. If the degree of aortic regurgitation is mild, there will be a persistent high differential between the aorta and the left ventricle throughout diastole and the trace will have a somewhat square appearance (see Fig. 34). In severe aortic regurgitation, there will be a rapid decrease in velocity in diastole due to the high end diastole pressure in the left ventricle and the low end diastolic pressure in

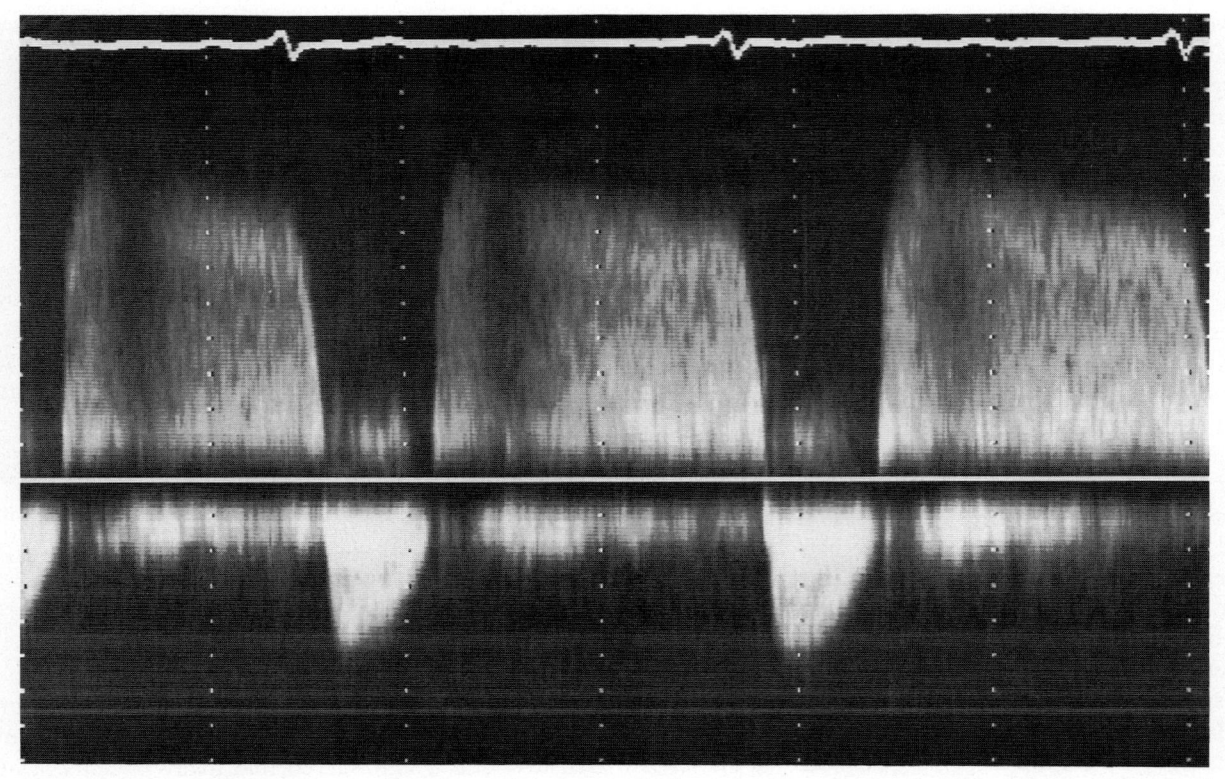

Fig. 34 **Apical continuous wave Doppler trace** showing mild aortic regurgitation and mild aortic stenosis. The aortic regurgitant trace has a square appearance due to the persistently high differential pressure between the aorta and left ventricle throughout diastole.

the aorta. There may be only a calculated pressure difference between the two of 5 mmHg. Reversal of flow in the descending thoracic aorta can also be assessed by continuous wave Doppler as well as pulsed wave Doppler from the suprasternal position but pulsed wave Doppler assessment can often be easier, as the cursor can be placed within the descending thoracic aorta rather than having to align this part of the aorta with the continuous wave probe.

TRICUSPID VALVE[35-38]

The tricuspid valve is much less commonly affected by primary valve disease than either the aortic or the mitral valve. Tricuspid stenosis is an extremely uncommon condition and tricuspid regurgitation though not uncommon, is more often functional than organic in nature. The two common settings for tricuspid regurgitation are as a trivial or mild jet found on some estimates in up to 15% of normal hearts and sometimes accounting for a 'murmur' in an otherwise normal heart. The other setting is of more significant tricuspid regurgitation found in pulmonary hypertension whether due to a cardiac cause such as mitral valve disease or a primarily pulmonary cause. The jet velocity of the regurgitant jet can be used to estimate the degree of pulmonary hypertension and this will be discussed in further detail below.

Normal tricuspid valve

The tricuspid valve is best seen in the apical four chamber view where its anterior and septal leaflets can be well seen (Fig. 35). The posterior leaflet is only seen on the long axis

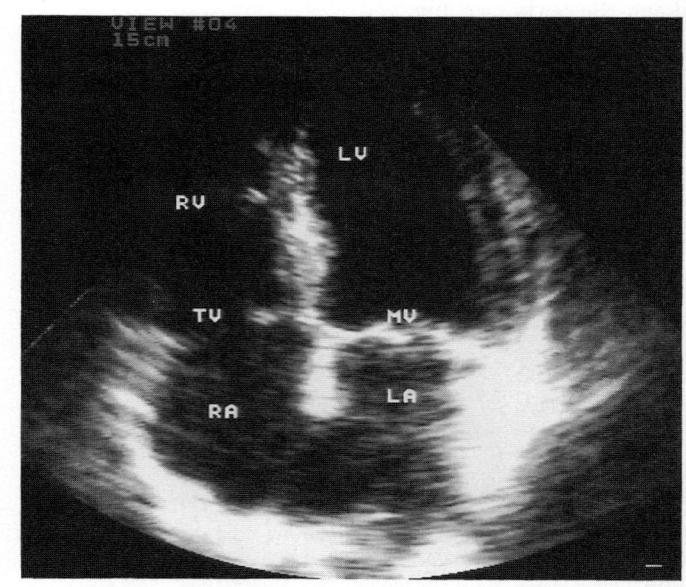

Fig. 35 **Apical four chamber view** showing a normal tricuspid valve.

parasternal view, but this is a poor window from which to assess the valve. The short axis parasternal view also demonstrates the valve well (Fig. 36).

M-mode tracings of the tricuspid valve are technically difficult to obtain and of little practical importance but when obtained appear essentially similar to those of the mitral valve although the orifice is slightly larger. Conditions in which right atrial and right ventricular dilatation occur will displace the valve to the left and this usually allows easier M-mode imaging.

Pulsed Doppler tracings of normal tricuspid flow are obtained by placing the sample volume between the tips of the open valve leaflets from the apical four chamber view or from a low left parasternal view. The trace again is similar in configuration to that of the mitral valve but the velocity of the flow is usually lower than that of the mitral valve because of the lower pressure in the right side of the heart (Fig. 37).

Colour flow Doppler examination is usually used to assess tricuspid regurgitation and this is best seen from the four chamber apical window and the left parasternal short axis view. A modified low left parasternal view is often useful in assessing the tricuspid valve.

The continuous wave cursor is placed through the tricuspid valve from the apical four chamber window, but sometimes the left parasternal short axis view provides an equally good, and in some patients better, window to assess the valve.

Tricuspid stenosis

Tricuspid stenosis is a rare condition and is usually rheumatic in origin, usually being associated with rheumatic mitral valve disease. Tricuspid stenosis can be congenital, but tricuspid atresia is more common than stenosis. Carcinoid syndrome may also affect the valve, but it usually causes regurgitation rather than stenosis. A right atrial myxoma may also cause obstruction of the tricuspid valve.

In rheumatic tricuspid stenosis there will be thickening of the valve cusps with restricted movement. The appearances are essentially the same as those of rheumatic mitral stenosis. Where there is a right atrial myxoma an echogenic mass will be noted in the right atrium which encroaches upon the tricuspid valve causing obstruction. It should be stated that many cases of right atrial myxoma do not cause tricuspid obstruction. In carcinoid syndrome, increased echogenicity of the valve cusps and adjacent structures may be seen.

As in mitral stenosis, tricuspid stenosis produces a characteristic high velocity flow through the valve which results in a turbulent jet in the right ventricle in diastole. This raised jet velocity is slow to decrease throughout diastole and in severe cases the pressure gradient will not drop to zero even at the end of diastole. Similar obstructive flow patterns may sometimes be noted in a patient who has had a previous tricuspid annuloplasty to correct tricuspid regurgitation. The flow characteristics of tricuspid stenosis are very similar to those of mitral stenosis but the velocities are lower due to the larger orifice size of the tricuspid valve and the smaller pressure difference on the right side of the heart. The diagnosis of tricuspid stenosis by Doppler technique is usually easy compared with the difficulties sometimes encountered in catheterisation. A patient can be symptomatic with only a small increase in valve gradient and therefore the Doppler technique is the most reliable and sensitive means of detecting tricuspid stenosis.

Colour flow Doppler examination is extremely useful in detecting turbulence and this will be seen in the right

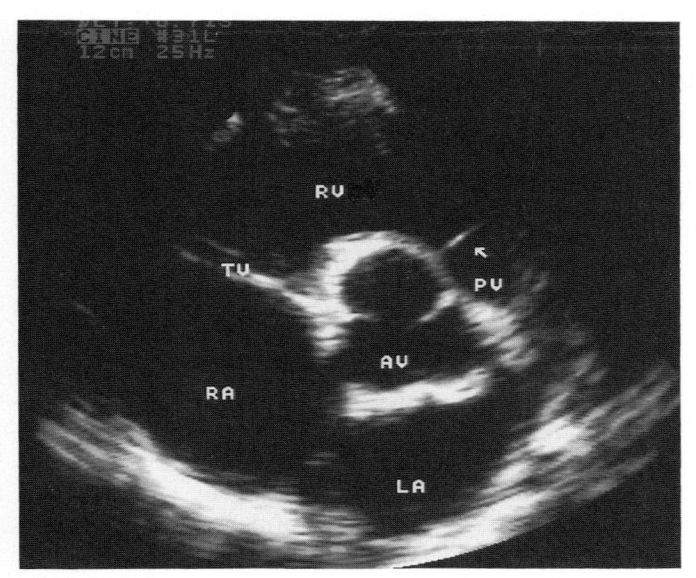

Fig. 36 Left parasternal short axis view of a normal tricuspid valve showing its relationship to the right ventricular outflow tract, right atrium and aortic root in this position.

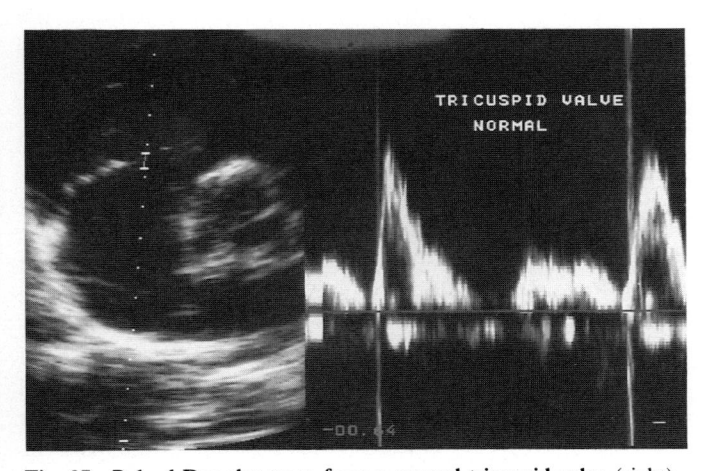

Fig. 37 Pulsed Doppler trace from a normal tricuspid valve (right) with the corresponding short axis parasternal images on the left.

ventricle in diastole just beyond the valve, due to the high velocity through the valve which has produced the turbulent jet. This is easily seen from the apical four chamber view.

Patients usually become symptomatic from tricuspid stenosis with relatively small increases in the valve gradient and thus continuous wave Doppler examination is rarely necessary in the diagnosis of tricuspid stenosis but if performed, the results are similar to those obtained using pulsed Doppler techniques. Doppler techniques are often more straightforward to interpret in this condition than catheter derived pressure data.

Tricuspid regurgitation

Tricuspid regurgitation can be functional or organic in origin. Functional tricuspid regurgitation is quite common and may be a normal finding in up to 15% of patients. Functional regurgitation of a more significant nature is seen frequently in mitral valve disease where there is dilatation of the right ventricle secondary to pulmonary hypertension. The jet size may be anything from mild to severe, depending on the degree of tricuspid annuluar dilatation. In the case of pulmonary hypertension it is not the severity of the regurgitation jet that is significant but the velocity of the jet and in some cases the jet may appear to be small in size but the velocity may be high which indicates a significant amount of pulmonary hypertension. Rheumatic heart disease may rarely involve the tricuspid as well as the mitral valve and can cause tricuspid regurgitation of an organic nature. In this situation, there will be thickening of the valve cusps. Carcinoid syndrome, infective endocarditis and valvular rupture secondary to trauma are other causes of acquired tricuspid regurgitation. Congenital tricuspid regurgitation is uncommon but is seen where there is an atrioventricular septal defect, Marfan's syndrome or in Ebstein's anomaly.

The valve cusps in tricuspid regurgitation often have a normal appearance especially where the tricuspid regurgitation is functional, though dilatation of the right ventricle causing stretching of the tricuspid valve annulus should raise one's suspicions as to the presence of regurgitation. There will be thickening of the valve cusps in rheumatic heart disease and in infective endocarditis vegetations may be seen on the valve. In malignant carcinoid disease, fibrous plaques may be seen on the ventricular side of the tricuspid valve which cause adhesions between the ventricular wall and the valve. Cross sectional imaging is particularly effective in diagnosing rupture of a valve cusp where there has been trauma and also in Marfan's syndrome where the cusps of the tricuspid valve will have a floppy appearance which may also be seen in the aortic and mitral valves.

The jet of tricuspid regurgitation is often centrally placed within the right atrium and this can be detected by pulsed Doppler sampling (Fig. 38). However, eccentric jets are not uncommon and the pulsed Doppler sample volume needs to be used carefully to map out the path of the regurgitant jet.

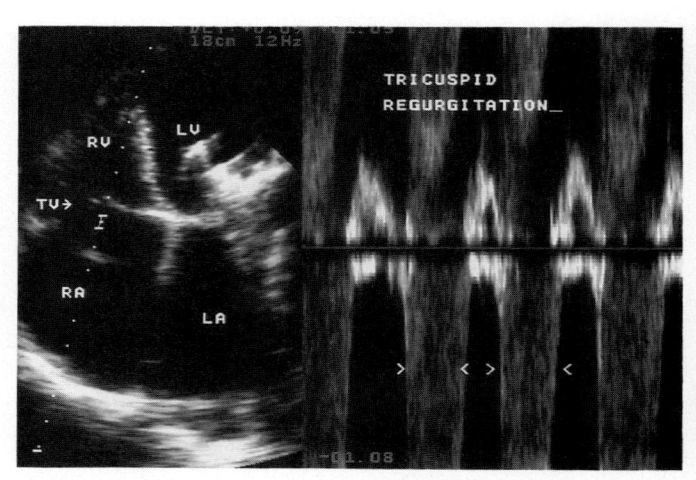

Fig. 38 Pulsed Doppler trace of tricuspid regurgitation (right) from the apical four chamber view (left). Note aliased trace.

Colour flow Doppler examination has greatly quickened and enhanced the assessment of tricuspid regurgitation and often negates the need to use pulsed Doppler techniques in assessing the presence and severity of a regurgitant jet. It is best assessed from the apical four chamber view (Plate 12) and is particularly useful where there is an eccentric jet or sometimes multiple jets (Plate 13). This is of importance when one wants to use continuous wave Doppler examination to assess the velocity of the jet, by locating the site and direction of the jet. In severe tricuspid regurgitation the colour flow jet can be seen to extend into the inferior vena cava and there will often be reversal of flow in the hepatic veins in ventricular systole.

Continuous wave Doppler examination is used to assess the velocity of the tricuspid jet and to establish the presence or absence of pulmonary hypertension and its severity. Pulmonary hypertension leads to pulmonary insufficiency and tricuspid regurgitation and though the regurgitant jets may be small in volume, their velocity in pulmonary hypertension will be quite high. The jet velocity is measured in metres per second and the calculation is performed using the modified Bernoulli equation which will give the systolic pressure drop across the tricuspid valve (Plate 14). If 10 mmHg is used as an approximate right atrial pressure (virtually all patients' right atrial pressure will lie between zero and 20 mmHg), the addition of the gradient across the tricuspid valve to the right atrial pressure will give the estimated peak systolic right ventricular pressure. If there is no pulmonary stenosis the pulmonary artery systolic pressure will be equal to this peak right ventricular systolic pressure.

VALVULAR DISEASE 173

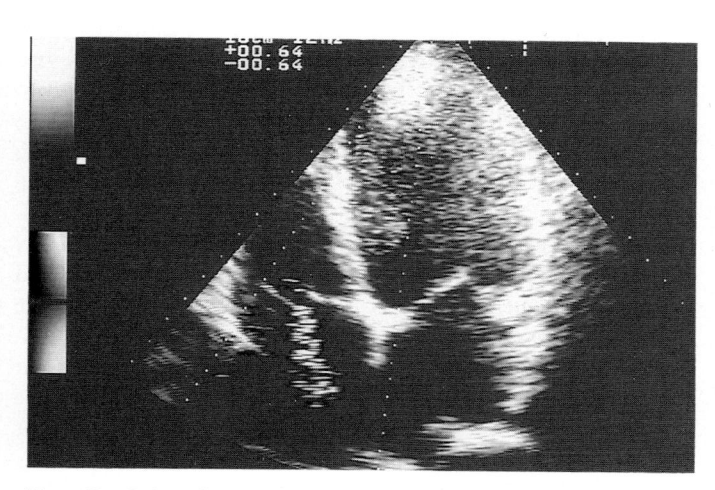

Plate 12 Colour flow Doppler image of tricuspid regurgitation showing a blue jet in the right atrium in this apical four chamber view. This figure is reproduced in colour in the colour plate section at the front of this volume.

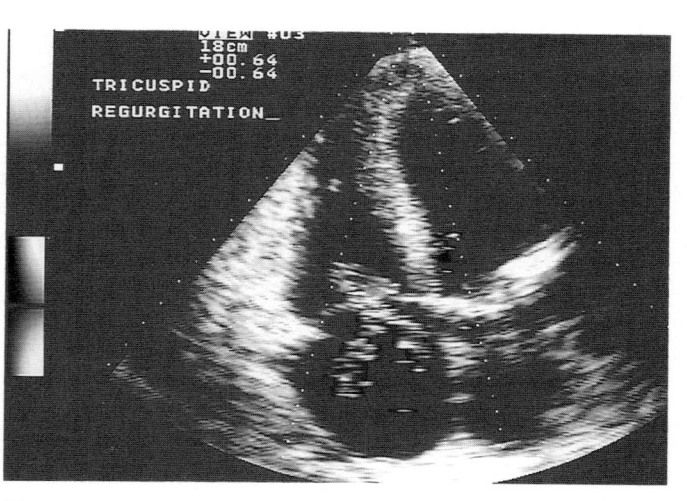

Plate 13 Colour flow Doppler image of tricuspid regurgitation from the apical four chamber window. In this case the jet is in two distinct and divergent streams. This figure is reproduced in colour in the colour plate section at the front of this volume.

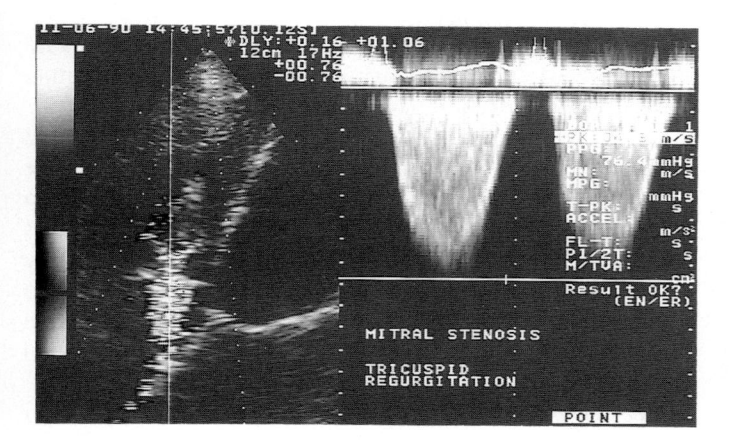

Plate 14 Apical colour flow image (left) in a patient with tricuspid regurgitation secondary to mitral stenosis. The colour flow jet has been used to direct a continuous wave beam. The spectral trace (right) shows a calculated peak jet velocity of 4.3 m/s (peak pressure drop of 76.4 mmHg). This figure is reproduced in colour in the colour plate section at the front of this volume.

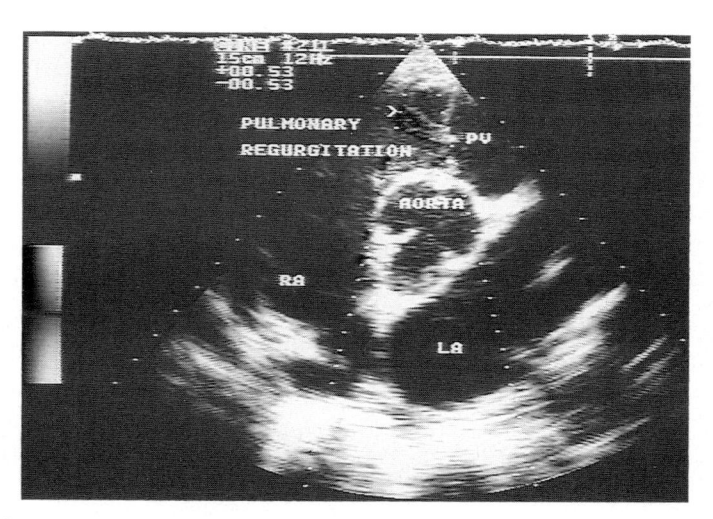

Plate 15 Colour flow Doppler image of mild pulmonary regurgitation seen as a 'red flame' in this left parasternal short axis view. This figure is reproduced in colour in the colour plate section at the front of this volume.

PULMONARY VALVE

The pulmonary valve is the least common of all the valves to warrant the echocardiographer's attention. Pulmonary valve stenosis is most commonly congenital and very rarely acquired. Pulmonary regurgitation is seen most often in pulmonary arterial hypertension, but a small amount of regurgitation is a normal finding in a minority of normal hearts.

Pulmonary stenosis

Congenital pulmonary stenosis may occur as an isolated phenomenon but it is often associated with other cardiac congenital abnormalities. Acquired causes of pulmonary stenosis include carcinoid syndrome and rheumatic heart disease, both of which are extremely rare.

The pulmonary valve is seen in the short axis left parasternal view (Fig. 39). In children and in a number of adults, it can be quite easily seen but in many adults, particularly those with less than optimal echo windows, the patient needs to be turned almost completely on the left side. Often suspended expiration improves the echo window in this position. In congenital pulmonary stenosis, the valve cusps may not be thickened but doming of the cusps will be seen. Post-stenotic dilatation of the pulmonary artery and right ventricular hypertrophy will be seen in long established congenital pulmonary stenosis.

Pulmonary stenosis will produce a high velocity turbulent jet in the pulmonary artery. Though continuous wave Doppler examination is more appropriate for assessing the velocity of this high velocity jet the cursor of the pulsed Doppler can be used to map the right ventricular outflow tract, pulmonary valve and beyond to assess the level of obstruction and is useful in differentiating an infundibular stenosis from an actual pulmonary valve stenosis. In valvular stenosis there is a relatively early rise to peak velocity due to the fixed obstruction, but in infundibular stenosis the maximum velocity occurs late in systole when the right ventricular outflow tract is at its narrowest. In pulmonary arterial hypertension there will be decrease in the acceleration time of the pulmonary flow. This is calculated by placing the pulsed Doppler sample volume just distal to the pulmonary valve, obtaining a clear trace and then measuring the time from the onset of systole to the time of peak velocity. In a normal patient with normal pulmonary circulation, this is usually well over 100 ms, but in pulmonary hypertension the acceleration time will be less than this. This is due to the increased resistance or impedence in the pulmonary circulation.

Colour flow Doppler examination will detect the turbulent jet of pulmonary stenosis but it is more especially useful where there is another level of obstruction such as an infundibular stenosis. The high jet velocity of pulmonary stenosis requires continuous wave Doppler examination to measure the pressure drop across the valve.

Pulmonary regurgitation[39,40]

The commonest cause of pulmonary regurgitation is pulmonary arterial hypertension, whether due to a cardiac cause such as severe mitral stenosis or a pulmonary cause such as recurrent pulmonary emboli. Other less common causes of pulmonary insufficiency include infective encarditis, pulmonary valvotomy or pulmonary stenosis and Marfan's syndrome. Carcinoid syndrome and syphilis are other rare causes of pulmonary regurgitation. It may also be seen as part of a congenital heart condition such as tetralogy of Fallot, ventricular septal defect or pulmonary stenosis itself. A trivial amount of pulmonary regurgitation may be detected in a significant minority of normal people and may be the cause of a 'murmur' in an otherwise normal heart.

In pulmonary hypertension, a dilated pulmonary artery may alert the echocardiographer to the possibility of pulmonary regurgitation. There may also be a dilated right ventricle and atrium, but the valve itself will most likely have a normal appearance. A vegetation may be noted on the valve in infective endocarditis and in Marfan's syndrome the valve may have a somewhat floppy appearance. In carcinoid syndrome, fibrous deposition on the endocardium of the valve may be seen and this may also extend to the right ventricle leading to fusing and restriction of these structures.

M-mode tracings have little to contribute to the diagnosis of pulmonary insufficiency. The pulsed wave Doppler sample volume should be placed just proximal to the pulmonary valve in the left parasternal short axis view to detect pulmonary regurgitation (Fig. 40). The regurgitant jet may well be eccentric and therefore mapping of the

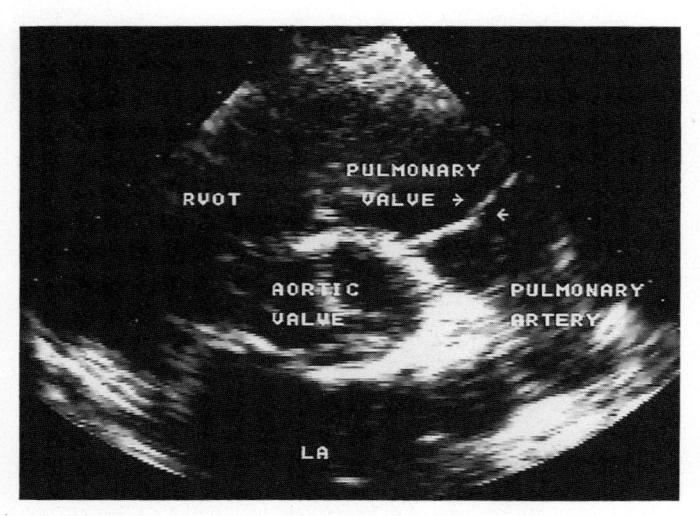

Fig. 39 This **left parasternal short axis view** shows the position of the pulmonary valve in relation to the aortic root and right ventricular outflow tract.

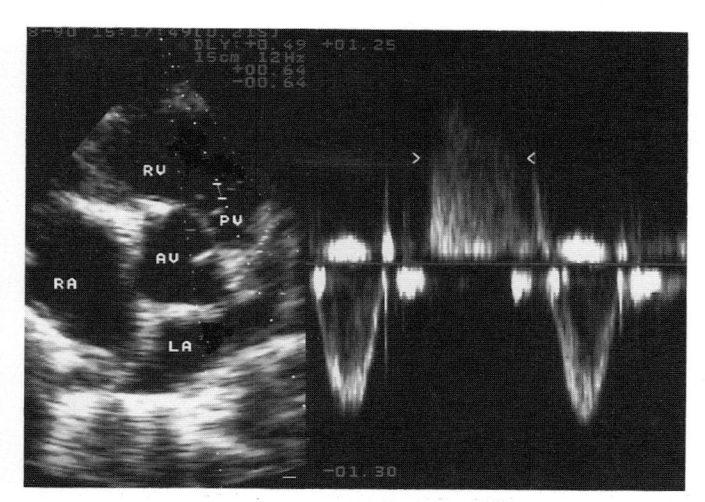

Fig. 40 Pulsed Doppler trace of mild pulmonary regurgitation (right) with the cursor placed just proximal to the pulmonary valve cusps from the left parasternal short axis position (left). The regurgitant jet is seen above the baseline (arrowed) with normal flow through the valve demonstrated as flow below the baseline.

pulmonary artery proximal to the valve will often be necessary to detect the actual jet itself. Quantitation of pulmonary reflux from the pulmonary artery signal alone is not very reliable as high flow into a compliant pulmonary artery can produce reverse flow pattern. A patent ductus arteriosus can also produce a reverse flow pattern.

Colour flow Doppler examination has made the detection of pulmonary regurgitation much easier and quicker than by conventional pulsed Doppler examination. The characteristic 'red flame' (Plates 15, 16) of mild pulmonary regurgitation may have little clinical importance and is often undetected by the stethescope. More significant pulmonary regurgitation will produce a larger jet back into the right ventricular outflow tract and beyond.

Continuous wave Doppler examination has little to add to the diagnosis of pulmonary regurgitation compared to colour flow and pulsed wave Doppler, except where there is poor cross sectional imaging and continuous wave Doppler can be used on the blind to do detect any abnormality in the pulmonary artery flow pattern.

CONCLUSION

Echocardiography has revolutionized the investigation and management of valvular heart disease. Prior to this, patients were managed by simple clinical assessment or by cardiac catheterisation. Echocardiography has the advantage of giving anatomical detail as well as haemodynamic information about the valves and the heart. The advent of Doppler techniques, particularly colour flow mapping, has greatly increased the ease with which regurgitant jets can be detected, particularly where those jets are eccentric. Quantitation of regurgitant jets still proves to be a major problem whereas quantitation of valvular stenosis has become highly accurate and compares well with cardiac catheterisation. Now that the number of patients with rheumatic heart disease is decreasing, degenerative aortic valve disease has become the commonest valvular stenosis seen by the echocardiographer. An accurate gradient across the aortic valve can be ascertained by continuous wave Doppler examination and left ventricular function can be assessed by two dimensional imaging; this leaves only the coronary arteries to be evaluated by invasive techniques.

Serial assessment can greatly help in the timing of surgical intervention, particularly in the management of chronic aortic regurgitation. Echocardiography also proves useful in infective endocarditis where a vegetation on a valve confirms the presence of established endocarditis. Of course, infective endocarditis is still a clinical diagnosis and the absence of a vegetation does not exclude this diagnosis. Further damage to the heart in endocarditis may be seen, for instance an aortic root abscess where the aortic valve is involved. The diagnosis of a ruptured chorda producing acute mitral regurgitation or the detection of aortic regurgitation secondary to aortic root dissection, can prove invaluable to a referring clinician. The use of the tricuspid jet in assessing the presence or absence of pulmonary arterial hypertension often negates the need for right heart studies to assess pulmonary pressure.

Echocardiography can nowadays produce a wealth of information on both the structural and haemodynamic aspects of the heart. The combination of state of the art equipment and an experienced operator will greatly reduce the need for more interventional investigative techniques.

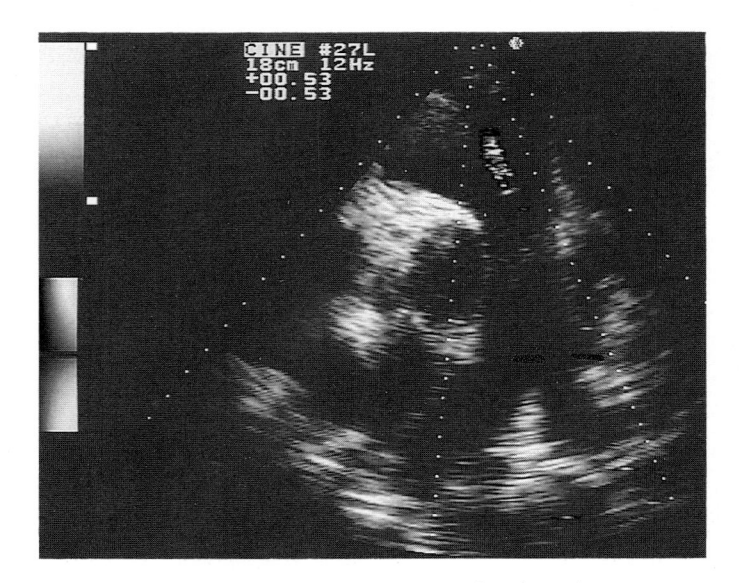

Plate 16 Modified left parasternal view showing the main pulmonary artery and its bifurcation. Pulmonary regurgitation is seen as a red jet. This figure is reproduced in colour in the colour plate section at the front of this volume.

Follow up studies on patients post surgery and intervention such as valvuloplasty continue to expand the role of this procedure. Studies with the transoesophageal probe are becoming more commonplace and this means that with ultrasound it is now possible to make a diagnosis, to assist the surgeon operating upon it and in the follow up of the progress of the patient whether the valve has been repaired or replaced by a prosthesis.

REFERENCES

1. Johnson S L, Baker D W, Lute R A, Dodge H T Doppler echocardiography. The localisation of cardiac murmurs. Circulation 1973; 48: 810
2. Kawabori I, Stevenson J G, Dooley T K, Guntheroth W G Evaluation of ejection murmurs by pulsed Doppler echocardiograph. British Heart Journal 1980; 43: 623
3. Hoffman A, Burckhardt D Evaluation of systolic murmurs by Doppler echocardiography. British Heart Journal 1983; 50: 337
4. Newburger J W, Rosenthal A, William R G, Fellows K, Miettinen O S Noninvasive tests in the initial evaluation of heart murmurs in children. New England Journal of Medicine 1983; 308: 61
5. Wilde P, Pitcher D Pulsed Doppler echocardiography in cardiac diagnosis. Journal of the Royal College of Physicians of London 1986; 20: 25
6. Holen J, Aaslid R, Landmark K, Simonsen S Determination of pressure gradient in mitral stenosis with a noninvasive ultrasound Doppler technique. Acta Medica Scandinavica 1976; 199: 455
7. Holen J, Simonsen S Determination of pressure gradient in mitral stenosis with Doppler echocardiography. British Heart Journal 1979; 41: 529
8. Hatle L, Angelsen B, Tromsdal A Noninvasive assessment of atrioventricular pressure half time by Doppler ultrasound. Circulation 1979; 60: 1096
9. Smith M D, Handshoe R, Handshoe S, Kwan O L, De Maria A N Comparative accuracy of two dimensional echocardiography and Doppler pressure half-time methods in assessing severity of mitral stenosis in patients with and without prior commisurotomy. Circulation 1986; 73: 100
10. Loperfido F, Laurenzi F, Gimigliano F et al A comparison of the assessment of mitral valve area by continuous wave Doppler and by cross sectional echocardiography. British Heart Journal 1987; 57: 348
11. Libanoff J, Rodbard S Atrioventricular pressure half-time. Measure of mitral valve orifice area. Circulation 1968; 38: 144
12. Nichol P M, Boughner D R, Persaud J A Non-invasive assessment of mitral insufficiency by transcutaneous Doppler ultrasound. Circulation 1976; 54: 656
13. Zhang Y, Ihlen H, Myrhe E, Levorstad K, Nitter-Hauge S Measurement of mitral regurgitation by Doppler echocardiography. British Heart Journal 1985; 54: 384
14. Blumlein S, Bouchard A, Schiller N B, Dae M, Byrd B F, Ports T, Botvinick E H Quantitation of mitral regurgitation by Doppler echocardiography. Circulation 1986; 74: 306
15. Helmcke F, Nanda N C, Hsuing M C, Soto B, Adey C K, Goyal R G, Gatewood R P Color Doppler assessment of mitral regurgitation with orthogonal planes. Circulation 1987; 75: 175
16. Stevenson J G, Kawabori I, Guntheroth W G Differentiation of ventricular septal defects from mitral regurgitation by pulsed Doppler echocardiography. Circulation 1977; 56: 14
17. Hatle L, Angelsen B, Tromsdal A Non-invasive assessment of aortic stenosis by Doppler ultrasound. British Heart Journal 1980; 43: 284
18. Hatle L Noninvasive assessment and differentiation of left ventricular outflow obstruction with Doppler ultrasound. Circulation 1981; 64: 381
19. Cannon S R, Richards K L, Rollwitz W T Digital Fourier techniques in the diagnosis and quantitation of aortic stenosis with pulsed Doppler echocardiography. Journal of Clinical Ultrasound 1982; 1: 1014
20. Simpson I A, Houston A B, Sheldon C D, Hutton I, Lawne T D V Clinical value of Doppler echocardiography in the assessment of adults with aortic stenosis. British Heart Journal 1984; 53: 636
21. Currie P J, Steard J B, Reeder G S et al Continuous wave Doppler echocardiographic assessment of severity of calcific aortic stenosis: a simultaneous Doppler-catheter correlative study in 100 patients. Circulation 1985; 71: 162
22. Skjaerpe T, Hegrenaes L, Hatle L Noninvasive estimation of valve area in patients with aortic stenosis by Doppler ultrasound and two dimensional echocardiography. Circulation 1985; 72: 810–818
23. Panidis I P, Mintz G S, Ross J Value and limitations of Doppler ultrasound in the evaluation of aortic stenosis; a statistical analysis of 70 consecutive patients. American Heart Journal 1986; 112: 150
24. Zoghbi W A, Farmer K L, Soto J G, Nelson J G, Quinones M A Accurate noninvasive quantification of stenotic aortic valve area by Doppler echocardiography. Circulation 1986; 73: 452
25. Veyrat C, Gourtchiglouian V, Dumora P, Abitbol G, Sainte Beuve D, Kalmanson D A new non-invasive estimation of the stenotic aortic valve area by pulsed Doppler mapping. British Heart Journal 1987; 57: 44
26. Boughner D R, Schuld R L, Persaud J A Hypertrophic obstructive cardiomyopathy assessed by echocardiographic and Doppler ultrasound techniques. British Heart Journal 1975; 37: 917
27. Gardin J M, Debestani A, Glascow G A, Butman S, Burn C S, Henry W C Echocardiographic and Doppler flow observations in obstructed and nonobstructed hypertrophic cardiomyopathy. American Journal of Cardiology 1985; 56: 614
28. Ciobanu M, Abbasi A S, Allen M, Spellberg R Pulsed Doppler echocardiography in the diagnosis and estimation of severity of aortic insufficiency. American Journal of Cardiology 1982; 49: 339
29. Diebold B, Peronnea P, Blanchard D Non-invasive quantitation of aortic regurgitation by Doppler echocardiography. British Heart Journal 1983; 49: 167
30. Kitabatake A, Ito H, Inoue M et al A new approach to noninvasive evaluation of aortic regurgitation fraction by two dimensional Doppler echocardiography. Circulation 1985; 72: 523
31. Touche T, Prasquier R, Nitenberg A, de Zuttere D, Gourgon R Assessment and follow up of patients with aortic regurgitation by an updated echocardiographic measurement of the regurgitant fracture in the aortic arch. Circulation 1985; 72: 819
32. Hoffman A, Pfisterer M, Stulz P, Schmitt H E, Burkart F, Burckhardt D Non-invasive gradient of aortic regurgitation by Doppler ultrasonography. British Heart Journal 1986; 55: 283
33. Masayama Y, Kodama K, Kitabatake A et al Noninvasive evaluation of aortic regurgitation by continuous wave Doppler echocardiography. Circulation 1986; 73: 460
34. Pridie R B, Benham R, Oakley C M Echocardiography of the mitral valve in aortic valve disease. British Heart Journal 1971; 33: 296
35. Waggoner A D, Quinones M A, Young J B, Brandon T A, Shah, Verani M S, Miller R R Pulsed Doppler echocardiographic detection of right-sided valve regurgitation. American Journal of Cardiology 1981; 472: 79
36. Veyrat C, Kalmanson D, Farjon M, Manin J P, Abitbot G Noninvasive diagnosis and assessment of tricuspid regurgitation and stenosis using one and two dimensional echo-pulsed Doppler. British Heart Journal 1982; 47: 596

37 Diebold B, Touati R, Blanchard D Quantitative assessment of tricuspid regurgitation using pulsed Doppler echocardiography. British Heart Journal 1983; 50: 443

38 Suzuki Y, Kambara H, Kadota K et al Detection and evaluation of tricuspid regurgitation using a real-time, two-dimensional, color-coded Doppler flow imaging system: comparison with contrast two-dimensional echocardiography and right ventriculography. American Journal of Cardiology 1986; 57: 811

39 Patel A K, Rowe G G, Dhaniani S P, Kosolcharoen P, Lyle L E W, Thomsen J H Pulsed Doppler echocardiography in diagnosis of pulmonary regurgitation: its value and limitations. American Journal of Cardiology 1982; 49: 19801

40 Masayama T, Kodama K, Kitabatake A, Sato H, Nanto S, Inoue M Continuous wave Doppler echocardiographic detection of pulmonary regurgitation and its application to noninvasive estimation of pulmonary artery pressure. Circulation 1986; 74: 484

11

Ischaemic heart disease

Coronary imaging
Pathological effects of left ventricular ischaemia and infarction
Tissue characterisation
Contrast echocardiography
Complications of ischaemic heart disease
Dysrhythmias and arrhythmias
Aneurysm

Rupture of the myocardium
   False or 'pseudo-aneurysm'
   Direct rupture into the pericardium
   Ventricular septal defect
Mitral regurgitation
Thrombus formation
Right ventricular infarction
Dressler's syndrome
Other complications

Jamie Weir

CORONARY IMAGING

The proximal 1 to 2 cm of the main coronary arteries can usually be imaged in adults, with the left coronary artery occasionally being seen beyond the origins of the left anterior descending and circumflex arteries. It may be possible to detect atheromatous plaques in the coronary walls in some cases but an accurate assessment of percentage narrowing is usually impossible. The vast majority of the echocardiographic signs of coronary artery disease arise from the effects of complications of that disease and detailed coronary assessment remains an angiographic exercise.

PATHOLOGICAL EFFECTS OF LEFT VENTRICULAR ISCHAEMIA AND INFARCTION

One of the most important factors to be aware of when studying patients with coronary artery disease is the poor discriminatory capacity of ultrasound. One patient may have severe triple vessel disease and yet have normal echocardiographic findings and ventricular function whilst another patient may have single vessel disease and an aneurysm. A third patient may have diffuse small vessel disease and present with a dilated cardiomyopathy. The lesson is that the absence of any echocardiographic abnormality does not indicate the absence of coronary artery disease.

Occlusion of the proximal left anterior descending (LAD) artery has been shown by some to produce marked septal dyskinesia or akinesia with septal excursion of less than 3 mm. In distal LAD occlusion, the septal excursion is more than 3 mm.[1]

When considering myocardial wall movement, certain terms are used and need comment. Hypokinesia refers to a segment of myocardium that moves in a normal direction but with reduced amplitude. Akinesia implies no movement or contraction at all. Dyskinesia occurs when a segment of myocardium responds and moves abnormally during contraction or relaxation. Aneurysm formation implies an area of infarcted myocardium bulging out from the cavity of the ventricle, often associated with outward wall movement during systole (i.e. 'paradoxical') and inward wall movement during diastole. Hyperkinesia is increased but normal movement of a ventricular wall, usually occurs in response to an akinetic segment on the opposite wall. A number of authors have looked at the development of a scoring points system for regional wall contraction patterns.[2-6] The requisites are for multiple views with good cross-sectional studies, factors not always easy to obtain in patients with ischaemic heart disease who are frequently overweight and have accompanying lung disease.

Whatever method is chosen, wall motion analysis should be performed by dividing the myocardium into segments and working out a wall motion index from the figures obtained using the four chamber apical view, the parasternal long axis view and three short axis views at the levels of the mitral valve leaflets, the papillary muscles and the apex. Right ventricular movement can also be assessed using these planes of reference. Analyses can either be performed by visual assessment alone or more accurately by digitisation techniques. The use of such methods makes it possible to follow up segmental wall abnormalities and relate changes to both the clinical aspect and the recovery or otherwise of the myocardium. Abnormal areas of contraction or relaxation may be due to ischaemia or infarction and it may not be possible to differentiate these in the early stages of the disease.

The practical clinical usefulness of extensive documentation of wall motion index scores is considered debatable by some but when combined with Doppler studies it does give an accurate global representation of movement that is most beneficial in individual patient studies. It has already been pointed out in Chapter 5 on ventricular function that abnormalities occur in the isovolumic contraction and relaxation phases of the cardiac cycle, as shown by M-mode echocardiography and synchronous apex-cardiography (Fig. 1).[7] The timing of changes in different parts of the ventricle may be asynchronous, with portions of the myocardium developing tension early and moving inwards with corresponding outward wall movement elsewhere during the period of isovolumic contraction (Fig. 2).[8] Digitised left ventricular dimension loops can be used to show dyskinetic myocardial segments in some patients with ischaemic heart disease and normal left ventricular angiograms. Patients with ischaemic heart disease may also have a marked delay in mitral valve opening and poor early diastolic filling indicating increased ventricular stiffness (Figs 3 and 4). Exercise recovery times in patients with coronary artery disease show that despite depression of resting left ventricular performance, functional recovery of the left ventricle is normal.[9] A further study[10] suggests that in patients with coronary artery disease, non-invasive diastolic pressure scales of both ventricles can be constructed from data obtained from

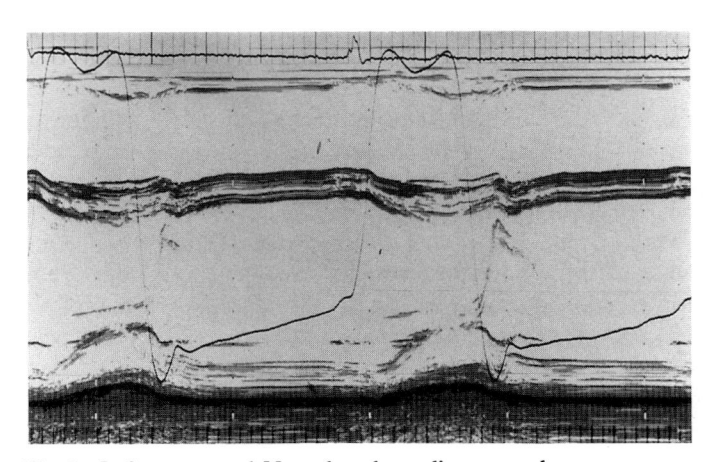

Fig. 1 Left parasternal M-mode echocardiogram and apexcardiogram of a patient with triple vessel disease but with normal echocardiographic parameters.

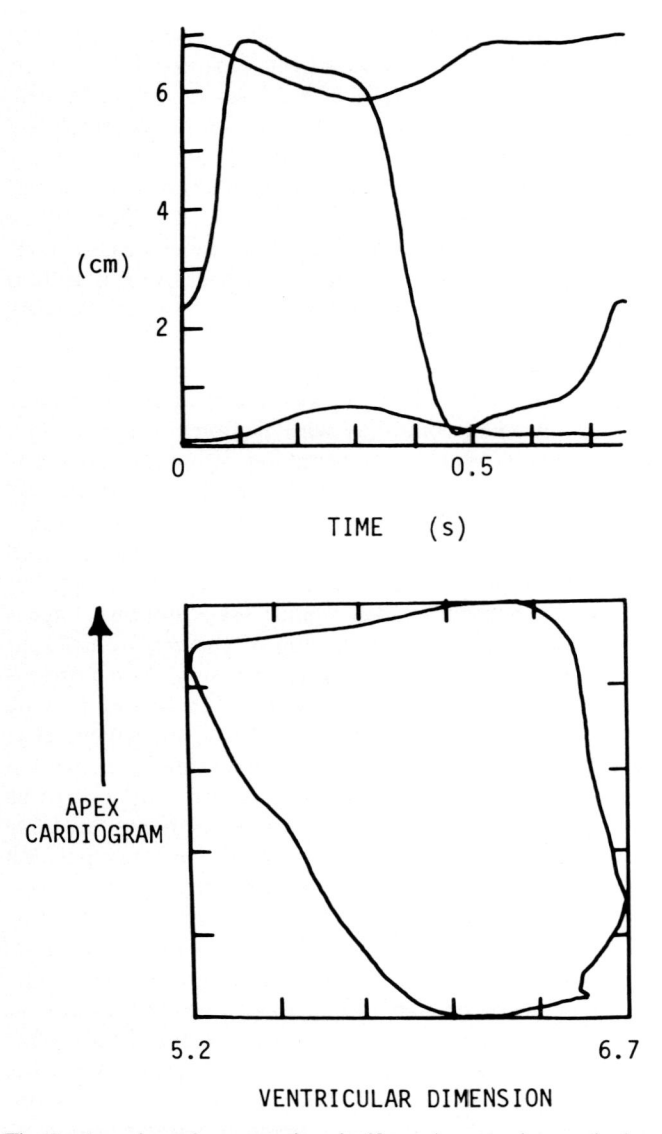

Fig. 2 Apex loop demonstrating significant increase in ventricular dimension (i.e. shape change) during isovolumic relaxation, in a patient with ischaemic heart disease and no evidence of mitral regurgitation.

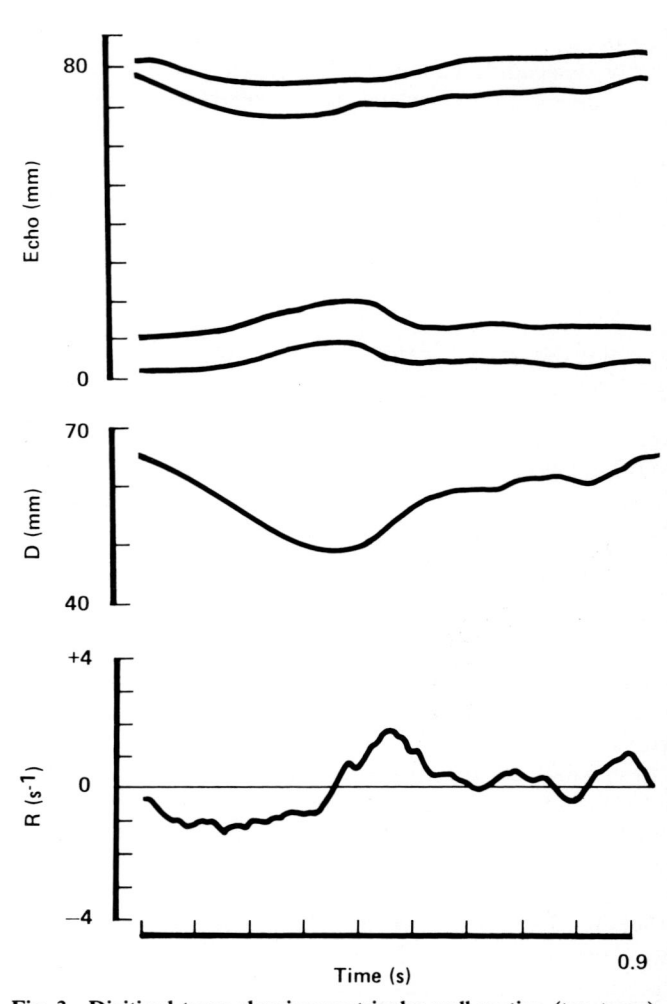

Fig. 3 Digitised trace showing ventricular wall motion (top trace), ventricular dimension (middle trace) and circumferential fibre shortening (bottom trace). The latter is reduced and there is poor and prolonged ventricular filling in a patient with extensive left ventricular ischaemia.

apexcardiograms, echocardiograms and cardiac catheterisation. This may well be of value when assessing causes and treatment of left heart failure with associated pulmonary venous hypertension.

It is of value to be able to detect necrotic from ischaemic areas of infarction, not only for selection of treatment but for predicting changes in ventricular function with time.[11] Necrotic zones of myocardial tissue have a wall thickness of 7 mm or less during the acute phase of the infarction with no improvement of movement with time. Those areas over 8 mm revealed improved wall movement even if they were akinetic originally and were thought to be ischaemic rather than necrotic in nature. There is also a relationship between the degree of ischaemic damage during infarction and the presence or absence of chest pain.[12] Patients with symptomatic attacks have greater wall motion abnormalities and larger functional impairment.

Doppler indices of left ventricular function in patients with ischaemic heart disease have been studied.[13,14] The additional information gained gives more insight into the function of the ventricles in patients with ischaemic heart disease, particularly relating to cardiac output and also the possibility of assessing left ventricular end diastolic pressure. Ascending aortic blood flow velocity has been used as an effective indicator of ventricular performance[15,16] in patients with myocardial ischaemia. In the absence of changes in blood pressure and heart rate, peak and mean velocities fall with coronary artery occlusion as shown

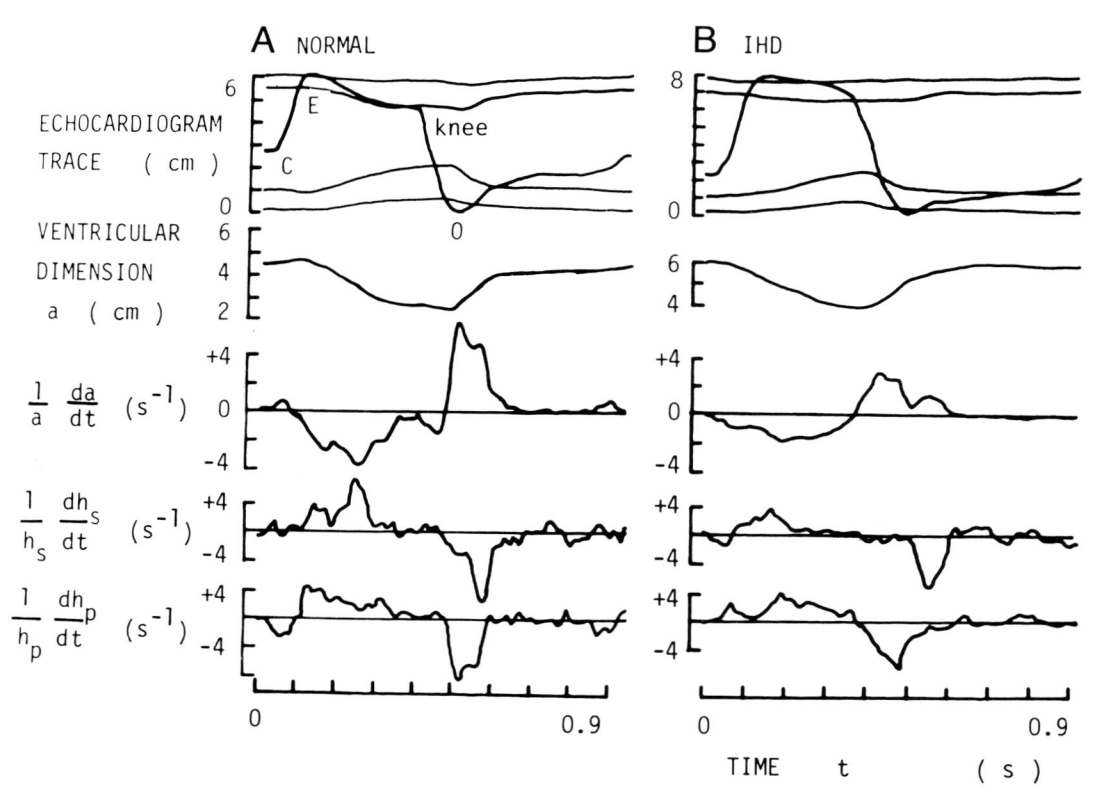

Fig. 4 Comparison of (A): normal and (B): abnormal (ischaemic heart disease) ventricles.

$\frac{1}{a}\frac{da}{dt}$ (s^{-1}) is the peak normalised rate of change of dimension.

$\frac{1}{h_s}\frac{dh_s}{dt}$ (s^{-1}) is the peak normalised rate of change of septal wall thickness.

$\frac{1}{h_p}\frac{dh_p}{dt}$ (s^{-1}) is the peak normalised rate of change of posterior wall thickness. The abnormalities of systolic and diastolic function are shown in the subject with ischaemic heart disease.

experimentally.[17] However, in patients with coronary occlusion, changes in blood pressure and heart rate do occur and much greater myocardial damage may be necessary before similar falls in aortic blood velocity indices are detected.

TISSUE CHARACTERISATION

The ability to detect abnormalities of the myocardium based on alteration of its acoustic properties has up to now been relatively poor. Constant movement makes it difficult to interrogate a section of myocardium over a reasonable time span. It is also difficult to set standards when there is so much variability of heart size, shape and depth (from the transducer). Several papers based on visual assessment ('eye-balling')[18] or quantitative texture analysis[19,20] have recently appeared and these suggest that some differentiation between infarcted and non-infarcted myocardium can be made. It is also possible to distinguish amyloid infiltration from normal heart. Milunski[20] goes further to suggest that ultrasonic tissue characterisation may show beneficial effects of coronary artery reperfusion even if wall motion remains abnormal. The need for ultrasound tissue characterisation may become diminished if magnetic resonance imaging becomes more widely available and sequences are developed which will analyse myocardial elements. Until such time, the ultrasonic characteristics of the normal and abnormal myocardium will continue to be studied and will play an important role in the understanding of ventricular function and pathology.

CONTRAST ECHOCARDIOGRAPHY

Prior to the advent of contrast echocardiography virtually all the indications for performing cardiac ultrasound in patients with coronary artery disease were to look for complications of myocardial infarction. Contrast echocardiography is not a new technique,[21] but its use has long been confined to the demonstration of shunts and flow abnormalities by outlining cardiac chambers. Recently however, myocardial perfusion scanning using sonicated material containing microbubbles has increasingly become used to detect perfusion abnormalities that may not be visible on coronary angiography.[22] It has been shown in dogs that there exists the ability to demonstrate variations in flow patterns throughout the myocardium in systole and diastole.[23] Coronary blood flow appears to be subendocardial in diastole and subepicardial in systole. The technique can be carried out only at cardiac catheterisation, with directional injection of sonicated fluid into the coronary arteries.[24] Videodensitometric analyses of regions of myocardium are performed to assess contrast enhancement, contrast defects and wash out time. The ability to be able to document coronary flow fully and relatively non-invasively by echocardiography is an important step in assessing functional myocardial perfusion and its relation to ischaemia and infarcted areas. There are no reported major side effects of this technique.

COMPLICATIONS OF ISCHAEMIC HEART DISEASE

Dysrhythmias and arrhythmias

A variety of rhythm disturbances occur in patients with myocardial ischaemia and infarction, some of which have a profound effect on echocardiographic parameters. Severe tachycardia may cause ventricular dilatation with reduction in the early rapid diastolic filling phase and lowered ejection fraction. Left bundle branch block shows characteristic appearances on an M-mode echocardiogram with an abnormal late anterior systolic movement of the interventricular septum.[25,26] Ectopic beats, pacemaker induced beats and septal ischaemia or infarction all produce abnormal septal movements.[26]

Aneurysm

An aneurysm of the left ventricle may occur at any site, most commonly at the apex (Fig. 5). Inferior aneurysm may involve the mitral apparatus and cause mitral regurgitation (Fig. 6). It is important to estimate size of the aneurysm and to determine the amount of viable myocardium, particularly if aneurysmectomy is to be contemplated. Cross-sectional imaging from the long axis parasternal position together with an apical four chamber view are essential if aneurysms are not to be missed. Septal and lateral wall aneurysms are better seen on echocardiography than on single plane angiography and cross-sectional echocardiography has a high sensitivity and specificity in the detection of all aneurysms.[27] Thrombus formation is frequently seen within the aneurysmal cavity.

Rupture of the myocardium

False or 'pseudo-aneurysm'

A false aneurysm results from a localised rupture of the left ventricular wall with containment by adherent pericardium. They have a high probability of rupture and like

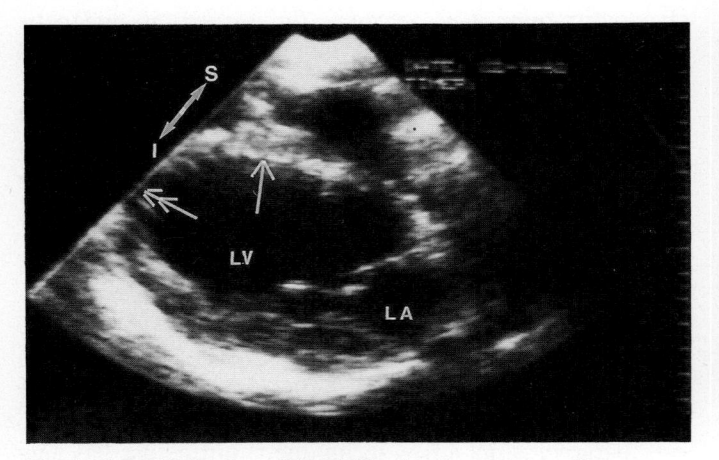

Fig. 5 **Septal infarction with calcification** (arrows) extending to involve the apex with a localised aneurysm (double arrows). Long axis parasternal view.

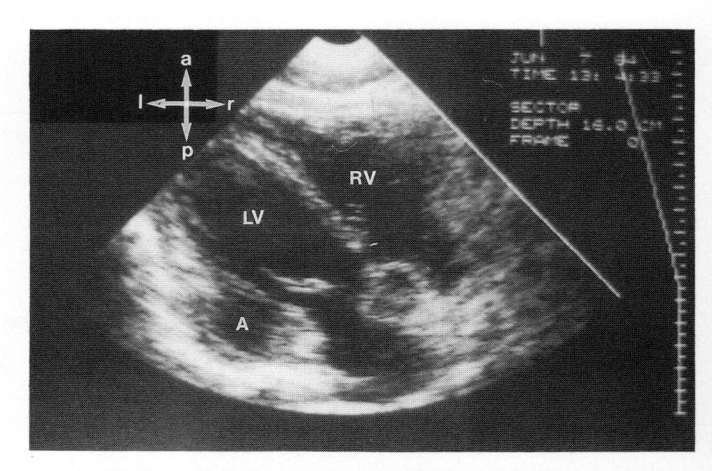

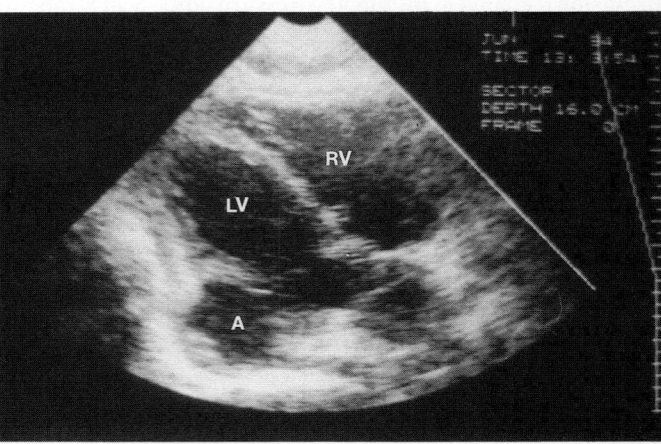

Fig. 6 **Inferior wall aneurysm.** (Subcostal view.) **A**: Diastole. Aneurysm (A) situated between the papillary muscles and the atrio-ventricular valve ring. **B**: Systole. The left ventricular cavity contracts but the aneurysm (A) increases in size.

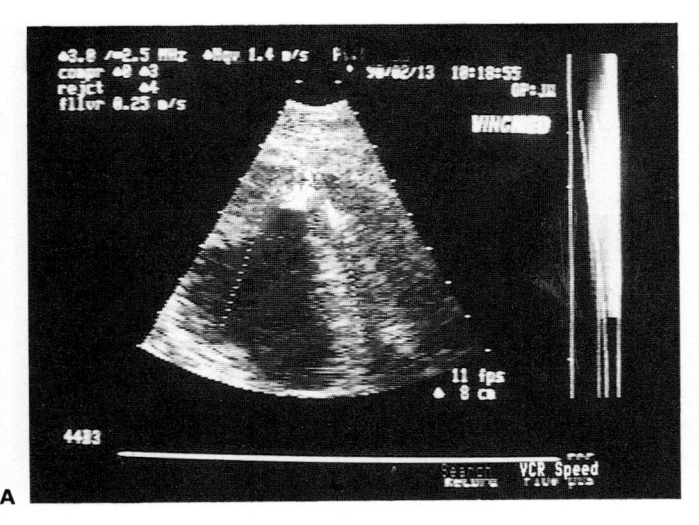

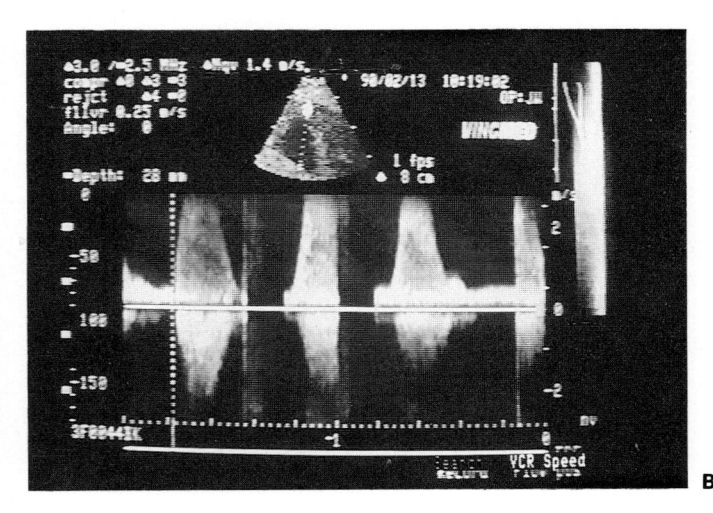

Plate 1 **A: VSD colour Doppler signal from apex of right ventricle** through the distal inter-ventricular septum. **B:** Pulsed Doppler signal from apex of right ventricle in the same patient. This figure is reproduced in colour in the colour plate section at the front of this volume.

true aneurysms they often contain thrombus. They are differentiated from a true aneurysm by their narrow neck, their overall contour and displacement mass effects.[28]

Direct rupture into the pericardium

This fatal outcome of a myocardial infarction is seldom a problem for echocardiographers. The patient rapidly succumbs to cardiac tamponade. It is only when loculation and containment of the rupture occurs producing a pseudo-aneurysm that echocardiography has anything to offer.

Ventricular septal defect

The finding of a harsh systolic murmur soon after a myocardial infarction suggests either a traumatic ventricular septal defect (VSD) or mitral regurgitation. Doppler echocardiography has made the differentiation easier and quicker than other procedures, which are often more invasive.[29] Acute septal rupture has a mortality rate greater than 50% in the early stages. The infarction may be anterior or postero-inferior with the ventricular septal defect commonly being found at the apex of the septum. Reliance on the ability to detect a traumatic VSD on cross-sectional imaging alone is unsatisfactory. Colour Doppler examination (Plate 1) has produced great benefits for the determination of septal defects and can be performed rapidly at the bedside. It is frequently the only investigation necessary prior to surgical repair. Occasionally small defects may be hard to detect and careful searching of all parts of the septum from multiple views is necessary in order not to miss a small jet. There may be associated mitral regurgitation if the infarct also involves the papillary muscles. Ventricular septal defect is a complicating factor in 1% to 2% of acute myocardial infarctions, with cardiogenic shock occurring in half of these cases. If the right ventricle is also affected by the infarct, the cardiac output may be severely impaired.

Mitral regurgitation

Three main causes of mitral regurgitation exist due to complications of myocardial infarction; a flail mitral valve leaflet, a papillary muscle infarct and dilatation of the mitral valve ring.

Complete rupture of a papillary muscle is fortunately a rare event and results in torrential mitral regurgitation and death. The postero-medial papillary muscle is the most commonly affected. Normally only part of a cusp is flail with prolapse of the affected part into the left atrium and failure of synaptic closure during systole (Fig. 7). Mitral regurgitation on Doppler examination often remains substantial in these circumstances. Early surgical intervention may improve prognosis.[30] An infarct that involves the papillary muscle will cause contraction abnormalities resulting in failure of normal mitral cusp movements.[31] The degree of mitral regurgitation is variable but is usually only mild to moderate and not as severe as that seen in papillary muscle rupture (Fig. 8).

In the healing phase of myocardial infarction, the fibrosis that may result can cause increase in valvular dysfunction. Depending on the leaflets involved, the mitral regurgitant jet will be seen to arise from the area concerned, usually at the edge of the valve ring. This contrasts to the central jet seen in the non-specific dilatation of the mitral annulus which is the third and last cause of mitral regurgitation.

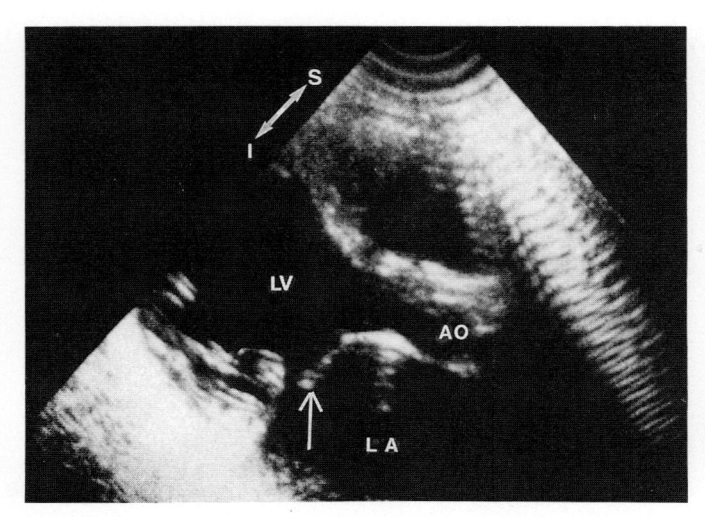

Fig. 7 Partial rupture of the anterior papillary muscle resulting in the anterior leaflet (arrow) prolapsing into the left atrium with failure of closure and torrential mitral regurgitation. Long axis parasternal view.

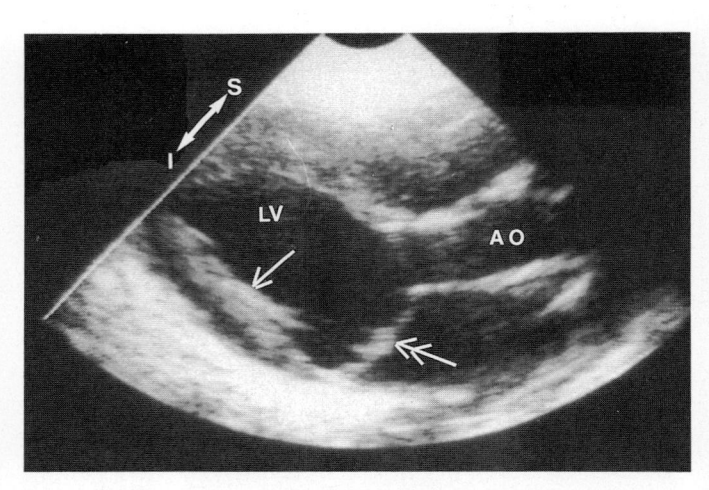

Fig. 8 Long axis parasternal view demonstrating an inferior infarction with papillary muscle involvement (arrow). Slight mitral prolapse has occurred as a result (double arrow).

Any condition that causes dilatation of the left ventricular cavity results in widening of the mitral annulus. The degree of regurgitation is usually small but may be clinically significant if there is a markedly dilated left ventricle with reduced ejection fraction and low cardiac output. It may be difficult to distinguish annulus dilatation from minor degrees of papillary muscle dysfunction and the two often coexist.

Thrombus formation

Left ventricular thrombus is a common finding in over 50% of patients with a trans-mural myocardial infarction. The percentage rises further if an aneurysm is present. Cross-sectional echocardiography has been shown to be a reliable method in the detection of thrombi[32,33] and is superior to angiography and radionuclide studies. Angiography is potentially hazardous in this situation.

There is a wide variation in the echogenicity of thrombi which depends partly on their longevity and partly on their composition.[34] Early thrombus may be relatively echolucent with only small scattered echoes present within the mass. As the thrombus consolidates, echogenicity increases.

Occasionally, the centre of a thrombus may become completely echolucent indicating liquefaction or, very rarely, infective abscess formation. A thrombus may have an extensive base and plaque-like configuration or it may project into the left ventricular cavity with a narrow base (Figs 9 to 11). It may be mobile (Fig. 12) or static (Fig. 13). Frond-like platelet thrombi with marked intracavity movement are at greater risk of embolisation

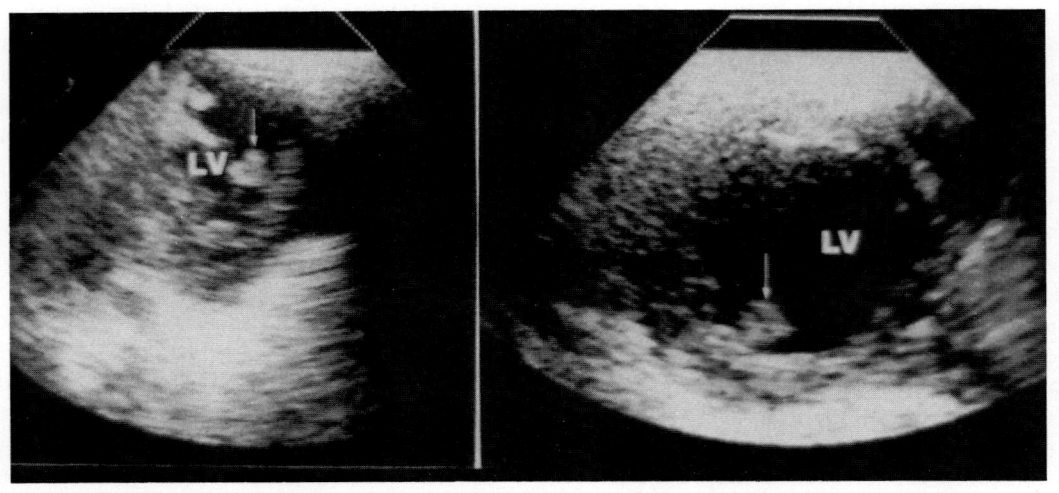

Fig. 9 Two cases (short axis views) demonstrating small friable narrow based thrombi (arrows) near the papillary muscles.

ISCHAEMIC HEART DISEASE 187

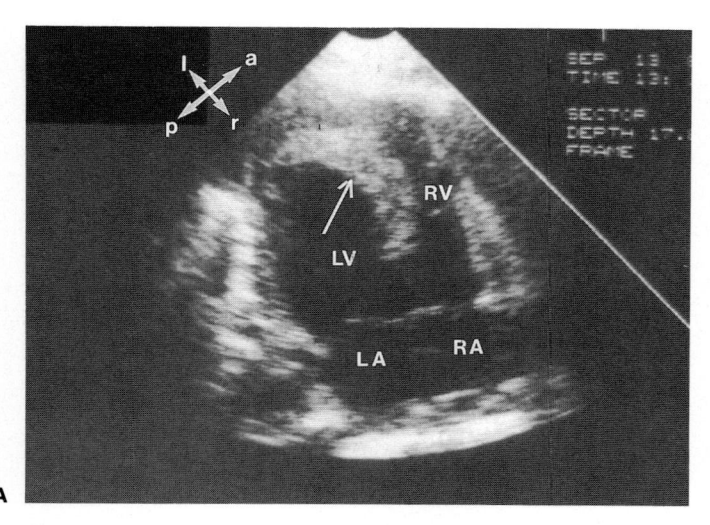

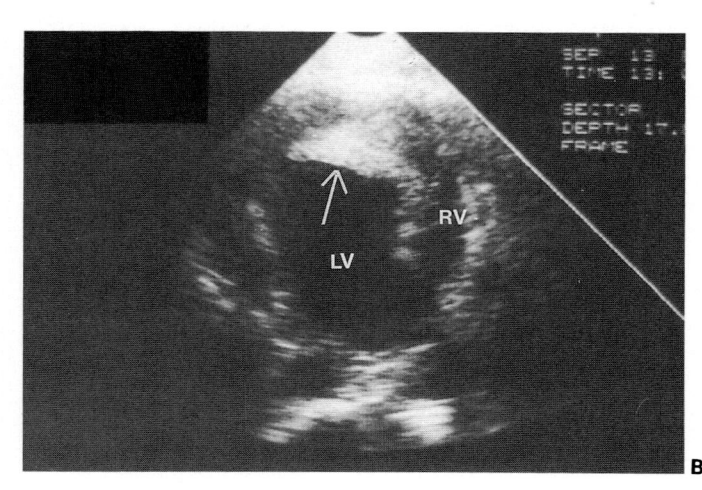

Fig. 10 **A: Apical four chamber view demonstrating a large curved echogenic thrombus** (arrow) attached to the inter-ventricular septum with extension into the apex. The internal echo pattern suggests organisation of the thrombus. **B:** Same patient, modified apical four chamber view, showing the densely echogenic apical extension of the thrombus (arrow).

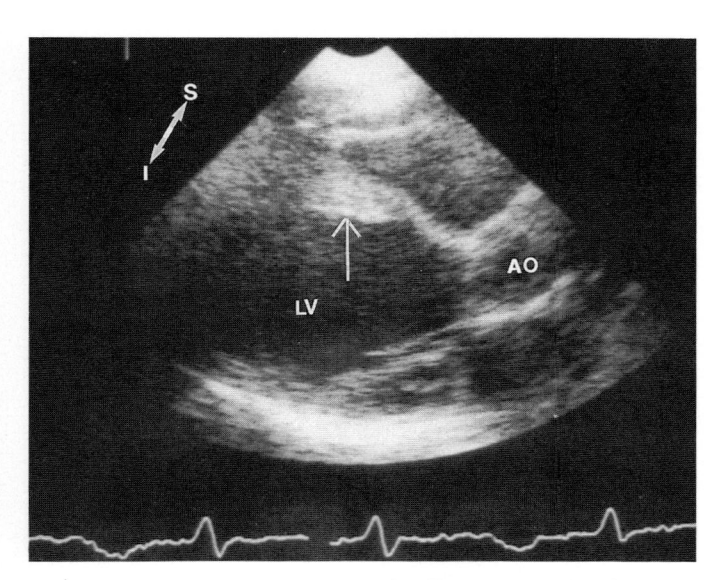

Fig. 11 **Parasternal long axis view of a dilated ischaemic left ventricle** with an adherent thrombus against the inter-ventricular septum (arrow). The thrombus has become covered with endothelium showing increased echogenicity (arrow).

than fixed echogenic lesions. The likelihood of emboli from thrombi have been studied by Lloret et al[35] who suggest that high-risk thrombi can be detected by cross-sectional echocardiography texture analysis and certain clinical features.

The surface of a thrombus also varies with time. Initially, the surface echogenicity is low, either similar to the internal echo structure, or slightly increased if the thrombus is echolucent. As the surface becomes covered with endothelium the echogenicity increases and it may be difficult to distinguish old thrombus from myocardium. There is, however, nearly always associated abnormal wall contraction and asynergy when a thrombus is present. Thrombi may occur anywhere in both the right and left ventricular cavities including attachments to the papillary muscles and chordae tendinae. They vary considerably in size, shape and texture and may cause both silent and clinically apparent emboli, depending on the tissue end point.

Right ventricular infarction

Approximately 40% of patients with an acute inferior myocardial infarction develop a right ventricular infarction as shown on cross-sectional echocardiography or radionuclide scanning,[36] although right ventricular failure occurs in only a small number of cases. Wall motion analysis using multiple views in a similar fashion to left ventricular studies can be applied to the right ventricle with equal results. As tricuspid regurgitation is present in many normal hearts, Doppler evaluation of the right ventricle and right atrium can be studied and indices of function compiled. The high mortality figures in patients with obvious clinical evidence of right ventricular infarction are probably due to the severity of the accompanying left heart disease.[37] If right ventricular infarction is only found on echocardiography with no clinical right ventricular failure, then mortality figures are low.[38]

Dressler's syndrome

The post-myocardial infarction (Dressler's) syndrome may develop about 2 to 4 weeks after a myocardial infarction and may recur.[39] It is diagnosed on clinical grounds and the presence of a pericardial effusion (Fig. 14). Cardiac

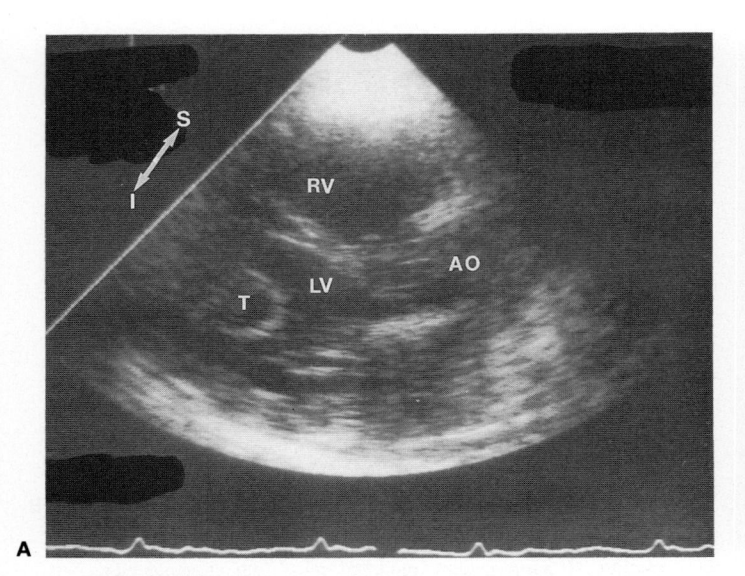

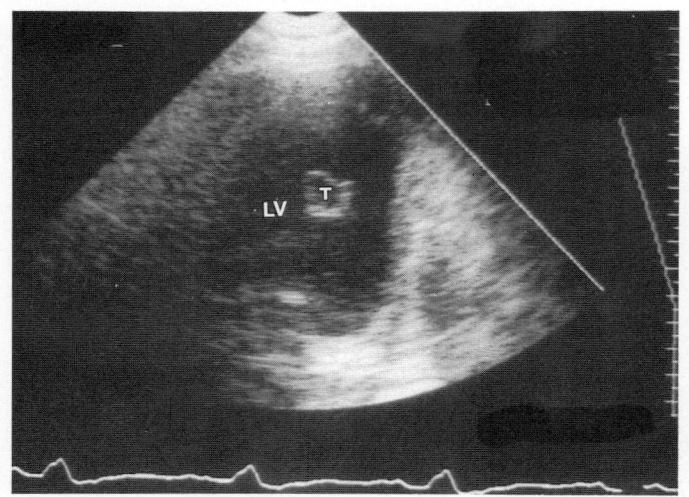

Fig. 12 **A: Long axis parasternal view. B: Apical two chamber view.** Large freely mobile jelly-like thrombus (T) floating in the left ventricular cavity. It embolised within a few hours with fatal results.

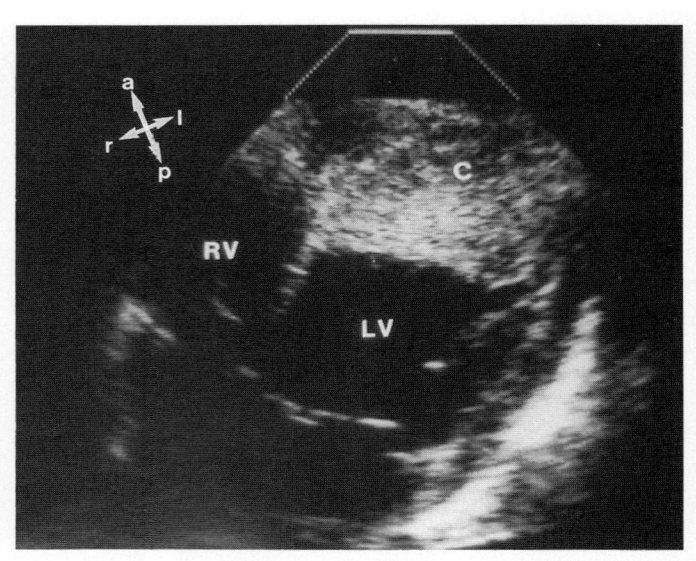

Fig. 13 **Apical four chamber view of a patient with evidence of a large clot (C) in the apex of the left ventricle.** There is evidence of endothelialisation.

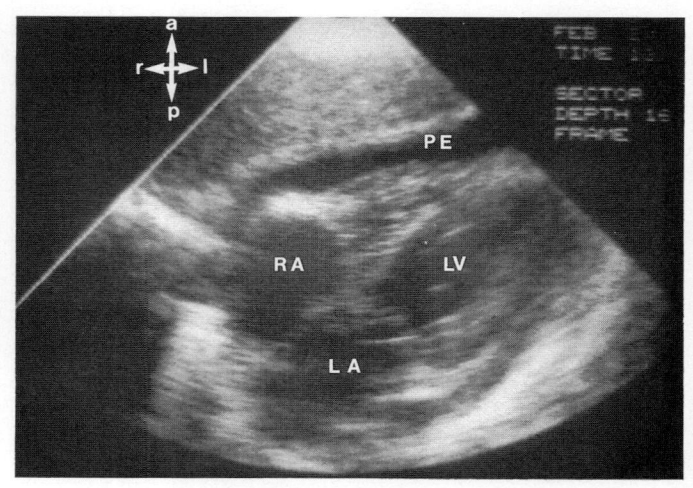

Fig. 14 **Subcostal four chamber view of a patient with Dressler's syndrome.** A small pericardial effusion (PE) is present.

tamponade is rare. It should not be confused with the small pericardial fluid collections that are often apparent immediately after a myocardial infarction. These may be due to haemorrhage or a sympathetic effusion augmenting the trace amount of pericardial fluid normally present. The fluid may be tapped under ultrasound guidance if necessary, particularly if the clinical picture is unclear or alternative causes for pericardial fluid are suspected.

Other complications

Rarely, bacterial infection may occur at the site of an infarct or in and around a mural thrombus. Septic emboli can result.

REFERENCES

1. Kureshi S A, Yonekura Y, Kambara H, et al. Interventricular septal motion in acute myocardial infarction with proximal and distal left anterior descending coronary lesions. Am Heart J 1987; 114: 1329–1333
2. Morganroth J, Chen C C, David D, et al. Exercise cross-sectional echocardiographic diagnosis of coronary artery disease. Am J Cardiol 1981; 47: 20
3. Hecht H S, Taylor R, Wang M, Shah P M. Comparative

evaluation of segmental asynergy in remote myocardial infarction by radionuclide angiography, two-dimensional echocardiography, and contrast ventriculography. Am Heart J 1981; 101: 740
4 Edwards W D, Tajik A J, Seward J B. Standardised nomenclature and anatomic basis for regional tomographic analysis of the heart. Mayo Clin Proc 1981; 56: 479
5 Kan G, Visser C A, Koolen J J, Dunning A J. Short and long term predictive value of admission wall motion score in acute myocardial infarction: a cross sectional echocardiographic study of 345 patients. Br Heart J 1986; 56: 422–428
6 Hagan A D, DeMaria A N. Clinical applications of two dimensional echocardiography and cardiac Doppler. Boston: Little, Brown & Co. 2nd Edition. 1989: pp 180–182
7 Martin C J, Weir J, Gemmell H G. Assessment of left ventricular function by synchronous echocardiography and apex cardiography. Br J Radiol 1982; 55: 342–351
8 Karliner J S, Bouchard R J, Gault J H. Dimensional changes in the human left ventricle prior to aortic valve opening. A cineangiographic study in patients with and without left heart disease. Circulation 1971; 44: 312–322
9 Vanderbossche J L, Taylor J E, Karliner J S. Left ventricular functional recovery from exercise in normals and patients with coronary heart disease. Cardiology 1987; 74: 111–115
10 Kekes E, Nadas I, Dekany M, Banyai F, Berentey E. Non invasive assessment of elevated ventricular diastolic pressures in patients with ischaemic heart disease. Cor Vasa 1987; 29: 20–28
11 Kashiro S, Simizu M, Hirata S, Ishikawa K. Two dimensional echocardiography in acute myocardial infarction — relationship between left ventricular wall thickness and wall motion abnormalities. Jpn Circ J 1988; 52: 1257–1267
12 Agati L, Penco M, Sciomer S, Fedele F, Neja C P, Dagianti A. Painless versus painful myocardial ischaemia: different left ventricular dysfunction detected by echocardiography. Int J Cardiol 1989; 22: 321–327
13 Mehta N, Bennett D, Mannering D, Dawkins K, Ward D E. Usefulness of non invasive Doppler measurement of ascending aortic blood velocity and acceleration in detecting impairment of the left ventricular functional response to exercise three weeks after acute myocardial infarction. Am J Cardiol 1986; 58: 879
14 Harrison M R, Smith M D, Friedman B J, DeMaria A N. Uses and limitations of exercise Doppler echocardiography in the diagnosis of ischaemic heart disease. J Am Coll Cardiol 1987; 10: 809
15 McLennan F M, Haites N E, Mackenzie J D, Daniel M K, Rawles J M. Reproducibility of linear cardiac output measurement by Doppler ultrasound alone. Br Heart J 1986; 55: 25–31
16 Haites N E, McLennan F M, Mowat D H R, Rawles J M. Assessment of cardiac output by the Doppler ultrasound technique alone. Br Heart J 1985; 53: 123–129
17 Mathias D W, Wann L S, Sagar K D, Klopfenstein H S. The effect of regional myocardial ischaemia on Doppler echocardiographic indexes of left ventricular performance: influence of heart rate, aortic blood pressure, and the size of the ischaemic zone. Am Heart J 1988; 116: 953–960
18 Kawamura K, Hishida H, Sakabe Y, et al. Analysis of myocardial texture in two-dimensional echocardiographic images. J Cardiol 1988; 18: 619–628
19 Chandrasekaran K, Aylward P E, Fleagle S R, et al. Feasibility of identifying amyloid and hypertrophic cardiomyopathy with the use of computerised quantitative texture analysis of clinical echo-cardiographic data. J Am Coll Cardiol 1939; 13: 832–840
20 Milunski M R, Mohr G A, Perez J E, et al. Ultrasonic tissue characterisation with integrated backscatter. Acute myocardial ischaemia, reperfusion, and stunned myocardium in patients. Circulation 1989; 80: 491–503

21 Gramiak R, Shah P M, Kramer D H. Ultrasound cardiography: contrast studies in anatomy and function. Radiology 1969; 92: 939
22 Lim Y J, Nanto S, Ikeda T, et al. Regional myocardial perfusion in ischaemic heart disease assessed by myocardial contrast echocardiography. J Cardiol 1988; 19: 21–30
23 Rovai D, L'Abbate A, Lombardi M, et al. Non uniformity of the transmural distribution of coronary blood flow during the cardiac cycle. In vivo documentation by contrast echocardiography. Circulation 1989; 79: 179–187
24 Reisner S A, Ong L S, Lichtenberg G S, et al. Myocardial perfusion imaging by contrast echocardiography with use of intracoronary sonicated albumin in humans. J Am Coll Cardiol 1989; 14: 660–665
25 Fujii J, Watanabe H, Watanabe T, Takahashi N, Ohta A, Kato K. M-mode and cross sectional echocardiographic study of the left ventricular wall motions in complete left bundle branch block. Br Heart J 1977; 93: 160
26 Weir J, Pridie R B. An atlas of clinical echocardiography. Edinburgh: Churchill Livingstone. 1984: p 149
27 Visser C A, Kan G, David G K, Lie K I, Durrer D. Echocardiographic cineangiographic correlation in detecting left ventricular aneurysm: a prospective study of 422 patients. Am J Cardiol 1982; 50: 337
28 Gatewood R P, Nanda N C. Differentiation of left ventricular pseudoaneurysm from true aneurysm with two dimensional echocardiography. Am J Cardiol 1980; 46: 869
29 MacLeod D, Fananapazir L, deBono D, Bloomfield P. Ventricular septal defect after myocardial infarction: assessment by cross sectional echocardiography with pulsed waved Doppler scanning. Br Heart J 1987; 58: 214–218
30 Wei J Y, Hutchins G M, Bulkley B H. Papillary muscle rupture in fatal acute myocardial infarction: a potentially treatable form of cardiogenic shock. Ann Intern Med 1979; 90: 149
31 Izumi S, Miyatake K, Beppu S, et al. Mechanism of mitral regurgitation in patients with myocardial infarction: a study using real-time two-dimensional Doppler flow imaging and echocardiography. Circulation 1987; 76: 777–785
32 Asinger R W, Mikell F L, Elsperger J, Hodges M. Incidence of left ventricular thrombosis after acute transmural myocardial infarction. Serial evaluation by two-dimensional echocardiography. N Engl J Med 1981; 305: 297
33 Keating E C, Gross S A, Schlamowitz R A, et al. Mural thrombi in myocardial infarctions. Prospective evaluation by two dimensional echocardiography. Am J Med 1983; 74: 989
34 Mikell F L, Asinger R W, Elsperger K J, Anderson W R, Hodges M. Tissue acoustic properties of fresh left ventricular thrombi and visualisation by two dimensional echocardiography: experimental observations. Am J Cardiol 1982; 49: 1157
35 Lloret R L, Cortada X, Bradford J, Metz M, Kinney E L. Classification of left ventricular thrombi by their history of systemic embolization using pattern recognition of two dimensional echocardiograms. Am Heart J 1985; 110: 761–765
36 Bellamy G R, Rasmussen H H, Nasser F, Wiseman J C, Cooper R A. Value of two dimensional echocardiography, electrocardiography, and clinical signs in detecting right ventricular infarction. Am Heart J 1986; 111: 304–309
37 Jugdutt B I, Sussex B A, Sivaram C A, Rossall R E. Right ventricular infarction: two dimensional echocardiographic evaluation. Am Heart J 1984; 107: 505
38 Cintron G B, Hernandez E, Linares E, Aranda J M. Bedside recognition, incidence and clinical course of right ventricular infarction. Am J Cardiol 1981; 47: 224
39 Dressler W, Leavitt S S. Pericarditis after acute myocardial infarction. JAMA 1960; 173: 129

12

Cardiomyopathy

Introduction
Hypertrophic cardiomyopathy
M-mode and two-dimensional imaging
  Myocardial features
  The mitral apparatus
Differential diagnosis of hypertrophic cardiomyopathy
Doppler findings in hypertrophic cardiomyopathy
  Diastolic events
  Systolic events

Dilated cardiomyopathy
Echocardiographic findings
Differential diagnosis of dilated cardiomyopathy
Intracardiac flow and embolisation
Indicators of prognosis
Restrictive cardiomyopathy
Amyloid heart disease
Endomyocardial fibrosis
Doppler echocardiography in restrictive cardiomyopathies

Petros Nihoyannopoulos

INTRODUCTION

Primary heart muscle disease results in a wide variety of derangements in cardiac structure and function. A major problem in the diagnosis of cardiomyopathies is the definition of the disorder causing the heart muscle disease, this often being of unknown aetiology.[1,2] Heart muscle disorders that are part of a general system disease must be considered.

The classification of cardiomyopathies based upon structural and functional disorders is currently grouped into three major categories; hypertrophic, dilated and restrictive cardiomyopathy.[1,2] While the boundaries between these categories are not completely distinct and may not always be respected by any given pathological process, they do provide a useful framework for describing the interrelationships between morphology and pathophysiology.

Dilated (congestive) cardiomyopathy consists of a marked destruction of ventricular myocardium that results in a severely dilated left ventricle with normal or thinned wall. Dilated cardiomyopathy is characterised by severe impairment of ventricular contractility which gives rise to marked generalised ventricular hypokinesis. Conversely, hypertrophic cardiomyopathy presents with a thick walled left ventricle often involving the ventricular septum alone, with a small cavity size and a supernormal contractile performance. Whereas the primary haemodynamic abnormality in hypertrophic cardiomyopathy often includes impaired left ventricular filling, the primary abnormality in dilated cardiomyopathy involves diminished left ventricular emptying.

Restrictive cardiomyopathy represents a hybrid of the previous two pathophysiological entities. Thus, the morphological picture of a restrictive process consists of a small left ventricular cavity and normal or near-normal myocardial thickness which contrasts with an enlarged left atrium. The impairment of left ventricular filling may be combined with a reduction in left ventricular emptying due to decreased contractility. There are several infiltrative disorders such as cardiac amyloidosis and endomyocardial fibrosis that produce a restrictive haemodynamic pattern and these are often described as restrictive cardiomyopathies.

Echocardiographically, the three main categories of cardiomyopathy may readily be distinguished by three simple measurements. The left ventricular internal dimensions, the left ventricular wall thickness and the left ventricular contractility (shortening fraction). Two-dimensional echocardiography has the capacity to image large sections of the heart, allowing recognition and differentiation of the regional myocardial thickness and segmental asynergy observed in patients with previous myocardial infarction. Two-dimensional echocardiography has also proven of great value in the recognition of left ventricular mural thrombi that may complicate dilated cardiomyopathy.

Two-dimensional and Doppler echocardiography are powerful non-invasive tools that permit comprehensive assessment of patients with cardiomyopathy. These techniques have a crucial place in the diagnosis, defining the morphological spectrum and pathophysiology and assessing the haemodynamic severity of the systolic or diastolic dysfunction. It is also just as important for detecting complications or improvement as the natural course of the disease is treated.

HYPERTROPHIC CARDIOMYOPATHY

Hypertrophic cardiomyopathy is an inherited disorder characterised by ventricular hypertrophy, impaired diastolic function and increased ventricular contraction. The first characterisation of hypertrophic cardiomyopathy was by the pathologist Donald Tear in 1958, from the autopsy examination of the hearts of nine adolescents and young adults who had died suddenly.[3] The gross pathology of hypertrophic cardiomyopathy is typically characterised by ventricular hypertrophy involving predominantly the left ventricle, but also the right ventricle in a significant number of patients. This hypertrophy can be asymmetrical, involving part of the ventricular septum, concentric involving the entire left ventricle or distal, affecting predominantly the cardiac apex. The functional abnormalities are now well-documented with forceful, over-active ventricular contraction often giving rise to complete emptying and achieving an ejection fraction of 80 to 100%. This powerful contraction and complete emptying of the ventricle often occurs in association with intraventricular pressure gradients. When the gradient is subaortic it occurs in association with abnormal systolic anterior movement of the mitral valve. These gradients are labile, variable and often absent and do not correlate well with prognosis.

M-mode and two-dimensional imaging

Myocardial features

The original M-mode recording techniques have been invaluable in developing echocardiographic diagnostic criteria for patients with hypertrophic cardiomyopathy.[4] These are: (a) the presence of asymmetrical hypertrophy of the ventricular septum (ASH), defined as the ratio of septal to posterior left ventricular wall thickness at end diastole being equal to or greater than 1.3:1,[5] (b) the systolic anterior motion of the mitral valve (SAM)[6] and (c) the premature midsystolic closure of the aortic valve.[7] SAM is seen in M-mode echocardiograms as a multilayered 'rainbow' occupying the ventricular space between the inward movement of the posterior wall and the relatively inert septum (Fig. 1).

The advent of two-dimensional echocardiography allowed anatomical sections of the heart to be obtained for the first time during life and the true size and shape of the valves and cavities could be ascertained. This also

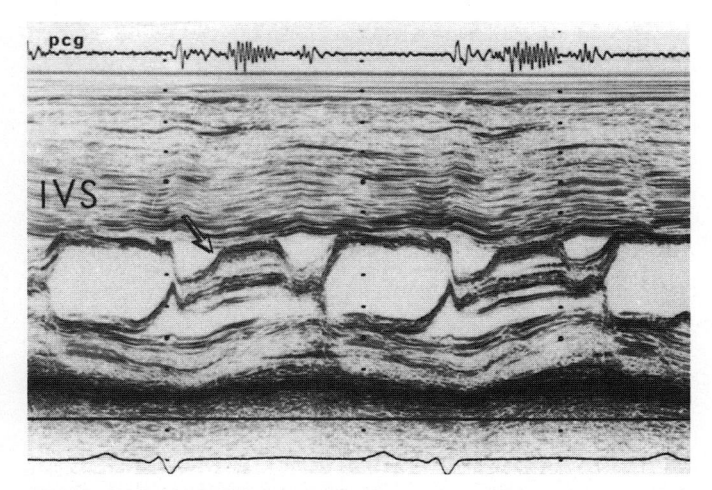

Fig. 1 M-mode left ventricular echocardiogram from a patient with hypertrophic cardiomyopathy showing systolic anterior motion of the mitral valve (arrowed), and asymmetrical septal hypertrophy. (IVS – ventricular septum, pcg – phonocardiogram.)

SAM and midsystolic closure of the aortic valve were pathognomonic of hypertrophic cardiomyopathy, have not been substantiated. Each one has been demonstrated to occur in a variety of other cardiac anomalies with no common pathophysiological mechanism.[8-12]

An inherent disadvantage of M-mode echocardiography is that only a small section of the left ventricle can be examined with the ultrasound beam, thus providing a one-dimensional, 'ice pick' view of the left ventricular anterior septum and posterior wall. Patients with hypertrophic cardiomyopathy may show a wide distribution of hypertrophy including the posterior septum and the lateral wall.[13] Consequently, it has become necessary for multiple two-dimensional echocardiographic sections to be obtained for comprehensive imaging of patients with hypertrophic cardiomyopathy.[14-16] These views include parasternal long and short axis, apical four and two chamber views, and subcostal projections.

The parasternal long axis view is particularly important in the visualisation of the profile of the interventricular septum and left ventricular outflow tract together with the mitral valve and its subvalvular apparatus. It is the view of choice for the detection of systolic anterior motion of the mitral valve and the presence of mid-systolic closure of the aortic valve. It is helpful to obtain simultaneous M-mode recordings of the mitral and aortic valve motion so that high frequency phenomena, such as SAM and midsystolic closure of the aortic valve, can be described more

permitted the realisation that oblique sections across the ventricles occurring with inappropriate transducer positions will tend to overestimate ventricular size and wall thickness. It is therefore not surprising that the detection of ASH, based on M-mode criteria alone, has been the cause of many false positive diagnoses of hypertrophic cardiomyopathy. Furthermore, the initial beliefs that ASH,

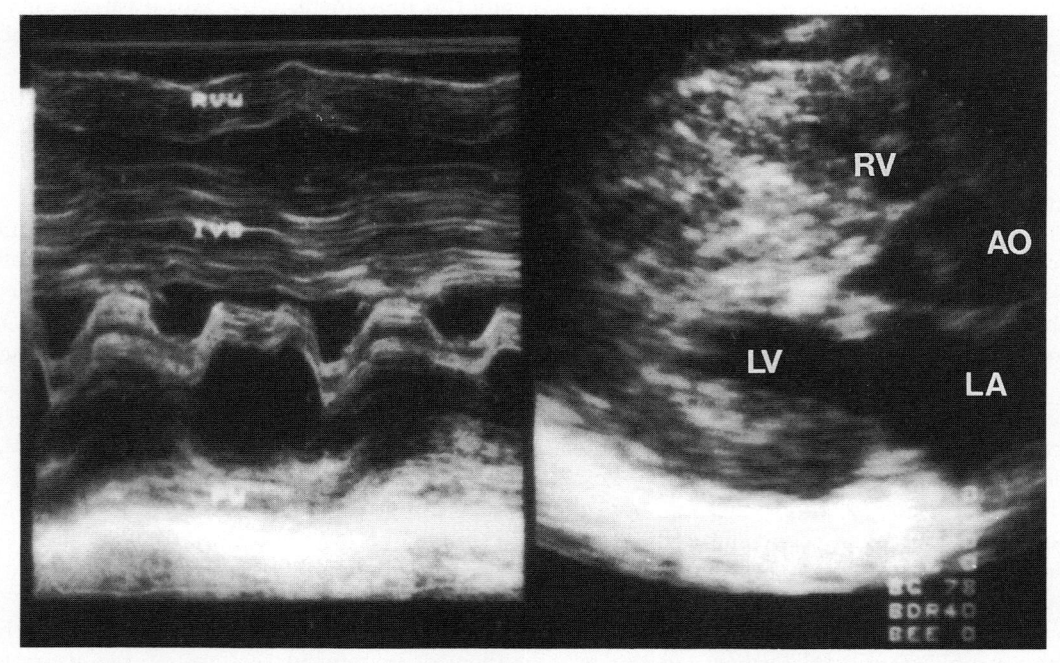

Fig. 2 M-mode echocardiogram (left) from a patient with hypertrophic cardiomyopathy obtained under direct supervision of the parasternal long axis two-dimensional image (right). Note the asymmetric septal hypertrophy and the systolic anterior motion of the mitral valve. Note that this patient also had a hypertrophied right ventricle. (IVS – ventricular septum, RVW – right ventricular free wall.)

accurately (Fig. 2). Left ventricular measurements can also be obtained from the parasternal long axis view. It is important however for those who interpret echocardiograms to be fully aware of the possible false diagnosis of ventricular septal hypertrophy, particularly when acute angulations of the ventricular septum occur (sigmoid septum), or indeed in the presence of right ventricular hypertrophy secondary to pulmonary stenosis or pulmonary hypertension.

The parasternal short axis views are probably the most important views for assessing ventricular hypertrophy as they provide serial tomographic sections of the ventricle, so that the complete distribution of the ventricular hypertrophy can be ascertained. These sections should pass across the mitral valve, papillary muscle level and the cardiac apex. Using this well-standardised approach, Shapiro and McKenna[17] defined three patterns of left ventricular hypertrophy; asymmetrical left ventricular hypertrophy encountered in 55% of their patients, symmetrical in 31% and distal in 14%.

Asymmetrical septal hypertrophy (ASH) is the most frequent form of left ventricular hypertrophy and has been regarded as the hallmark of hypertrophic cardiomyopathy (Fig. 3).[5] Although this hypertrophy usually involves the anterior septum to various extents and severities, it may also involve only the apical, mid or posterior septum and the lateral wall.[16] In approximately 50% of the patients with proximal ASH, the hypertrophy extends into the anterior left ventricular free wall. Frequently, wall thickening is strikingly heterogeneous and contiguous segments of the left ventricle may differ greatly in thickness. Figure 4 is from a patient with hypertrophic cardiomyopathy in whom only the lateral wall is hypertrophied.

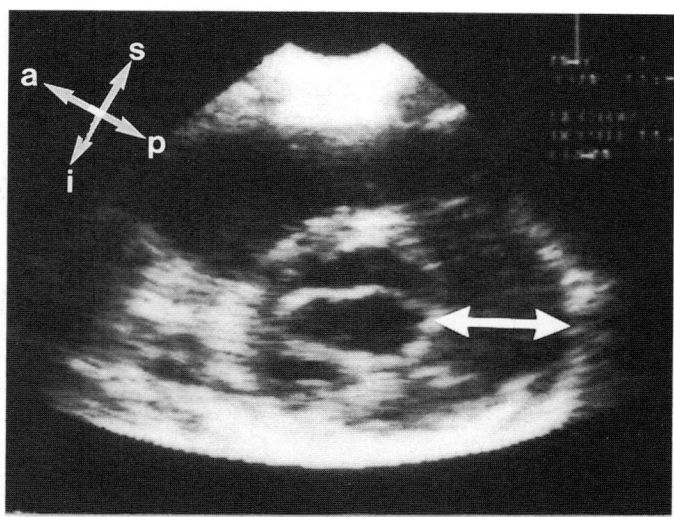

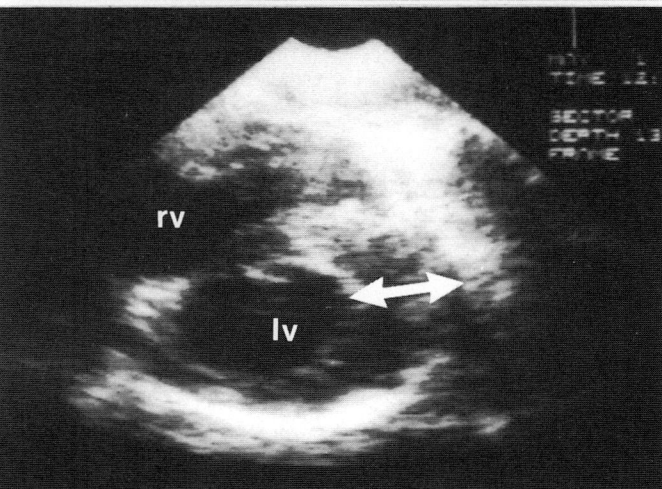

Fig. 4 Parasternal short axis views from a patient with hypertrophic cardiomyopathy. This patient clearly shows marked lateral wall hypertrophy (arrows) beginning proximally, at the mitral valve level (top) and extending all the way down to the apex (bottom). This pattern of hypertrophy could not be visualised from parasternal long axis projections.

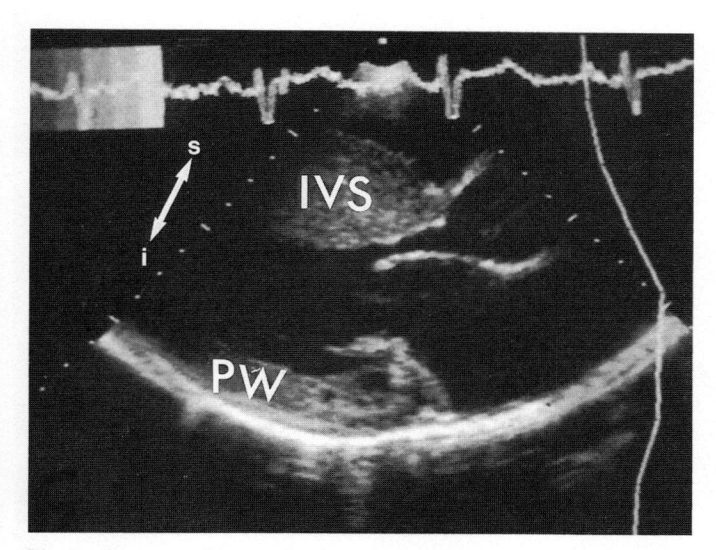

Fig. 3 Parasternal long axis view during diastole showing marked hypertrophy of the ventricular septum contrasted with the only mildly hypertrophied posterior wall. (IVS – interventricular septum, PW – posterior wall.)

Concentric or symmetrical left ventricular hypertrophy is also frequently encountered in patients with hypertrophic cardiomyopathy and when this occurs, the echocardiographic differentiation from secondary causes of left ventricular hypertrophy may be very difficult. Figure 5 is from a patient with hypertrophic cardiomyopathy showing marked concentric left ventricular hypertrophy also involving the right ventricular wall. This patient exhibited decreased overall ventricular contraction and relaxation (Fig. 6) which simulates that seen in cardiac amyloidosis.

Predominantly distal (apical) distribution of left ventricular hypertrophy has also been noted in a substantial number of patients. Japanese authors indicate that patients with giant negative T-waves have hypertrophy confined to

196 CARDIAC ULTRASOUND

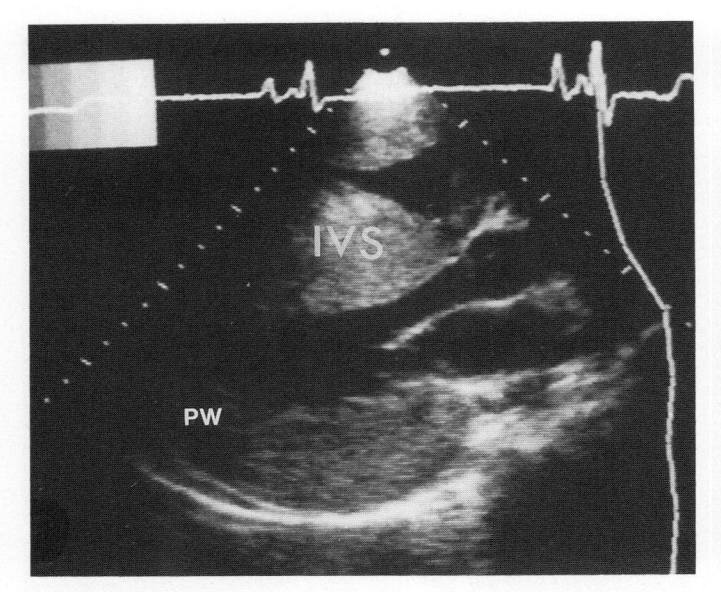

Fig. 5 **Parasternal long axis view from a patient with hypertrophic cardiomyopathy.** Note that this patient shows marked concentric left ventricular hypertrophy with small internal cavity dimensions.

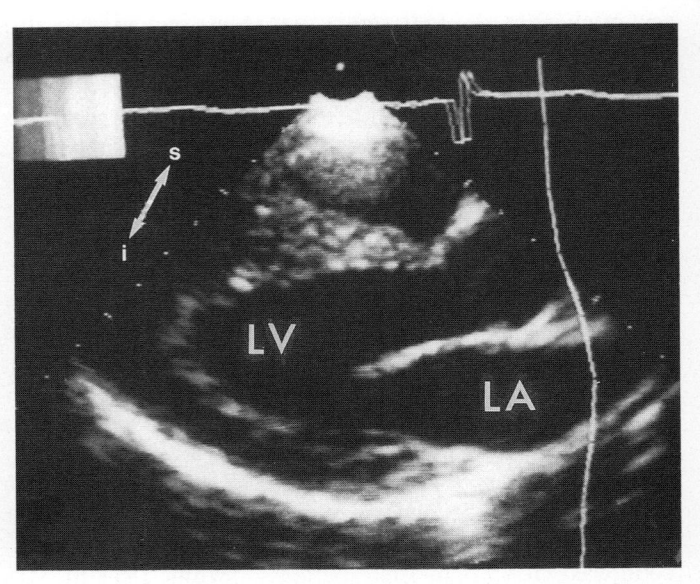

Fig. 7 **Parasternal long axis view from a patient with hypertrophic cardiomyopathy and giant T waves on the electrocardiogram.** Note the 'spade' configuration of the left ventricular cavity.

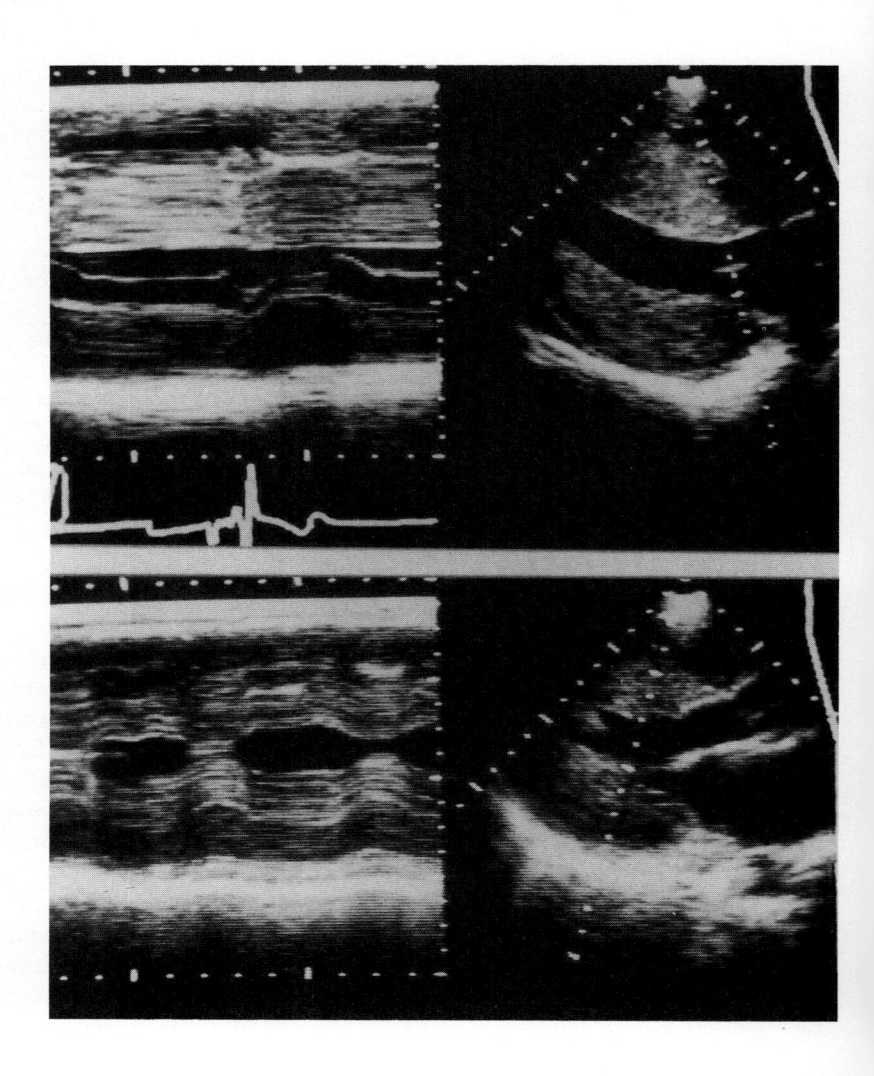

Fig. 6 **Serial M-mode echograms from the same patient as in Fig. 5 demonstrating the global impairment of the ventricular function.** Note again the small left ventricular internal dimensions hardly reaching 4 cm in end diastole. The ventricular septum measured 5 cm in thickness.

the left ventricular apex, mild symptoms and few adverse prognostic features.[18] In a recent study involving Western patients with hypertrophic cardiomyopathy, we have described a wider clinical and echocardiographic spectrum.[19] The overall prevalence of giant T-waves in these series was 15% and was associated with greater left ventricular hypertrophy at mid-ventricular level and beyond. Figure 7 is from a patient with giant negative T-waves associated with left ventricular hypertrophy confined to the true left ventricular apex below the level of the papillary muscles. This distribution of hypertrophy characteristically creates a 'spade' deformity or shortening of the left ventricular cavity, best seen from parasternal long axis projections. Serial short axis projections however are of pivotal importance in order to avoid a false positive diagnosis of apical hypertrophy caused by oblique cuts of the left ventricular cavity that may be obtained in the long axis views (Fig. 8).

The right ventricle can also be involved in hypertrophic cardiomyopathy (Figs 2 and 9). The whole of the right ventricle can be imaged using standardised views across the right ventricular inflow tract, right ventricular outflow tract and apical and subcostal views.[20] In a recent study we have found that 44% of patients with hypertrophic cardiomyopathy also had right ventricular hypertrophy to a variable extent.[21] It is also of interest that the finding of right ventricular hypertrophy was related to clinical and echocardiographic features of severe disease, particularly dyspnoea on exertion, severe left ventricular hypertrophy and supraventricular and ventricular arrhythmias.

Hypertrophic cardiomyopathy has been reported with increasing frequency in the elderly. Only a limited number of patients however have the 'classical' clinical and echocardiographic features with left ventricular outflow tract obstruction. Many cases are discovered incidentally when patients undergo investigations for coronary artery disease or hypertension. An association in elderly patients of hypertrophic cardiomyopathy and mitral annular calcification has also been reported (Fig. 10).[22] These authors found a greater prevalence of mitral annular calcification in patients with hypertrophic cardiomyopathy when compared with age-matched control subjects who did not have hypertrophic cardiomyopathy.

In patients with hypertrophic cardiomyopathy, the thickness of the ventricular septum is not related to the presence of left ventricular outflow tract obstruction or the occurrence of systolic anterior motion of the mitral valve (SAM). Another abnormality of the ventricular septum often seen in patients with hypertrophic cardiomyopathy is the occurrence of a short linear, localised thickening of the proximal endocardial surface immediately opposite the mitral valve. This corresponds to a fibrous thickening of the mural endocardium resulting from the repeated contact between the valvular and mural endocardium during systole (SAM) or diastole.

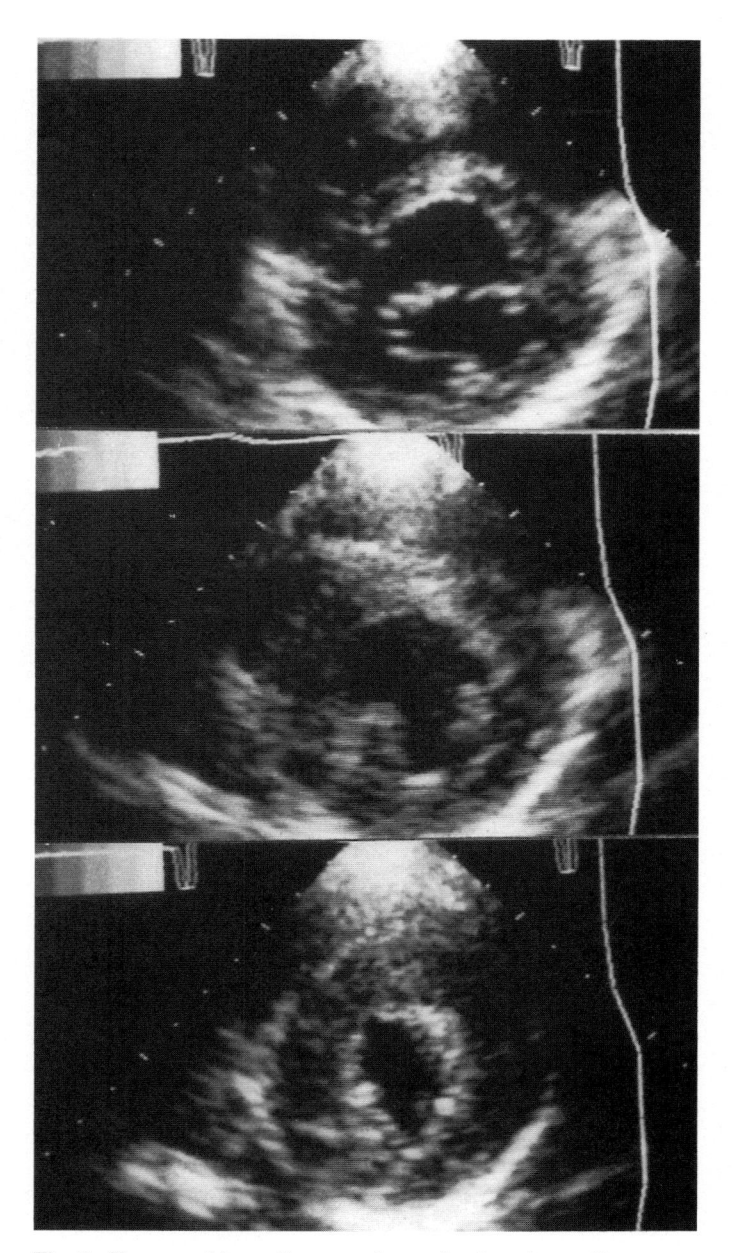

Fig. 8 Hypertrophic cardiomyopathy confined to the cardiac apex. Serial parasternal short axis views of the left ventricle at mitral valve level (top), papillary muscle level (middle) and apex (bottom). Note the absence of ventricular hypertrophy at the base of the heart, contrasted with the hypertrophied apex.

The mitral apparatus

The mitral apparatus is visualised in its integrity from parasternal and apical long axis projections and consequently these represent the optimal views for the visualisation and assessment of SAM.

Controversy still exists as to the mechanisms of SAM. There are now three major explanations of SAM, these being: (a) a Venturi effect resulting in the mitral valve

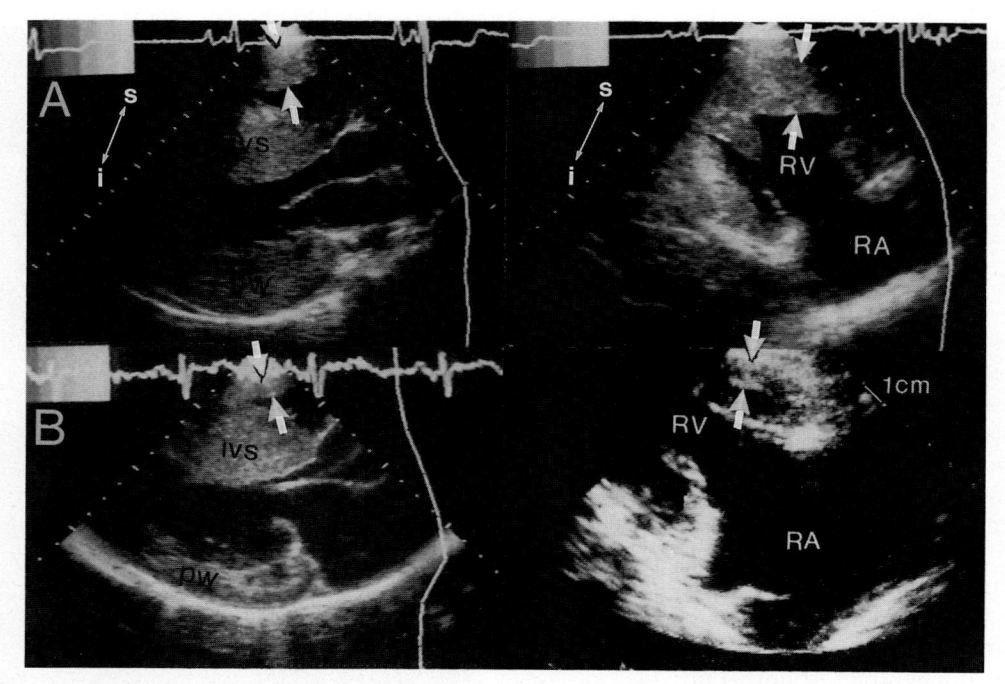

Fig. 9 Hypertrophic cardiomyopathy with right ventricular involvement (arrows) as shown from parasternal long axis views (left panels) and right ventricular inflow tract views (right panels). **A:** Patient with concentric left ventricular hypertrophy and marked right ventricular involvement, and **B:** Patient with asymmetrical left ventricular hypertrophy and moderate right ventricular involvement (IVS – interventricular septum, pw – posterior left ventricular wall).

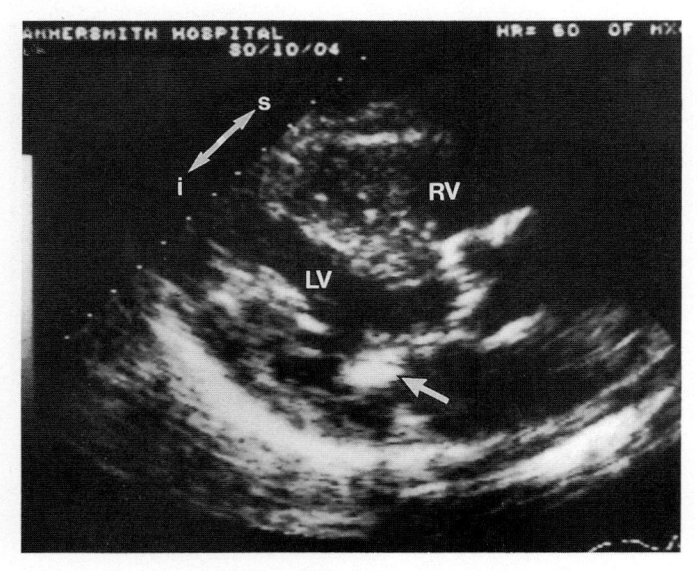

Fig. 10 Parasternal long axis view of the left ventricle showing asymmetrical septal hypertrophy and posterior mitral annular calcification (arrowed) from an 88-year-old patient.

cusps being aspirated into the relatively low pressure left ventricular outflow tract by the high velocity of blood flow through the region,[23] (b) abnormal mitral valve cusp coaptation at the onset of systole in association with a small left ventricular cavity[24] and (c) secondary to abnormal position-ing of the papillary muscles which are displaced forward and medially during systole.[25]

The significance of SAM is also under debate. There has been no doubt that the presence and the duration of SAM has been associated with the presence of a left ventricular outflow tract gradient measured at cardiac catheterisation.[26,27] SAM by itself is not pathognomonic of hypertrophic cardiomyopathy.[12] Whether or not the presence of SAM reliably indicates left ventricular outflow tract obstruction remains under considerable debate.

Differential diagnosis of hypertrophic cardiomyopathy

Other entities that simulate hypertrophic cardiomyopathy must be recognised. These include misinterpretations of normal variants of left ventricular shape and the presence of predominant right ventricular hypertrophy. Furthermore, although left ventricular asymmetry (ASH) is a characteristic morphological feature of hypertrophic cardiomyopathy, a significant number of patients with hypertrophic cardiomyopathy have diffuse myocardial thickening similar to that encountered with secondary causes of ventricular hypertrophy and this makes the differential diagnosis more difficult (Figs 5 and 6).

One of the commonest interpretative errors of asymmetrical septal hypertrophy is encountered in older patients where the ventricular septum is bent. In some elderly patients the ventricular septum comes off with an acute angle as it continues down from the anterior aortic wall (angled or sigmoid septum). This angulation appears to form a localised septal thickening which can easily be misinterpreted as ASH and thus hypertrophic cardiomyopathy. Left ventricular wall thickening, small outflow tract dimensions and a small incomplete SAM, may complete the illusion of hypertrophic cardiomyopathy.

Asymmetrical septal hypertrophy may occur in conditions causing thinning or thickening of the left ventricular posterior wall relative to the septum. The most common cause of preferential posterior wall thinning is transmural myocardial infarction, while the most common cause for preferential septal thickening is right ventricular pressure overload secondary to pulmonary stenosis or hypertension.

Hypertensive heart disease, aortic stenosis and cardiac amyloidosis may sometimes simulate hypertrophic cardiomyopathy. Patients with chronic renal failure or cardiac amyloidosis may have an echocardiographic appearance mimicking that of hypertrophic cardiomyopathy. The vigorous left ventricular systolic contraction in patients with hypertrophic cardiomyopathy should, in the majority of cases, differentiate these patients from those with cardiac infiltration where ventricular contraction is depressed.

Another major diagnostic difficulty occurs in some athletes who may present with symmetrical or even asymmetrical left ventricular hypertrophy involving the septum more than the free wall, often associated with bradycardia. Perhaps the essence of the discrimination between hypertrophic cardiomyopathy and physiological adaptation lies in the cavity dimensions rather than in the wall thickness, whether asymmetrical or not. In hypertrophic cardiomyopathy the cavity dimensions tend to be at the lower end of the normal limits, particularly at end systole, whereas the athlete is vagotonic with resting bradycardia and the ventricular dimensions are at the upper limits of normal.

Doppler findings in hypertrophic cardiomyopathy

The addition of Doppler techniques to two-dimensional and M-mode echocardiography has provided comprehensive haemodynamic information on patients with hypertrophic cardiomyopathy. Pulsed wave Doppler has proved to be particularly useful in the assessment of the left ventricular filling, allowing the measurement of diastolic blood flow velocities and flow times.[28-30] Systolic events are predominantly characterised by the presence of increased intraventricular flow velocities and the presence or absence of intraventricular pressure drops. Continuous wave Doppler has proved to be a reliable method for measuring the peak systolic pressure drop (gradient) across the left ventricular outflow tract using the simplified Bernoulli equation ($\Delta P = 4V^2$).[31,32] The recent introduction of colour flow imaging complements the anatomical information obtained by two-dimensional echocardiography[33] and facilitates further the understanding of the underlying pathophysiological changes occurring in hypertrophic cardiomyopathy as well as drawing attention to the site of obstruction.

Diastolic events

The basic functional disorder in hypertrophic cardiomyopathy occurs during diastole with impaired relaxation, filling and compliance of the ventricles. Far from being uniform, myocardial dysfunction is patchy and irregular depending upon the extent and distribution of the myofibrillar lesions. Early studies using M-mode echocardiography have shown that the rates of filling and relaxation of the left ventricle were abnormal in patients with hypertrophic cardiomyopathy. Although these measurements are sensitive, they are entirely non-specific, are time consuming and require excellent quality recordings which may be obtainable only in a small number of patients. No single or even combination of M-mode echocardiographic criteria is diagnostic.[34] Doppler echocardiography on the other hand provides a direct estimate of diastolic filling abnormalities of the left ventricle and has been proven a reliable technique in distinguishing normal from abnormal diastolic filling.[29]

Diastolic flow velocity waveforms may be recorded with pulsed wave Doppler by positioning the sample volume in the inflow region of the left ventricle. From this position the following indices are commonly abnormal in patients with hypertrophic cardiomyopathy: (a) the early diastolic peak (E wave) is reduced and prolonged with slow deceleration, (b) the late diastolic peak (A wave) is increased, (c) the ratio E/A is reduced (Fig. 11). As with early M-mode diastolic indices, however, these Doppler parameters are sensitive but lack specificity, as they are determined by multiple factors including the intrinsic properties of the cardiac muscle and the loading conditions of the left ventricle.[35]

Colour flow imaging can readily distinguish the high presystolic inflow velocity (A wave) from the lower velocity of the early diastolic filling flow (E wave) by the increased brightness of the red-orange colour occurring in late diastole, which also often aliases. The higher velocity in late diastole may be seen extending far into the left ventricular cavity and even on occasions reaching the cardiac apex, because patients with hypertrophic cardiomyopathy usually have small left ventricular cavity dimensions.

Systolic events

The systolic events in patients with hypertrophic cardiomyopathy may be categorised into two main groups. Firstly, those occurring in the left ventricular cavity and outflow tract, in which the highlight is the presence or ab-

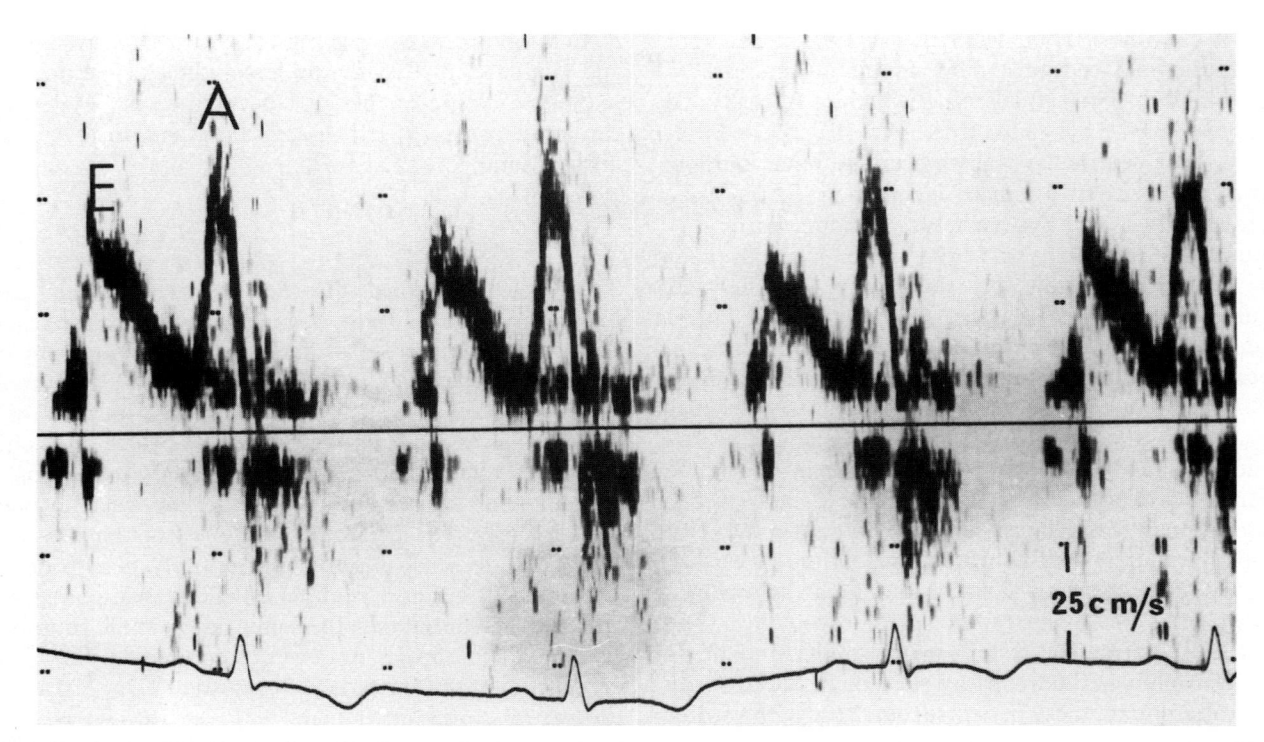

Fig. 11 **Pulsed wave Doppler tracing with the sample volume placed in the left ventricular inflow,** showing the reduced early filling flow velocity (E wave) and the increased late filling flow velocity (A wave).

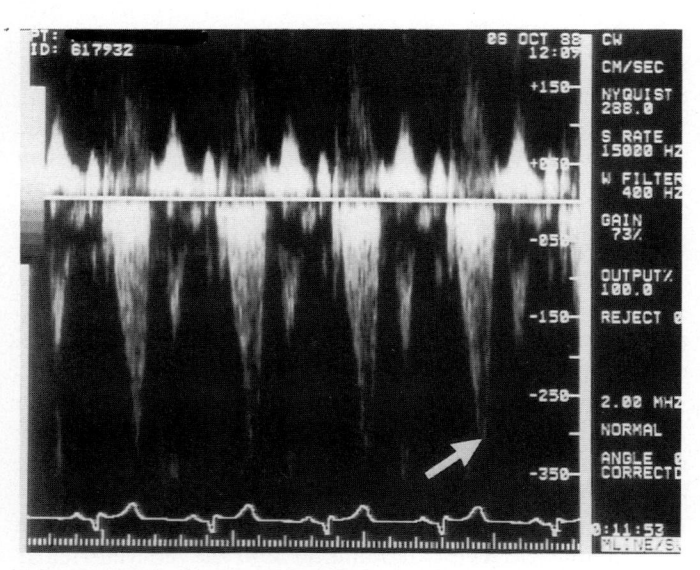

Fig. 12 **Continuous wave Doppler echocardiogram of left ventricular outflow velocity from a patient with hypertrophic cardiomyopathy.** The maximal left ventricular outflow tract velocity (arrow) is 3.2 m/s reflecting a peak instantaneous pressure drop of 41 mmHg.

sence of an intraventricular gradient, and secondly the presence or absence of mitral regurgitation.

Doppler echocardiography has been used to measure blood flow velocities within the heart, particularly for calculating pressure gradients across stenotic valves, using the modified Bernoulli equation: $\Delta P = 4v^2$, in which ΔP = pressure gradient and v = peak velocity in metres per second. This technique has also proved valid for calculating the dynamic gradient across the left ventricular outflow tract in patients with hypertrophic cardiomyopathy.[31] In contrast with fixed obstruction, the flow velocity profile in patients with hypertrophic cardiomyopathy, as obtained with continuous wave Doppler examination, presents a slow and gradual increase and only reaches maximal velocity late in systole so that the overall shape of the flow velocity is markedly different (Fig. 12). The intensity of the signal is highest during early systole and becomes lowest during late systole, when the velocity is greatest. Flow velocities in the various parts of the left ventricle can be recorded with pulsed wave Doppler. Work from our institution[33] has shown the presence of a gradual increase in velocity commencing at the region of the cardiac apex and progressively becoming higher, usually reaching its peak in the subaortic area.

Colour flow imaging can identify readily the uniformity or non-uniformity of the intraventricular flow. In apical four-chamber and two-chamber projections in normal individuals, the ventricular flow coded in blue (blood flow directed away from the transducer) becomes progressively brighter as it moves from the apex towards the left ventricular outflow tract. At this position it will alias and the flow map will demonstrate a central red zone (colour reversal) immediately below the aortic valve. In patients with hypertrophic cardiomyopathy, the intraventricular colour flow map during systole is characterised by a non-homogeneous blue colour with a lighter than normal hue which usually aliases at mid-ventricular level, at the level of the hypertrophied papillary muscles or at the level of the mitral valve. When systolic anterior motion of the mitral valve occurs, the systolic flow at this level becomes turbulent with a 'mosaic' colour pattern. When the flow crosses the aortic valve into the ascending aorta laminar flow is re-established.

Better timing of the intraventricular systolic events can be obtained with the superimposition of colour-coded blood flow on M-mode echocardiograms. This provides a higher temporal resolution and a wider range of velocities displayed in colour so that an accurate analysis of timing and direction of the blood flow can be performed. The M-mode ultrasound beam will be directed along the mitral valve from the parasternal long axis projection to record the systolic anterior motion of the mitral valve, together with the colour flow imaging. High velocity turbulent flow usually occurs at the time when the mitral valve leaflets impinge on the ventricular septum during systole.

The events occurring at this time are not fully understood. It is conceivable that the mitral valve causes narrowing of the outflow tract preventing blood from passing through. It is more likely that powerful ventricular contraction squeezes the blood quickly out of the left ventricle. This increased intraventricular acceleration of the blood flow during systole appears to have its origin at the cardiac apex,[33] and at papillary muscle level. This flow is further accelerated without losing its physiological laminar characteristics because of the natural 'obstacle' produced by the hypertrophied papillary muscles. When it then reaches the outflow tract, it encounters the anteriorly displaced mitral leaflets (SAM) and loses its laminar flow, becoming turbulent with the characteristic mosaic pattern on colour flow imaging. At this level further flow acceleration occurs with velocities reaching as high as 5 to 6 m/s. This progressive step up in intraventricular systolic flow velocity may be responsible for the pressure drop between left ventricular outflow tract and the rest of the ventricle.

Occasionally in a sub-group of patients with hypertrophic cardiomyopathy, turbulent flow and an abnormal pressure drop can be seen in the middle of the left ventricle or even at the apex. It is this inhomogeneity of the intraventricular flow during systole that appears to be fairly specific in distinguishing most of the patients with hypertrophic cardiomyopathy from secondary causes of left ventricular hypertrophy.[36]

Mitral regurgitation is a well-recognised component of the complex pathophysiology encountered in patients with hypertrophic cardiomyopathy. Its association with the systolic anterior motion of the mitral valve and the magnitude of the intraventricular gradient has also been well documented.[37-40] Patients who do not have systolic anterior motion of the mitral valve rarely have mitral regurgitation.

Colour flow imaging can detect readily the presence of mitral regurgitation with high sensitivity and specificity. The most useful views are the apical four-chamber and two-chamber projections, but the parasternal long- and short-axis views may also be very useful in detecting jets directed posteriorly. Mitral regurgitation in patients with hypertrophic cardiomyopathy is noted as a mosaic pattern (turbulent flow) present in the left atrium during systole. The jet is usually directed anteriorly and may easily be confused with the turbulent jet of the left ventricular outflow tract, as they can be separated by as little as 1 cm at their origin. It can be very difficult to separate these two high velocity jets with continuous wave Doppler alone and a great deal of expertise is required in both the recording and the interpretation. The frequency of mitral regurgitation, as assessed by colour flow imaging, appears to be related to the presence of SAM of the mitral valve and is more severe in patients with resting outflow tract gradients.

The exact mechanism of mitral regurgitation in patients with hypertrophic cardiomyopathy remains controversial. Some early studies suggested an 'eject, obstruct, leak' theory in which mitral regurgitation results from left ventricular outflow tract 'obstruction'.[41] It has also been suggested that mitral regurgitation is initiated as a result of distortion of the mitral apparatus which begins in early systole.[37,38] This is supported by the Doppler studies showing that mitral regurgitation begins early, before the occurrence of SAM–septal contact and when there is no significant gradient across the left ventricular outflow tract.[40] In this study the onset of mitral regurgitation was 94 ± 29 ms after the electrocardiographic R-wave, whereas the onset of systolic anterior motion of the mitral valve was 120 ± 20 ms after the R-wave. As systole progresses there is a further decrease in left ventricular systolic dimensions and mitral valve distortion increases following the anterior mitral leaflet–septal contact. This would therefore result in an increased amount of mitral regurgitation occurring later in systole.

A third cause of mitral regurgitation is secondary to the presence of mitral annular calcification. This pattern, as mentioned earlier on, is particularly encountered in the older patients with hypertrophic cardiomyopathy.

DILATED CARDIOMYOPATHY

Dilated (congestive) cardiomyopathy is primarily a disease of the systolic function of the heart. It is characterised by a reduction in systolic ventricular function and chamber dilatation involving both ventricles. Rare forms of dilated cardiomyopathy solely involving the right ventricle also have been reported. Congestive heart failure of unknown cause is the hallmark of this disorder. An association with alcohol, hypertension, pregnancy and puerperium has been established but causal links have not yet been defined, except perhaps in case of alcohol which produces dilated cardiomyopathy but by definition is not an idiopathic (or primary) cardiomyopathy. The diagnosis of idiopathic dilated cardiomyopathy is basically one of exclusion.

Echocardiographic findings

The echocardiographic findings in patients with dilated cardiomyopathy are those of a dilated, poorly contracting ventricle. Early M-mode studies clearly showed that diastolic dimensions were significantly increased compared with the normal population and the extent of systolic myocardial thickening was reduced, reflecting the reduction in left ventricular systolic function. Generally, the left ventricular wall thickness is normal or slightly reduced when compared with normal individuals, although the total left ventricular mass[42] is markedly increased consequent upon ventricular dilatation. The left atrial dimensions are also increased compared with normal individuals, an indirect sign of elevated left ventricular filling pressures. Another common M-mode echocardiographic finding in patients with dilated cardiomyopathy is early closure of the aortic valve which reflects the patient's decreased stroke volume. This finding is progressively more marked with increasing severity of the cardiomyopathy.

Two-dimensional echocardiography has largely confirmed the early M-mode echocardiographic findings in patients with dilated cardiomyopathy. This modality can provide imaging of the entire left ventricle and will demonstrate the diffuse pattern of left ventricular hypokinesis (Fig. 13).

Over the past few years, considerable interest has been centred on the right ventricle as a potential source of life-threatening arrhythmia and occasionally a distinct cardiomyopathy can be seen which involves solely the right ventricle. This can readily be recognised with two-dimensional echocardiography although other causes producing right ventricular dilatation such as atrial septal defects, tricuspid regurgitation, pulmonary hypertension should be considered first. It is likely that a variety of conditions are involved, including isolated right ventricular cardiomyopathy,[43] Uhl's disease[44] and arrhythmogenic right ventricular dysplasia.[45-47] In a group of patients who presented to our institution with ventricular tachycardia of right ventricular origin, those with adverse clinical and electrophysiological features had generalised right ventricular dilatation and normal left ventricles. This study suggested that surveillance of the right ventricle in patients presenting with serious arrhythmias may define isolated right ventricular abnormalities, which in turn may identify patients at particularly high risk of sudden death.[47]

Generalised dilatation with poor function of the ventricles, relatively normal wall thickness and secondary enlargement of the atria, in the absence of significant

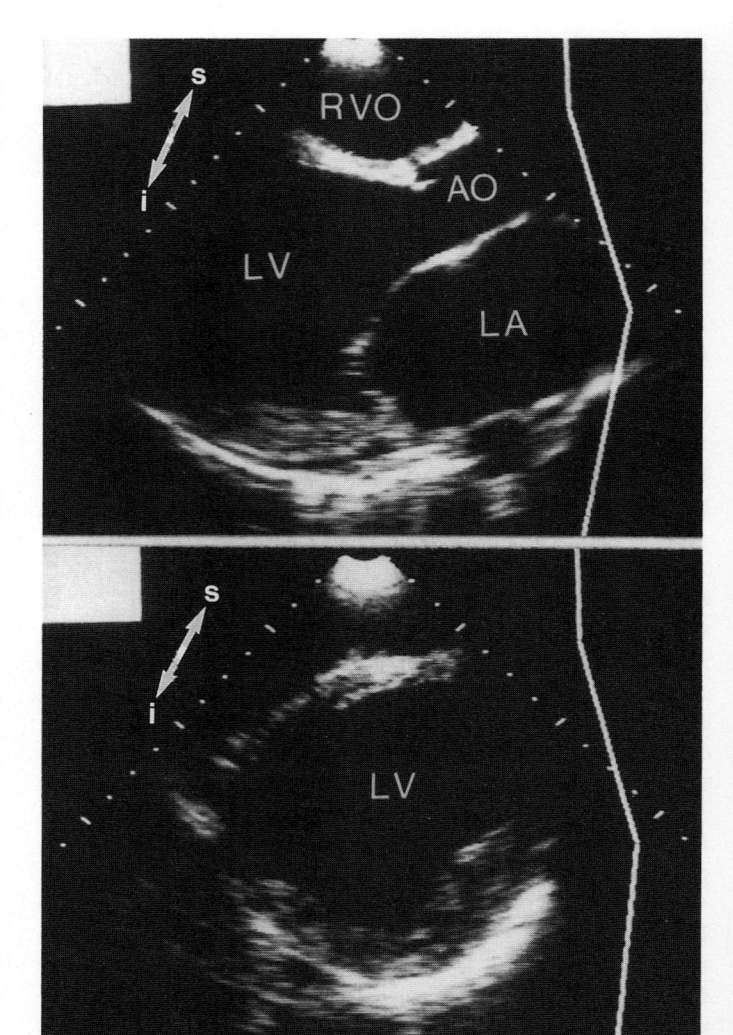

Fig. 13 Parasternal long axis (top) and short axis (bottom) views from a patient with dilated cardiomyopathy. Note the marked increase of chamber dimensions and the normal left ventricular wall thickness. (RVO – right ventricular outflow tract.)

valvular or congenital heart disease, are strongly supportive of a heart muscle disorder. However, the differential diagnosis between primary (idiopathic) and secondary heart muscle disorder will remain a clinical task.

Differential diagnosis of dilated cardiomyopathy

Patients with dilated and poorly contracting left ventricles can only be diagnosed as having dilated cardiomyopathy if other cardiac conditions resulting in left ventricular failure are excluded. Two-dimensional and Doppler echocardiography have been extremely useful in accomplishing this task as they represent the primary non-invasive technique for diagnosing left ventricular volume overload conditions due to valvular regurgitation which may lead ultimately to a dilated and hypocontractile left ventricle. Functional atrio-ventricular valve regurgitation commonly accompanies ventricular dilatation due to the geometrical distortion of the subvalvular apparatus and the stretched atrio-ventricular annular ring. It is important to map carefully the spatial extent of this regurgitant jet using colour flow imaging. Often however it is difficult to exclude a causal link between valvular regurgitation and ventricular impairment. In our own experience the direct morphological appearance of the valve with two-dimensional imaging (or preferably using the transoesophageal approach), will contribute most to the differential diagnosis. When the valve appears entirely normal it is most unlikely that it will be leaking sufficiently to cause ventricular dysfunction, despite the presence of a regurgitant jet on colour flow, and so the jet can be explained as a secondary or 'functional' leak due to stretching of the annulus.

Perhaps one of the most challenging tasks to the echocardiographer is to separate patients with dilated cardiomyopathy from patients with left ventricular failure secondary to coronary heart disease (coronary heart failure). In contrast to dilated cardiomyopathy, coronary disease usually results in regional differences in myocardial perfusion and function. Some investigators have assumed that the demonstration of segmental wall motion abnormalities of systolic myocardial thickening using two-dimensional echocardiography reliably indicates an ischaemic aetiology, but controversies still exist as to whether or not this is the case.

If a patient with ischaemic heart disease has sustained a single transmural myocardial infarction in a localised segment of the left ventricle and the remaining left ventricle is normal, the differential diagnosis from dilated cardiomyopathy is easy. If on the other hand the patient has sustained several myocardial infarctions in different sites which have damaged a large myocardial area and have led to ventricular dilatation, the distinction from dilated cardiomyopathy is very difficult.[48] Although it has been proposed that the presence of biventricular enlargement aids in distinguishing patients with dilated cardiomyopathy from coronary heart failure, work from our group[49] failed to demonstrate any significant differences between the two groups.

It is well known that patients with acute myocarditis may develop discrete wall motion abnormalities prior to the subsequent evolution of diffuse myocardial depression,[50] a finding which makes the distinction from an ischaemic origin difficult on echocardiography. It seems likely that other, as yet unidentified infectious pathogens, may affect the myocardium regionally and thus might explain the observation of heterogeneity of systolic regional ventricular wall motion in some patients.

Myocardial texture may be different in patients with dilated cardiomyopathy and coronary heart failure. Occasionally, myocardial scarring following extensive transmural myocardial infarction can be visualised as a highly echogenic, akinetic and thin wall involving the territory of a coronary artery. In Chagas disease[51] and myocardial sarcoidosis,[52] the myocardium can be highly reflective, making the differential diagnosis from coronary artery disease difficult. Myocardial tissue characterisation currently constitutes a rapidly expanding area of interest and is beginning to be applied clinically to the assessment of the various reflected ultrasound patterns that may characterise particular pathological changes.

Intracardiac flow and embolisation

Reduced systolic ventricular function and chamber dilatation produce a characteristic flow pattern which is commonly seen in patients with dilated and poorly contracting ventricles. Swirling of the intracardiac flow can often be visualised at the cardiac apex with two-dimensional echocardiography. This reflects the high intracardiac filling pressures and the decreased flow velocity profile which are predisposing factors for cellular aggregation, spontaneous echo contrast and consequent thrombus formation.

The pattern of intracavitary flow velocity profile can be characterised with colour flow imaging and can be used to predict those patients in which regional stasis may occur. A series of short boluses of flow can be visualised during diastole from apical four chamber projections, giving the appearance of 'puffs of smoke'. The velocity of flow is low because of the low output state, so that the usual colour flow map of intraventricular inflow is shown by darker shades of red. In systole the left ventricular outflow tract velocity will also be low, sometimes without the usual colour aliasing.

Ventricular dilatation, diffuse hypokinesis and the consequent low intraventricular velocities constitute a major risk for the development of intraventricular thrombi and the concurrent risk of systemic embolisation. Echocardiography can identify readily the presence of intraventricular thrombus and this can lead to prompt anticoagulant treatment. In contrast to thrombus formation in patients following myocardial infarction, intraventricular thrombus in patients with dilated cardiomyopathy is likely to embolise and the prompt recognition of low intraventricular flow velocities may be of value in selecting patients for anticoagulant treatment.

Indicators of prognosis

The recent advances in medical treatment and the successes of cardiac transplantation represent tremendous advances in modern cardiovascular care. Consequently, it has become apparent that patients with dilated cardiomyopathy need careful assessment before any major therapeutic decisions are made. Although the long-term survival in these patients is generally poor, the disease affects a diverse population with many subsets. Not only may there be multiple causes, as yet unknown, but mortality may vary widely within the subsets. Ventricular function as assessed by the ejection fraction or stroke volume appear to be the major physiological determinants of survival.

In several reports some additional clinical and haemodynamic variables have been advocated as useful predictors of the clinical course. Low voltage on the electrocardiogram, conduction system defects, ventricular arrhythmias and high left ventricular end diastolic pressures have been associated with poor prognosis in the past. On the other hand atrial fibrillation and left ventricular hypertrophy have been associated with longevity. Some pathological studies have also suggested that patients with thinner walls also have lower survival rates. Unfortunately, there are no more specific echocardiographic parameters associated with survival rate. In particular the severity of left ventricular dilatation does not appear to be a reliable predictor of mortality.

RESTRICTIVE CARDIOMYOPATHY

Restrictive cardiomyopathy is the term used to describe the form of heart muscle disease in which there is restriction or resistance to ventricular inflow. The ventricles fill rapidly during the early part of diastole and are halted abruptly later in diastole as the non-elastic chambers fail to stretch further to accommodate any additional blood volume. As with the rest of the primary cardiomyopathies, there are no known causes of restrictive cardiomyopathy. There are however several other types of diseases infiltrating the myocardium, causing a similar restrictive physiology and these are described under the same generic term of restrictive cardiomyopathy.[2]

Restrictive cardiomyopathy is the rarest form of cardiomyopathy. The important echocardiographic feature of patients with restrictive cardiomyopathy is the presence of small, well-contracting ventricles with bi-atrial enlargement and normal pericardium. During diastole it may be possible to observe an abrupt halt of the ventricular filling with two-dimensional real time imaging but this is more easily seen on the M-mode echocardiogram (Fig. 14). In the normal individual, the diastolic phase is characterised by smooth and progressive increase of the left ventricular cavity dimensions from early to late diastole. The ventricular septum and posterior wall also exhibit a brief posterior displacement in early and late diastole respectively. In patients with restrictive cardiomyopathy, the entire diastolic phase becomes horizontal with fading of the various dips seen on the M-mode echocardiogram. Furthermore, the rate of decline of the movement of the posterior wall is reduced, giving a more gradual slope than normal.

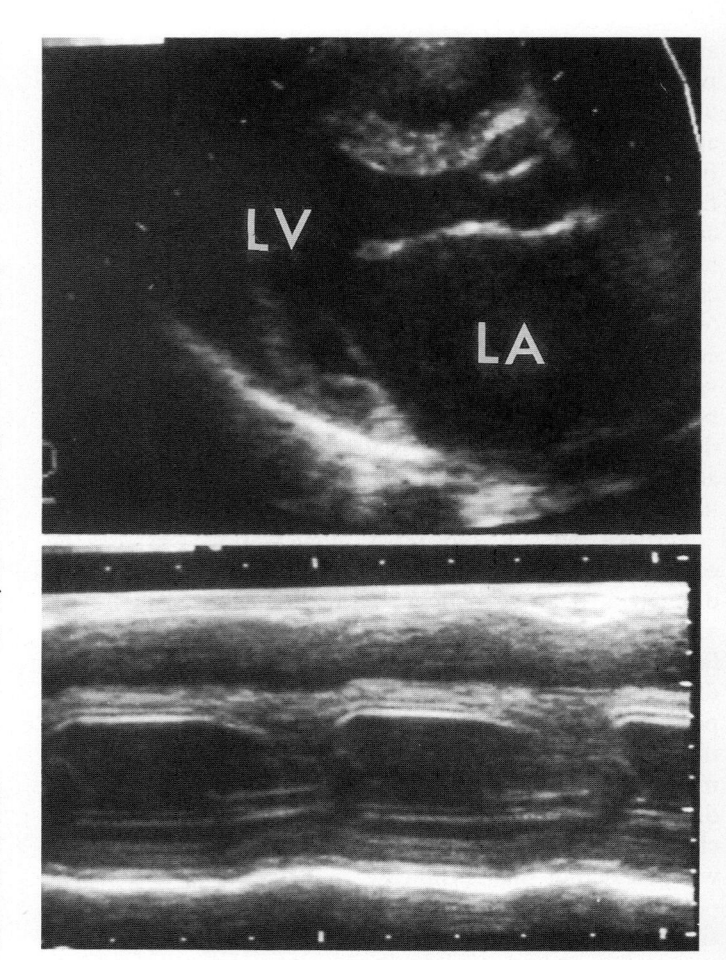

Fig. 14 Parasternal long axis (top) and simultaneous M-mode echocardiogram (bottom) from a patient with restrictive cardiomyopathy. Note the normal size ventricle contrasting with the large atrium. On the M-mode echocardiogram the diastolic phase is flat and the wall thickness is normal.

Amyloid heart disease

The commonest type of cardiac infiltration is cardiac amyloidosis. Here, a restrictive haemodynamic state is used to describe the effects of widespread amyloid disease in which ventricular filling is severely reduced. Cardiac amyloidosis may be primary or it may be secondary to myeloma or a large number of inflammatory disorders. It may also be of familial or senile aetiology.[53] Significant cardiac involvement is most commonly seen in the primary or myeloma related groups.

Amyloid deposition begins as a focal subendocardial accumulation between the muscle fibres of the myocardium. Expansion of these myocardial deposits eventually causes pressure atrophy and separation of myocardial fibres. This mechanism is responsible for the marked thickening of the left and right ventricular walls, normal or decreased left ventricular cavity size, and reduced left ventricular diastolic and systolic function. The walls of intramural coronary arteries and veins, as well as the conducting system may also be infiltrated and this accounts for the electrocardiographic abnormalities encountered in some patients. The endocardium is also involved and this may lead to thrombus formation. Amyloidosis also causes a focal or diffuse thickening of valves and the atrial septum but clinical valvular dysfunction is rare.

The echocardiographic diagnosis of cardiac amyloidosis relies upon a constellation of findings consisting of biventricular hypertrophy, with a granular sparkling (ground glass appearance) of the myocardium, normal or small ventricular cavities and enlarged atria (Figs 15 and 16). The associated depressed myocardial function (both systolic and diastolic) is almost pathognomonic of the amyloid infiltrate and may greatly facilitate the differential diagnosis from hypertrophic cardiomyopathy.

Endomyocardial fibrosis

This type of cardiac infiltration was originally described by Löffler in 1936 and is associated with intense eosinophilia. There is an initial stage of inflammatory exudates in the endocardium which is often packed with eosinophils. In the later stages, granulation tissue develops followed by fibrosis and endarteritis obliterans. As the disease advances, the fibrosis and added thrombus obliterates the apices of the ventricles. Endomyocardial fibrosis, by limiting the distensibility of the endocardium, produces haemodynamic changes very similar to restrictive cardiomyopathy (Fig. 17).[54]

Two-dimensional echocardiographic features in patients with endomyocardial fibrosis include a thickened

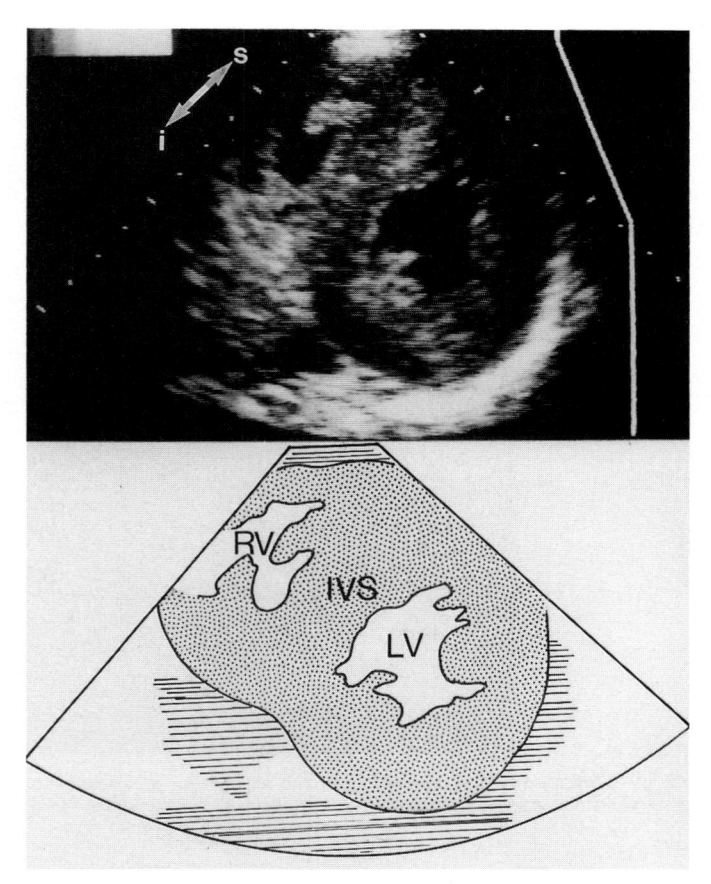

Fig. 16 Parasternal short axis view from a patient with cardiac amyloidosis. Note the concentric left ventricular hypertrophy with a highly reflective and granular, sparkling appearance.

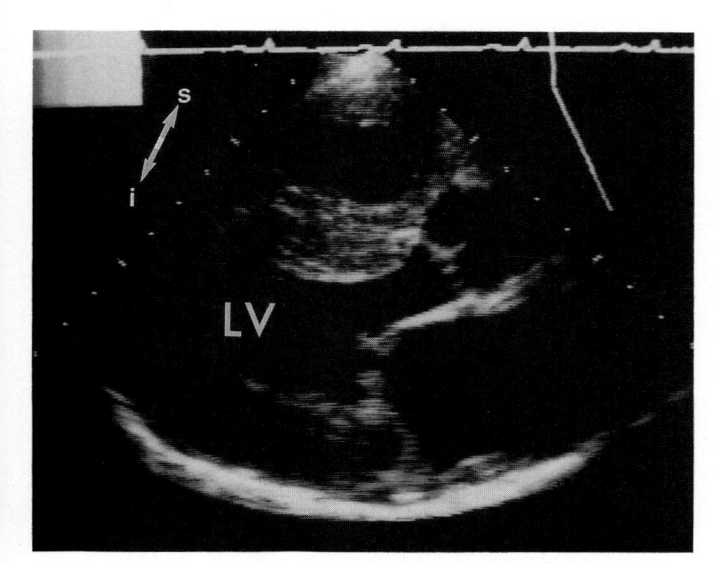

Fig. 15 Parasternal long axis view from a patient with cardiac amyloidosis. There is marked concentric left and right ventricular hypertrophy with the mitral and aortic valves also being homogeneously thickened without affecting their mobility.

posterobasal left ventricular wall with tethering of the posterior mitral leaflet. Typically, the posterior mitral leaflet becomes incorporated into the thickened fibrotic posterior left ventricular wall, leading to mitral regurgitation which may become severe enough to require valve replacement (Fig. 18). Two-dimensional imaging from the apical four-chamber projection shows characteristic space occupying lesions (thrombus) in the apices of both ventricles. In severe cases virtually the whole of the inflow tract of the ventricles may be obliterated, leaving only a small outflow tract portion. This obliteration persists in systole and diastole, and is quite unlike the elimination of the left ventricular cavity in systole produced by the powerfully contracting hypertrophied muscle in patients with hypertrophic cardiomyopathy. Bi-atrial enlargement is also found in the majority of these patients as a result of the restrictive ventricular filling imposed by the non-compliant ventricles.

Doppler echocardiography in restrictive cardiomyopathies

The restrictive haemodynamic pattern seen in symptomatic

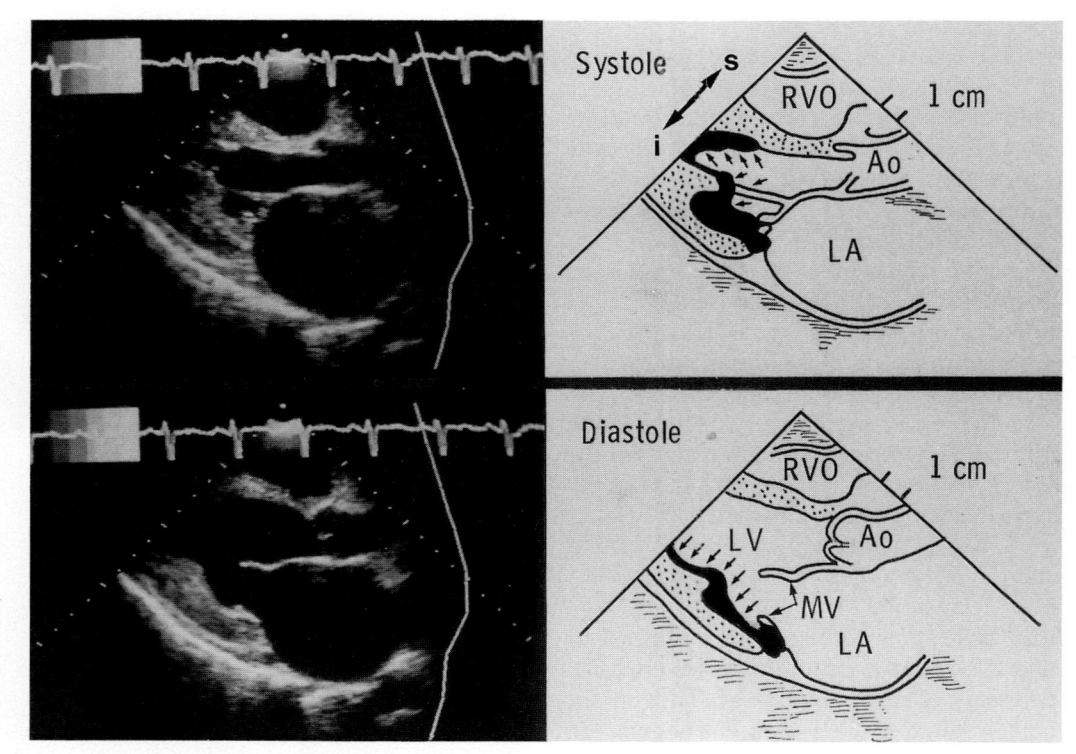

Fig. 17 Parasternal long axis views of the heart from a patient with hypereosinophilic syndrome. Note the typical 'restrictive pattern' with small ventricle and large atrium. Also the left ventricular endocardium is thickened (arrows) obliterating the cardiac apex during systole.

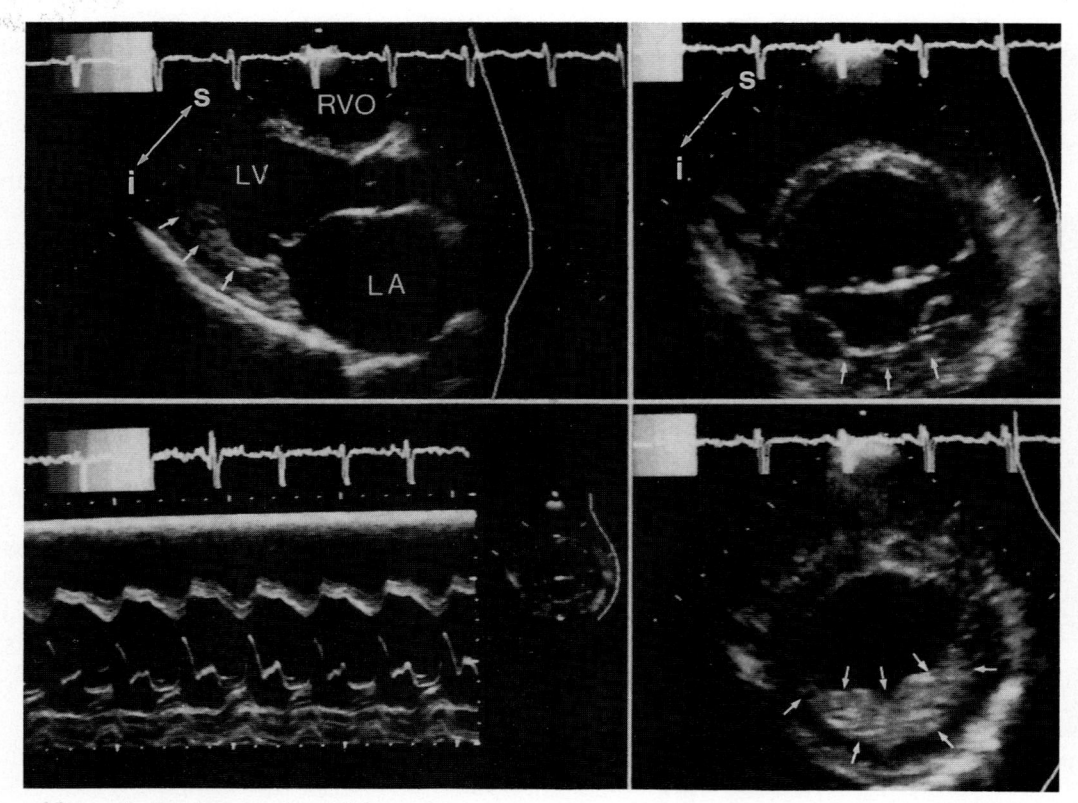

Fig. 18 Parasternal long axis (top left panel) and M-mode echocardiogram (bottom left panel) and short axis views (right panels) from a patient with endomyocardial fibrosis. Note the thickened endocardium posteriorly (arrows) with the posterior mitral valve leaflet becoming tethered and incorporated into it (RVO – right ventricular outflow).

patients with restrictive cardiac filling of various aetiologies can be recognised with Doppler echocardiography.[55] Shortened mitral and tricuspid deceleration times, and central venous flow velocity patterns with increased flow reversal in inspiration, all suggest restrictive physiology. These findings are nonspecific however and do not permit the distinction between patients with restrictive cardiomyopathy and constrictive pericarditis. In a recent study from Stanford, Hatle and her associates[56] showed that despite indistinguishable baseline haemodynamics, patients with constrictive pericarditis can be differentiated from patients with restrictive cardiomyopathy by comparing respiratory variation in transvalvular flow velocity patterns as recorded by Doppler ultrasound. In patients with constrictive pericarditis, marked respiratory variation in left ventricular isovolumic relaxation time and peak mitral flow velocity in early diastole was observed, which disappeared after surgery and was not present in patients with restrictive cardiomyopathy or normal individuals. The deceleration time of early mitral and tricuspid flow velocity was shorter than normals in both groups, indicating an early cessation of ventricular filling, but only patients with restrictive cardiomyopathy showed a further shortening of tricuspid deceleration time with inspiration.[56]

Doppler with colour flow imaging can depict the presence of mitral or tricuspid regurgitation and assess its severity. In most patients the severity of the valvular regurgitation is mild to moderate. However in patients with endomyocardial fibrosis, mitral regurgitation is often severe and difficult to assess on clinical grounds alone because of the presence of restrictive physiology. Most patients with restrictive cardiomyopathy have normal ventricular systolic function except patients with cardiac amyloidosis where both the systolic and the diastolic ventricular function are depressed, resulting in a low intraventricular flow velocity profile. This impaired ventricular function with colour flow imaging will be represented as homogeneous dark red and blue colours similar to that commonly seen in dilated cardiomyopathy.

REFERENCES

1 Goodwin J F, Oakley C M. The cardiomyopathies. Br Heart J 1972; 34: 545
2 Goodwin J F. The frontiers of cardiomyopathy. Br Heart J 1982; 48: 1–18
3 Tear R D. Asymmetrical hypertrophy of the heart in young adults. Br Heart J 1958; 20: 1
4 Rossen R M, Goodman D J, Ingham R E, Popp R L. Echocardiographic criteria in the diagnosis of idiopathic hypertrophic subaortic stenosis. Circulation 1974; 50: 747
5 Henry W L, Clark C E, Epstein S E. Asymmetric septal hypertrophy: echocardiographic identification of the pathognomonic anatomic abnormality of IHSS. Circulation 1973; 47: 225–233
6 Shah P M, Gramiak R, Kramer D H. Ultrasound localisation of left ventricular outflow tract obstruction in hypertrophic obstructive cardiomyopathy. Circulation 1969; 40: 3–11
7 Feigenbaum H. Clinical applications of echocardiography. Prog Cardiovasc Dis 1976; 53: 258–268
8 Aziz K U, Paul M H, Muster A J. Echocardiographic assessment of left ventricular outflow tract in d-transposition of the great arteries. Am J Cardiol 1978; 41: 543–551
9 Maron B J, Gottdiener J S, Perry L W. Specificity of systolic anterior motion of the anterior mitral leaflet for hypertrophic cardiomyopathy: prevalence in large population of patients with other cardiac diseases. Br Heart J 1981; 45: 206–212
10 Larter W E, Allen H D, Sahn D J, Goldberg S J. The asymmetrical hypertrophied septum: further differentiation of its causes. Circulation 1976; 53: 19–27
11 Mintz G S, Kotler M N, Segal B L, Parry W R. Systolic anterior motion of the mitral valve in the absence of asymmetric septal hypertrophy. Circulation 1978; 57: 256
12 Boughner D R, Rakowski H, Wigle D. Mitral valve systolic anterior motion in the absence of hypertrophic cardiomyopathy. Circulation 1978; 57: 256
13 Maron B J, Gottdiener J S, Bonow R O, Epstein S E. Hypertrophic cardiomyopathy with unusual locations of left ventricular hypertrophy undetectable by M-mode echocardiography. Identification by wide-angle two-dimensional echocardiography. Circulation 1981; 63: 409–418
14 Fezi O, Emmanuel R. Echocardiographic spectrum of hypertrophic cardiomyopathy. Br Heart J 1975; 37: 1286
15 Martin R P, Rakowski H, French J, Popp R L. Idiopathic hypertrophic subaortic stenosis viewed by wide-angle, phased array echocardiography. Circulation 1979; 59: 1216–1217
16 Maron B J, Gottdiener J S, Epstein S E. Patterns and significance of distribution of left ventricular hypertrophy in hypertrophic cardiomyopathy. A wide angle, two-dimensional echocardiographic study of 125 patients. Am J Cardiol 1981; 48: 418–428
17 Shapiro L M, McKenna. Distribution of left ventricular hypertrophy in hypertrophic cardiomyopathy: a two-dimensional echocardiographic study. J Am Coll Cardiol 1983; 2: 437
18 Yamaguchi H, Ishimura T, Nishiyama S, et al. Hypertrophic non-obstructive cardiomyopathy with giant, negative T-waves (apical hypertrophy); ventricular and echocardiographic features in 30 patients. Am J Cardiol 1979; 44: 401–412
19 Alfonso F, Nihoyannopoulos P, Stewart J, Dickie S, Lemery R, McKenna W J. Clinical significance of giant negative T-waves in hypertrophic cardiomyopathy. J Am Coll Cardiol 1990; 15: 965–971
20 Foale R A, Nihoyannopoulos P, McKenna W J, et al. The echocardiographic measurement of the normal adult right ventricle. Br Heart J 1986; 56: 33–44
21 McKenna W J, Kleinebenne A, Nihoyannopoulos P, Foale R. Echocardiographic measurement of right ventricular wall thickness in hypertrophic cardiomyopathy: relation to clinical and prognostic features. J Am Coll Cardiol 1988; 11: 351–358
22 Kronzon I, Glassman E. Mitral ring calcification in idiopathic hypertrophic subaortic stenosis. Am J Cardiol 1978; 42: 60–66
23 Henry W L, Clark C E, Griffith J M, Epstein S E. Mechanism of left ventricular obstruction in patients with obstructive asymmetric septal hypertrophy (idiopathic hypertrophic subaortic stenosis). Am J Cardiol 1975; 35: 337–345
24 Shah P M, Taylor R D, Wong M. Abnormal mitral valve coaptation in hypertrophic obstructive cardiomyopathy: proposed role in systolic anterior motion of the mitral valve. Am J Cardiol 1981; 48: 258–263
25 Levine R, Vlachakes G J, Gieseking E, et al. New insights into the mechanism of obstruction in hypertrophic cardiomyopathy: experimental models. Circulation 1989; (supplement II) 80: II-662
26 Henry W L, Clark C E, Glancy D L, Epstein S E. Echocardiographic measurement of the left ventricular outflow gradient in idiopathic hypertrophic subaortic stenosis. N Engl J Med 1973; 288: 989
27 Pollick C, Rakowski H, Wigle E D. Muscular subaortic stenosis:

the quantitative relationship between systolic anterior motion and the pressure gradient. Circulation 1984; 69: 43

28 Gidding S S, Suider A R, Pocchini A P, Peters J, Farnsworth R. Left ventricular diastolic filling in children with hypertrophic cardiomyopathy. Assessment with pulsed Doppler echocardiography. J Am Coll Cardiol 1986; 8: 310

29 Spirito P, Maron B J, Bonow R O. Non-invasive assessment of left ventricular diastolic function: comparative analysis of Doppler echocardiographic and radionuclide angiographic techniques. J Am Coll Cardiol 1986; 7: 518–526

30 Maron B J, Spirito P, Green K J, Wesley Y E, Bonow R O, Arce J. Non-invasive assessment of left ventricular diastolic function by pulsed Doppler echocardiography in patients with hypertrophic cardiomyopathy. J Am Coll Cardiol 1987; 10: 733–742

31 Sasson Z, Yock P G, Hatle L K, Alderman E L, Popp R L. Doppler echocardiographic determination of the pressure gradient in hypertrophic cardiomyopathy. J Am Coll Cardiol 1988; 11: 752–756

32 Hatle L. Non-invasive assessment of differentiation of left ventricular outflow tract obstruction with Doppler ultrasound. Circulation 1981; 64: 381–387

33 Nihoyannopoulos P, Yonezawa Y, McKenna W J, Oakley C M. Intracavitary flow patterns in hypertrophic cardiomyopathy. A pulsed and continuous wave Doppler study with colour flow mapping. Br Heart J 1987; 57: 592 (abstract)

34 Doi Y L. M-mode echocardiography in hypertrophic cardiomyopathy. Diagnosis, criteria, prediction of obstruction. Am J Cardiol 1981; 45: 6

35 Grossman W, McLaurin L P. Diastolic properties of the left ventricle. Ann Intern Med 1976; 84: 316–326

36 Nihoyannopoulos P, Yonezawa Y, Dickie S, McKenna W J, Oakley C M. Accelerated intraventricular systolic flow differentiates patients with hypertrophic cardiomyopathy from those with secondary causes of hypertrophy. Br Heart J 1988; 59: 127 (abstract)

37 Wigle E D, Adelman A G, Auger P, Marquis Y. Mitral regurgitation in muscular subaortic stenosis. Am J Cardiol 1969; 24: 698–706

38 Pridie R B, Oakley C M. Mechanism of mitral regurgitation of hypertrophic obstructive cardiomyopathy. Br Heart J 1970; 32: 203–208

39 Kinoshita N, Nimura Y, Okamoto M, Miyatake K, Nagata S, Sakakibara H. Mitral regurgitation in hypertrophic cardiomyopathy: non-invasive study by two-dimensional Doppler echocardiography. Br Heart J 1983; 49: 574–583

40 Yonezawa Y, Nihoyannopoulos P, McKenna W J, Doi Y L, Ozawa T. Mitral regurgitation in hypertrophic cardiomyopathy. A colour Doppler echocardiographic study. Am J Noninvas Cardiol 1988; 2: 195–198

41 Adelman A G, McLoughlin M J, Marquis Y, Auger P, Wigle E D. Left ventricular cineangiographic observations in muscular subaortic stenosis. Am J Cardiol 1969; 24: 689–697

42 Devereux R B, Reicheck N. Echocardiographic determination of left ventricular mass in man. Circulation 1977; 55: 613

43 Fitchet D H, MacArthur C G, Oakley C M, Krikler D M, Goodwin J F. Right ventricular cardiomyopathy presenting with recurrent ventricular tachycardia. Am J Cardiol 1981; 47: 402

44 Child J S, Perloff J K, Francoz R, et al. Uhl's anomaly (parchment right ventricle): clinical, echocardiographic, radionuclear, hemodynamic and angiographic features in two patients. Am J Cardiol 1984; 53: 635

45 Rowland E, McKenna W J, Sugrue D, Barcley R, Foale R A, Krikler D M. Ventricular tachycardia of left bundle block configuration in patients with isolated right ventricular dilatation: clinical and electrophysiological features. Br Heart J 1984; 51: 15–24

46 Rossi P, Massumi A, Gillette P, Hall R J. Right ventricular dysplasia: clinical features, diagnostic techniques and current management. Am Heart J 1982; 103: 415–420

47 Foale R A, Nihoyannopoulos P, Ribeiro P, et al. Right ventricular abnormalities in ventricular tachycardia of right ventricular origin: Relation to electrophysiological features. Br Heart J 1986; 56: 45–54

48 Diaz R A, Foale R A, Nihoyannopoulos P, et al. Regional wall motion abnormalities in dilated cardiomyopathy: an echocardiographic study. Chest 1986; 89: 526S

49 Athanassopoulos G, Saad C, Diaz R A, Oakley C M, Nihoyannopoulos P. Can Doppler derived parameters of left ventricular diastolic function differentiate dilated cardiomyopathy from coronary heart failure? Eur Heart J 1989; 10: (suppl)

50 Pasquini J A, Gottdiener J S, Cutler D J, et al. Myocarditis with transient left ventricular apical dyskinesis. Am Heart J 1985; 109: 371

51 Acquatella H, Schiller N B, Puigbo J J et al. M-mode and two-dimensional echocardiography in chronic Chagas' heart disease. A clinical pathologic study. Circulation 1980; 62: 787

52 Valentine H, McKenna W J, Nihoyannopoulos P, et al. Sarcoidosis. A pattern of clinical and morphological presentation. Br Heart J 1987; 57: 256–263

53 Nihoyannopoulos P. Amyloid heart disease. Current Opinion in Cardiology 1987; 2: 371–376

54 Gottdiener J S, Maron B J, Schooley R T, et al. Two-dimensional echocardiographic assessment of the idiopathic hypereosinophilic syndrome: Anatomic basis of mitral regurgitation and peripheral embolisation. Circulation 1983; 67: 572–578

55 Appleton C P, Hatle L K, Popp R L. Demonstration of restrictive ventricular physiology by Doppler echocardiography. J Am Coll Cardiol 1988; 11: 757–768

56 Hatle L K, Appleton C P, Popp R L. Differentiation of constrictive pericarditis and restrictive cardiomyopathy by Doppler echocardiography. Circulation 1989; 79: 357–370

13

Infective endocarditis

Introduction
The role of echocardiography
Underlying heart disease
Native valve endocarditis
Evidence of valvular damage
Risks of embolisation
Lesions that mimic valvular vegetations
Perivalvular damage
Pericardial effusion
Haemodynamic effects
Prosthetic valve endocarditis
Follow-up of patients with endocarditis

Petros Nihoyannopoulos

INTRODUCTION

Bacteraemia from any cause may be followed by the development of infective endocarditis but its diagnosis may be hampered by the absence of a constant diagnostic criterion. It is therefore apparent that the single most important diagnostic tool is the high index of clinical suspicion, particularly when a patient is known to have congenital heart disease or valvular disease (including prosthetic valves) and has fever and malaise.

The development of effective antibiotic treatment and advances in cardiac surgery have dramatically improved survival in patients with infective endocarditis but the key to significant reduction of mortality and morbidity is early diagnosis.[1]

The advent of two-dimensional echocardiography has provided additional accuracy to the non-invasive assessment of patients with known or suspected infective endocarditis. It can confirm the clinical suspicion of endocardial infection, it can depict complications and it may contribute to the patients' management. The absence of echocardiographic findings, however, does not exclude the possibility of infection, this remaining a clinical task.

The role of echocardiography

Since the first description of valvular vegetations detected by M-mode echocardiography,[2,3,4] cardiac ultrasound has assumed increased importance in the assessment and management of patients with known or suspected infective endocarditis. The advent of two-dimensional echocardiography and more recently transoesophageal echocardiography, has provided additional accuracy to the ultrasonic detection, localisation and characterisation of valvular lesions and complications from the infection.

The role of echocardiography in patients with infective endocarditis can be divided into three main categories, namely the description of the underlying cardiac pathology, the detection of evidence of valvular and/or paravalvular destruction (vegetations, abscess) and thirdly the assessment of the individual patient's clinical course.

Underlying heart disease

The detailed description of the intracardiac anatomy is the primary role of two-dimensional echocardiography, preceding attempts to diagnose vegetations or perivalvular infection. All the conventional echocardiographic views[5] must be obtained to assess the valves and chambers from different projections.

Non-rheumatic pathology of the cardiac valves now constitutes the most frequent underlying heart disease in patients with infective endocarditis. In a recent study[1] we found that only 25% of patients with infective endocarditis had rheumatic valve disease prior to the infection, whereas the majority of patients with native valve endocarditis had either non-rheumatic valve disease or a congenital abnormality of the heart. It was also important to note that in a substantial number of patients (17%) no underlying cardiac pathology could be identified, either clinically or echocardiographically. In this category of patients were included drug addicts with tricuspid valve endocarditis who had a structurally normal tricuspid valve.

Cardiac valve replacement and the use of other intravascular prostheses has increased dramatically over the past 25 years and now prosthetic valve endocarditis accounts for approximately 30% of patients.[1] It is here that traditional echocardiography has its greatest limitations and transoesophageal echocardiography its major applications.

NATIVE VALVE ENDOCARDITIS

Evidence of valvular damage

Infective endocarditis may produce varying degrees of valvular damage such as rupture of chordae tendinae with a flail mitral leaflet (Fig. 1), perforation of an aortic cusp or mitral valve aneurysm. Two-dimensional echocardiography can readily identify these abnormalities while Doppler interrogation and colour flow imaging can assess the resulting valvular regurgitation.

Valvular vegetations are the hallmark of infective endocarditis. It is believed that endocardial damage sets the scene, determining the site where platelets, red cells and fibrin adhere to develop a non-bacterial vegetation. This may then be colonised by circulating bacteria with subsequent bacterial multiplication and further growth of the now infected vegetation. The echocardiographic description of this pathological process has been well-described. Vegetations are intracardiac mass lesions, adherent to a valve with a 'shaggy', irregular appearance which does not impair the motion of the valve. Some vegetations are discrete, sessile masses closely adherent to the valve (Fig. 2), while others are pedunculated (Figs 3 and 4), or friable with free prolapse into a cardiac cavity (Fig. 5). The minimum size of a vegetation that can be detected by echocardiography varies according to technique but is approximately 2 mm. Two-dimensional echocardiography is by far superior in the detection of valvular vegetations when compared with M-mode echocardiography (Fig. 6).[6-12] Table 1 summarises a number of studies which have compared the sensitivity of M-mode and two-dimensional echocardiography in the detection of valvular vegetations. Interestingly, the smaller series evaluating all patients with suspected endocarditis report the highest sensitivities and the larger series the lowest sensitivities. This may be due to the fact that the underlying pathology varied greatly from one study to another.

The valves in patients with rheumatic heart disease or floppy mitral valve may have similar acoustic properties to the vegetations, making the differential diagnosis difficult. The recent addition of transoesophageal echocardiography

212 CARDIAC ULTRASOUND

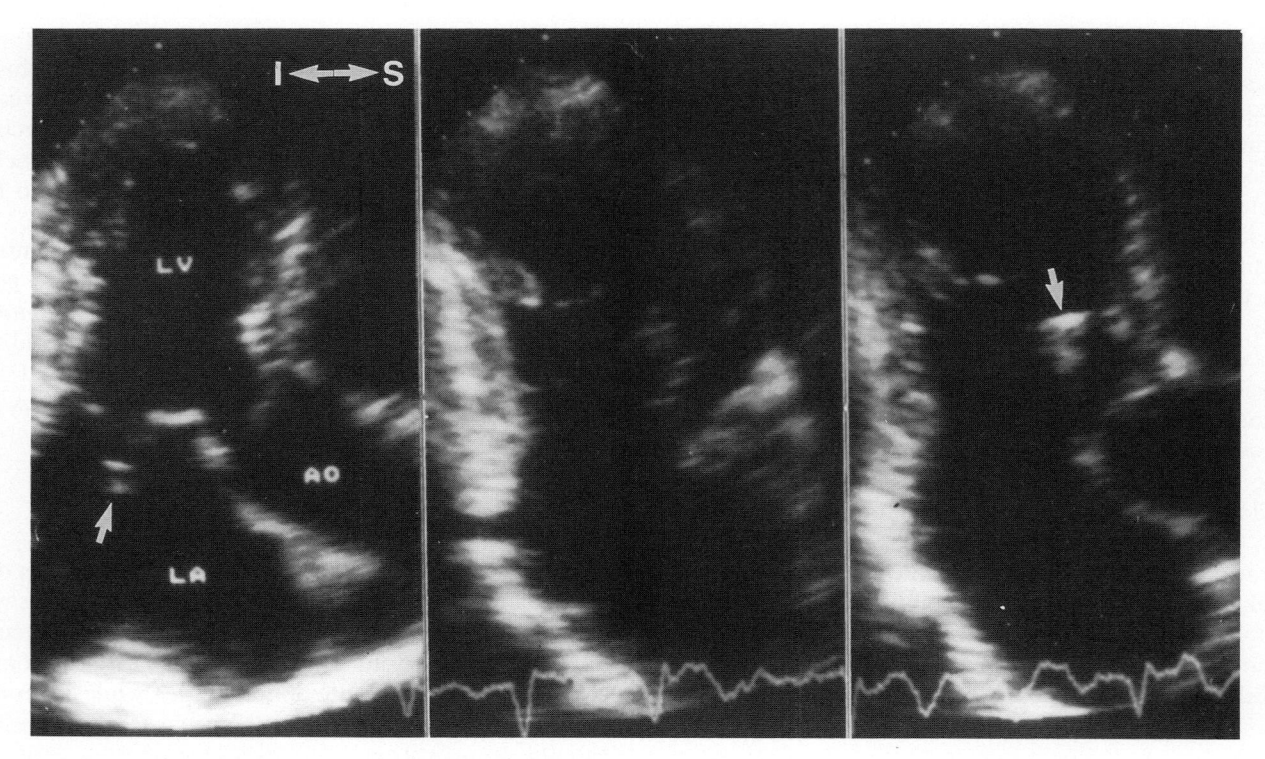

Fig. 1 Apical long axis view of the heart during systole (first panel), early diastole (middle) and late diastole (right panel) showing a vegetation (arrowed) attached to the mitral valve and projecting into the left atrium during systole and into the left ventricle in diastole. (AO = aorta, LA = left atrium, LV = left ventricle.)

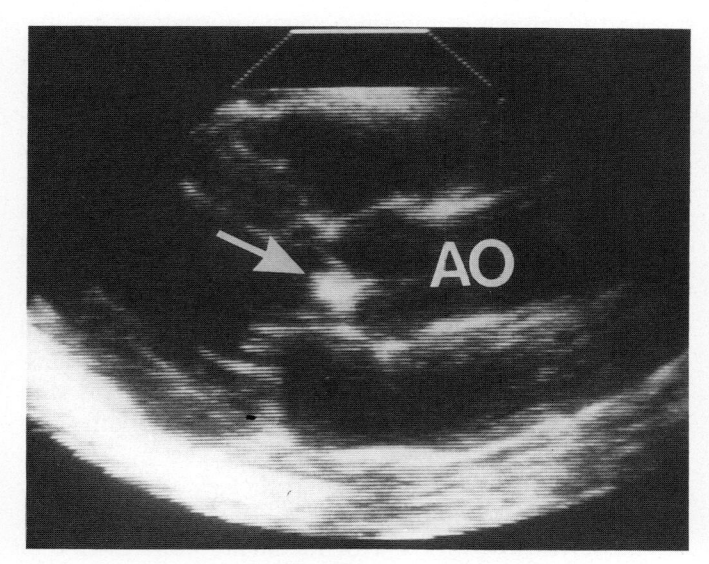

Fig. 2 Long axis parasternal view from a 68-year-old patient with streptococcal aortic valve endocarditis. The vegetation (arrow) is closely attached to the aortic valve, and showed little independent mobility.

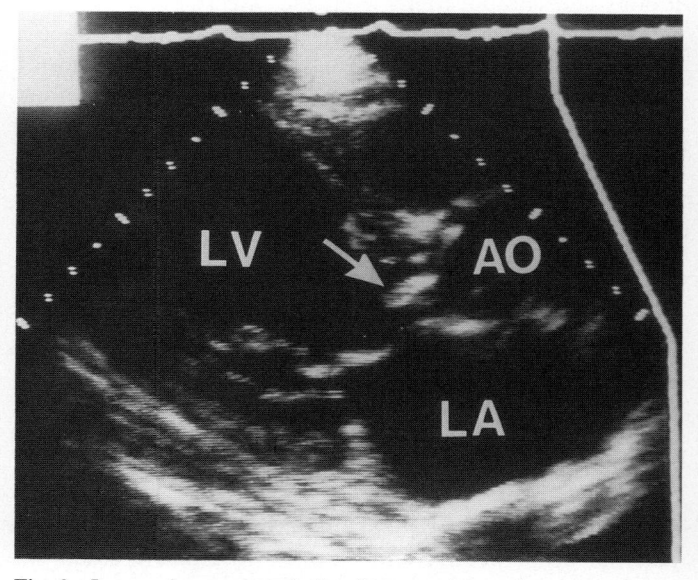

Fig. 3 Long axis parasternal view from another patient with aortic valve endocarditis. In this patient the aortic valve vegetation (arrow) was highly mobile, clearly protruding into the left ventricular outflow tract during diastole.

INFECTIVE ENDOCARDITIS 213

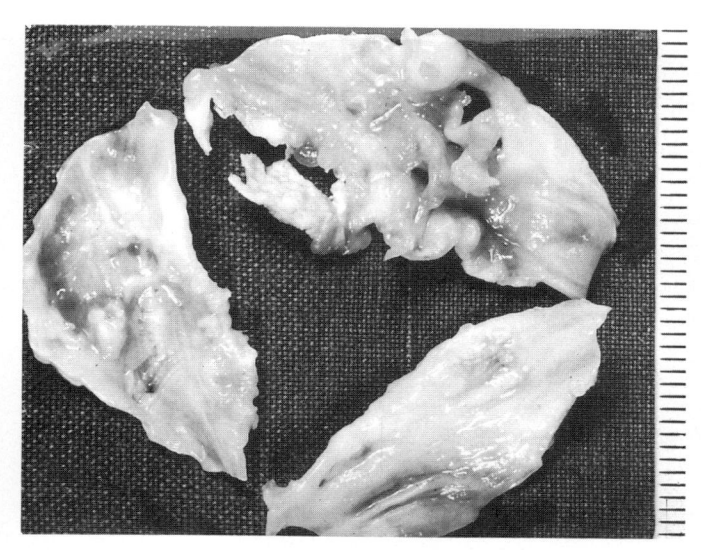

Fig. 4 **Aortic valve with vegetation in the same patient of Fig. 3, removed at the time of surgery for aortic valve replacement.** Note the vegetation attached to the left coronary cusp with secondary erosion and destruction of the cusps.

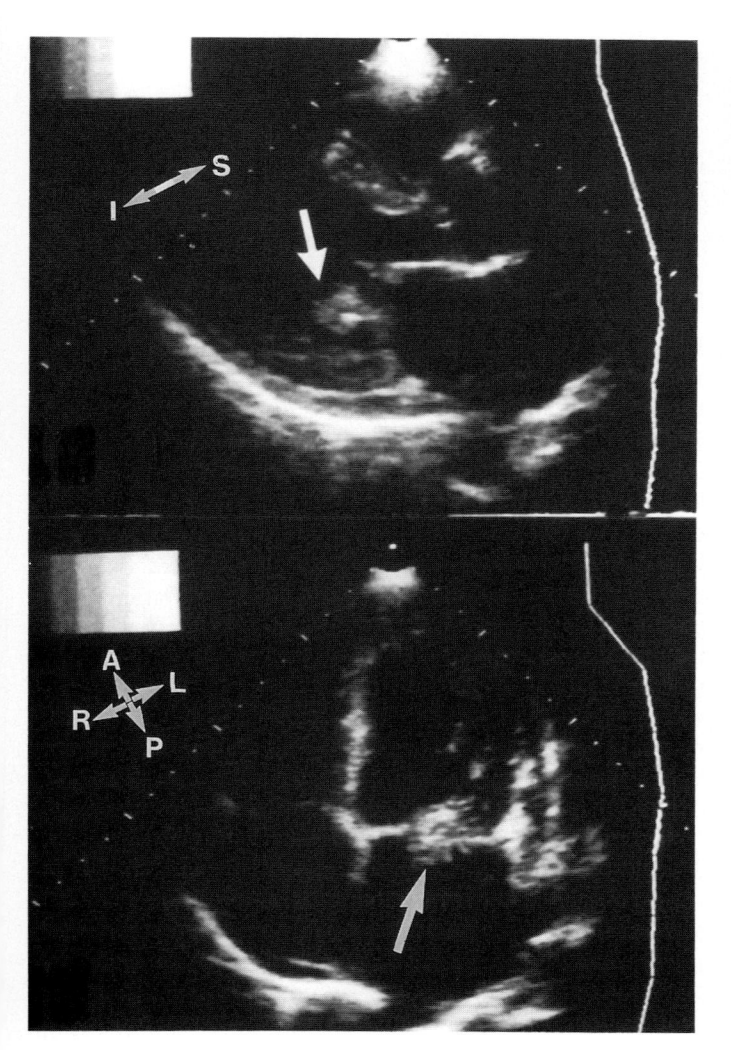

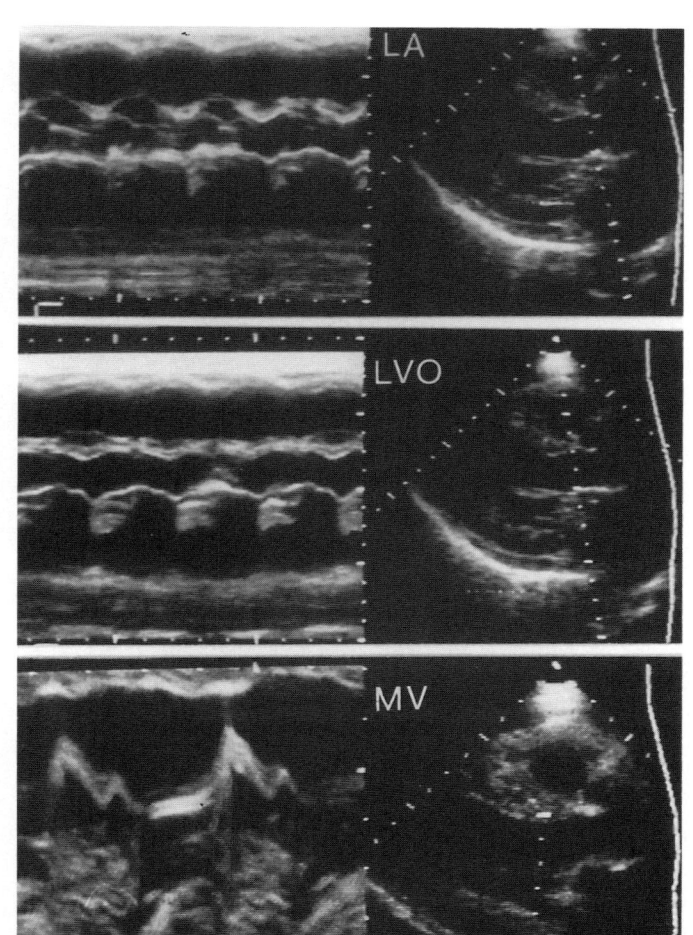

Fig. 6 **Simultaneous M-mode and parasternal long axis two-dimensional echocardiogram from a patient with a large vegetation on the mitral valve.** The two-dimensional image helps to guide and position the M-mode beam across the vegetation throughout the cardiac cycle, along the left atrium during systole (top), left ventricular outflow tract (middle) and mitral valve during diastole (bottom). (LVO = left ventricular outflow tract.)

Table 1 Comparative studies of echocardiographic detection of vegetations

Study	Date	Number of patients	Sensitivity (%) M-mode	2D
Gilbert[6]	1977	7	85	100
Wann[7]	1979	23	78	83
Berger[8]	1980	12	50	83
Martin[9]	1980	43	14	81
Stewart[10]	1980	87	—	54
Strom[11]	1980	24	84	100
Rubenson[12]	1981	11	45	100

Fig. 5 **Long axis parasternal (top) and apical four chamber (bottom) views** showing a large, friable vegetation (arrow) attached to the posterior mitral leaflet.

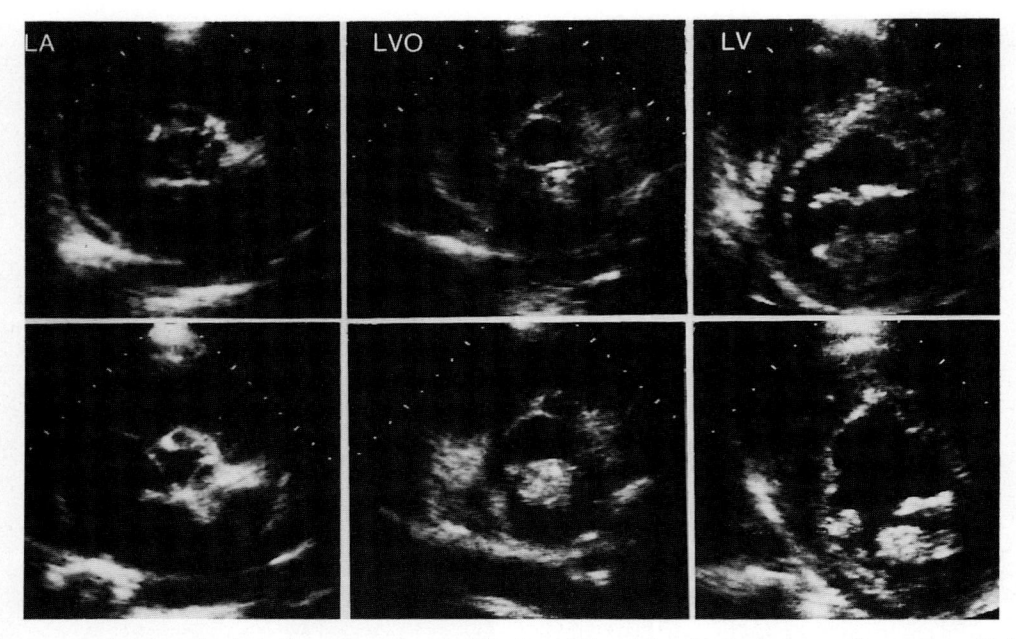

Fig. 7 Sequential parasternal short axis views from the patient in Fig. 6, at left atrial, left ventricular outflow tract and left ventricular levels. The vegetation is seen protruding into the left atrium during mitral ring (LVO, top and bottom) and into the left ventricle during systole (LA, top and bottom) and then coming forward through the diastole (LV, top and bottom). (LVO = left ventricular outflow tract.)

can help in distinguishing valvular vegetations from the surrounding tissues by demonstrating a mobile sessile mass on the atrial side (in the presence of mitral valve disease), or the left ventricular outflow tract (in the presence of aortic valve disease).[13] Conversely, when there is no underlying valvular pathology the detection of vegetations is a lot easier (Fig. 7). The best example is in tricuspid valve endocarditis where vegetations are usually larger than in left sided endocarditis and the tricuspid valve is structurally normal. With two-dimensional echocardiography, right sided vegetations can readily be detected and the best echocardiographic views are those of the parasternal right ventricular inflow tract view (Fig. 8), apical four chamber and right ventricular outflow tract view, where the pulmonic valve can be visualised. Right sided endocarditis has until recently comprised only 5% of cases but in one recent study this figure has risen to over 12%, reflecting increasing intravenous drug abuse and the increased medical use of indwelling catheters.

Patients with small muscular ventricular septal defects may develop right sided endocarditis and vegetations are commonly developed at the site of the jet lesion on the tricuspid leaflets. Figure 9 is from a 28-year-old patient with a moderate size ventricular septal defect and a vegetation on the tricuspid valve. Although several studies have shown the increased frequency of tricuspid valve involvement, pulmonic valve involvement is still rare.[14] A dense echogenic and mobile mass can be clearly seen on the pulmonic valve leaflets by two-dimensional echocardiography, often protruding into the right ventricular outflow tract during diastole (Fig. 10).

Risks of embolisation

Large vegetations are more prone to embolise.[15] Patients with tricuspid valve vegetations often experience pulmonary embolic events, most of them being subclinical. In acute tricuspid endocarditis with large vegetations secondary to a coagulase positive staphylococcus, valvulectomy may be indicated to reduce the risk of multiple pulmonary embolisation with abscess formation in the lungs. Of potentially more serious consequences are those patients who have emboli from left sided vegetations. The greatest frequency of major systemic embolic events occur in association with infections that produce large mobile vegetations such as *Haemophilus parainfluenza*, fungal, slow-growing Gram negative bacilli (aspergillus) and nutritionally variant *viridans streptococci*.[16,17] Patients with no history of embolisation who have large vegetations seen on two-dimensional echocardiography are worrisome, but this condition by itself does not usually justify valve replacement.

The proximity of the coronary ostia to the infected aortic valve puts the coronary circulation at risk of embolisation. If fragments of vegetation embolise to the coronary arterial tree they will usually lead to myocardial infarction. Two-dimensional echocardiography is a useful tool for assessing

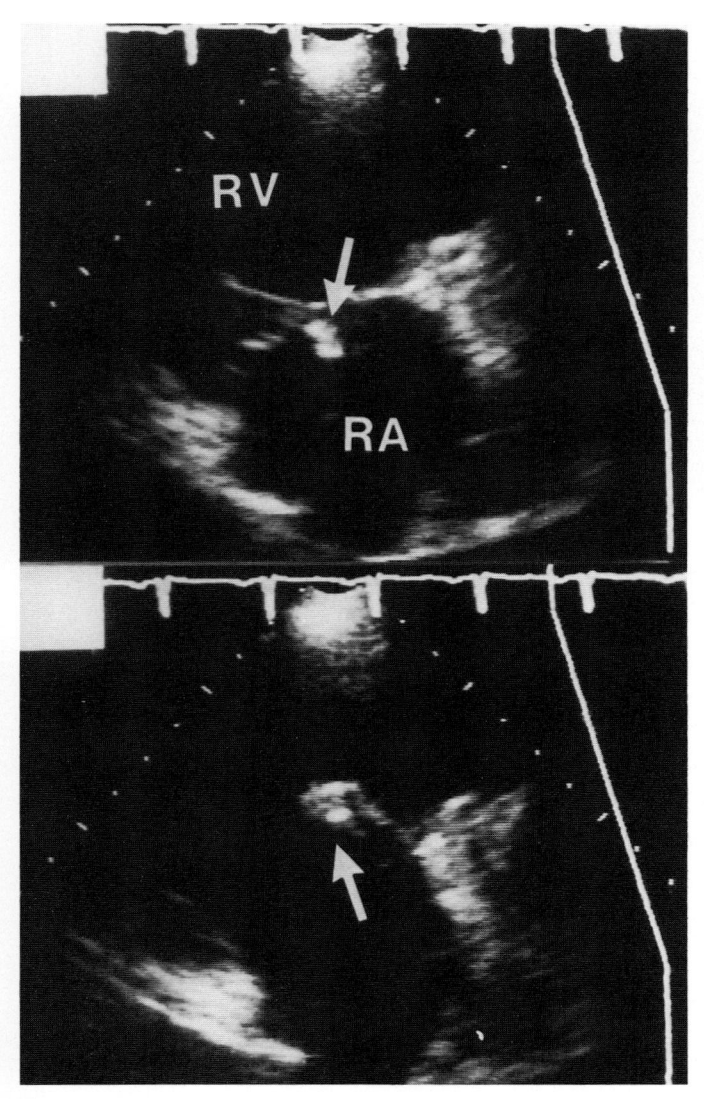

Fig. 8 Parasternal right ventricular inflow tract from a patient with a right sided endocarditis during systole (top) and diastole (bottom). The vegetation (arrow) is seen as an irregular mass attached at the tip of the anterior tricuspid leaflet and protruding into the right atrium during systole.

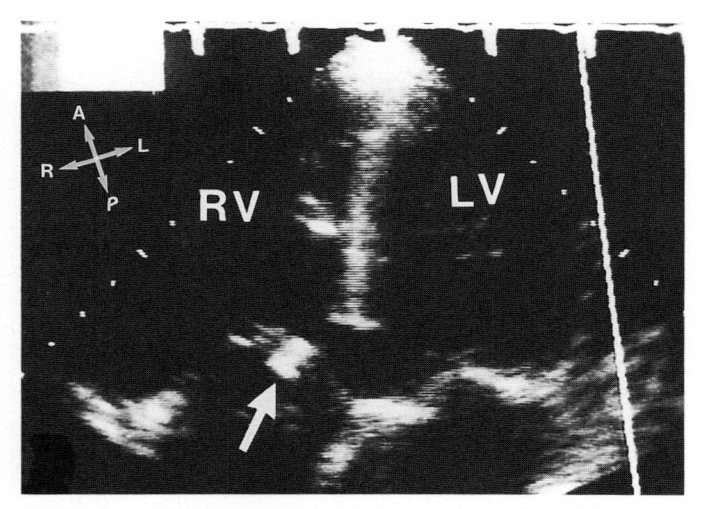

Fig. 9 Apical four chamber view from a young patient with a muscular ventricular septal defect and right sided endocarditis showing vegetations attached to the tricuspid leaflets. All chamber sizes are normal.

segmental wall motion abnormalities in this setting. Occasionally, coronary embolisation may be the patient's main clinical presentation and this obscures the infection. Figure 11 is from a 30-year-old male who was urgently admitted to the coronary care unit with the diagnosis of acute myocardial infarction. A two-dimensional echocardiogram was performed because of his young age and a large vegetation on the mitral valve was readily recognised. A localised antero-apical left ventricular akinesis was also seen, implying a transmural myocardial infarction. Once coronary embolisation from the infected mitral valve was recognised, the patient underwent urgent mitral valve replacement without further complication. A *streptococcus viridans* endocarditis was diagnosed.

In addition to cardiac valves, other intracardiac structures may be the site of vegetations. These include the right side of the ventricular septum in patients with small muscular ventricular septal defects, the right ventricular free wall, usually opposite the site of the ventricular septal defect and the pulmonary artery in patients with patent ductus arteriosus. The increased spatial resolution of two-dimensional echocardiography allows these sites of infection to be recognised in most cases.

Lesions that mimic valvular vegetations

Considerable attention must be paid to technical detail to avoid false positive and false negative studies. All the conventional echocardiographic views must be obtained in each patient without diagnostic bias, so that each valve will be assessed from different projections to minimise the risk of misinterpretations. Proper gain settings are crucial to the diagnosis of vegetations and paravalvular abscesses. It is often helpful to start the recording with the gain all the way up and turn the gain gradually down until an optimum picture of any vegetations is obtained. The gain should be turned down even further so that complications such as pericardial effusion or paravalvular abscess can be detected.

There are several conditions in which infected vegetations can be wrongly diagnosed. Valvular structures involved with marked irregularities and leaflet thickening are often so thickened that they can easily simulate vegetations. Figure 12 is from a patient with rheumatic heart disease without infective endocarditis. The markedly thickened and irregular mitral and aortic valve leaflets are indistinguishable from vegetations. The distinction of pre-existing valvular pathology from infective pathology with images obtained from multiple projections is the essential

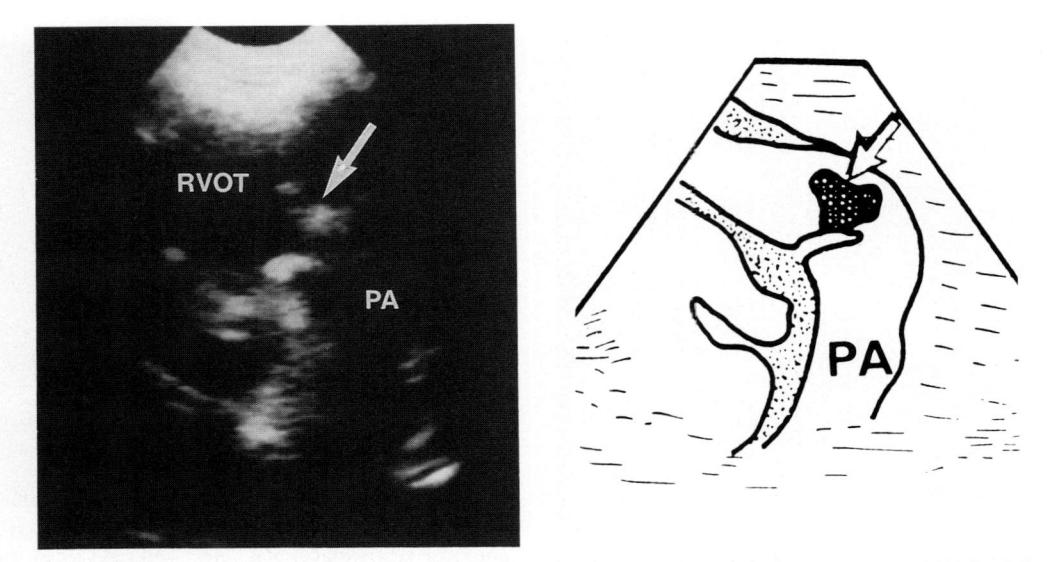

Fig. 10 Parasternal right ventricular outflow tract view visualising the pulmonary valve and main pulmonary artery during diastole. Note the vegetation (arrow) on the pulmonary valve protruding into the right ventricular outflow tract (RVOT).

part of the diagnosis. Floppy mitral valve is perhaps the commonest cause of misinterpretation and misdiagnosis of valvular vegetations (Fig. 13). In our experience, the short axis projection of the left ventricle at the mitral valve level provides images that can usually differentiate pedunculated vegetations from marked mitral leaflet irregularities (degeneration). Libman-Sacks vegetations (non-bacterial vegetations) encountered in patients with systemic lupus erythematosus are very similar to the infective endocarditis lesions and may be difficult to distinguish, but these vegetations are often firmly attached to the proximal or middle portion of the leaflet without exhibiting any independent movement (Fig. 14), in contrast to the more mobile and often pedunculated fresh infected vegetations which typically occupy the leaflet tips. The knowledge of the systemic disorder may be of some additional help for the differential diagnosis between infected and sterile vegetations. These non-bacterial vegetations can also get infected, particularly as some of these patients are immunosuppressed. In this case they are almost impossible to differentiate. Intracardiac masses other than vegetations can also be great mimics of vegetations. Thrombus formation on cardiac implants such as prosthetic valves, pacing wires or central lines reaching the right atrium may become indistinguishable from infected material. A final diagnostic problem occurs in elderly patients with sclerotic lesions in the mitral and aortic valves, as small areas of leaflet degeneration can simulate vegetations.

A previously obtained echocardiographic study, in the absence of any suspicion of infection, can be of considerable assistance. If the patient presents at a later date with a condition that seems to be infective endocarditis, the previously obtained echocardiographic examination will serve as a baseline comparative study and it will prove crucial for the differential diagnosis between vegetations and underlying pathology.

It is therefore emphasised that the diagnosis of infective endocarditis is a clinical task and the echocardiographic detection of vegetations should play a strong supportive role. Vegetations may be impossible to visualise in patients with structurally very abnormal valves or they may be invisible because they are too small, laminar or spread over the valve surface and adjacent endocardium rather than being protuberant and mobile. Whilst two-dimensional echocardiography is an excellent diagnostic tool, it is by no means easy in this condition and its accurate performance and interpretation require considerable training and experience.

Perivalvular damage

Although vegetations are the hallmark of infective endocarditis, echocardiography also provides clinically important information regarding the presence of perivalvular infection. Spread of the infection from the valve to adjacent structures may result in severe suppurative complications. Aortic ring abscesses are reported to occur more frequently than mitral ring abscesses[17,18] and two-dimensional echocardiography may help in the detection of these complications (Fig. 15). Perivalvular damage is more common when more aggressive organisms such as staphylococci or enterococci are involved.

Echocardiographically, a perivalvular abscess formation appears as an echo-free space at the base of the aortic root or in the upper part of the inter-ventricular septum.[19–21] A double shadow is noted in the aortic wall adjacent to the

INFECTIVE ENDOCARDITIS 217

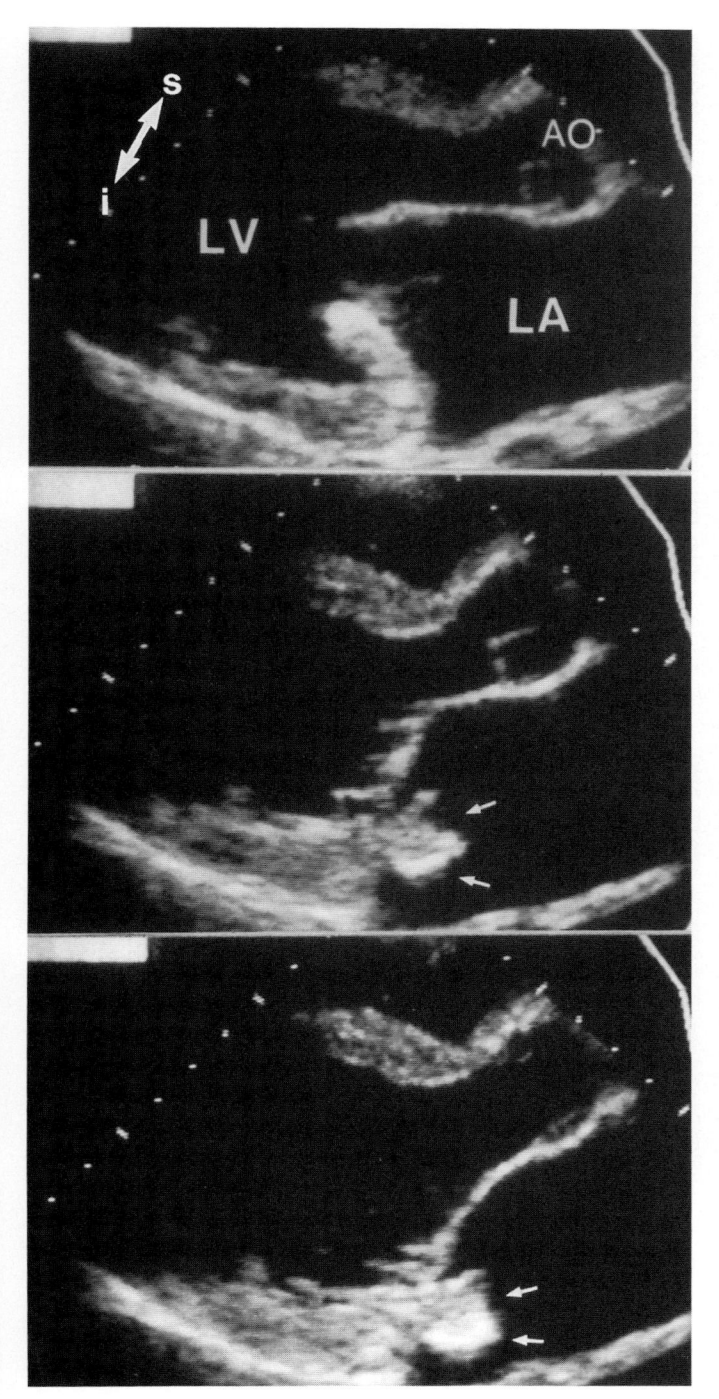

Fig. 11 Parasternal long axis view during diastole (top), late diastole (middle) and systole (bottom) from a 30-year-old patient with a large vegetation (arrows) on the posterior mitral leaflet. Note also that the left ventricle is dilated.

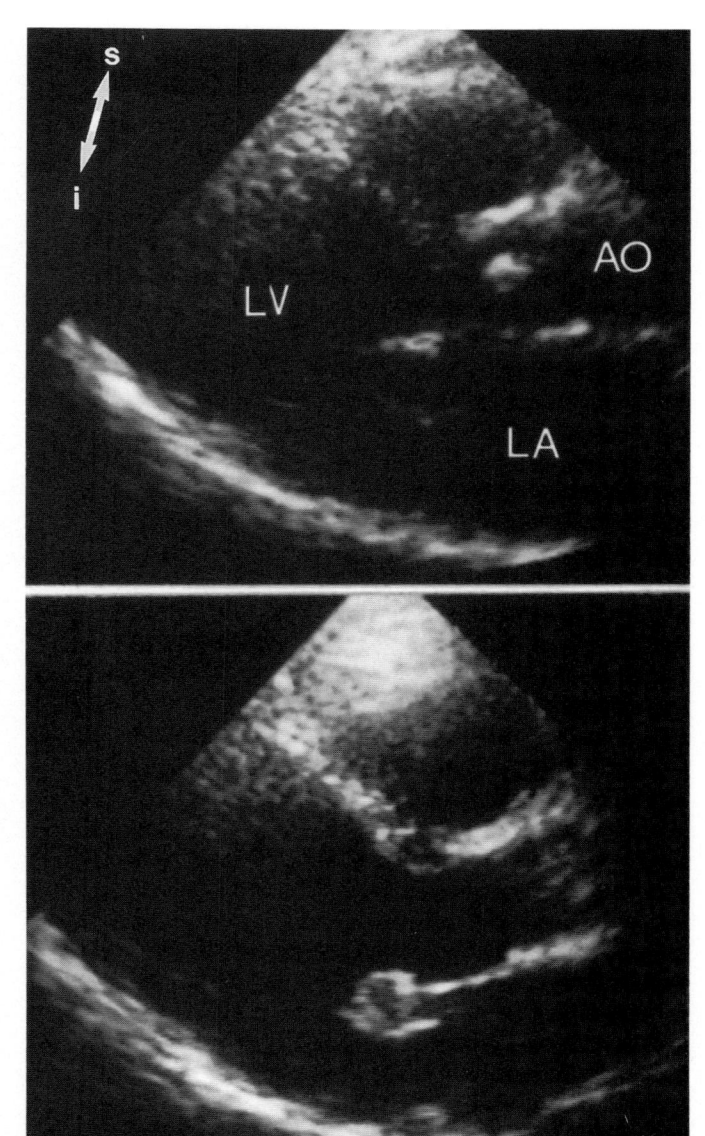

Fig. 12 Parasternal long-axis view during diastole (top) and systole (bottom) from a patient with rheumatic heart disease. This patient had never had endocarditis. Note that the mitral and aortic valve appearances can easily be misinterpreted as having vegetations. This 'lumpy' valve appearance, however, is not seen from short axis projections.

diseased valve (Figs 16 and 17). If this shadow is seen in the anterior aortic wall, an area of reduced echo density may be discerned extending into the upper interventricular septum, representing downward extension of the abscess. When aortic root abscess involves the sinus of Valsalva, aneurysmal enlargement and perforation may occur creating a left-to-right shunt from the aorta to the right ventricle. The haemodynamic consequences of this complication can often be appreciated as enlargement of the right ventricle and a hyperdynamic left ventricle. This abnormal flow is detectable on colour flow echocardiography.

Progression of the infection into the adjacent interventricular septum resulting in abscess formation can be suspected clinically by the new onset of conduction disturbances, particularly complete heart block. Extensive abscess formation involving the region of the left ventricular out-

218 CARDIAC ULTRASOUND

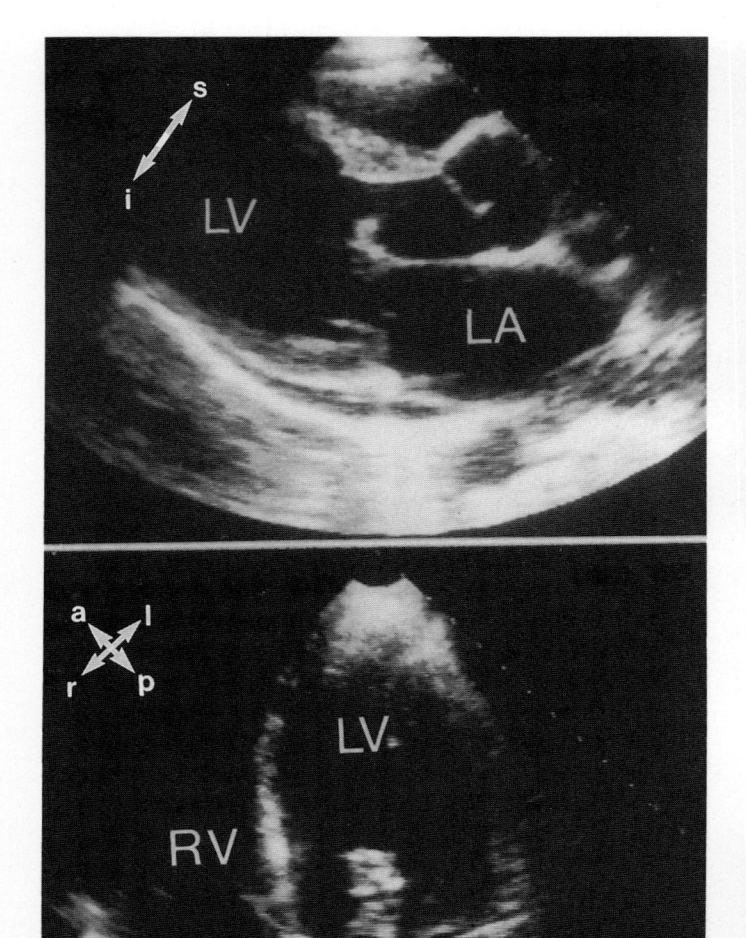

Fig. 13 Parasternal long axis (top) and apical four chamber (bottom) views from a patient with floppy mitral valve and vegetation. This patient underwent surgery for mitral valve replacement. The mitral valve was largely disorganised and had a large, friable vegetation up on the anterior mitral leaflet.

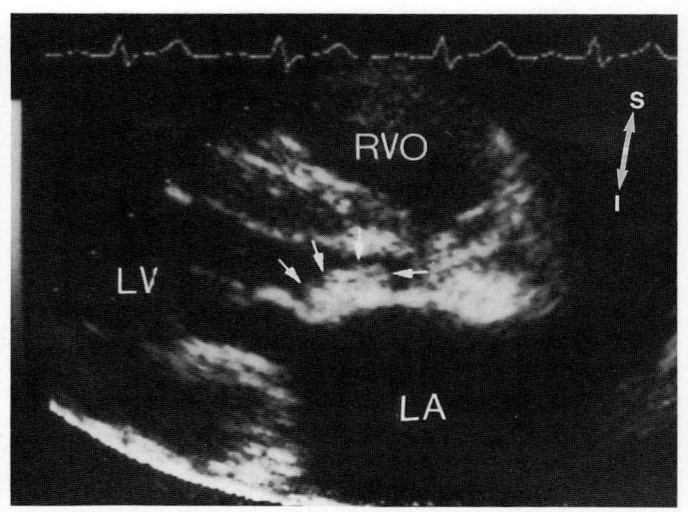

Fig. 14 Parasternal long axis view from a patient with systemic lupus erythematosus, showing a large vegetation (arrows) on the anterior mitral leaflet. Note that the lesion occupies the middle portion of the leaflet, sparing the leaflet's tip. Furthermore, this mass did not exhibit any independent movement from that of the leaflet. (RVO = right ventricular outflow tract.)

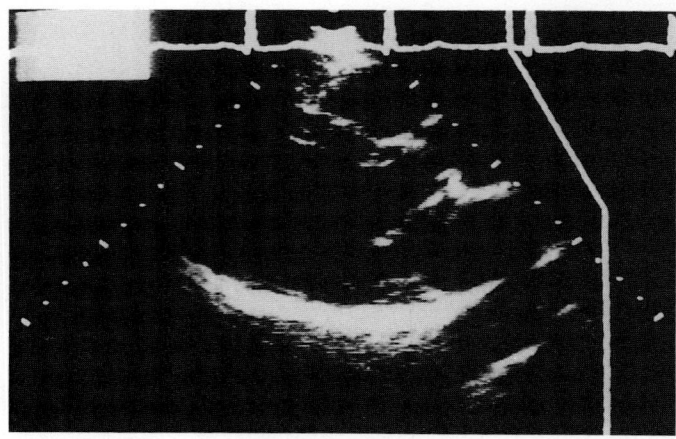

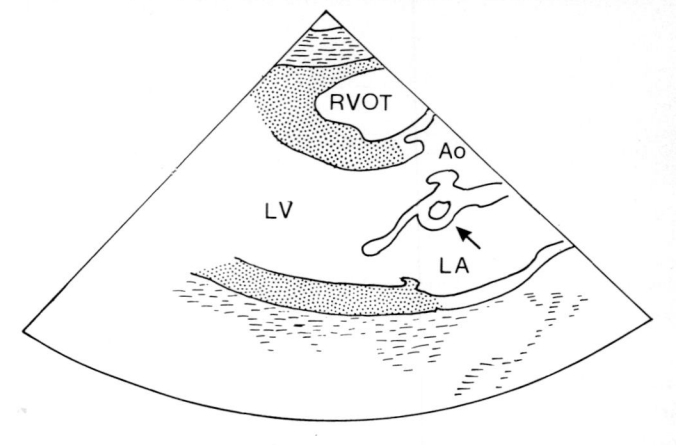

Fig. 15 Parasternal long axis view showing an abscess cavity (arrows) between the origin of the anterior mitral leaflet and the posterior aortic wall. (RVOT = right ventricular outflow tract.)

flow tract is an indication for early surgical intervention. The full echocardiographic description of the extension of the perivalvular damage is therefore of major importance for the surgeons in the pre-operative planning of the surgical procedure, namely aortic valve replacement versus composite aortic valve and root replacement.

Pericardial effusion

Pericardial involvement in infective endocarditis is rare. In our recent series, pericardial effusion occurred in less than 3% of consecutive patients with a first episode of endocarditis.[22] Pericarditis is often associated with *Staphylococcus aureus* infective endocarditis and results from bacteraemia

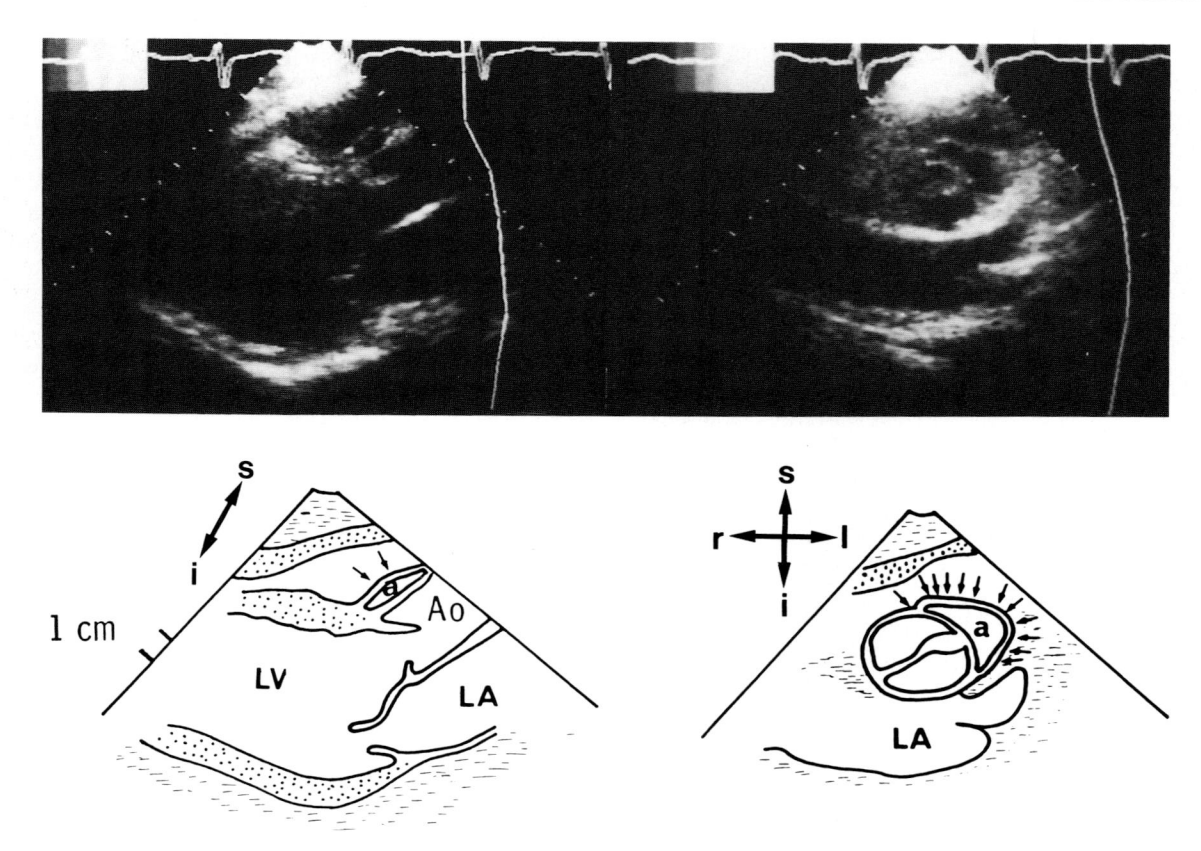

Fig. 16 **Parasternal long axis (left) and short axis (right) views,** showing a large abscess cavity (arrows) anterior to the aortic root. (a = abscess cavity.)

or direct extension of a myocardial abscess into the pericardial cavity, constituting a grave complication. Acute pericarditis may also be the initial presentation of infective endocarditis. This is a more benign form of pericardial effusion, usually being sterile and regressing with antibiotic treatment. The cause is unknown but it is probably a manifestation of the altered immune state of the patient. The presence of pericardial fluid can easily be detected with two-dimensional echocardiography but the diagnosis of purulent pericarditis should be established by pericardiocentesis.

Haemodynamic effects

One of the major complications of infective endocarditis is the patient's acute haemodynamic deterioration. The clinical course of patients with infective endocarditis involving the aortic valve differs significantly from that involving the mitral valve. These patients may deteriorate quickly and consequently treatment should be in an institution where emergency surgery is available. Acute aortic regurgitation may follow sudden prolapse of an aortic cusp, tearing of a cusp or perforation of a leaflet in a patient with a previously competent or near competent aortic valve. The patient is ill, vasoconstricted, tachycardic and may be hypotensive and restless, making the clinical diagnosis very difficult. Doppler echocardiography, particularly with colour flow imaging, is extremely helpful in the assessment of the patient's haemodynamic status. Acute aortic regurgitation into a non-compliant left ventricle results in a rapid rise of left ventricular diastolic pressure which exceeds the left atrial pressure in late diastole with consequent premature mitral closure and sometimes 'diastolic' mitral regurgitation seen on Doppler. If continuous wave Doppler is used, the aortic regurgitant flow pattern will show a rapid decrease in the maximal velocity which will reflect the rapid rise of left ventricular diastolic pressures and the rapid drop in aortic diastolic pressure. The superimposition of M-mode recording is helpful in timing the diastolic events and it will show the early closure of the mitral valve preceding the P wave of the electrocardiogram and markedly preceding the hyperkinetic inward movement of the left ventricular posterior wall.[23]

Acute mitral regurgitation usually results from chordal rupture or destruction of leaflet tissue.[24] The left atrium is usually small and non-compliant, leading to rapid rise of left atrial pressures and to pulmonary oedema. The presence and severity of mitral regurgitation can also be directly ascertained with colour flow imaging from multiple views, by the visualisation of a widespread high velocity

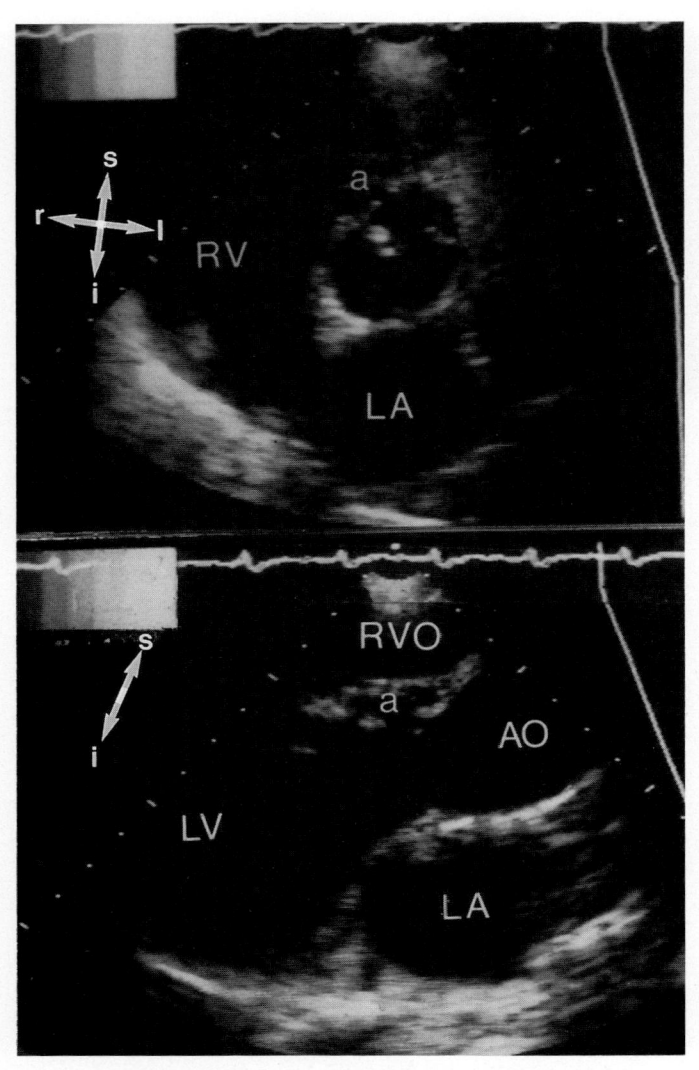

Fig. 17 Parasternal short axis (top) and long axis (bottom) from another patient with endocarditis and an aortic root abscess. Note here that the aortic valve is tricuspid with a samll localised vegetation. (a = abscess cavity, AO = aortic root, LA = left atrium, LV = left ventricle, RVO = right ventricular outflow tract.)

and high intensity turbulent jet in the left atrium, reaching the pulmonary veins. In patients who have chronic mitral regurgitation following an episode of infective endocarditis, serial echocardiographic examinations have proved helpful in predicting which patient will do well after mitral valve replacement. In a group of patients who had surgery for chronic mitral regurgitation, a higher 5 year mortality was seen in patients with left ventricular internal systolic dimensions of greater than 50 mm.[25]

In addition to the obvious value of Doppler echocardiography for assessing severity of valvular regurgitation in patients with infective endocarditis, Doppler and colour flow imaging are also helpful when looking for rare fistulous communications from a sinus of Valsalva aneurysm or a perivalvular abscess to the right or left heart chamber.[26,27]

PROSTHETIC VALVE ENDOCARDITIS

The development of valve replacement for the management of patients with valvular heart disease provided a new opportunity for the development of endocarditis. A prosthetic valve can become infected by organisms introduced at the time of surgery, through wound infection and mediastinitis after surgery. It can also occur at any later time, following spontaneous bacteraemia or bacteraemia following instrumentation in the same way that native valves become infected. The causal organisms are different in early infections from those found in later infections so it is helpful to distinguish 'early' from 'late' prosthetic valve endocarditis. Most early onset prosthetic valve endocarditis occurs within 2 weeks of surgery but some organisms may take as long as 2 or 3 months to show themselves. Fungal or other indolent infections (for example klebsiella) may take even longer to appear. Although it is customary to define the cut-off of early versus late prosthetic valve endocarditis at a postoperative time of three months, this time may vary according to the organism involved so that it is preferable if possible to refer to early or late prosthetic valve endocarditis without stipulating an exact time.

In major cardiac centres, prosthetic valve endocarditis now accounts for about one-third of all cases with endocarditis. It still carries a high mortality but this excess mortality is largely confined to cases with early prosthetic valve endocarditis, while the mortality of late prosthetic valve endocarditis is now comparable with that of infections of native valves. The incidence of infection does not differ between mechanical and tissue valves. Both are more susceptible to infection if there is a paravalvular leak. Echocardiography now plays a vital role in the detection of valve malfunction when infection is suspected. Traditional precordial two-dimensional echocardiographic examination is very limited in its ability to detect infected material surrounding the prosthetic valve, as the prosthetic material generates multiple reflections and reverberations which obscure the visualisation of the much more subtle echogenicity of vegetations and/or perivalvular abscess formation. This applies to all types of prosthesis. In patients with bioprosthetic valves, vegetations can occasionally be detected, as these valves have thin leaflets, often echocardiographically transparent, mounted on thin stents (Fig. 18).

Recently with the introduction of the transoesophageal approach, the diagnostic value of echocardiography has been dramatically improved in the context of prosthetic valve endocarditis.[13,28,29] Imaging the heart from the oesophagus provides a clear visualisation of virtually all cardiac structures without disturbance by bones, lungs and the precordial chest wall. The close relationship between the oesophagus and the heart allows higher transducer frequencies to be applied, leading to improved image resolution. More accurate assessment of the prosthetic ring

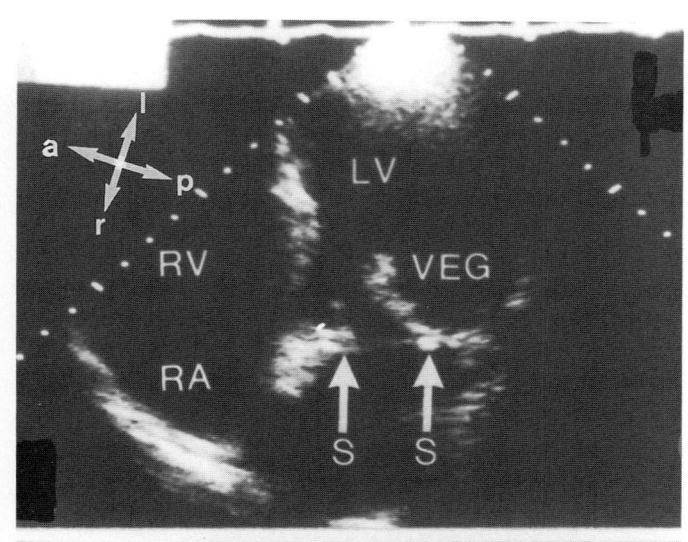

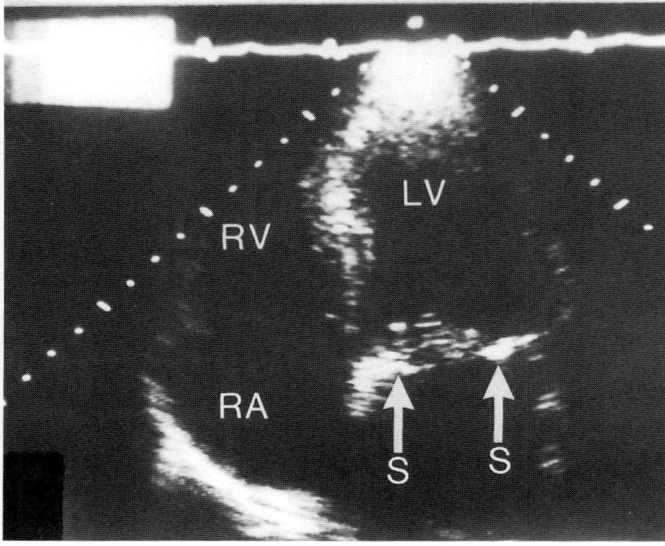

Fig. 18 Apical four chamber view during diastole (top) and systole (bottom) from a patient with a Mitroflow pericardial bioprosthesis. A large, highly mobile and echogenic mass is clearly visualised, attached to the valve leaflets. (S = stents of the artificial valve, VEG = vegetation.)

and the presence or absence of vegetations can be obtained without interference of the prosthetic material. If there is a discrete vegetative mass with motion distinct from the underlying prosthesis, detection is enhanced. Often, infection may result in disruption of sutures or supporting tissues, allowing the prosthetic ring to move. This partial dehiscence of the prosthetic valve ring can readily be identified with transoesophageal echocardiography and constitutes one of the major indications of this technique, although this can occasionally be seen precordially. Perhaps the most clinically valuable information that echocardiography can provide in prosthetic valve endocarditis is the presence or absence of a ring abscess. These occur a lot more frequently in patients with aortic prostheses[30] and may be suspected clinically in the presence of persisting unexplained pyrexia. The usual trans-thoracic echocardiographic examination is extremely poor in the detection or exclusion of paravalvular abscess in the presence of a prosthetic valve and may mislead or delay crucial therapeutic decisions, in the case of false negative findings. Transoesophageal echocardiography provides excellent imaging of the aortic and mitral annulus and the presence of a ring abscess can be identified promptly. Furthermore, patients with suspected prosthetic valve endocarditis can be followed up easily with transoesophageal echocardiography, so that further potentially serious complications can be detected early.

The improved image resolution of the transoesophageal approach has also enhanced greatly the detection and assessment of regurgitant lesions with colour Doppler mapping. The positioning of the transducer against the left atrial wall means that the ultrasound is reflected from atrial blood and tissue without being attenuated by atrioventricular prostheses, thus facilitating the detection of paravalvular leaks. The superior diagnostic accuracy of the transoesophageal approach for two-dimensional imaging and colour Doppler flow velocity mapping, has been shown in patients with prosthetic valve malfunction.[31] When prosthetic mitral regurgitation is severe, the jet reaches the posterior wall of the left atrium and pulmonary veins, producing a flow reversal into the pulmonary veins displayed as a multicolour variance jet on some types of colour flow imaging.

FOLLOW-UP OF PATIENTS WITH ENDOCARDITIS

Echocardiography now plays a vital role after the diagnosis of infective endocarditis has been made. The ready availability of this technique together with its non-invasive nature, constitutes the ideal technique of serial assessment and the progression or regression of the infected valve. Doppler echocardiography with colour flow imaging evaluates the valvular regurgitation, while two-dimensional imaging shows the change in size and shape of the vegetations. The serial measurement of left ventricular function is the third important assessment that echocardiography can provide. Left ventricular function may be seriously affected for a short time during the acute phase of infective endocarditis.[32] The early detection of left ventricular dysfunction with echocardiography may alert the clinicians to the potential danger of the occurrence of arrythmias.

Vegetations almost invariably change in their echocardiographic appearance. The majority of vegetations become smaller with increased echodensity as they heal. This eventually makes them indistinguishable from other localised degenerative valvular lesions. Some vegetations may actually increase in size, but this constitutes a rather early assessment during the hyperacute phase of the infection.

Lastly, a few more vegetations will remain unchanged in size following bacteriological cure, but compared with the initial mobile and fluffy appearance of the fresh vegetation they will become more echogenic and virtually immobile.

There are obviously problems with attempting to size vegetations on serial echocardiographic studies. Sizing these lesions requires strict technical and interpretative expertise. The same operator, interpreter and instrument must be used when studying the patient serially. Slight differences in transducer positions or in the instrument, can markedly alter the apparent size of the vegetation. We commonly advocate weekly serial assessment when the diagnosis of infective endocarditis has been established and the patient is clinically stable, so that changes in size of vegetations or the development of new vegetative lesions and/or paravalvular abscess can be recognised promptly.

Lastly, a pre-discharge echocardiogram is very important, as it will assess the degree of valve destruction and the resulting valvular leaks after bacteriological cure. This echocardiographic study will also serve as a baseline for further assessment of the medium- and long-term haemodynamic consequences of the infection and for further evaluation, if recurrence of infective endocarditis is suspected.

REFERENCES

1. Nihoyannopoulos P, Oakley C M, Exadactylos N, Ribeiro P, Westaby S, Foale R A. Duration of symptoms and the effects of a more aggressive surgical policy; two factors affecting prognosis of infective endocarditis. Eur Heart J 1985; 6: 380-390
2. Dillon J C, Feigenbaum H, Konecke L L, et al. Echocardiographic manifestations of valvular vegetations. Am Heart J 1973; 86: 698
3. Schelbert H R, Muller O F. Detection of fungal vegetations involving Starr-Edwards mitral valve prosthesis by means of ultrasound. Vasc Surg 1972; 6: 20
4. Spangler R D, Johnson M L, Holmes J H, et al. Echocardiographic demonstration of bacterial vegetations in active infective endocarditis. JCU 1973; 1: 126
5. Tajik A J, Hagler D J, Mair D D, Lie J T. Two-dimensional real-time ultrasonic imaging of the heart and great vessels. Technique, image orientation, structure identification and validation. Mayo Clin Proc 1978; 53: 271-303
6. Gilbert B W, Haney R S, Crawford F. Two-dimensional echocardiographic assessment of vegetative endocarditis. Circulation 1977; 55: 346
7. Wann L S, Hallam C C, Dillon J C, et al. Comparison of M-mode and cross-sectional echocardiography in infective endocarditis. Circulation 1979; 60: 728
8. Berger M, Delfin L S, Jelveh M, et al. Two-dimensional echocardiographic findings in right-sided infective endocarditis. Circulation 1980; 61: 855
9. Martin R P, Meltzer R S, Chia B L, et al. Clinical utility of two-dimensional echocardiography in infective endocarditis. Am J Cardiol 1980; 46: 379
10. Stewart J A, Silimperi D, Harris P, et al. Echocardiographic documentation of vegetative lesions in infective endocarditis: clinical implications. Circulation 1980; 61: 374
11. Strom J, Becker R, Davis R, et al. Echocardiographic and surgical correlations in bacterial endocarditis. Circulation 1980; 62: 164
12. Rubenson D S, Tucker C R, Stinson E B, et al. The use of echocardiography in diagnosing culture-negative endocarditis. Circulation 1981; 64: 641
13. Taams M A, Gussenhoven E J, Bos E, de Jaegere P, Roelandt T R T C, Sutherland G R. Enhanced morphological diagnosis in infective endocarditis by transoesophageal echocardiography. Br Heart J 1990; 63: 109-113
14. Andy J J, Sheikh M U, Ali N, et al. Endocardiographic observations in opiate addicts with active infective endocarditis: frequency of involvement of the various valves and comparison of echocardiographic features of right and left-sided cardiac valve endocarditis. Am J Cardiol 1977; 40: 17
15. Nasser F N, Gura G M, Sewart J B, Tajik A J. Embolism and infective endocarditis: identification of high risk group by two-dimensional echocardiography. Circulation 1980; 62: 100
16. Geraci J E, Wikowske G J, Wilson W R, Washington J A II. Haemophilus endocarditis: a report of 14 patients. Mayo Clin Proc 1977; 52: 209-215
17. Merchant R K, Louria D B, Geisler P H, Edgecomb J H, Utz J P. Fungal endocarditis: a review of the literature and report of three cases. Ann Int Med 1958; 48: 242-266
18. Arnett E R, Roberts W C. Valve ring abscess in active infective endocarditis. Frequency, location and clues to clinical diagnosis from the study of 95 necropsy patients. Circulation 1976; 54: 140-145
19. Scanlon J C, Seward J B, Tajik A J. Valve ring abscess in infective endocarditis: visualisation with wide angle two-dimensional echocardiography. Am J Cardiol 1982; 49: 1794
20. Pollak S J, Felner J M. Echocardiographic identification of an aortic valve ring abscess. J Am Coll Cardiol 1986; 7: 1167
21. Saner H E, Asinger R W, Homans D C, Helseth H K, Hosperger K J. Two-dimensional echocardiographic identification of complicated aortic root endocarditis: implications for surgery. J Am Coll Cardiol 1987; 10: 859
22. Ribeiro P, Shapiro L, Nihoyannopoulos P, Gonzalez A, Oakley C M. Pericarditis in infective endocarditis. Eur Heart J 1985; 6: 975-978
23. Mann T, McLaurin L, Grossman C E. Acute aortic regurgitation due to infective endocarditis. N Engl J Med 1975; 293: 108
24. Mintz G S, Kotler M N, Segal B L, et al. Two-dimensional echocardiographic recognition of ruptured chordae tendinae. Circulation 1978; 57: 244
25. Brandenburg R O, Giuliani E R, Wilson W R, et al. Infective endocarditis: a 25 year overview of diagnosis and therapy. J Am Coll Cardiol 1983; 1: 280-291
26. Shaffer E M, Snider A R, Beekman R H, Behrendt D M, Peschiera A W. Sinus of Valsalva aneurysm complicating bacterial endocarditis in an infant: diagnosis with two-dimensional and Doppler echocardiography. J Am Coll Cardiol 1987; 9: 588
27. Fisher E A, Estioko M R, Stern E H, Goldman M E. Left ventricular to left atrial communication secondary to a para-aortic abscess: colour flow Doppler documentation. J Am Coll Cardiol 1987; 10: 222
28. Daniel W G, Schroder E, Muge A, Lichtlen P R. Transoesophageal echocardiography in infective endocarditis. Am J Cardiac Imaging 1988; 2: 78-85
29. Erbel R, Rohmann S, Drexter M, et al. Improved diagnostic value of echocardiography in patients with infective endocarditis by transoesophageal approach: a prospective study. Eur Heart J 1988; 1: 43-53
30. Wilson W R, Danielson G K, Giuliani E R, et al. Prosthetic valve endocarditis. Mayo Clin Proc 1982; 57: 75-81
31. Nellessen U, Schnittger I, Applleton C P, et al. Transoesophageal two-dimensional echocardiography and colour Doppler flow velocity mapping in the evaluation of cardiac valve prostheses. Circulation 1988; 78: 848-855
32. Hackett D, Nihoyannopoulos P, Weston C, Oakley C M. Myocardial depression and nephrotic syndrome in streptococcus sanguis endocarditis. Quart J Med 1985; 57: 867-873

14

Prosthetic valves

Introduction
Types of prosthetic valve
Mechanism of prosthetic valve failure
M-Mode and cross-sectional echocardiography of prosthetic heart valves
Normal prosthetic valve function
Abnormal prosthetic valve function
Bacterial endocarditis

Doppler evaluation of prosthetic heart valves
Technical problems and limitations
Theoretical considerations
In vitro studies
In vivo studies
Aortic prostheses
　Normal function
　Abnormal function

Mitral prostheses
　Normal function
　Abnormal function
Tricuspid prostheses
Transoesophageal echocardiogram in the assessment of prosthetic valve disease

James Nolan and Peter Bloomfield

INTRODUCTION

Patients who have undergone heart valve replacement commonly have associated clinical problems such as coronary artery disease or abnormalities of ventricular function and may also have lung disease such as chronic obstructive airways disease. It may be difficult to assess symptoms such as breathlessness using clinical examination alone. Cardiac catheterisation presents problems, especially in patients with multiple prostheses, and it carries an additional small risk if they are taking anticoagulants. Echocardiography which includes Doppler examination is established as a valuable technique in the assessment of patients with prosthetic heart valves. Careful evaluation of patients using all ultrasound modalities can usually identify abnormal prosthetic valve function and may thus avoid the need for invasive investigations.

In the last 20 years the enthusiasm for biological valve prostheses has produced a large cohort of patients with valves implanted 10 or more years ago. These patients commonly present with heart failure due to bioprosthetic valve failure.[1] Prompt and accurate diagnosis of bioprosthetic valve failure facilitates early surgery for prosthetic valve replacement at lower operative risk before further clinical deterioration has occurred.

There are technical limitations to the use of ultrasound in assessing patients with prosthetic valves, the structure of which may be highly reflective. This causes reverberation of signals which makes it difficult to identify the motion of component parts of the prosthesis. There may also be 'acoustic shadowing' of an area behind the prosthesis which cannot be interrogated by ultrasound either for imaging or for Doppler evaluation.

The different ultrasound techniques used in the assessment of patients with prosthetic valves are complementary to each other, and also to clinical findings and other non-invasive techniques. If a deductive approach is used and all of the information is collated, then an accurate assessment of the patient with a prosthetic valve can usually be made without resorting to cardiac catheterisation. An ultrasound examination taken in isolation may lead to the diagnosis of prosthetic valve dysfunction being missed because of the limitations of the technique.

The aims of this chapter are to describe the findings with each ultrasound modality in normal and abnormal prosthetic valve function. These findings will be described with respect to the different types of valve prosthesis in common use.

TYPES OF PROSTHETIC VALVE

The original mechanical heart valve prosthesis designed by Albert Starr was a ball and cage design and this type of prosthesis with minor modifications is still in use today (Fig. 1). The other principal type of mechanical prosthesis

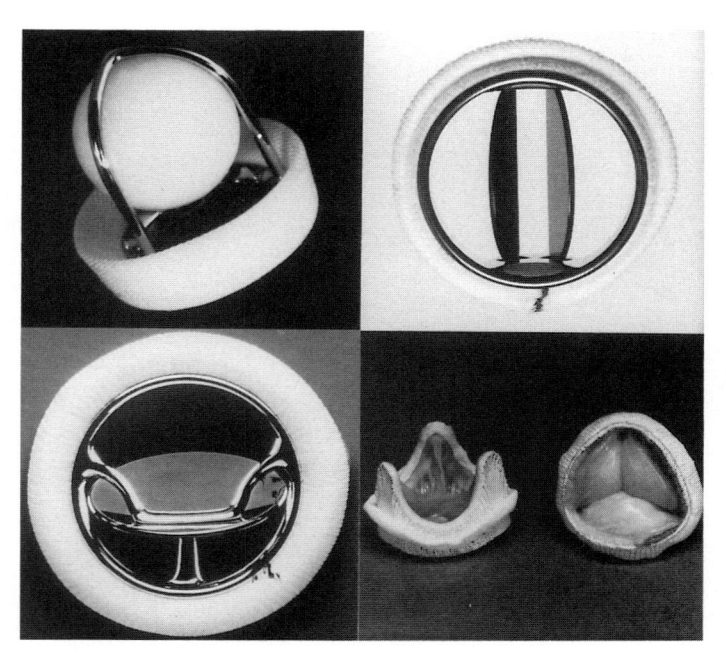

Fig. 1 Examples of commonly used prosthetic heart valves. Top left, Starr–Edwards ball and cage valve; bottom left, Bjork–Shiley monostrut single tilting disc valve; top right, St Jude valve with two tilting discs; and bottom right, Carpentier–Edwards porcine bioprosthetic valve.

is a tilting disc design. A single disc is used in the Bjork–Shiley prosthesis popular in Europe and two tilting discs are used in the St Jude valve which is widely used in North America (Fig. 1). Prosthetic valves made from biological tissue are commonly made from glutaraldehyde treated pig's aortic valves mounted on a wire stent. An example of this is the Carpentier–Edwards valve shown in Figure 1. Bioprosthetic valves have also been fabricated from bovine pericardium, as with the Ionescu–Shiley prosthesis. Antibiotic sterilized human aortic valves are also used for valve replacement in some centres.

MECHANISM OF PROSTHETIC VALVE FAILURE

All prosthetic heart valves are mildly stenotic. Many mechanical prostheses are also designed to have some regurgitant flow to ensure constant blood flow across the prosthetic components in the hope of reducing the risk of thrombosis. These features must be distinguished from valve failure.

Failure of mechanical prosthetic valves is very rarely due to failure of a component but when this does occur the consequences may be dramatic and are often fatal. The tilting disc of a prosthesis may break free from its retaining strut, causing sudden disastrous valve failure and embolisation of valve components into the systemic circulation.[2] Thrombosis interfering with the mechanical action of the prosthesis may occur and rapidly cause severe obstruction.

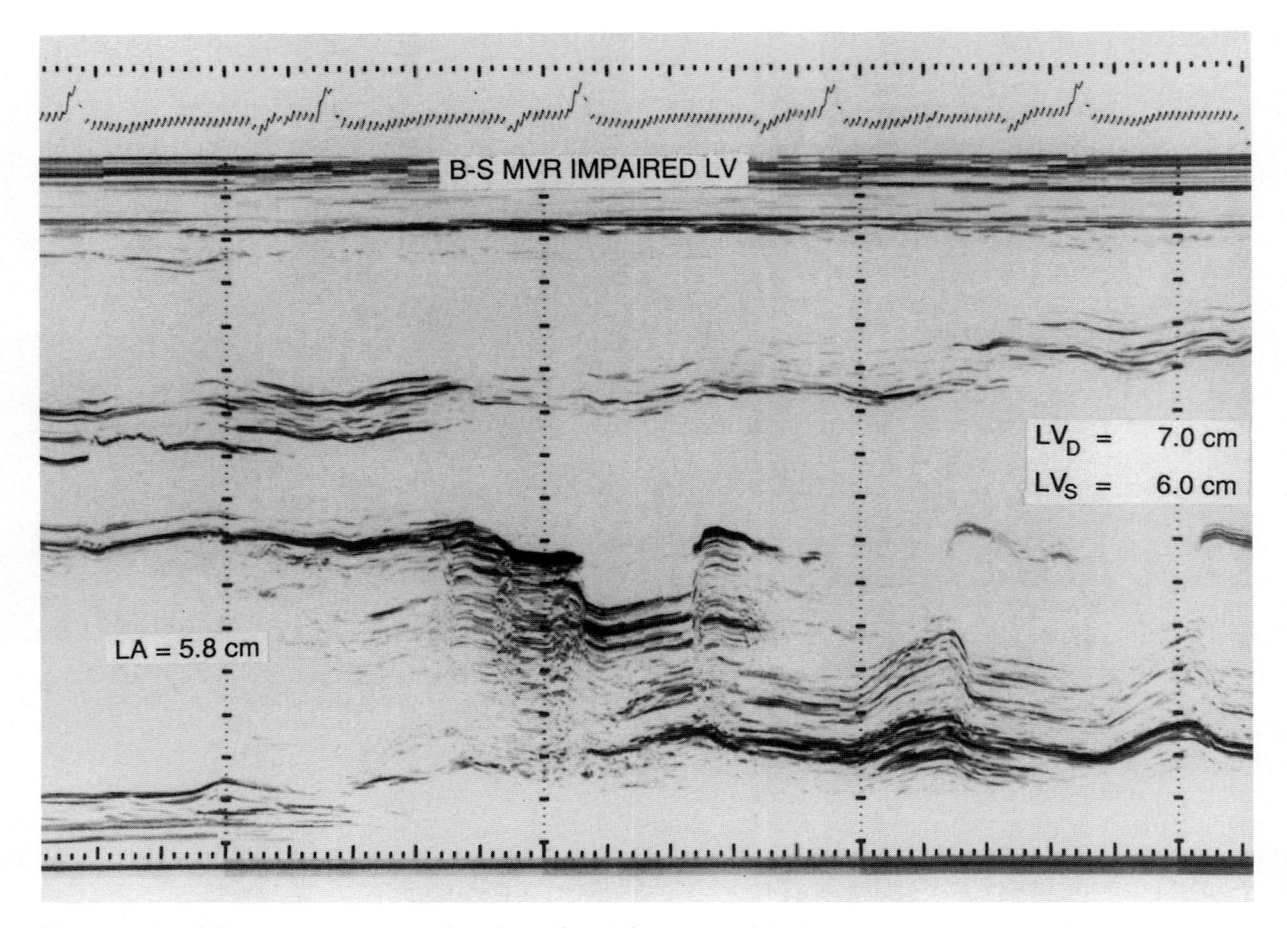

Fig. 2 M-mode echocardiogram scanning from left atrium (left) to left ventricle (right) in a patient with a Bjork–Shiley tilting disc prosthesis and severely impaired ventricular function. The left atrium is enlarged at 5.8 cm and the left ventricle is dilated and hypocontractile with an end diastolic dimension of 7.0 cm and end systolic dimension of 6.0 cm.

An ingrowth of fibrous material or a pannus may gradually occur causing gradual and progressive obstruction to flow.

Intrinsic failure of biological prosthetic valves is most commonly due to rupture of one or more of the cusps of the prosthesis. This may cause the gradual development of symptoms. If cusp rupture occurs rapidly and is severe the patient may become acutely and severely ill with heart failure. The cusps of biological prosthetic valves may calcify and stiffen, rendering the valve functionally stenotic. This mode of failure more commonly occurs in children and young adults and in very young children can occur within one or two years of implantation.

The prosthetic valve may fail to function adequately not because of an intrinsic failure of the prosthesis but because it is inadequately secured to the surrounding tissues. This may occur because of imperfect surgical technique, dehiscence of sutures from friable tissues or erosion of tissue by infection. The end result may be a paraprosthetic leak which if small may cause haemolysis of blood cells in a high velocity jet, and if large enough may cause heart failure.

M-MODE AND CROSS SECTIONAL ECHOCARDIOGRAPHY OF PROSTHETIC HEART VALVES

Normal prosthetic valve function

M-mode echocardiography remains a simple and reliable way of quantitating left ventricular function in patients who do not have wall motion abnormalities due to ischaemic heart disease. It is thus useful for identifying the left ventricular dysfunction that can commonly occur in patients with prosthetic heart valves. As precise measurement of left ventricular dimensions can be made it is also useful in the serial evaluation of patients before and after valve replacement. An example from a patient with severely impaired left ventricular function and a Bjork–Shiley mitral valve prosthesis is shown in Figure 2.

Motion of the disc or ball in a mechanical valve is best appreciated from the apical position in patients with mitral or aortic valve prostheses as motion of these structures is axial to the ultrasound beam. The degree of excursion of the disc or ball and the rate of opening and closing can be

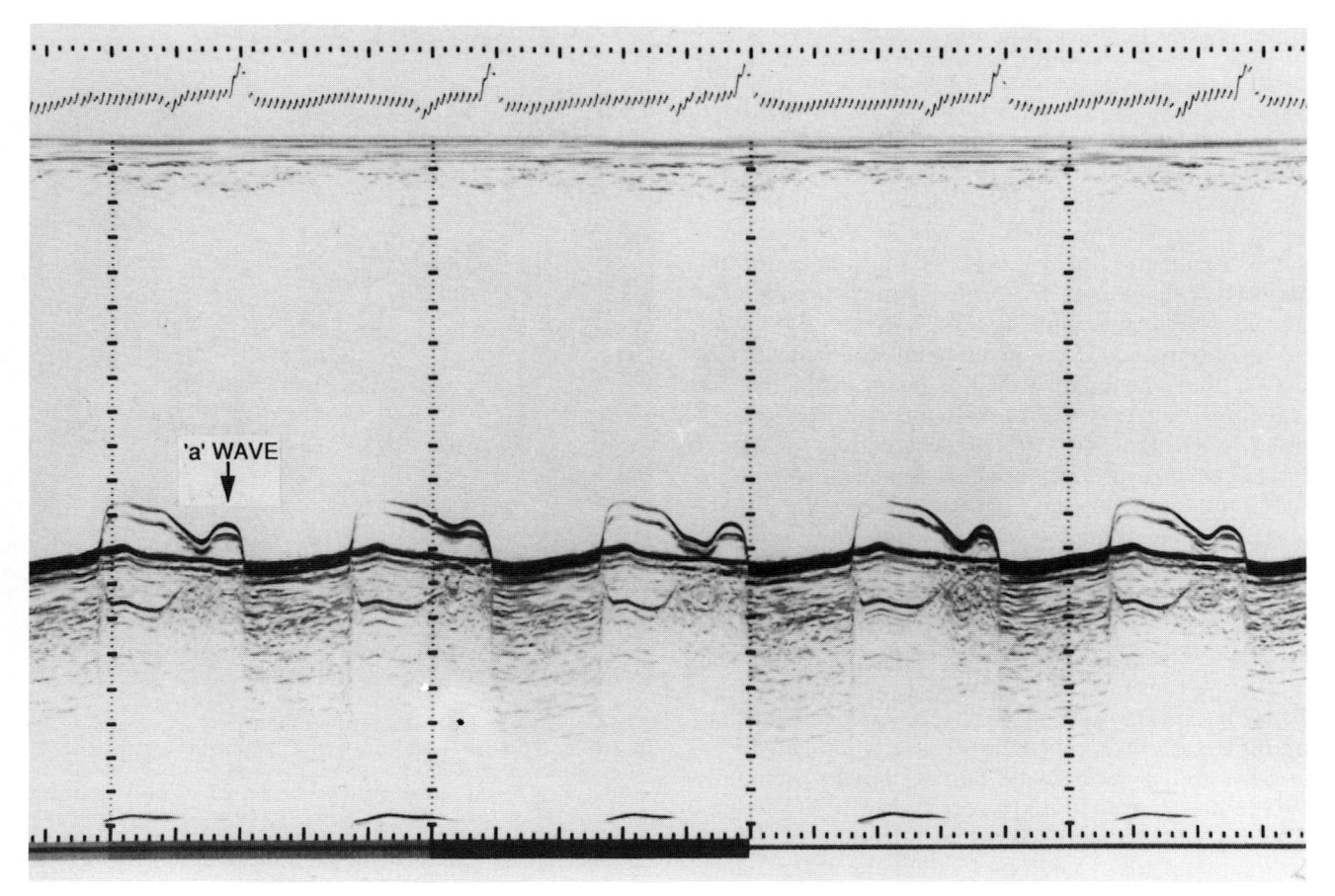

Fig. 3 M-mode echocardiogram recorded from the apex in the same patient shown in Fig. 2. The disc of the Bjork–Shiley prosthesis opens towards the apex with the onset of diastole and starts to close again in mid-diastole reflecting a high left ventricular diastolic pressure. The disc is thrown open again with atrial systole, a wave. Heart failure in this patient was due to impaired left ventricular function and the prosthetic valve was functioning normally.

measured. Overall excursion of the disc can be diminished due to a low cardiac output secondary to impaired ventricular function, but the rate of opening of the disc is normal in these circumstances. Figure 3 is an M-mode recording taken from the apex of the same patient as shown in Figure 2. The disc opens normally but can be seen to close partially before atrial systole which reflects the high left ventricular end diastolic pressure. The prosthesis opens fully again following atrial systole. This can be compared with the motion of the disc in a patient with a Bjork–Shiley mitral valve prosthesis and normal ventricular function shown in Figure 4. The leaflets of bioprosthetic valves can occasionally be identified by M-mode echocardiography, their movements normally giving rise to the typical box-shaped pattern of mild mitral stenosis.

The movement of the component parts of the prosthesis and of the sewing ring can be readily identified by cross-sectional echocardiography. The leaflets of bioprosthetic valves used in the mitral and tricuspid positions can be best imaged from the apical four chamber view. There is a tendency for leaflets to thicken with increasing age of the prosthesis and it is important to recognise this as

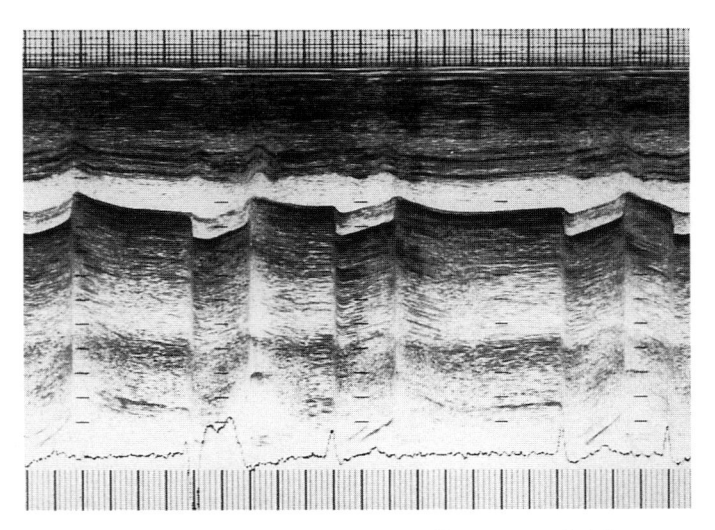

Fig. 4 Left parasternal M-mode echocardiogram recorded from a patient with a normally functioning Bjork–Shiley tilting disc prosthesis.

these changes may erroneously give rise to the suspicion that infective endocarditis is affecting the cusps of the prosthesis.[1,2,3]

Abnormal prosthetic valve function

The assessment of left ventricular function is essential in the evaluation of patients with prosthetic valves who have symptoms or signs of congestive heart failure. Left ventricular dysfunction as described above is common, and may be due to the longstanding deleterious effects of volume loading lesions such as aortic incompetence, associated rheumatic involvement of the myocardium, coronary artery disease, or myocardial damage occurring at the time of valve replacement surgery. It is important clinically to identify patients with severely impaired ventricular function as they can be identified as being unsuitable for further cardiac surgery even if prosthetic valve dysfunction is present. Such patients may also benefit from treatment with vasodilating drugs such as the angiotensin converting enzyme inhibitors. Younger patients with severely impaired ventricular function may be identified as being potential candidates for cardiac transplantation.

Evidence of left ventricular volume overload in a patient with a prosthetic valve may indicate significant prosthetic regurgitation. The appearance of a 'snappy' left ventricular contraction pattern in a patients with a mitral valve prosthesis may be the only easily identifiable ultrasonic imaging feature of severe mitral prosthetic regurgitation (Fig. 5).

Patients who have undergone cardiac surgery commonly have abnormal or even frankly paradoxical septal motion on M-mode echocardiography which is probably due to altered motion of the whole heart within the chest following cardiac surgery. Previously abnormal septal motion

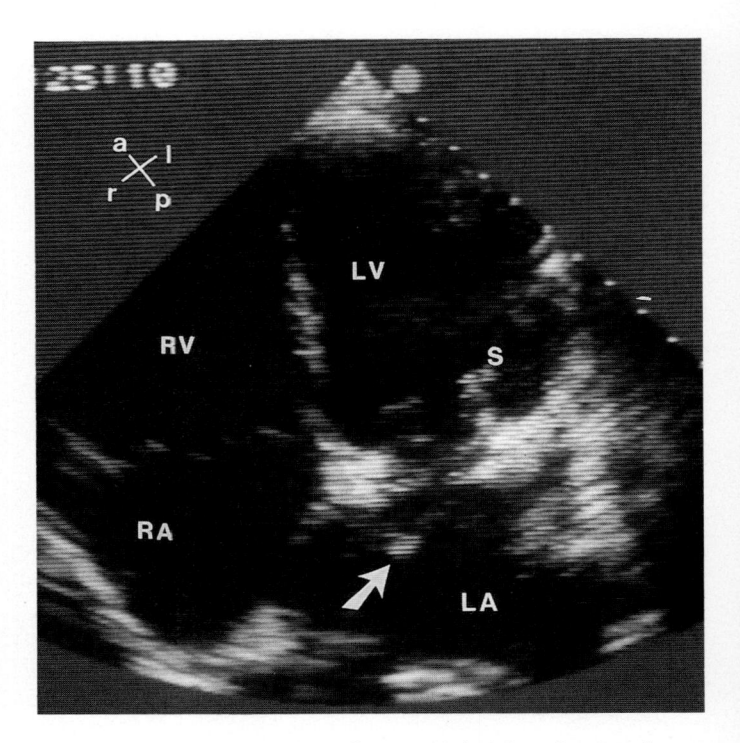

Fig. 6 Cross-sectional echocardiogram. Apical four chamber view of a patient with a porcine mitral valve prosthesis in whom one of the cusps of the prosthesis had torn causing acute prosthetic mitral regurgitation. In this image the cusp can be seen to have prolapsed on the atrial side of the prosthesis (arrow). Such appearances are more dramatic in real time and a derived M-mode recording of the flail cusp showing the motion of the cusp is shown in Fig. 7. One of the stents of the prosthesis is clearly seen in this image (S).

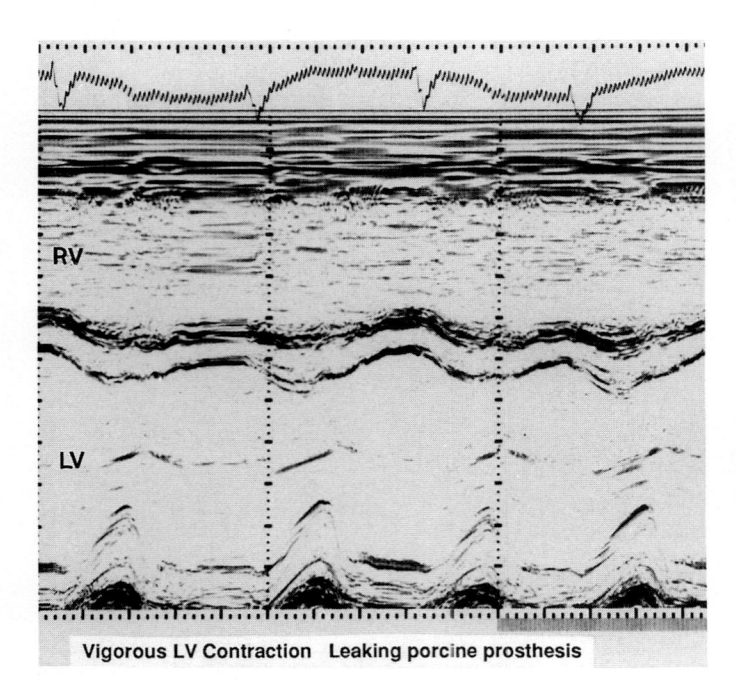

Fig. 5 M-mode echocardiogram showing vigorous left ventricular contraction in a patient with severe prosthetic mitral regurgitation.

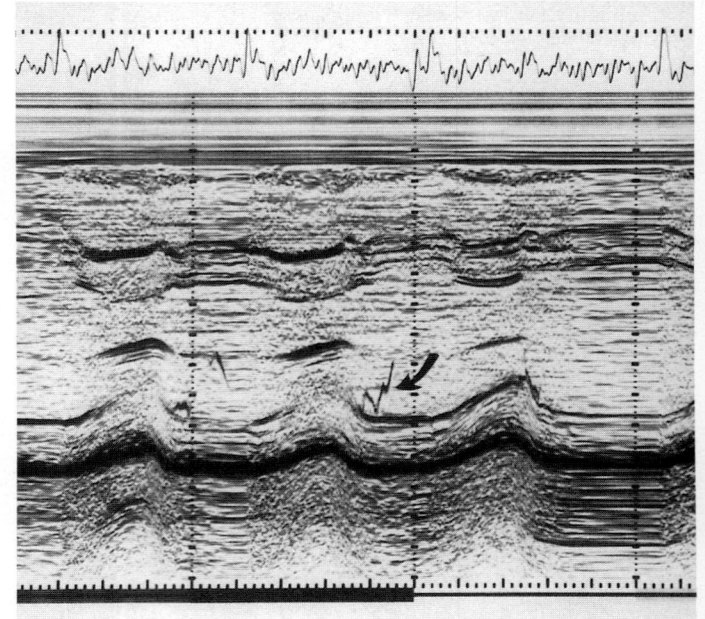

Fig. 7 M-mode echocardiogram from the patient shown in Fig. 6. The torn cusp was highly mobile and is shown here moving rapidly in early diastole (arrow). It can also be appreciated from this recording that the pattern of left ventricular contraction is vigorous suggesting volume overload.

may become normal with the vigorous septal contraction associated with prosthetic valve regurgitation.

Phonocardiography in conjunction with M-mode echocardiography has been used in the past to identify patients with prosthetic valve dysfunction but these techniques are time consuming, lack specificity and have been superseded by cross-sectional echocardiography and Doppler techniques.

The sewing ring of both biological and mechanical prosthetic valves is highly reflective of ultrasound and abnormal rocking motion of the sewing ring in patients with dehiscence of the prosthesis from the surrounding cardiac structures can usually be identified. This problem is most likely to occur early after prosthetic valve implantation and is often associated with infective endocarditis. In almost all prosthetic valves the sewing ring is radio-opaque and an abnormal rocking motion may be more readily identified by fluoroscopy than by cross sectional echocardiography. A notable exception is the Wessex bioprosthetic valve in which the sewing ring is completely radiolucent. In this type of valve the sewing ring is still strongly echogenic.

Abnormalities of the leaflets of bioprosthetic valves are most easily detected when the ultrasound beam is directed in a plane perpendicular to the leaflets without the interference of the sewing ring and valve stents.[3,4,5] Thus mitral prostheses are best evaluated from the apical view and in Figures 6 and 7 prolapse of one of the leaflets of a mitral bioprosthesis can be identified. This is often best appreciated in real time when motion of the abnormal leaflet can be compared to that of the other leaflets.

A derived M-mode (Fig. 7) of the patient illustrated in Figure 6 shows the rapid motion of the ruptured cusp. Vegetations due to infective endocarditis[4] may also be identified as shown in Figure 8.

The evaluation of mechanical prosthetic valves by cross-sectional echocardiography is hampered by the reverberation of ultrasound signals from the metal, silastic, and pyrolite carbon components of these valves and it is thus important to be aware of the radiographic appearance of different prosthetic valves as fluoroscopy and echocardiography are frequently complementary. All models of the Bjork–Shiley valve made after 1975 have a radio-opaque

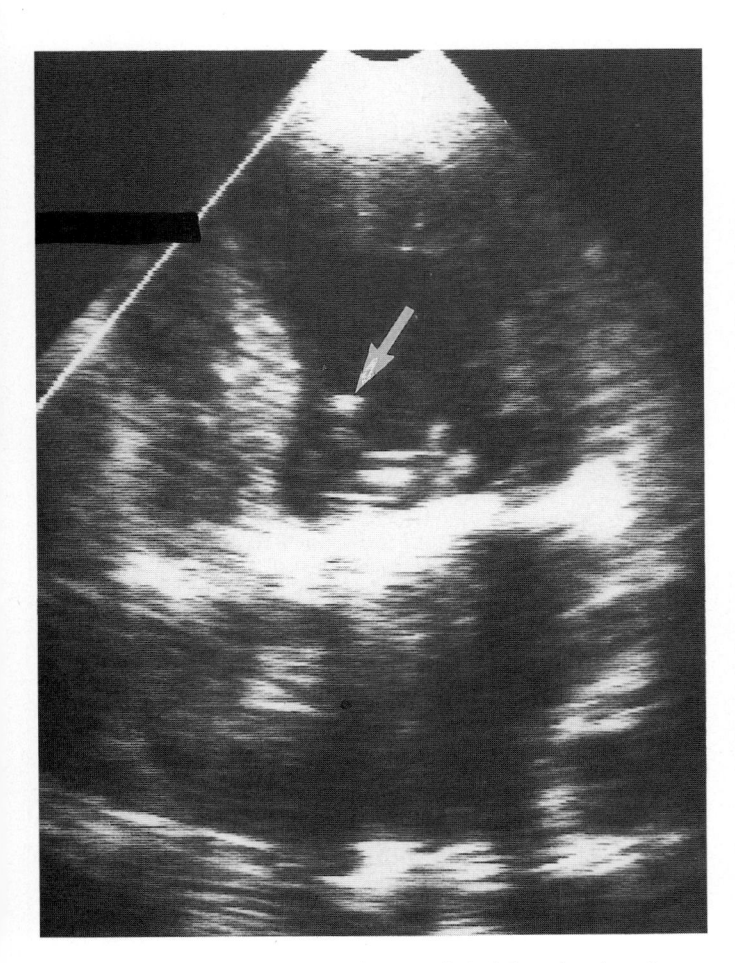

Fig. 8 Cross-sectional echocardiogram. Apical four chamber view from a patient with endocarditis affecting the leaflets of a porcine mitral prosthesis. A vegetation was suspected to be present on one of the leaflets (arrow). The patient had several positive blood cultures and was treated with antibiotics.

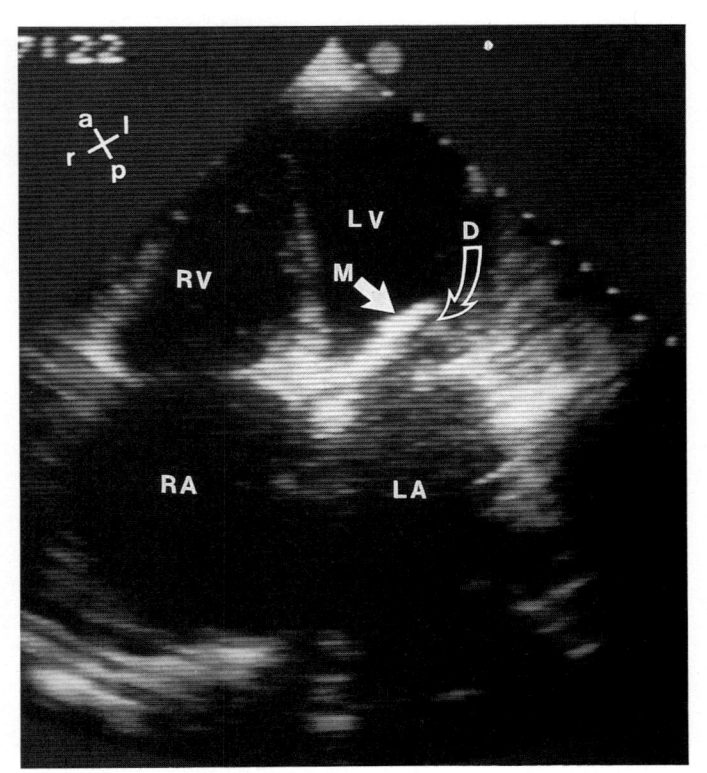

Fig. 9 Cross-sectional echocardiogram. Apical four chamber view from a patient with calcified pannus ingrowth across the ventricular side of the Bjork–Shiley mitral valve prosthesis. It was suspected from the real time images that the mass (M) may be interfering with the motion of the disc (D) but as the mass and disc were both highly reflectant of ultrasound it was difficult to be certain of this.

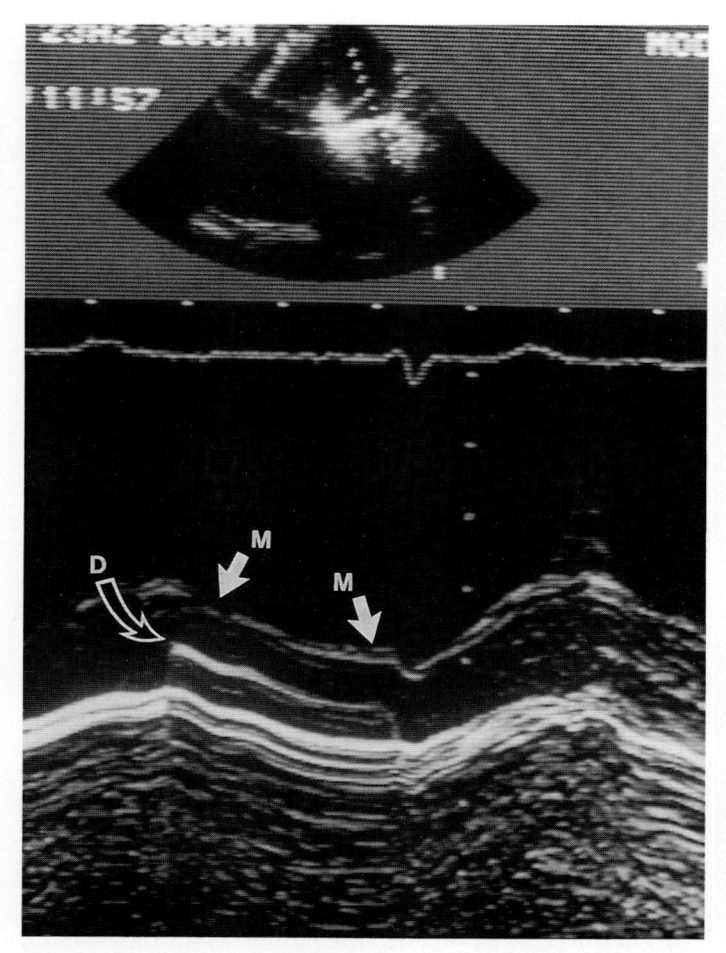

Fig. 10 Derived M-mode echocardiogram from the patient shown in Fig. 9. In diastole the disc (D) opens to a position close to the mass (M) within the left ventricle. Fluoroscopy demonstrated that the disc excursion was limited by the mass (see Fig. 11).

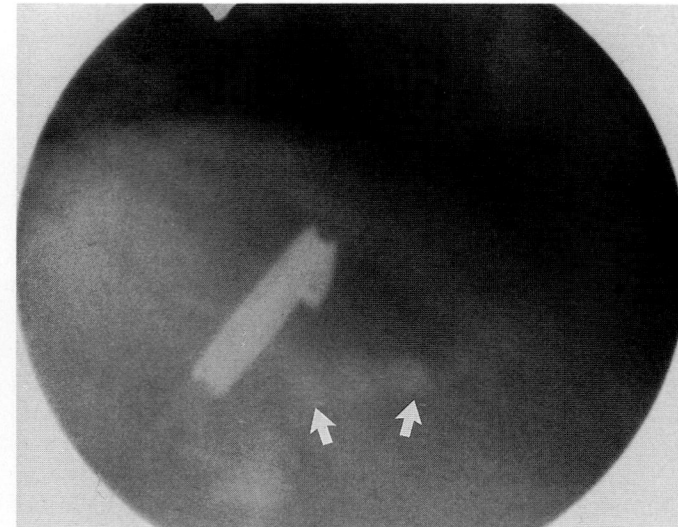

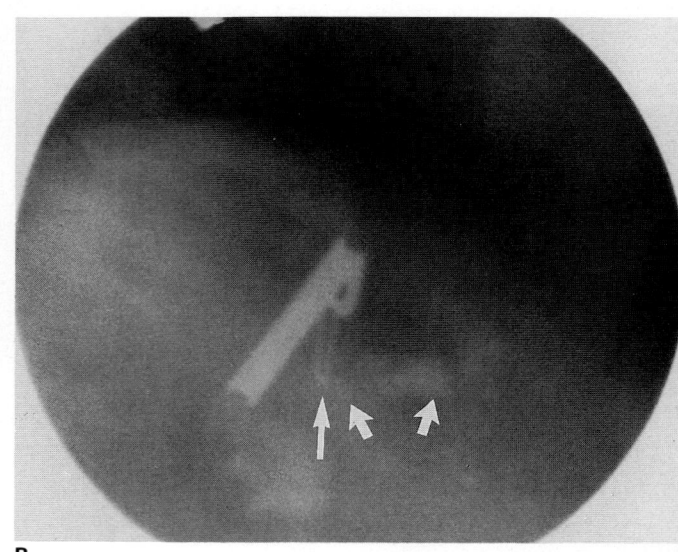

Fig. 11 A: Fluoroscopy of the patient with the Bjork–Shiley mitral valve prosthesis shown in Figs 9 and 10 (right anterior oblique projection). The systolic image is shown with the disc closed. The calcified mass on the ventricular side of the prosthesis is indicated by the two arrows. **B:** In diastole the disc is open to an angle of only about 30° (thin arrow). Normally the disc opens to an angle of about 60° but in this case motion of the disc is clearly limited by the calcified mass (thick arrows).

marker in the rim of the disc which makes identification of its motion easy.[6] The St Jude valve has a sewing ring which is radiolucent and the two discs are only faintly radio-opaque making fluoroscopic assessment difficult. After many years of implantation it is not uncommon for a pannus of fibrous and endothelial tissue to overgrow the structures of the prosthesis but this may be very difficult to demonstrate by echocardiography. Thrombus formation may rarely occur in association with mechanical prostheses causing severe impairment of function. The degree of excursion of the disc of a tilting disc prosthesis may be more accurately determined by fluoroscopy than by cross sectional echocardiography. Figures 9, 10 and 11 show these different imaging modalities in the assessment of a patient with a Bjork–Shiley mitral valve prosthesis. In Figure 9 a mass of echo dense material lies within the left ventricular cavity adjacent to the Bjork–Shiley prosthesis. From the derived M-mode trace in Figure 10 the disc of the valve can be seen to move to a position close to the mass in diastole and there is a suspicion that the degree of disc excursion is limited. On fluoroscopy the calcified mass can be seen to limit full opening of the disc which only opens to 30° instead of the usual 60° (Fig. 11).

Bacterial endocarditis

The identification of vegetations in association with prosthetic heart valves is notoriously difficult by cross-sectional echocardiography. Vegetations may be identified on bioprosthetic valve leaflets as shown above, but these appearances may be confused with the thickening of leaflets that tends to occur some years after implantation as a natural ageing process affecting these prostheses.[3,4,5] Vegetations affecting the moving components of mechanical prostheses have to be very large to allow them to be differentiated from the motion of the disc or ball. Furthermore an infected abscess lying beneath the sewing ring in either the mitral or the aortic position is commonly not identified using conventional transthoracic cross-sectional echocardiography. Indeed it is our own experience that an aortic root abscess in association with a prosthetic valve has only rarely been shown by transthoracic echocardiography. Transoesophageal echocardiography has brought the ultrasound transducer closer to the prosthetic valve especially in the mitral position and has enhanced the ability of echocardiography to detect such lesions.[7] The vegetations of infective endocarditis, structural abnormalities of bioprosthetic valve leaflets and thrombus formation in association with prosthetic valves, are much more readily detected using the transoesophageal technique.[8,9,10] Magnetic resonance imaging may well prove to be an important additional modality in the assessment of these difficult conditions.

DOPPLER EVALUATION OF PROSTHETIC HEART VALVES

Technical problems and limitations

All prosthetic valves are relatively obstructive in comparison to normally functioning native valves. If the prosthetic valve lies at some distance from the ultrasound transducer, then aliasing of the Doppler signal can occur with both pulsed wave Doppler and with colour flow mapping techniques. Continuous wave Doppler examination therefore is often the most accurate method of obtaining velocities of blood across prosthetic valves. The motion of the component parts of mechanical prostheses can produce an impressive artefact which may impair definition of the velocity profile generated from blood moving across the valve. In particular the initial inscription of the Doppler velocity waveform may be difficult to separate from the artefact. If continuous wave Doppler without imaging is used the audio signal from the opening and closing clicks of mechanical valves can make the identification of the Doppler velocity profile time consuming and tedious although this problem has been reduced by the development of steerable continuous wave Doppler in conjunction with cross-sectional echocardiographic imaging. Colour flow Doppler examination is useful in identifying the direction of flow through the prosthesis and facilitating proper alignment of the continuous wave Doppler beam. All Doppler techniques are limited by the acoustic shadowing that is created by the solid components of mechanical prosthetic valves. This latter problem has been elegantly shown by Sprecher et al[11] in which turbulent flow in a phantom model could not be detected behind closed tilting disc or ball and cage prosthetic valves and was partly obscured by the sewing ring of a porcine valve, but was readily detected behind the closed cusps of a porcine valve.

Theoretical considerations

In theory the use of the modified Bernoulli equation should be applicable to the evaluation of prosthetic valves. Flow patterns across prosthetic valves are, however, fundamentally different from those found across native valves with considerable variation being found between different types of prosthesis. Flow through porcine prosthetic valves might be expected to be similar to that through native valves, but flow beyond mechanical valves would be expected to be considerably different with semi-central flow in tilting disc valves and peripheral flow through ball and cage valves. The modified Bernoulli equation is applicable to flow across prosthetic valves if three conditions are fulfilled:

1. Flow must be incompressible, i.e. the density of blood does not change.
2. Flow must be frictionless, i.e. pressure loss due to viscose resistance is negligible.
3. Flow velocities must be measured along streamlines of the flow.

The first condition can be considered to be true at pressures found within the heart. Flow through a prosthetic valve may however occur through an irregularly shaped orifice, and therefore create significant viscous resistance. Flow through a prosthetic valve may not be parallel to the streamlines of flow especially in those mechanical valves with tilting discs or moving parts which would be expected to change the major direction of flow and thereby to create turbulent flow.

In vitro studies

Yoganathan et al[12] have performed a series of flow visualisation studies in a phantom model of fluid passing through the St Jude and Bjork–Shiley mechanical valves and the Carpentier–Edwards porcine valve. The use of a laser light source and the addition of tracer particles to the fluid in the phantom to obtain photographs of flow patterns beyond the prosthesis, allowed them to show that with these prostheses flow was principally streamlined, and indeed in the porcine prosthetic valve flow was central and similar to that through human aortic valves. The tilting disc prosthesis produced only a modest change in the overall direction of flow. These results suggest that on theoretical grounds Doppler methods could accurately be used to measure pressure gradients across prosthetic valves. Some investigators have measured pressure gradients by continuous wave Doppler examination and compared these with direct manometric measurements across a variety of irregular stenotic orifices including those of prosthetic valves. An excellent correlation has been found in these studies between mean pressure gradient derived by Doppler methods and by direct manometric measurement.[13]

In vivo studies

The pressure gradient across prosthetic valves has been measured in vivo simultaneously by means of cardiac catheterisation techniques and by Doppler ultrasound. Holen demonstrated a close correlation between peak instantaneous pressure gradient and mean pressure gradient simultaneously measured by these two techniques across newly implanted Bjork–Shiley and Hancock porcine prosthetic valves.[14,15] Similarly Wilkins et al studied 12 patients with mechanical or porcine prosthetic mitral or tricuspid valves which were thought to be stenotic.[16] They performed simultaneous continuous wave Doppler examination and cardiac catheterisation measurements using direct measurement of atrial and ventricular pressure by transeptal catheterisation or direct left ventricular puncture.

In these patients with stenotic prosthetic valves there was a highly significant correlation between peak instantaneous pressure gradient and mean pressure gradient measured simultaneously by both techniques. Burstow et al[17] have reproduced these findings in both patients with mitral and aortic prosthetic valves. It is important to appreciate that the mean pressure gradient should be calculated from the sum of multiple measurements of instantaneous velocity along the Doppler velocity profile. This is because in the modified Bernoulli equation there is a squared relationship between velocity and pressure at any one instant, as illustrated in Figure 12. Manual calculation using this formula is impractical and for use in clinical practice this calculation is usually done by computer, often within the measurements package of commercially available ultrasound equipment.

Wilkins et al also compared valve area calculated by cardiac catheterisation using the Gorlin formula to that obtained by two Doppler methods; the pressure half-time method of Hatle et al,[18] and that of Holen et al.[19] The latter method derives valve area by measuring cardiac output by catheterisation and the velocity of blood flowing across the valve by simultaneously obtained Doppler tracings. Correlation of prosthetic valve area calculated by the Gorlin and the two Doppler methods was poor. This might have been expected on theoretical grounds because the Doppler methods measure blood velocity directly and the Gorlin equation assumes a relationship between velocity of blood across a stenotic orifice (which cannot be measured at catheterisation), and the measured pressure difference. Wilkins found the correlation between the two Doppler methods was better than between either Doppler method

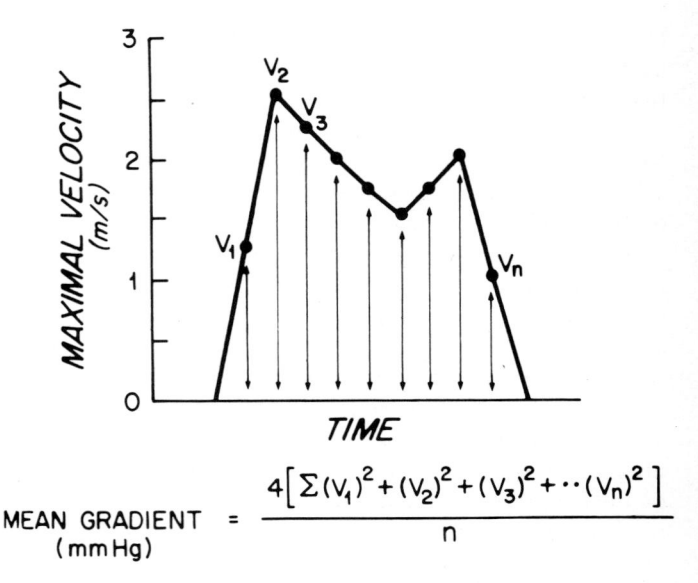

$$\text{MEAN GRADIENT (mmHg)} = \frac{4\left[\Sigma (V_1)^2 + (V_2)^2 + (V_3)^2 + \cdots (V_n)^2\right]}{n}$$

Fig. 12 Calculation of mean pressure gradient from the Doppler velocity profile across a mitral prosthetic valve. Maximal velocity is measured at multiple points along the Doppler velocity profile (V1, V2, V3 etc) and the mean gradient derived from integration of the pressure gradient calculated by the modified Bernoulli equation at each point on the Doppler trace. Most computer programmes designed to derive mean pressure gradient calculate peak instantaneous pressure gradient at 5 or 10 millisecond intervals along the Doppler spectral profile. From Wilkins G T et al, Circulation 1986; 74: 786, with permission of the American Heart Association.

and catheterisation method. In practical terms this means that Doppler is a very useful method for measuring mean gradient across a prosthetic valve accurately. The measurement of effective valve area is, however, based on a number of assumptions whether measured by Doppler or catheterisation methods and values obtained by the two different methods correlate poorly.

Another approach to measuring the effective orifice area of a prosthesis uses the continuity equation which simply states that laminar flow through a conduit is equal to the product of the mean velocity and the cross-sectional area of the conduit. With flow remaining constant, the ratio of cross sectional areas at two different sites is inversely proportional to the ratio of the respective mean velocities:

$$Q = A_1 \times V_1 = A_2 \times V_2$$

Where Q is flow, A_1 is the cross-sectional area of a normal part of the heart, V_1 is mean velocity through A_1, A_2 is the cross-sectional area of the stenosis (or prosthetic valve) and V_2 is the mean velocity of blood through A_2. If A_1, V_1 and V_2 are known then A_2 the stenotic area can be derived:

$$A_2 = \frac{A_1 \times V_1}{V_2}$$

In practice in patients with mitral prosthetic valves V_1 is measured by pulsed wave Doppler in the aortic root and A_2 is the cross-sectional area of the aortic root measured by two-dimensional echocardiography. V_2 would be the mean velocity measured across the mitral prosthesis, and the effective prosthetic mitral valve area can therefore be calculated. This calculation assumes that no significant valve regurgitation is present. In patients with aortic valve prostheses the cross-sectional area of the left ventricular outflow tract can be taken as A_1, and the velocity of profile of blood V_1 is obtained by pulsed wave Doppler just below the prosthetic valve. In practice this is done by placing the sample volume so that the valve clicks are easily obtained and then moving the sample volume towards the body of the left ventricle until the clicks almost disappear. V_2 is obtained by continuous wave Doppler and aortic valve area calculated by the equation above. The diameter of the left ventricular outflow tract is very nearly the same as the diameter of the aortic prosthetic valve and a simpler method of assessing aortic prosthetic valve area is to compare the ratio of Doppler spectral velocity profile above and below the prosthetic valve.

Rothbart et al[20] found that in patients with significant prosthetic aortic valve obstruction the ratio of left ventricular outflow velocity to peak aortic velocity was always 0.35 or less.

Aortic prostheses

Normal function

Continuous wave Doppler examination without imaging can easily be applied to obtain a velocity profile across the aortic prosthesis in most patients. Ideally the velocity trace should be obtained from at least two separate anatomical sites to ensure that peak velocities are accurately recorded. The mean pressure drop correlates well with the peak instantaneous pressure drop. Figure 13 shows the correlation for Bjork–Shiley valves used in the aortic position in a group of patients studied in our department; the mean pressure drop was approximately half the peak instantaneous pressure drop. In practice peak instantaneous velocity is the most frequent measurement made. There is a trend towards higher velocities across smaller prostheses,[21] but there is a wide range of velocities across prostheses of the same size and considerable overlap of velocities across prostheses of different sizes.[22-27] Figure 14, for example, depicts peak instantaneous velocity recorded from patients attending our department for routine review and who had a Bjork–Shiley or porcine valve implanted in the aortic position approximately 10 years previously. There is considerable overlap in peak instantaneous pressure drop in patients with the same and different size of prosthesis. Three patients with impaired ventricular function were included and peak instantaneous pressure drop in these patients was similar to those with normal ventricular function. Patients with very small aortic

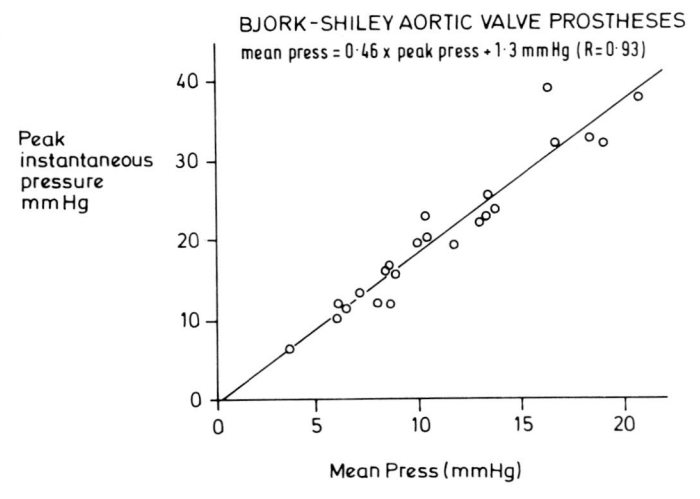

Fig. 13 Mean and peak instantaneous pressure gradient in a series of patients with Bjork–Shiley aortic valve prosthesis. There is a close correlation between the two with mean pressure gradient being approximately one half peak instantaneous pressure (authors' data).

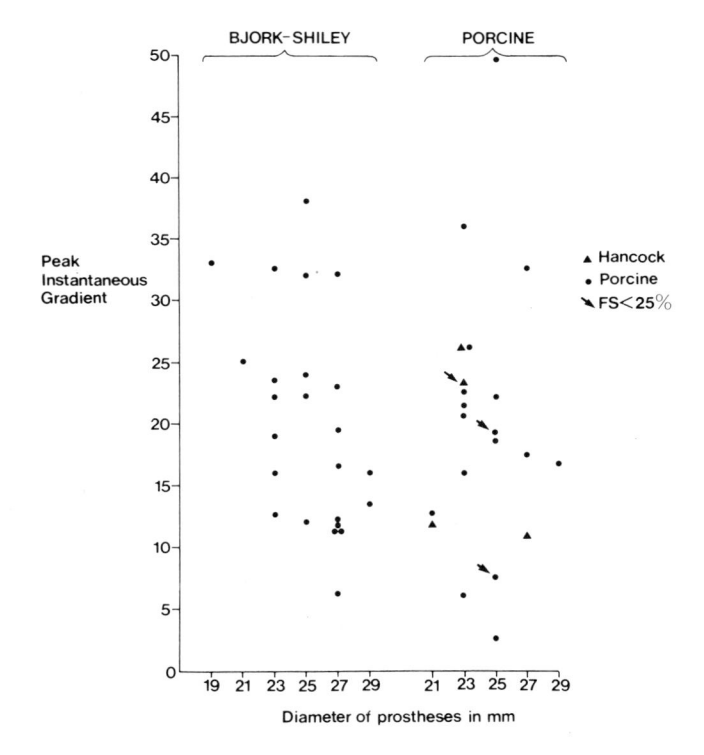

Fig. 14 Doppler peak instantaneous pressure gradient in mmHg measured across Bjork–Shiley and porcine aortic prostheses implanted 10 or more years previously and studied in the authors' department. Values for Hancock prostheses are identified with a triangle and other porcine prostheses were all Carpentier–Edwards. There is a wide range of values across prostheses of the same size. One 25 mm porcine prosthesis has a peak instantaneous gradient of 50 mmHg but the patient remained asymptomatic. Patients with impaired ventricular function on M-mode echocardiography with a fractional shortening (FS) of less than 25% are identified by a small arrow.

Table 1 Aortic prostheses: normal values (± SD) for Doppler measurements of different types of prosthetic valve

	Peak velocity (m/s)	Peak pressure drop (mmHg)	Mean pressure drop (mmHg)
Mechanical			
Starr–Edwards	3.10 ± 0.47	38.6 ± 11.7	24.0 ± 4.0
St Jude	2.37 ± 0.27	25.5 ± 5.1	12.5 ± 6.4
Bjork–Shiley	2.62 ± 0.42	23.8 ± 8.80	14.3 ± 5.3
Biological			
Carpentier–Edwards	2.37 ± 0.46	23.2 ± 8.7	14.4 ± 5.7
Hancock	2.38 ± 0.35	23.0 ± 6.7	11.0 ± 3.3
Ionescue–Shiley	2.49 ± 1.71	24.7 ± 7.7	14.0 ± 4.3

(Adapted from Reisner and Meltzer, J Am Soc Echo 1988; 1:201–210, with permission)

prostheses (19 mm in diameter or less) may have significantly higher velocities.

The range of normal values for normally functioning aortic prostheses is shown in Table 1 which is derived from Reisner and Meltzer's review of eighteen published studies.[21] The range of values for any one prosthesis is wide and it may not be accurate to identify prosthetic valve malfunction by a value falling outside the normal range for that prosthesis. Therefore there is some merit in obtaining a velocity profile in each individual patient soon after implantation of the prosthesis for future comparison should prosthetic dysfunction be suspected at a later date.

Abnormal function

Abnormally functioning aortic prostheses which are stenotic may be identified because the peak velocity recorded over the valve is outside the normal range for that prosthesis or has increased significantly over that obtained from previous recordings in the same patient. It is important to remember that prostheses of 19 mm or less in size can produce much higher velocities than larger prostheses. It should also be appreciated that patients with impaired left ventricular function and diminished cardiac output may have a normal velocity across a stenotic aortic prosthesis because the flow across it is diminished. Similarly patients with regurgitant aortic prostheses may have higher velocities across the prosthesis because of the increased flow (Fig. 15). Regurgitation through an aortic prosthesis is easily detected by both continuous wave, pulsed wave and colour flow mapping techniques as the orientation of the aortic prostheses is such that regurgitant flow is easily detected from the parasternal or apical positions. Quantitation of the degree of regurgitation is more difficult. The intensity of the Doppler signal may provide a rough guide and also the extent to which the regurgitant jet can be detected within the body of the left ventricle by pulsed wave Doppler or colour flow mapping techniques from the apical view can also give an impression of the degree of regurgitation.

Severe prosthetic aortic regurgitation is indicated if the width or height of the regurgitant jet fills more than two-

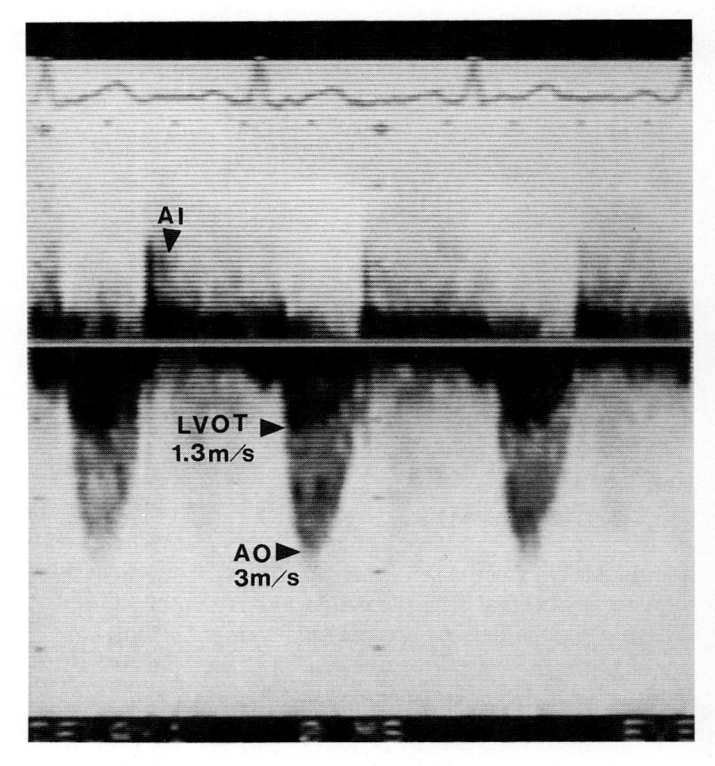

Fig. 15 Continuous wave Doppler recording from a patient with a porcine aortic prosthesis and associated paraprosthetic leak. Peak instantaneous velocity is 3 m/s giving a peak instantaneous gradient of 35 mmHg which is at the high end of the normal range. There is aortic regurgitation (AI) present and the velocity profile of the left ventricular outflow tract is discernible within the aortic velocity trace (LVOT), and is increased at 1.3 m/s indicating increased systolic flow across the prosthetic valve due to the aortic regurgitation.

thirds of the left ventricular outflow tract, and the length of the jet extends beyond the papillary muscles. Colour flow mapping may underestimate the severity of regurgitation in patients with mechanical or bioprosthetic aortic valves.[27,28] The slope of the aortic regurgitant spectral profile recorded by continuous wave Doppler examination, and the end diastolic pressure difference between aorta and left ventricle may give an indication of severity of aortic reflux as is the case with severe regurgitation of a native

Table 2 Mitral prostheses: normal values (± SD) for Doppler measurements of different types of prosthetic valve

	Peak velocity (ms)	Peak pressure drop (mmHg)	Mean pressure drop (mmHg)	Half time (ms)	Valve area (cm^2)
Mechanical					
Starr–Edwards	1.97 ± 0.42	15.5 ± 5.8	4.5 ± 2.4	113 ± 29	1.95 ± 0.50
St Jude	1.56 ± 0.29	10.0 ± 3.6	3.5 ± 1.3	77 ± 17	2.88 ± 0.64
Bjork–Shiley	1.62 ± 0.30	10.7 ± 2.7	2.9 ± 1.6	90 ± 27	2.40 ± 0.62
Biological					
Carpentier–Edwards	1.76 ± 0.74	12.5 ± 3.6	6.5 ± 2.1	90 ± 25	2.45 ± 0.74
Hancock	1.54 ± 0.26	9.2 ± 3.2	4.3 ± 2.1	129 ± 31	1.71 ± 0.41
Ionescue–Shiley	1.46 ± 0.27	8.5 ± 2.9	3.3 ± 1.2	93 ± 25	2.36 ± 0.75

(Adapted from Reisner and Meltzer, J Am Soc Echo 1988; 1:201–210, with permission)

aortic valve. The rate of fall of velocities in the aortic regurgitant jet can be measured in a manner analogous to the measurement of pressure half time in mitral stenosis. In both circumstances the left ventricle is filling through a stenotic orifice. With mild prosthetic aortic regurgitation the pressure half time of the regurgitant jet will be long and with severe regurgitation it will be short. In practice a pressure half time of the aortic regurgitant jet of less than 300 milliseconds usually indicates a significant leak and one of less than 250 milliseconds, a severe leak.

Mitral prostheses

Normal function

Continuous wave Doppler recordings of velocities across mitral prostheses are easily obtained from the apical position in most subjects. Occasionally the orientation of the prosthesis is such that peak velocities are obtained from the lower left sternal edge. Velocities across normally functioning prostheses are usually low enough for the velocity profile to be recorded adequately with pulsed wave Doppler examination. Colour flow mapping produces characteristic appearances with different types of prosthesis.

A mosaic of turbulent flow is seen passing through the central orifice, with porcine and other bioprosthetic valves. The mosaic of turbulent flow may be somewhat eccentric with tilting disc prostheses, and two eccentric jets of turbulent flow are usually seen with ball and cage prostheses. The cross-sectional echocardiographic images and corresponding colour flow mapping images are illustrated in Figure 16 and Plate 1. Identification of the location and direction of the flow through the prosthesis with colour flow mapping facilitates the proper orientation of the continuous wave beam to obtain the optimal spectral profile.

Maximum velocity and pressure half-time are easily calculated from the velocity profiles, and mean pressure drop can be calculated as described above under 'In vivo studies'. A range of normal values for commonly seen prostheses is given in Table 2, also derived from Reisner & Meltzer's review.[21]

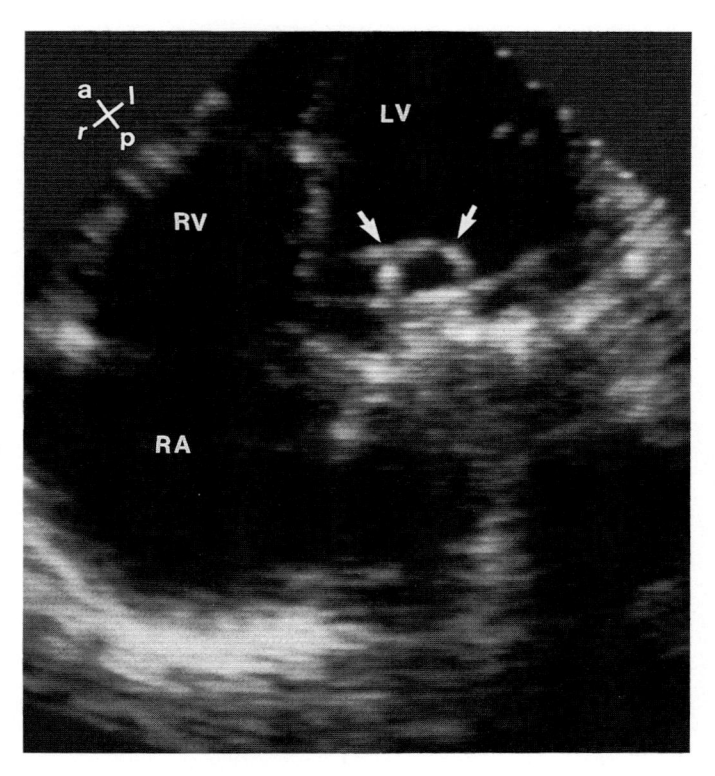

Fig. 16 Cross-sectional echocardiogram. Apical four chamber view of a patient with a Starr–Edwards mitral prosthesis. This image taken in early systole shows the prosthesis in the closed position with the empty cage indicated by arrows.

Abnormal function

Stenosis of a bioprosthetic or mechanical prosthetic mitral valve may be recognised by abnormal prolongation of the pressure half-time or an abnormally high mean gradient. Recognition of such an abnormality is important in patients with a mechanical prosthesis as thrombotic obstruction is a life-threatening condition requiring urgent intervention.

Regurgitation through a bioprosthesis is usually easy to demonstrate and the regurgitant jet can frequently be demonstrated by continuous wave Doppler examination and the location of the regurgitant jet can be indicated by

236 CARDIAC ULTRASOUND

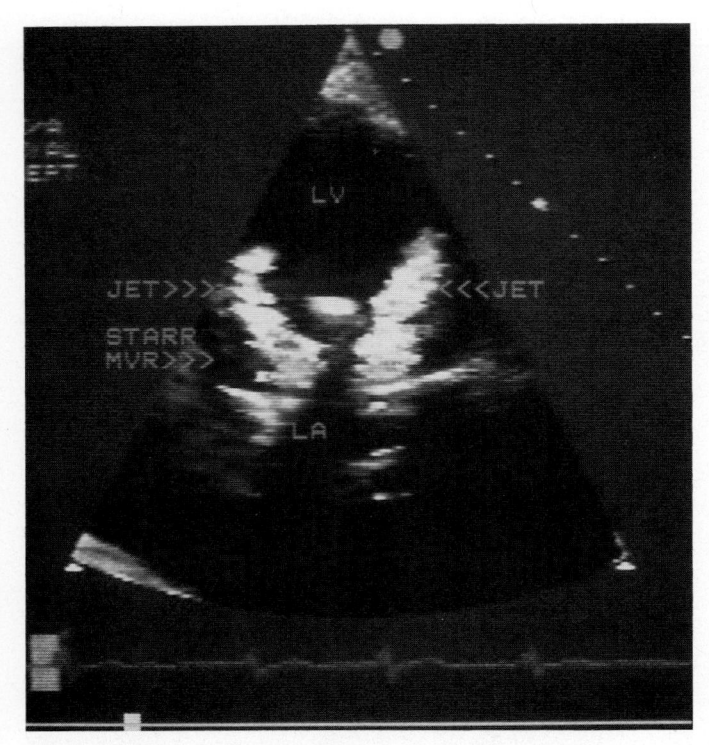

Plate 1 Doppler colour flow mapping superimposed on the cross-sectional echocardiographic image shown in Fig. 16. This frame in early diastole demonstrates the two characteristic jets of turbulent flow at the edge of the Starr–Edwards prosthesis (MVR). This figure is reproduced in colour in the colour plate section at the front of this volume.

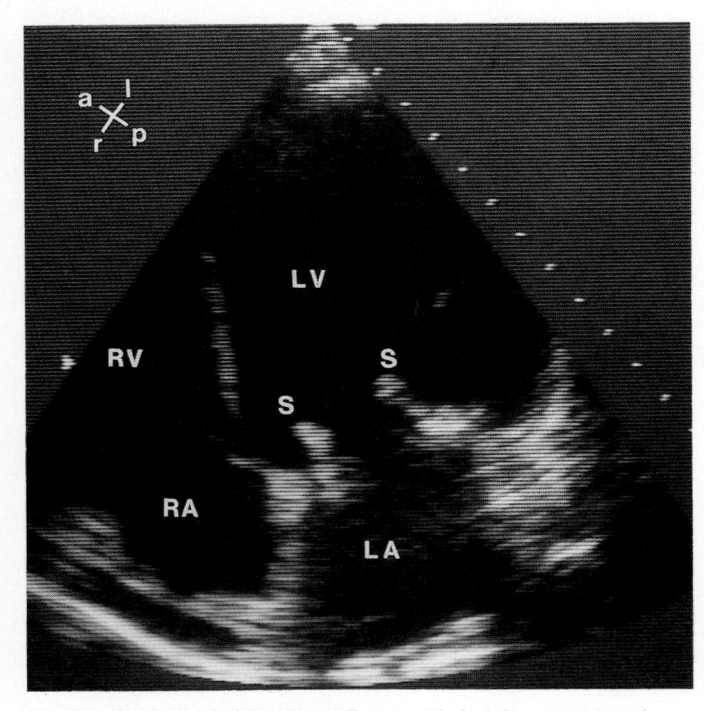

Fig. 17 Cross-sectional echocardiogram. Apical four chamber view of a patient with a Carpentier–Edwards mitral prosthesis. The prosthesis used may have been too large for the patient as it can be seen to sit at an angle within the mitral annulus with the two stents (S) out of alignment.

pulsed wave Doppler or colour flow mapping. Figures 17, 18 and Plates 2A, B, and C are recordings from a patient with a regurgitant porcine mitral prosthesis. In the cross-sectional echocardiographic four chamber view the prosthetic valve appears to sit at an angle within the mitral annulus, suggesting that the prosthesis used was large in relation to the size of the patient's heart.

The superimposed colour Doppler images show a jet of turbulent flow in diastole directed towards the interventricular septum. The valve is also stenotic as well as regurgitant and forward flow within the left atrium aliases from red to blue as blood accelerates towards the prosthetic mitral valve (Plates 2A and 2B). In systole the regurgitant jet fills half of the left atrium, probably indicating severe regurgitation (Plate 2C). The mitral regurgitant jet is easily detected on continuous wave Doppler examination. Forward velocities are increased above 2 m/s, and the pressure half time is prolonged indicating some associated prosthetic valve stenosis. The severity of regurgitation may be underestimated by mapping the extent of the turbulent jet within the left atrium.[28,29] The regurgitant jet may also be eccentric and difficult to detect at all. Abnormally high peak velocities across a mitral bioprosthetic valve in diastole with a normal pressure half-time are an important clue to the presence of prosthetic regurgitation. The abnormally high velocities across the valve in diastole are due to the increased flow created by the regurgitant lesion. If the regurgitant jet is not detected, increased flow velocities in diastole may be the only sign of prosthetic regurgitation in the Doppler examination.

Regurgitant bioprosthetic valves in the mitral position may produce a characteristic Doppler signal which sounds like a honk on the audio signal and appears as striations in the spectral profile. Chambers et al[30] have described this finding as being pathognomonic of bioprosthetic valve cusp rupture and we have also found this in our own experience. An example of this phenomenon is shown in Figure 19, a recording made from a patient who suddenly developed heart failure and severe intravascular haemolysis due to rupture of a cusp of a porcine prosthetic valve. The striated spectral profile is thought to be a harmonic due to the rapid vibration of the torn cusp within the regurgitant jet.

Some of our patients have actually complained of a honking noise emanating from their chest as the first indication of prosthetic valve failure.

Regurgitation through a mechanical mitral prosthesis can be exceedingly difficult to detect. This is because of the acoustic shadowing in the left atrium created by the prosthesis. This may mask the regurgitant jet from continuous wave, pulsed wave and colour flow mapping Doppler techniques.[28] The greater beam width of the continuous wave Doppler signal often makes this a more useful technique than pulsed wave Doppler examination for detecting regurgitant lesions. Stand alone continuous wave Doppler is best used from a number of different anatomical

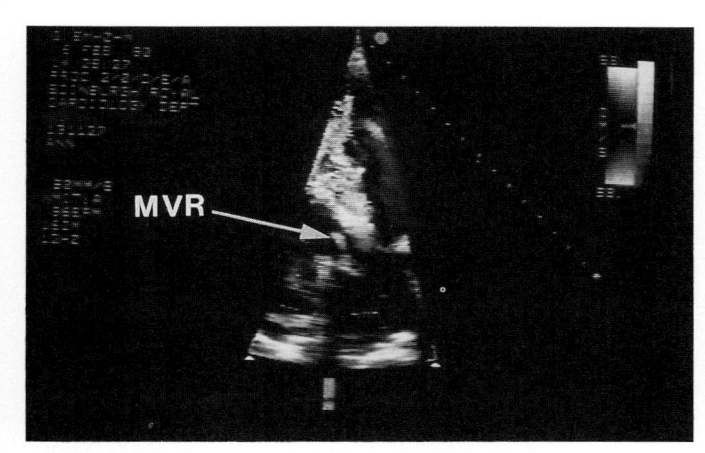

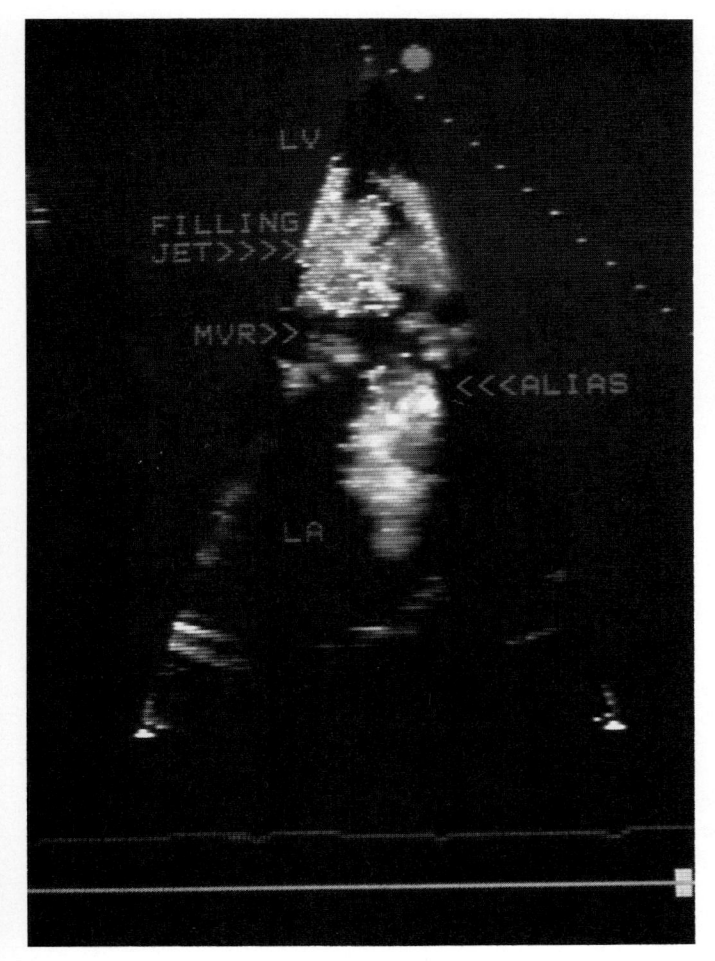

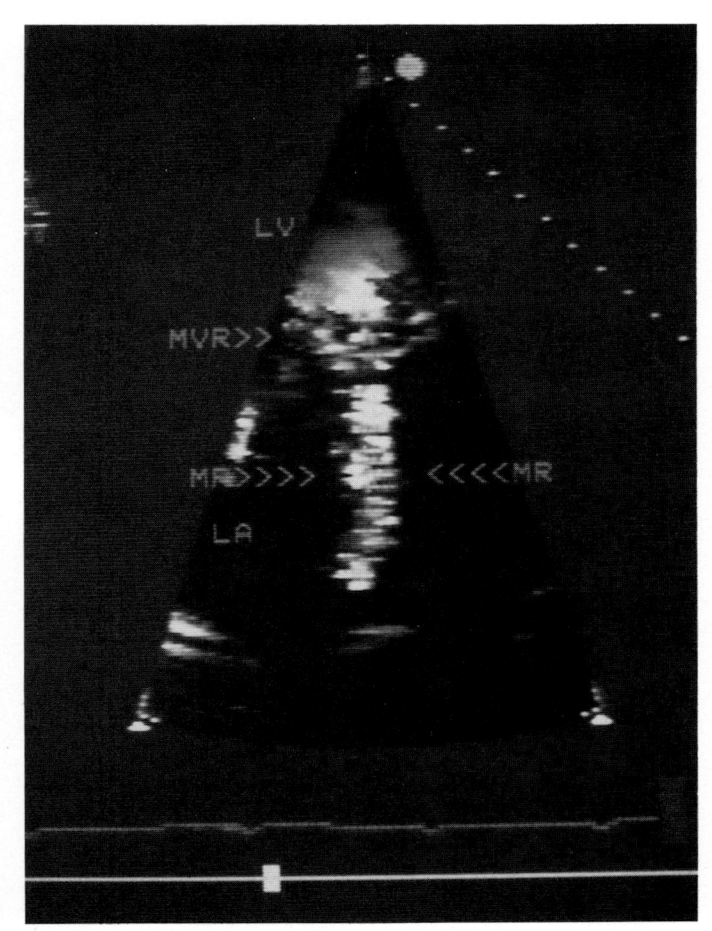

Plate 2 A: Doppler colour flow mapping superimposed on the cross-sectional echocardiographic image shown in Fig. 17. This frame in diastole shows turbulent flow through the centre of the prosthesis (MVR) directed towards the intraventricular septum because of the angle at which the prosthesis lies. **B:** Doppler colour flow mapping from the same patient as in A showing that the valve is also relatively stenotic and the colour aliases from red to blue within the left atrium as blood accelerates from the left atrium towards the prosthesis.
C: Doppler colour flow mapping superimposed on the cross-sectional echocardiographic image shown in Fig. 17. This frame in systole shows a turbulent mosaic of flow (jet) directed through the centre of the regurgitant prosthetic valve (MVR) in systole filling half of the left atrium. This figure is reproduced in colour in the colour plate section at the front of this volume.

positions such as the lower and upper left sternal edge and the axilla. This requires a careful and painstaking examination by an experienced operator. Increased forward flows across a mechanical mitral prosthesis may be an important clue to the presence of important regurgitation. As a general rule the finding of a maximum velocity across a mitral prosthesis of any sort of greater than 2 m/s should raise the suspicion of important prosthetic regurgitation. Figure 20 is a recording from a patient with a Bjork–Shiley mitral valve prosthesis with a significant paraprosthetic

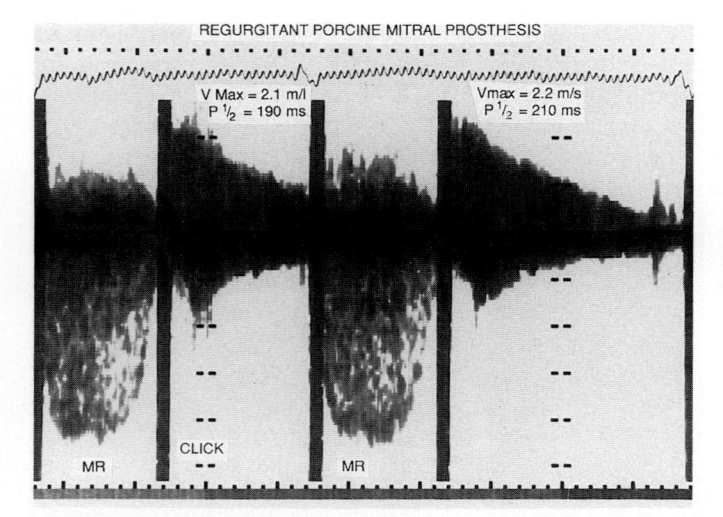

Fig. 18 **Continuous wave Doppler recording** from the patient shown in Fig. 17 and Plates 2A, B, and C with a severely regurgitant porcine mitral prosthesis in whom a high intensity jet of mitral regurgitation is seen. Peak forward velocity (V_{max}) is greater than 2 m/s, and the pressure half time is also prolonged at 190–210 milliseconds. In this patient the porcine prosthesis had degenerated with cusp calcification and partial rupture of one of the cusps so that the prosthesis was both stenotic and regurgitant. The calcified cusps also produced a click on opening and closing. The gain settings are quite high in this recording which tends to increase the intensity of the Doppler spectral profile of the regurgitant jet.

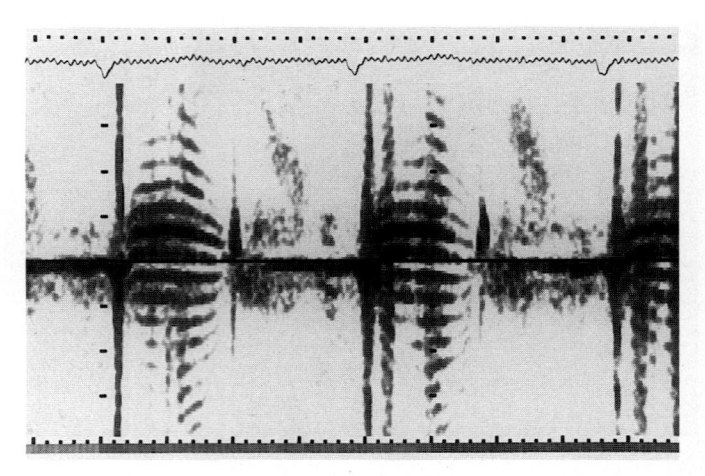

Fig. 19 **Continuous wave Doppler recording** from a patient with rupture of a cusp of a porcine mitral valve prosthesis. The striated spectral recordings in systole represent harmonic summation of the ultrasound signal and are probably produced by vibrations of the torn cusp. This finding is virtually pathognomonic for rupture of a cusp, and such patients frequently have a honking or musical murmur.

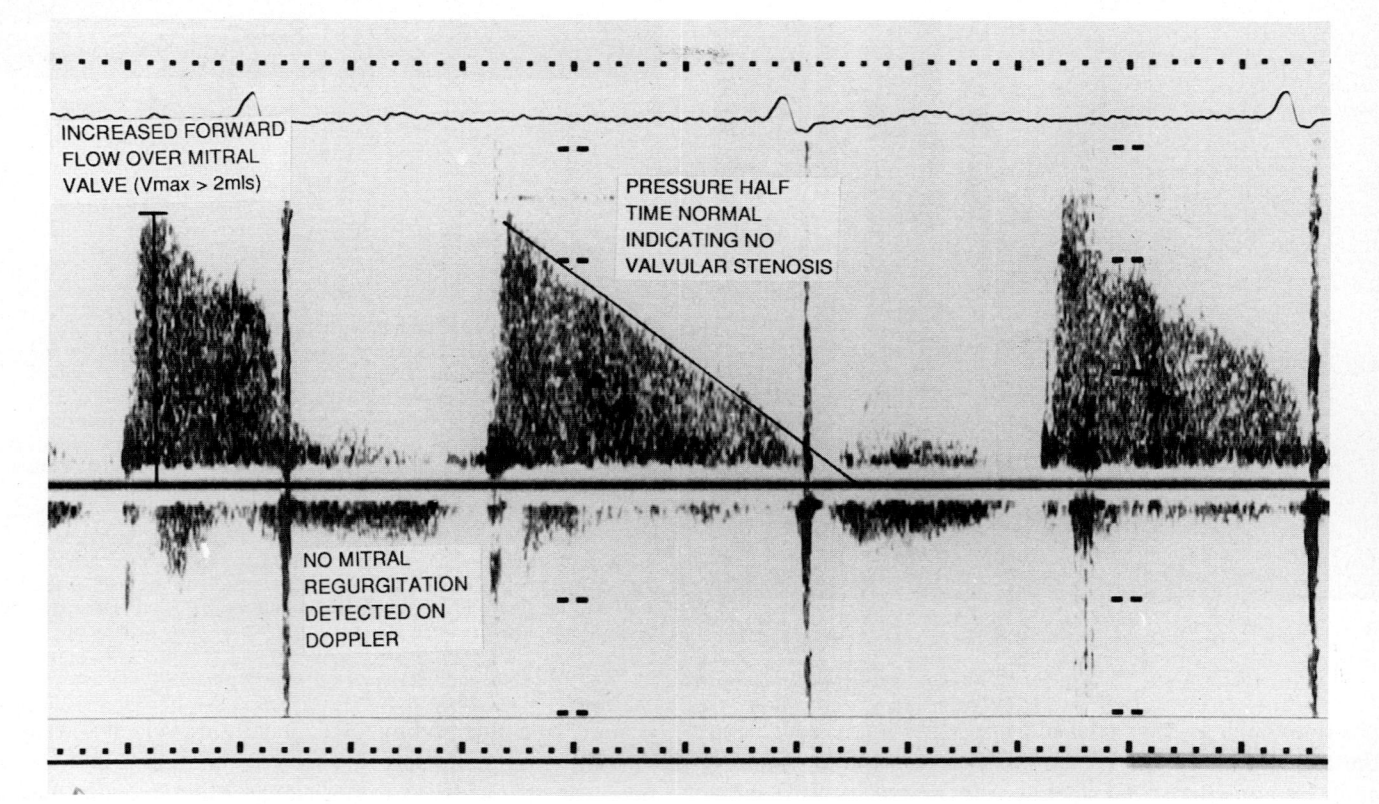

Fig. 20 **Continuous wave Doppler recording** from a patient with a regurgitant Bjork–Shiley mitral prosthesis. Peak velocities across the prosthesis are increased at more than 2 m/s and the pressure half time is normal but no mitral regurgitation could be detected. At left ventricular angiography prosthetic mitral regurgitation was easily demonstrated. Presumably the regurgitant jet could not be detected by the interrogating continuous wave Doppler ultrasound beam because of acoustic shadowing behind the closed mechanical prosthesis.

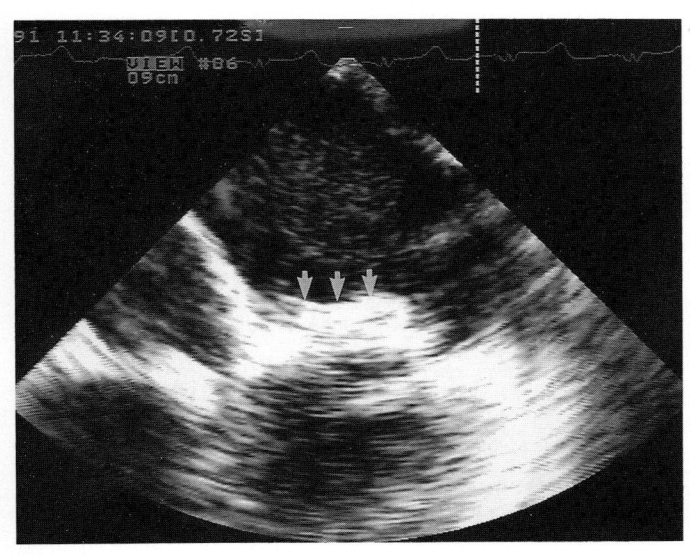

leak. A peak velocity in diastole of more than 2 m/s is recorded, the pressure half-time is normal but no mitral regurgitant jet could be detected presumably because of acoustic shadowing behind the prosthetic valve.

The problem of acoustic shadowing in the left atrium by mechanical prosthetic valves is overcome by the use of a transoesophageal transducer.[9] The regurgitant jet may also be more easily detected by colour flow mapping using this technique. The degree of the regurgitation is difficult to document accurately by any of the Doppler techniques.

The strength of the signal for regurgitant flow on continuous wave Doppler examination is a good qualitative guide to the degree of regurgitation but the intensity of the spectral signal may also be high in patients with a small regurgitant jet due to a paraprosthetic leak with very turbulent flow and when gain settings on the echocardiography machine are high.

Pulsed wave and colour flow mapping can be used to plot the degree of regurgitation by mapping the depth to which turbulent flow can be detected posteriorly within the left atrium but this has proved to be useful only as a qualitative guide to its haemodynamic severity.[28,29]

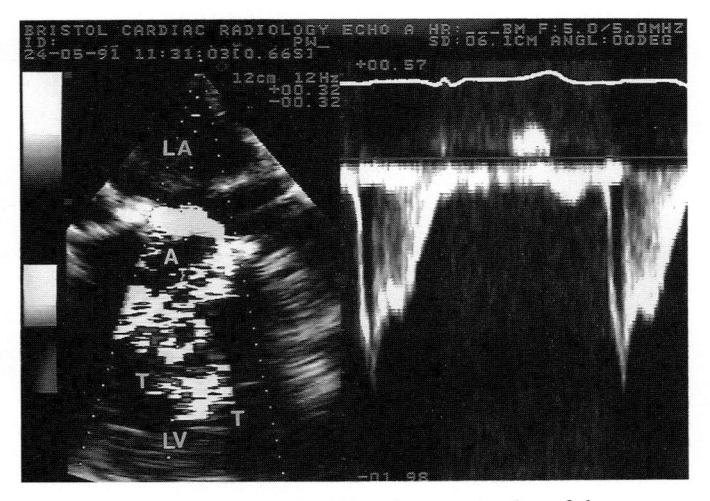

Plate 3 **Colour flow and pulsed Doppler examination** of the same prosthetic valve shown in Fig. 21. Diastolic high velocity colour flow with central blue aliasing (A) and turbulent dissipation of the jet in the left ventricle (T) are clearly seen within the colour sector. The pulsed Doppler recording of the same flow is shown on the right, the sample volume lying in the central blue aliased flow. This figure is reproduced in colour in the colour plate section at the front of this volume.

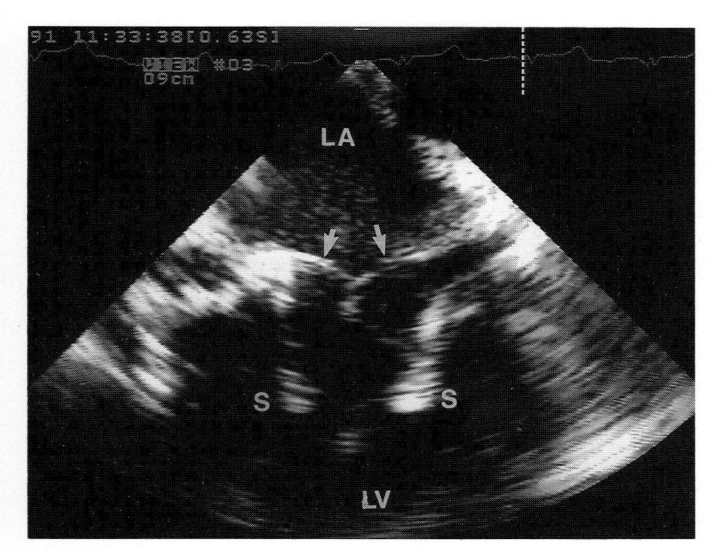

Fig. 21 **A: Transoesophageal image** from a patient with suspected endocarditis and a porcine mitral prosthesis. The supporting stents of the valve (S) and the closed leaflets (arrowed) are clearly seen in this systolic image which reveals no abnormality. **B:** Diastolic transoesophageal image from the same patient shown in **A** taken in a slightly more cranial plane which shows the echogenic superior sewing ring of the prosthesis (arrowed). **C:** Systolic transoesophageal image from the same position and cardiac cycle as **B**. A 1.0 cm diameter vegetation (arrowed) has prolapsed into the left atrium. This mobile vegetation was not visible on the precordial examination.

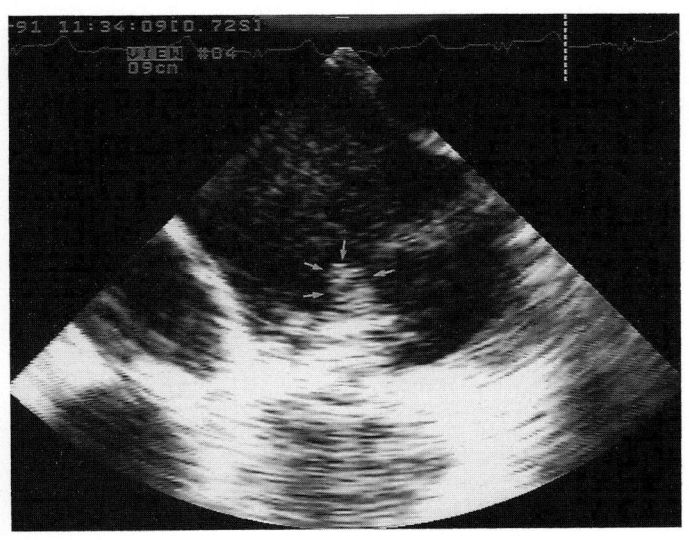

Tricuspid prostheses

The Doppler echocardiographic characteristics of prosthetic valves in the tricuspid position are similar to those used in the mitral position. However, the pressure half-time of similar prostheses implanted in the mitral and tricuspid positions in the same patient are significantly longer across the tricuspid prosthesis. The normal range of pressure half-time for Carpentier–Edwards and Bjork–Shiley valves in the mitral position is therefore not applicable to the same valves in the tricuspid position.

Pye et al[31] found in a small series of patients with both tricuspid and mitral prostheses that a peak velocity of more than 1.6 m/s in the absence of regurgitation and a pressure half-time in excess of 200 milliseconds indicated significant obstruction of the tricuspid prosthesis.

TRANSOESOPHAGEAL ECHOCARDIOGRAPHY IN THE ASSESSMENT OF PROSTHETIC VALVE DISEASE

The dramatic increase in the use of transoesophageal transducers in recent times has been of particular value in the assessment of valve prostheses, particularly those in the mitral position. High quality image detail can be achieved which is considerably superior to that possible from the precordial approach (Fig. 21A, B and C). Colour flow and pulsed Doppler techniques can also be used from this position (Plate 3) but continuous wave studies are not as yet generally available with these transducers. In cases of suspected prosthetic valve malfunction which are not confidently assessed by the precordial technique, the use of the endoscopic approach is becoming routine in those centres where the equipment and skills are available.

REFERENCES

1. Rahimtoola S H. Perspective on valvular heart disease: an update. J Am Coll Cardiol 1989; 14: 1–23
2. Taylor K. Acute failure of artificial heart valves. Br Med J 1988; 297: 996–997
3. Alam M, Lakier J B, Pickard S B, Goldstein S. Echocardiographic evaluation of porcine bioprosthetic valves: experience with 309 normal and 59 dysfunctioning valves. Am J Cardiol 1983; 52: 309–315
4. Effron M K, Poop R C. Two dimensional echocardiographic assessment of bioprosthetic valve dysfunction and infective endocarditis. J Am Coll Cardiol 1983; 2: 597–606
5. Alam M, Rosmanm H S, Lakier J B, Kemp S, Khaja F, Hautamaki K, Magilligan D J, Stein P D. Doppler and echocardiographic features of normal dysfunctioning bioprosthetic valves. J Am Coll Cardiol 1987; 10: 851–858
6. Bjork V O, Henze A, Hindmarsh T. Radio opaque marker in the tilting disc of the Bjork–Shiley heart valve. Evaluation of in vivo prosthetic valve function by cine radiography. J Thorac Cardiovasc Surg 1977; 73: 563–574
7. Daniel W G. Nellessen V, Schroder E, Nikutta P, Nonnast-Daniel B, Mugge A. Transoesophageal echocardiography as the method of choice for the detection of endocarditis-associated abscesses. Circulation 1986; 74 (Suppl II): II–55
8. Mugge A, Daniel W G, Frank G, Lichtlen P R. Echocardiography in infective endocarditis: re-assessment of the prognostic implications of vegetation size determined by the transthoracic and the transoesophageal approach. J Am Coll Cardiol 1989; 14: 631–638
9. Nellessen U, Schnittger I, Appleton C P, Masuyama T, Bolger A, Fischell T A, Tye T, Poop R L. Transesophageal two-dimensional echocardiography and color Doppler flow velocity mapping in the evaluation of cardiac valve prostheses. Circulation 1988; 78: 848–855
10. Daniel W G, Mugge A, Frank G. Improved diagnosis of prosthetic valve malfunction by transoesophageal echocardiography. Circulation 1988; 78 (Suppl II): II-606
11. Sprecher D L, Adamick A, Adams D, Kisslo J. In vitro colour flow and continuous wave Doppler ultrasound masking of flow by prosthetic valves. J Am Coll Cardiol 1987; 9: 1306–1310
12. Yoganathan A P, Chaux A, Gray R J, Woo Y R, De Robertis M, Williams F P, Matloff J M. Bileaflet, tilting disc and porcine aortic valve substitutes: in vitro haemodynamic characteristics. J Am Coll Cardiol 1984; 3: 313–320
13. Redquarth J A, Goldberg S J, Vasko S D, Allen H D. In vitro verification of Doppler prediction of transvalve pressure gradient and orifice area in stenosis. Am J Cardiol 1984; 53: 1369–1378
14. Holen J, Simonsen S, Froysaker T. An ultrasound Doppler technique for the non-invasive determination of the pressure gradient in the Bjork–Shiley mitral valve. Circulation 1979; 59: 436–442
15. Holen J, Simonsen S, Froysaker T. Determination of the pressure gradient in the Hancock mitral valve from non-invasive ultrasound Doppler data. Scand J Clin Lab Invest 1981; 41: 177–182
16. Wilkins G T, Gillam L D, Kritzer G L, Levine R A, Palacios I F, Weyman A E. Validation of continuous-wave Doppler echocardiographic measurements of mitral and tricuspid prosthetic valve gradients: a simultaneous Doppler-catheter study. Circulation 1986; 74: 786–795
17. Burstow D J, Nishimura R A, Bailey K R, Reeder G S, Homes D R, Seward J B, Tajik A J. Continuous wave Doppler echocardiographic measurement of prosthetic valve gradients: a simultaneous Doppler-catheter correlative study. Circulation 1989; 80: 505–511
18. Hatle L, Angelsen B, Tromsdal A. Non-invasive assessment of atrioventricular pressure half time by Doppler ultrasound. Circulation 1979; 60: 1096–1104
19. Holen J, Aashid R, Landmark K, Simonsen S, Ostrem T. Determination of effective orifice area in mitral stenosis from non-invasive ultrasound Doppler data and mitral flow rate. Acta Med Scand 1977; 201: 83–88
20. Rothbart R M, Castriz J L, Harding L V, Russo C D, Teague S M. Determination of aortic valve area by two dimensional and Doppler echocardiography in patients with normal and stenotic bioprosthetic valves. J Am Coll Cardiol 1990; 15: 817–824
21. Reisner S A, Meltzer R S. Normal values of prosthetic valve Doppler echocardiographic parameters: a review. J Am Soc Echo 1988; 1: 201–210
22. Williams G A, Labvitz A J. Doppler hemodynamic evaluation of prosthetic (Starr–Edwards and Bjork–Shiley) and bioprosthetic (Hancock and Carpentier–Edwards) cardiac valves. Am J Cardiol 1985; 56: 325–332
23. Sagar K B, Wann L S, Paulsen W H J, Romhilt D W. Doppler echocardiographic evaluation of Hancock and Bjork–Shiley prosthetic valves. J Am Coll Cardiol 1986; 7: 681–687
24. Gibbs G L, Wharton G A, Williams G T. Doppler echocardiographic characteristics of the Carpentier–Edwards xenograft. Eur Heart J 1986; 7: 353–356
25. Panidis I P, Ross J, Mintz G S. Normal and abnormal prosthetic valve function as assessed by Doppler echocardiography. J Am Coll Cardiol 1986; 8: 17–326
26. Cooper D M, Stewart W J, Schiavone W A, Lombardo H P, Lytle

B W, Loop F D, Salcedo E E. Evaluation of normal prosthetic valve function by Doppler echocardiography. Am Heart J 1987; 114: 576–582
27 Ramirez M C, Wong M, Sadler N, Shah P M. Doppler evaluation of bioprosthetic and mechanical aortic valves: data from four models in 107 ambulatory patients. Am Heart J 1988; 115: 418–425
28 Alam M, Rosman H S, McBroom D, Graham L, Magilligan D J, Khaja F, Stein P D. Colour flow Doppler evaluation of St Jude Medical prosthetic valves. Am J Cardiol 1989; 64: 1387–1389
29 Alam M, Rosman H S, Hautamaki K, Graham L, Magilligan D J, Khaja F, Stein P D. Colour flow Doppler evaluation of cardiac bioprosthetic valves. Am J Cardiol 1989; 64: 1389–1392
30 Chambers J B, Monaghan M J, Jackson G, Jewitt D E. Doppler echocardiographic appearances of cusp tears in tissue valve prostheses. J Am Coll Cardiol 1987; 10: 462–466
31 Pye W, Weerasana N, Bain W H, Hutton I, Cobbe S M. Doppler echocardiographic characteristics of normal and dysfunctioning prosthetic valves in the tricuspid and mitral position. Br Heart J 1990; 63: 41–44

# Cardiac masses

Introduction
Primary cardiac tumours
Benign cardiac tumours
  Myxoma
  Rhabdomyoma
  Fibroma
  Other benign primary tumours
Malignant primary tumours of the heart

Secondary cardiac tumours
Carcinoid disease
Intracardiac thrombi
Ventricular thrombi
Atrial thrombi
Differential diagnosis

Petros Nihoyannopoulos

INTRODUCTION

Cardiac tumours, although rare, represent a continuing diagnostic challenge, particularly as surgery now offers complete cure in many cases. Primary cardiac tumours are exceedingly rare with an autopsy incidence of approximately 1 in 10 000. The great majority of these tumours are benign with myxomas being the most frequent type.[1] Metastatic tumours occur 20 to 40 times more frequently than primary cardiac tumours and are observed in 10–12% of patients with malignancy. Cardiac involvement and distribution are usually related to the tumour's overall incidence and its propensity to spread via direct extension as opposed to vascular or lymphatic channels. The most frequent cardiac metastases are related to lung and breast carcinomas, followed by oesophageal carcinoma, melanoma, leukaemia, lymphoma, renal cell carcinoma and hepatoma. Some patients with acquired immunodeficiency syndrome (AIDS) have also been found to have intracardiac involvement with Kaposi's sarcoma and lymphoma.[2]

Detection of intracardiac masses has always been one of the most fascinating uses of echocardiography. Until the early 1950s the diagnosis of an intracardiac mass could only be made at autopsy. In 1952 the antemortem diagnosis of a left atrial myxoma was made for the first time using angiography[3] and in 1954 the first atrial myxoma was excised using cardiopulmonary by-pass.[4] The presence of therapeutic options for the patients with a cardiac tumour has accordingly placed more emphasis on early diagnosis.

The advent of M-mode echocardiography brought the first major step in non-invasive recognition of cardiac tumours. The introduction of two-dimensional echocardiography provided a new dimension in the diagnosis of intracardiac tumours during life and it has now become the diagnostic test of choice.[5] Comprehensive imaging of all four intracardiac chambers and valves, as well as of the immediate extracardiac spaces, affords greater overall reliability in the diagnosis of cardiac masses than cardiac catheterisation or even other non-invasive investigations, with the possible exception of magnetic resonance imaging.

The recent introduction of transoesophageal echocardiography has overcome some major obstacles in ultrasound imaging of the heart.[6,7] The more posterior chambers and structures can be visualised even in difficult subjects as the technique avoids the lungs, bones and muscles which so often hinder ultrasound transmission.

PRIMARY CARDIAC TUMOURS

Primary cardiac tumours of the heart are rare, with an incidence of less than 0.25%. They are of great clinical interest since they are often benign, occur predominantly in children and are often attached by a slender stalk that makes them amenable to surgical removal.[8,9] They are, however, very difficult to diagnose clinically, because of their rarity and because they often present as a mysterious cause of cardiac decompensation. Table 1 shows the most common types of primary tumours of the heart. Myxomas, rhabdomyomas and fibromas are seen in decreasing order of frequency and comprise 66% of all primary neoplasms. Fibromas and myxomas tend to be solitary lesions, whereas rhabdomyomas are often multiple. Neither the patient's age nor the tumour distribution is predictive of the histological type. A family history or physical evidence of tuberous sclerosis[10] may suggest the diagnosis of rhabdomyoma, which may be found in 50% of individuals with tuberous sclerosis. While rhabdomyomas and fibromas are the most frequently encountered primary cardiac tumours in children, myxomas are by far the most frequent in adults. Malignant primary tumours of the heart are usually sarcomas (Table 1) and cannot be distinguished with certainty from benign tumours by echocardiography.

Table 1 Common types of primary cardiac tumours

BENIGN
  Myxoma
  Rhabdomyoma
  Fibroma
  Lipoma
  Papillary fibroelastoma
  Haemangioma

MALIGNANT
  Angiosarcoma
  Rhabdomyosarcoma
  Fibrosarcoma

Benign cardiac tumours

Myxoma

Of all benign cardiac tumours, myxomas are by far the commonest and they occur most often in the left atrium (75%). They can, however, occur in the right atrium (20%), the left ventricle (2.5%) and the right ventricle (2.5%).[11–13] Myxomas are usually pedunculated, solitary tumours but occasionally they can involve more than one cardiac chamber. A 'syndrome myxoma' has also been described in a subset of patients who have myxoma associated with pigmented skin lesions and peripheral and endocrine neoplasms.[14] Although the pathological origin of these tumours has long been debated, recent studies support the argument that they have an endothelial or endocardial origin.[12]

Left atrial myxoma may remain undiagnosed for many years and can produce a wide spectrum of non-specific signs. They can mimic almost any cardiovascular disorder and may produce symptoms and signs that direct attention away from the heart.[15] A left atrial myxoma can be of two main types, the first and commonest form being that of a translucent, friable, slightly lobulated or villous mass with a frog-spawn texture (Fig. 1). The second, more rare form

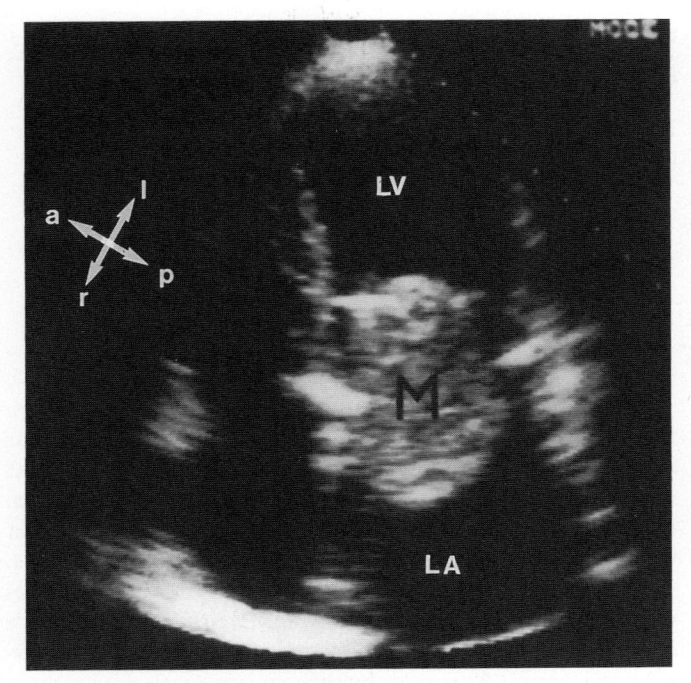

Fig. 1 Apical four chamber view from a patient with left atrial myxoma (M) during diastole. Note that the myxoma is protruding into the left ventricle through the mitral annulus.

of left atrial myxoma is smooth, spherical and solid in appearance, exhibiting little movement (Fig. 2). Both types can remain clinically silent for many years until they reach a sufficient size to produce signs of obstruction to the left ventricular inflow when the myxoma is solid or, more frequently, embolise to the brain, peripheral vessels or coronary arteries. Left atrial myxomas are generally pedunculated and attached by a fibrovascular stalk of various thickness and length. Most commonly, the stalk is attached to the atrial septum at the level of the foramen ovale. Right atrial myxomas are less likely to arise from the atrial septum and ventricular myxomas tend to arise from the lateral wall rather than the inter-ventricular septum.

The first echocardiographic diagnosis of atrial myxoma was reported in 1961 by Edler and associates, using M-mode techniques.[16] The M-mode echocardiographic recording of left atrial myxoma is usually represented by a cloud of echoes behind the anterior mitral leaflet in diastole, as well as abnormal systolic echoes in the left atrium, behind the posterior aortic wall (Fig. 3). Pechaceck et al[13] however found that only 59% of patients with left atrial myxomas are diagnosed with M-mode techniques alone, as this modality lacks spatial resolution and the ultrasonic beam may fail to traverse the mass, or even may produce atypical intra-atrial echoes indistinguishable from artefacts or other cardiac structures. Two-dimensional echocardiography has become the definitive imaging modality for the diagnosis of intracardiac tumours. Its diagnostic accuracy arises from its ability to examine all

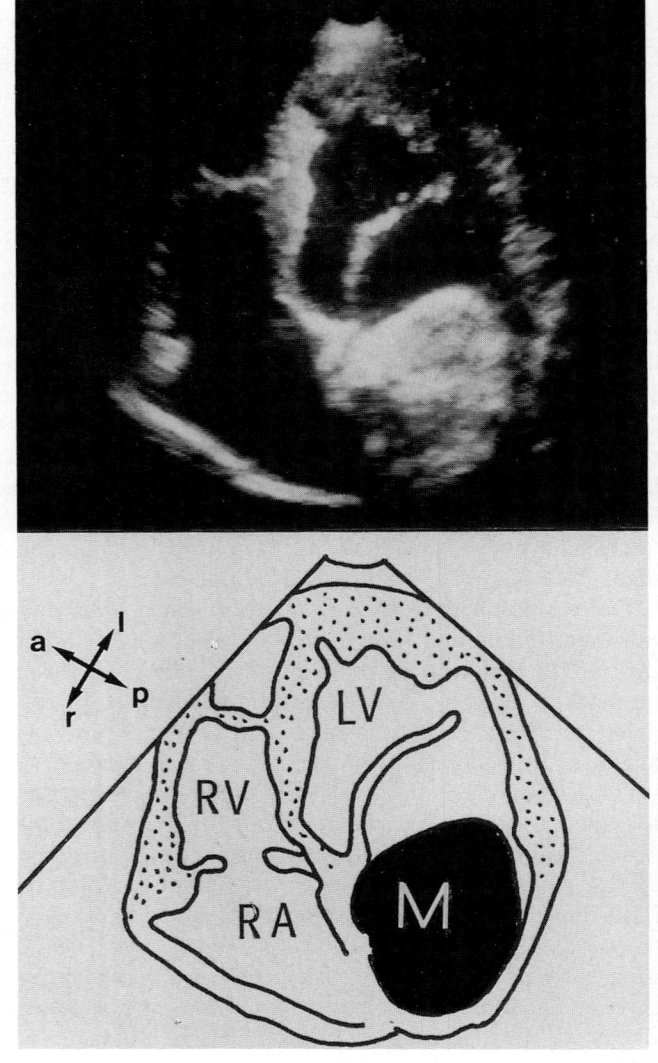

Fig. 2 Apical four chamber view from a patient with a solid myxoma. In contrast with the myxoma in Fig. 1, during diastole this tumour remains immobile without crossing the mitral annulus. (M = myxoma.) (Reproduced with permission.[15])

four intracardiac chambers from multiple planes (Fig. 4). This has made cardiac catheterisation, which can be potentially hazardous and delay surgery, both unnecessary and unjustifiable. Two-dimensional echocardiography permits firstly the detection, and secondly the characterisation of the tumour by assessing its size, its points of attachment, its degree of mobility and its consistency (Fig. 5). Particular attention must be given to comprehensive imaging of the left atrium and its appendage from multiple views and transducer positions. In addition to diagnosing a left atrial myxoma, a concomitant right atrial myxoma or myxomas in other sites, should be excluded.[17,18] With the advent of transoesophageal echocardiography, left atrial myxomas can be visualised even more clearly and their attachment to the surrounding atrial walls can be better

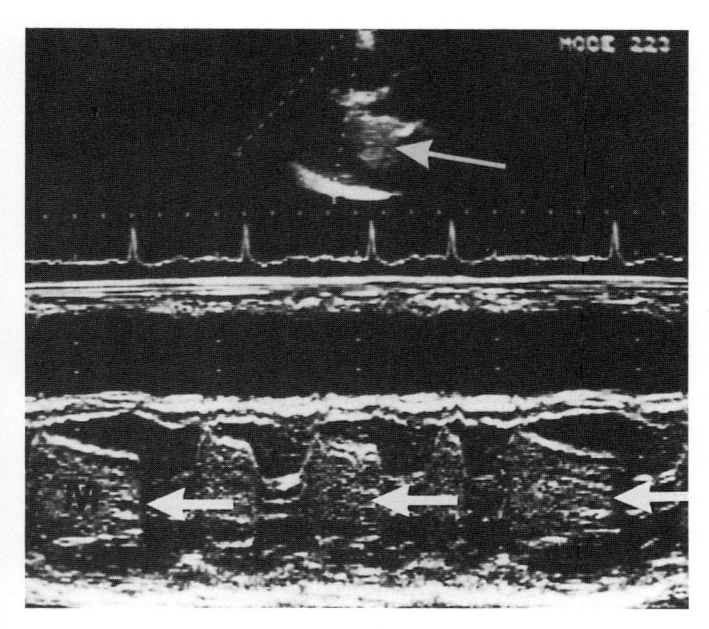

Fig. 3 Parasternal long axis view (top) and simultaneous M-mode echocardiogram (bottom), showing a left atrial myxoma as a cloud of echoes behind the mitral valve (arrows). Note also the 'stenotic' appearance of the mitral valve motion.

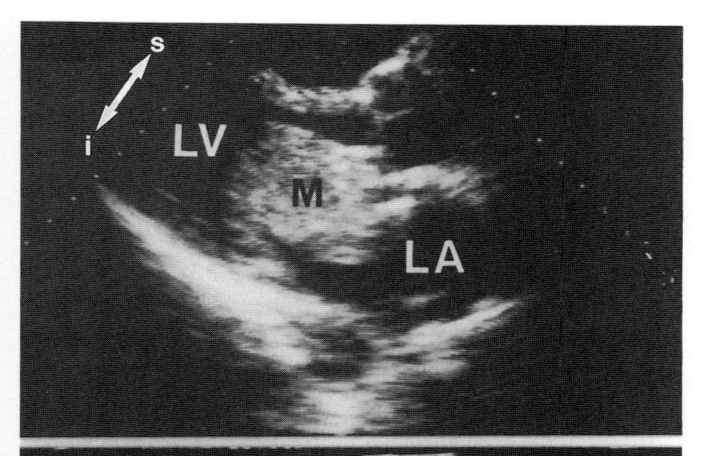

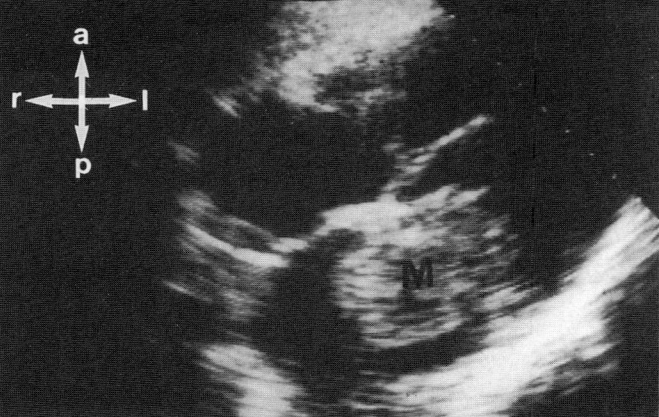

Fig. 4 Long axis parasternal (top) and subcostal (bottom) views from a patient with left atrial myxoma. Note that during diastole the myxoma is engaging the left ventricular inflow. (M = myxoma.)

described.[19] Figure 6 is from a patient with a typical frog-spawn texture of left atrial myxoma of a rather small size, tending to protrude into the left ventricular inflow through the mitral annulus during diastole. The point of attachment of this tumour could not be visualised from the transthoracic approach. Figure 7 illustrates the transoesophageal approach to the same tumour during diastole, where its attachment to the fossa ovalis can now be clearly visualised (arrow). Figure 8 shows the tumour after surgical excision.

Left atrial myxomas vary in size and can virtually fill the left atrium. A large myxoma can obstruct the mitral valve orifice and impede diastolic flow into the ventricle. The myxoma in Figure 2 reached 7 cm in diameter and was virtually immobile, producing clinical signs typical of mitral stenosis. The softer and more mobile type of myxoma is often contained within the back of left atrium during systole. During diastole, it protrudes into the left ventricle through the mitral annulus (Fig. 5). In early diastole the myxoma hits the atrial surface of the anterior mitral leaflet which becomes thickened and more echogenic with time. Long-standing atrial myxomas may calcify and very occasionally the tumour can be detected on a chest X-ray. With the concurrent recording of the M-mode echocardiogram, which provides a better time resolution, it is easier to appreciate the initial opening of the mitral leaflet followed by the sudden forward move of the myxoma against the anterior mitral leaflet. The myxoma in Figure 9 is from a 33-year-old patient following massive cerebral and peripheral embolisation. At autopsy (Fig. 10), the size of the myxoma hardly reached 15 mm in its longest diameter but interestingly, the atrial surface of the anterior mitral leaflet was eroded, implying that this myxoma was of a much larger size before embolising.

Left atrial myxomas are typically attached by a thin stalk to the atrial septum, at the level of the fossa ovalis. This attachment, however, may vary and can be at any site within the left atrium or even on the mitral valve. The pre-operative recognition of the tumour's attachment may aid the surgeons to choose the appropriate surgical technique for its removal. It is customary for the surgeon to excise a full thickness of wall surrounding the pedicle and patch the defect created, but if the tumour is near a pulmonary vein or the mitral valve, this may be difficult to perform. Echocardiography is the only pre-operative investigation required nowadays and surgery should follow without delay, in order to avoid potentially disastrous embolisation.

Right atrial myxomas comprise about 20% of all myxomas and cardiac symptoms, when present, may mimic tricuspid valve abnormalities such as tricuspid stenosis, Ebstein's anomaly or pulmonary hypertension. The patient may present with unexplained heart failure.[8] Although it is relatively easy to image most myxomas in the left atrium with M-mode echocardiography, it is considerably more difficult to image tumours in the right atrium. A minimum

248 CARDIAC ULTRASOUND

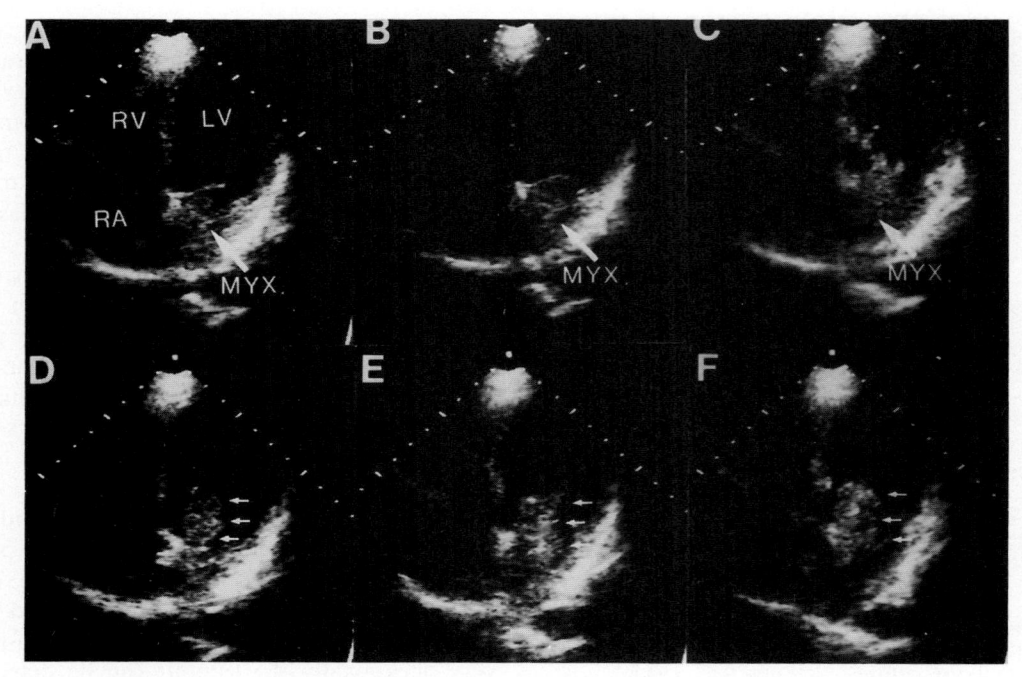

Fig. 5 Serial apical four chamber views during systole (A,B), early diastole (C) and late diastole (D–F), demonstrating the mobility of a typical, frog spawn type of myxoma (arrows). During systole, the tumour is packing the back of the left atrium. In early diastole, the mitral valve opens fully, while the tumour is lagging behind. Later in diastole, the myxoma crosses the mitral annulus and enters the left ventricular inflow. (Reproduced with permission.[15])

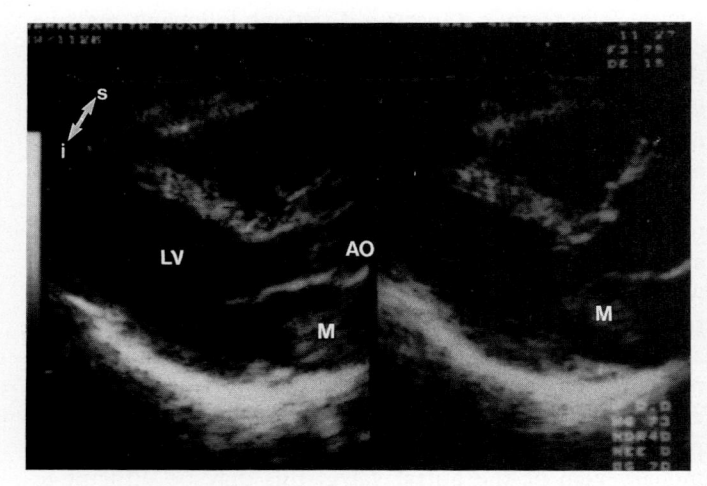

Fig. 6 Parasternal long axis views during systole (left) and diastole (right), demonstrating a typical left atrial myxoma. Note that its attachment to the atrial wall is not visualised. (AO = aorta, LV = left ventricle, M = myxoma.)

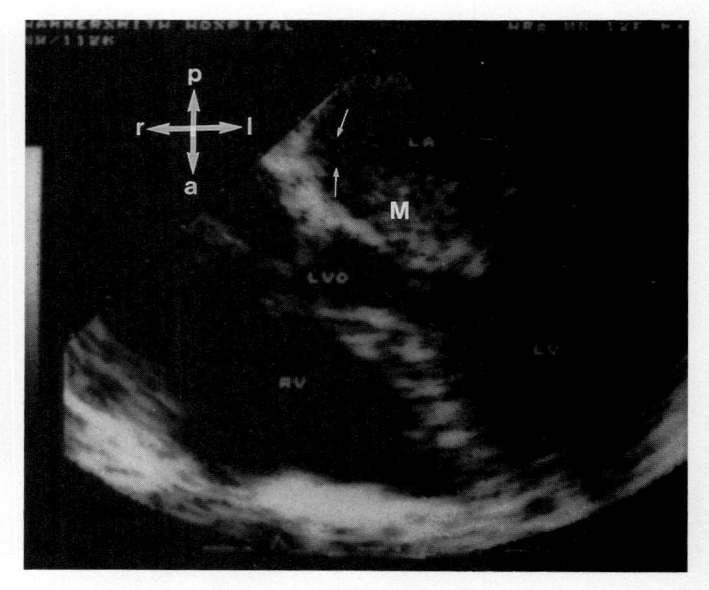

Fig. 7 The same myxoma from Fig. 6 viewed from the transoesophageal approach. The tumour is seen lying along the anterior mitral leaflet, while posteriorly it is attached by a thin stalk at the fossa ovalis (arrowed). (LVO = left ventricular outflow tract, M = myxoma.)

of five two-dimensional planes should be performed for complete evaluation of the right atrium and adjoining structures:

(1) long axis parasternal right ventricular inflow tract view;
(2) short axis parasternal view at the base (aortic root);
(3) apical four chamber view;
(4) subcostal four chamber (atrial) view;
(5) subcostal short axis at the base (superior vena cava-right atrium-right ventricle).

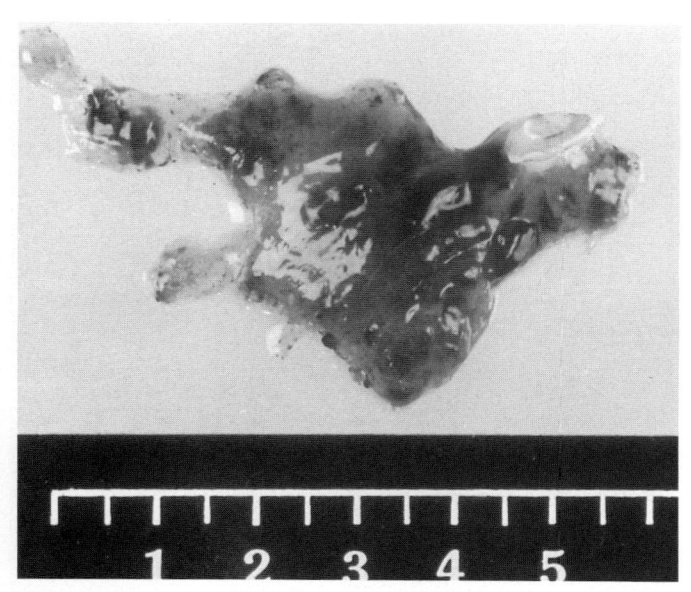

Fig. 8 The myxoma from Figs 6 and 7 after surgical removal. Note the gelatinous, frog spawn appearance of the tumour.

Transoesophageal echocardiography provides yet another echocardiographic window, particularly when the transthoracic approach is of suboptimal quality. It also helps enormously for the visualisation of the right side of the atrial septum and the region of the coronary sinus.[7]

Ventricular myxomas are extremely rare. About 5% of all myxomas arise from the ventricles with equal distribution between right and left. Right ventricular myxomas become symptomatic predominantly through obstruction to blood flow, whereas left ventricular myxomas may become symptomatic through obstruction or systemic embolisation. Two-dimensional echocardiography is significantly more effective than M-mode echocardiography for the detection, localisation and sizing of ventricular masses. The optimal visualisation of the right and left ventricular free walls, using all the conventional echocardiographic projections, is of pivotal importance in distinguishing between a ventricular myxoma and ventricular thrombus. Ventricular myxomas are commonly attached to the ventricular free walls with the adjacent myocardium contracting normally. Conversely, thrombi in the ventricles are often attached to the apex or along the ventricular septum with the adjacent myocardial contraction usually being impaired (hypokinetic or akinetic).

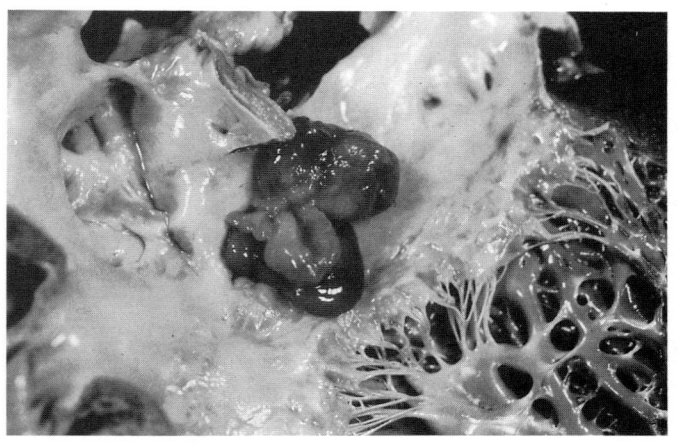

Fig. 10 The myxoma from Fig. 9 at autopsy. It measured 2.5 × 1 cm.

Rhabdomyoma

These are benign tumours and constitute the most common primary tumour of the heart in infancy and childhood.[20-23] 85% are seen in children below the age of 15, while the great majority of these tumours occur in children less than 1 year of age. Rhabdomyomas are frequently multiple and are found with equal frequency in both ventricles. The tumours are variable in size and cause symptoms either by

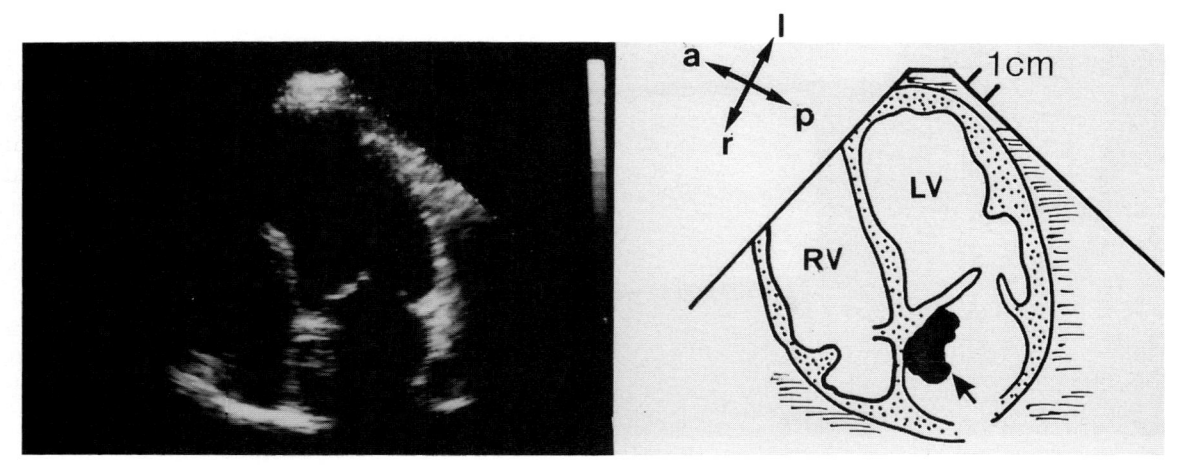

Fig. 9 Apical four chamber view from a patient with a left atrial myxoma. Despite the small size of the mass (arrow), the atrial surface of the anterior mitral leaflet was eroded, implying that the myxoma had previously been a lot bigger, reaching the mitral valve during diastole.

obstructing intracardiac blood flow or by interfering with the normal cardiac conduction. A diffuse form of the disease that affects the entire heart and leads to global heart failure is more rare.[24]

Although the neoplastic nature of rhabdomyomas remains controversial, it is believed that these are tumours originating from cardiac muscle cells and are hamartomas rather than true tumours. They have a congenital origin and have limited potential for growth.

The differential diagnosis of rhabdomyomas is usually suggested by two-dimensional echocardiography when the child is referred for investigation of arrhythmias, heart failure or signs of obstruction of any of the cardiac valves. Indeed, the diagnosis of cardiac arrhythmias in a child should prompt a careful echocardiographic examination of the entire heart, including the tip of the cardiac apex. Figure 11 is from a 2-year-old child with rhabdomyoma, originally referred for a two-dimensional echocardiogram, to investigate the cause of progressive heart failure. The apical four chamber view shows the presence of an intracardiac mass on the lateral left ventricular wall. The serial parasternal short axis views defined the localisation and the extent of myocardial involvement of the tumour better (Fig. 12). These views demonstrate the tumour involving the distal portion of the left ventricular lateral and inferior walls, commencing immediately below the level of papillary muscles and reaching the cardiac apex. Localised left ventricular hypokinesis of the tumour-infiltrated muscle was also apparent in the real time imaging of the heart. This localised myocardial thickening may resemble the two-dimensional echocardiographic appearance of hypertrophic cardiomyopathy, particularly when the tumour infiltrates the ventricular septum.

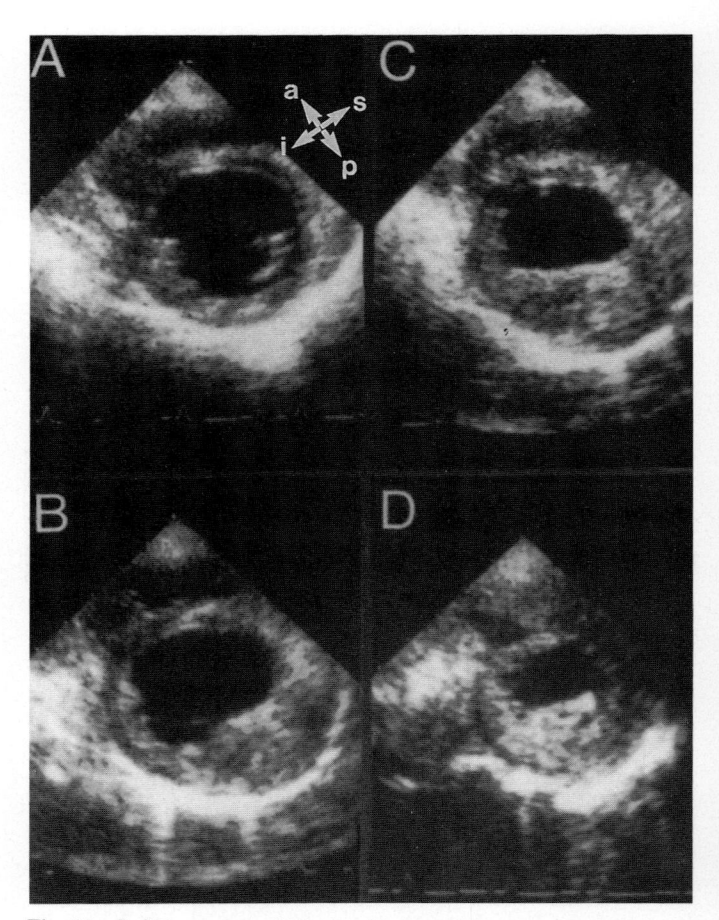

Fig. 12 **Serial parasternal short axis views from the same patient as in Fig. 11,** from the papillary muscle level (A) down to the apex (B, C, D). The tumour is shown to occupy the inferolateral left ventricular wall.

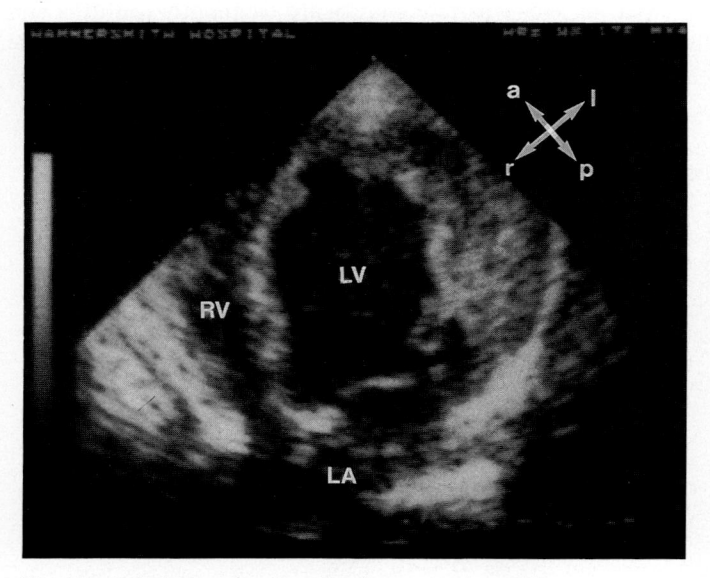

Fig. 11 **Apical four chamber view from a patient with a rhabdomyoma.** Note the thickened and lobulated appearance of the lateral left ventricular wall.

Fibroma

Fibromas are benign tumours of the heart that can be found in patients of any age, but in the overwhelming majority they are seen in patients younger than 10 years of age, constituting the second most common paediatric cardiac tumour.[25] Fibromas may grow slowly to a large size and usually present as circumscribed solid, firm and highly echogenic mass lesions. These tumours are virtually always solitary and are located in the left ventricular free wall or the inter-ventricular septum, similar to rhabdomyomas. Patients present with arrhythmias or obstructive symptoms and have a high risk of sudden death. Congestive failure is usually related to interference with myocardial contraction.

Cardiac fibromas are frequently located in the interventricular septum and often present with arrhythmias producing an 'asymmetrical septal hypertrophy' which must not be confused with true hypertrophic cardiomyopathy.

Although complete resection of the fibroma is the therapeutic goal of the cardiac surgeon, it is often difficult to resect the entire tumour so the potential for sudden death in these patients remains. Two-dimensional echocardiography is an excellent means of observing these patients for possible regrowth of the tumour. Cardiac transplantation remains an alternative surgery particularly for the very large and unresectable fibromas.[26]

Other benign primary tumours

Other rarely seen benign tumours of the heart include lipomas, papillary fibroelastomas and haemangiomas.

Intracardiac lipomas usually appear as small lobulated subendocardial masses and are often a coincidental finding at autopsy. They can be found throughout the heart.

Myocardial or endocardial lipomas can become symptomatic through interference with cardiac conduction or through obstruction to intracardiac blood flow.[27]

Papillary fibroelastomas are also uncommon intracardiac tumours and their diagnosis is rarely made during life. These benign cardiac tumours often have a sessile base and have a superficial similarity to viral warts of the skin. They usually arise from the mitral and aortic valves or the endocardium (Fig. 13). They are rarely of any clinical significance but they may be the cause of syncope, cerebral embolisation, coronary emboli or even sudden death. With the wide use of two-dimensional echocardiography, papillary fibroelastomas can now be depicted during life, usually as an incidental finding.

The significance of these benign intracardiac masses is perhaps greater in the confusion they can create to the echocardiographers on their first encounter with the lesion. It is therefore of great clinical importance, when such a lesion has been discovered, to review the recorded video tape with an appropriate experienced physician, relating the finding to the patient's clinical context, before rushing into major surgical decisions.

Malignant primary tumours of the heart

Most of these malignant tumours of the heart are sarcomas and usually associated with poor prognosis (Table 1). There are no specific echocardiographic features that can distinguish between the various types of the malignant cardiac tumours. There are, however, some characteristics, such as the associated pericardial collection, that allow two-dimensional echocardiography to distinguish between benign and malignant primary tumours.

Angiosarcoma is the most frequently encountered cardiac sarcoma, with the overwhelming majority involving the right side of the heart or pericardium.[28,29] These tumours usually invade the vena cava, tricuspid valve and pericardium. It is therefore very common for them to present clinically with pericardial effusion or acute tamponade, right heart failure, or with signs of obstruction to right atrial filling. Many of these patients will also have signs of metastatic lesions at the time of presentation.

Echocardiography is the most valuable tool in suggesting the diagnosis of angiosarcoma. When the lesion is demonstrated early, echocardiography may show only a persistent pericardial effusion, predominantly anteriorly. At a later stage the anterior pericardial space is associated with marked thickening of the anterior right ventricular free wall which is also markedly hypokinetic. Occasionally, extension of the tumour inside the right atrium or the right ventricular cavities, may also occur. Figure 14 is a parasternal long axis view from a 29-year-old patient who was initially referred because of persistent pericardial effusion. It shows a large mass occupying the entire right

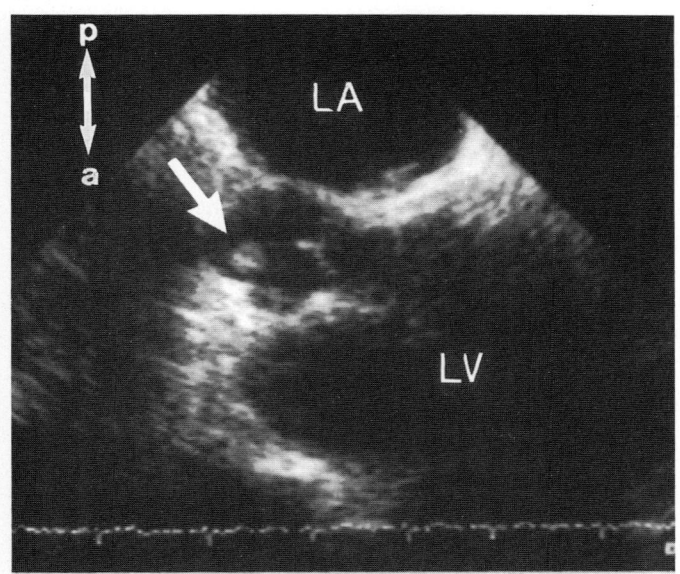

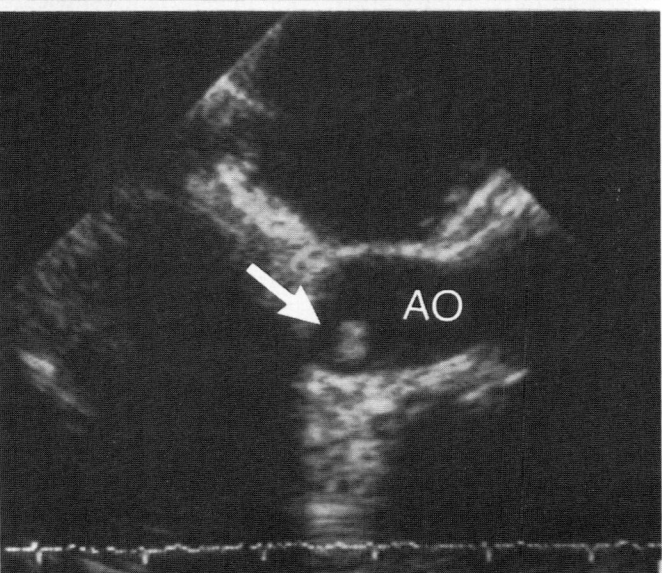

Fig. 13 Apical five chamber view from the transoesophageal approach showing a spherical mass (arrow), possibly a papillary fibroelastoma, in the aortic root.

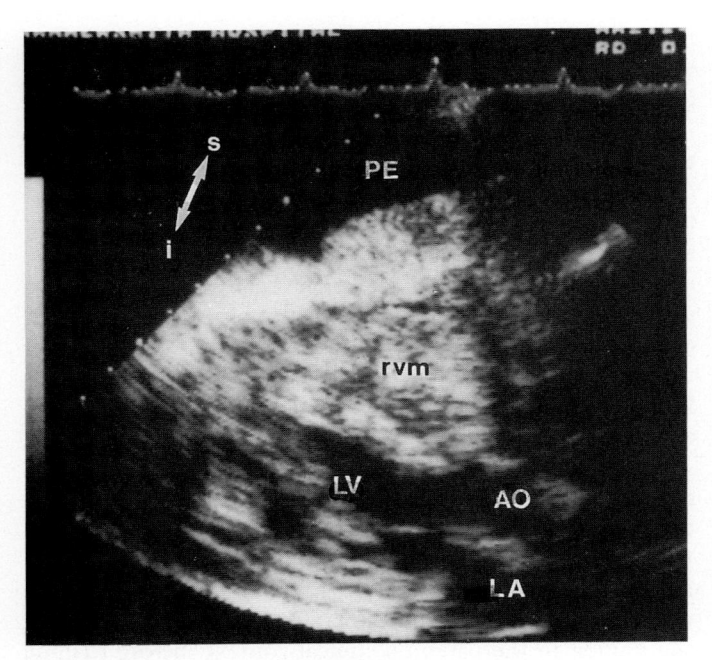

Fig. 14 Parasternal long axis view from a patient with angiosarcoma. The right ventricle is filled with a large tumour mass. Note also a moderate pericardial effusion with extensive thickening of the pericardium, projecting into the pericardial space (PE = pericardial effusion, RVM = right ventricular mass).

ventricle and extending anteriorly into the pericardial space.

Mesotheliomas may originate primarily from the pericardium. These tumours show a wide range of histological appearances. The tumour may grow by superficial spread and usually invades the myocardium superficially. Eventually, the tumour may spread circumferentially encapsulating a major part of the heart and leading to constrictive pericardial disease.

SECONDARY CARDIAC TUMOURS

Secondary tumours of the heart are common and are virtually all malignant. Almost any tumour in the body may metastasise to the heart with the exception of most cerebral neoplasms. The most common site of tumour spread is the pericardium, leading to tamponade which may require immediate treatment. Myocardial or endocardial metastases are less common but are important to recognise promptly, as they may have decisive prognostic implications in patients with malignancy.

Secondary invasion of the heart by metastatic tumours often remains undiagnosed before death but two-dimensional echocardiography is of great value in the demonstration of cardiac metastasis, as well as for the on-going assessment of patients with secondary cardiac malignancies. It is particularly sensitive in the detection of pericardial effusion, which is the commonest echo-cardiographic finding in patients with cardiac metastases

and is extremely helpful in excluding the presence of biventricular dysfunction, which can be clinically confused with haemodynamic compromise from cardiac tamponade.

Secondary tumours can spread to the heart by direct extension from surrounding intrathoracic structures, by haematogenous spread via the vascular bed or by lymphatic spread. Direct extension occurs most often in the setting of a bronchogenic carcinoma, through the pericardium into the right ventricular free wall or the atria. Other mediastinal tumours can behave in the same manner. Indirect extension to the heart via the vascular bed or the lymphatic network, can theoretically occur from any malignant tumour. The embolised tumour cells lodge in the myocardium as it has the greatest blood supply. The endocardium and valves are less frequently affected by metastatic tumours.

The most frequently encountered echocardiographic findings in malignant cardiac involvement are pericardial effusion, with or without pericardial thickening, myocardial thickening with possible different myocardial texture to the surrounding healthy myocardium and with concomitant myocardial hypokinesis or akinesis. Endocardial invasion is rare but it can occur, particularly in the very advanced stages.

The clinical suspicion of pericardial effusion is often the main reason for requesting an echocardiographic examination. Chandraratna and Aronow[30] reported several patients with malignant pericardial effusion, where two-dimensional echocardiography demonstrated 'cauliflower-like masses' extending from the parietal or epicardial surface into the pericardial space. Popovic[31] described the case of a breast carcinoma spreading through the pericardium into the anterior wall of the right ventricle which eventually caused an intracavitary obstruction of the right ventricular outflow tract. Although the right ventricular free wall can be visualised well with two-dimensional echocardiography when there is a pericardial effusion, this might not be so easy in the absence of any pericardial collection or indeed when the pericardial space has been infiltrated with tumour. From parasternal long axis projections the right ventricular free wall is very close to the ultrasound transducer, so that the near gain resolution is often insufficient to differentiate between artefact, myocardium or tumour infiltrate.

Myocardial involvement by metastatic tumour is rare and more commonly will represent primary cardiac tumour. It can result in congestive heart failure, arrhythmia, outflow tract obstruction or peripheral emboli. The two-dimensional echocardiogram usually shows a focal area of myocardial thickening, sometimes with increased reflectivity or localised wall motion abnormality.[32]

Intracavitary metastases are the least common type of secondary cardiac tumours, generally presenting as intracavitary or valvular obstruction. Melanoma has the propensity to metastasise to the endocardium and to project as an intracavitary mass.³³⁻³⁵ Occasionally, metastatic tumours can be seen to invade the right atrium, usually entering it via the inferior vena cava. Hepatomas, renal cell carcinomas, Wilm's tumour and various uterine tumours have been known to grow up the inferior vena cava and invade the right atrium.³⁶ Intracavitary metastases can readily be detected with two-dimensional echocardiography using multiple projections, as space-occupying lesions, but it is often very difficult to differentiate between primary and secondary cardiac tumour. As a general rule, intracavitary or mural masses demonstrated by two-dimensional echocardiography are more likely to represent a primary rather than a secondary cardiac tumour.³³,³⁴

Carcinoid disease

One particular tumour involving the intracardiac valves that deserves particular attention is carcinoid disease. The primary carcinoid tumour can spread into the heart via the inferior vena cava into the right atrium and the right ventricle, where it involves the tricuspid valve, pulmonary valve and the right ventricular endocardium. Typically, carcinoid spread into the heart involves the right ventricular endocardium together with the tricuspid and pulmonary valves, with immobilisation of the valves at one point during the cardiac cycle, thus producing predominantly tricuspid and pulmonary regurgitation.³⁷,³⁸ Occasionally, these valves may be stenotic when the immobilisation of the leaflets occurs early in diastole for the tricuspid valve or early in systole for the pulmonary valve. The subvalvular tricuspid apparatus together with the thickened endocardium will create multiple bright echoes, demonstrating a web-like formation. Figure 15 is an apical four-chamber view from a patient with carcinoid involvement of the heart showing the resultant deformity of the tricuspid valve together with the web-like formation of the right ventricular endocardium.

INTRACARDIAC THROMBI

Ventricular thrombi

Intracardiac thrombi can occur in any chamber where blood flow is stagnant or where a thrombogenic surface is exposed to blood flow. Clinically, one encounters ventricular thrombi following myocardial infarction, in patients with dilated cardiomyopathy, or in patients with cardiac implants. Ventricular thrombus is rarely suspected with M-mode echocardiography, as this technique is insensitive due to the lack of spatial resolution. Two-dimensional echocardiography is the technique of choice in the detection of intracardiac thrombi. Of all the cardiac chambers, the right ventricle may be the most difficult to evaluate in this context. When considering the diagnosis of right ventricular thrombus, it is important to

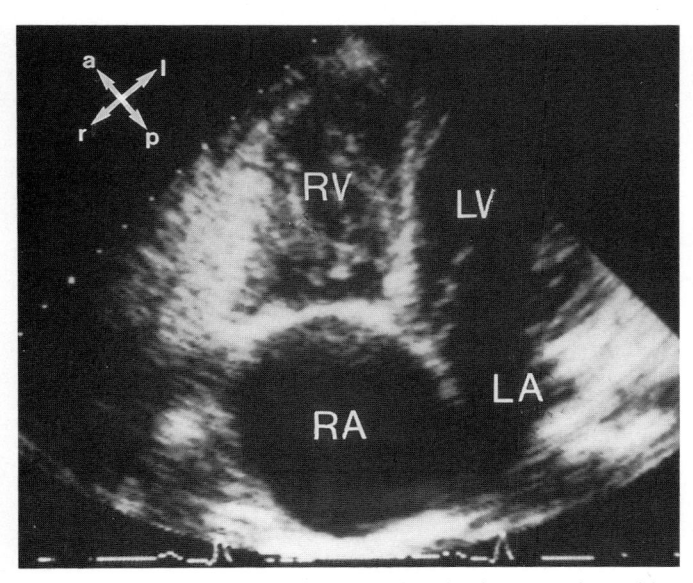

Fig. 15 Apical four chamber view in diastole, from a patient with carcinoid heart disease. Note the thickened and stenotic tricuspid valve together with the web-like formation of the sub-valvular tricuspid apparatus.

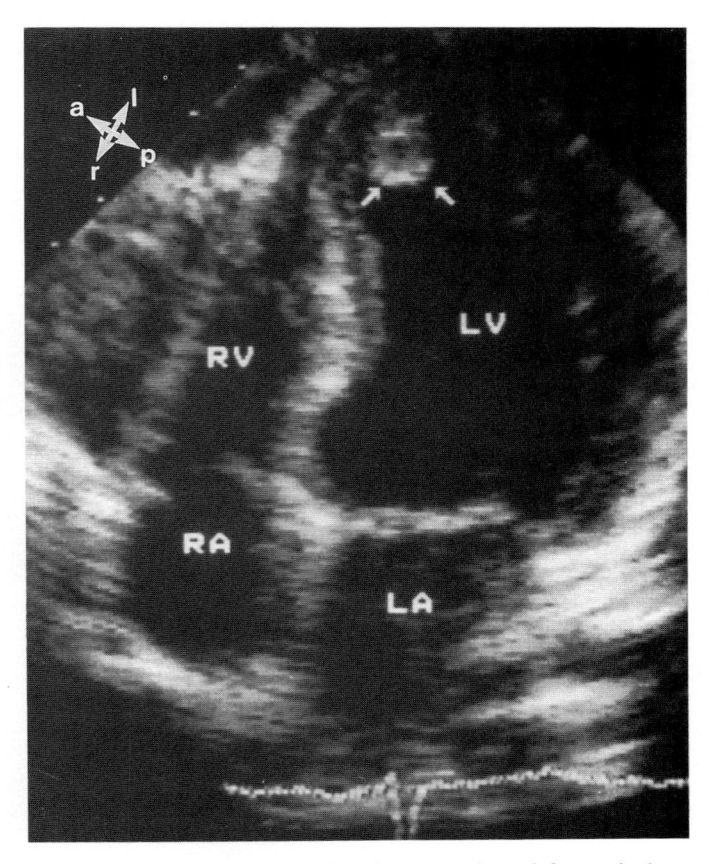

Fig. 16 Apical four chamber view demonstrating a left ventricular thrombus at the apex (arrows), in a patient with recent myocardial infarction. The apex was akinetic. The thrombus is quite reflective and protrudes from a broad base into the left ventricular cavity.

keep in mind the normal intracavitary structures of the ventricle as well as the echocardiographic features of any prosthetic device that might be present.

Left ventricular thrombus is a common autopsy finding in patients with myocardial infarction and dilated cardiomyopathy. In experienced hands two dimensional echocardiography has the ability to provide thorough imaging of the left ventricular apex, the site where the majority of left ventricular thrombi occur, as well as to provide information on the motion of thrombi.

All the available echocardiographic views can and should be used to visualise a left ventricular thrombus, but the apical and parasternal short axis projections are the most useful. Particular care must be taken to obtain optimal images of the cardiac apex from both long- and short-axis projections with use of the depth of field setting to minimise potential near field artefacts, while maintaining optimal left ventricular wall resolution and in particular, resolving the endocardial boundaries.[39]

The echocardiographic diagnosis of left ventricular thrombus is made when an echogenic mass, distinct from the adjacent ventricular wall, is seen in association with a wall motion abnormality from at least two echocardiographic projections (Fig. 16). The thrombus should appear similar in location and size from each view. If this is not so, then the findings should be interpreted with extreme caution. Although two-dimensional echocardiography is now generally recognised as the reference standard for the in vivo diagnosis of left ventricular thrombus, there are several technical considerations that may lead to false diagnosis and misinterpretations. Increased echodensities originating from structures close to the transducer may obscure the presence of the thrombus when viewed from the apical four-chamber projection. Also a transducer-related fixed artefact in the near field may give the false impression of a rounded apical mass.[40] Assinger[41] emphasised the danger of false positive diagnoses and suggested strict echocardiographic criteria for diagnosing left ventricular thrombus. These are the serial identification of an echo-dense mass, with a margin distinct from the ventricular wall and an apical location with associated akinesia or hypokinesia of the adjacent myocardial wall.

Left ventricular thrombi are usually stationary, although at times portions of them may show considerable random motion. It remains uncertain whether adherent but partially mobile thrombi are more likely to embolise. Despite conflicting reports, it is our experience that thrombi following myocardial infarction do not often embolise whether or not they might show any degree of mobility,[39] in contrast with thrombi occurring in patients with dilated cardiomyopathy which are more prone to embolise.

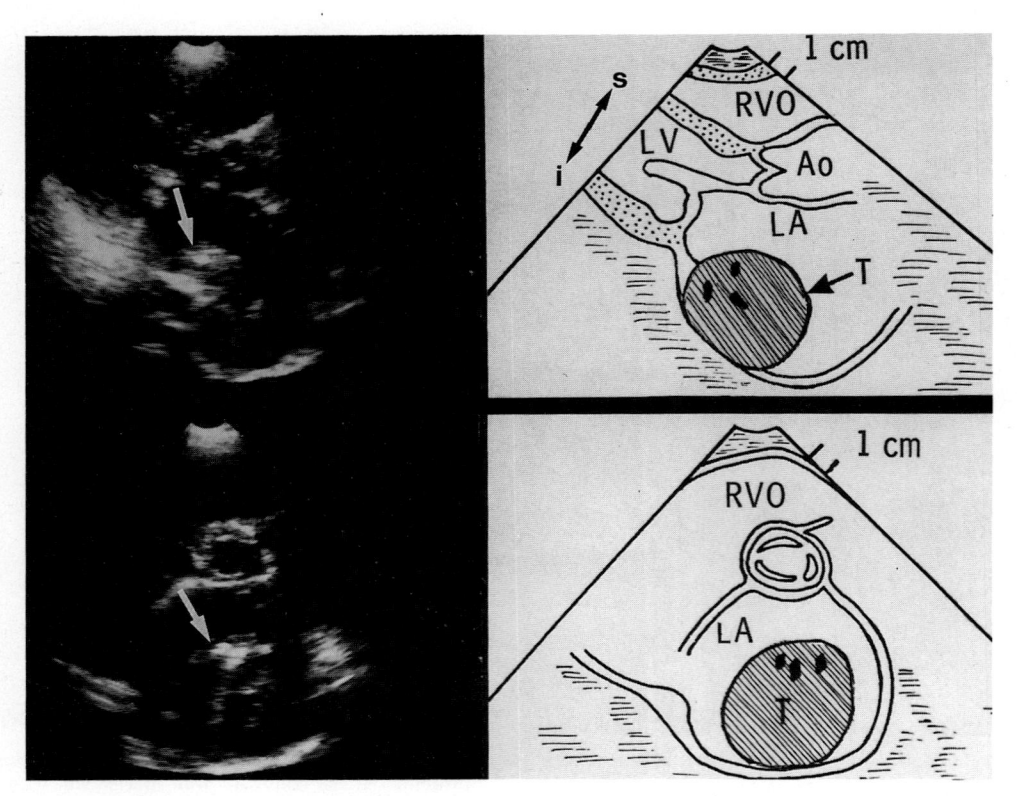

Fig. 17 Parasternal long axis (top) and short axis (bottom) views from a patient with rheumatic heart disease, demonstrating a large thrombus attached to the posterior wall of the left atrium (arrowed). (RVO = right ventricular outflow tract, T = thrombus.)

Atrial thrombi

The atrium, particularly in patients with atrial fibrillation, is a frequent site for thrombus formation. The location, size and motion of left atrial thrombi are variable. Two-dimensional echocardiography is again an excellent tool for the depiction of atrial thrombi. A thrombus fully adherent to the atrial wall, as seen in Figure 17, does not have any independent motion. Thrombi without a firm attachment to the atrial wall may show a jiggling motion during the cardiac cycle. There are, however, major limitations in the detection of left atrial thrombi during a routine transthoracic echocardiographic examination. A thrombus attached to the sewing ring of a prosthetic mitral valve will be very difficult to detect and these thrombi frequently are missed, due to the highly echogenic prosthetic material that obscures the visualisation of the much less echogenic thrombus. A great number of thrombi lodge in the left atrial appendage, which is usually invisible from the transthoracic approach. With the transoesophageal approach however, the left atrial appendage can be explored in full, so that even small atrial thrombi can readily be shown.

Right atrial thrombi occur much less frequently than left atrial thrombi (Fig. 18). They are usually present in association with intracardiac catheters, central lines or pacing wires and it is often difficult to distinguish between thrombus and vegetation, particularly as both can coexist. The most useful views to detect right atrial thrombi are the apical four chamber and subcostal views, particularly as the latter provides imaging of both the inferior and superior vena cava. Figure 19 is an apical four-chamber and subcostal view from a patient with right atrial thrombus. The thrombus was highly mobile, protruding through the tricuspid valve into the right ventricle in diastole. The attachment of this thrombus at the superior vena cava, however, could only be visualised from the subcostal view.

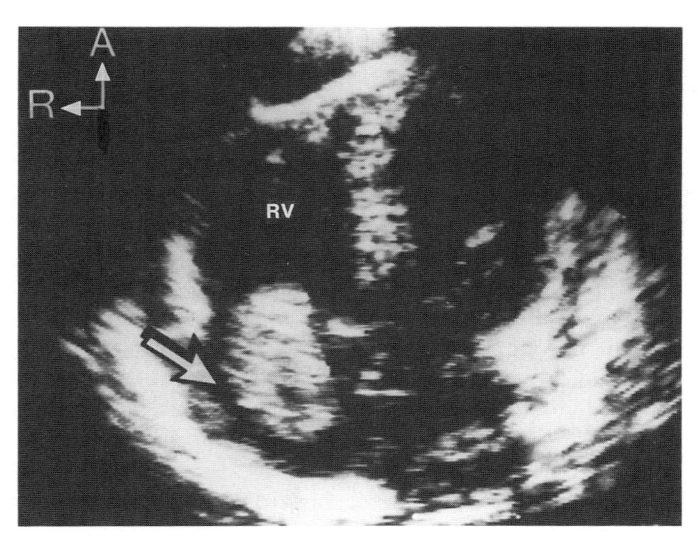

Fig. 18 Apical four chamber view from a patient with a large right atrial thrombus (arrow).

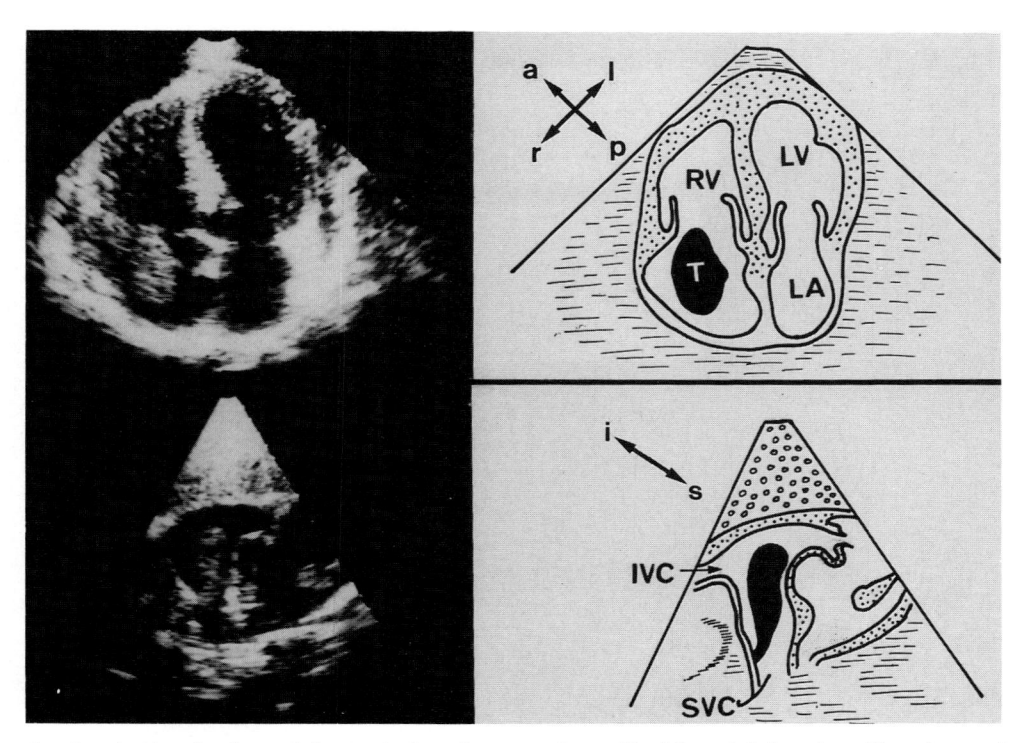

Fig. 19 Apical four chamber (top) and subcostal (bottom) views from a patient with right atrial thrombus. Note the attachment of the thrombus at the origin of the superior vena cava. (IVC = inferior vena cava, LA = left atrium, LV = left ventricle, RV = right ventricle, SVC = superior vena cava, T = thrombus.) (Reproduced with permission.[44])

Often, right atrial thrombi appear as a poorly reflective mass with a sling-like appearance, moving randomly within the atrium or right ventricle but with clear separation from the tricuspid valve. These thrombi usually develop in situ in the inferior or superior vena cavae and appearing as a cast of the vein.

Differential diagnosis

As the use of two-dimensional echocardiography has extended beyond the patients who present with specific cardiological symptoms, the chance of unexpected intracardiac 'discoveries' of mass lesions has dramatically increased. Because of the potential serious clinical implications for the patient, it is imperative for the individuals performing and interpreting echocardiograms to be familiar with the large variations of the normal intracardiac structures. A number of patients have been referred to our echocardiography laboratory with the diagnosis of right atrial thrombus or even tumours and on repeat echocardiographic examination it was shown that they did not have any intracardiac mass. Occasionally, a prominent Eustachian valve or Chiari network will produce prominent echoes within the right atrium that easily can be confused with an atrial tumour or thrombus.[42] These normal structural variants can usually be identified correctly by scanning the inferior vena cava up to the right atrial junction, seeking to identify the Eustachian valve and all three tricuspid leaflets from multiple projections. These should include the parasternal right ventricular inflow tract, apical four chamber and subcostal views. The right atrial appendage which is often very mobile, can also be confused occasionally with a right atrial mass. Experience with the many normal variations and the use of multiple views should eliminate this confusion.

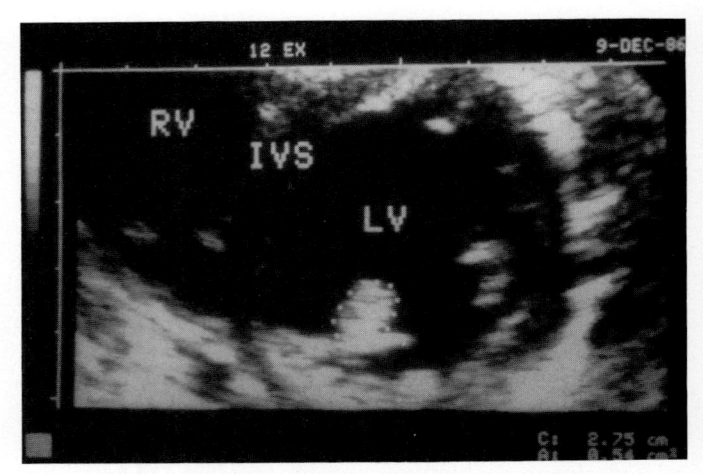

Fig. 20 Parasternal short axis view from a normal patient. Note that the posteromedial papillary muscle is obliquely cut, a finding that can be misinterpreted as intraventricular tumour (IVS = ventricular septum).

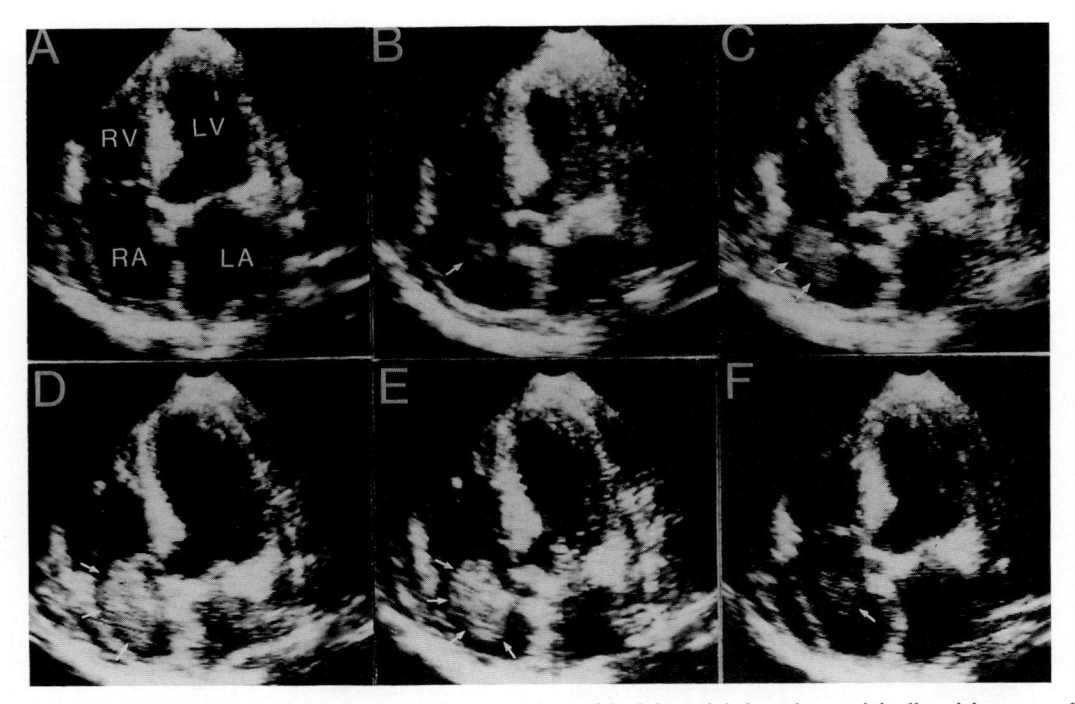

Fig. 21 Sequential frames of the apical four chamber view from a patient with right atrial thrombus, originally misinterpreted to be a myxoma. During systole (A) no intra-atrial mass is visualised. In early diastole (B, C), the mass appears within the right atrium (arrows), while later in diastole (D, E) it appears engaging the tricuspid annulus, before disappearing again in the back of the right atrium during systole (F). Note the similarities of this mass with a myxoma. (Reproduced with permission.)

In the left ventricle heavy trabeculations at the apex, which frequently occur in hypertrophied ventricles, may present confusion when attempting to explore the apex for possible thrombus. These trabeculations may appear as muscle bridges and can present in different arrangements in the left ventricle. Echo-free areas on either side of these bridges and lack of any wall motion abnormality will help in distinguishing these structures from thrombi. Chordal structures, also called false tendons, that inter-connect muscle trabeculations usually present in the left ventricle and can similarly simulate or even hide small thrombi. An abnormally orientated papillary muscle, or an oblique orientation of the echocardiographic plane through a papillary muscle, can also be confused with an intracardiac thrombus or tumour. Figure 20 is from a patient referred to our laboratory with the presumptive diagnosis of left ventricular tumour. On repeat examination the study was entirely normal (and the patient reassured) but the 'left ventricular mass', previously misinterpreted, could easily be reproduced by cutting obliquely the posteromedial papillary muscle.

The differential diagnosis of intracavitary masses include vegetations (infected or sterile), thrombi, or cardiac tumours which may be primary or secondary. A mobile intracardiac mass may be either a thrombus or a tumour. Often specific masses have fairly characteristic appearances and locations into the intracardiac cavities which helps in making a suggestive diagnosis. Examples of these are the left atrial myxomas, valvular vegetations and thrombi located at the left ventricular apex following myocardial infarction or dilated cardiomyopathy. When, however, the lesions are atypical, the differential diagnosis is very difficult and lesions should be interpreted with caution. The echocardiographic features of a pedunculated thrombus are essentially the same as those of a tumour mass and cannot necessarily distinguish a tumour from thrombus (Fig. 21). Levisman[43] reported a case of a pedunculated tumour in the left ventricle that appeared from gross morphological features to be a myxoma, although the pathological diagnosis was pedunculated thrombus.

Intra-atrial thrombi are far more frequent than myxomas and other tumours and should be suspected first when a mobile intracardiac mass is visualised. It may be difficult, however, to determine the aetiology of a solid reflectile mass within the left atrium, as thrombi may appear the same as a tumour on two-dimensional echocardiography. Up to now, neither echocardiography nor magnetic resonance imaging or any other imaging technique, have been useful in distinguishing the various histological types. We have previously described[44] the incidental detection of a right atrial thrombus, which was misinterpreted as being a myxoma, both on echocardiography but also at surgery, emphasising the ultrasonic and macroscopic similarities that some of these masses may acquire. The incidental diagnosis of this atrial thrombus initiated further investigations leading to the diagnosis of bronchial adenocarcinoma.

REFERENCES

1 Prichard R W. Tumors of the heart: review of the subject and report of 150 cases. Arch Pathol 1951; 51: 98
2 Fink L, Reicheck N, St John Sutton M G. Cardiac abnormalities in acquired immunodeficiency syndrome. Am J Cardiol 1984; 54: 1161–1163
3 Goldberg H P, Glenn F, Dotter C T, Steinberg I. Myxoma of the left atrium: diagnosis made during life with operative and post-mortem findings. Circulation 1952; 6: 762
4 Neumann H A, Cordell A R, Prichard R W. Intracardiac myxomas: literature review and report of six cases, one successfuly treated. Am Surgeon 1966; 32: 219
5 Fyke F E III, Seward J B, Edwards W D, et al. Primary cardiac tumours: experience with 30 consecutive patients since the introduction of two-dimensional echocardiography. J Am Coll Cardiol 1985; 5: 1465–1473
6 Schluter M, Hinrichs A, Thier W, et al. Transoesophageal two-dimensional echocardiography: Comparison of ultrasonic and anatomic sections. Am J Cardiol 1984; 53: 1173
7 Seward J B, Khandheria B K, Oh J K, et al. Transesophageal echocardiography: technique, anatomic correlations, implementations and clinical applications. Mayo Clin Proc 1988; 63: 649–680
8 Nihoyannopoulos P. Cardiac tumours. Current Opinion In Cardiology 1986; 1: 286–291
9 Goldberg H, Steinberg I. Primary tumours of the heart. Circulation 1955; 11: 963
10 Bass J L, Breningstall G N, Swaiman K F. Echocardiographic incidence of cardiac rhabdomyoma in tuberous sclerosis. Am J Cardiol 1985; 55: 1379
11 Meller J, Teichholtz L E, Pichard A D, Matta R, Litwak R, Herman M V. Left ventricular myxoma: echocardiographic diagnosis and review of the literature. Am J Med 1977; 63: 816
12 Bulkley B H, Hutchins G M. Atrial myxomas: a fifty year review. Am Heart J 1979; 97: 639–643
13 Pechaceck L W, Gonzalez-Camid F, Hall R J, Garcia E G, de Castro C M, Leachman R D, Montiel-Amoroso G. The echocardiographic spectrum of atrial myxoma: A ten year experience. Tex Heart Inst J 1986; 13: 179–195
14 Vidaillet H J Jr. Cardiac tumours associated with hereditary syndromes. Am J Cardiol 1988; 61: 1455
15 Nihoyannopoulos P, Venkatesan P, David J, Hackett D, Valantine H, Oakley C M. Left atrial myxoma: new perspectives in the diagnosis of murmur free cases. Br Heart J 1986; 56: 554–560
16 Edler I. The use of ultrasound as a diagnostic aid and its effects on biological tissues: continuous recording of the movements of various heart-structures using an ultrasound echo method. Acta Med Scand 1961; 370 (suppl): 1–65
17 Fitterer J D, Spicer M J, Nelson W P. Echocardiographic demonstration of bilateral atrial myxomas. Chest 1976; 70: 282–284
18 De Maria A N, Vismara L A, Miller R R, Neumann A, Mason D T. Unusual echographic manifestations of right and left heart myxomas. Am J Med 1975; 59: 713–720
19 Their W, Schluter M, Krebber H J, et al. Cysts in left atrial myxomas identified by transoesophageal cross-sectional echocardiography. Am J Cardiol 1983; 51: 1793
20 Fisher D R, Beerman L B, Park S C, et al. Diagnosis of cardiac rhabdomyoma by two-dimensional echocardiography. Am J Cardiol 1984; 53: 978

21 Houser S, Forbes N, Stewart S. Rhabdomyoma of the heart: a diagnosis and therapeutic challenge. Ann Thorac Surg 1980; 29: 373–377
22 Nadas A S, Ellison R C. Cardiac tumours in infancy. Am J Cardiol 1968; 21: 363
23 Van Der Hauwaert L G. Cardiac tumours in infancy and childhood. Br Heart J 1971; 33: 125
24 Shrivastava S, Jacks J J, White R S, et al. Diffuse rhabdomyomatosis of the heart. Arch Pathol Lab Med 1977; 101: 78–80
25 Feldman P S, Meyer M W. Fibroelastic hamartoma (fibroma) of the heart. Cancer 1976; 38: 314–323
26 Jamieson S W, Gandani V A, Reitz B A, et al. Operative treatment of an unresectable tumour of the left ventricle. J Thorac Cardiovasc Surg 1981; 81: 797
27 Arciniegas E, Hakimi M, Farooki Z Q, et al. Primary cardiac tumours in children. J Thorac Cardiovasc Surg 1980; 79: 582
28 Panella J S, Milton L P, Victor T A, Semerjian R A, Hueter D C. Angiosarcoma of the heart. Diagnosis by echocardiography. Chest 1979; 76: 221–223
29 Duncan W J, Rowe R D, Freedom R M, Izukawa T, Olley P M. Space-occupying lesions of the myocardium: role of two-dimensional echocardiography in detection of cardiac tumours in children. Am Heart J 1982; 104: 780–785
30 Chandraratna P A N, Aronow W S. Detection of pericardial metastases by cross-sectional echocardiography. Circulation 1981; 63: 197
31 Popovic A D, Harrigan P, Sanfilippo A J, Weyman A E. Echocardiographic diagnosis of cardiac metastases secondary to breast malignancy. Echocardiography: A Jrnl. of CV Ultrasound & Allied Tech. 1989; 6: 283–288
32 Lestuzzi C, Biasi S, Nicolosi G L, et al. Secondary neoplastic infiltration of the myocardium diagnosed by two-dimensional echocardiography in seven cases with anatomic confirmation. J Am Coll Cardiol 1987; 9: 439
33 Ports T A, Cogan J, Schiller N B, Rapaport E. Echocardiography of left ventricular masses. Circulation 1978; 58: 528
34 Ports T A, Schiller N B, Strunk B L. Echocardiography of right ventricular tumours. Circulation 1977; 56: 439
35 Glancy D L, Roberts W C. The heart in malignant melanoma: A study of 70 autopsy cases. Am J Cardiol 1968; 21: 555
36 Farooki Z Q, Henry J G, Green E W. Echocardiographic diagnosis of right atrial extension of Wilm's tumour. Am J Cardiol 1975; 36: 363
37 Callahan J A, Wroblewski E M, Reeder G S, Edwards W D, Seward J B, Tajik A L. Echocardiographic features of carcinoid heart disease. Am J Cardiol 1982; 50: 762
38 Howard R J, Drobac M, Rider W D, et al. Carcinoid heart disease: diagnosis by two-dimensional echocardiography. Circulation 1982; 66: 1059
39 Nihoyannopoulos P, Smith G C, Maseri A, Foale R A. The natural history of left ventricular thrombus in myocardial infarction: a rationale in support of masterly inactivity. J Am Coll Cardiol 1989; 14: 903–911
40 Meltzer R S, Guthaner D, Rakowski H, Popp R L, Martin R P. Diagnosis of left ventricular thrombi by two-dimensional echocardiography. Br Heart J 1979; 42: 261
41 Assinger R W, Mikel F L, Sherma B, et al. Observations on detecting left ventricular thrombus with two-dimensional echocardiography: emphasis on avoidance of false-positive diagnoses. Am J Cardiol 1981; 47: 145–156
42 Werner J A, Cheitlin M D, Gross B W, Speck S M, Ivey T D. Echocardiographic appearance of the Chiari network: Differentiation from right-heart pathology. Circulation 1981; 63: 1104–1109
43 Levisman J A, MacAlpin R N, Abbasi A S, Ellis N, Eber L M. Echocardiographic diagnosis of a mobile, pedunculated tumour in the left ventricular cavity. Am J Cardiol 1975; 36: 957
44 Nihoyannopoulos P, Isaacs J, Bidstrup B, Oakley C M. Right atrial thrombus mimicking myxoma. J Cardiovasc Ultrason 1988; 7: 263–267

16

Pericardium

Normal appearances
Pericardial effusion
Diagnosis of a pericardial effusion
Cardiac tamponade
Pericardial aspiration
Specific types of pericardial effusion
   Tuberculous pericarditis
   Pyopericardium
   Pericardial effusions in heart failure
   Myocardial infarction and Dressler's syndrome
   Post traumatic and post surgical
   Aortic disease
Pericardial thickening and constriction
Pericardial tumours
Congenital abnormalities of the pericardium
Pericardial cysts
Absence of the pericardium

George Hartnell

The diagnosis of pericardial effusion was one of the earliest uses of echocardiography and has been the most useful technique for assessing the majority of cases of pericardial disease, in particular those patients with pericardial effusions. Although magnetic resonance imaging has now become established as the most accurate method for imaging many types of pericardial disease[1] its limited availability and considerable expense mean that echocardiography should be the initial and often the only investigation required in patients with pericardial disease. Echocardiography is useful in the diagnosis of pericardial effusions, the assessment of cardiac tamponade and pericardial constriction, the diagnosis of tumour invasion and the diagnosis of congenital defects.

NORMAL APPEARANCES

The normal pericardium consists of two layers (visceral or serous pericardium and parietal or fibrous pericardium) which are separated in normal patients by a few (up to 20) millilitres of pericardial fluid which is not visible on echocardiography. The visceral pericardium is very thin and the normal parietal pericardium has a maximum thickness of 2–3 mm. The two layers cannot be separated by echocardiography in normal patients and appear as a single echogenic layer on the surface of the heart.

The fibrous pericardium is a conical fibrous sac which surrounds the heart and is fused with the bases of the great vessels as they enter the heart. Inferiorly it is continuous with the central tendon of the diaphragm and it also has connections with the upper and lower ends of the sternum. The serous pericardium is reflected over the bases of the great vessels to cover almost the whole of the surface of the heart and is reflected over the origins of the pulmonary veins so that there is no pericardial space directly behind the left atrium.

The pericardium forms an oblique sinus between the pulmonary veins, usually separated from the left atrium, which is seldom seen on echocardiography. The transverse sinus passes above the pulmonary veins and posterior to the ascending aorta and pulmonary artery but anterior to the superior vena cava and left atrium.

The pericardium can be affected by many conditions but these have only a limited number of effects on the pericardium, namely pericardial effusions (Table 1), pericardial thickening and pericardial masses. Echocardiography is useful in showing all of these and should be the first investigation in any patient with suspected pericardial disease.

PERICARDIAL EFFUSION

Echocardiography should give more than just the diagnosis of pericardial effusion and should answer the following questions:

Table 1 Causes of pericardial effusion (commonest causes listed first)

Viral pericarditis
Tuberculous pericarditis
Purulent infection
Myocardial infarction*
Dressler's Syndrome
Malignancy*
Rheumatoid arthritis*
Systemic lupus eythematosus*
Uraemia
Heart failure*
Myxoedema
Radiation
Trauma (including surgery)*
Aortic dissection*
Myocarditis*
Anticoagulants
Rheumatic fever

* These causes may have other echocardiographic abnormalities

Is there a pericardial effusion?
How large is the effusion?
What is the nature of the effusion fluid?
What is the underlying cause of the effusion?
Where is the effusion and is it in a position where it is accessible to percutaneous drainage if necessary?
Are there any features to suggest that the effusion is causing haemodynamic impairment (cardiac tamponade)?
Is the underlying cardiac function abnormal for any other reason?
In sequential studies has there been any change?

Diagnosis of a pericardial effusion

Separation of the visceral and parietal layers of pericardium by pericardial fluid usually produces an echo-free space surrounding the heart. This is usually well seen on both M-mode (Fig. 1) and cross sectional echocardiography (Fig. 2). Errors are most likely with an isolated M-mode examination which may show a number of echo-free spaces

Table 2 Echo free spaces mimicking pericardial effusion on echocardiography[3]

Pericardial fat
Subepicardial fat[2]
Pleural effusion
Ascites
Descending aorta
Extension of large left atrium behind left ventricle
Laminated thrombus in aneurysm/infarct/pseudoaneurysm
Morgagni hernia
Mitral annulus calcification
Pericardial tumours[8]
Coronary artery fistulae[3]

Causes of false negative echocardiogram in pericardial effusion
Inappropriately high gain setting
Loculated effusion
Asymmetric effusion[5]
Echogenic effusions (pyopericardium/haemopericardium)

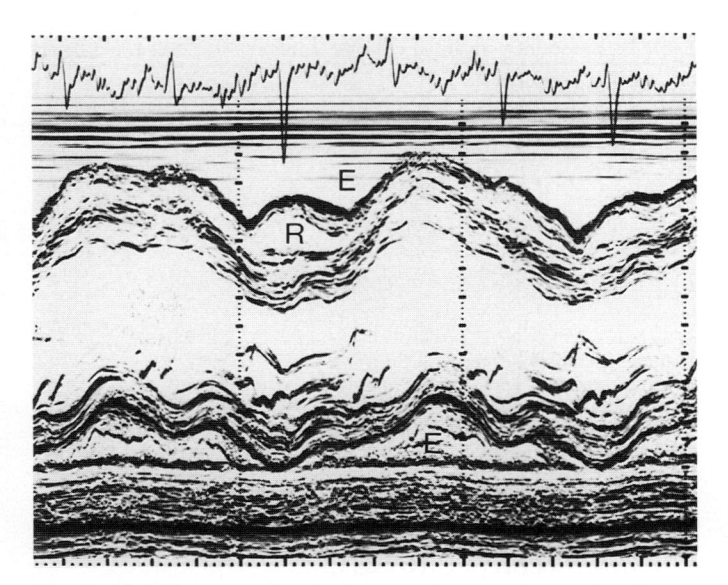

Fig. 1 **M-mode image** showing large, mainly anterior, pericardial effusion (E), 'swinging heart' and compressed right ventricle (R).

which can be confused with a pericardial effusion (Table 2). These may result from exaggerated variations of normal structures, such as epicardial or pericardial fat pads,[2] or large low echogenicity pathological structures such as tumours,[3] pleural effusions and aneurysms.

Differentiation from pleural fluid is important as there is often a common aetiology (i.e. heart failure, malignancy, uraemia). On cross sectional echocardiography the distinction should be clear as the abnormal contour of pleural fluid does not surround the heart and it is often possible to see collapsed lung moving in the pleural effusion. If there are pleural and pericardial effusions the two are separated by an echogenic layer of pleura and pericardium (Fig. 3). Pericardial effusions may also be mimicked by areas of acoustic shadowing which can be caused by areas of abnormal calcification such as mitral annulus calcification.[4]

Many of these sources of error are more clearly differentiated from pericardial fluid by cross sectional echocardiography and this should be the standard for diagnosing a pericardial effusion.[5] On the basis of M-mode echocardiography it was stated that an anterior echo free space is unlikely to represent a pericardial effusion unless there is a posterior echo free space.[6] This is not now considered to be accurate because cross sectional echocardiography has shown that some pericardial effusions, especially small or chronic effusions, can be very localised (Fig. 4).

Pericardial effusion may be missed or hard to define on both cross sectional M-mode echocardiography if the effusion has a similar echogenicity to adjacent myocardium. This may be due to echogenic material in the effusion in patients with haemopericardium, pyopericardium and tuberculous pericarditis. In a few patients with pyopericardium a purulent 'peel' forms over the surface of the heart which is echogenic and may either obliterate the signs of a pericardial effusion or obscure its size.[7]

Quantitation of the size of pericardial effusions has been attempted using both cross sectional and M-mode echocardiography but this is inaccurate as the distribution of fluid can vary with position and is often asymmetric. Most echocardiographic methods for estimating the volume of a pericardial effusion make assumptions about symmetrical distribution of the effusion around the heart and these are

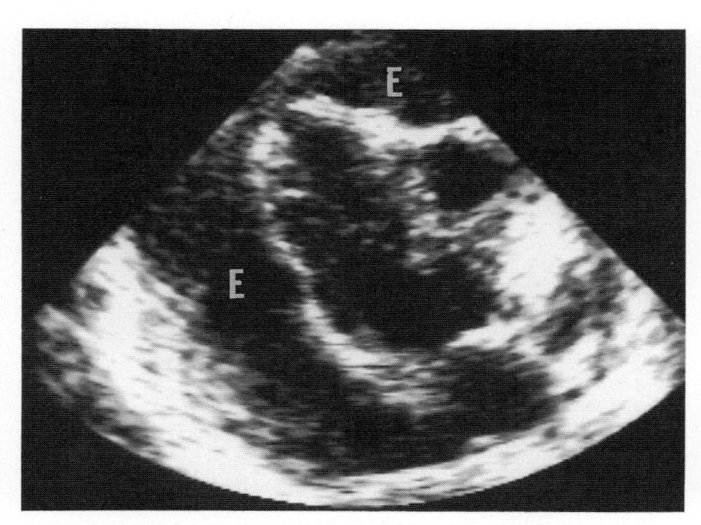

Fig. 2 Apical long axis image of a huge (up to 5 cm thick) pericardial effusion (E) surrounding compressed left ventricle (note concavity on free wall).

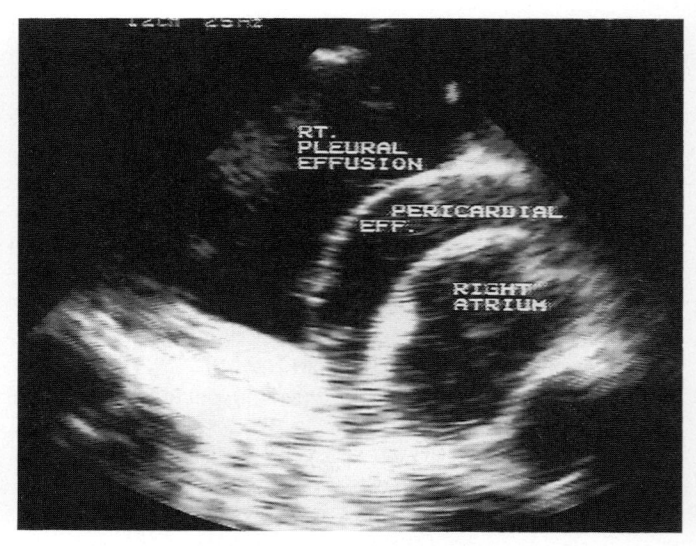

Fig. 3 Low right parasternal view of a pericardial effusion surrounding the right atrium and separated from a large right pleural effusion.

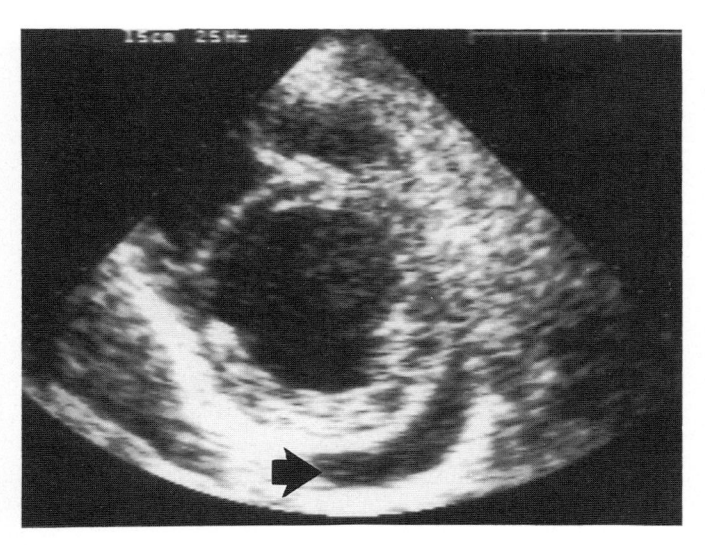

Fig. 4 **Parasternal short axis view showing a small localised pericardial effusion** (arrowed) confined to the posterior border of the left ventricle.

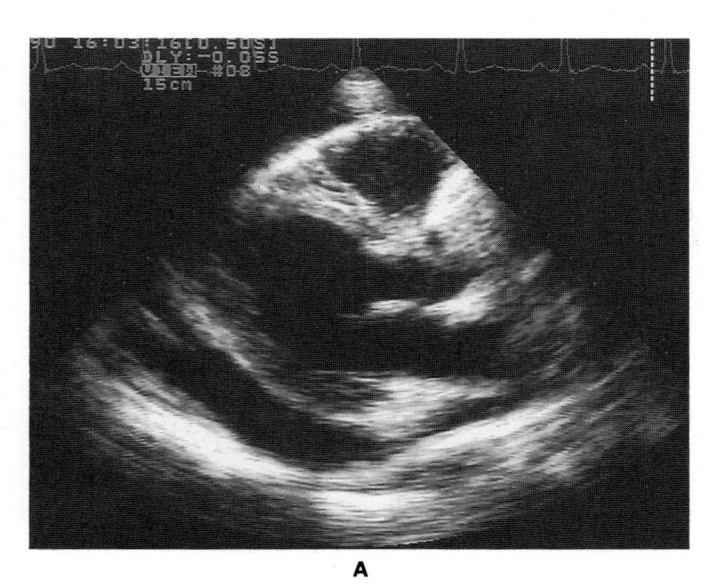

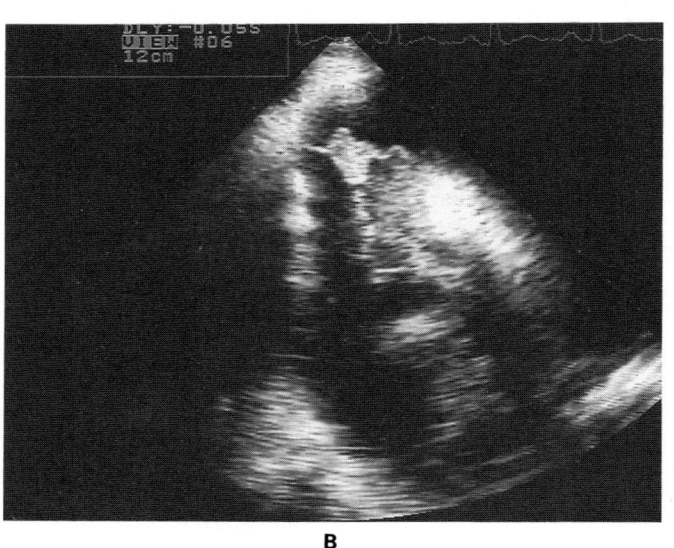

Fig. 5 **A: Parasternal long axis view in a patient with a large pericardial effusion** due to tuberculous pericarditis. **B:** Irregular mass and fibrinous strands in the same patient shown in A.

assumptions that are usually not valid. The best that usually can be achieved is the distinction between small (Fig. 4), moderate or large effusions (Fig. 2). If it is necessary to estimate accurately the size of a pericardial effusion then magnetic resonance imaging or pericardial drainage are more accurate.

Apart from the features relating to isoechogenic pericardial effusions mentioned above there are a variety of features which may give an indication of the underlying cause of a pericardial effusion. Inflammatory changes occurring in patients with tuberculous pericarditis produce an irregular, thickened surface, especially of the visceral pericardium, from which strands of echogenic material project into the pericardial effusion bridging the space between the pericardial surfaces (Fig. 5A and B). Although this appearance is probably most commonly due to tuberculosis it is not pathognomonic and a similar inflammatory response can occur in patients with malignant pericardial effusions (which can be inflammatory or haemorrhagic),[8] inflammatory effusions (such as in rheumatoid arthritis[9]) and idiopathic pericardial effusions.[10] This evidence of inflammation may predict a risk of progression to pericardial constriction. In patients with malignant pericardial effusions there may occasionally be evidence of direct pericardial invasion by tumour (Figs 6, 7A and B), although this is usually a late feature. Often the site of tumour invasion (particularly extension from mediastinal secondary deposits) is difficult to see by cross sectional echocardiography and alternative imaging techniques may be required to demonstrate this.

CARDIAC TAMPONADE

The haemodynamic importance of a pericardial effusion depends not only on its size but also on the speed with which it has accumulated, the elasticity of the pericardium and the presence or absence of any coexisting cardiac disease. Thus rapid development of a small effusion may lead to cardiac tamponade while the slow accumulation of a large effusion, as sometimes occurs with tuberculous pericarditis, may have little apparent haemodynamic effect. Although the need for pericardial drainage is often clinically obvious there are a number of echocardiographic signs which it is claimed may be helpful to indicate the relative haemodynamic importance of a pericardial effusion (Table 3). These signs mainly reflect impairment of cardiac filling but are not necessarily specific.

The accuracy of any echocardiographic method for detecting cardiac tamponade depends not only on the

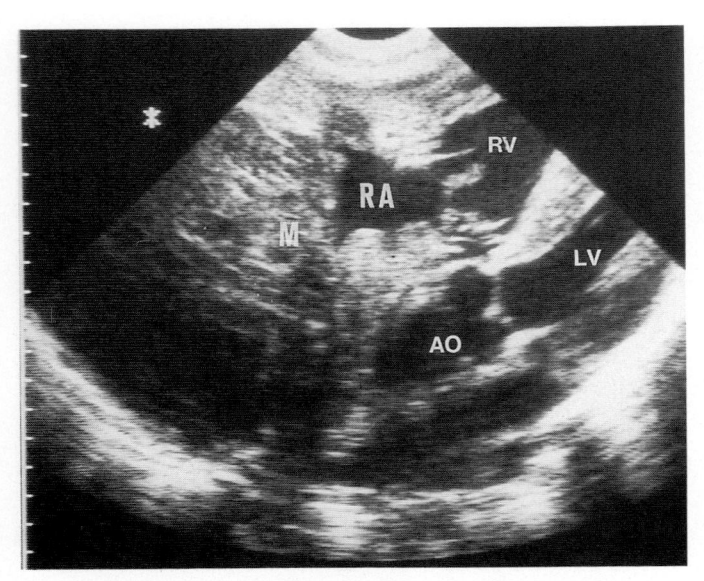

Fig. 6 Subcostal four chamber view showing pericardial invasion from a mediastinal secondary malignancy (M) invading the right atrium.

Table 3 Echocardiographic signs suggesting cardiac tamponade[11]

Small right ventricle or right atrium relative to left ventricle or left atrium
Large respiratory variation in chamber dimensions
Right ventricular early diastolic collapse or free wall inversion
Right or left atrial free wall collapse or inversion
Overactive interventricular septal motion compared with left ventricular free wall motion
Short ventricular filling phase
Early systolic notching of right ventricular free wall
Marked respiratory variation in pulmonary or tricuspid flow
Inspiratory decrease in mitral EF slope
Decreased inspiratory mitral opening
Abnormal inspiratory increase in tricuspid flow
Abnormal inspiratory decrease in mitral flow
Inspiratory changes in left ventricular isovolumic relaxation and ejection time

A large effusion or a 'swinging heart' are not signs of tamponade

echocardiographic criteria used but also on the other methods for validating the diagnosis. Cardiac tamponade is part of a continuum in patients with varying degrees of cardiac compression and the accuracy of the various methods for detecting tamponade will depend on the diagnostic criteria used to define tamponade. Some haemodynamic criteria (such as right atrial pressure exceeding 12 mmHg) correlate well with some echocardiographic features such as diastolic collapse of the free wall of the right atrium but both sets of criteria will exclude patients with 'low pressure' tamponade.[11] In addition some of the signs described can be produced in other conditions in which there is elevation of right heart pressure and impaired right heart filling, such as congestive cardiac failure or pericardial effusions with constrictive pericarditis.[12] The absence of clear cut echocardiographic signs of tamponade in a patient with a pericardial effusion and clinical signs of tamponade should not prevent urgent pericardial drainage.

The majority of echocardiographic signs which have been described as indicating the presence of cardiac tamponade due to pericardial effusion are those relating to poor filling of the right atrium and right ventricle. Diastolic left or right atrial compression[13] or right ventricular compression[14] seen on either M-mode (Fig. 8) or cross sectional echocardiography has been reported to be a sensitive in-

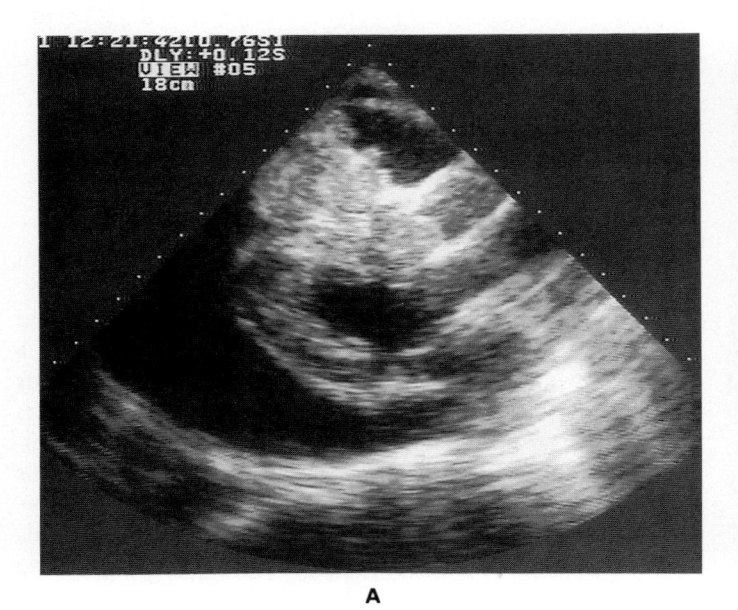

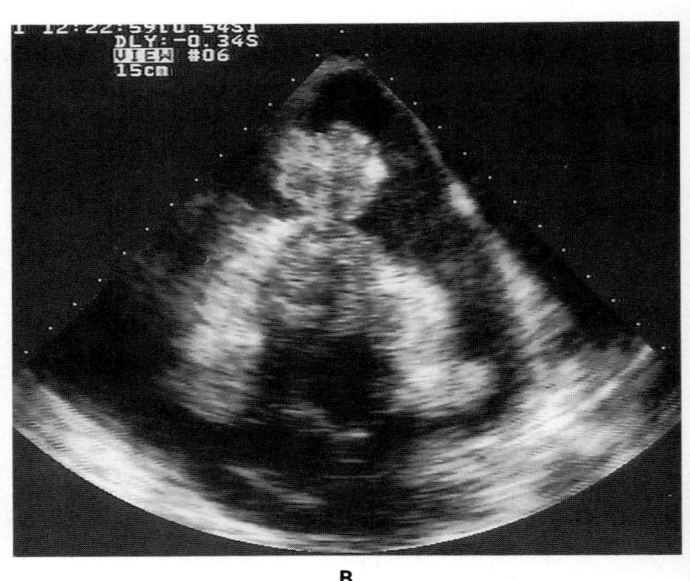

Fig. 7 A: Parasternal long axis view in a patient with a large pericardial effusion and a secondary pericardial deposit from a spindle cell sarcoma. **B:** Apical deposit in the same patient as A.

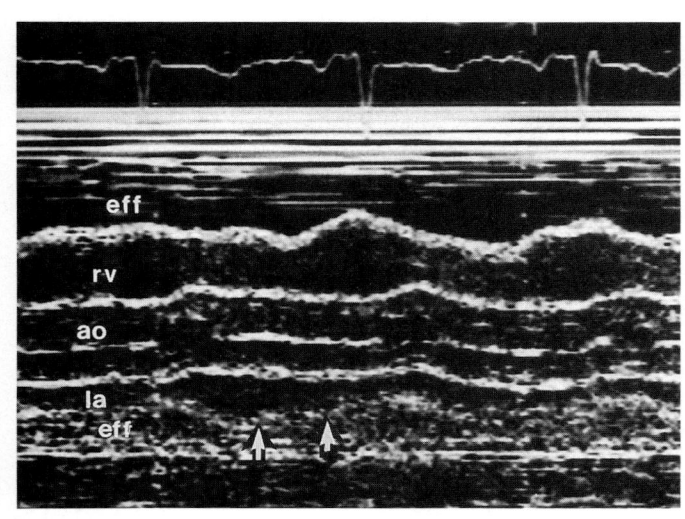

Fig. 8 M-mode tracing showing diastolic left atrial compression (note narrowing of atrial cavity during diastole). eff = effusion.

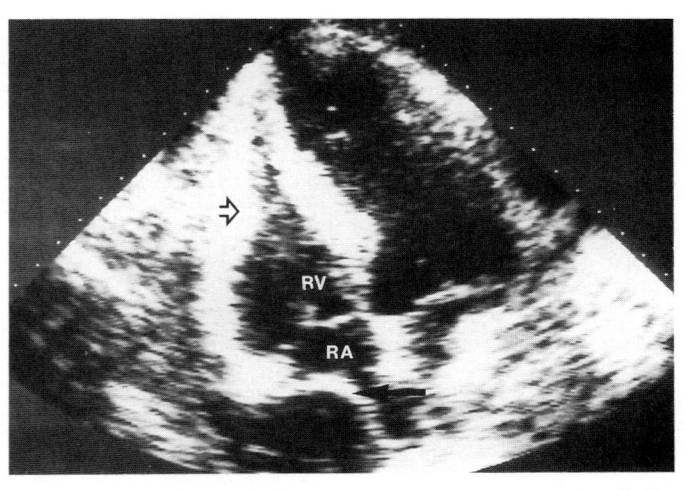

Fig. 10 Apical four chamber view in a patient with a smaller effusion than in Fig. 9 showing a compressed right ventricle and right atrial collapse.

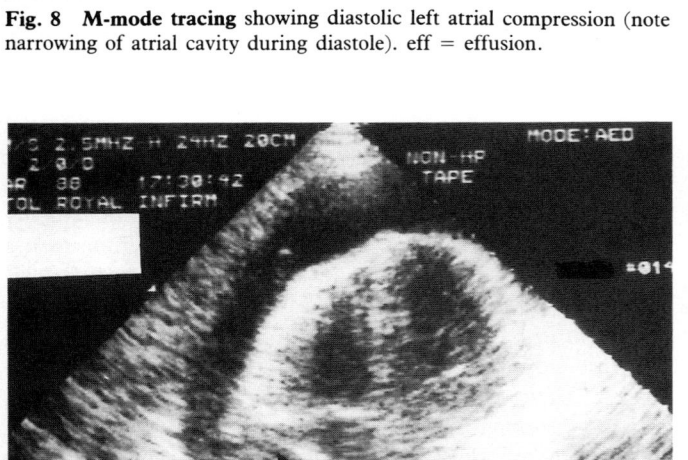

Fig. 9 Apical four chamber view showing right atrial inversion (arrowed) in a patient with a large pericardial effusion and clinical tamponade.

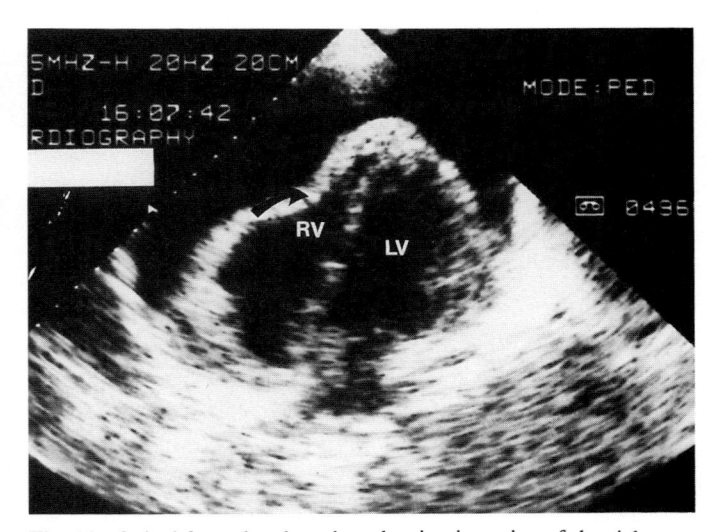

Fig. 11 Apical four chamber view showing inversion of the right (curved arrow) ventricular free wall in a patient with tamponade.

dicator of tamponade and is caused by compression of the low pressure chambers as the ventricles fill during diastole. In particular right atrial inversion (Fig. 9) has been reported to be accurate in the diagnosis of tamponade (sensitivity 100%, specificity 82%, predictive value 50%.)[15] The use of an empirical cut off to the ratio of time of inversion to cardiac cycle length (0.34) improved specificity and predicitive value to 100% with a small loss of sensitivity (94%).[15]

Diastolic right ventricular compression[16] (Fig. 10) or collapse[17] (Fig. 11) has also been reported to be a sensitive indicator of cardiac tamponade which is reversed as tamponade is relieved. The cyclical reversal of the right ventricular wall collapse is a characteristic finding as shown in Figure 12A and B. There are other causes of abnormal right ventricular wall motion which may mimic these abnormalities but the presence of normal right ventricular wall motion seems to be a reliable indicator that a pericardial effusion is not causing impairment of cardiac function.

In some patients with tense pericardial effusions but without haemodynamic signs of tamponade both right ventricular early diastolic collapse and right atrial late diastolic collapse may be present indicating that abnormal cardiac filling is occurring without the development of clinical cardiac tamponade.[18]

Although changes in right heart chamber size and diastolic collapse are useful indicators of cardiac tamponade in some patients these may be difficult to see clearly. This is

Impaired right atrial and right ventricular filling in patients with cardiac tamponade may be reflected in abnormal changes in the diameter of the inferior vena cava in response to respiration. This has led to the description of inferior vena cava plethora, with an abnormal respiratory response, as a sensitive indicator of cardiac tamponade.[12] In this method inferior vena cava plethora is defined as a decrease in upper inferior vena caval diameter of less than 50% after deep inspiration or a sniff. The percentage decrease in inferor vena caval diameter after inspiration (the 'caval respiratory index') was closely correlated with central venous pressure. This method has been reported to be more sensitive but much less specific for cardiac tamponade than right atrial or right ventricular diastolic collapse. Caval plethora is a non-specific marker of raised central venous pressure and should only be used in the diagnosis of cardiac tamponade in an appropriate clinical context as it may also occur in patients with pericardial constriction and congestive cardiac failure.[11] This seriously limits its application as a useful sign of tamponade.

Abnormal cardiac filling in patients with pericardial effusions has been investigated with M-mode echocardiography to investigate changes in systolic time intervals in response to inspiration.[20] The recognition of pulsus paradoxus is a common clinical method for monitoring changes in the haemodynamic effects of a pericardial effusion and it is a reflection of an exaggerated inspiratory reduction in left ventricular function. It might be expected that this would be reflected in changes in systolic time intervals. However it has been shown that even in patients without tamponade but with a pericardial effusion there is an exaggerated decrease in left ventricular ejection time and an increase in pre-ejection period.[20] This indicates that even in the absence of tamponade pericardial effusions can still have a significant effect on ventricular performance and may explain why some of the echocardiographic imaging signs of tamponade are not completely specific. Patients with abnormal systolic time intervals may represent an intermediate group of severity in cases of pericardial effusion which may be at a higher risk of developing tamponade, possibly due to less pericardial elasticity than in other cases.

Abnormalities of cardiac filling are reflected by abnormal transvalvar flow which can be detected by pulsed wave Doppler examination. Various parameters of cardiac filling have been investigated and have been reported to show abnormalities related to significant cardiac tamponade.[21] In patients with tamponade there is an inspiratory increase in left ventricular isovolumic relaxation time, a reduction in early mitral flow velocity and a reduction in mitral flow velocity during atrial systole. These abnormalities are reversed by pericardiocentesis. In the same patients there was an increase in tricuspid flow velocity in early diastole and during atrial contraction, which also reverted to normal after pericardiocentesis. Left ventricular ejection time,

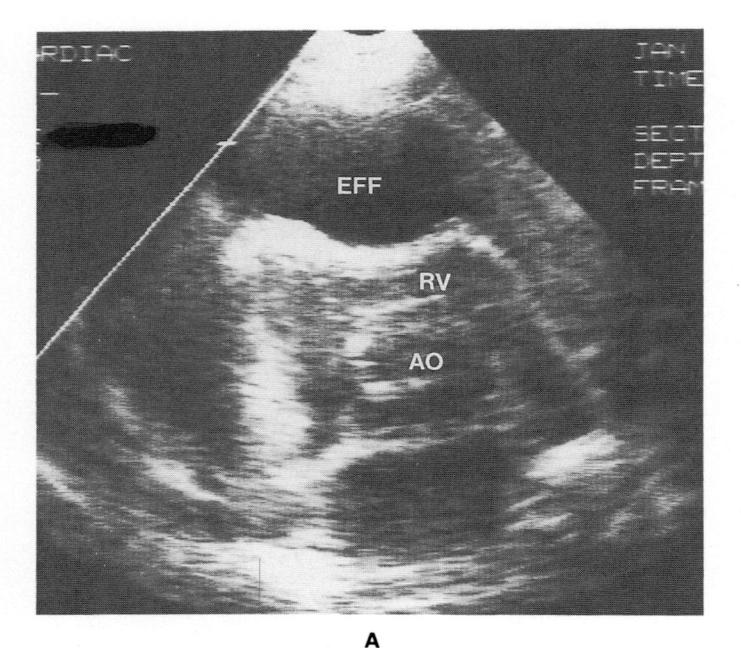

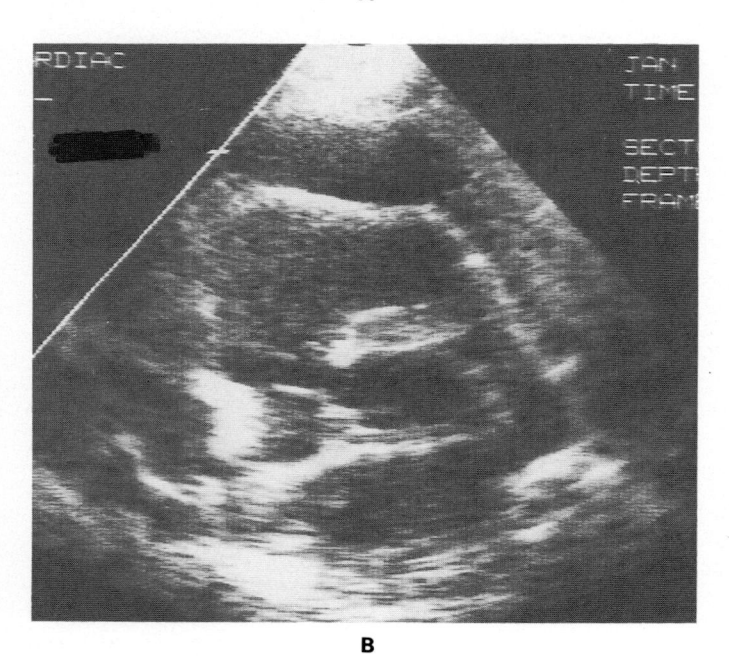

Fig. 12 A: Parasternal short axis view showing early diastolic collapse of the right ventricular free wall in a patient with tamponade. **B:** Late diastolic recovery of the right ventricular free wall in the same patient as A.

especially so in sick and shocked patients who may be unable to cooperate and in whom echocardiographic imaging of the right side of the heart is difficult. The right ventricle may also be so compressed that it cannot be identified and in these circumstances the injection of venous echocontrast will increase the echogenicity of the chambers of the right atrium and right ventricle and will assist in their identification.[19]

and aortic flow velocity decreased more on inspiration in patients with tamponade as expected from the results of measurement of systolic time intervals discussed above,[20] and these changes were also reversed after pericardiocentesis. There was an increase in pulmonary artery flow velocity in the tamponade group. Flow abnormalities were also recorded in the superior and inferior vena cava and hepatic veins. Although it has been suggested that these findings may be useful in the diagnosis of cardiac tamponade they are relatively insensitive and non-specific indicators of tamponade should not be used to diagnose pericardial tamponade in isolation.[22]

PERICARDIAL ASPIRATION

Pericardial aspiration is often required in patients with a pericardial effusion in order to relieve tamponade or to provide samples for diagnosis. Preliminary echocardiography should be used to determine the most accessible route for aspiration, either by the subcostal route or through the chest wall, and should be used to indicate the depth at which the effusion will be encountered. If a subcostal approach is being used, cross sectional echocardiography makes it possible to ensure that an aspirating needle will not inadvertently puncture the left lobe of the liver (Fig. 13). Cross sectional echocardiography allows the selection of what may seem to be unusual puncture sites if it can show that there is no lung between the pericardial effusion and the skin puncture site. Ultrasonically guided pericardiocentesis can be performed reliably and with a very low incidence of complication.[23] In patients where a catheter needs to be left in place to drain a large or viscous effusion the position of the drainage catheter should be visible on cross sectional echocardiography and this will ensure a satisfactory position (Fig. 14).

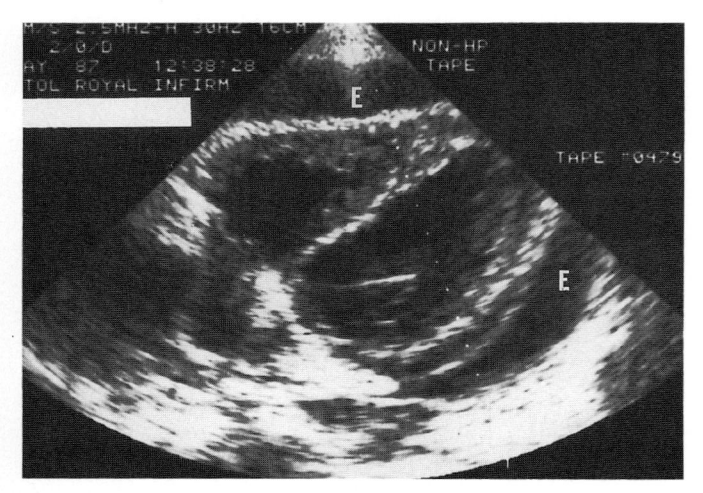

Fig. 13 Subcostal four chamber view showing the short distance between the pericardial effusion (E) and the surface of the chest. There is no intervening liver.

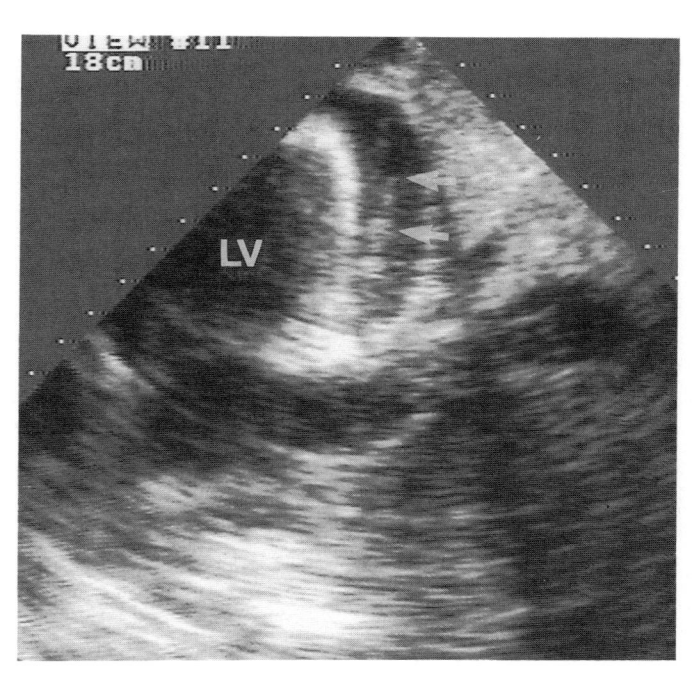

Fig. 14 Apical view showing an indwelling catheter (arrowed) draining a pericardial effusion.

In some difficult cases, especially if the effusion is loculated or viscous, simultaneous echocardiography should be used to guide the insertion of the drainage needle. The scan plane should be orientated parallel to the long axis of the needle to give the clearest indication of the position of the tip of the needle. The transducer should be positioned over a good echo window remote from the skin puncture so that the needle is imaged in the best focused zone for that transducer. If possible a transducer frequency should be chosen to optimise imaging at the level where the pericardium will be entered. If there is doubt about whether or not the needle is in the pericardial effusion, a small amount of saline or echocardiographic contrast medium can be injected which will show the position of the needle tip. In difficult cases, especially with echogenic effusions, an angiographic J-guide wire can be inserted and its movement in the pericardial effusion can be sought on cross sectional echocardiography.

A miniaturised echocardiographic transducer has been developed which can be mounted on the tip of a pericardiocentesis needle to indicate the position of the needle to the pericardial effusion and the surface of the heart.[24] This seems to be an unnecessarily sophisticated approach to a procedure which is usually satisfactorily performed using more conventional imaging methods.

Specific types of pericardial effusion

Tuberculous pericarditis

Tuberculous pericarditis is always secondary to infection

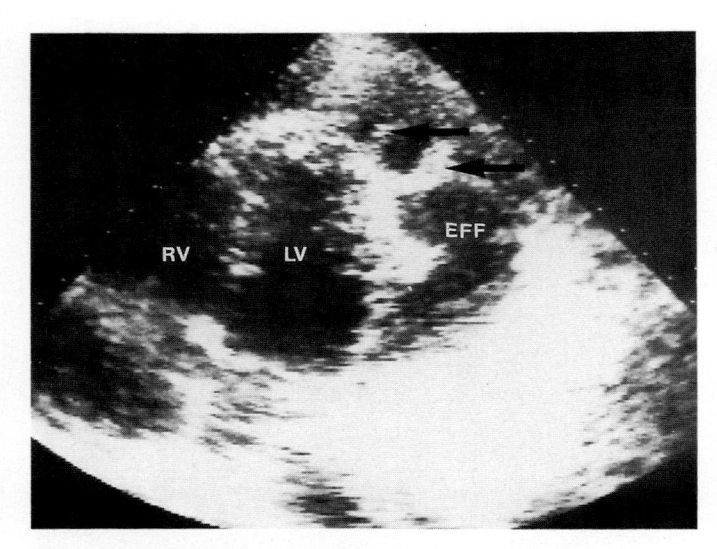

Fig. 15 Apical view from a patient with acute pericarditis with thickened pericardium and fibrinous strands (arrowed) passing through an effusion (EFF).

elsewhere but may be the first indication of that infection. Presentation may be with acute pericarditis, pericardial effusion or pericardial constriction. At the time of diagnosis a tuberculous pericardial effusion may be very large and may produce signs of tamponade, although the rate of deterioration is usually slower than with other causes of pericardial effusion leading to tamponade.

The echocardiographic features include surface irregularity of the pericardium, strands crossing the pericardial space[5] and irregular thickening of the pericardium[25] (Fig. 15) but these are not specific for a tuberculous aetiology. Drug treatment produces a reduction in the size of the effusion but there is often a slow progression in the thickening of the pericardium to cause pericardial constriction.

Pyopericardium

Pyopericardium is uncommon and can be a consequence of direct spread from adjacent structures (most commonly lobar pneumonia) or haematogenous spread from a distant source of infection. Pericardial tamponade may develop rapidly and can require urgent drainage, often with an indwelling drainage catheter which can be inserted under ultrasonic contol. Pyopericardium is often echogenic and can be difficult to see clearly on echocardiography. In these circumstances injection of saline or the passage of a J-guide wire into the effusion may clarify the position of an aspirating needle. In an intermediate stage an echogenic pericardial 'peel' may develop. This is separate from the thickened pericardium and it lies within the pericardial effusion.[7]

In spite of drainage and treatment with antibiotics, pyopericardium may reaccumulate rapidly and become loculated, which may necessitate separate drainage catheters. Progression to constriction is common but unpredictable and follow-up by echocardiography over several years may be necessary. In some cases constriction develops very quickly so that aspiration becomes ineffective and measurement of systolic time intervals shows deteriorating left ventricular function which, in the appropriate context, may indicate a need for early surgical intervention.[26]

Pericardial effusions in heart failure

Pericardial effusions of varying size are a common incidental finding in patients with heart failure. Although significant sized effusions can occur these are unlikely to cause tamponade and the main role of echocardiography is in the assessment of underlying cardiac function. Apart from evidence of associated poor cardiac function (Fig. 16) or valve dysfunction there are no other diagnostic features.

Myocardial infarction and Dressler's syndrome

Pericarditis (as indicated by the presence of a pericardial friction rub) may occur in up to 16% of cases of acute myocardial infarction. Assessment by M-mode echocardiography shows that about half of these cases have a pericardial effusion but it has also been shown that pericardial effusions develop in up to 37%[27] of patients with myocardial infarction. Most of these effusions are small and cause no symptoms. In another series using cross sectional echocardiography, 26% of cases of acute myocardial infarction developed a pericardial effusion, of which the majority were small.[28] The development of a pericardial effusion was related to the size of the myocardial infarct and a

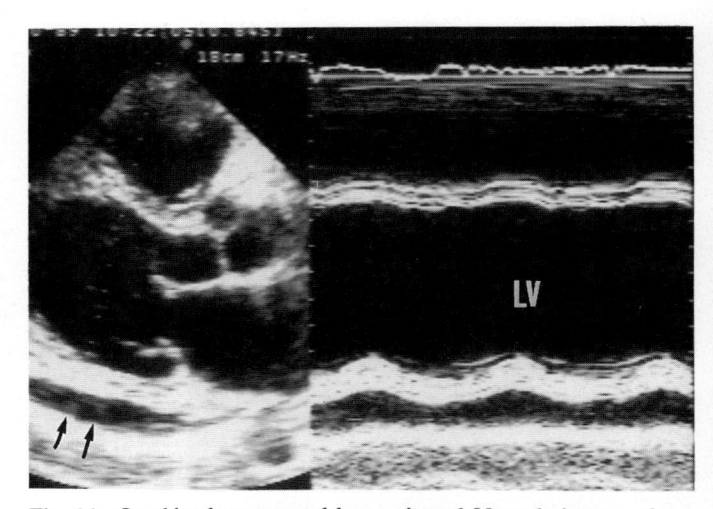

Fig. 16 Combined parasternal long axis and M-mode images of a patient with poor left ventricle (seen on M-mode, LV) and a secondary posterior effusion (arrowed).

poorer prognosis. Treatment with anticoagulants may occasionally precipitate haemorrhage which can rapidly lead to tamponade requiring urgent echocardiographic confirmation and drainage.

Post-infarction haemopericardium due to myocardial rupture is usually rapidly fatal but there have been cases where the diagnosis has been made and surgical repair has been successful. The haemopericardium has a low level echo pattern compared with the echo free ventricular chambers. This is due to clot formation and in the context of acute myocardial infarction followed by sudden deterioration this finding should suggest the diagnosis and indicate the need for urgent repair.[29]

Pericardial effusion is common in Dressler's syndrome but usually does not require drainage and only very rarely progresses to constriction.

Post traumatic and post surgical

Haemopericardium can complicate both penetrating and non-penetrating chest injury. The rapid collection of even a small amount of pericardial blood can rapidly lead to severe tamponade and the development of signs of tamponade should be urgently investigated with a view to open repair of the site of injury. In cases of penetrating trauma (i.e. knife wounds) there may also be evidence of local contraction abnormalities due to coronary artery damage. Haemopericardium can also complicate blunt chest trauma, most commonly following road traffic accidents. In a patient with hypotension following blunt trauma there may be a haemopericardium but the echocardiographic examination should also specifically seek other causes of hypotension such as aortic rupture. The latter condition occurs most commonly at the aortic isthmus which is difficult to see with echocardiography and next most commonly at the aortic root which should be easily visible. Mitral valve rupture, acute ventricular septal defect and myocardial infarctation due to coronary artery damage can also complicate blunt trauma.

Cardiac tamponade is a not uncommon complication of cardiac surgery and its development may be delayed for some time (up to three months) after surgery.[30] In some cases cross sectional echocardiography shows a conventional type of non-loculated pericardial effusion which may have features suggesting tamponade. In other cases the effusion may be loculated, especially posteriorly, and be associated with local compression of the left ventricle and abnormal paradoxical motion of the posterior wall.[30] Other cases may be associated with a loculated effusion which can compress the right atrium or superior vena cava and may be visible on cross sectional echocardiography.[31] In all these situations the loculated fluid is more echogenic than blood in the ventricles and should be separated from the cardiac chambers by a layer of myocardium.

Aortic disease

Although ascending aortic disease is an uncommon cause of a pericardial effusion, its recognition is important as urgent surgical treatment is effective and there is often very little time to make the diagnosis. Haemopericardium can complicate aortic dissection or rupture of the aorta, usually through an aortic sinus in patients with Marfan's Syndrome or similar types of annuloaortic ectasia. The development of a haemopericardium, possibly containing low level echoes (Fig. 17), in these circumstances usually causes tamponade which can develop very rapidly. The echocardiographic features are those of tamponade due to any other cause, although there will usually be other echocardiographic features of the precipitating aortic disease (aortic regurgitation, ascending aortic dilatation and a dissection flap). Urgent echocardiography should not delay surgery and is aimed at confirming the diagnosis, the underlying cause and other complications, such as aortic incompetence. There is little to be gained by inserting a percutaneous drain as this is likely to be unhelpful and will delay definitive surgical treatment.

PERICARDIAL THICKENING AND CONSTRICTION

Pericardial thickening is usually the consequence of pericarditis or haemopericardium (of whatever cause) and can develop over a period which may vary from a few weeks to several years following the original episode. Pericardial thickening can also result from invasion by tumour such as mesothelioma, metastases and lymphoma.

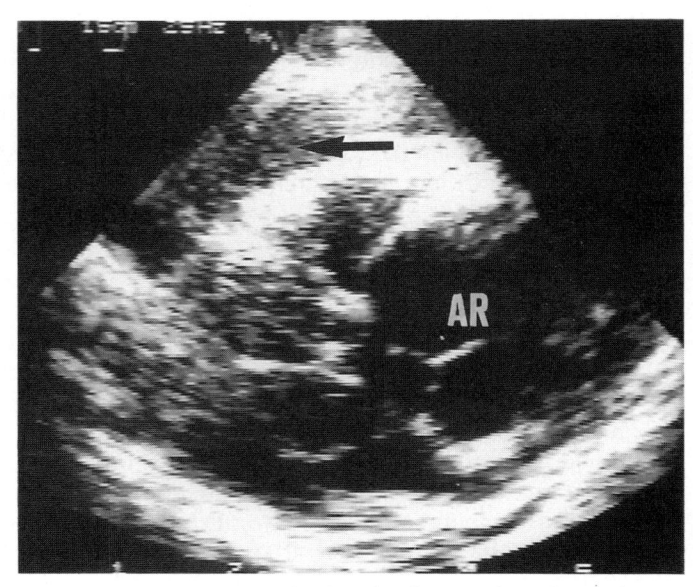

Fig. 17 Parasternal long axis view showing an echogenic anterior hemopericardium (arrowed) and a dissection flap in a dilated aortic root (AR).

Table 4 Echocardiographic features reported in pericardial constriction

Thickened pericardium
Abrupt end to ventricular filling or flat endocardial motion
Rapid early diastolic filling
Overactive septal motion
Early diastolic septal kick
Early closure of mitral valve
Left atrial enlargement
Dilated inferior vena cava and hepatic veins
Premature opening of pulmonary valve
Displacement of ventricular and atrial septa to left on inspiration
Shortened filling phase on Doppler examination
Increased transmitral flow velocity in early diastole
Angle <150° between posterior walls of left ventricle and atrium

Pericardial constriction is the syndrome which develops when pericardial thickening impairs cardiac filling, leading to distension of the systemic and pulmonary veins and eventually to a reduction in cardiac output. In all cases of constrictive pericarditis there is fusion of the two layers of the pericardium, which become thickened, non-distensible and, in about 30% of cases, calcified.

Chronic pericarditis and pericardial constriction probably still most commonly occur as a complication of tuberculous pericarditis although the echocardiographic features of pericardial thickening and constriction apply to all aetiologies. Many patients with a history of tuberculous pericarditis also have chronic lung and pleural disease as a result of their tuberculosis which may make them particularly difficult to examine by echocardiography.

Although thickening of the pericardium can be demonstrated by various imaging methods its presence does not necessarily indicate that there is haemodynamically important constriction. Echocardiography is relatively insensitive in detecting pericardial thickening in experimental models[32] and when compared with computerised tomography in patients with constrictive pericarditis (detecting only 29% of cases of thickened pericardium).[33] Even the use of a carefully standardised technique of echocardiographic measurement of pericardial thickness is a poor method of differentiating normal from thickened pericardium.[34] Although there is no single reliable echocardiographic sign of constriction there are a number of features which may indicate that there is haemodynamically important restriction of cardiac filling and therefore constriction. There features are useful in the evaluation of patients with suspected pericardial constriction when combined with an alternative method for demonstrating pericardial thickening such as magnetic resonance imaging.[1,33]

M-mode features of constriction are useful in assessing the functional significance of pericardial thickening. The most sensitive findings are said to include exaggerated movement of the septum compared with the free wall of the left ventricle (very non-specific), an early end to ventricular filling with flattening of the posterior wall movement in diastole[34] and an early diastolic septal kick[33] or early diastolic septal notch which is said to be present in up to 92% cases of pericardial constriction.[35] Other workers have also reported associated enlargement of the left atrium, premature pulmonary valve opening and an atrial systolic notch[36] although the latter is claimed to be a very insensitive sign.[35] Cross sectional echocardiography adds little to the M-mode examination but shows a normal sized heart with reduced wall motion (affecting both ventricles) or a sudden stop to ventricular filling early in diastole. Whilst there may be other reasons which might explain these appearances in one ventricle, when both ventricles are affected the diagnosis of constriction is likely. Although no echocardiographic sign alone is diagnostic of pericardial constriction, in most appropriate clinical situations, especially when pericardial thickening is confirmed by computerised tomography or magnetic resonance imaging, the presence of several of these signs is good evidence for the presence of constriction.

One of the more difficult differential diagnoses to make is that between restrictive cardiomyopathy and pericardial constriction. Even at cardiac catheterisation the haemodynamic findings may be similar.

It has been reported that it is possible to distinguish between the two diagnoses with digitised M-mode echocardiography.[37] In this study patients with pericardial constriction had significantly reduced peak left ventricular filling and posterior wall diastolic thinning rates. Patients with restrictive cardiomyopathy had reduced fractional shortening, decreased left ventricular filling and emptying rates, decreased percentage posterior wall thickening and decreased posterior wall thickening and thinning rates. Comparing the features of pericardial constriction with those of restrictive cardiomyopathy it was found that there were significant differences in peak left ventricular emptying rate, decreased percentage posterior wall thickening and decreased peak left ventricular posterior wall thickening and thinning rates. The differentiation between these two conditions is important as pericardial constriction is treatable by pericardectomy whilst restrictive cardiomyopathy is not. In the absence of alternative reliable methods for demonstrating pericardial thickening in difficult cases this may be a useful method for making the distinction between these conditions.

Another method for detecting pericardial constriction relates to the differential effect of the thick pericardium on the left ventricle (surrounded by pericardium) and left atrium (not constrained by pericardium).[38] Enlargement of the left atrium produces an angle between the posterior walls of the left ventricle and left atrium. An angle of less than 150 degrees in an appropriate clinical situation suggests the presence of pericardial constriction. Mitral valve disease will also cause reduction of this angle.

In some cases of pericardial constriction a pericardial effusion may also be present and this may be loculated and relatively echogenic. In some cases the distinction between a thick fibrinous effusion causing tamponade and acute constriction may be difficult, although this is usually not important as the treatment of both conditions is similar.

Following pericardectomy the echocardiographic features of pericardial constriction should return to normal. If this does not happen this may indicate that the original diagnosis was wrong and that the haemodynamic findings could be due to a restrictive cardiomyopathy.[37] Trans-oesophageal echocardiography has been used during pericardectomy to monitor the response to removal of the pericardium and a return to normal diastolic blood flow.[39]

PERICARDIAL TUMOURS

Benign pericardial tumours are rare and are often of mesenchymal origin. They usually have a good prognosis unless they are complicated by pericardial effusion or become very large, these complications being most common with teratomas. Other benign tumours include fibromas, lipomas, angiomas and neurofibromas.

Malignant tumours involving the pericardium are common, although they are often only diagnosed at post-mortem. They are usually metastatic (especially from lung or breast) (Fig. 7), lymphomatous or local tumours invading from the adjacent mediastinum (Fig. 6). They may present with pericardial effusions, which are often haemorrhagic and complicated by tamponade, or with pericardial thickening and the rapid development of constriction. The features of these are the same as for other causes of effusions and thickening. There may be associated pleural effusions and pleural involvement with tumour (Fig. 18).

The commonest primary malignant tumour of the pericardium is mesothelioma but this is a very rare tumour and pleural mesotheliomas invading the pericardium are commoner. Pericardial mesothelioma may present as constrictive pericarditis, haemorrhagic pericarditis, acute pericarditis, vena caval obstruction and even as an asymptomatic pericardial effusion.[8] Mesothelioma may produce widespread pericardial thickening or local plaques. The diagnosis is often made late and usually has a very poor prognosis, although in a few cases survival may be for six months or more.[8]

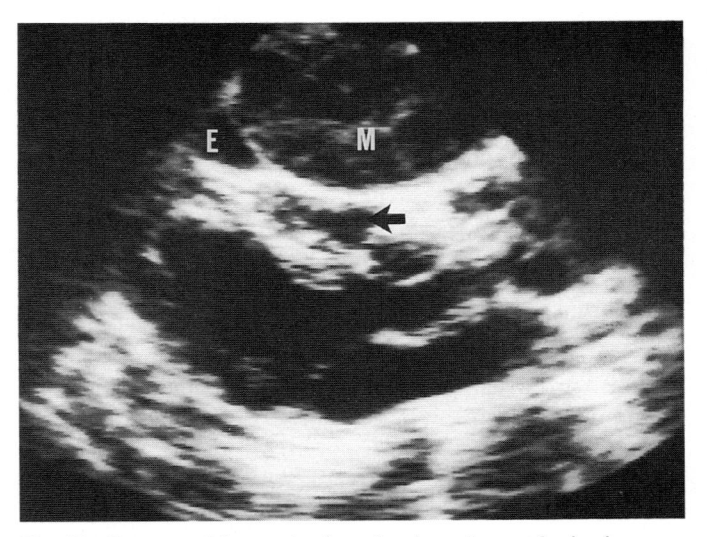

Fig. 19 Parasternal long axis view showing a low and mixed echogenicity anterior mass (M) compressing the right ventricle (arrowed) and a small pericardial effusion (E). The mass was found to be a lymphoma at thoracotomy.

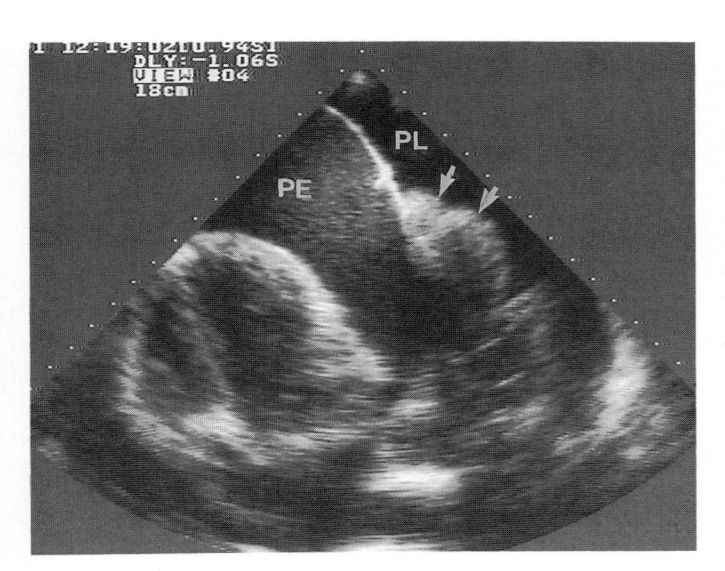

Fig. 18 Apical view of a patient with multiple pericardial and pleural secondary malignant deposits. The pleural deposits are arrowed. (PE = pericardial effusion. PL = pleural effusion.)

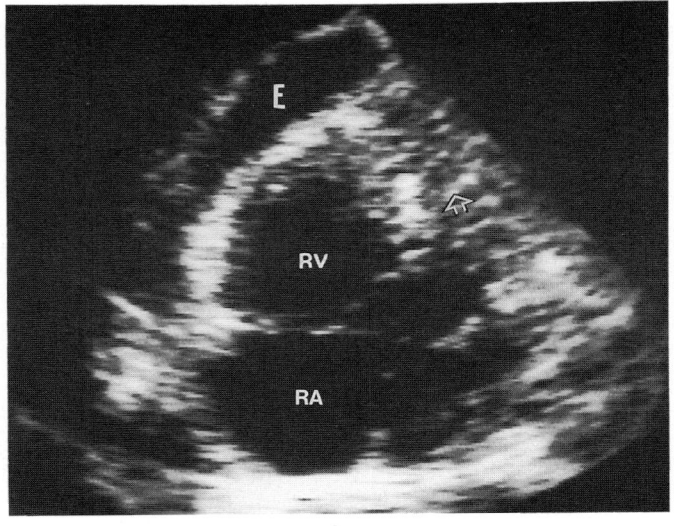

Fig. 20 Oblique apical four chamber view showing a pericardial effusion (E) and pericardial invasion and thickening by lymphoma (arrowed).

Pericardial involvement by lymphoma is not uncommon, occurring in up to 25% of cases and in particular in patients with non-Hodgkins lymphoma[40] as a result of spread from the mediastinum. Primary cardiac lymphoma is rare. Presentation can be with pericarditis, pericardial effusion or cardiac tamponade. The pericardial effusion may be haemorrhagic and can lead to tamponade. Two-dimensional echocardiography will show any pericardial effusion and may show either a discrete mass of lymphoma (Fig. 19) or thickening of involved pericardium or myocardium (Fig. 20). Following treatment cross sectional echocardiography can demonstrate resolution of the pericardial or myocardial involvement.[41]

Patients with pericardial lymphoma are at risk of developing pericardial constriction either due to haemopericardium complicating the lymphoma or as a result of mediastinal irradiation, although current radiotherapy regimes make this relatively uncommon.

CONGENITAL ABNORMALITIES OF THE PERICARDIUM

Pericardial cysts

Pericardial cysts are collections of fluid surrounded by tissue of pericardial origin, although the majority do not communicate with the pericardium. Congenital cysts most commonly occur in the cardiophrenic recess (70% in the right recess, 20% in the left, 10% elsewhere). Other cysts with an identical appearance can be seen in hydatid disease and pericardial cysts can also be due to pericardial teratoma.[42]

Pericardial cysts are not imaged reliably by M-mode examination but they are well seen on cross sectional echocardiography where they are seen as well defined echo free masses located close to the heart but clearly separated from any cardiac chamber by a definite layer of myocardium.[42] Pericardial cysts can be large and compress adjacent cardiac structures leading to intracardiac obstruction and pressure gradients detectable on Doppler. The echo free nature of pericardial cysts allows differentiation from solid tumours, fat pads and lipomas although differentiation from bronchogenic cysts may be impossible.[43]

Absence of the pericardium

Absence of the pericardium is a rare and usually benign condition, although some patients do experience pain. In cases of partial absence of the pericardium there is a risk of strangulation of the left ventricle in the defect.

Other associated congenital abnormalities such as bronchogenic cysts, atrial septal defect, Fallot's tetralogy, hiatus hernia, lung sequestration and ectopia cordis occur in up to 30% of cases. Usually there is partial or complete absence of the left sided pericardium. Right sided or total absence of the pericardium is very rare.

In congenital absence of the pericardium, M-mode and cross sectional echocardiography shows an enlarged right ventricle with abnormal septal motion (varying from paradoxical to flat septal motion depending on the phase of respiration).[44] These features are non-specific but it has been stated[45] that a large left atrial appendage passing around the lateral border of the pulmonary artery may be diagnostic.

In most cases of acquired absence of the pericardium following pericardectomy, the right ventricle is enlarged and abnormal septal motion develops that was not present preoperatively.[44]

REFERENCES

1 Hartnell G G, Rozkovec A, Waring J, Vann Jones J, Wilde R P H, Goddard P R. Magnetic resonance imaging in the assessment of pericardial disease. Br J Radiol 1988; 61: 779.
2 Rifkin R D, Isner J M, Carter B L, Bankoff M S. Combined posteroanterior subepicardial fat simulating the echocardiographic diagnosis of pericardial effusion. JACC 1984; 3(5): 1333–1339.
3 Come P C, Riley M F, Fortuin N J. Echocardiographic mimickry of pericardial effusion. Am J Cardiol 1981; 47: 365–370.
4 Dashkoff N, Karacuschansky M, Come P C, Fortuin N J. Echocardiographic features of mitral annulus calcification. Am Heart J 1977; 94: 585–592.
5 Windle J R, Felix G, Pinsky W W, Kugler J D. False-negative findings in pericardial effusion using M-Mode echocardiography. Pediatr Cardiol 1983; 4: 225–228.
6 Williams G. Echocardiography of pericardial disease. In: Hunter S, Hall R, eds Clinical echocardiography. Tunbridge Wells, Castle House, 1986; p 96.
7 Wolf W J. Echocardiographic features of a purulent pericardial peel. Am J Heart 1986; 111: 990–992.
8 Coplan N L, Kennish A J, Burgess N L, Deligdish L, Goldman M E. Pericardial mesothelioma masquerading as a benign pericardial effusion. JACC 1984; 4 (6): 1307–1310.
9 Lam D, Rapaport E. Two-dimensional echocardiographic demonstration of intrapericardial fibrinous strands in rheumatoid pericarditis. Am Heart J 1987; 114 (2): 442–444.
10 Kessler K M, Bilsker M S, Manasa M, Laignhold M, Myerburg R J. Pericardial web: extensive pericardial adhesions associated with idiopathic pericarditis. Am Heart J 1986; 111 (3): 602–603.
11 Fowler N O. Inferior vena cava plethora as an echocardiographic sign of cardiac tamponade. JACC 1988; 12 (6): 1478–1479.
12 Himelman R B, Kircher B, Rockey D C, Schiller N B. Inferior vena cava plethora with blunted respiratory response: a sensitive echocardiographic sign of cardiac tamponade. JACC 1988; 12 (6): 1470–1477.
13 Kronzon I, Cohen M L, Winer H E. Diastolic atrial compression; a sensitive echocardiographic sign of cardiac tamponade. JACC 1983; 2 (4): 770–775.
14 Singh S, Wann S, Schuchard G H, Klopfenstein H S, Leimgruber P P, Keelan M H, Brooks H L. Right ventricular and right atrial collapse in patients with cardiac tamponade – a combined echocardiographic and hemodynamic study. Circulation 1984; 70 (6): 966–971.
15 Gillam L D, Guyer D E, Gibson T C, King M E, Marshall J E, Weman A E. Hydrodynamic compression of the right atrium: a

new echocardiographic sign of cardiac tamponade. Circulation 1983; 68(2): 294–301.
16. Schiller N B, Botvinik E H. Right ventricular compression as a sign of cardiac tamponade. An analysis of echocardiographic ventricular dimensions and their clinical implications. Circulation 1977; 56 (5): 774–779.
17. Armstrong W F, Schilt B F, Helper D J, Dillon J C, Feigenbaum H. Diastolic collapse of the right ventricle with cardiac tamponade: an echocardiographic study. Circulation 1982; 65 (7): 1491–1496.
18. Naggar C Z, Dillon W D, Butterly J R, Malacoff R F. Echocardiographic manifestations of tense pericardial effusion. JACC 1985; 6 (2): 467–470.
19. Stratienko A A, Pollock S G, Keller M W, Sarembock I J. Use of venous contrast echocardiography for diagnosis of cardiac tamponade. Am J Cardiol 1989; 64: 691–692.
20. Spodick D H, Paldino D, Flessas A P. Respiratory effects on systolic time intervals during pericardial effusion. Am J Cardiol 1983; 51: 1033–1035.
21. Appleton C P, Hatle L K, Popp R L. Cardiac tamponade and pericardial effusion: respiratory variation in transvalvular flow velocities studied by Doppler echocardiography. JACC 1988; 11 (5): 1020–1030.
22. Fowler N O. The significance of echocardiographic-Doppler studies in cardiac tamponade. JACC 1988; 11 (5): 1031–1033.
23. Callahan J A, Seward J B, Nishimura R A, Miller F A, Reeder G S, Shub C, Callahan M J, Schattenberg T T, Tajik A J. Two-dimensional echocardiographically guided pericardiocentisis: experience in 117 consecutive patients. Am J Cardiol 1985; 55: 476–479.
24. Meilman H, Kronzon I, Krasnow N. A new ultrasonic device for safer pericardiocentesis (abstract). Circulation 1984; 80 (4): II–395 (abst 1578).
25. Chia B L, Choo M, Tan A, Ee B. Echocardiographic abnormalities in tuberculous pericardial effusion. Am Heart J 1984; 107 (5): 1034–1035.
26. Bjorkhem G, Lundstrom N R, Vitarelli A. Sequential study of echocardiographic changes in purulent pericarditis. Pediatr Cardiol 1984; 5: 317–332.
27. Kaplan K, Davison R, Parker M, Przybylet J, Light A, Bresnahan D, Ribner H, Talano J V. Frequency of pericardial effusion as determined by M-mode echocardiography in acute myocardial infarction. Am J Cardiol 1985; 55: 335–337.
28. Pierard L A, Albert A, Henrard L, Lemperuer P, Sprynger M, Carlier J, Kulbertus H E. Incidence and significance of pericardial effusion in acute myocardial infarction as determined by two-dimensional echocardiography. JACC 1986; 8 (3): 517–520.
29. Garcia-Fernandez M A, Moreno M, Rossi P N, Lopez-Sendon J L, Banuelos F. Echocardiographic features of hemopericardium. Am Heart J 1984; 107: 1035–1036.
30. D'Cruz I A, Kensey K, Campbell C, Replogle R, Jain M. Two-dimensional echocardiography in cardiac tamponade occurring after cardiac surgery. JACC 1985; 5 (5): 1250–1252.
31. Fyke F E, Tancredi R G, Shub C, Julsrud P R, Sheedy P F II. Detection of intrapericardial hematoma after open heart surgery: the roles of echocardiography and computed tomography. JACC 1985; 5(6): 1496–1499.
32. Pandian N G, Skorton D J, Kieso R A, Kerber R E. Diagnosis of constrictive pericarditis by two-dimensional echocardiography: studies in a new experimental model and in patients. JACC 1984; 4 (6): 1164–1173.
33. Sutton F J, Whitley N O, Applefield M M. The role of echocardiography and computed tomography in the evaluation of constrictive pericarditis. Am Heart J 1985; 109 (2): 350–355.
34. Voelkel A G, Pietro D A, Folland E D, Fisher M l, Parisi A F. Echocardiographic features of constrictive pericarditis. Circulation 1978; 58 (5): 871–875.
35. Candel-Riera J, Gutierrez-Palau L, Garcia-Del-Castillo H, Permanyer-Milralada G, Soler-Soler J. Atrial systolic notch and early diastolic notch on the interventricular septal echogram in constricted pericarditis. JACC 1985; 5 (4): 1020–1021.
36. Engel P J, Fowler N O, Tei C, Shah P M, Driedger H J, Shabetai R, Harbin A D, Franch R H. M-Mode echocardiography in constrictive pericarditis. JACC 1985; 6 (2): 471–474.
37. Morgan J M, Raposo L, Clague J C, Chow W H, Oldershaw P J. Restrictive cardiomyopathy and constrictive pericarditis: non-invasive distinction by digitised M-mode echocardiography. Br Heart J 1989; 61: 29–37.
38. D'Cruz I A, Dick A, Gross C M et al. Abnormal left ventricular-left atrial posterior wall contour: a new two-dimensional echocardiographic sign in constrictive pericarditis. Am Heart J 1989; 118 (1): 128–132.
39. Kyo S, Takamoto S, Matasumura M, Asano H, Yokote Y, Motoyama T, Omoto R. Immediate and early postoperative evaluation of results of cardiac surgery by transoesophageal two-dimensional Doppler echocardiography. Circulation 1987; 76 (V): 113–121.
40. Roberts W C, Glancy D L, De Vita V T. Heart in malignant lymphoma (Hodgkins disease, lymphosarcoma, reticulum cell sarcoma and mycosis fungoides). A study of 196 autopsy cases. Am J Cardiol 1968; 22: 85.
41. Armstrong W F, Buck J D, Hoffman R, Waller B F. Cardiac involvement by lymphoma: detection and follow-up by two-dimensional echocardiography. Am Heart J 1986; 112 (3): 627–631.
42. Pezzano A, Belloni A, Faletra F, Binaghi G, Colli A, Rovelli F. Value of two-dimensional echocardiography in the diagnosis of pericardial cysts. Eur Heart J 1983; 4: 238–246.
43. Gomes M N, Hufnagel C A. Intrapericardial bronchogenic cysts. Am J Cardiol 1975; 36: 817–822.
44. Payvandi M N, Kerber R E. Echocardiography in congenital and acquired absence of the pericardium. An echocardiographic mimic of right ventricular volume overload. Circulation 1976; 53 (1): 86–92.
45. Ruys F, Paulus W, Stevens C, Brutsaert D. Expansion of the left atrial appendage is a distinctive cross-sectional echocardiographic feature of congenital defect of the pericardium. Eur Heart J 1983; 4: 738–741.

17

Thoracic aorta

Introduction
Dilatation and aneurysms of the thoracic aorta
Aortic dissection
Traumatic aortic aneurysms and aortic rupture
Mycotic aneurysms
Annuloaortic ectasia
Sinus of Valsalva aneurysms

George Hartnell

INTRODUCTION

The thoracic aorta is not part of the heart but it is examined, at least in part, in any routine echocardiographic examination. Disease of the thoracic aorta frequently affects cardiac function and similar disease processes can affect both structures. Echocardiography is particularly useful for investigating thoracic aortic disease in spite of some constraints imposed by restricted echo windows. More recently, trans-oesophageal echocardiography has enhanced the precision of ultrasonic diagnosis of aortic disease.

In normal patients the aorta, seen from a left parasternal approach, arises from the aortic valve ring and extends to the right and anteriorly as it passes up to the aortic arch. It is lost to view behind the sternum before reappearing when viewed from the suprasternal notch where it curves posteriorly to the left and then caudally. It is seldom possible in adults to follow it beyond the origin of the left subclavian artery from this approach. The lower descending thoracic aorta is seen in a sagittal projection through the left atrium (usually most clearly from a parasternal approach) in up to 92% of patients[1] and then can be seen entering the abdomen from a subcostal approach. In some patients a right parasternal view can be used to demonstrate the mid ascending aorta, particularly if the patient is rotated towards their right side. If the view of the aorta is inadequate from a transthoracic approach, transoesophageal echocardiography can be used to provide a very clear view of much of the thoracic aorta[2] (see Ch. 9).

The potential transthoracic echocardiographic views for imaging the thoracic aorta include:

Left parasternal: Long and short axis views of the aortic root, ascending aorta and lower descending aorta.

Right parasternal: Variable visualisation of the ascending aorta. Particularly useful if the ascending aorta is dilated.

Suprasternal notch: Aortic arch and the origins of the common carotid and subclavian arteries. Variable length of the descending aorta.

Supraclavicular fossae: Proximal subclavian arteries and sometimes distorted or dilated aortic arch.

Apical: Aortic root and part of descending aorta.

Subcostal: Long and short axis for lower descending thoracic aorta and continuation into abdominal aorta. Sometimes the aortic root, especially if the lungs are overinflated (Fig. 1).

The aorta is easily recognised on M-mode or cross sectional echocardiography as a pair of parallel lines moving together, with slight separation in systole. The range of normal diameters for the aorta varies at different levels, between the sexes[3] and also with the size of the patient. The ranges of normal values on cross sectional and M-mode examination are given in Table 1.[3,4] There is good correlation with these values when compared with the results obtained by measurement at surgery.[5] There are other similar parallel sided structures which can be mistaken for the aorta on M-mode examination if anything but the parasternal approach is used and therefore cross sectional echocardiography should be used in conjunction with this for imaging the thoracic aorta.[6]

Aortic disease can affect the heart and the major branches of the aorta so these structures must be examined when performing an ultrasound examination of the aorta to assess aortic regurgitation, left ventricular function, possible haemopericardium and examination for possible disease extension into the subclavian and common carotid arteries and the abdominal aorta.

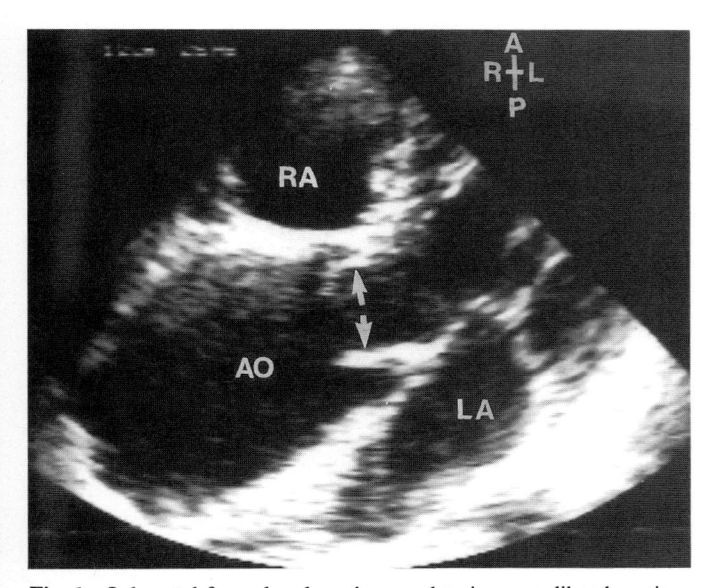

Fig. 1 Subcostal four chamber view used to image a dilated aortic root in a patient with poor views from other approaches. Aortic valve leaflets are arrowed.

Table 1 Normal aortic diameters in adults: cross sectional and M-mode

Cross-sectional measurements at end-diastole, from the leading edge of each aortic wall in centimetres.[4]

	Mean	SD	Range
Aortic valve annulus	1.9	0.2	1.4–2.6
Widest point of aortic root (Level of sinuses of Valsalva)	2.8	0.3	2.1–3.5
Ascending aorta	2.4	0.4	1.7–3.4
Mid-ascending aorta	2.6	0.3	2.1–3.4

M-Mode
Measurements (end-diastole) from the leading edge of each aortic wall echo in centimetres[5]

	Mean	Range
Widest point of aortic root	2.7	2.0–3.7
Corrected for body surface area	1.5 (cm/m^2)	1.2–2.2 (cm/m^2)
Measurements from internal echo of each aortic wall in centimetres[3]	2.4	1.7–3.3
Corrected for body surface area	1.4 (cm/m^2)	0.9–1.9 (cm/m^2)
Mean diameter males = 2.5 cm (SD 0.35), females = 2.24 (SD 0.33)		

DILATATION AND ANEURYSMS OF THE THORACIC AORTA

Localised dilatation can result from weakening and stretching of the wall (true aneurysm) (Fig. 2) or perforation of the vessel wall, which is contained by connective tissue or thrombus around the perforation (false aneurysm). There are many causes of aortic aneurysm (Table 2) but in Western societies the commonest cause is atherosclerosis (70% cases) and about 25% of these aneurysms involve the thoracic aorta. Atherosclerotic aneurysms are commoner in men and are especially common in hypertensive patients. Aneurysms can develop as diffuse areas of dilatation forming a fusiform aneurysm or as a localised area of dilatation, often eccentric, forming a saccular aneurysm. Dilatation can also be associated with aortic dissection.

Echocardiography confirms the diagnosis by demonstrating the size of the lumen of the aneurysm and is useful for assessing, in combination with Doppler examination, associated valvar or left ventricular disease[7] (Fig. 2).

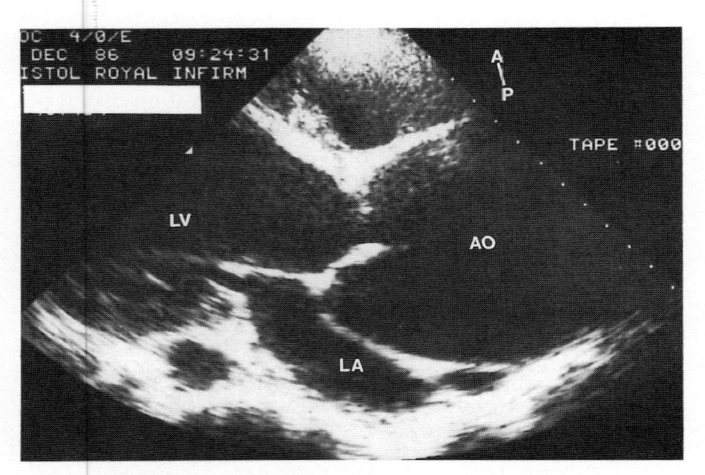

Fig. 2 Parasternal long axis view showing an aneurysmally dilated (8.5 cm) aortic root. The dilated left ventricle is due to chronic aortic regurgitation and the left atrium is distorted by the aorta.

Table 2 Causes of true thoracic aortic aneurysms

Atherosclerosis
Trauma
Cardiac surgery
Marfan's syndrome
Ehler's Danlos syndrome
Mycotic (including post-operative)
Tertiary syphilis
Takayasu's aortitis
Inflammatory aortitis syndromes (i.e. Reiter's syndrome, giant cell arteritis)
False aneurysms
   Trauma
   Infection
   Following rupture of a true aneurysm
   Rupture of aortic ulcer (usually atheromatous)

Although these associated changes have been well documented by M-mode[7] examination, cross sectional echocardiography is quicker, easier and more accurate.[8] Several of the important causes of aortic aneurysm specifically cause aortic regurgitation, in particular Marfan's Syndrome, tertiary syphilis and Ehler's Danlos Syndrome. Passive dilatation of the aortic root by an aneurysm can also cause aortic regurgitation. This should be evaluated by pulsed wave or colour flow Doppler examination. Two-dimensional echocardiography demonstrates about 85% of saccular aneurysms but some are missed or incompletely seen, especially in the descending aorta. In these situations the diagnosis can be obtained by further imaging using computerised tomography[9] or magnetic resonance imaging.[10] The majority of thoracic aortic aneurysms visible with echocardiography are fusiform and usually start in the ascending aorta close to the aortic valve (Fig. 3A). They should be traced as far distally as possible to define their length (Fig. 3B) and extension into major branches. More localised saccular aneurysms may contain mural thrombus (Fig. 3C) but the majority of fusiform aneurysms do not contain significant thrombus on echocardiography. In the case of saccular aneurysms particular attention should be given to the size of the aneurysm, the width of its mouth from the aorta and its relationship to other structures, which may be compressed or may complicate a surgical procedure.

False aneurysms of the thoracic aorta are rare due to the very high mortality of aortic rupture but a few cases survive and cross-sectional echocardiography may show these well. Flow through the mouth of the false aneurysm can be shown by Doppler techniques to establish that there is a communication with the lumen of the aorta.[11]

AORTIC DISSECTION

Dissection of the aorta occurs as a result of weakening of the connective tissues which form the media of the aortic wall. It is associated with a variety of conditions of which hypertension and atherosclerosis are the most common (Table 3). A tear in the intimal part of the wall allows blood rapidly to enter the potential space in the weakened tissue plane of the aortic wall. Dissections may be localised or very extensive, can remain in the plane of the media, can re-enter the aortic lumen or can rupture into the surrounding tissues. The majority of dissections start in the thoracic aorta close to the aortic valve (Fig. 4) or in the upper part of the descending aorta. Symptoms and signs depend on the site and rate of progression of the dissection. Many acute dissections extend rapidly and by the time of diagnosis extend from the aortic root into the brachiocephalic arteries (Fig. 4B and 4C) or down into the abdominal aorta (Fig. 5). Improvements in the medical and surgical management of patients with acute dissection have led to great improvements in prognosis[12] but accurate diagnosis and staging are essential to assign the patient to the appropriate treatment as the results of inappropriate treatment are poor.

When the dissection starts in the ascending aorta (Type A[13] or De Bakey Types 1 and 2,[14] 58%–70% of cases) surgery is usually the best treatment.[12] If the dissection starts distal to the origin of the left subclavian artery (type B or De Bakey Type 3, 30%–42% of cases) medical control of hypertension is usually the best treatment. The aim of echocardiography in patients with suspected dissection (especially with an acute presentation) is to make a diagnosis, to stage the dissection and demonstrate any complications which may affect management. These include haemopericardium, aortic regurgitation, poor left ventricular function and branch vessel dissection. It is often not possible to get all of this information by precordial echocardiography alone and supplementary imaging by transoesophageal echocardiography, computerised tomography[15] or magnetic resonance imaging[10,16] is often necessary.

The diagnosis of aortic dissection is primarily based on the visualisation of the dissection flap but a number of criteria have to be satisfied for the diagnosis to be certain because artefactual appearances can be deceptive on occasion. The intimal flap should be visible in at least two views (Fig. 6A and B), although this may be difficult if the flap is orientated parallel to the echo beam. The apparent flap will have a different motion to that of adjacent cardiac structures[17] (i.e. aortic wall or aortic cusps) consistent with

Table 3 Conditions associated with aortic dissection

Atherosclerosis
Hypertension
Marfan's syndrome
Pregnancy
Coarctation of aorta
Bicuspid aortic valve
Trauma (including aortic catheterisation)
Cardiac or aortic surgery (particularly aortic valve replacement)
Ehler's Danlos syndrome (and similar connective tissue disorders)

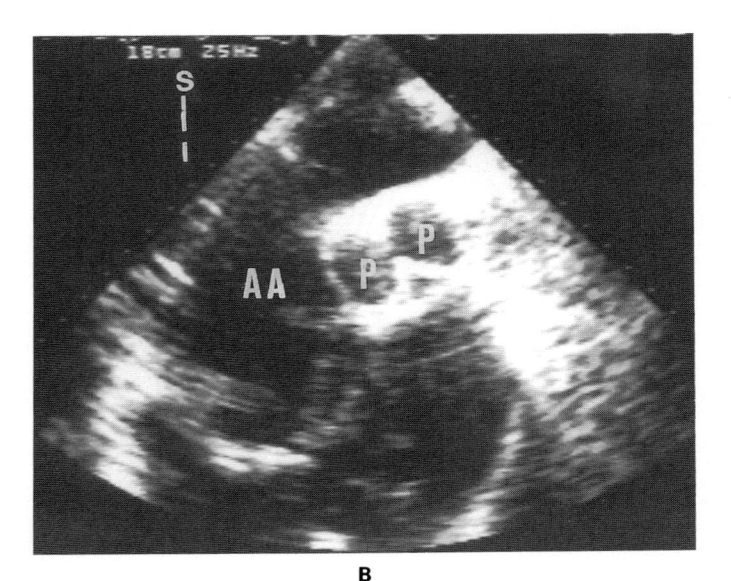

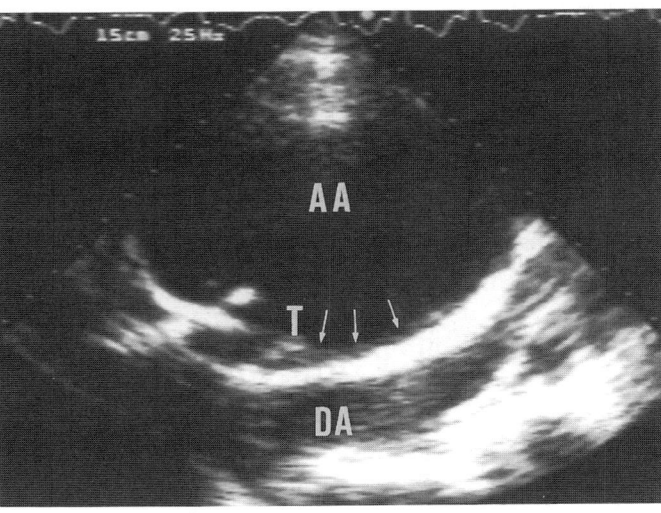

Fig. 3 A: Apical four chamber view showing huge aortic root but a normal diameter aortic valve ring. B: Suprasternal view in same case as A showing the dilated ascending aorta (AA) merging into a normal calibre aortic arch. Compare the aortic diameter with that of the right and left pulmonary arteries (P). C: Sagittal parasternal view in same case as A showing the dilated ascending aorta (AA), mural thrombus (T) and normal calibre descending aorta (DA).

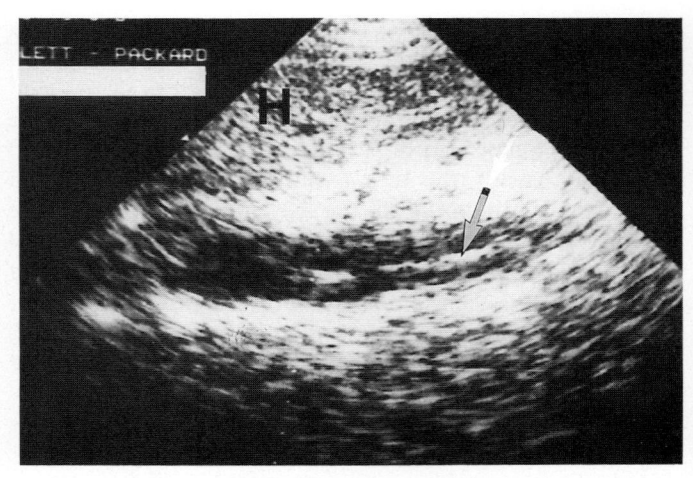

Fig. 5 Sagittal upper abdominal view showing a dissection flap (arrowed) in the abdominal aorta imaged through the liver (H).

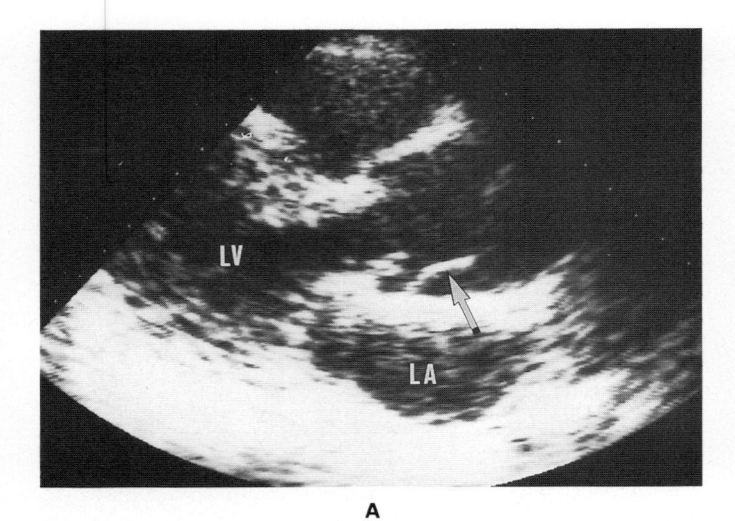

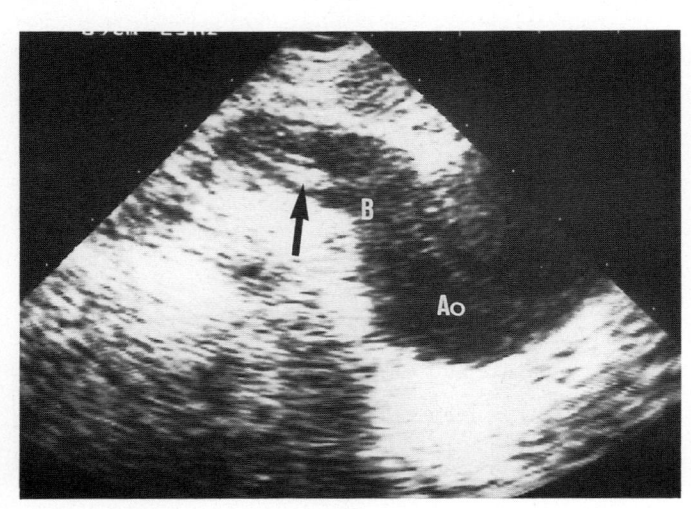

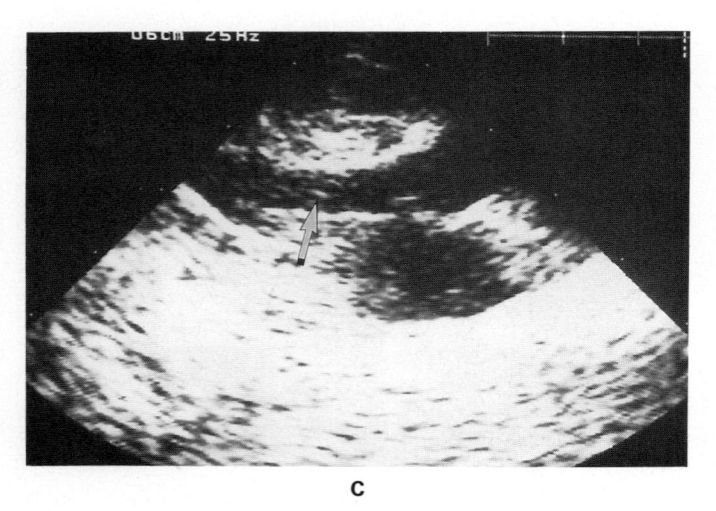

Fig. 4 A: Parasternal long axis view showing dissection flap (arrowed) arising within 1 cm of the aortic valve. **B:** Oblique view through the aortic arch in the same patient as **A** showing the dissection flap (arrowed) extending into the origin of the brachiocephalic artery (B). **C:** Dissection flap (arrowed) in same case as **A** in the right common carotid artery.

a moving flap which defines a false channel.[6] The flap should be differentiated from multipath echoes from other structures and should be a consistent finding separating true and false lumens. Other confirmatory signs include sinuous movement of the flap or varying orientation of the flap. The aorta may be very dilated in some cases of dissection, an aortic diameter of >42 mm being reported to be a strong indicator of dissection[17] but a normal aortic diameter does not exclude the diagnosis.

If colour flow Doppler is used it should be possible to demonstrate different flow patterns in the true and false lumen (Plates 1A, 1B, 2A, 2B, 3A, 3B) (antegrade in the true lumen and retrograde or no flow in the false lumen).[18] This can also be achieved with pulsed wave Doppler examination but this is technically more difficult. In some cases slow moving blood in the false lumen may have low level, mobile, intracavitary echoes[19] similar to those seen elsewhere where there is slow moving blood in a large cavity (i.e. in left ventricular aneurysms) (Fig. 7). The mobility of the echoes allows differentiation from thrombus. In patients with distal dissection the flap may be orientated parallel to the echo beam and may therefore not be visible. In this situation colour flow Doppler examination may sometimes show the absent or reduced flow across part of the diameter of the affected aorta corresponding to the false lumen. In cases of more distal dissection image clarity is reduced and other aortic pathology, such as atherosclerotic plaque, may mimic a flap.[20]

A number of other less common M-mode and cross sectional echocardiography signs of dissection have been described. Mid-systolic closure of the aortic valve, possibly due to disruption of the aortic valve attachments, has been described but does not appear to be very specific for aortic dissection.[21] Apparent duplication of an aortic cusp may be seen on the M-mode trace. Cross sectional echocardiography shows this to be due to dehiscence of the dissection

THORACIC AORTA 281

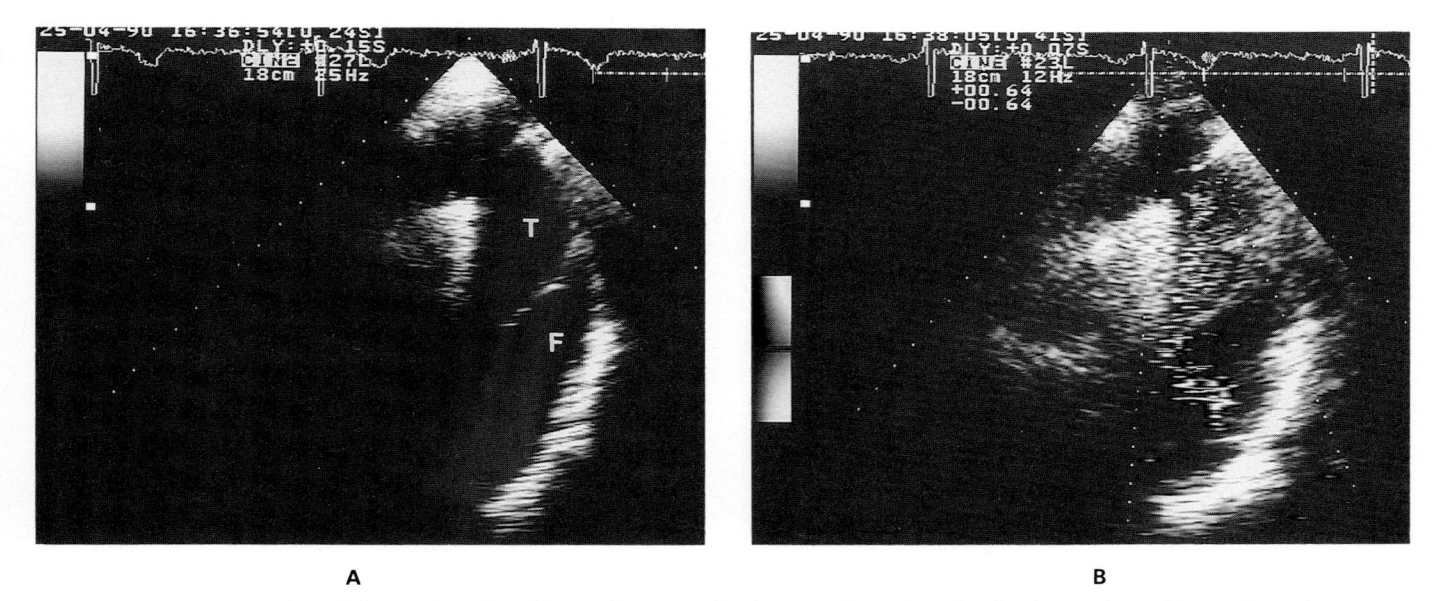

Plate 1 **A: Suprasternal view of the aortic arch** and descending aorta showing an oblique dissection flap in a patient with type B aortic dissection. T — true lumen; F — false lumen. **B:** Colour flow image in the same section as **A**. The flow in the true lumen (blue, away from the transducer) is seen to alias as it passes through a tear into the false lumen. This figure is reproduced in colour in the colour plate section at the front of this volume.

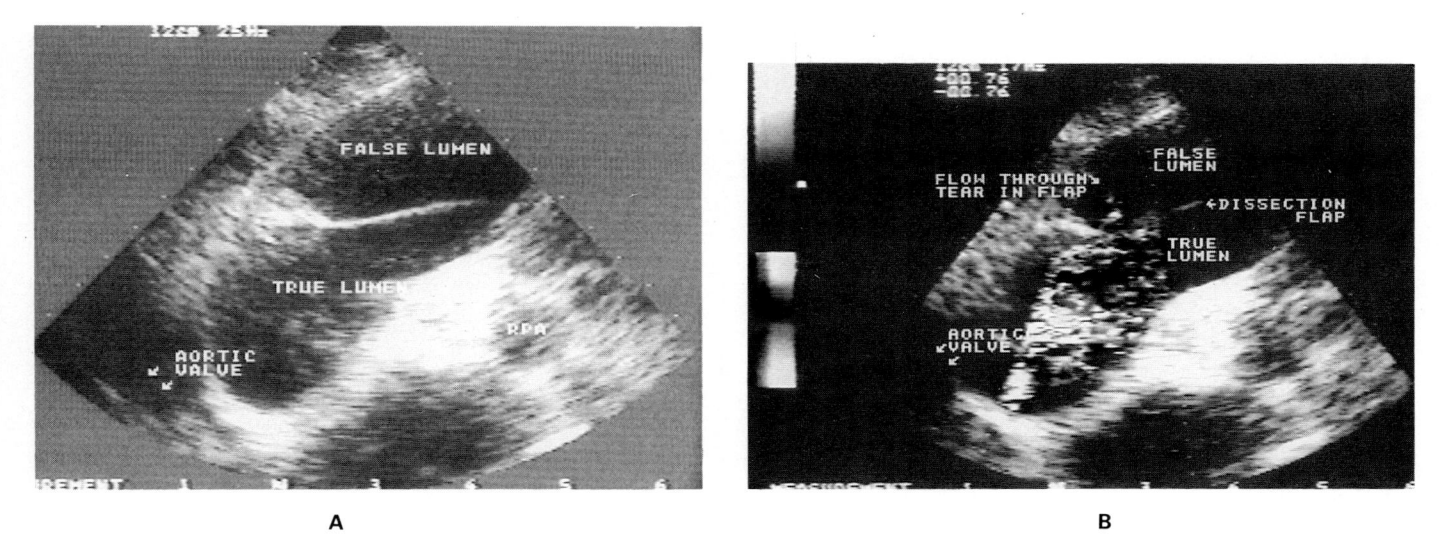

Plate 2 **A: Modified right parasternal view** of a dissection flap in the ascending aorta. **B:** Colour flow imaging of the same section showing flow in the true lumen (with central aliasing) passing through a small tear into the false lumen. Colour imaging is confined to a central sector. This figure is reproduced in colour in the colour plate section at the front of this volume.

282 CARDIAC ULTRASOUND

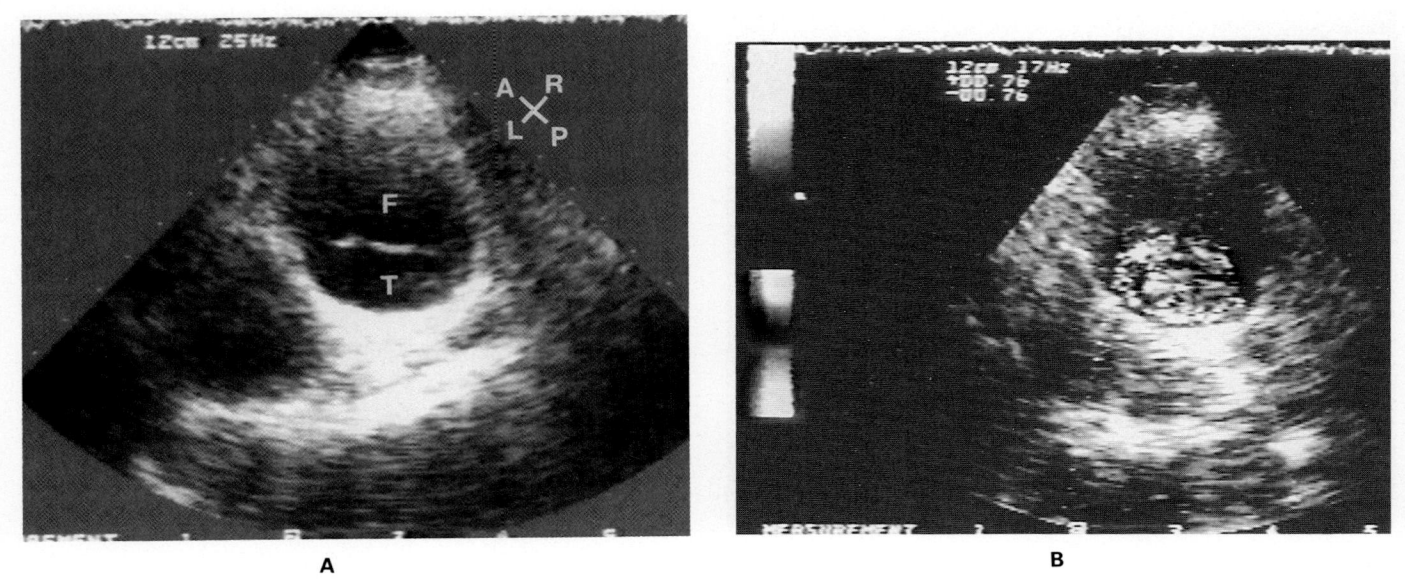

Plate 3 A: Transoesophageal image of the descending aorta showing a dissection flap separating the true lumen (T) from the false lumen (F). **B:** Colour flow image of the same section as **A** showing flow in the true lumen and no detectable flow in the false lumen. This figure is reproduced in colour in the colour plate section at the front of this volume.

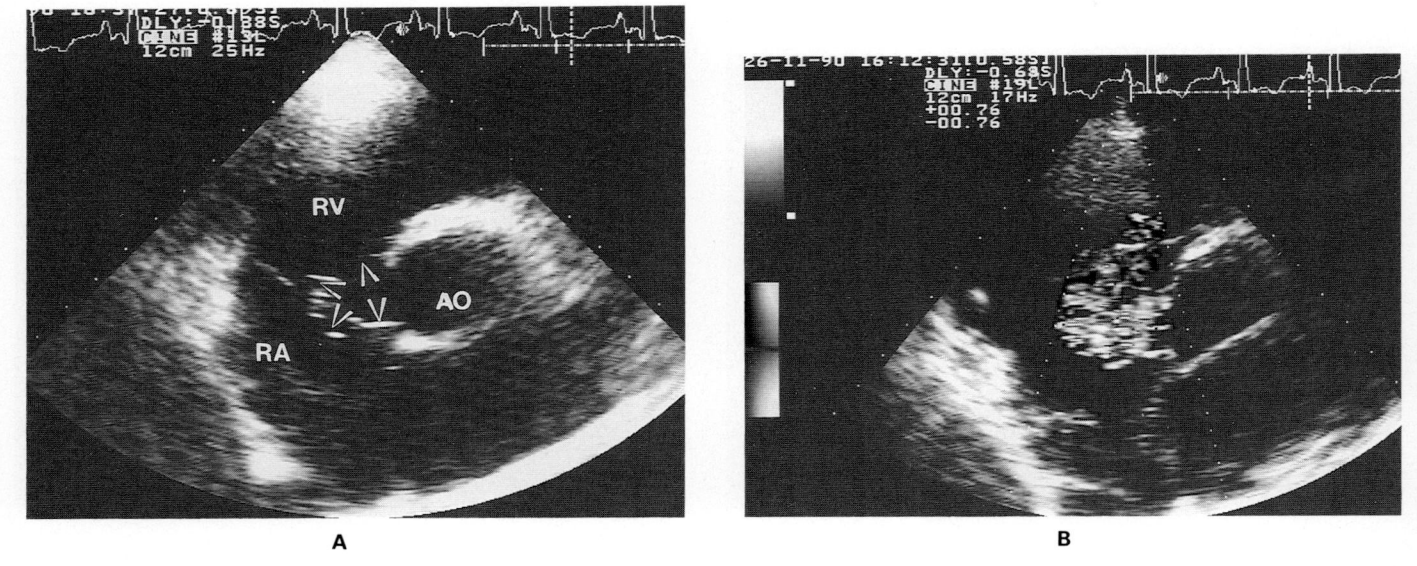

Plate 4 A: Ruptured sinus of Valsalva aneurysm (arrowed) seen from a modified parasternal short axis view. **B:** Colour flow image of the same section as Figure 11A showing turbulent flow through the ruptured sinus of Valsalva aneurysm from aortic root to right ventricle. This figure is reproduced in colour in the colour plate section at the front of this volume.

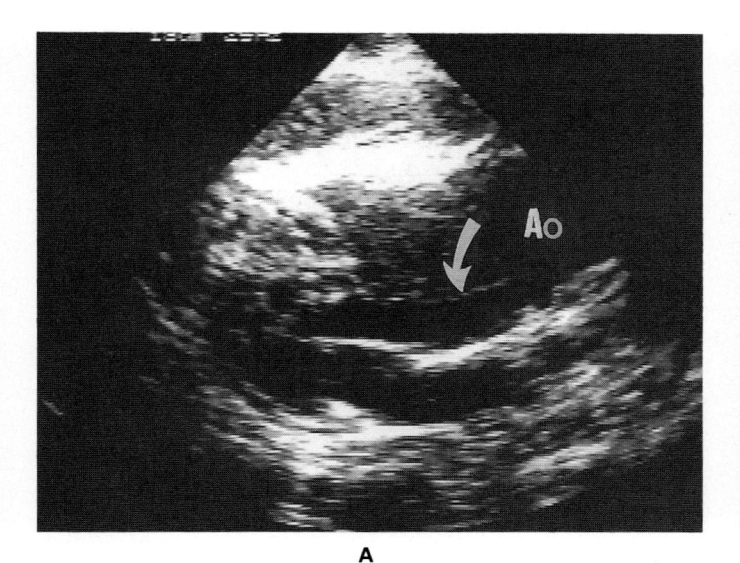

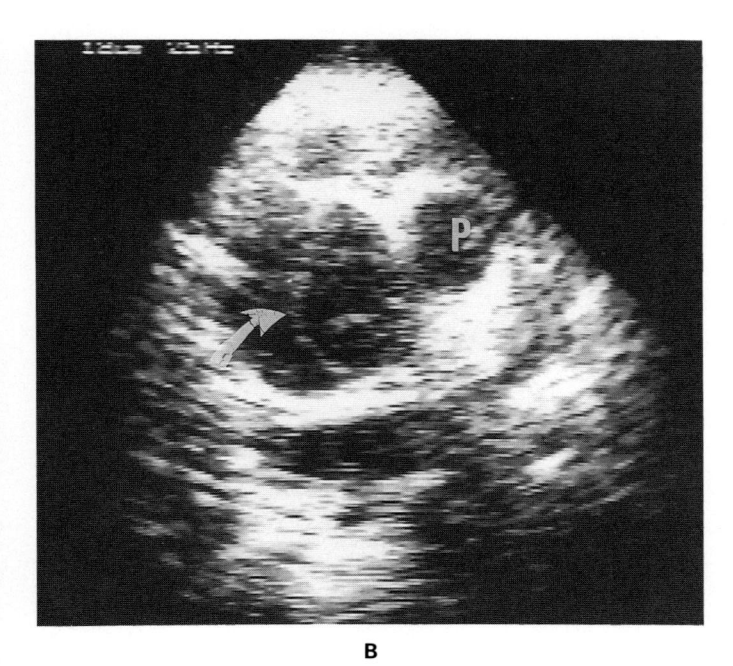

Fig. 6 **A: Parasternal long axis view giving a poor view of a dissection flap (arrowed) in the ascending aorta. B:** Short axis parasternal view taken from same position as in **A** clearly showing the curved dissection flap (arrowed) in the ascending aorta. P = right pulmonary artery.

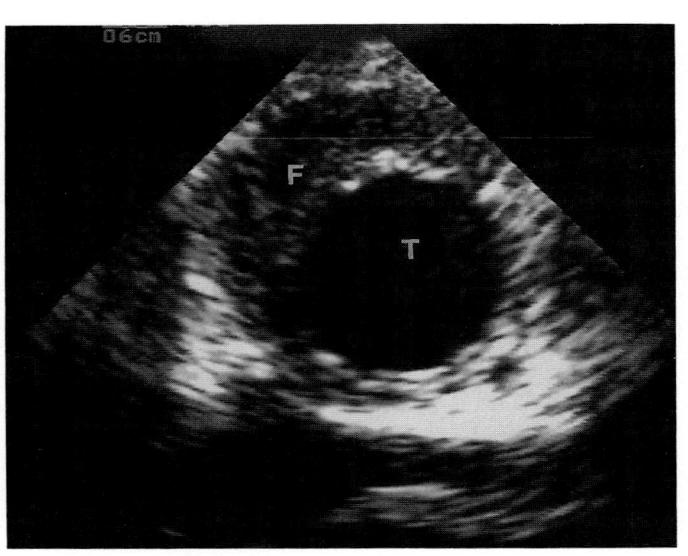

Fig. 7 **Transoesophageal image of the descending aorta** showing a circular true lumen (T) and a crescentic false lumen (F) containing low level echoes.

Table 4 Reported causes of false positive diagnosis of aortic dissection

Calcific aortic valve
Reverberation artefacts
Aortic root abscess
Monitoring catheter in right heart or pulmonary artery
Imaging venous valves in innominate vein
Atherosclerotic plaque

flap through the aortic valve[22] which may also be associated with prolapse of an aortic cusp involved in the dissection.[23] In some cases the dissection flap extends to the root of the aortic valve cusps but not through the valve rings and multiple echoes are seen at the level of the aortic valve which may cause confusion by mimicking the movement of an aortic cusp.[24]

Although M-mode examination can be used to make the diagnosis of dissection,[25] cross sectional echocardiography is much more accurate,[6,17] especially in the diagnosis of distal dissection and extension into branch arteries. M-mode examination is also more prone to false positive diagnoses (Table 4). Some reports show good accuracy for the cross sectional echocardiographic diagnosis of aortic dissection in selected series (up to 100% sensitivity[17] for ascending aortic dissection and up to 94% specificity[6]) but this can be difficult to achieve in practice. The accuracy of echocardiography depends on the proportion of cases with ascending aortic dissections which are easier to see by echocardiography, the number of patients investigated without dissection and the technical and interpretative skill of the operator. There are considerable practical difficulties in examining sick patients who are restless, in pain and unable to cooperate. Many patients are obese and are smokers which makes accurate examination even more difficult. Thus although cross sectional echocardiography is very useful in diagnosing acute dissections[21] it should never, except in exceptionally clear cases where a positive diagnosis is made, be the sole imaging investigation of patients with possible aortic dissection. Contrast enhanced computerised tomography is probably the most appropriate complementary investigation[9,26] although magnetic resonance imaging, if available, may be suitable if the patient is fit enough to enter the scanner. Angiography is rarely necessary if these non-invasive techniques are available.

Doppler abnormalities in the aortic arch have been reported using continuous wave Doppler in patients with aortic dissection. There may be an early systolic notch on the Doppler flow profile from aortic arch branches in patients[27] without loss of pulses while there is a widened wave form in patients with branch artery occlusion.

Once an aortic dissection has been diagnosed there are further specific questions that need to be answered about staging and the presence of complications. The full extent of the dissection, in particular its relationship to the left subclavian artery (separating Type A from Type B), should be demonstrated. Extension into the common carotid,[21] subclavian, renal and mesenteric arteries should be excluded if possible, augmented by pulsed wave and colour flow Doppler if available, as such extension may need surgical attention. In patients with loss of pulses but no evidence of dissection the origins of the affected arteries should be examined in the same way to establish an alternative cause for an absent pulse, most commonly an arterial stenosis.

Complicating aortic regurgitation due to aortic annulus dilatation or dissection through the attachment of the aortic valve should be quantified by Doppler examination. Left ventricular function may be impaired acutely by severe aortic regurgitation or by the dissection of the origin of a coronary artery. Chronic impairment of left ventricular function may result from chronic aortic regurgitation, hypertension or coexistent ischaemic heart disease and should be assessed at the same time. The presence of haemopericardium is often obvious but if it is not seen immediately, a specific search should be made as the presence of even a small pericardial effusion may indicate leakage into the pericardium which can rapidly increase and lead to tamponade.

Transoesophageal echocardiography (see Ch. 9) improves visualisation considerably (Fig. 8A, B and C) and is an important although more invasive supplementary method of imaging acute dissection and can be used in difficult cases.[28] In some centres this is becoming the

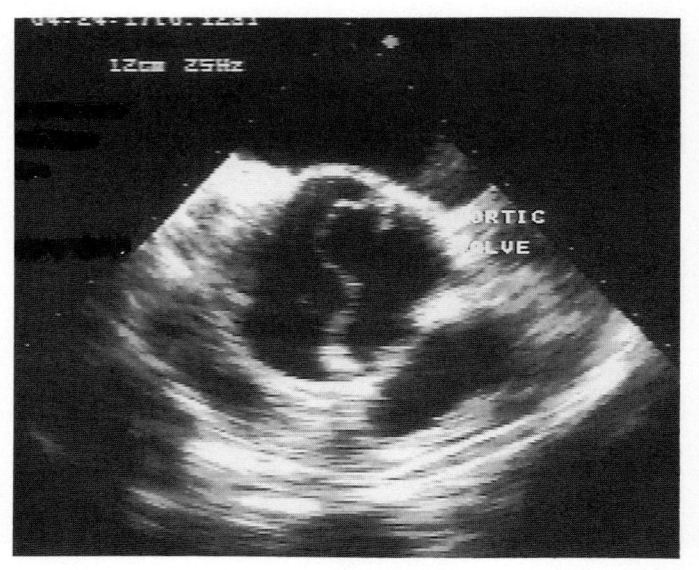

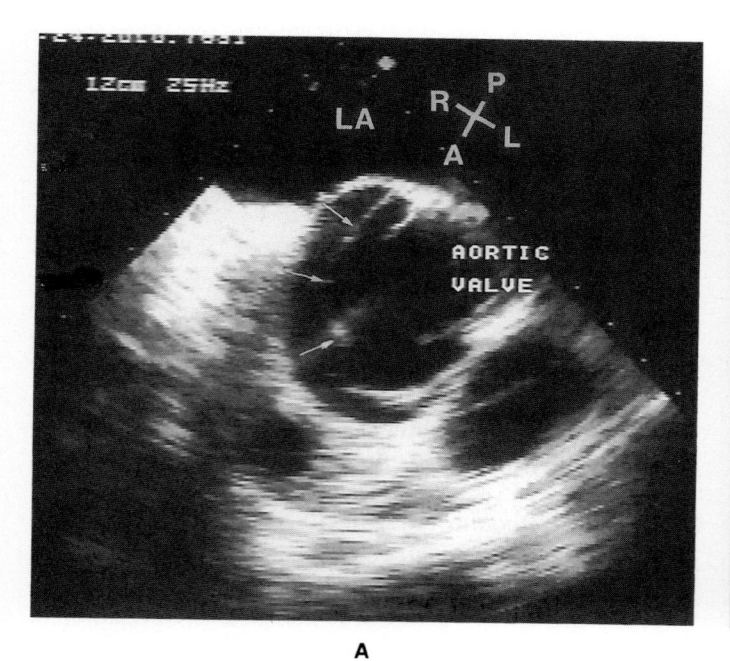

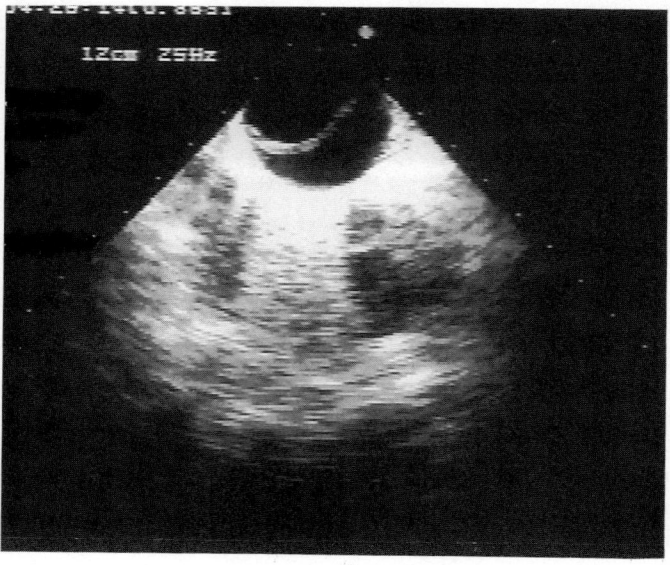

Fig. 8 **A:** Transoesophageal image at aortic root level showing the aortic valve leaflets in systole and a dissection flap (arrowed) in the dilated aortic root. **B:** A section just cranial to that in A showing the tortuous flap in the aortic root. **C:** Descending aorta in the same patient as A and B showing extension of the flap. The patient had a successful operation immediately after this emergency examination.

examination of choice for patients with suspected aortic dissection. When transthoracic and transoephageal echocardiography are combined, the overall diagnostic accuracy for diagnosing acute dissection exceeds that of computerised tomography or angiography alone.[29]

The untreated mortality rate of patients presenting with acute aortic dissection is up to 50% in the first four days.[30] Over 90% of cases can be diagnosed antemortem[12] but this should be done quickly and safely as well as accurately. Echocardiography and other examinations should be organised so that delay in diagnosis and instituting definitive treatment is kept to an absolute minimum.

TRAUMATIC AORTIC ANEURYSMS AND AORTIC RUPTURE

Traumatic aortic aneurysms and aortic rupture most commonly follow blunt trauma to the thorax, usually in a road traffic accident. Complete or partial transection of the aorta leads to death before arrival at hospital in over 80% of cases. Of those patients that do reach hospital alive the majority have a partial rupture of the distal arch of the aorta and aortography is probably still the most appropriate investigation. Echocardiography is useful in patients with partial ruptures at the second most common site (just above the aortic valve) when cross sectional echocardiography will show assymetry of the aorta and a step in the line of the aortic wall. In some cases Doppler examination may show associated aortic regurgitation or flow into a false aneurysm. There may also be a haemopericardium in these cases.

MYCOTIC ANEURYSMS

Mycotic aneurysms of the thoracic aorta may complicate infective endocarditis of the aortic valve or coarctation, local thoracic sepsis, intravenous drug abuse and cardiac or aortic surgery. In the latter situation there is often evidence of previous local infection but no active infection at the time of surgical repair. On M-mode examination there may be a double border to the affected segment of aorta but the diagnosis is much more reliably made by cross sectional echocardiography which shows a localised eccentric dilatation of the affected aorta, sometimes with a layer of infected material within it, or thickening of the aortic wall.[31] An echo free cavity is relatively rare in aneurysms complicating endocarditis[31] but it is commoner in other types of mycotic aneurysm. Pulsed wave or colour flow Doppler will show flow into the aneurysm and abnormal flow patterns within the aneurysm, as in any saccular aneurysm.

ANNULOAORTIC ECTASIA

Annuloaortic ectasia describes aneurysmal dilatation of the ascending aorta starting at the aortic valve ring and extending, according to the original definition,[30] to the origin of the innominate artery. This may be secondary to hypertension, coarctation of the aorta or aortic valve disease, these conditions usually determining the prognosis. In other cases where there is no apparent predisposing cause, the annuloaortic ectasia is probably the result of cystic medical necrosis. In some patients this may be associated with other features of Marfan's syndrome but in many cases it is an isolated finding and is regarded by some as being a 'forme fruste' of Marfan's syndrome.[33] Dilatation of the aorta begins just above the aortic valve (Fig. 9) and extends for a variable distance into the ascending aorta and aortic arch. Less commonly the descending aorta and coronary arteries[34] may be involved. The aorta can become very large and when the aortic diameter exceeds 5 cm there is an increasing risk of acute aortic dissection or rupture. Even at lesser diameters there is a lower but still significant risk of dissection. Dilatation of the aortic root leads to aortic regurgitation and is also related to a worsening of prognosis.[34]

Patients with Marfan's syndrome, and probably their first degree relatives, should be screened at regular, if infrequent, intervals in order to recognise dilatation at an early stage. If this is detected the frequency of examination should be increased as there is good evidence that surgical repair is more successful if it is performed as a planned rather than as an emergency procedure. Echocardiography is the most acceptable method for doing this and it should also be used to monitor development of aortic regurgitation. Mitral regurgitation due to mitral prolapse is also common in Marfan's Syndrome.

Screening and follow up examinations should follow a standard protocol to reduce technical inter-examination variations. Aortic diameters should be measured at the level of the aortic valve annulus, the widest segment of the

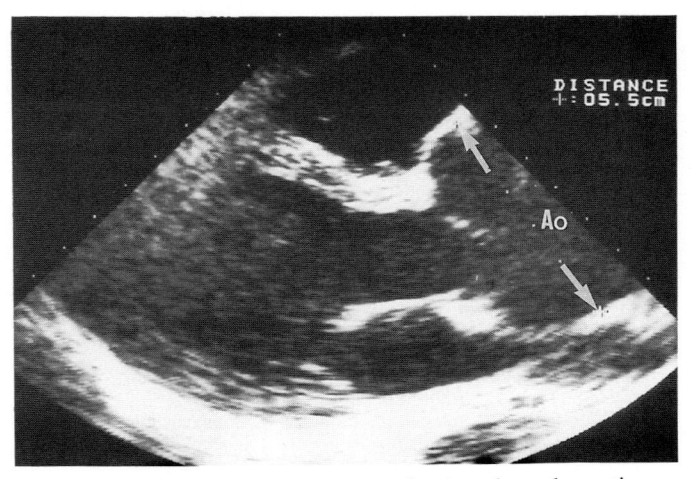

Fig. 9 Dilatation of the aortic root starting just above the aortic valve in patient with Marfan's syndrome. Note the thickening of the aortic wall.

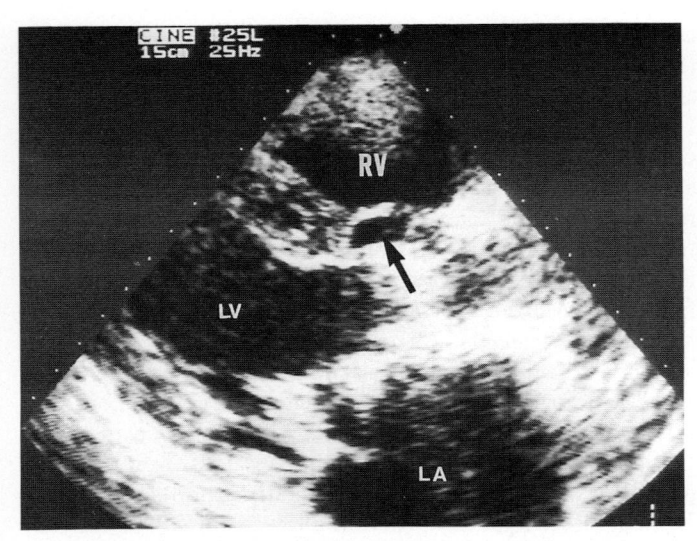

Fig. 10 Parasternal long axis view showing an unruptured sinus of Valsalva aneurysm (arrowed) extending into the base of the interventricular septum and projecting into the right ventricle.

aortic root, the mid-ascending aorta, the apex of aortic arch and the descending aorta behind the heart. The development of significant aortic regurgitation, left ventricular dilatation or an aortic diameter of greater than 5 cm should lead to consideration of aortic root replacement to prevent progression to heart failure or acute rupture or dissection of the aorta.[35]

SINUS OF VALSALVA ANEURYSMS

Sinus of Valsalva aneuryms may be congenital or they may be acquired secondary to endocarditis, atherosclerosis, syphilis or aortic dissection. They have long been recognisable by M-mode examination[36] and cross sectional echocardiography.[37] Usually only one sinus is affected but sometimes multiple sinuses can be affected.[38] On M-mode echocardiography there is a localised increase in aortic diameter, exaggerated and eccentric motion of the aortic valve and a structure may be seen adjacent to the interventricular septum but moving independently of it.[36] Two-dimensional echocardiography shows an abnormal thin-walled sac (Fig. 10) projecting from the aortic root into a right heart chamber[39] if the right sinus is affected or posteriorly mimicking aortic dissection[40] if the non-coronary sinus is affected. In cases complicating bacterial endocarditis there may be echogenic material in the cavity of the aneurysm, presumably due to the presence of vegetations.[37] The use of echocardiographic contrast media increases the ability of 2-dimensional echocardiography to detect such aneurysms increasing the sensitivity from 58% to 75%.[40] Two-dimensional echocardiography is poor at demonstrating rupture of a sinus of Valsalva aneurysm and this is much better demonstrated by pulsed wave or colour flow Doppler examination[40] which shows turbulent, high velocity flow through the ruptured segment into a right heart chamber (Plates 4A and B). In unruptured cases there is no flow abnormality.

The differential diagnoses of sinus of Valsalva aneurysm include ventricular septal aneurysm, coronary arteriovenous fistula, coronary artery aneurysm and Fallot's tetralogy. The diagnosis should be clear in most cases but sometimes non-echocardiographic methods may be necessary to exclude alternative diagnoses.[40]

REFERENCES

1. Come P C. Improved cross-sectional echocardiographic technique for visualisation of the retrocardiac descending aorta in its long axis. Am J Cardiol 1983; 51: 1029–1032.
2. Erbel R, Borner N, Steller D, Brunier J, Thelen M, Pfeiffer C, Mohr-Kahaly S, Iversen S, Oelert H, Meyer J. Detection of aortic dissection by transoesophageal echocardiography. Br Heart J 1987; 58: 45–51.
3. Triulzi M, Gilliam L, Gentile F, Newell J B, Weyman A E. Normal adult cross-sectional echocardiographic values: linear dimensions and chamber areas. Echocardiography 1984; 1: 403–426.
4. Feigenbaum H. Echocardiography. Philadelphia, Lea and Febiger, 1983, p 551.
5. Francis G S, Hagan A D, Oury J, O'Rourke R A. Accuracy of echocardiography for assessing aortic root diameter. Br Heart J 1975; 37: 376–378.
6. Victor M F, Mintz G S, Kottler M N, Wilson A R, Segal B L. Two dimensional echocardiographic diagnosis of aortic dissection. Am J Cardiol 1981; 48: 1155–1159.
7. Moohart R W, Spangler R D, Blount S G. Echocardiography in aortic root dissection and dilatation. Am J Cardiol 1975; 36: 11–16.
8. Matthew T, Nanda N C. Two-dimensional and Doppler echocardiographic evaluation of aortic aneurysm and dissection. Am J Cardiol 1984; 54: 379–385.
9. Bruno L, Prandi M, Colombi P, La Vecchia L. Diagnostic and surgical management of patients with aneurysms of the thoracic aorta with various causes. Br Heart J 1986; 55: 81–91.
10. Hartnell G G, Wisheart J D, Wilde R P H, Goddard P R. MR Imaging of thoracic aortic disease provides useful extra information (Abstract). Radiology 1989; 173 (P): 148.
11. Wendel C H, Cornman C R, Dianzumba S B. Diagnosis of pseudoaneurysm of the ascending aorta by pulsed Doppler cross sectional echocardiography. Br Heart J 1985; 55: 567–570.
12. Wolfe W G, Moran J F. The evolution of medical and surgical management of acute aortic dissection. Circulation 1977; 56 (4): 503–505.
13. Daily P O, Trueblood H W, Stinson E B, Wuerflein R D, Schumway N E. Management of acute aortic dissections. Ann Thorac Surg 1970; 10: 237–247.
14. De Bakey M E, Menly W S, Cooley D A, Morris G C, Crawford E S, Beall A C. Surgical management of dissecting aneurysm of the aorta. J Thorac Cardiovasc Surg 1965; 49: 130–149.
15. Goldman A P, Kotler M N, Scanlon M H, Ostrum B, Parameswaran R, Parry W R. The complementary role of magnetic resonance imaging, Doppler echocardiography and computed tomography in the diagnosis of dissecting thoracic aneurysms. Am Heart J 1986; 111 (5); 970–981.
16. Goldman A P, Kotler M N, Scanlon M H, Ostrum B J, Parameswaran R, Parry W R. Magnetic resonance imaging and

two-dimensional echocardiography. Am J Med 1986; 80: 1225–1229.
17 Granato J E, Dee P, Gibson R S. Utility of two-dimensional echocardiography in suspected ascending aortic dissection. Am J Cardiol 1985; 56: 123–129.
18 Liu M W, Louie E K, Levitsky S. Color flow Doppler assessment of aortic regurgitation complicated by aneurysmal dilatation and dissection of the ascending aorta in the Marfan syndrome. Am Heart J 1988; 115 (5): 1118–1119.
19 Panidis I P, Kotler M N, Mintz G S, Ross J. Intracavitary echoes in the aortic arch in Type III aortic dissection. Am J Cardiol 1984; 54: 1159–1160.
20 Nestico P, Panidis I P, Kotler M N, Mintz G S, Mattleman S, Ross J. Atherosclerotic plaque simulating aortic dissection by echocardiography and angiography. Am Heart J 1985; 109(3): 607–609.
21 McLeod A A, Monaghan M J, Richardson P J, Jackson G, Jewitt D E. Diagnosis of acute aortic dissection by M-mode and cross-sectional echocardiography: a five year experience. Eur Heart J 1983; 4: 196–202.
22 Cohen I S, Wharton T P. 'Duplication' of aortic cusp. New M-mode echocardiographic sign of intimal tear in aortic dissection. Br Heart J 1982; 47: 173–176.
23 Come P C, Bivas N K, Sacks B, Thurer R L, Weintrub R M, Axelford P. Unusual echographic findings in aortic dissection: diastolic prolapse of intimal flap into left ventricle. Am Heart J 1984; 107 (4): 790–792.
24 Steriotis J, Athanasopoulos K, Aravanis C. Unusual echocardiographic image of ascending aortic aneurysm dissection. Am Heart J 1984; 107 (5): 1023–1025.
25 Brown O R, Popp R L, Kloster F E. Echocardiographic criteria for aortic root dissection. Am J Cardiol 1975; 36: 17–20
26 Tottle A J, Wilde R P H, Hartnell G G. Diagnosis of aortic dissection using echocardiography and computed tomography (Abstract). Br J Radiol 1989; 62: S100–101.
27 Dany F, Bensaid J, Blank P, Virot P, Christides C, Kim M. Contribution of continuous wave Doppler ultrasound to the diagnosis of aortic dissection (Abstract). Circulation 1989; 80(4): II–395 (abst 1580).
28 Borner N, Erbel R, Braun B, Henke B, Meyer J, Rumpelt J. Diagnosis of aortic dissection by transoesophageal echocardiography. Am J Cardiol 1984; 54: 1157–1158.
29 Erbel R, Daniel W, Visser C, Engberding R, Roelandt J, Rennollet H. Echocardiography in diagnosis of aortic dissection. Lancet i: 1989; 457–460.
30 Anagnostopoulos C E, Prabhakar M J, Kittle C F. Aortic dissection and dissecting aneurysms. Am J Cardiol 1972; 30: 263–273.
31 Ellis S G, Goldstein J, Popp R L. Detection of endocarditis-associated perivalvular abscesses by two-dimensional echocardiography. JACC 1985; 5(3): 647–653.
32 Ellis P R, Cooley D A, De Bakey M E. Clinical considerations and surgical treatment of annulo-aortic ectasia. J Thorac Cardiovasc Surg 1961; 42: 363–370.
33 Emmanuel R, Ng R A C, Marcomichedlakis J, Moores E C, Jefferson K E, MacFaul P A, Withers R. Formes frustes of Marfan's syndrome, presenting with severe aortic regurgitation. Clinicogenetic study of 18 families. Br Heart J 1977; 39: 190–197.
34 Becker A E, Van Mantgem J-P. The coronary arteries in Marfan's syndrome: a morphologic study. Am J Cardiol 1975; 36: 315–321.
35 Fox R, Ren J F, Pandidis I P, Kotler M N, Mintz G S, Ross J. Anuloaortic ectasia: a clinical and echocardiographic study. Am J Cardiol 1984; 54: 177–181.
36 Rothbaum D A, Dillon J C, Chang S, Feigenbaum H. Echocardiographic manifestation of right sinus of Valsalva aneurysm. Circulation 1974; 69: 768–771.
37 Lewis B S, Agathangelou N E. Echocardiographic diagnosis of unruptured sinus of Valsalva aneurysm. Am Heart J 1984; 107 (5): 1025–1027.
38 Chamsi-Pasha H, Musgrove C, Morton R. Echocardiographic diagnosis of multiple congenital aneurysms of the sinus of Valsalva. Br Heart J 1988; 59: 724–726.
39 Terdjman M, Bourdarias J P, Farcot J C, Gueret P, Dubourg O, Ferrier A, Hanania G. Aneurysms of sinus of Valsalva: Two-dimensional echocardiographic diagnosis and recognition of rupture into the right heart cavities. JACC 1984; 3 (5): 1227–1235.
40 Chiang C W, Lin F C, Fang B R, Kuo C T, Lee Y S, Chang C H. Doppler and two-dimensional echocardiographic features of sinus of Valsalva aneurysm. Am Heart J 1988; 116 (5): 1283–1288.

Echocardiography in the developing world

Introduction
Instrumentation
Summary of applications
Pericardial disease
Pericardial effusion
Constrictive pericarditis
Effusive constrictive pericarditis
Rheumatic heart disease
Dilated cardiomyopathy
Infective endocarditis
Miscellaneous conditions
Summary

George Strang

INTRODUCTION

Cardiovascular disease is common in the developing world, where the lack of resources makes its full assessment impossible. The development of health care, which involves recognition of patterns of disease and planning of preventive, medical and surgical services, depends on accurate diagnosis. The speed and relative simplicity of echocardiography compared with more sophisticated methods of assessing heart disease make it ideal for the developing world where it has been shown to be cost effective.

The infrequency of ischaemic heart disease and the presence of geographical difficulties make echocardiography particularly useful. Many ultrasound machines incorporate facilities for the examination of intra-abdominal organs and the heads of neonates in addition to echocardiography, which increases their value in the Third World. The technique can be learned relatively quickly by clinicians and it becomes an appropriate extension of their clinical skills which is important in practices where there is no department of radiology. Portable ultrasound machines enable the physician to complete his assessment of patients with heart disease on visits to outlying hospitals. There is a constant need to practise with appropriate technology in the Third World, because economic constraints are felt more keenly than in developed countries and diagnostic ultrasound can be considered a form of appropriate technology, because of its ease of use for the doctor and patient and its wide application.

The majority of the African population of southern Africa are good echocardiographic subjects as obesity is uncommon, and views from four standard positions can be obtained in the majority; i.e. parasternal long axis and short axis, apical and subcostal 4 chamber views. It is very unusual to see a patient from whom no useful information can be obtained.

Many practices in the developing world are far from cardiothoracic centres and need the ability to diagnose and manage cardiac problems locally and refer selected patients for open heart surgery. The development of cardiac surgery in the local centres, for example closed mitral valvotomy and pericardiectomy, is more likely if the physician can support his clinical findings with echocardiography. It follows that the number of referrals to major centres for diagnosis can be reduced and these referrals can be specifically for open heart surgery, thus reducing the cost and inconvenience of transporting patients over long distances.

Experience in southern Africa over 14 years, in which echocardiography has been available for 7 years, has indicated that in terms of confirming or reaching a diagnosis, clinical assessment followed by echocardiography is far more useful than clinical assessment followed by conventional chest radiography and electrocardiography.[1] The frontal chest radiograph remains useful in demonstrating the overall heart configuration, the lung fields and the pulmonary vasculature but the commonly employed lateral view with a barium swallow becomes redundant since the non-specific finding of left atrial enlargement seen on barium swallow is unhelpful. Echocardiography will give definitive information.

Rheumatic, myopathic and hypertensive heart disease are common in southern Africa[2] and there is a high prevalence of tuberculosis as in many other developing countries. Tuberculous pericarditis is such a common cause of the clinical picture of 'congestive heart failure' in Transkei, that it has been named 'Transkei heart'.[3] The rarity of ischaemic heart disease and the very 'anatomical' or 'structural' nature of most of the heart disease, make echocardiography particularly relevant.

INSTRUMENTATION

The type of echocardiography required will depend on the practice and on the time available to the physician. In a peripheral centre two-dimensional echocardiography alone will suffice, but with the addition of M-mode, a remarkable amount of information can be obtained and patients with rheumatic heart disease requiring open heart surgery can be assessed accurately before referral.[4] Doppler echocardiography[5] is desirable but not essential in the developing world and its benefits should be balanced against the time and funds available to the physician, whose practice is likely to encompass general medicine in addition to cardiology. Usually, patients in the developing world present late, when physical examination is valuable in reaching a diagnosis, and imaging echocardiography alone is usually adequate for reaching a diagnosis.

The choice of ultrasound machine will depend on availability and on after-sales service. In remote areas it is essential to have access to skilled help in the event of faults and a service contract may be advisable. Recordings illustrated in this article were made with four machines, i.e. an ATL 100 two-dimensional sector scanner, an ATL 300C, an ADR 4000 portable machine and an Aloka echocamera. All were found to be reliable and robust. Doppler facilities were not available on any of the instruments.

Contrast echocardiography[6] can be undertaken without special contrast media by using a mixture of the patient's blood, normal saline and air. Air is drawn through a sterile swab, into a syringe containing the blood and saline and the mixture is shaken vigorously for a few minutes. After decanting visible bubbles, it is injected rapidly into a vein in the antecubital fossa. The technique is a simple way of improving diagnostic ability and can often be used to confirm the presence of a right to left intracardiac shunt, a left to right shunt and tricuspid regurgitation.

SUMMARY OF APPLICATIONS

Echocardiography has been found helpful in the following ways:

1. Diagnosis and monitoring of pericardial disease;
2. Assessment of patients with clinically diagnosed rheumatic heart disease for surgery locally, or referral elsewhere for open heart surgery;
3. Rapid diagnosis of serious intra-cardiac problems which cannot be diagnosed clinically;
4. For the confirmation of clinical diagnoses and the elucidation of difficult or unusual problems, such as congestive cardiac failure of unknown cause and large heart of unknown cause.

The following list shows an analysis of echocardiographic examinations made over an 18 month period in Umtata, Transkei.

Pericardial disease	
Tuberculous	682
Amoebic	4
Pyogenic	1
Rheumatic heart disease	133
Dilated cardiomyopathy	69
Cor pulmonale	27
Congenital heart disease	17
Infective endocarditis	15
Post-operative	12
Normal	9
Calcific aortic stenosis	7
Extracardiac	4
Miscellaneous	24

The high number of studies of pericardial disease is explained by an ongoing research study into pericardial disease which necessitated frequent restudy of 89 patients presenting with pericardial effusion and 78 patients with constrictive pericarditis.

PERICARDIAL DISEASE

Pericarditis is usually tuberculous in origin and occurs in three forms, pericardial effusion, constrictive pericarditis and effusive-constrictive pericarditis, a combination of the other two. In Umtata, at least 100 new patients with these conditions are seen annually.[1] Echocardiography is important in the management of pericarditis, by confirming the diagnosis, differentiating the three types, and in differentiating the disease from other causes of apparent congestive cardiac failure. It may also provide information on the aetiology of the pericarditis and is useful in monitoring the progress of the disease during treatment. On occasion, the mechanism of pulsus paradoxus can be seen at echocardiography.

Pericardial effusion

Two-dimensional and M-mode features of pericardial effusion are well described.[7] The two-dimensional technique is easier and even an inexperienced operator can learn quickly to diagnose a pericardial effusion. Typically a tuberculous pericardial effusion is moderate or large in size and fibrinous strands extend into it from the visceral and parietal surfaces (Fig. 1).

In an area where tuberculosis is prevalent, *Mycobacterium tuberculosis* can be cultured from many of these patients[8] and echocardiography can be used to demonstrate whether or not percutaneous pericardiocentesis will be safe. If a pericardial friction rub is heard (in approximately 20%)[9] it is inadvisable to perform percutaneous pericardiocentesis before echocardiography, since in many such patients the anterior surface of the heart can be seen rubbing against the parietal pericardium. Under these circumstances, if examination of the fluid is required, or if drainage is necessary to relieve tamponade, an inferior pericardiotomy and drainage is safer.[10,11]

Confirmation of a pericardial effusion by echocardiography may give no clue as to its aetiology and since amoebiasis occurs in populations affected by tuberculous pericarditis, it is essential to scan the liver in the subcostal view during echocardiography, to exclude an amoebic liver abscess as the cause.[12] Amoebic abscess may cause tamponade, before penetrating the diaphragm, during the 'sympathetic' or 'pre-suppurative' stage. The fluid may be straw coloured, making differentiation from other causes difficult.[13]

A 40-year-old man presented in tamponade and a pericardial effusion was confirmed by echocardiography, but a liver scan was not done at the same time. Straw coloured fluid was drained at pericardiocentesis. Tam-

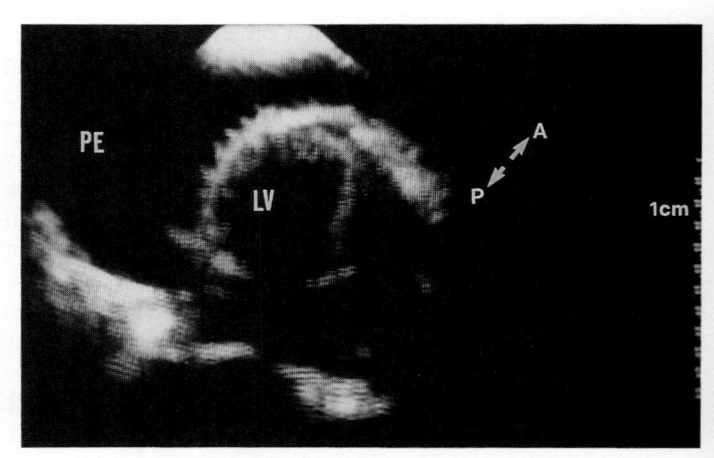

Fig. 1 Tuberculous pericardial effusion. Two-dimensional echocardiogram, apical 4-chamber view. Note the large pericardial effusion (PE) and the fibrinous strands extending into it, from the visceral pericardium.

ponade recurred three times over the next few days and was relieved by repeated pericardiocentesis. After the fourth drainage, inferior pericardiotomy was undertaken with underwater tube drainage. Discharge from the pericardium, which usually stops after 48 hours, continued for 3 weeks, at which time it had an anchovy sauce appearance. At this stage, echocardiography was repeated with a liver scan and showed an amoebic liver abscess communicating with the pericardial sac (Fig. 2). The patient received metronidazole and after a period of severe constriction, lasting 4 months, the disease resolved completely. The rubber drain in the pericardium almost certainly saved him from fatal tamponade, when the abscess ruptured through the diaphragm and was decompressed by it.

The proximity of many amoebic liver abscesses to the pericardium, noted during liver scanning, should be an indication to drain them (Fig. 3). Amoebic abscesses may cross the diaphragm, even when the patient is receiving metronidazole.[14] For every patient with amoebic pericarditis in Transkei, 100 are seen with tuberculous pericarditis. Although uncommon, amoebic pericarditis is a condition likely to be fatal if not treated specifically.[1]

While there may be disagreement about what constitutes tamponade, there are occasions when echocardiography indicates clearly the need for pericardiocentesis. Figure 4 is an echocardiographic examination of a teenage boy who had a pericardial effusion with pulsus paradoxus of 30 mmHg. Both two-dimensional and M-mode examinations showed a marked swing of the interventricular septum to the left during inspiration, when the right ventricle accommodated venous return at the expense of the left ventricle. During inspiration, the diastolic separation of the mitral valve cusps was incomplete and the duration of mitral valve opening was reduced. This ex-

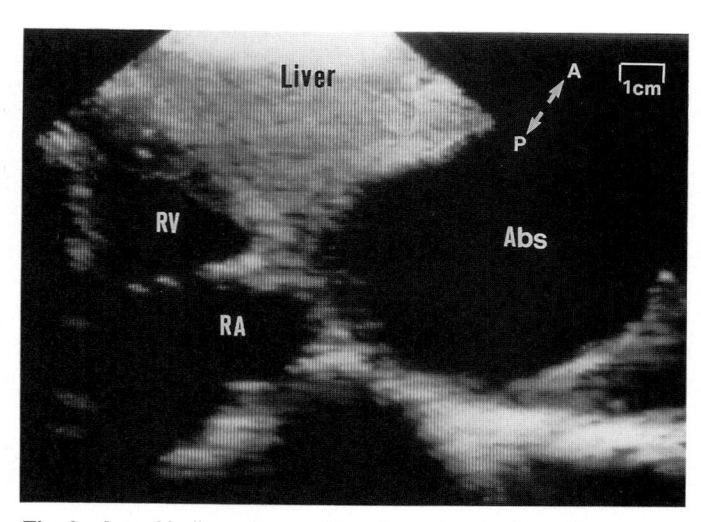

Fig. 3 Amoebic liver abscess. Two-dimensional echocardiogram, sub-costal view. Note the proximity of the liver abscess (Abs) to the heart. The abscess did not communicate with the pericardium in this case.

plains the mechanism of pulsus paradoxus,[15] and was an indication for pericardiocentesis, which reduced the pulsus paradoxus and improved the echocardiographic findings.

Constrictive pericarditis

In southern Africa sub-acute constrictive pericarditis is much more common than chronic calcific constrictive pericarditis, which is seen in less than 5% of patients with constriction.[1] The absence of radiological calcification, means that if the condition is missed clinically, it may also be missed on the chest radiograph. The electrocardiographic findings serve to indicate a cardiac abnormality only and are non-specific.[16] Echocardiography is particularly valuable in identifying this condition. Typically, a thick fibrinous exudate surrounds the heart, filling the pericardial sac. It may contain small loculi of fluid. The surface movements of the heart are diminished (Fig. 5), its chambers are normal sized and there is no sign of valvular disease or of myocardial hypertrophy. The inferior vena cava and intrahepatic veins are greatly dilated (Fig. 6). On anti-tuberculosis treatment the exudate may resolve with return of normal cardiac movement, or it may condense into a thick skin imprisoning the heart.[1] Usually, this can be distinguished from myocardium. Movement of the interventricular septum to the left on inspiration is seen commonly in constrictive pericarditis and may be responsible in part for pulsus paradoxus (Fig. 7).[1] The pericardial knock, the palpable equivalent of the early third heart sound due to rapid diastolic filling of the constricted ventricles, can be demonstrated by M-mode echocardiography (Fig. 8). Obviously the diagnosis is more difficult

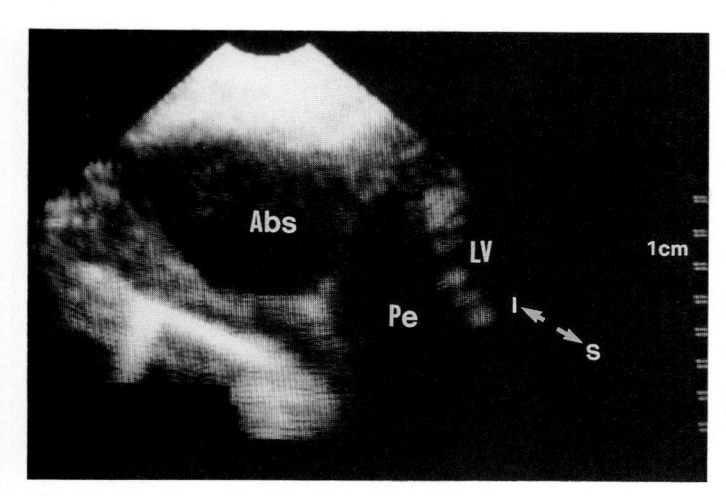

Fig. 2 Amoebic pericarditis. Two-dimensional echocardiogram, sub-costal view. Liver abscess cavity (Abs) is seen in communication with the pericardial sac (Pe).

294 CARDIAC ULTRASOUND

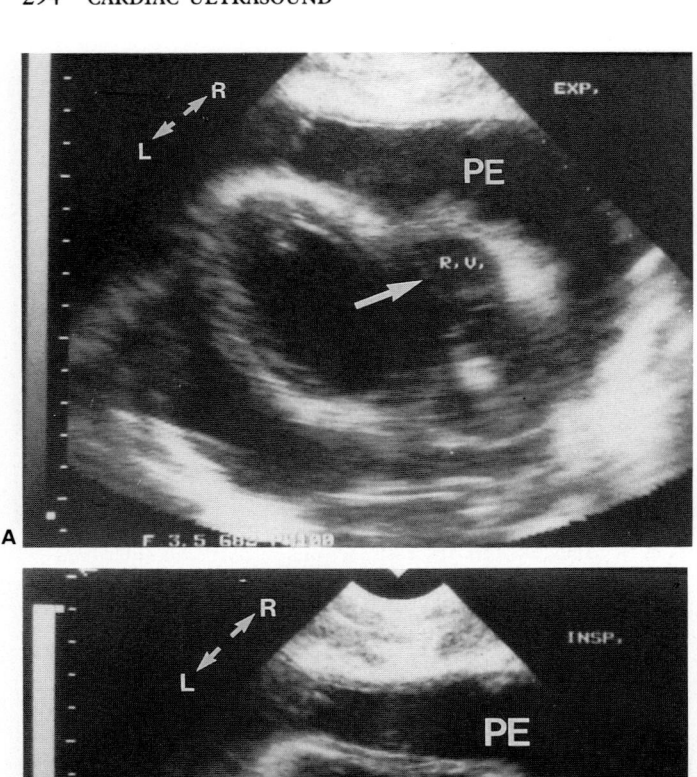

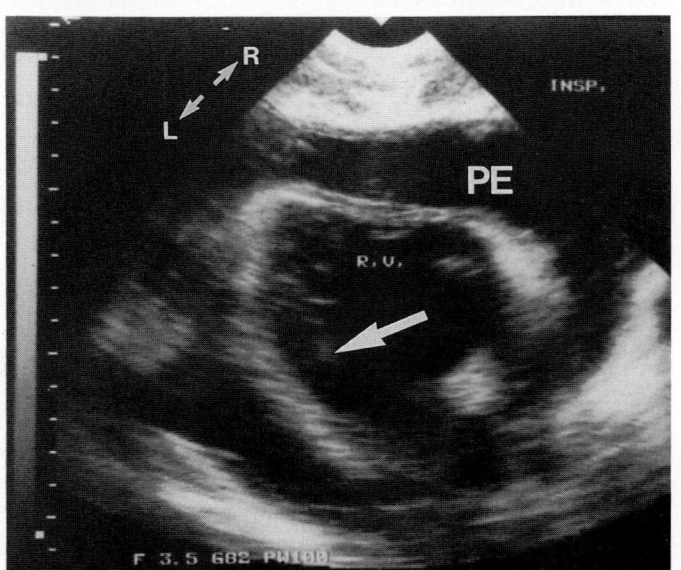

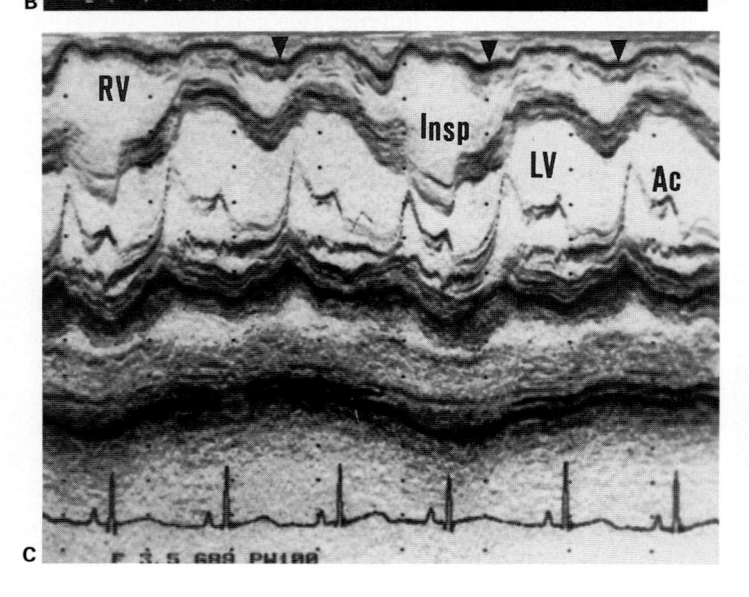

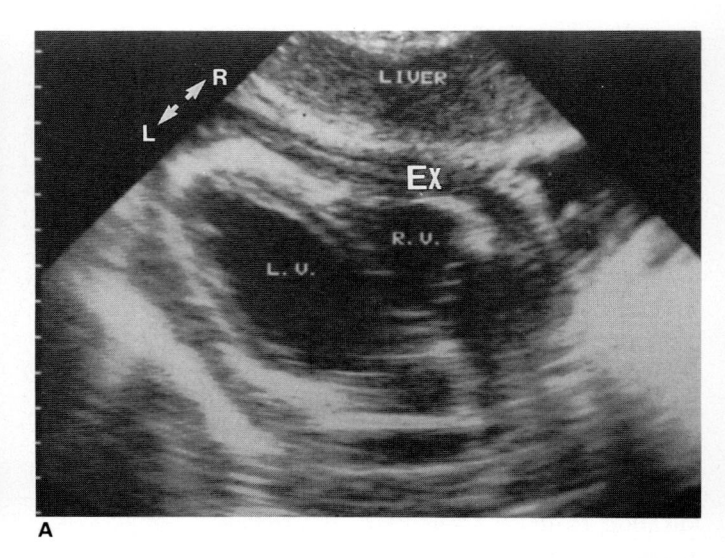

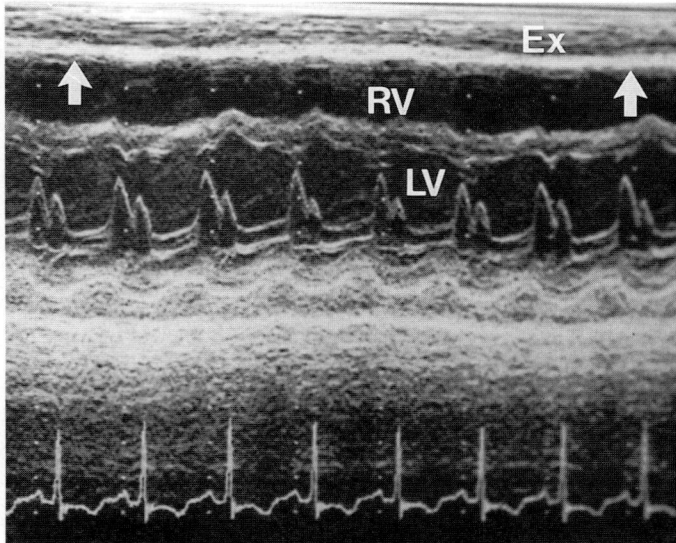

Fig. 5 (above) **Sub-acute constrictive pericarditis.** Same patient as Fig. 4, after one month. **A:** Two-dimensional echocardiogram, sub-costal view. Note the thick exudate (Ex) which fills the pericardial sac. **B:** M-mode echocardiogram of the same patient, parasternal long axis view. Note the reduced mobility of the anterior surface of the heart (arrowed), and the thick exudate (Ex), covering the visceral pericardium.

Fig. 4 (left) **Tuberculous pericardial effusion (PE) associated with significant pulsus paradoxus. A:** Two-dimensional echocardiogram, sub-costal view in expiration and **B:** same view in inspiration. Note the marked swing of the inter-ventricular septum (arrowed) to the left, on inspiration. **C:** M-mode echocardiogram of the same patient. In inspiration (Insp), the interventricular septum moves to the left, reducing the size of the left ventricle. The mitral valve opens to a lesser extent and for a shorter time in inspiration. (Ac = ant cusp of mitral valve.) Note the active movements of the surface of the heart (arrowed).

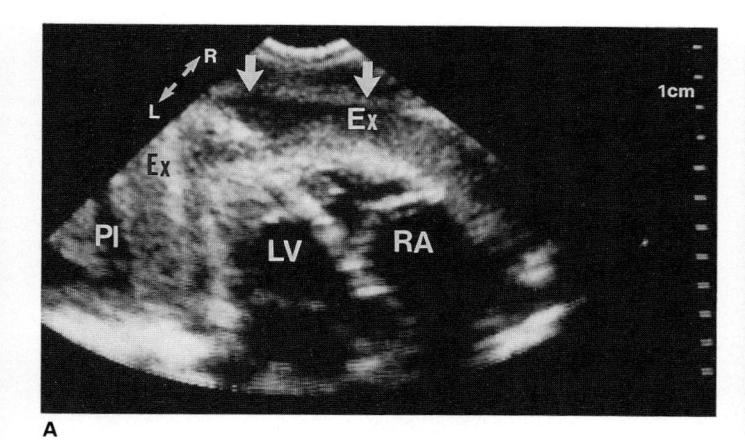

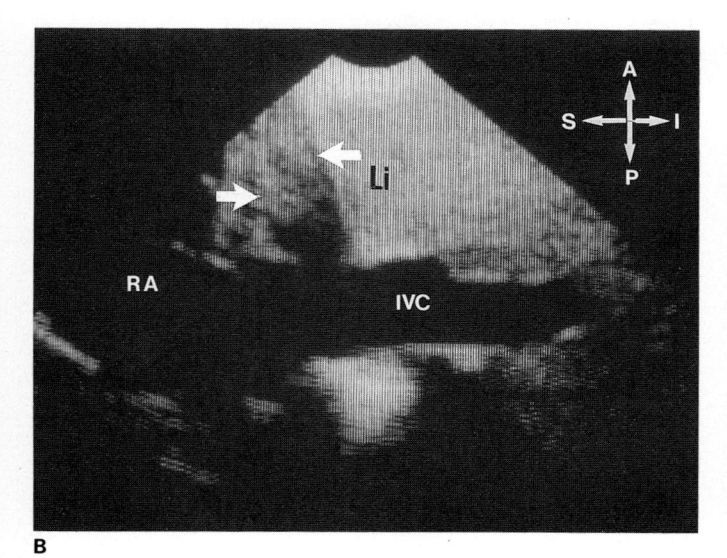

Fig. 6 Sub-acute constrictive pericarditis. A: Two-dimensional echocardiogram, sub-costal 4-chamber view. Note the thick exudate (Ex) in the pericardial sac (PL = left pleural space). **B:** Sub-costal longitudinal view in the same patient. Arrows mark the visceral and parietal pericardium. (Li = liver, IVC = inferior vena cava.)

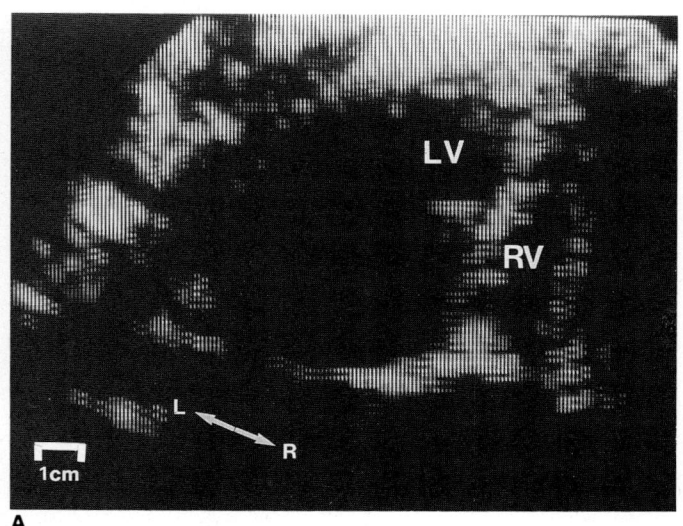

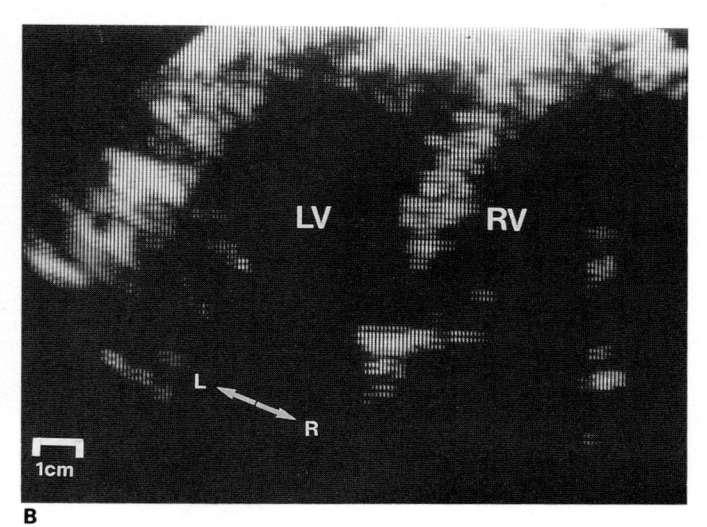

Fig. 7 Constrictive pericarditis. Two-dimensional echocardiogram, apical 4-chamber views. **A:** In expiration. Note the small volume of the right ventricle. **B:** Same view in inspiration. Note the considerable increase in size of the right ventricle as a result of movement of the interventricular septum to the left.

if a patient has not been followed through the exudative phase of constriction and presents with constrictive pericarditis due to a pericardial skin. The clinical features[9] and echocardiographic findings will normally allow differentiation from a restrictive cardiomyopathy, an unusual type of cardiomyopathy in southern Africa. Occasionally, thoracotomy is required to settle the matter when all investigations fail to make a clear diagnosis. This is justified since surgically remediable constrictive pericarditis should not be missed. If a restrictive cardiomyopathy is found, an adequate biopsy can be taken. Recent reports suggest that M-mode echocardiography[17] and Doppler echocardiography[18] can differentiate the two clearly, but confirmation in larger numbers of patients is required.

Effusive constrictive pericarditis

Echocardiography is the most useful investigation in confirming the coexistence of pericardial effusion and constriction, because although the cardiac shadow may be enlarged radiographically, due to a pericardial effusion (Fig. 9), the circulatory disturbances due to constriction of the visceral pericardium may not be suspected. Therefore, in addition to a pericardial effusion, thickening of the visceral pericardium is seen and the surface movements of the heart are diminished (Fig. 10). The pericardial knock is sometimes seen and the inferior vena cava is dilated.

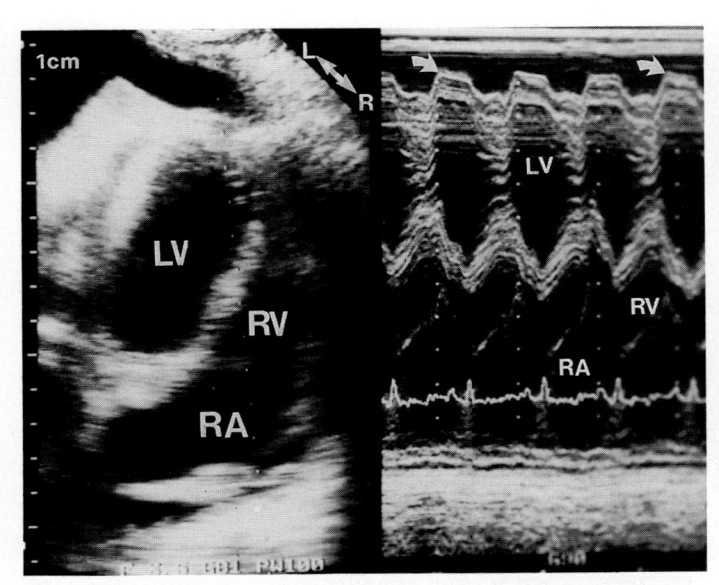

Fig. 8 Constrictive pericarditis with pericardial knock. Simultaneous two-dimensional and M-mode recordings. The cursor crosses the tricuspid valve (two-dimensional view, left) and in the M-mode recording (right), a marked outward movement of the surface of the heart occurs early in diastole (arrowed).

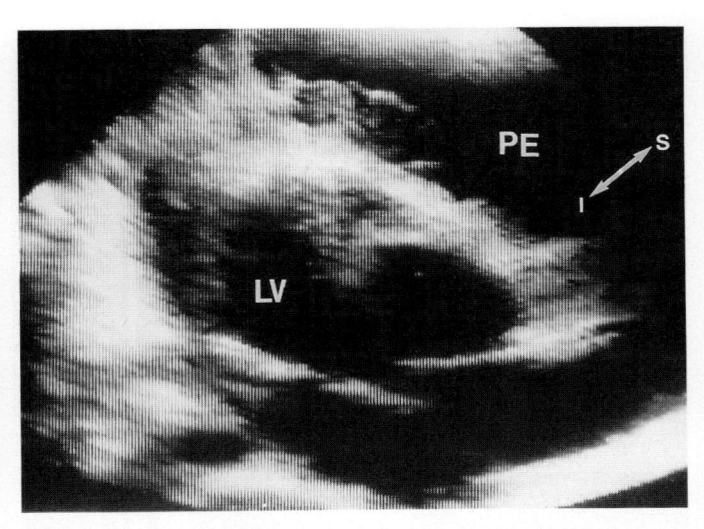

Fig. 10 Effusive–constrictive pericarditis. Two-dimensional echocardiogram, apical long axis view. Note the extensive fibrinous exudate in the pericardial sac. The posterior surface of the heart is stuck to the parietal pericardium and the anterior surface and apex are covered in a thick fibrinous exudate. Surface movements were diminished. Eventually, the patient required pericardiectomy (PE = pericardial effusion).

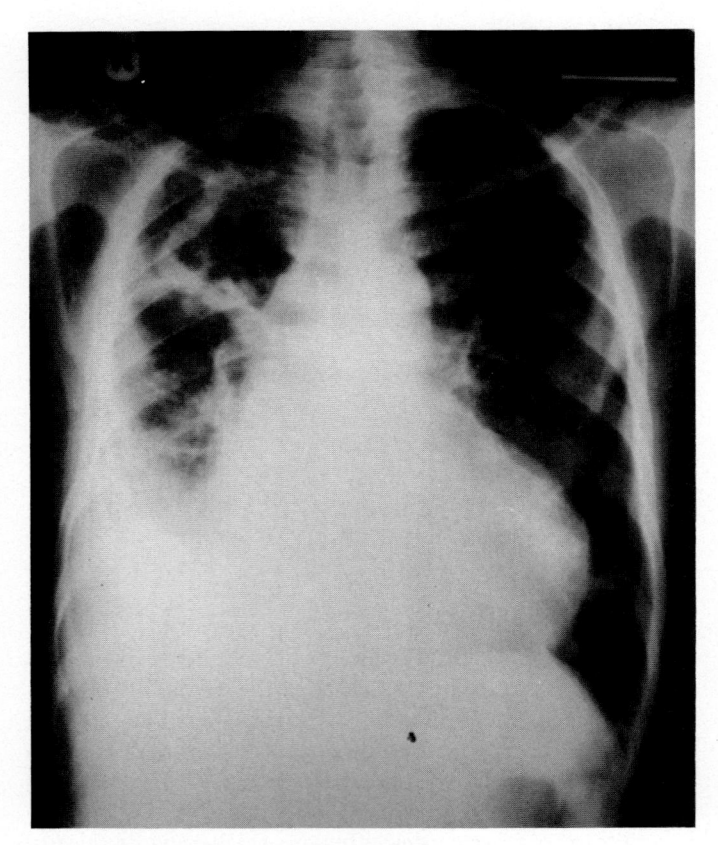

Fig. 9 Effusive–constrictive pericarditis. Chest X-ray. Note the enlarged cardiac shadow with an appearance more in keeping with cardiac enlargement or a pericardial effusion than with constrictive pericarditis. The patient had clinical features of constriction, including a pericardial knock and echocardiographic features of constrictive–effusive pericarditis.

Pericardiocentesis does not relieve the circulatory problem, because of visceral constriction. Serial echocardiography in sub-acute constriction and in effusive-constrictive pericarditis will indicate the development of a pericardial skin, amenable to surgical stripping, which cannot be undertaken for a fibrinous exudate. Pericardiectomy for constrictive pericarditis was undertaken 17 times in Umtata, over 18 months.

RHEUMATIC HEART DISEASE

Echocardiography is helpful in assessing patients with chronic rheumatic heart disease, with a view to performing closed mitral valvotomy locally, referral for open heart surgery elsewhere and in monitoring complications and progress in patients on long-term medical treatment. On a number of occasions when the suitability of a stenotic mitral valve for closed valvotomy has been in doubt clinically, echocardiography has indicated that it is suitable.

Figure 11 shows the mitral valve of a young woman referred in the mid-trimester of pregnancy, with a large haemoptysis and signs of severe mitral stenosis with mobile valve cusps. Echocardiography confirmed this and closed mitral valvotomy was undertaken successfully.

The decision to perform a closed valvotomy on a patient who has had a similar operation previously, requires confirmation that the valve remains suitable. This was the case

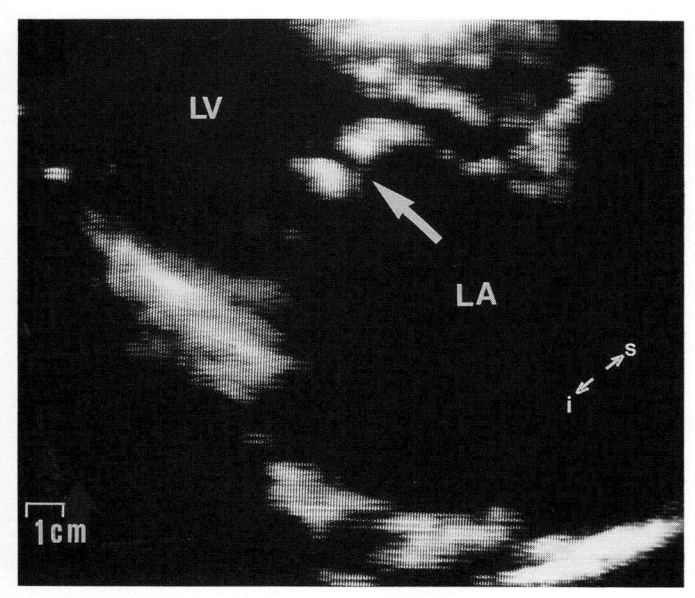

Fig. 11 Mobile mitral stenosis. Two-dimensional echocardiogram. Parasternal long axis view, in diastole. The left atrium is enlarged and a very narrow gap (arrowed) is seen between the thickened, mobile mitral valve cusps. The posterior cusp shows echo fall-out. The anterior mitral cusp is bowed.

in the example of a young woman who had undergone closed mitral valvotomy at another hospital seven years previously. She re-presented with increasing breathlessness on exertion, and physical examination revealed an opening snap and a loud first sound. Echocardiography (Fig. 12) suggested that the valve was amenable to closed valvotomy as the valve tissues remained thin and mobile. This procedure was undertaken successfully.

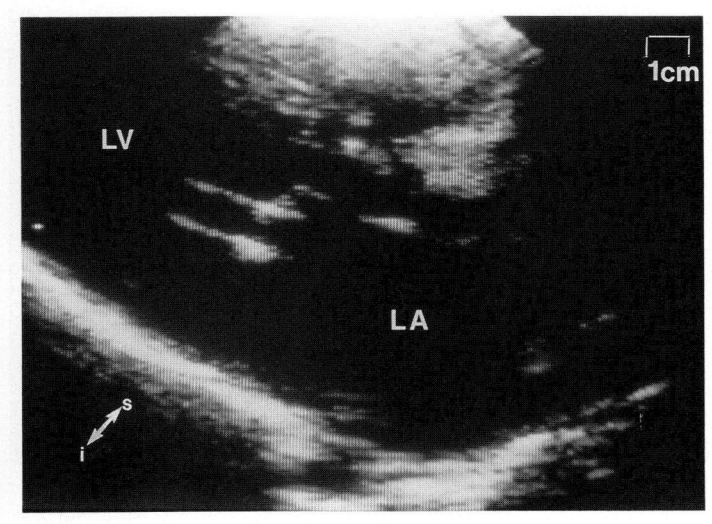

Fig. 12 Re-stenosis of mitral valve. Two-dimensional echocardiogram, parasternal long axis view. There is thickening of the mitral valve cusps and the chordae tendinae, but the cusps are mobile.

Figure 13 shows a recording made pre-operatively and at 1 year post-operatively of a teenage boy referred with a history of episodes of pulmonary oedema and congestive heart failure. On examination he was found to have severe mitral stenosis, pulmonary hypertension, functional tricuspid regurgitation and minimal aortic regurgitation. Repeated physical examination failed to elicit an opening snap, but two-dimensional echocardiography suggested a mobile valve and closed mitral valvotomy was undertaken. A year later he was well and echocardiography confirmed the adequacy of the operation.

Figure 14 shows the mitral valve of an elderly man, disabled by chronic rheumatic heart disease, in whom physical examination suggested an immobile mitral valve which would be unsuitable for closed valvotomy. This was confirmed by echocardiography which showed a very thick and rigid valve. He was referred for mitral valve replacement which was carried out successfully, using a bioprosthetic valve.

Atrial fibrillation associated with rheumatic mitral valve disease is an accepted indication for prophylactic anticoagulation. Since embolism can complicate mitral stenosis even in the presence of sinus rhythm,[19] some would consider mitral stenosis per se to be an indication for anticoagulation. In a developing country supplies of the anticoagulant, attendance for assessment and laboratory control of the drug cannot be guaranteed. Local practice which has proved to be safe, is to prescribe a fixed dose of Warfarin 5 mg or 2.5 mg daily[2] for those who can obtain it. The beneficial effects of anticoagulant treatment were seen in a young woman with severe mitral stenosis and atrial fibrillation who was found to have a large left atrial thrombus at echocardiography (Fig. 15). After 10 days of treatment with heparin she started warfarin therapy and the thrombus was shown to have disappeared on echocardiography performed three months later. No embolism occurred before or after the administration of warfarin and at subsequent closed valvotomy no thrombus was found in the left atrium.

Over an 18-month period after the acquisition of two-dimensional echocardiography, 17 closed mitral valvotomies were undertaken in Umtata, the referral centre of Transkei.[1]

There are clear indications for referral for mitral valve replacement and for aortic valve replacement for aortic stenosis, but patients with asymptomatic aortic regurgitation present a problem, since irreversible damage to the left ventricle may occur while the patient remains free of symptoms. This condition can be monitored by echocardiography and changes in the end systolic diameter and left ventricular fractional shortening can guide the decision to refer the patient for aortic valve replacement.[20]

Over an 18-month period, during which two-dimensional echocardiography was available in Umtata, 55 patients were referred to the nearest cardiothoracic centre

298 CARDIAC ULTRASOUND

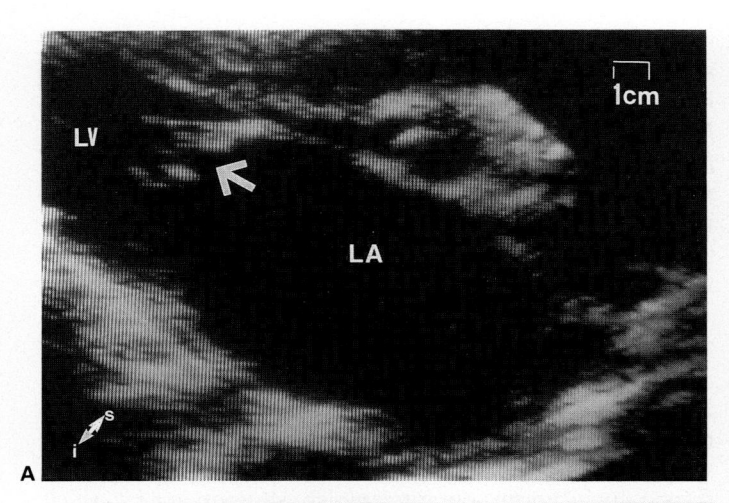

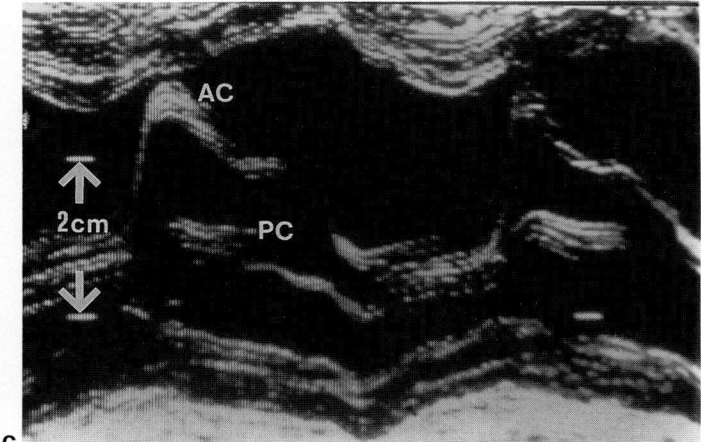

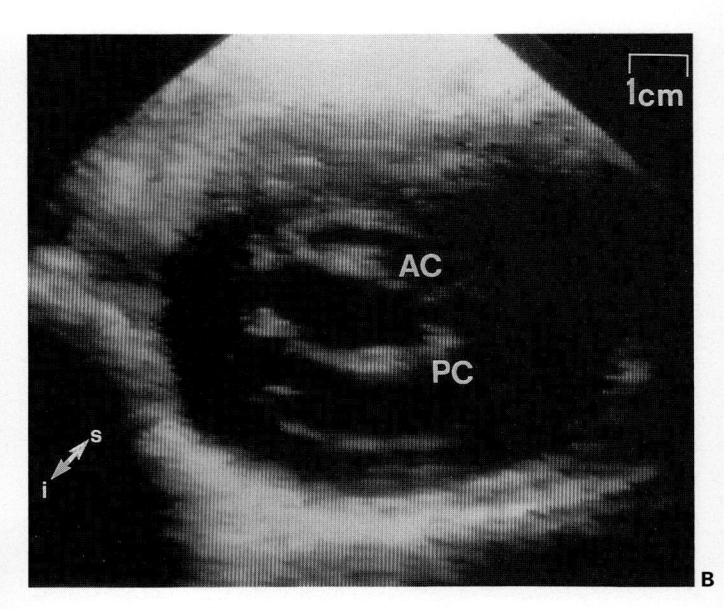

Fig. 13 **Mobile mitral stenosis, pre- and 1 year post-operative records. A:** Pre-operative echocardiogram two-dimensional parasternal long axis view, in which an enlarged left atrium, thickened mitral valve cusps and bowing of the anterior cusp are seen. The narrow orifice of the mitral valve is arrowed. **B:** Same patient 1 year post-operatively. Two-dimensional parasternal short axis view of the mitral valve in diastole. Although the cusps are thickened, a reasonable orifice has been obtained by closed mitral valvotomy (AC = anterior cusp, PC = posterior cusp). **C:** Same patient, post operative M-mode echocardiogram of the mitral valve. Although thickened, adequate separation of the cusps is noted. NB in this recording, the divisions indicate a distance of 2 cm (AC = anterior cusp, PC = posterior cusp).

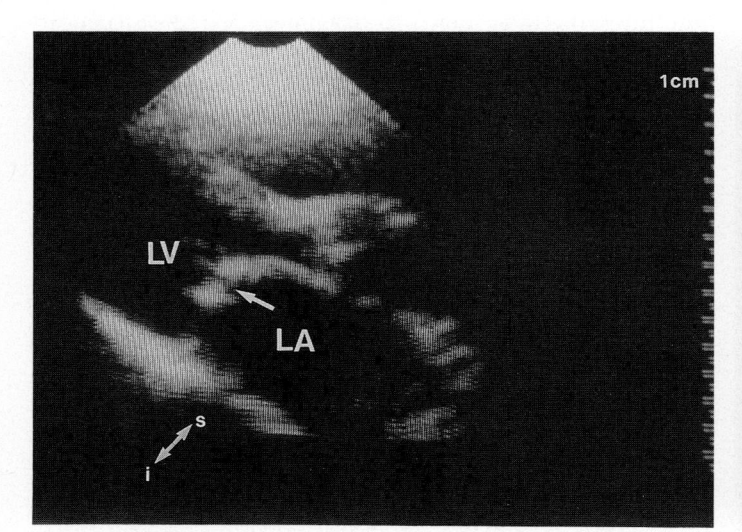

Fig. 14 **Fibrotic mitral stenosis.** Two-dimensional parasternal long axis view, in diastole. Note the marked thickening of the mitral valve cusps and co-existent thickening of the aortic valve cusps. The narrow orifice between the mitral valve cusps is arrowed.

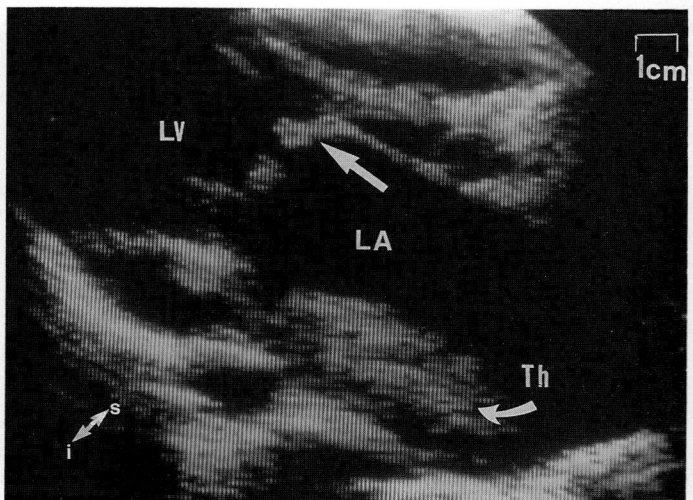

Fig. 15 **Mobile mitral stenosis, thrombus in the left atrium.** Two-dimensional parasternal long axis view, in diastole. The thrombus (Th, arrowed) is adherent to the posterior wall of the left atrium; there is a narrow orifice between the cusps of the mitral valve (arrow). The posterior cusp shows echo fall-out.

in South Africa; the great majority for valve replacement for rheumatic heart disease.

DILATED CARDIOMYOPATHY

Dilated cardiomyopathy is common in southern Africa and since it is often associated with functional mitral regurgitation, a surgically remediable cause such as rheumatic mitral valve disease must be excluded. Although physical examination is helpful in the differentiation, echocardiography allows a definitive diagnosis. With modern medical treatment, including the use of angiotensin converting enzyme inhibitors, much can be done to give symptomatic relief to patients with dilated cardiomyopathy. Two-dimensional echocardiography shows a dilated left ventricle with greatly reduced contractility and anatomically normal valves. Often there is enlargement of all cardiac chambers. M-mode measurements indicate a decreased fractional shortening of the left ventricle.

Dilated cardiomyopathy is common and cannot always be diagnosed with certainty by clinical examination alone. Echocardiography allows clear differentiation of several other conditions with similar clinical presentations and therefore appropriate management. Figure 16 shows features of a sub-mitral aneurysm in a teenage girl whose congestive heart failure was attributed to dilated cardiomyopathy. Sub-mitral aneurysm can be associated with mitral regurgitation and can be treated surgically. It may be associated with peripheral embolism and with angina pectoris, both of which are indications for echocardiography in the African population.[21] Figure 17 is another example of a congenital sub-mitral aneurysm in a 2-year-old child whose congestive heart failure was attributed to viral myocarditis.

Advanced calcific aortic stenosis may mimic dilated cardiomyopathy and the differentiation is important since aortic valve replacement is indicated for such disease even in the presence of left ventricular dysfunction.[22] Figure 18 illustrates the aortic valve of a middle-aged woman presenting in congestive heart failure who was thought to have a dilated cardiomyopathy. Calcific aortic stenosis with impaired left ventricular function was diagnosed with two-dimensional echocardiography and she was referred for surgery and received a prosthetic aortic valve.

Most patients with dilated cardiomyopathy die of congestive heart failure without peripheral embolism and in view of the difficulties of administering therapy, routine anticoagulation is not advised for such patients. However, the presence of an intracardiac thrombus such as is seen in Figure 19 suggests the need for long term anticoagulation. It is not uncommon to see spontaneous contrast in the

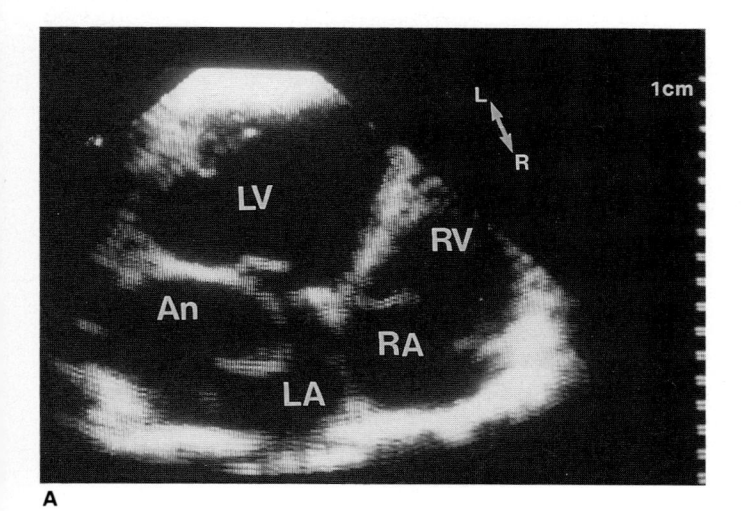

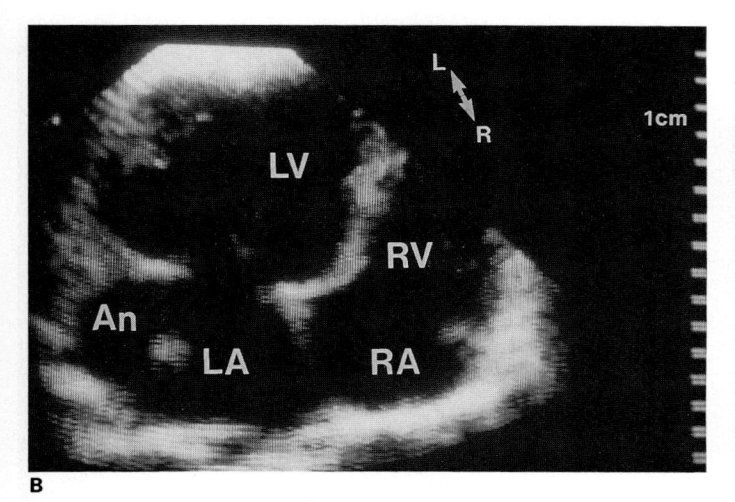

Fig. 16 Congenital sub-mitral aneurysms. Two-dimensional echocardiogram. **A:** In systole. Apical 4-chamber view in which the left atrium is compressed by the sub-mitral aneurysm (An) in systole. Mitral valve cusps closed. **B:** In diastole. Apical 4-chamber view in which the compression of the left atrium is less, as the sub-mitral aneurysm (An) empties in diastole. The mitral valve cusps are open.

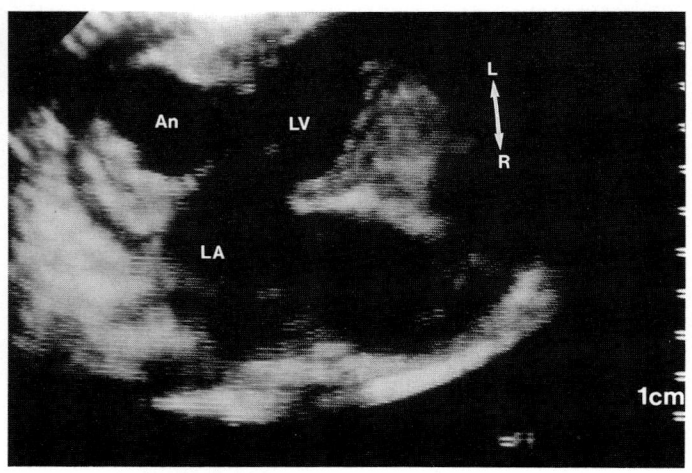

Fig. 17 Congenital sub-mitral aneurysms. Two-dimensional echocardiogram, apical 4-chamber view. The aneurysm (An) is seen arising from the posterior wall of the left ventricle.

300 CARDIAC ULTRASOUND

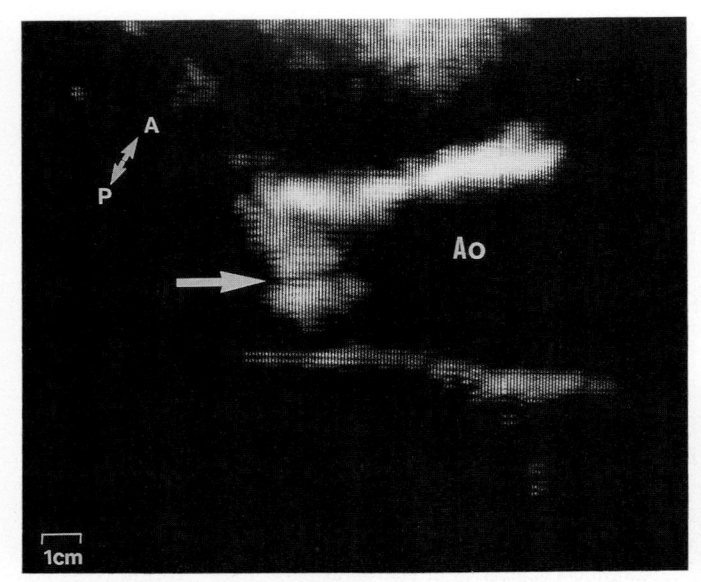

Fig. 18 Calcific aortic stenosis. Two-dimensional echocardiogram, parasternal long axis view in systole. The aortic cusps are very thick with impaired mobility and the aortic orifice (arrowed) is small.

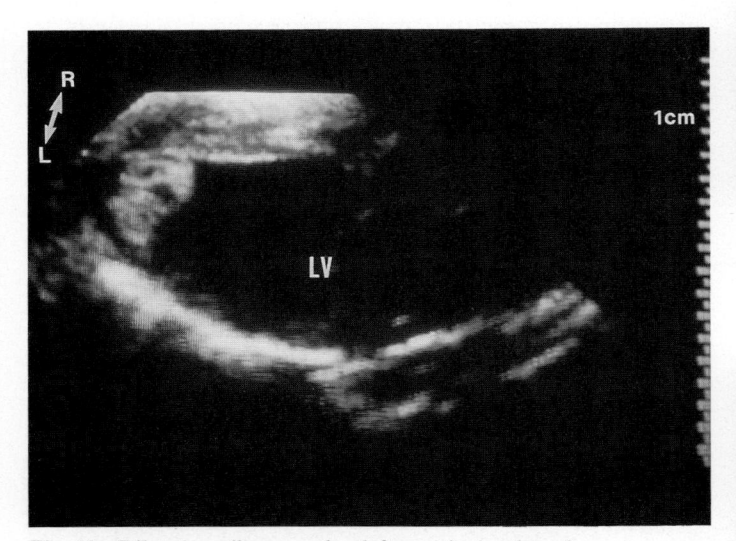

Fig. 19 Dilated cardiomyopathy, left ventricular thrombus. Two-dimensional echocardiogram, sub-costal view. Note the dilated left ventricle (LV) with a large thrombus in the apex.

dilated chambers of these hearts, which may indicate the likelihood of subsequent thrombus formation, but this has not been proved.

INFECTIVE ENDOCARDITIS

Patients with infective endocarditis may not show typical clinical features of the disease, and the clinical diagnosis may often be in doubt. Blood cultures in a developing country may be unavailable or unreliable. Echocardio-graphy is thus very valuable in confirming the diagnosis[23] and in assessing the need for surgical management. In most patients with infective endocarditis seen in Transkei, the disease complicated severe rheumatic heart disease, which would require surgery in its own right in the near future. The diagnosis of infective endocarditis becomes an indication for early referral for surgery after starting antibiotic treatment, since both the haemodynamic problem and the infection can be treated simultaneously. Figure 20 was recorded from a teenage boy known to have asymptomatic

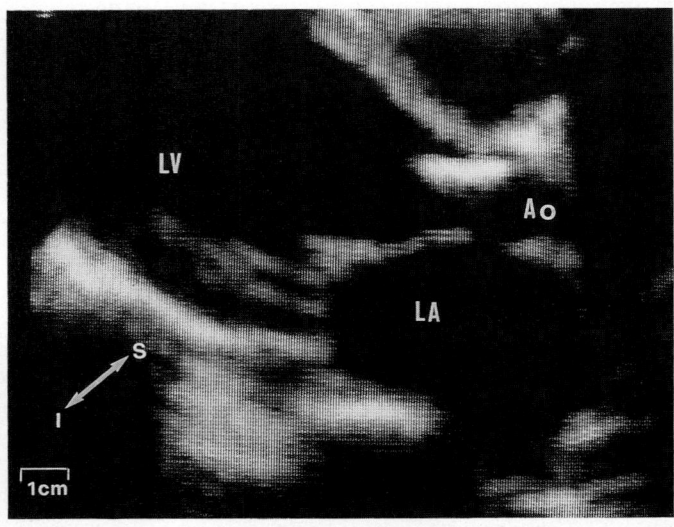

Fig. 20 Infective endocarditis. Two-dimensional parasternal long axis view, in which a large mobile vegetation is seen on an aortic valve cusp.

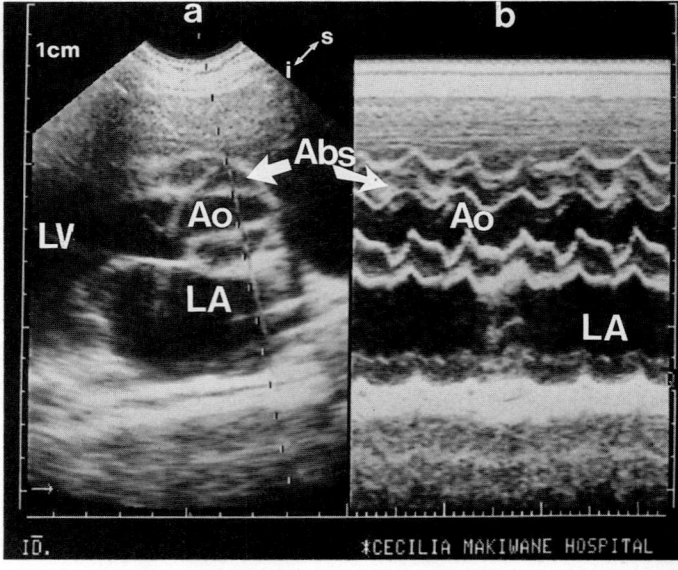

Fig. 21 Infective endocarditis with root abscesses. Two-dimensional (left) and M-mode (right) echocardiograms. Note the double-walled ascending aorta. The abscess cavities are arrowed (Abs = root abscess).

aortic regurgitation. He was admitted with a short history of increasing breathlessness and had developed pulmonary oedema. Equivocal finger clubbing was the only sign supporting the diagnosis of infective endocarditis. He was referred for aortic valve replacement.

Figure 21 is the record of a young woman in congestive heart failure who was found to have severe aortic regurgitation and peripheral signs supporting the diagnosis of infective endocarditis. The echocardiogram showed aortic root abscesses complicating infective endocarditis and she was referred for urgent surgery. Aortic valve replacement and replacement of part of the ascending aorta were undertaken as an emergency, following which there was a marked improvement in her condition.

With M-mode echocardiography, the findings of premature closure of the mitral valve and of premature opening of the aortic valve are additional reasons to refer a patient with infective endocarditis for early aortic valve replacement, since they indicate gross aortic regurgitation into a relatively non-compliant left ventricle, with a rapid and severe rise in left ventricular diastolic pressure.[24]

MISCELLANEOUS CONDITIONS

Figure 22 was recorded from a middle-aged woman with open pulmonary tuberculosis who was thought to have cor pulmonale, but had some signs suggestive of an ostium secundum atrial septal defect. A defect was seen in the interatrial septum with echocardiography, but a contrast study was done to exclude echo-fall-out. This indicated a right to left shunt at atrial level.

The 'negative jet' contrast technique seen in left to right shunting[25] is illustrated in Figure 23. A young man was admitted with a right ventricular stab wound which was repaired surgically. After several days, he was noted to have a cardiac murmur, suggestive of a ventricular septal defect. Plain echocardiography supported this, and the diagnosis was confirmed by contrast echocardiography, the bubbles of contrast in the right ventricle being displaced by the jet of blood from the left ventricle. The defect was repaired surgically.

Significant tricuspid regurgitation can be suggested by the appearance of contrast in the inferior vena cava after injection into an arm vein. Contrast echocardiography can also be used to assess cardiac output and pulmonary resistance.[26]

A middle-aged woman with nephrosis was found to have raised jugular venous pressure and non-specific cardiac signs. Echocardiography (Fig. 24) showed the typical myocardial features of cardiac amyloid[27] and the diagnosis of amyloidosis was confirmed by rectal biopsy.

An elderly woman who had upper abdominal pain for several weeks was referred for echocardiography because her chest radiograph showed a slight increase in the heart size. A barium meal had been done to exclude upper

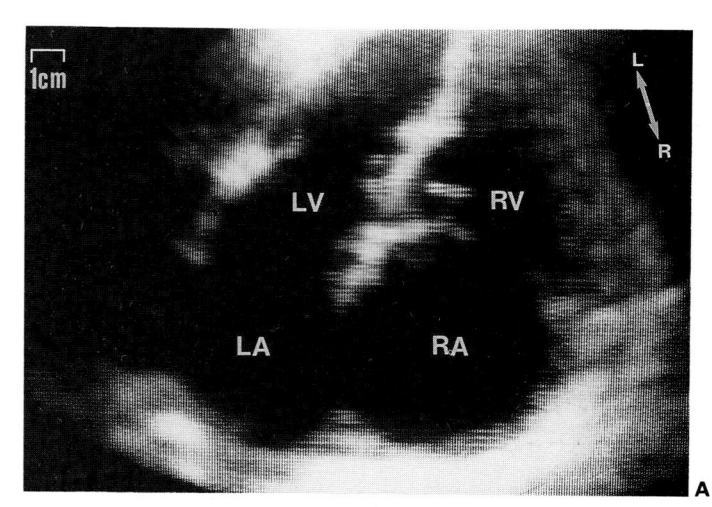

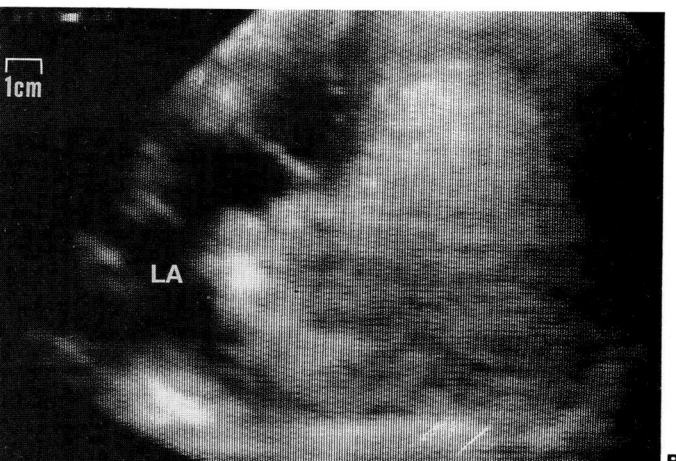

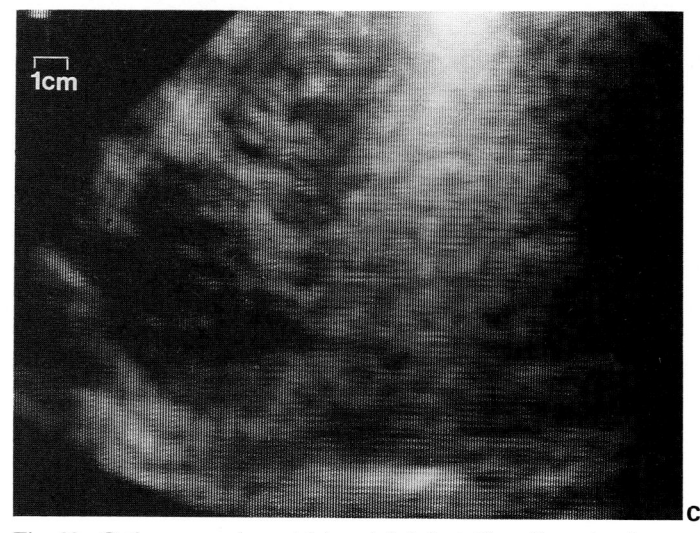

Fig. 22 Ostium-secundum atrial septal defect. Two-dimensional echocardiograms. **A:** Apical 4-chamber view, showing possible echo fall-out in the inter-atrial septum. **B:** Atrial septal defect. The same study after injection of echo-contrast medium. Opacification of the right atrium and right ventricle have occurred and the contrast is crossing the intra-atrial septum into the left atrium. **C:** Opacification of all four chambers is apparent at a later stage of the recording.

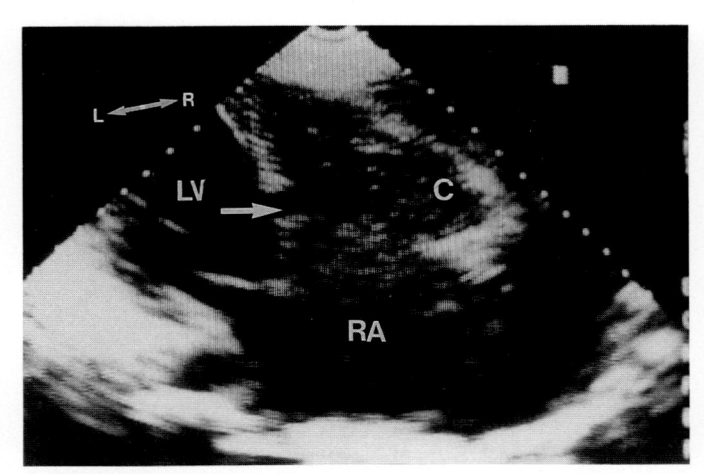

Fig. 23 Traumatic ventricular septal defect. Negative contrast study. Two-dimensional echocardiogram, apical 4-chamber view. Bubbles of contrast (C) are pushed away from the ventricular septal defect (arrowed) by the left to right shunt.

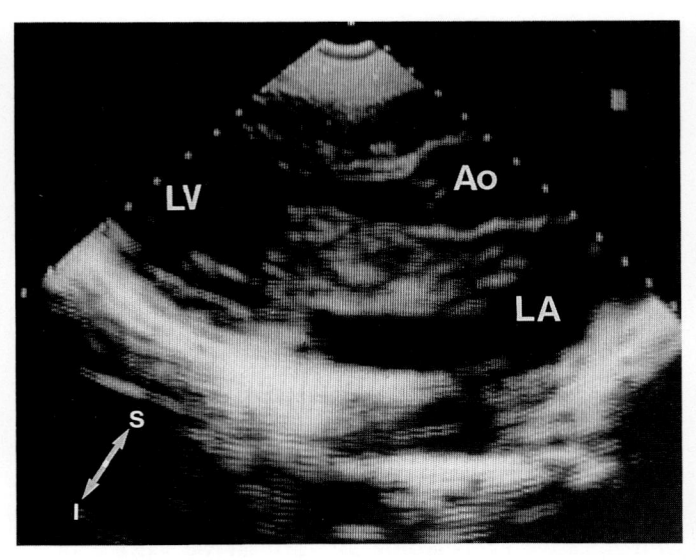

Fig. 25 Left atrial myxoma. Two-dimensional echocardiogram, parasternal long axis view, in diastole. The myxoma, which arises from the inter-atrial septum, can be seen obstructing the mitral valve orifice.

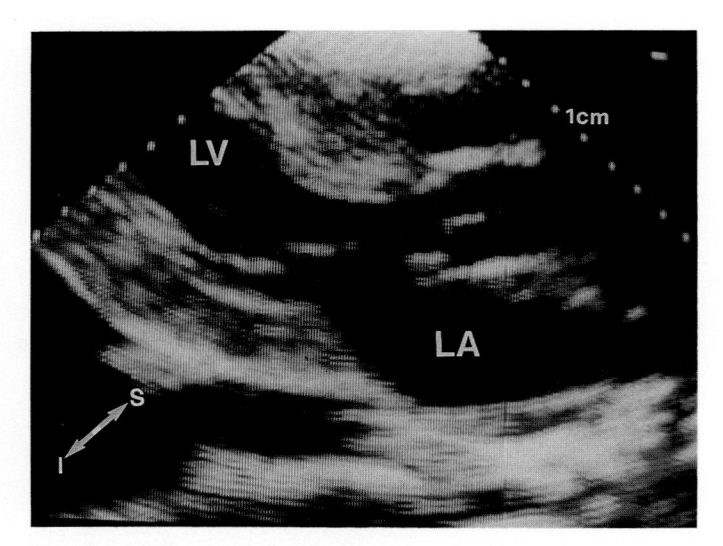

Fig. 24 Cardiac amyloid. Two-dimensional echocardiogram, parasternal long axis view. Note the small chambers, the greatly thickened inter-ventricular septum and left ventricular free wall and the glistening appearance of the myocardium.

gastrointestinal pathology. Physical examination suggested mitral valve obstruction and echocardiography led to an immediate diagnosis of left atrial myxoma (Fig. 25). The tumour was resected successfully and the upper abdominal pain which had resulted from liver congestion also resolved.

SUMMARY

The simplicity and rapidity with which echocardiography can be done results in an early and thorough assessment of many cardiac problems seen in the developing world. Since the management and prognosis of most conditions depends on correct diagnosis, the case for echocardiography in the developing world is strong. The differentiation of dilated cardiomyopathy, cor pulmonale, especially if acyanotic, and pericarditis, can be difficult even for the experienced physician, but it is exceptional not to obtain useful information from echocardiography. Experience has shown that echocardiography is far more sensitive at detecting cor pulmonale than electrocardiography.

The acquisition of echocardiographic equipment is likely to lead to a reduction in expenses, since appropriate management of patients can be started early and the numbers of patients referred to cardiothoracic centres for full assessment are reduced. Similarly, those referred are likely to have been assessed correctly and to require little further investigation before cardiac surgery.

ACKNOWLEDGEMENTS

I thank Dr D. G. Gibson of the Department of Cardiology, Brompton Hospital, London who taught me the technique of two dimensional echocardiography.

The patients with tuberculous pericarditis were studied with support by Grant 14290/1.5/BMO/CDJS/slp from the Wellcome Trust, London.

I thank Mrs M. S. Frauenstein for typing the manuscript.

REFERENCES

1. Strang J I G. Echoes from the Third World – two dimensional echocardiography in a developing country. S Afr Med J 1990; 77: 85–91
2. Wilkins E G L, Strang J I G. The cardiologist in the Third World. BMJ 1984; 289: 609–611
3. Gelfand M. The Sick African. 3rd ed. Cape Town: Juta & Co. 1957: p 494
4. St. John Sutton M G, St. John Sutton M, Oldershaw P et al. Valve replacement without pre-operative cardiac catheterisation. N Eng J Med 1981; 305: 1233–1238
5. Peller O G, Wallerson D C, Devereux R B. Role of Doppler and imaging echocardiography in selection of patients for cardiac valvular surgery. Am Heart J 1987; 114: 1445–1461
6. Seward J B, Tajik A J, Hagler D J, Ritter D G. Peripheral venous contrast echocardiography. Am J Cardiol 1977; 39: 202–212
7. Feigenbaum H. Echocardiography. 4th ed. Philadelphia: Lea & Febiger. 1986: p 548.
8. Strang J I G, Kakaza H H S, Gibson D G et al. Controlled trial of complete open surgical drainage and of prednisolone in treatment of tuberculous pericardial effusion in Transkei. Lancet 1988; 2: 759–764
9. Strang J I G. Tuberculous pericarditis in Transkei. Clin Cardiol 1984; 7: 667–670
10. Hofmeyr G J, Purry N A. Inferior pericardiotomy in the treatment of pericardial effusions. S Afr Med J 1979; 55: 280–284
11. Cassell P, Cullum P. The management of cardiac tamponade: drainage of pericardial effusions. Br J Surg 1967; 54: 620–626
12. Strang J I G. Two-dimensional echocardiography in the diagnosis of amoebic pericarditis. S Afr Med J 1987; 71: 328–329
13. Adams E B, MacLeod N. Invasive amoebiasis: II. Amoebic liver abscess and its complications. Medicine (Baltimore) 1977; 56: 325–334
14. Adams E B. The management of invasive amoebiasis. S Afr J Hosp Med 1976; 6: 327–335
15. Feigenbaum H. Echocardiography. 4th ed. Philadelphia: Lea & Febiger. 1986: p 561
16. Strang J I G, Kakaza H H S, Gibson D G, Girling D J, Nunn A J, Fox W. Controlled trial of prednisolone as adjuvant in treatment of tuberculous constrictive pericarditis in Transkei. Lancet 1987; 2: 1418–1422
17. Morgan J M, Rapaso L, Clague J C, et al. Restrictive cardiomyopathy and constrictive pericarditis: non-invasive distinction by digitised M-mode echocardiography. Br Heart J 1989; 61: 29–37
18. Hatle L K, Appleton C P, Popp R L. Differentiation of constrictive pericarditis and restrictive cardiomyopathy by Doppler echocardiography. Circulation 1989; 79: 357–370
19. Wood P. An appreciation of mitral stenosis. I. Clinical features. BMJ 1954; 1: 1051–1063
20. Nishimura R A, McGoon M D, Schaff H V, Giuliani E R. Chronic aortic regurgitation: Indications for operation — 1988. Mayo Clin Proc 1988; 63: 270–280
21. Chesler E. Aneurysms of the left ventricle. Cardiovasc Clin 1972; 4: 188–217
22. Smith N, McAnulty J H, Rahimtoola J H. Severe aortic stenosis with impaired left ventricular function and clinical heart failure: results of valve replacement. Circulation 1978; 58: 255–264
23. Martin R P, Meltzer R S, Chia B L, Stinson E B, Rakowski H, Popp R L. Clinical utility of two-dimensional echocardiography in infective endocarditis. Am J Cardiol 1980; 46: 379–385
24. Gibson D G. Oxford Textbook of Medicine. 2nd ed. Oxford: Oxford University Press. 1987: 13. p 297
25. Weyman A E, Wann L S, Caldwell R L, Hurwitz R A, Dillon J C, Feigenbaum H. Negative contrast echocardiography: a new method for detecting left to right shunts. Circulation 1979; 59: 498–505
26. Gibson D G. Oxford textbook of medicine. 2nd ed. Oxford: Oxford University Press. 1987: 13. p 40
27. Nicolosi G L, Pavan D, Lestuzzi C, Burelli C, Zardo F, Zanuttini D. Prospective identification of patients with amyloid heart disease by two-dimensional echocardiography. Circulation 1984; 70: 432–437

SECTION 3

Congenital heart disease

19

Segmental approach

Introduction
Practical considerations
Image orientation
Atrial situs
Venous connections
Atrioventricular connection
Ventriculo-arterial connection
The cardiac chambers
Atrial septum
Atrioventricular septum
Ventricular septum
The great arteries
The coronary arteries
Acquired abnormalities
Conclusion

Ian D. Sullivan and Vanda M. Gooch

INTRODUCTION

Clinical practice in paediatric cardiology has altered radically in the decade since the introduction of cross-sectional echocardiography because analysis of structural heart disease in infants and children is ideally suited to imaging in the infinite number of 'tomographic slices' available to the echocardiographer. This chapter will describe an approach to cross-sectional echocardiographic imaging in congenital heart disease based on sequential segmental analysis.[1] While the vast majority of congenital heart defects occur in hearts with normal connections, this approach simplifies and standardises the description of more complicated abnormalities. The position of the heart in the thorax, together with information about atrial arrangement, atrioventricular and ventriculo-arterial connections is used as the framework upon which the detailed description of structural abnormality is based. This facilitates a systematic approach to each examination, making it less likely that an important abnormality will receive close attention while subsidiary additional problems are overlooked. Adherence to a pattern of examination within an institution also means that studies of complex heart disease performed by another operator will be easier to interpret. This 'overview' is illustrated with selected abnormalities which might be sought at each phase of the integrated examination. These specific lesions are dealt with separately in detail in the chapters which follow.

Normal cardiac anatomy and standard echocardiographic techniques are considered in Chapter 4. Some specific morphological features, important in the assessment of congenital heart defects, are highlighted in this chapter. More detailed morphological considerations have been reviewed elsewhere.[1,2]

Practical considerations

Infants and small children generally have excellent acoustic windows. The heart is also close to the scanhead. This enables the use of transducers with high carrier frequency to give optimal images. A 7.5 MHz mechanical sector scanhead, suitable for use in neonates and small infants, may have axial resolution of less than 0.35 mm at shallow depths.[3] A 5 MHz transducer has sufficient penetration to provide satisfactory images in most children.

The examination should be performed in a warm environment. Sedation may be required in infants and young children to facilitate a full examination but is not usually necessary if the examination is performed just after a feed. A teat dipped in a mixture of brandy and fruit elixir is usually very suitable for neonates and other young infants. Oral chloral hydrate, 30 to 50 mg/kg by mouth, is effective and safe in older infants and toddlers. Small toys or other suitable distractions may also be helpful in the latter group. Parents frequently provide important reassurance and the images displayed may be a useful visual aid in the description of what is 'wrong' with their child's heart.

While the standard echocardiographic planes familiar to adult cardiologists are employed, there are several important differences. The best acoustic window in children is usually the subcostal one, more diagnostic information being obtained from this site than from any other. In this way the paediatric examination is very different from the usual adult examination. In order that a three-dimensional description of cardiac structure is obtained from a series of two-dimensional images, the scanhead is moved in 'sweeps' from each transducer position, so that the real time image conveys information about the relationships of adjacent structures which are not apparent from photographs of single frames. The operator must correlate the real time images with the movement of the transducer head and scanning plane to describe the anatomy. An image memory loop, or a recorder which allows single frame video tape analysis, is essential to appreciate details of morphology which may not be evident in the real time display. As a memory loop facility is also essential for optimal analysis of colour flow Doppler information, most modern machines now include this feature.

The sequence of examination normally consists of abdominal views of the great vessels, followed by subcostal, apical, parasternal and suprasternal views in turn. A frightened child may be more amenable to an apical or parasternal transducer position than a subcostal one in the first instance and the sequence of examination should be altered accordingly. Children of body weight less than 20 kg usually can be examined supine; in larger patients improved precordial images may be obtained with the patient rolled to the left (assuming there is levocardia). Suprasternal imaging is facilitated by placing a pad or pillow under the scapulae to extend the neck. Even so, access to the suprasternal notch may be difficult if the transducer is bulky. This posture is unpleasant for some children and suprasternal imaging should be left until last whenever possible. Examination techniques may require modification in special circumstances, for example chest drains and surgical dressings may limit transducer access after open heart surgery. Extension of the neck for suprasternal imaging is contra-indicated in the days immediately following primary repair of oesophageal atresia. Premature babies require expeditious examination with 'minimal handling'.

Doppler assessment is often best left until the imaging study is completed. The nature of the Doppler information required should then be apparent. It may be preferable to use a scanhead with a lower transmission frequency for pulsed Doppler interrogation to minimise aliasing of the signal, whether this is a colour flow map or conventional spectral Doppler. This approach will also facilitate the positioning of a non-imaging continuous wave Doppler transducer when high velocity signals, so common in structural heart disease, are sought. The small size and offset crystals of commercially available non-imaging continuous wave transducers continue to be attractive in paediatrics, even when imaging transducers which incorporate 'steerable continuous wave Doppler' are available. Inevitably, if good alignment with an anticipated flow signal is obtained during imaging, it may be opportune to perform Doppler interrogation, especially if continuing patient co-operation cannot be guaranteed. It is also noteworthy how often a restless neonate may be soothed by the Doppler audio signal!

Image orientation

The anatomical coronal, sagittal and transverse planes of the body cannot be used conveniently in the description of tomographic cardiac structure. The conventional long axis, short axis and four chamber views of the heart each describes a 'family' of planes at varying degrees of obliquity to the standard anatomical planes.[4] The presentation format of these cross-sectional images in congenital heart disease can be confusing.

There is general uniformity in the orientation of parasternal long axis, parasternal short axis and suprasternal images. However, a number of formats are employed in the presentation of subcostal and apical views, none of which is absolutely right or wrong.

In adults, most echocardiographers present images from these sites so that the part of the heart closest to the transducer is at the top of the image display, with left sided structures on the right of the screen. This is an option approved by the American Heart Association,[4] and has the advantage that the image is 'continuous' with the conventional parasternal short axis orientation as the transducer is slid from the apex to a parasternal short axis position. There has been advocacy of the 'anatomical display'[5,6] by some paediatric echocardiographers who present subcostal and apical images so that the cardiac apex or anterior free wall is at the bottom of the image display, with left sided structures to the right as the observer views the screen. This is also a format option approved by the American Heart Association.[4] While this format may be intuitively appealing to some, it has the disadvantage that the image must be 'reinverted' at some arbitrary location to convert an apical to a conventional parasternal short axis image format. In addition, inverting the image for part of the examination, as necessitated by the use of the anatomical format, may complicate Doppler assessment, especially colour flow mapping, because the variation in transducer location at either the top or bottom of the image must be incorporated into the assessment of Doppler flow information.

In a third approach, some operators prefer not to invert the image on the screen when a subcostal or apical imaging position is chosen, keeping the transducer position at the top of the screen. Left sided structures, however, are displayed on the left of the screen. Photographs of single video frames in this format can be inverted to provide 'anatomical' display.

There is no uniformity of practice, with some experienced operators using a combination of these display orientations.

It is crucial that, whatever format is chosen, there is consistency within an institution, and orientation is provided in image display for publication. We have chosen to display subcostal and apical images in anatomical format. Long axis, short axis and suprasternal views are displayed according to convention.[4] When the imaging plane is close to the coronal, sagittal or transverse plane of the body, we use superior, inferior, anterior or posterior labels as appropriate for orientation purposes. When the imaging plane is oblique to the standard anatomical planes, only one axis is identified.

Atrial situs

Atrial arrangement, or situs, may be usual (solitus), mirror image (inversus) or ambiguous (right or left isomerism). Whilst the vast majority of patients will have normal atrial situs, the unusual cardiac positions and structural abnormalities within the chest which accompany isomeric atrial arrangements, are much easier to elucidate if the abnormal atrial arrangement has been established at the outset. Images of the atrial appendages as they 'clasp' the great arteries, obtained from a modified parasternal short axis position, may allow right atrial morphology to be distinguished from left atrial morphology (Fig. 1). In practice,

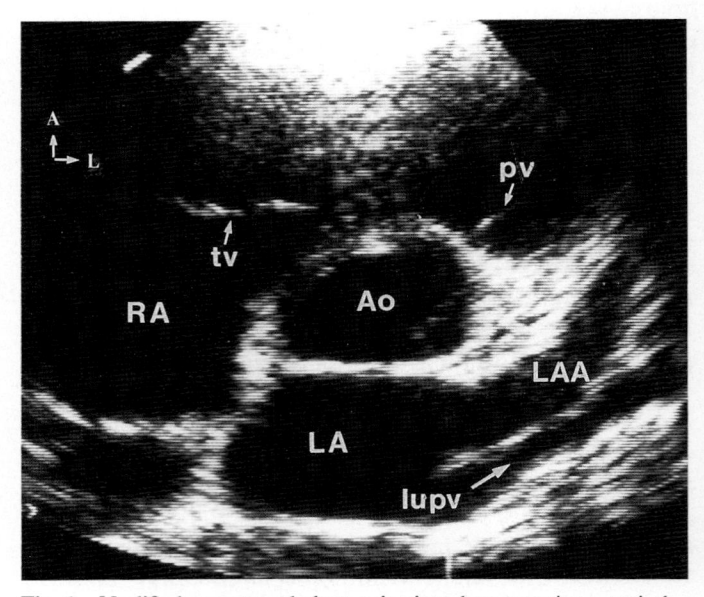

Fig. 1 Modified parasternal short axis view demonstrating a typical finger-like left atrial appendage with narrow base and tubular appendage. LAA – left atrial appendage, lupv – left upper pulmonary vein.

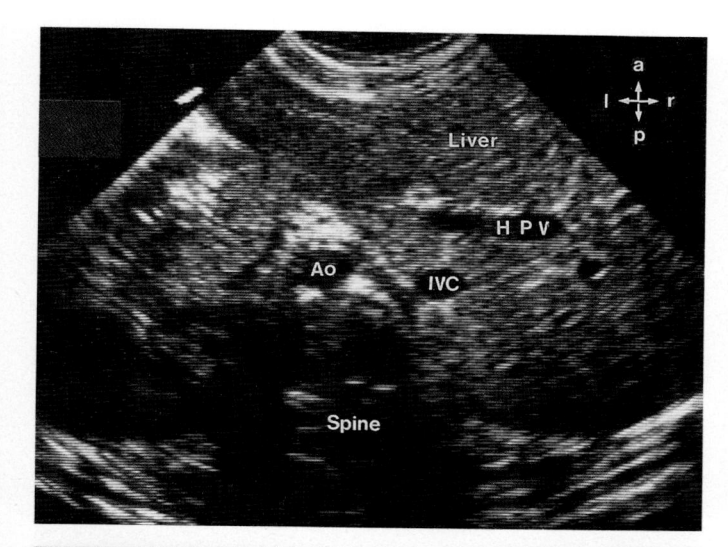

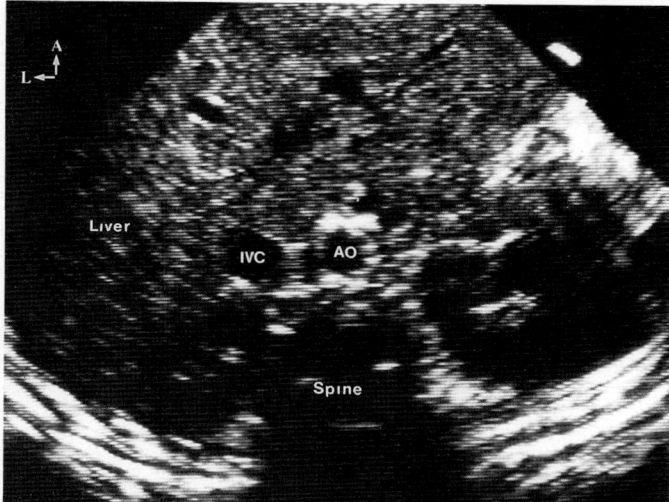

Fig. 2 Transverse sections of the abdomen just below the diaphragm. **Top:** Normal arrangement of the great vessels, with the inferior caval vein to the right indicating usual atrial arrangement. HPV – hepatic portal vein. **Lower:** The inferior caval vein is to the left in a patient with mirror image atrial arrangement.

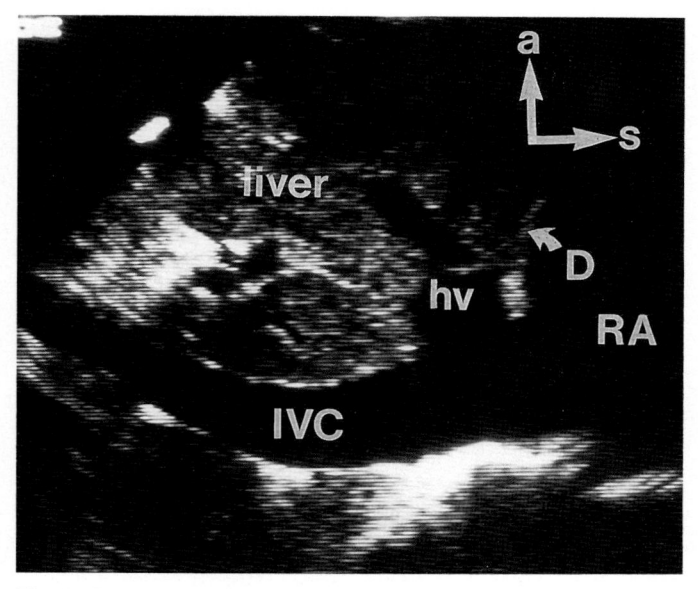

Fig. 3 Right parasagittal abdominal view showing normal hepatic veins joining the inferior caval vein at its junction with the right atrium. D – diaphragm, hv – hepatic veins.

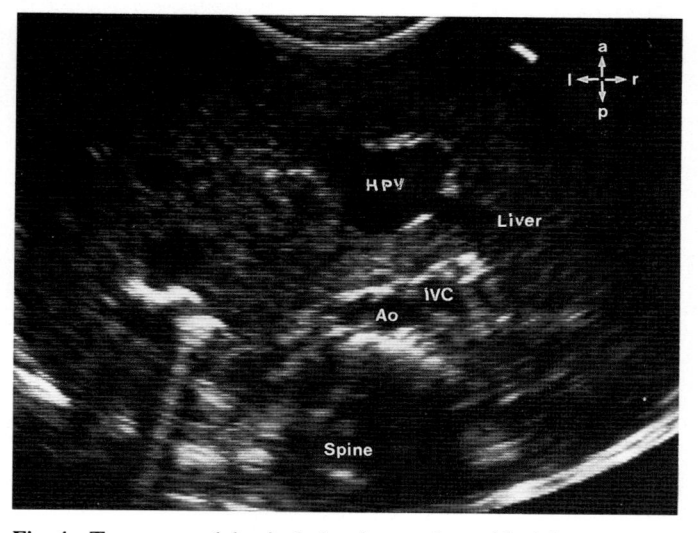

Fig. 4 Transverse abdominal view in a patient with right isomerism. HPV – hepatic portal vein.

it is much easier to infer atrial arrangement from the abdominal great vessels. Transverse and longitudinal sections of the great vessels just below the diaphragm provide an indirect but accurate indication of atrial arrangement.[7,8]

In usual atrial arrangement, the inferior caval vein is positioned to the right of the spine. The descending aorta is usually to the left but may be close to the midline (Fig. 2). The opposite applies in mirror image arrangement when the inferior caval vein is to the left (Fig. 2). Hence the morphologic right atrium is lateralised to the same side as the inferior caval vein. Hepatic veins join the inferior caval vein just below the diaphragm at its junction with the right atrium (Fig. 3). With right atrial isomerism, both the descending aorta and inferior caval vein are usually to one side of the midline, with the inferior caval vein anterior to the descending aorta (Fig. 4). The inferior caval vein drains into the heart, together with hepatic veins, from below. In left atrial isomerism, the suprarenal portion of the inferior caval vein is usually absent and there is azygos or hemiazygos continuation of the inferior caval vein behind the heart to join either the right or left sided superior caval vein respectively (Fig. 5). The azygos channel lies posterolateral to the descending aorta below the diaphragm. The descending aorta is often in the midline (Fig.

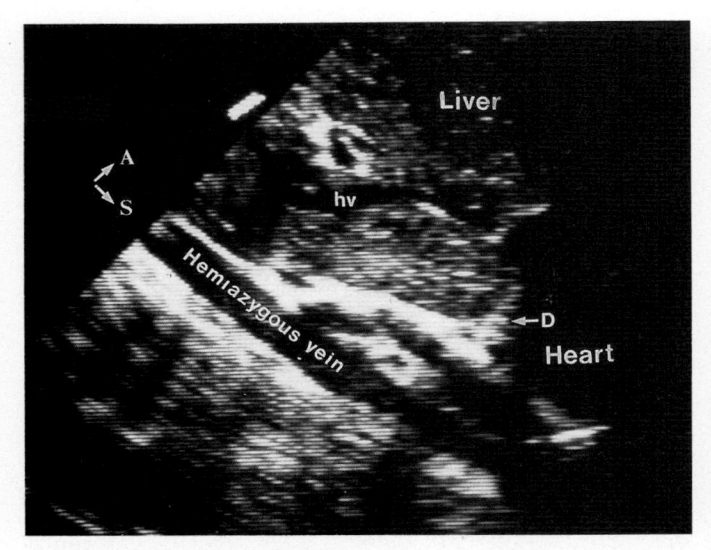

Fig. 5 **Parasagittal subcostal view** in a patient with left isomerism. There is a hemiazygous vein which ascends posterior to the heart to join the left superior caval vein. D – diaphragm, hv – hepatic vein.

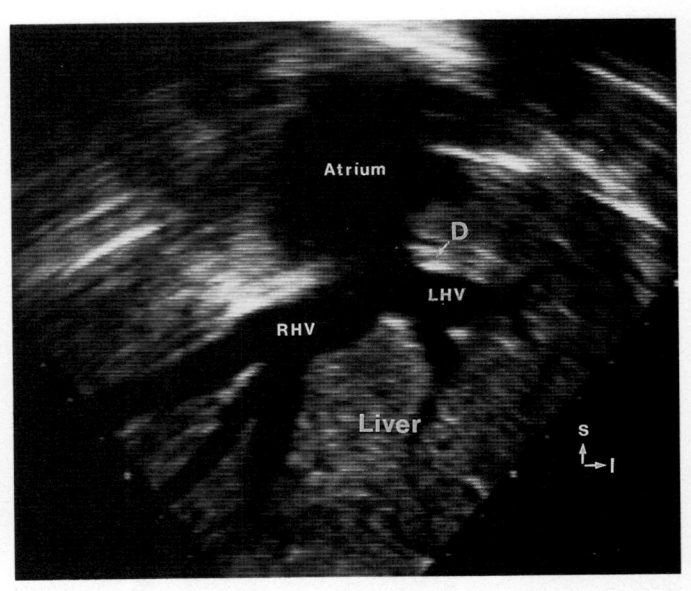

Fig. 7 **Subcostal paracoronal view** in left isomerism demonstrating right and left heptaic veins draining directly to the heart. D – diaphragm, L – left hepatic vein, R – right hepatic vein.

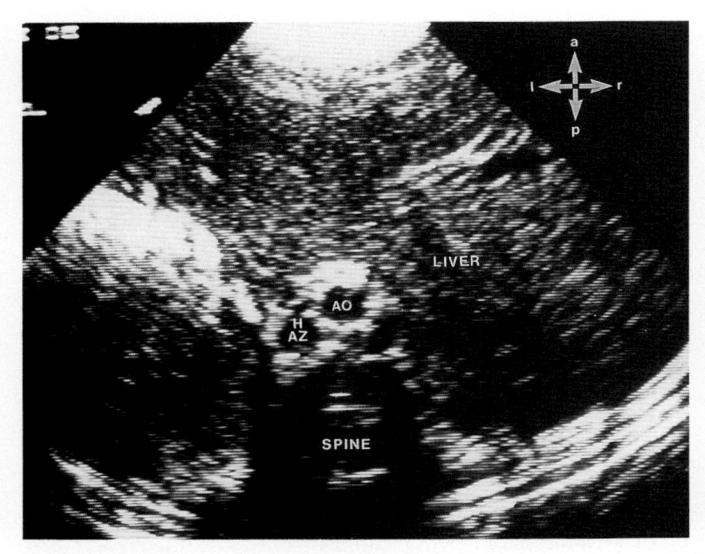

Fig. 6 **Transverse abdominal view** in a patient with left isomerism. The hemiazygos continuation of the inferior caval vein is posteriorly situated. HAZ – hemiazygos vein.

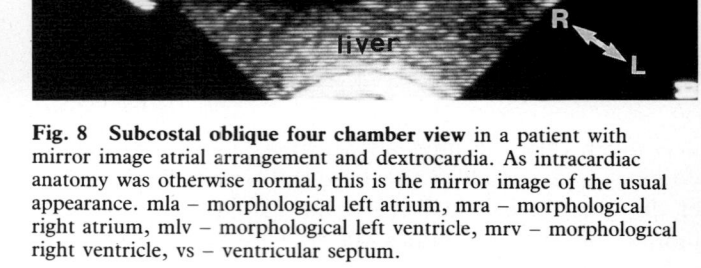

Fig. 8 **Subcostal oblique four chamber view** in a patient with mirror image atrial arrangement and dextrocardia. As intracardiac anatomy was otherwise normal, this is the mirror image of the usual appearance. mla – morphological left atrium, mra – morphological right atrium, mlv – morphological left ventricle, mrv – morphological right ventricle, vs – ventricular septum.

6). The separate drainage of the hepatic veins directly into the heart which occurs in most, but not all, cases of left isomerism[9] can also be demonstrated (Fig. 7). The position of the liver, which is usually a midline structure in isomeric atrial arrangement,[8] should also be noted.

Cardiac position is most easily confirmed from the subcostal position. This is usually levocardia: the cardiac apex to the left. When the heart is in the right chest, or the midline (dextrocardia or mesocardia) this will be readily apparent, as will be the direction of the cardiac apex (Fig. 8). All subsequent transducer positions can be modified according to this information. Hence, the standard echocardiographic approach to the child with suspected congenital heart disease should start with transverse and sagittal abdominal views. Questions from accompanying parents as to the anatomic location of their child's heart are to be expected!

Venous connections

Systemic venous drainage from below the diaphragm has already been described. It is equally important to demonstrate the pattern of superior caval vein drainage. Normally the right internal jugular and innominate veins join to form the right sided superior caval vein. This is readily demonstrated from a suprasternal paracoronal cut (Fig. 9). The innominate vein courses superior to the transverse part of the aortic arch, and passes immediately anterior to the origin of the innominate artery (Fig. 10). A small or absent innominate vein suggests the possible presence of an additional left sided superior caval vein. When this is present it usually drains to the coronary sinus (Fig. 11), but may drain directly to an atrium, especially if there is atrial isomerism (Fig. 12). Conversely, a large innominate vein and right sided superior caval vein suggests high right atrial pressure or excessive venous flow in these vessels. Exceptionally, the innominate vein will pass posterior to the ascending part of the aortic arch so that it is 'retro-aortic' (Fig. 13). Prior knowledge of this unusual anatomy is important surgically if haemorrhage resulting from damage to

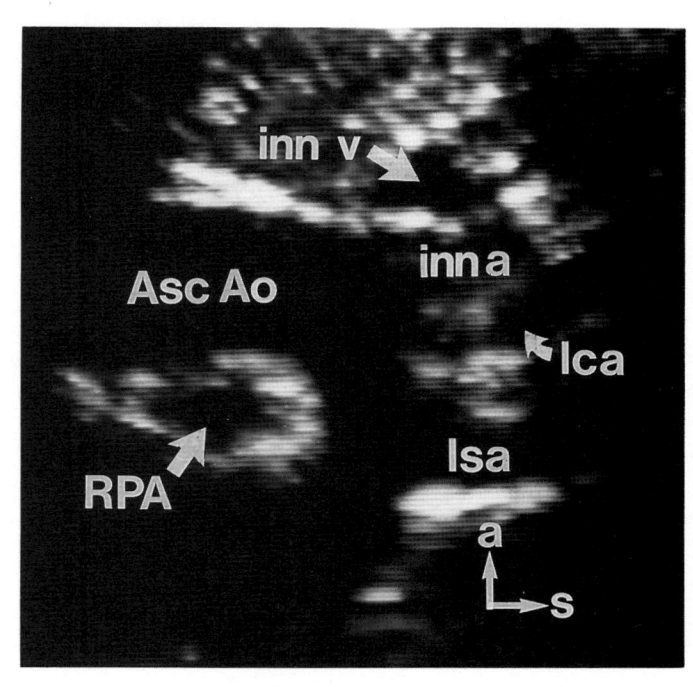

Fig. 10 High parasternal view in the long axis of the aortic arch. The innominate vein passes anterior to the innominate artery. Asc Ao – ascending aorta, inn a – innominate artery, lca – left carotid artery, lsa – left subclavian artery, RPA – right pulmonary artery, inn v – innominate vein.

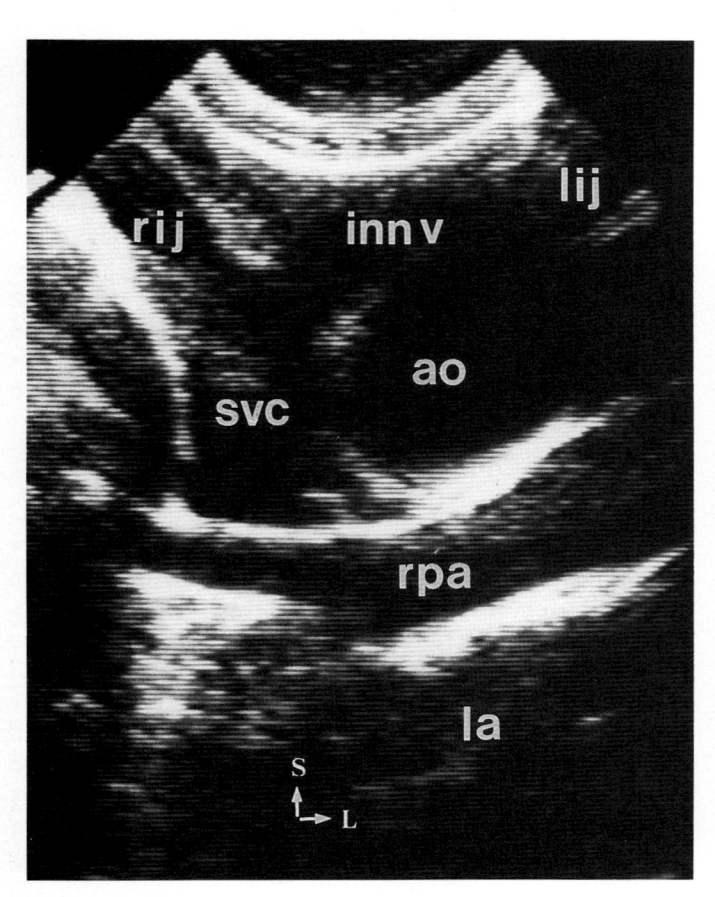

Fig. 9 Normal suprasternal paracoronal view. lij – left internal jugular, rij – right internal jugular, inn v – innominate vein, rpa – right pulmonary artery.

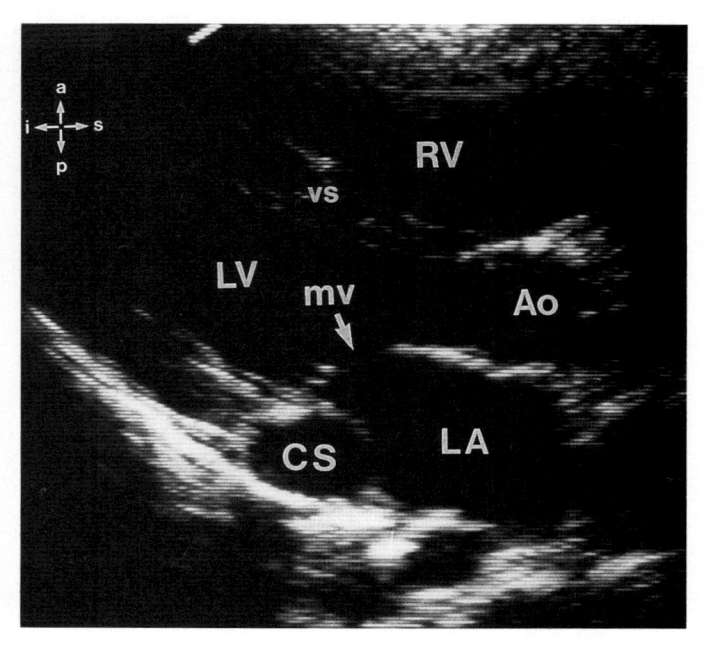

Fig. 11 Parasternal long axis view of a left caval vein showing an enlarged coronary sinus. The left caval vein drains to the coronary sinus as an isolated abnormality. cs – coronary sinus, vs – inter-ventricular septum.

314 CARDIAC ULTRASOUND

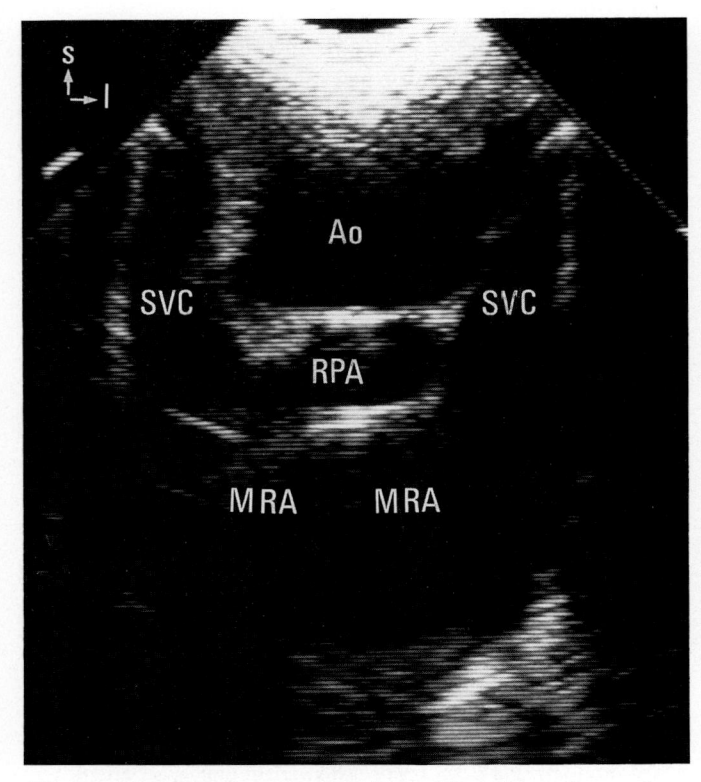

Fig. 12 Suprasternal paracoronal view – bilateral superior caval veins (no bridging vein). Both superior caval veins drain to ipsilateral atria in this patient with right atrial isomerism. MRA – morphological right atrium, RPA – right pulmonary artery.

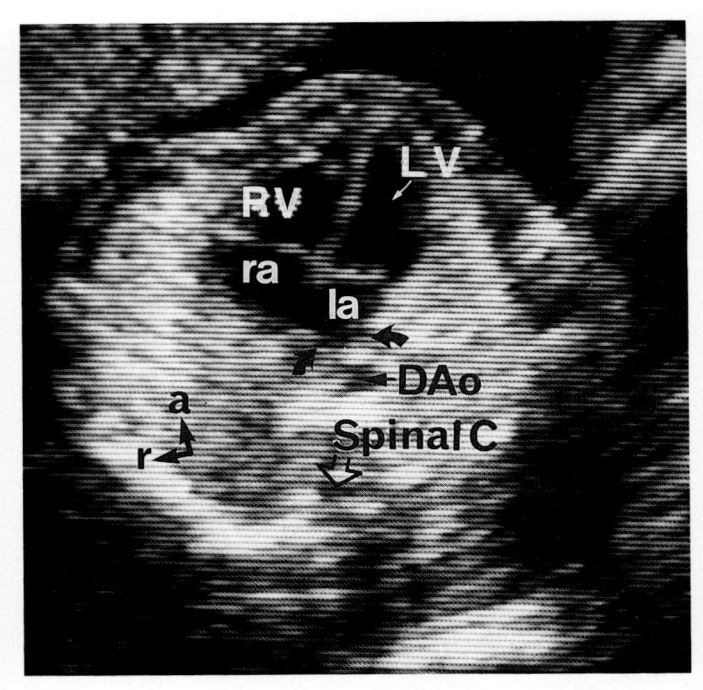

Fig. 14 Transverse thoracic four chamber view – normal fetus. Normal pulmonary veins (curved arrows) are demonstrated passing on either side of the descending aorta to enter left atrium. DAo – descending aorta, Spinal C – spinal canal.

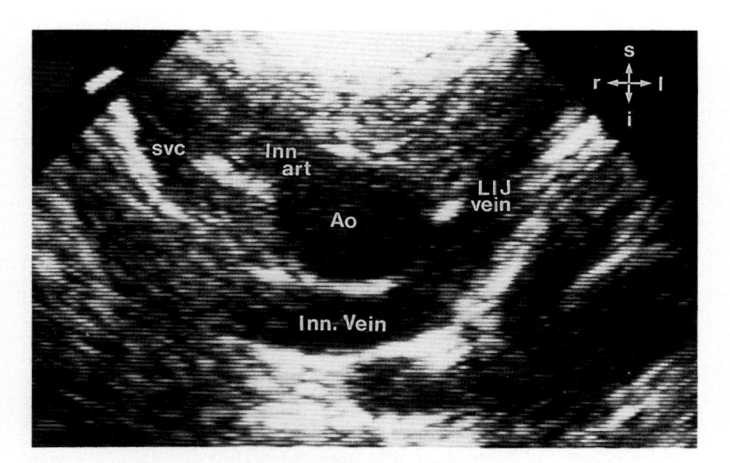

Fig. 13 Suprasternal paracoronal view – retro-aortic innominate vein. Inn art – innominate artery, Inn vein – innominate vein, LIJ – left internal jugular.

the innominate vein is to be avoided during dissection of the great arteries.

The details of systemic venous drainage are crucial with isomeric atrial arrangements, as the nature of the associated intracardiac abnormalities means that definitive surgery may only be possible with sophisticated modifications of the Fontan operation.[10,11] Classification of these hearts as 'polysplenia' or 'asplenia'[11] gives no information about the specific venous connections and this terminology is probably better avoided. Bilateral superior caval veins are common in many structural heart abnormalities in addition to those which include atrial isomerism. Knowledge of this is important for venous cannulation technique in all such hearts requiring cardiopulmonary by-pass surgery.

Normal pulmonary veins pass on either side of the descending aorta to enter the back of the left atrium (Fig. 14). Each of the four pulmonary veins usually enters the left atrium separately, but ipsilateral pulmonary veins may join at their junction with the left atrium. While flow into the left atrium from the right and left pulmonary veins respectively can be confirmed by Doppler interrogation from a subcostal or apical position, separate identification of each of the four pulmonary veins may be difficult. The right upper and left lower pulmonary veins may be imaged from the subcostal position (Fig. 15), while the connection of each pulmonary vein to the left atrium can be often visualised from the suprasternal position (Fig. 16). Identification of pulmonary veins may be facilitated by conventional pulsed or colour flow Doppler imaging. Partial or total anomalous venous connection must be suspected if normal pulmonary veins cannot be identified.

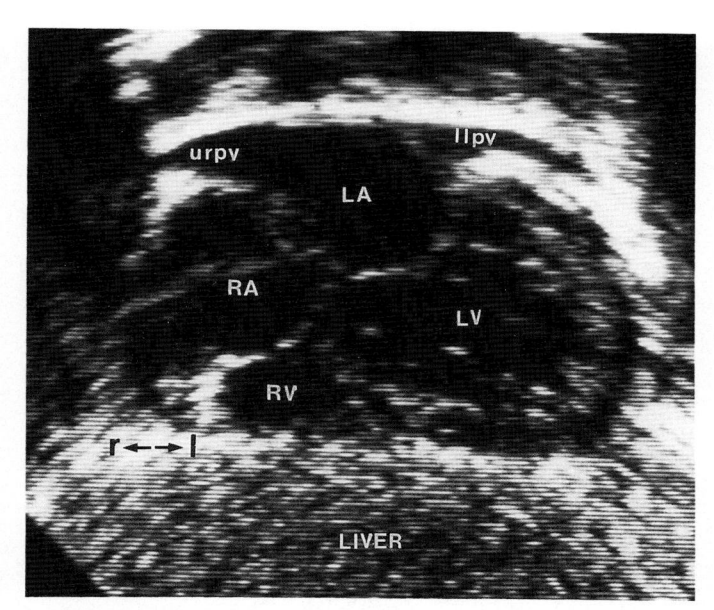

Fig. 15 **Subcostal oblique four chamber view** showing upper right and left lower pulmonary veins draining to left atrium. llpv – lower left pulmonary vein, urpv – upper right pulmonary vein.

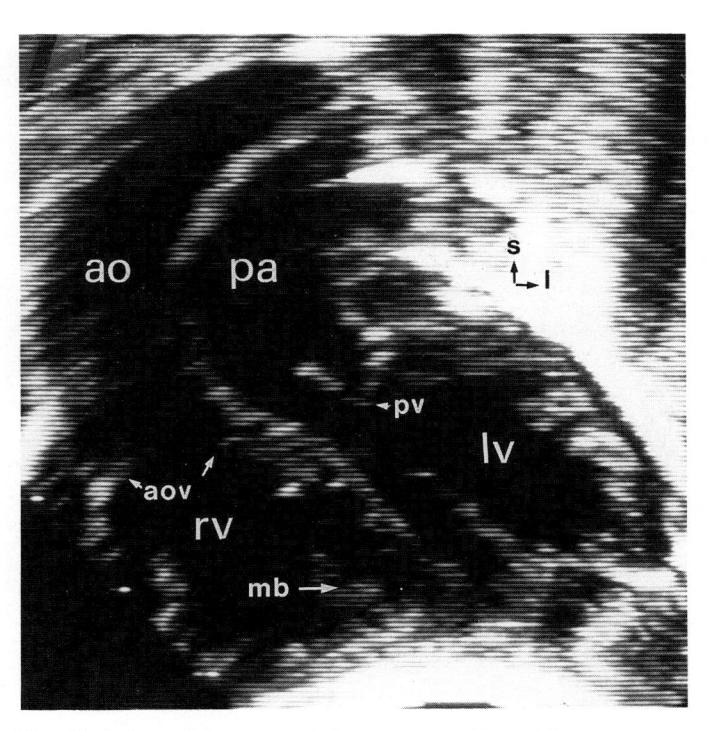

Fig. 17 **Subcostal paracoronal view** – transposition of the great arteries. The distinctive moderator band is demonstrated at the apex of the right ventricle in a patient who has transposition of the great arteries. aov – aortic valve, mb – moderator band.

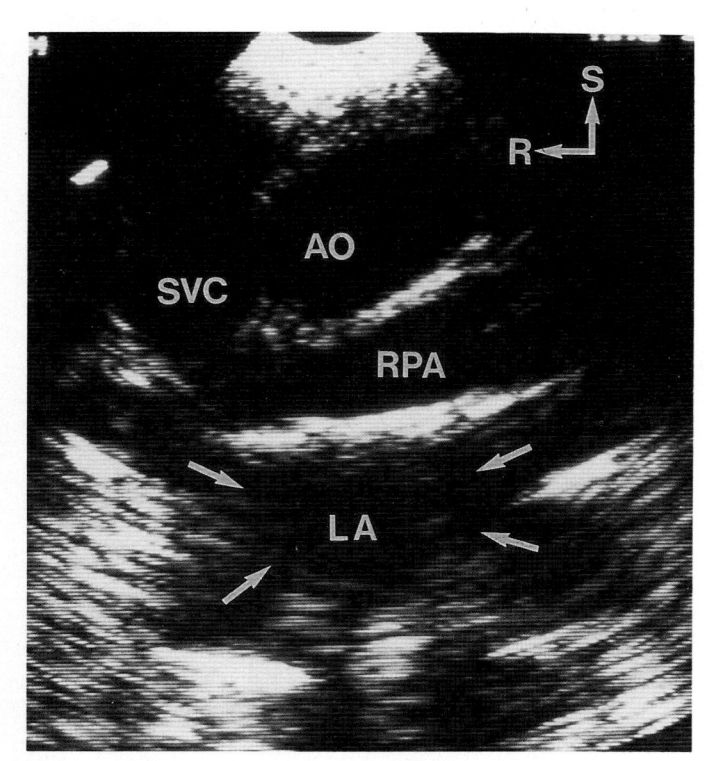

Fig. 16 **Suprasternal paracoronal view** showing normal pulmonary veins (arrows) connecting to left atrium. RPA – right pulmonary artery.

Atrioventricular connection

Echocardiographic assessment of atrioventricular connection depends on the recognition of atrial and ventricular morphology. Atrial arrangement has been discussed above. Right ventricular morphology is usually recognised by a) the coarse apical and septal trabecular pattern, especially the distinctive moderator band near the apex (Figs 14 and 17); b) features which distinguish the morphology of the tricuspid valve from that of the mitral valve, the septal origin of the normal tricuspid valve being slightly more apically positioned than that of the mitral valve (Figs 14 and 18); and c) part of the tricuspid valve tension apparatus is attached to the ventricular septum, whilst the mitral valve chordae are not attached to the septum but are anchored by anterolateral and posteromedial papillary muscles attached to the free wall of the ventricle (Fig. 19). It is an exaggeration of the apical displacement of the attachments of the septal and mural leaflets of the tricuspid valve which makes severe examples of Ebstein's anomaly of the tricuspid valve easy to recognise (Fig. 20).

The normal connection of morphological right atrium to morphological right ventricle, and morphological left atrium to morphological left ventricle results in atrioventricular concordance (Fig. 18, left). The connection is discordant if right atrium connects to morphological left ventricle and left atrium to morphological right ventricle (Fig. 18, right). The connection is ambiguous if isomeric atria are each connected to a ventricle, because, in this situation, one half of the atrioventricular connection is 'concordant' and the other half 'discordant'. When the

316 CARDIAC ULTRASOUND

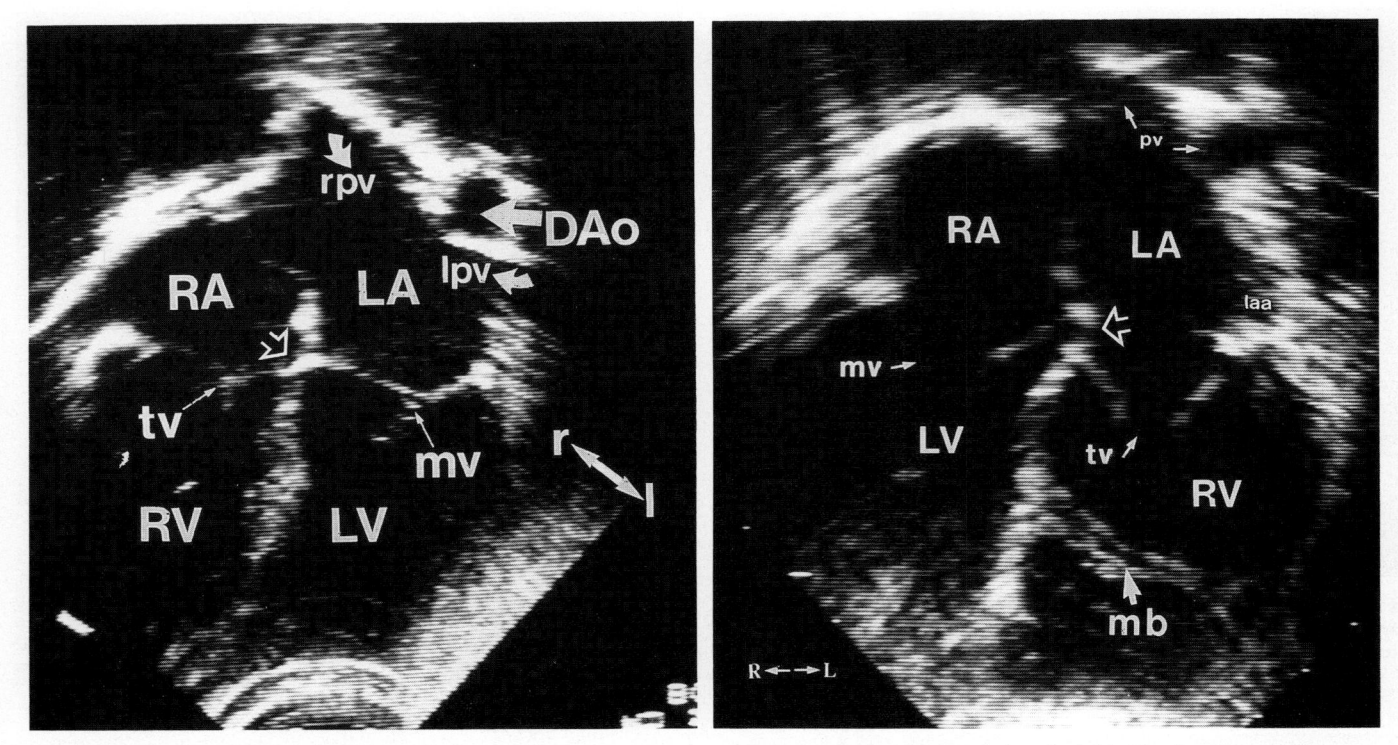

Fig. 18 **Apical four chamber view. Left:** Atrioventricular concordance. Note that the septal origin of the tricuspid valve is more apically positioned than that of the mitral valve. **Right:** Atrioventricular discordance. Note the 'reverse off-setting' of the atrioventricular valves, and the moderator band in the left sided ventricle, which in this situation is a morphological right ventricle. The open arrow indicates the muscular atrioventricular septum. mb – moderator band, rpv – right pulmonary vein, lpv – left pulmonary vein, DAo – descending aorta, laa – left atrial appendage, pv – pulmonary vein.

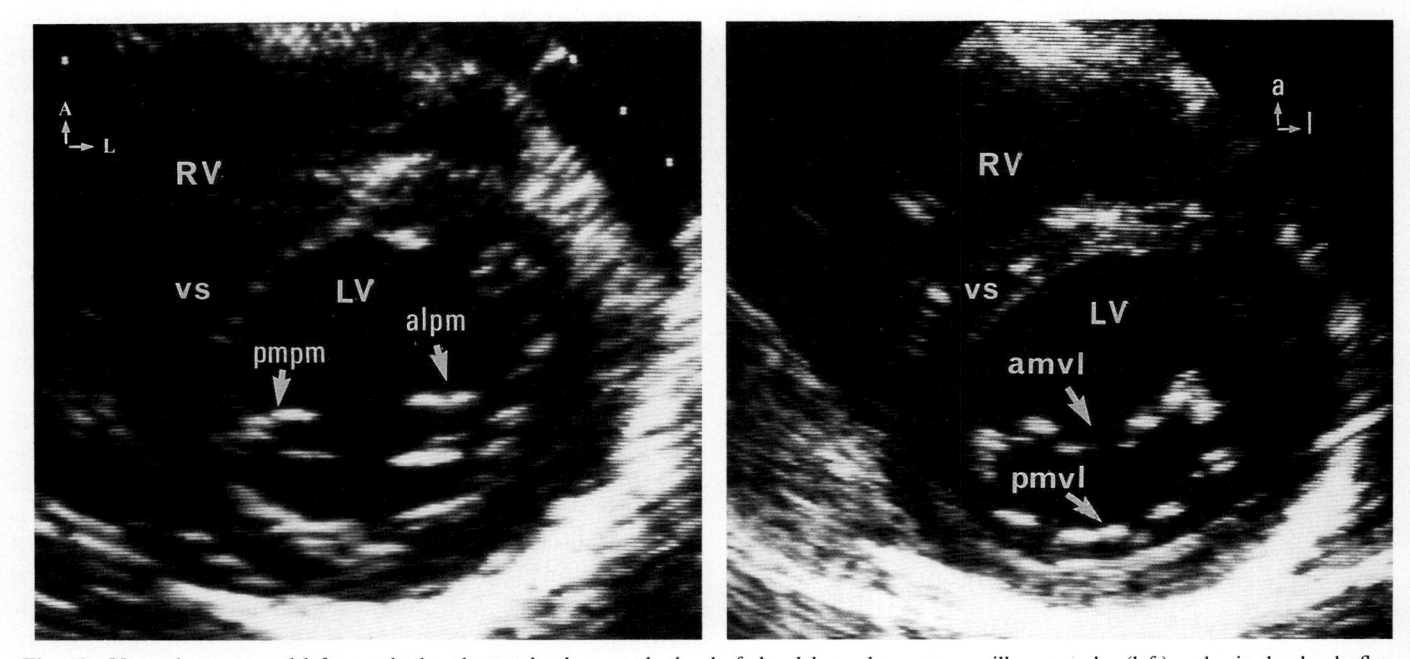

Fig. 19 **Normal parasternal left ventricular short axis views** at the level of chordal attachment to papillary muscles (left) and mitral valve leaflets (right). alpm – anterolateral papillary muscle, amvl – anterior mitral valve leaflet, pmpm – posteromedial papillary muscle, pmvl – posterior mitral valve leaflet, vs – inter-ventricular septum.

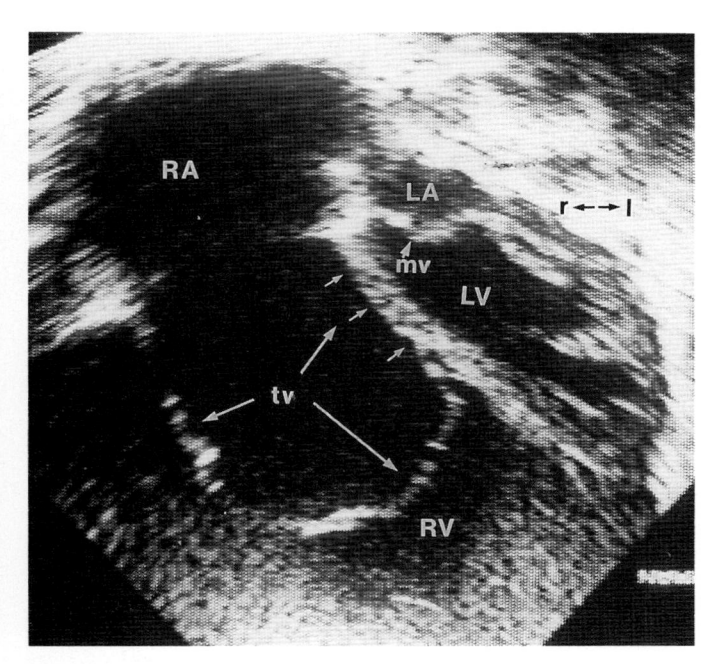

Fig. 20 Apical view – **Ebstein's anomaly** of the tricuspid valve, showing gross apical displacement of the attachment of the septal leaflet of the tricuspid valve (small arrows).

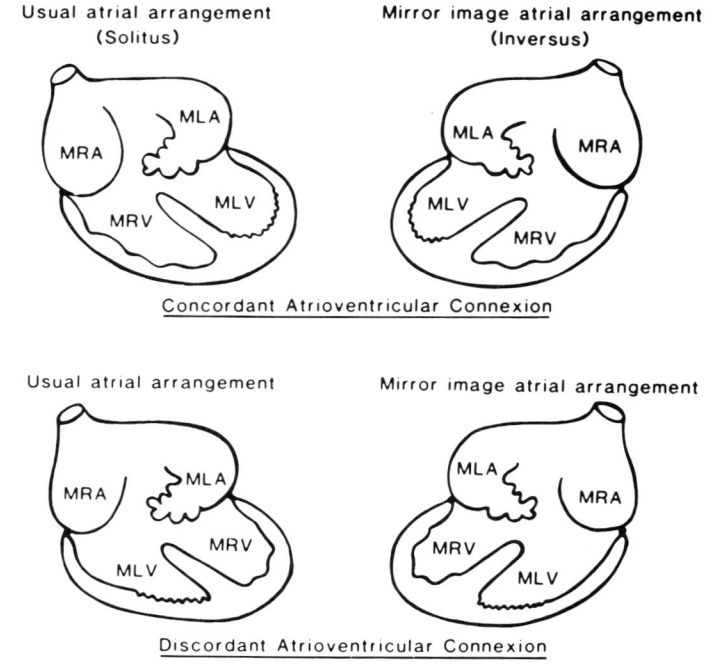

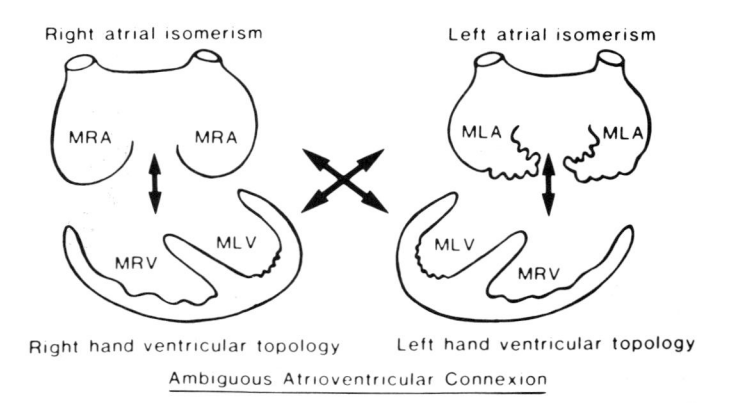

Fig. 21 Types of biventricular atrioventricular connection (reproduced with permission from Reference 1). M – morphological, R – right, L – left, A – atrium, V – ventricle.

atrioventricular connection is ambiguous, ventricular topology or looping, which describes the manner in which the right ventricle is wrapped around the left ventricle, must be considered (Fig. 21). This may be ascertained by the imaginary placement of the palm of the observer's hand against the septal surface of the morphological right ventricle, with the thumb positioned in the inlet portion of the ventricle and the fingers in the outlet as described by Van Praagh.[12] In the normal heart, the right hand can be so positioned, indicating a right hand pattern of ventricular topology or D-looping (Fig. 18, left). There is a left hand pattern when it is the left hand which can be positioned in this way with respect to the morphological right ventricle, giving rise to L-looping. This occurs, for example, in hearts with usual atrial arrangement and atrioventricular discordance (Fig. 18, right).

When the atria are connected to only one ventricle, there is a univentricular atrioventricular connection (Fig. 22). If both atria connect to one ventricle there are usually two atrioventricular valves (Fig. 23), although sometimes a common atrioventricular orifice drains both atria (Fig. 24). Alternatively, either the right or left atrioventricular connection may be absent, giving rise to 'tricuspid atresia' or 'mitral atresia' respectively (Fig. 25).

When there is a univentricular atrioventricular connection, ventricular morphology can usually be deduced from chamber position. An anterior ventricle will be a morphological right ventricle and a posterior ventricle a morphological left ventricle, no matter whether it is the main ventricle or a rudimentary ventricle. If only a single ventricle can be identified, it may be of indeterminate morphology (Fig. 22).

An apical transducer position is sufficient to identify a normal atrioventricular connection. However, analysis of the atrioventricular connection in other circumstances will require a series of 'sweeps' from subcostal and precordial positions.

Ventriculo-arterial connection

The usual connection of morphological left ventricle to aorta and morphological right ventricle to pulmonary artery

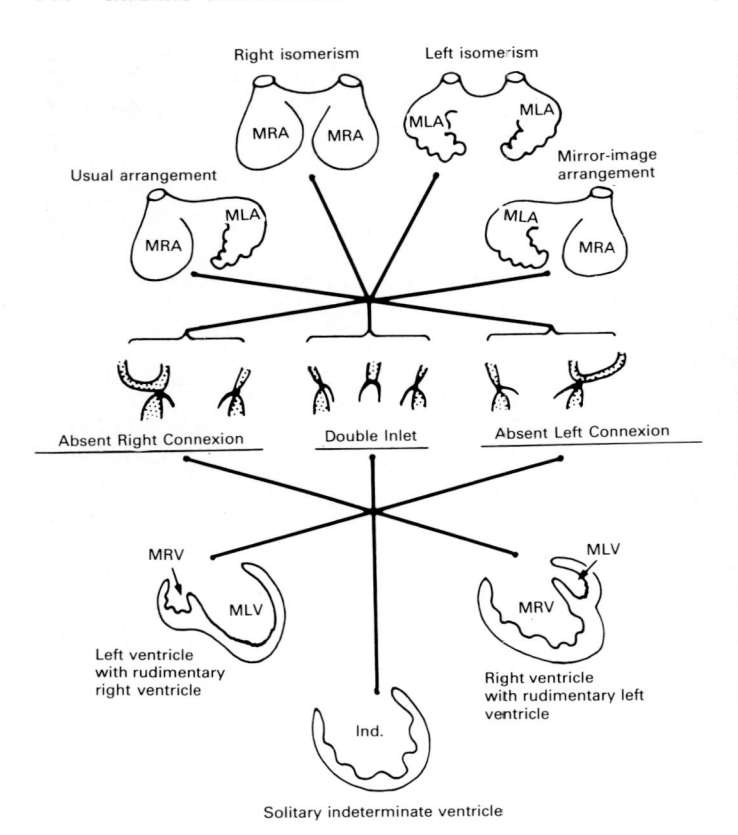

Fig. 22 Types of univentricular atrioventricular connection (reproduced with permission from Reference 1). M – morphological, R — right, L – left, A – atrium, V – ventricle.

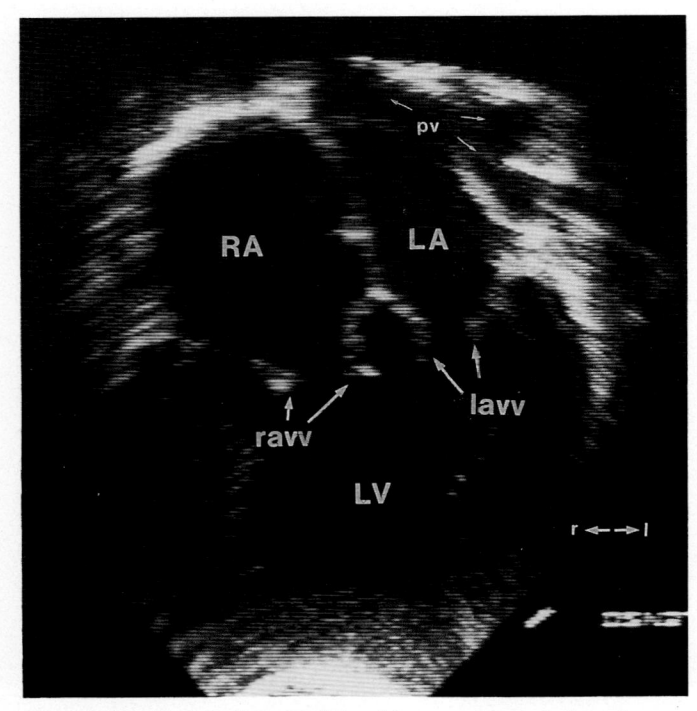

Fig. 23 Double inlet left ventricle with two atrioventricular valves. Apical view in diastole. ravv – right atrioventricular valve, lavv – left atrioventricular valve, pv – pulmonary veins.

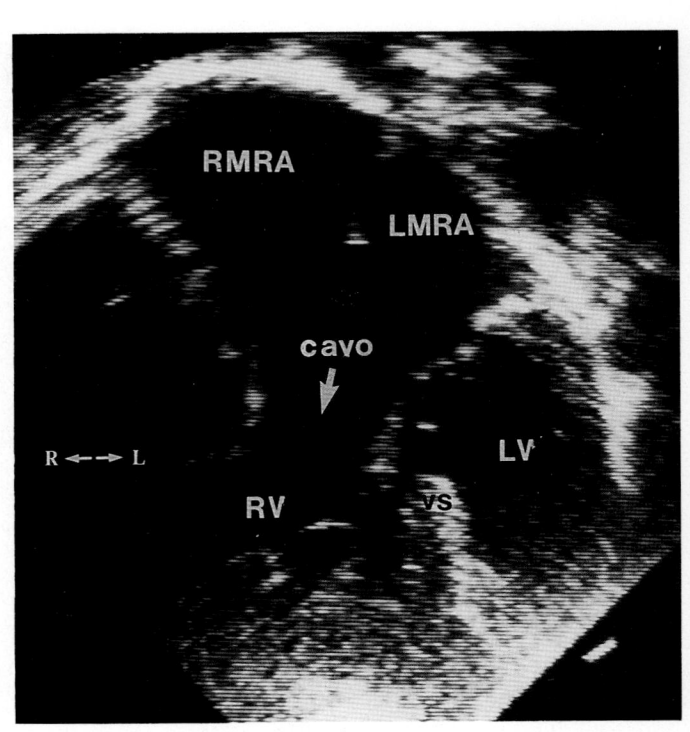

Fig. 24 Double inlet right ventricle. Apical view in diastole demonstrating a common atrioventricular orifice in a patient with right atrial isomerism. Note the malalignment between the atrial septum and ventricular septum. RMRA – right sided morphological right atrium, LMRA – left sided morphological right atrium, cavo – common atrioventricular orifice, vs – inter-ventricular septum.

results in ventriculo-arterial concordance. The other possible types of ventriculo-arterial connection are ventriculo-arterial discordance (transposition of the great arteries), double outlet ventricle or single outlet from the heart. The great arteries are normally distinguished by early branching of the pulmonary trunk, and the origins of the head and arm vessels from the aorta (Fig. 26).

The normal concordant ventriculo-arterial connection is characterised by a more cephalad position of the pulmonary valve compared to the aortic valve and 'cross-over' of the proximal great arteries which gives rise to the normal short axis appearance (Fig. 27). The more cephalad position of the pulmonary valve results from the presence of the 'septal' aspect of the subpulmonary infundibulum.[13]

Complete transposition of the great arteries is characterised by a more or less parallel course of the proximal great arteries (Fig. 17). Double outlet right ventricle (DORV) is a convenient term for the heterogeneous group of hearts which have both great arteries largely or completely arising from the morphological right ventricle. These hearts are usually subdivided on the basis of the location of the ventricular septal defect (VSD) in relation to the great arteries.[14] When one or other arterial valve overrides the trabecular part of the ventricular septum, the

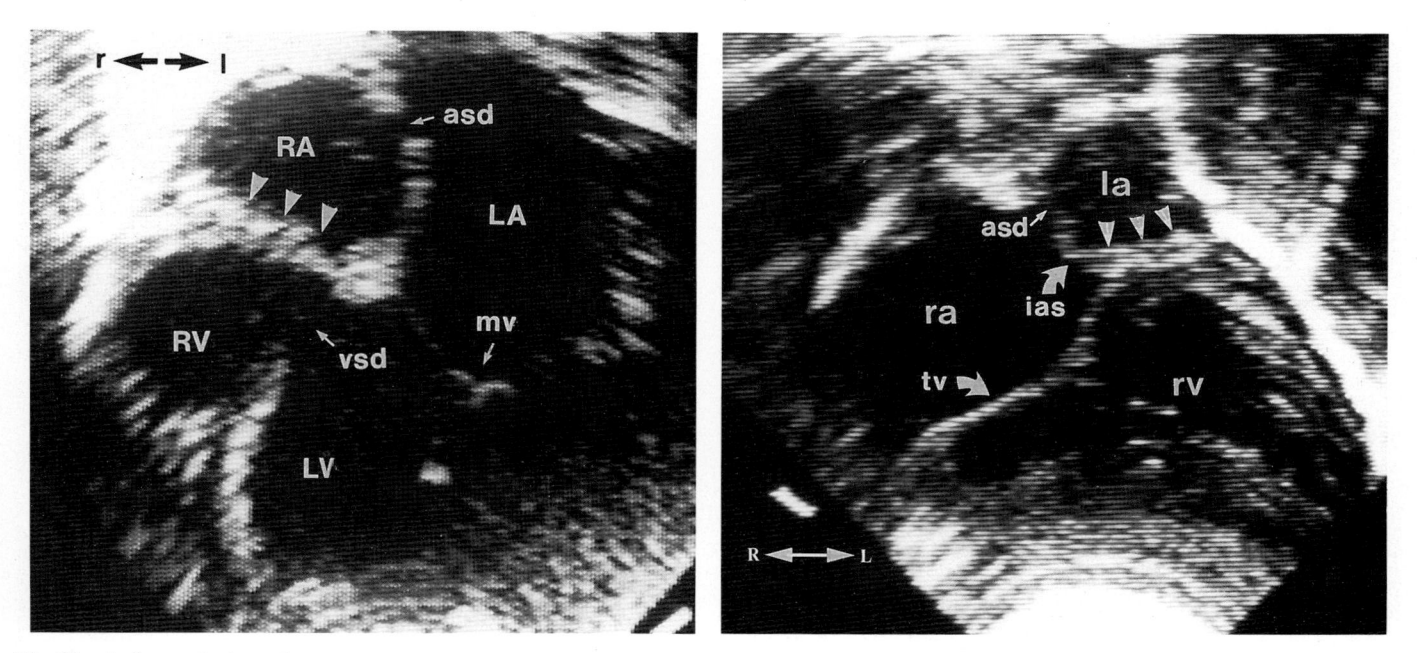

Fig. 25 **Atrioventricular valve atresias. Left:** Apical view showing absent right atrioventricular connection (arrowheads), with left atrioventricular valve to left ventricle (tricuspid atresia). **Right:** Subcostal oblique view demonstrating absent left atrioventricular connection (arrowheads) with right atrioventricular valve to right ventricle (mitral atresia). asd – atrial septal defect, ias – interatrial septum, tv – tricuspid valve, vsd – ventricular septal defect.

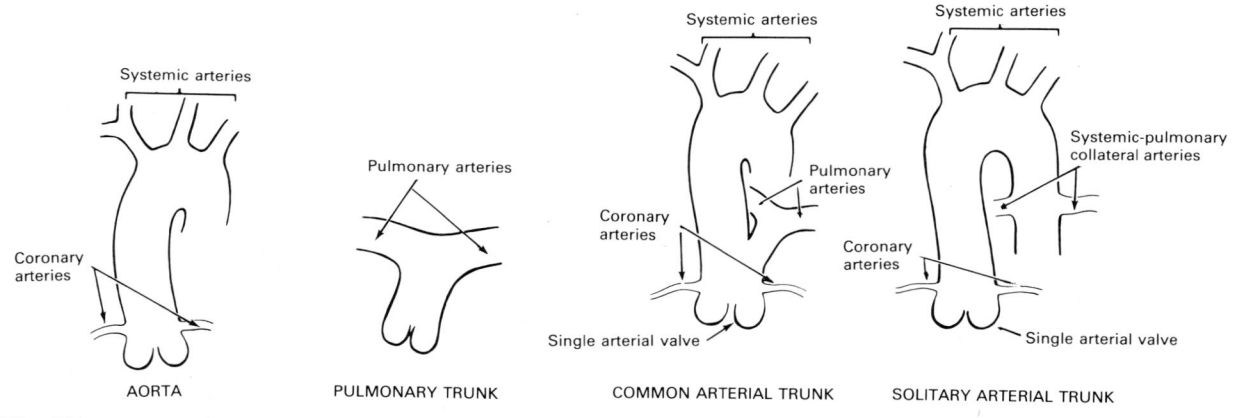

Fig. 26 **The different types of great arteries.** Reproduced with permission from reference 1.

appropriate great artery is deemed to connect to whichever ventricle it 'overrides' by more than 50%. This should be assessed from the parasternal long axis plane and not from a subcostal or apical position. Consequently, tetralogy of Fallot with more than 50% of the aortic diameter overriding the right ventricle is classified as DORV with a subaortic VSD (Fig. 28). The degree of pulmonary valve 'override' will determine whether a heart with an anterior aorta and a subpulmonary VSD should be classified as ventriculo-arterial discordance or DORV with a subpulmonary VSD (Taussig Bing anomaly) (Fig. 29). In other cases of DORV, the VSD may be at a distance from both great arteries, in which case it is non-committed. Double outlet left ventricle is very rare (Fig. 30).

A single outlet from the heart may be a common arterial trunk (truncus arteriosus), or a solitary arterial trunk which occurs in some cases of pulmonary atresia with VSD (Fig. 26). A common arterial trunk almost invariably overrides the ventricular septum. The pulmonary arteries can be identified arising from the left posterior aspect of the common trunk (Fig. 31) although the branching pattern can vary. The truncal valve is often dysplastic and regurgitant (Fig. 32). Pulmonary atresia with VSD is characterised by an atretic right ventricular outflow tract, and may be

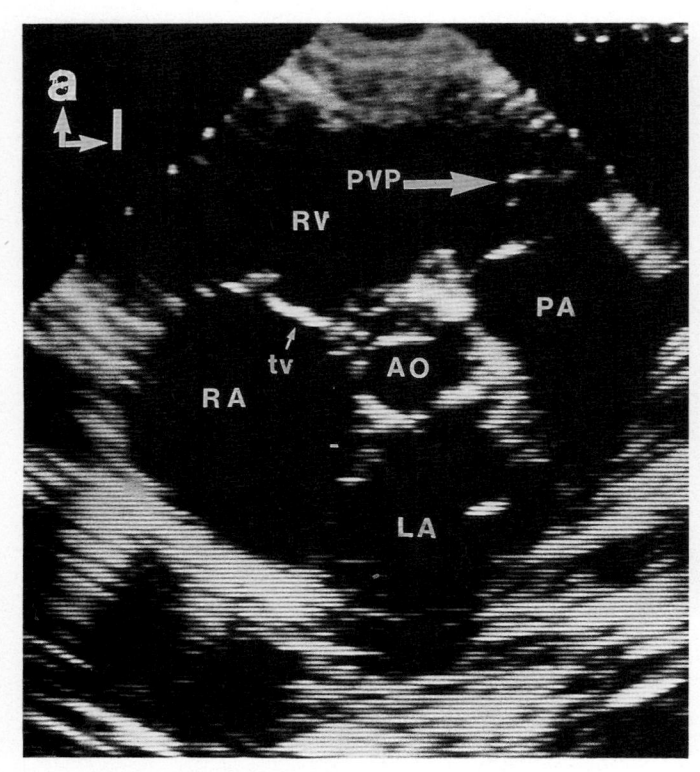

Fig. 27 Normal parasternal short axis – great arteries. The right ventricular outflow tract and pulmonary trunk 'cross over' the proximal ascending aorta. PVP – prolapsing pulmonary valve cusp.

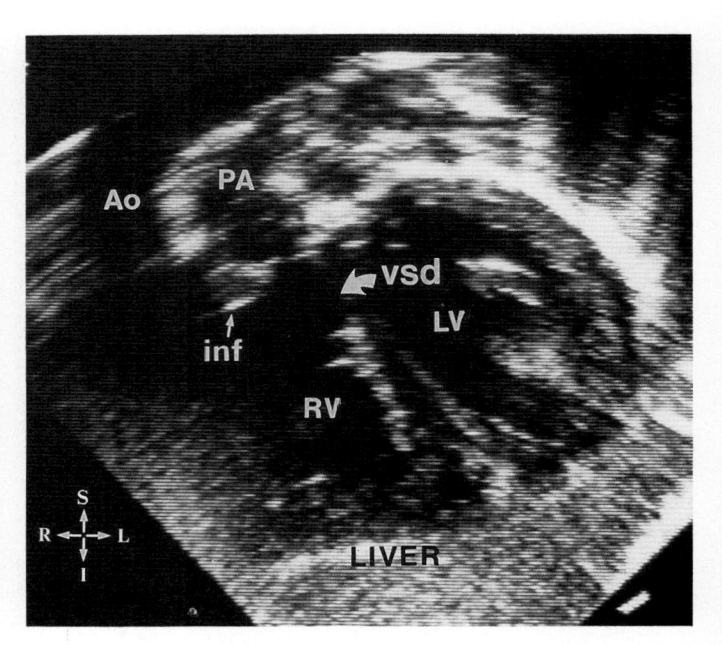

Fig. 29 Subcostal paracoronal view – double outlet right ventricle and subpulmonary VSD. Parasternal long axis views in the same patient confirmed that the pulmonary artery had more than 50% of its diameter committed to right ventricle. Note the infundibular muscle separating the roots of the aorta and pulmonary trunk. inf – infundibular muscle, vsd – ventricular septal defect.

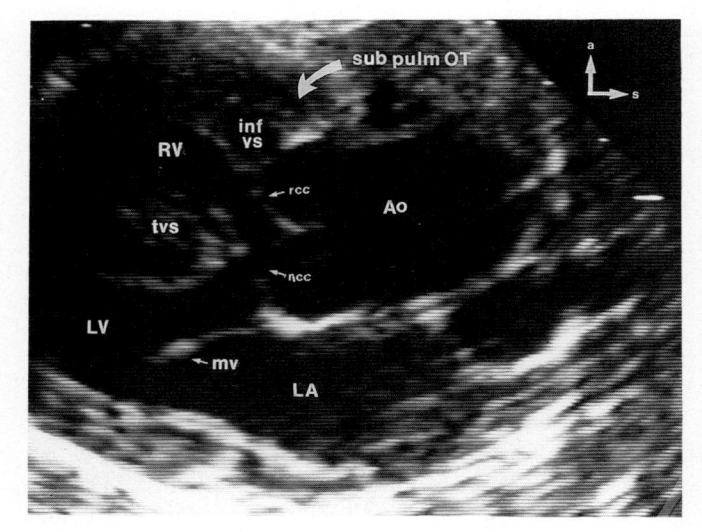

Fig. 28 Parasternal long axis – tetralogy of Fallot. There is a subaortic VSD. The aorta overrides the trabecular septum by slightly more than 50% so, strictly speaking, the ventriculo-arterial connection is double outlet right ventricle. There is anterocephalad deviation of the infundibular septum resulting in obstruction to pulmonary flow. inf vs – infundibular septum, sub pulm OT – subpulmonary outflow tract, tvs – trabecular ventricular septum, ncc – non-coronary aortic cusp, rcc – right coronary aortic cusp.

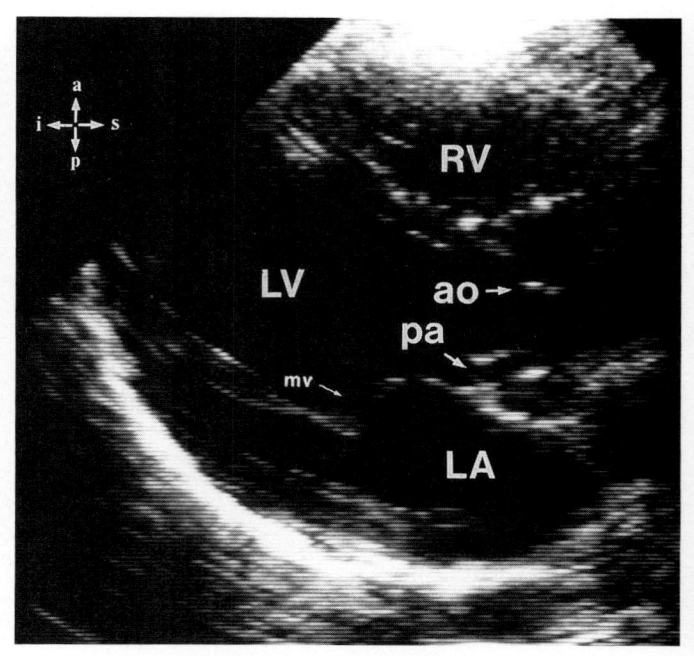

Fig. 30 Modified parasternal long axis – double outlet left ventricle. The aorta is anterior to the pulmonary trunk in this very rare anomaly. There is subvalvar and valvar pulmonary stenosis. The VSD also present is not shown in this plane.

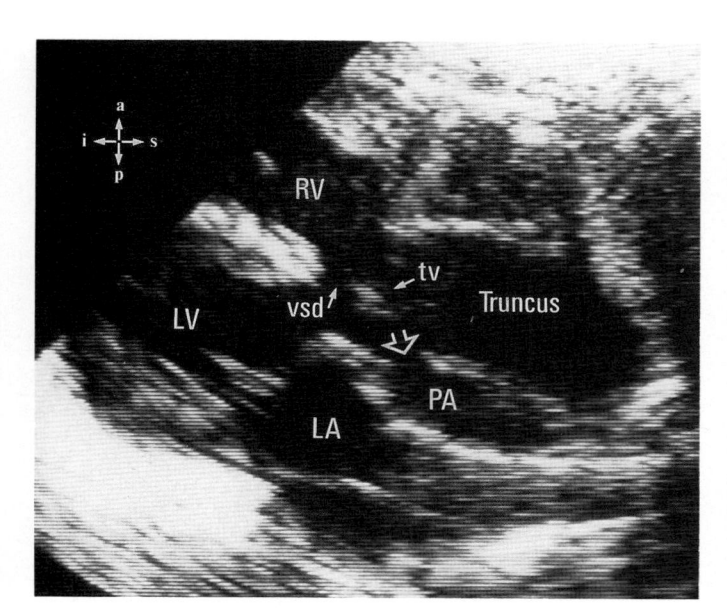

Fig. 31 Parasternal long axis view – common arterial trunk. The arterial trunk overrides the ventricular septum. The pulmonary arteries share a common origin from the posterior and left aspect of the common trunk (open arrow). vsd – ventricular septal defect, tv – truncal valve.

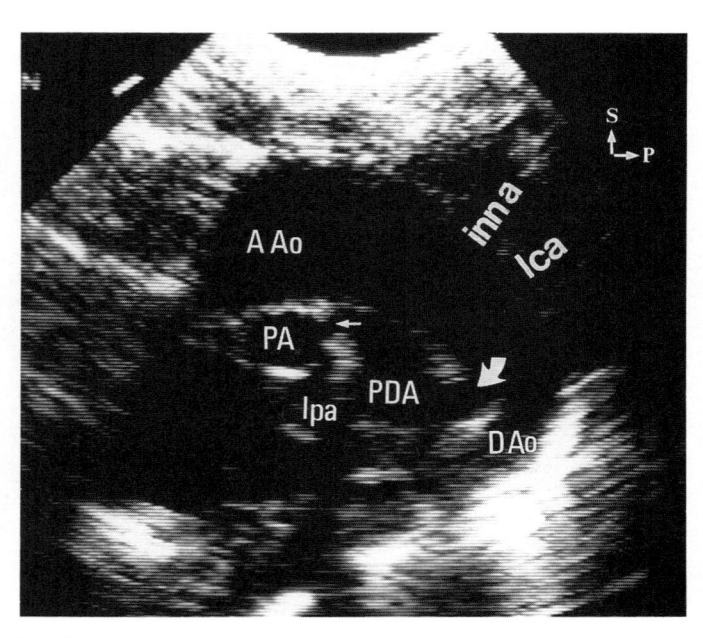

Fig. 33 Suprasternal oblique view – tortuous arterial duct with a vertical origin from the aorta (big arrow) supplying hypoplastic central pulmonary arteries. The duct inserts at the origin of the left pulmonary artery (small arrow). AAo – ascending aorta, DAo – descending aorta, PDA – persistent arterial duct, lpa – left pulmonary artery, inn a – innominate artery, lca – left carotid artery.

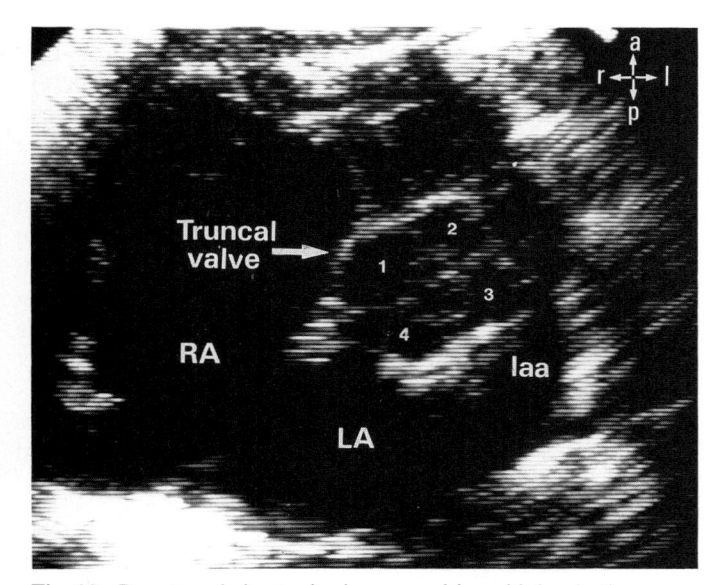

Fig. 32 Parasternal short axis view – quadricuspid dysplastic truncal valve in a patient with common arterial trunk. laa – left atrial appendage.

thought of as the extreme form of tetralogy of Fallot. Central pulmonary arteries, when present, are perfused by an arterial duct or major aortopulmonary collateral arteries. The central pulmonary arteries may be extremely hypoplastic (Fig. 33), or even completely absent. In the latter situation, there is a solitary arterial trunk (Fig. 26) which, like a common trunk, almost invariably overrides the ventricular septum. Demonstration of an atretic right ventricular outflow tract is possible in pulmonary atresia with VSD, whereas there is no right ventricular outflow tract in hearts with a common arterial trunk (compare Figs 28 and 31).

The cardiac chambers

Fundamental to cross-sectional echocardiography in congenital heart disease is recognition of the expected relative dimensions of cardiac chambers and great vessels, as well as haemodynamic inferences obtained from the motion of cardiac structures. It is important to bear in mind that normal appearances will evolve from prenatal to neonatal to later post-natal life. Alterations from normal provide a marker for the disturbed flow characteristic of various structural defects. A simple example is the right heart volume overload which occurs because of left to right shunting via an atrial septal defect. This is characterised by enlargement of the right heart cavities (Fig. 34) and 'paradoxical' motion of the ventricular septum because of the excessive volume of blood entering the right ventricular cavity during diastole. Conversely, if the atrial septum bulges into the left atrium, it can be inferred that right atrial pressure exceeds that in the left atrium and any shunting at atrial level will be from right to left (Figs 25, left and 35). When left ventricular volume overload is apparent in childhood,

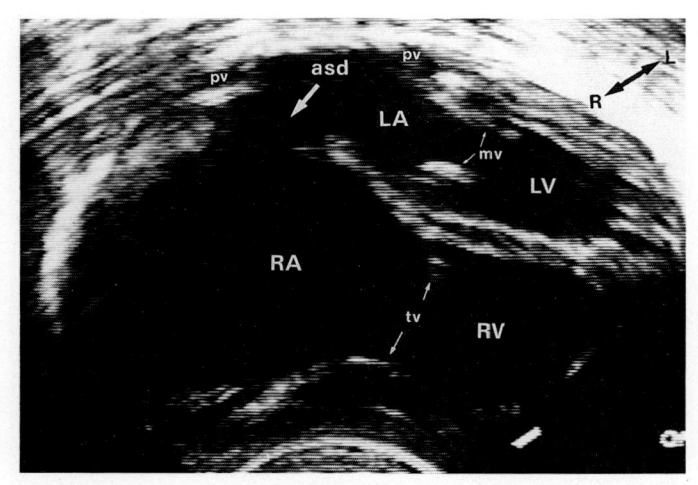

Fig. 34 Subcostal oblique four chamber view – secundum atrial septal defect with marked enlargement of right atrium and right ventricle. pv – pulmonary vein, asd – atrial septal defect.

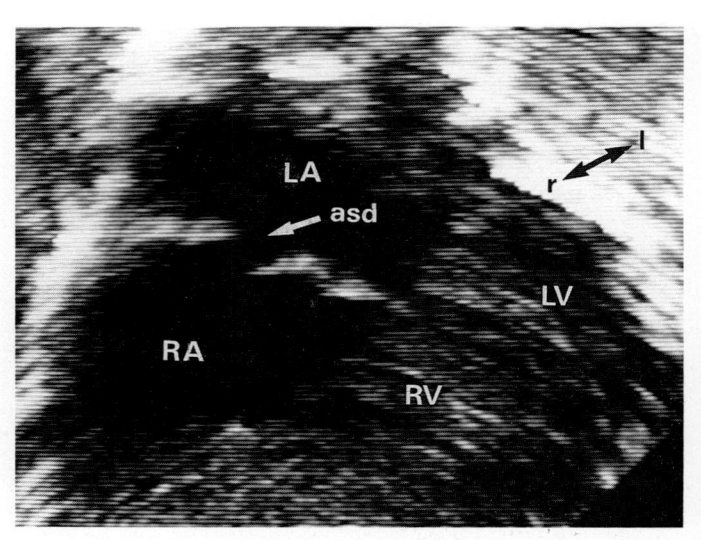

Fig. 36 Subcostal oblique view – secundum atrial septal defect. The surface of the atrial septum is perpendicular to the axial plane of the ultrasound beam to demonstrate a secundum atrial septal defect. asd – atrial septal defect.

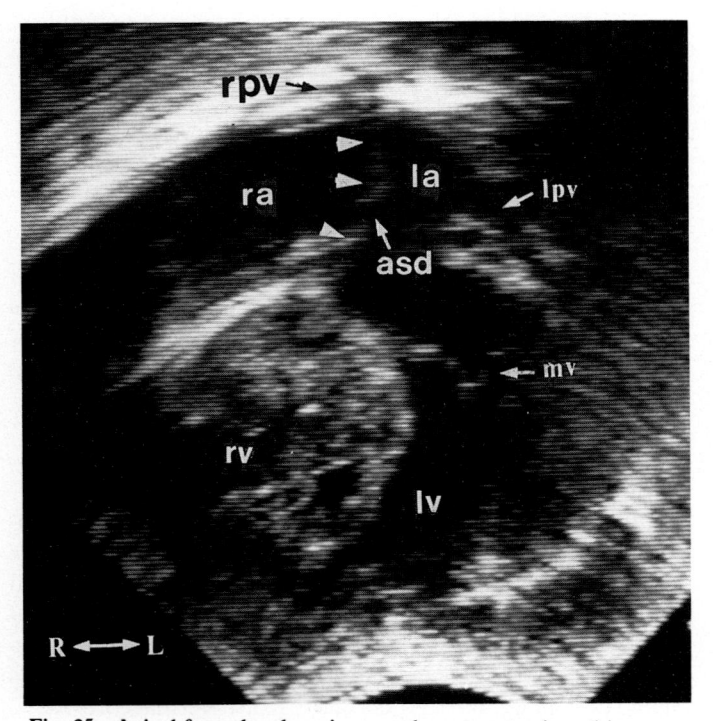

Fig. 35 Apical four chamber view – pulmonary atresia and intact ventricular septum. The interatrial septum (arrowheads) bulges into the left atrium because of obligatory flow from right atrium to left atrium via the atrial septal defect. Note the tiny right ventricular cavity with massive myocardial hypertrophy. asd – atrial septal defect, rpv – right pulmonary vein, lpv – left pulmonary vein.

Atrial septum

In the normal heart, the left atrium is posterior and to the left of the right atrium. Hence, the atrial septum is obliquely orientated. As a result, the most common interatrial communication, a hole at the foramen ovale (secundum atrial septal defect), is best assessed from a subcostal position (Fig. 36), because the surface of the atrial septum then lies more or less perpendicular to the axial plane of the ultrasound beam. From an apical view, the atrial septum is more or less in the axial plane of the ultrasound beam and 'drop out' from the region of the foramen ovale, which is the thinnest part of the atrial septum, may be misleading unless 'T' artefacts are evident at the margins of the hole (Fig. 37). The so-called sinus venosus atrial septal defect is an interatrial communication which occurs at the junction of the superior caval vein and the heart. This is also recognised from the subcostal position. The superior caval vein appears to override the atrial septum (Fig. 38).

Atrioventricular septum

The atrioventricular septum may be thought of as the region where the atrial septum and ventricular septum 'overlap', and it effectively separates the left ventricle from the right atrium.[2] There are two components. Posteriorly (or caudad), a muscular portion lies between the septal attachments of the mitral valve and a more apically positioned septal attachment of the tricuspid valve (Figs 18, left and 39A). Immediately anterior (or cephalad) to this, a fibrous (or membranous) portion of the atrioventricular septum separates the subaortic outflow tract of the left ventricle from the right atrium (Fig. 39B).

the most likely causes are left to right shunting via a VSD or a persistent arterial duct, followed by a long list of increasingly rare lesions. Consequently, the most likely structural defect is often apparent as soon as the heart is imaged.

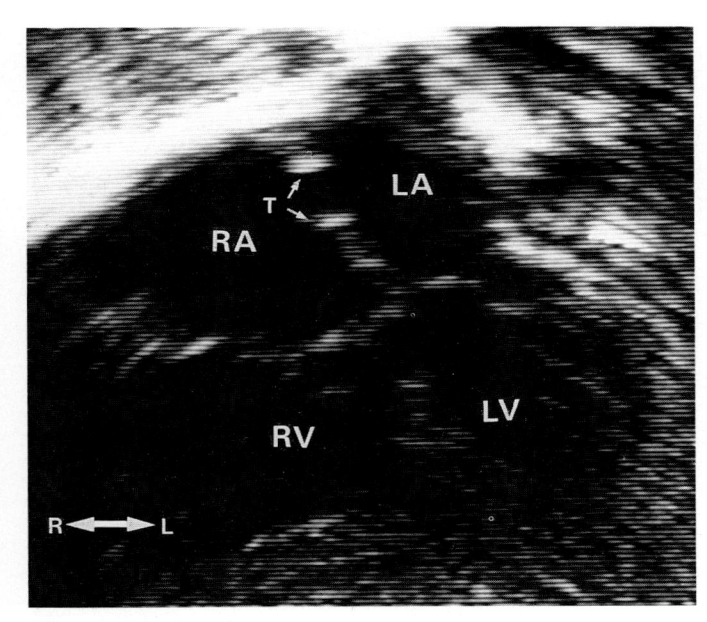

Fig. 37 Apical four chamber view – 'T' artefacts (T) at the margins of a secundum atrial septal defect.

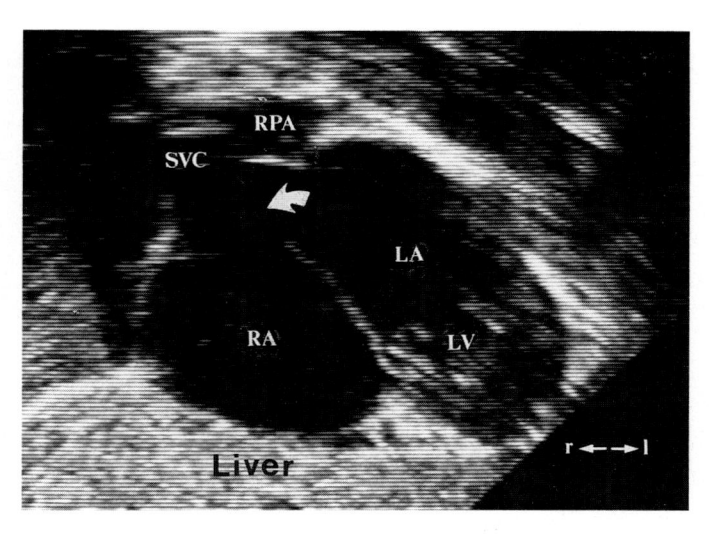

Fig. 38 Subcostal oblique view – so-called 'sinus venosus atrial septal defect' (arrow). Note that the superior caval vein appears to override the interatrial septum. RPA – right pulmonary artery.

The third common form of interatrial communication occurs in atrioventricular septal defects. As the name implies, this is an abnormality which occurs because of failure of normal development of the atrioventricular septum. Consequently, in the presence of an atrioventricular septal defect there is interatrial communication below the true atrial septum (although this may be deficient as well), atrioventricular valve morphology is altered, and there is frequently an inter-ventricular communication immediately below the atrioventricular valve leaflets. A complete atrioventricular septal defect occurs when communications exist at both atrial and ventricular levels (Fig. 40). A partial atrioventricular septal defect, or 'ostium primum atrial septal defect' occurs when there is no ventricular component to the communication (Fig. 41).

Detailed atrioventricular valve morphology in atrioventricular septal defects is best assessed in subcostal short axis planes[15] so that the plane of the ultrasound beam is in the

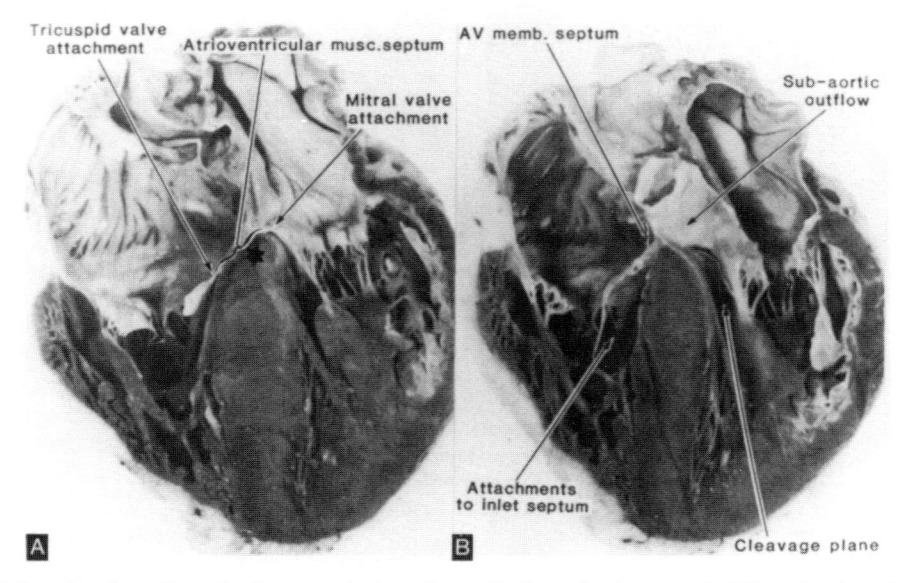

Fig. 39 Apical four and five chamber slices. **A:** An anatomical specimen sliced to stimulate an apical four chamber view demonstrates the atrioventricular muscular septum (star) between the septal attachments of the mitral and tricuspid valves. **B:** A slightly more anterior plane (simulating an echocardiographic apical 'five chamber' plane) demonstrates the atrioventricular membranous septum. (Reproduced with permission from Reference 2.)

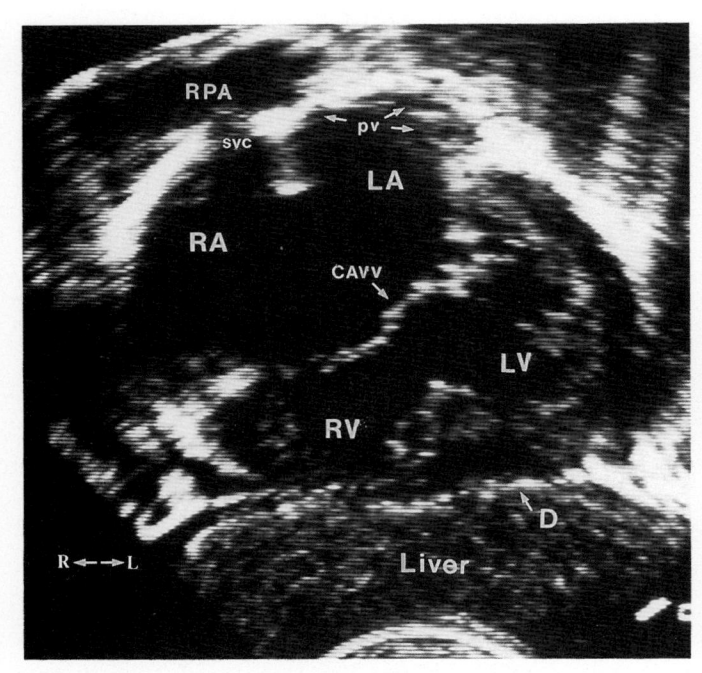

Fig. 40 Subcostal oblique four chamber systolic frame – complete atrioventricular septal defect. There is a common atrioventricular valve, with large atrial and ventricular communications above and below the valve respectively. RPA – right pulmonary artery, pv – pulmonary veins, CAVV – common atrioventricular valve, D – diaphragm.

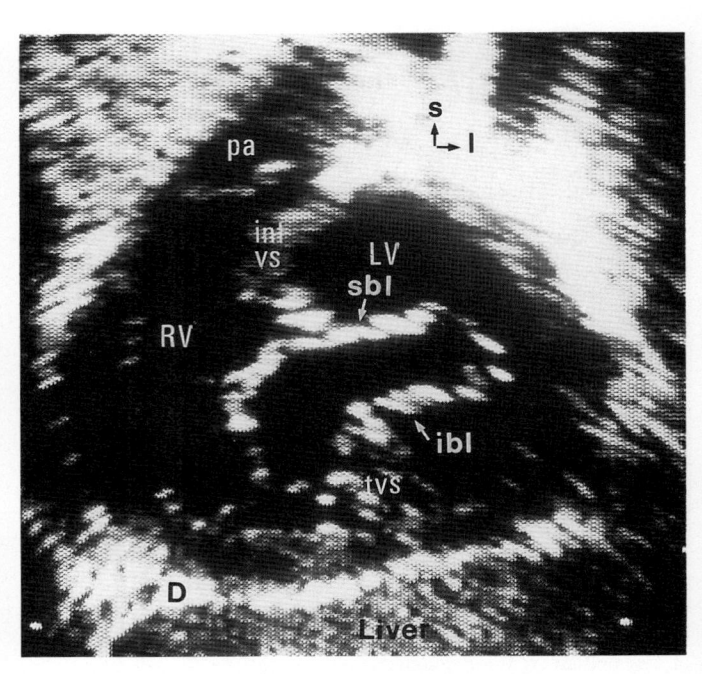

Fig. 42 Subcostal oblique view through the atrioventricular valve annulus in a patient with a complete atrioventricular septal defect with common atrioventricular orifice. ibl – inferior bridging leaflet, inf vs – infundibular ventricular septum, sbl – superior bridging leaflet, tvs – trabecular ventricular septum, D – diaphragm.

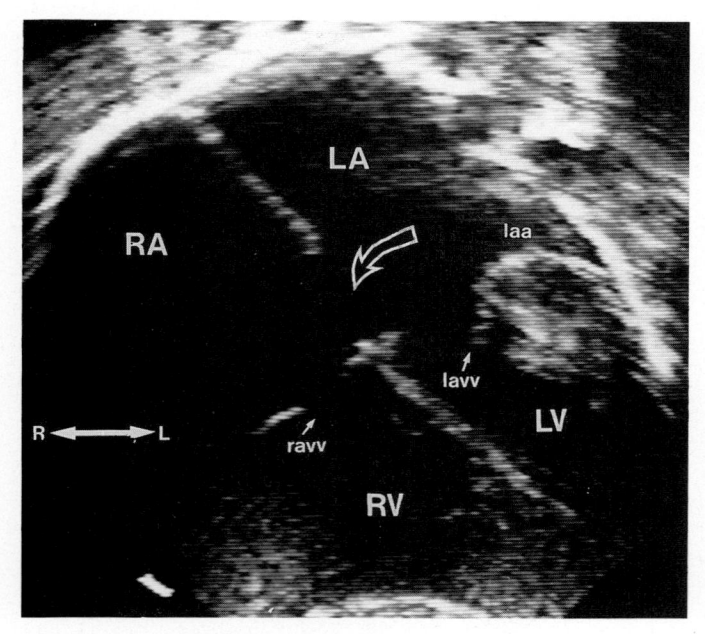

Fig. 41 Subcostal oblique four chamber view – partial atrioventricular septal defect ('primum ASD'). There is a partitioned atrioventricular orifice. There is an atrial communication above the partitioned valve (large arrow). ravv – right atrioventricular valve, lavv – left atrioventricular valve, laa – left atrial appendage.

plane of the atrioventricular valve annulus. There may be a common atrioventricular orifice, usually with five leaflets, draining both atria (Fig. 42), or, if there is tissue connecting the superior and inferior bridging leaflets, a partitioned atrioventricular orifice. The superior bridging leaflet of the atrioventricular valve bulges into the left ventricular outflow tract in ventricular diastole and gives rise to the so-called 'goose neck' appearance on angiography (Fig. 43). The left side of the commissure between superior and inferior bridging leaflets (Fig. 44), often erroneously referred to as a 'cleft mitral valve' should not be confused with a genuine isolated cleft in the anterior leaflet of a mitral valve (Fig. 45).

Ventricular septum

In the normal heart, the right ventricle wraps itself around the front of the left ventricle (Fig. 27), so that the ventricular septum is a complicated, curved structure. As might be expected, ventricular septal morphology varies considerably with different structural abnormalities. In atrioventricular discordance, for example, the ventricles are usually side by side so the ventricular septum is straighter, with a more or less sagittal orientation (Fig. 18, right).

The central fibrous body of the normal heart is the area of fibrous continuity between tricuspid, aortic and mitral valves (Fig. 39B). The normal ventricular septum has a small membranous and much a larger muscular portion.

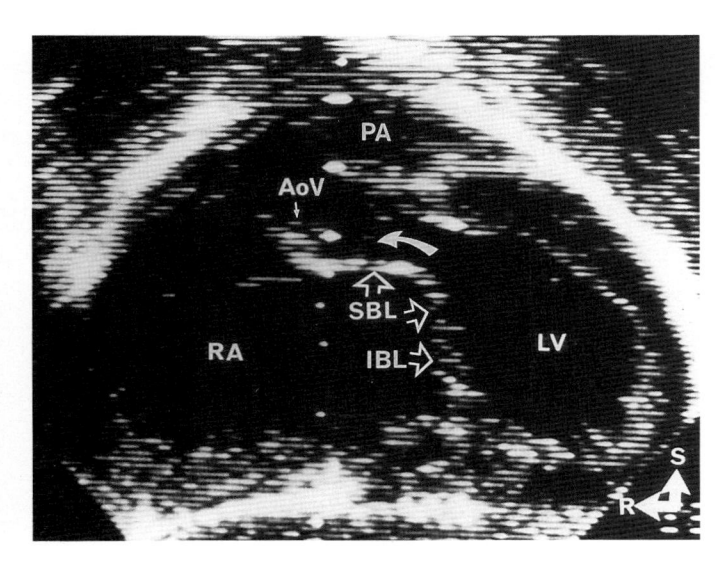

Fig. 43 Subcostal paracoronal view – atrioventricular septal defects. Left: The superior bridging leaflet protrudes into the left ventricular outflow tract (curved arrow) giving rise to the 'goose neck' appearance. **Right:** The equivalent right anterior oblique angiographic projection. AAo – ascending aorta, AoV – aortic valve, SBL – superior bridging leaflet, IBL – inferior bridging leaflet, lca – left coronary artery.

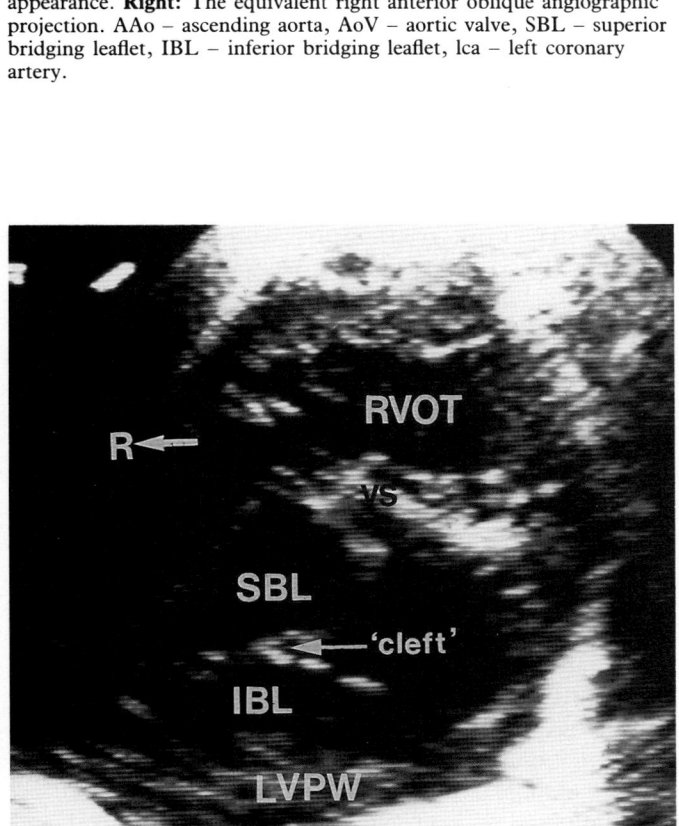

Fig. 44 Parasternal short axis view – atrioventricular septal defect. The section is taken at the level of the atrioventricular valve annulus. The commissure between the superior and inferior bridging leaflets is sometimes called a 'cleft'. LVPW – left ventricular posterior wall, RVOT – right ventricular outflow tract, SBL – superior bridging leaflet, IBL – inferior bridging leaflet, vs – inter-ventricular septum.

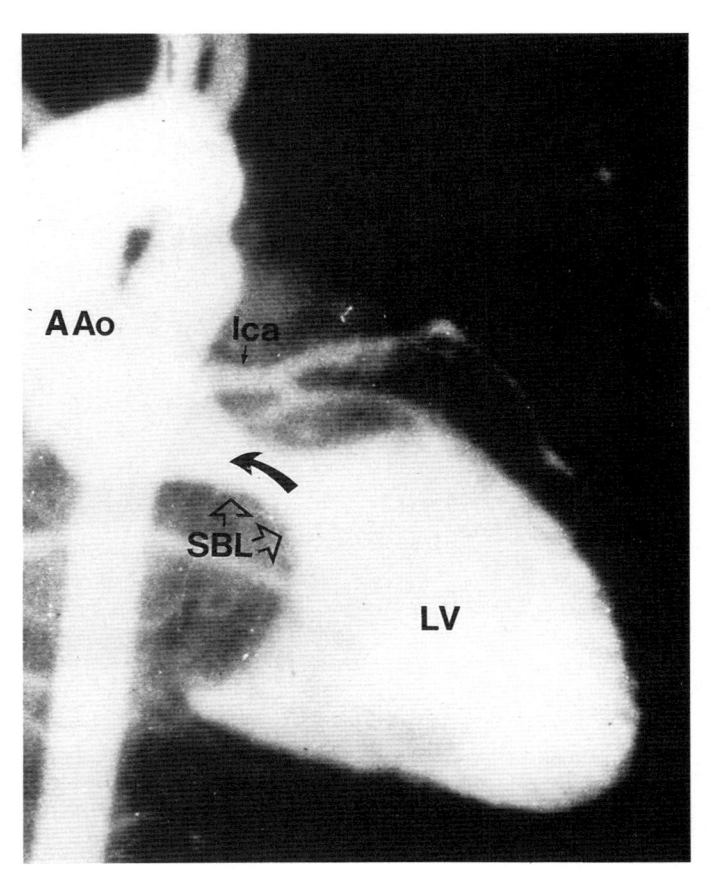

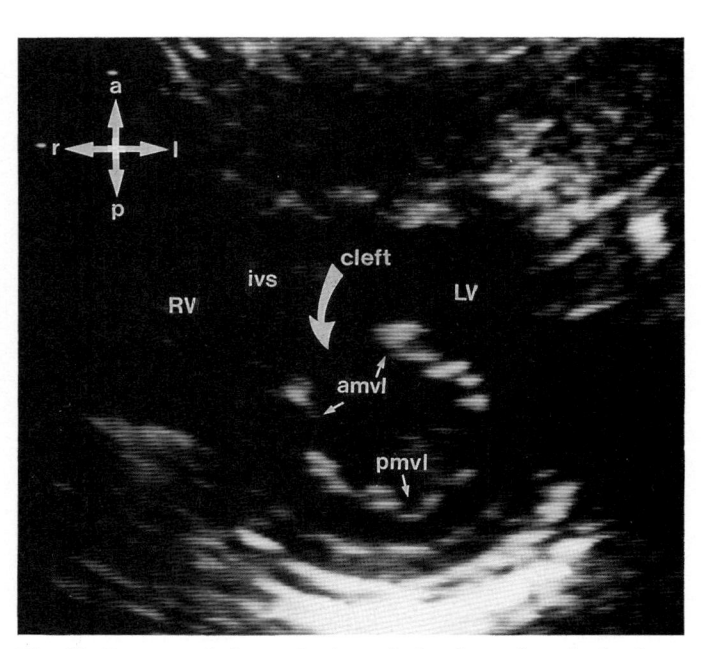

Fig. 45 Parasternal short axis view – isolated anterior mitral valve leaflet cleft. amvl – anterior mitral valve leaflet, ivs – inter-ventricular septum, pmvl – posterior mitral valve leaflet.

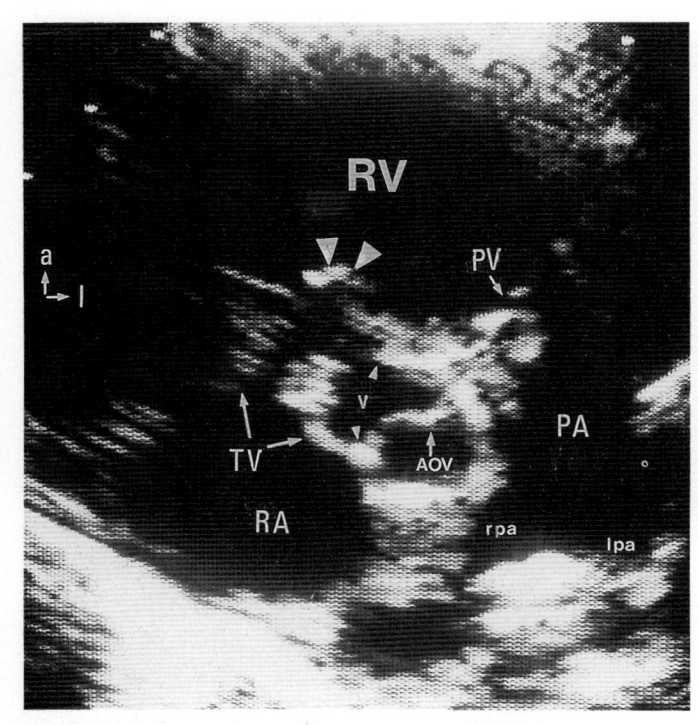

Fig. 46 Parasternal short axis view – perimembranous VSD. The margins of the VSD are delineated by small arrowheads. There is fibrous continuity between the tricuspid valve and the aortic valve at the lower arrowhead. The VSD is partly plugged on its right ventricular aspect by fibrous tissue (large arrowheads). AOV – aortic valve, v – ventricular septal defect, rpa – right pulmonary artery, lpa – left pulmonary artery.

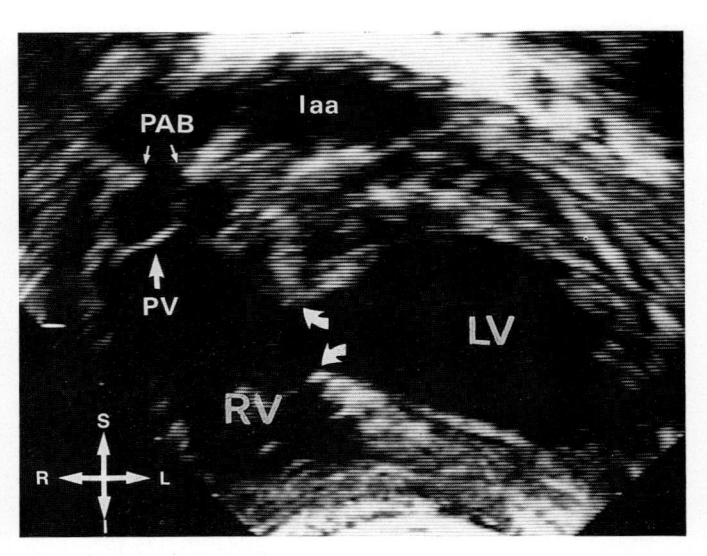

Fig. 48 Subcostal paracoronal view – large muscular trabecular ventricular septal defect (curved arrows). Palliative surgery (pulmonary artery banding) has been performed. PAB – pulmonary artery band, laa – left atrial appendage.

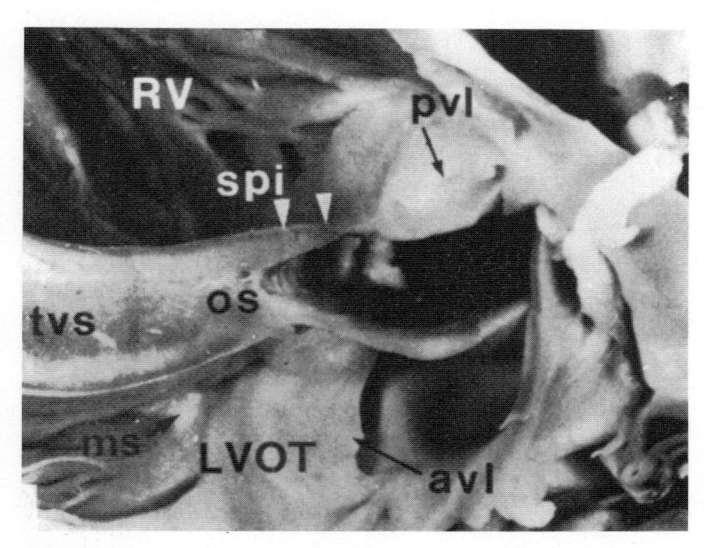

Fig. 47 Normal heart sectioned to simulate a modified parasternal long axis view. The left aspect of the membranous septum can be seen from the left ventricular outflow tract. The pulmonary valve is supported on a sleeve of subpulmonary infundibular muscle. The true outlet septum is small. avl – aortic valve leaflet, ms – membranous septum, os – outlet septum, pvl – pulmonary valve leaflet, spi – subpulmonary infundibulum, tvs – trabecular ventricular septum, LVOT – left ventricular outflow tract. Adapted from Reference 12.

The membranous septum is continuous with the central fibrous body. The septal leaflet of the tricuspid valve is usually attached to the membranous septum on its right ventricular aspect, dividing it into atrioventricular (Fig. 39B) and ventricular components, above and below this line of attachment respectively. The importance of the membranous septum is that the majority of ventricular septal defects abut this area, so that part of their margin is composed of fibrous tissue.[16] Recognition that such a defect is membranous or perimembranous (extending beyond the strict limits of the membranous septum) allows identification of the region of the penetrating bundle of cardiac conducting tissue in the postero-inferior rim of the defect, which must not be damaged during surgical closure of the hole if heart block is to be avoided. An isolated perimembranous ventricular septal defect is most easily recognised by showing fibrous continuity between the tricuspid valve and aortic valve at the margin of the defect in a normally connected heart (Fig. 46), usually from a subcostal or parasternal short axis cut. The left ventricular aspect of the membranous septum is just below the aortic valve (Figs 39B and 47), so that perimembranous ventricular septal defects which extend towards the outlet septum may be demonstrated in parasternal long axis views.

A minority of ventricular septal defects are not perimembranous and are either muscular or doubly committed subarterial defects,[16] although most of the latter group are perimembranous as well.[13] Muscular defects, with entirely muscular rims, are typically in the trabecular septum (Fig. 48). Interrogation of the normal curved trabecular septum requires a combination of subcostal, apical and precordial sweeps. The inlet portion is best imaged from an apical position, although this term may be confusing, as the

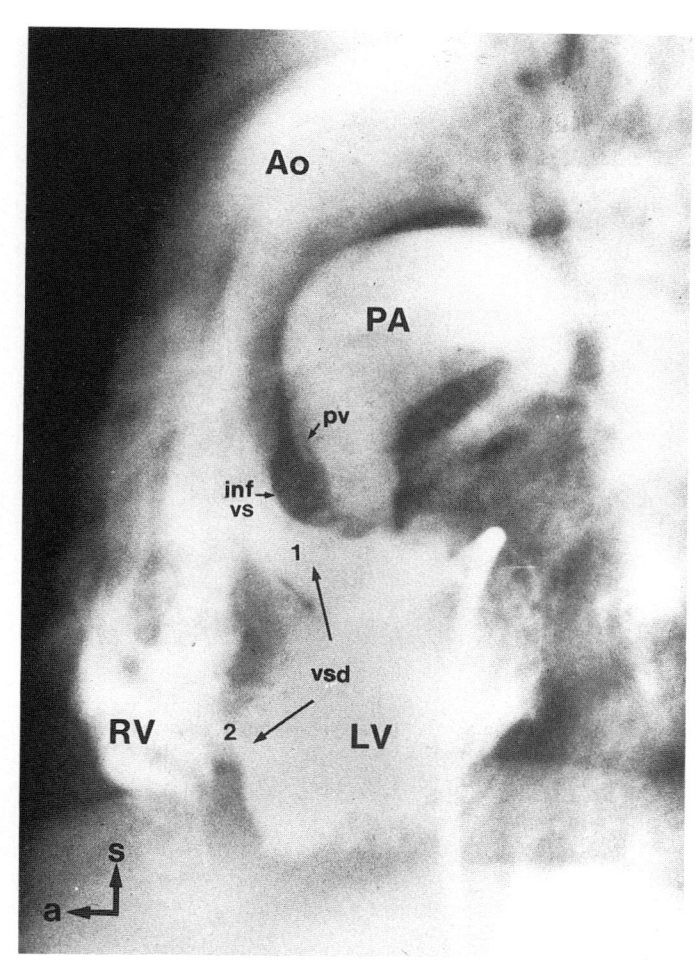

Fig. 49 Angiogram in ventriculo-arterial discordance. Lateral projection left ventricular cine-angiogram in a patient with ventriculo-arterial discordance and two ventricular septal defects (vsd 1 and 2). The infundibular (or outlet), ventricular septum is an extensive area of muscle (compare with Fig. 47). vsd 1 is an outlet muscular defect and vsd 2 is in the mid-muscular septum. inf vs – infundibular ventricular septum.

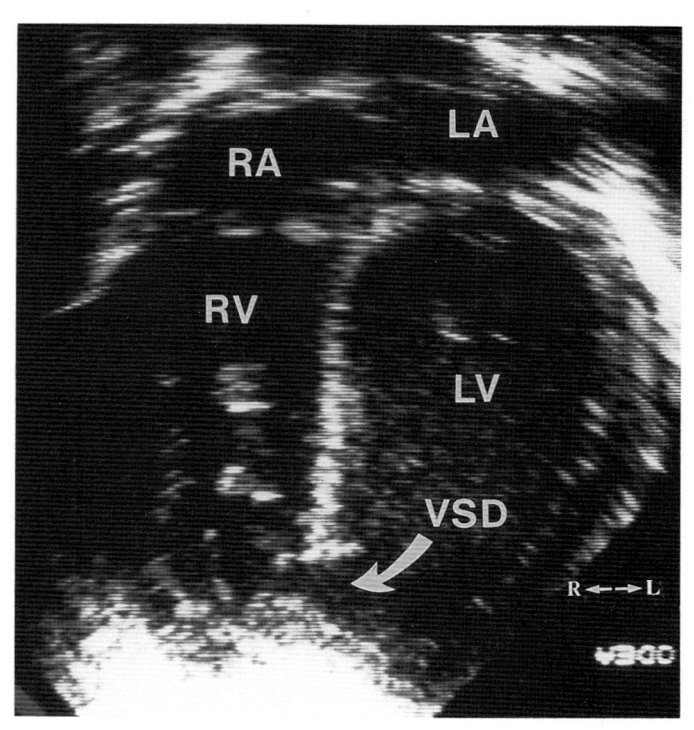

Fig. 50 Apical muscular ventricular septal defect. Apical view with the transducer directed more posteriorly than for a four chamber cut, demonstrating an apical muscular ventricular septal defect. VSD – ventricular septal defect.

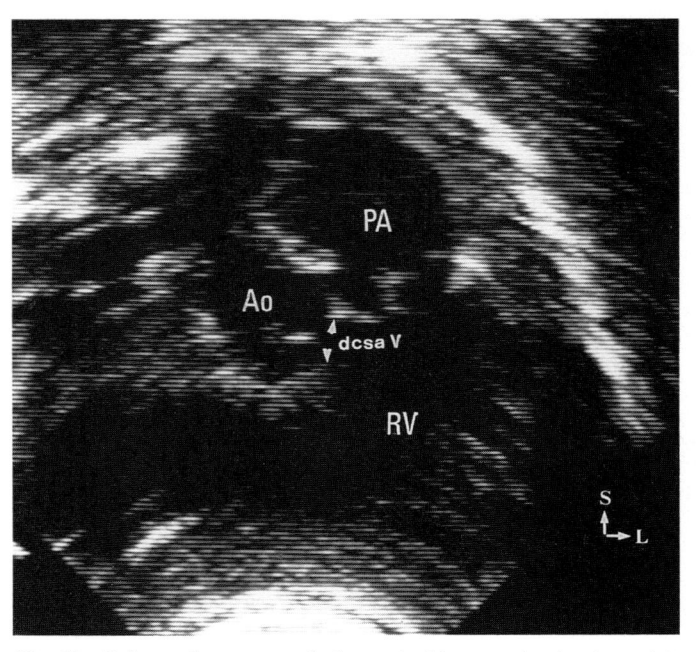

Fig. 51 Subcostal paracoronal view – doubly committed subarterial ventricular septal defect (dcsa V). The margins of the defect are delineated by arrowheads. The point of fibrous continuity between the aortic valve and the pulmonary valve is indicated by the upper arrowhead.

'inlet' septum actually separates the inflow part of the right ventricle from the left ventricular outflow tract (Fig. 39B). The outlet portion of the ventricular septum is small in hearts with a concordant ventriculo-arterial connection (Fig. 47), but larger in hearts with ventriculo-arterial discordance (Fig. 49) and other abnormalities such as Fallot's tetralogy or DORV (Fig. 28). Consequently, ventricular septal defects in ventriculo-arterial discordance are often outlet muscular in position (Fig. 49).

Important ventricular septal defects at the extreme poles of the ventricular septum are easily overlooked. Apical trabecular defects require good image resolution in the near field if they are to be visualised from an apical position (Fig. 50). Alternatively, the transducer may be directed anteriorly towards the apex from a subcostal position, which requires a relaxed abdominal wall! Multiple small defects may be present, sometimes being identifiable by Doppler

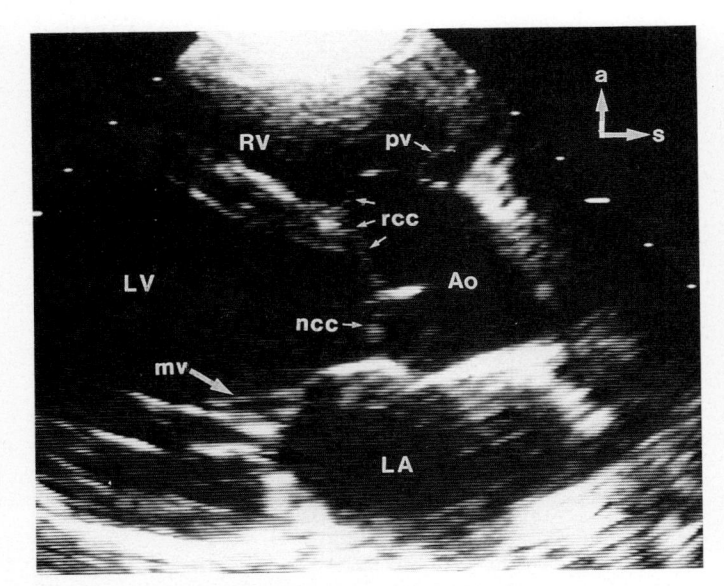

Fig. 52 Parasternal long axis view – ventricular septal defect. Prolapse of the right coronary cusp of the aortic valve into a doubly committed subarterial ventricular septal defect is demonstrated. Note the fibrous continuity between the aortic valve and pulmonary valve. ncc – non-coronary cusp, rcc – right coronary cusp.

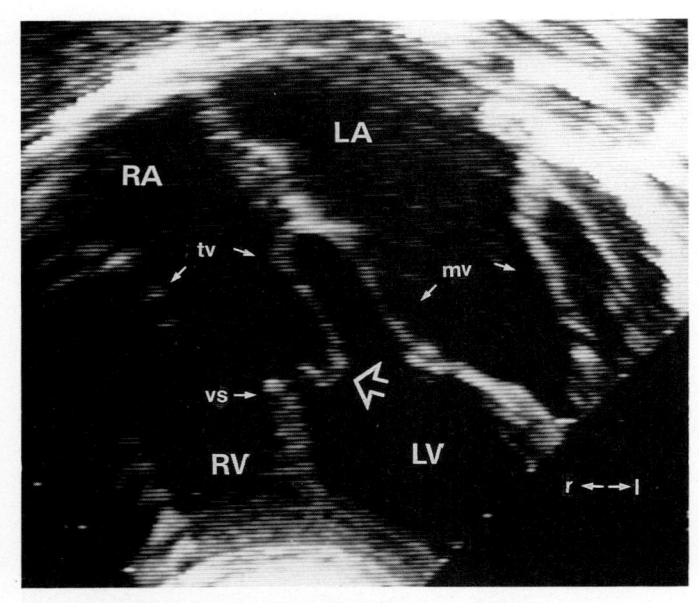

Fig. 53 Apical four chamber view – large perimembranous ventricular septal defect. The tricuspid valve straddles the ventricular septum, so part of its tension appartus is anchored to the left ventricular aspect of the septum (large arrow). vs – ventricular septum.

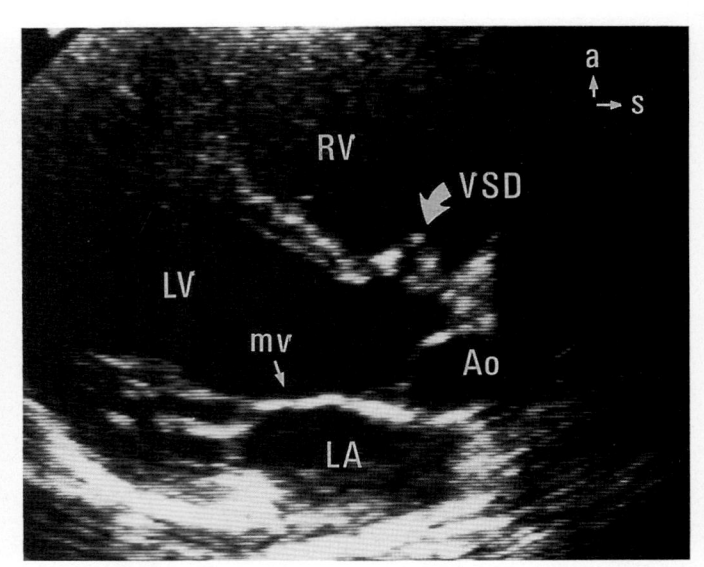

Fig. 54 Parasternal long axis view – perimembranous ventricular septal defect partly plugged by fibrous tissue on its right ventricular aspect. VSD – ventricular septal defect.

pulmonary infundibulum as is normally the case.[13] While relatively rare in Caucasians, this abnormality is common in Oriental populations. The defects are usually best identified from a subcostal position with the scan plane aligned with the right ventricular outflow tract to show the arterial valves in fibrous continuity (Fig. 51). Similar features may be also recognised from the parasternal short axis. Prolapse of the right coronary cusp of the aortic valve into a doubly committed or other perimembranous defect may occur during childhood (Fig. 52).

It is important to detect if the tension apparatus from an atrioventricular valve passes through a ventricular septal defect to be anchored in the 'wrong' ventricle. When this occurs, the tension apparatus of an atrioventricular valve being tethered in both ventricles, the valve is said to straddle the ventricular septum (Fig. 53). This may complicate surgical closure. Also of importance in the assessment of a ventricular septal defect is the presence of fibrous tissue adjacent to the right ventricular aspect of the defect. This tissue, sometimes termed an aneurysm, arises from the membranous septum or adjacent tricuspid valve apparatus and may 'plug' the hole. The presence of this tissue may predict spontaneous closure of the defect (Figs 46 and 54).[17]

The great arteries

Identification of the great arteries is necessary as described above (Fig. 26). The relative diameters of the great arteries correlate approximately with the blood volume flowing in each vessel, especially in fetal or early post-natal life. The broad disparity which may occur is evident in hypoplastic left heart syndrome when the only ascending aortic perfu-

colour flow mapping when the defects themselves have not been imaged. Doubly committed subarterial ventricular septal defects are at the other end of the ventricular septum, being roofed by the aortic and pulmonary valves. In this situation the arterial valves are in fibrous continuity, rather than being separated by the septal aspect of the sub-

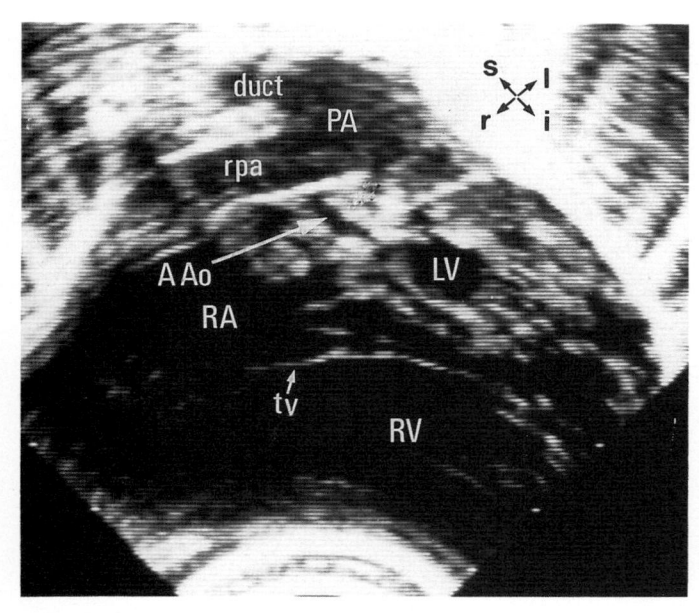

Fig. 55 Subcostal oblique cut – hypoplastic left heart syndrome. The left ventricular cavity and ascending aorta in this neonate are extremely small whereas the right ventricle and pulmonary artery are large. AAo – ascending aorta, rpa – right pulmonary artery.

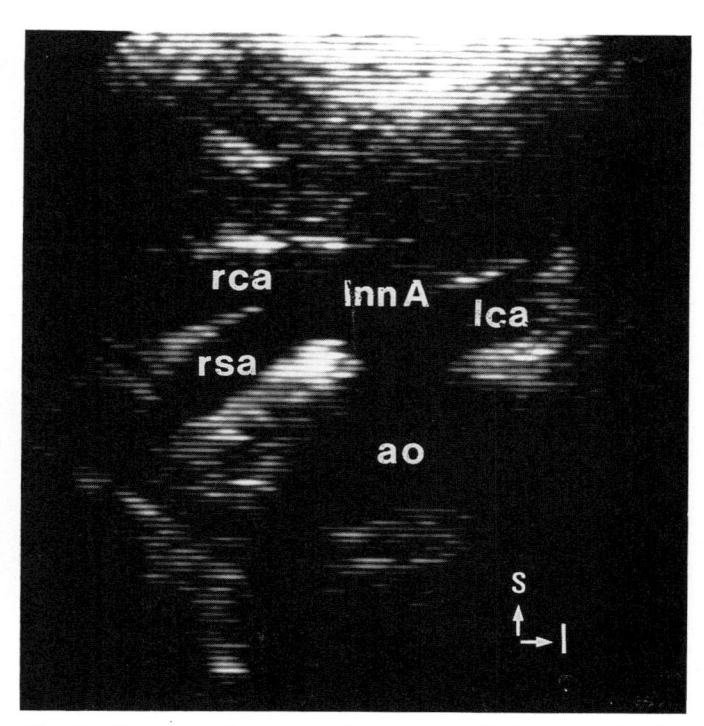

Fig. 56 Suprasternal paracoronal cut – normal left aortic arch. The first branch is the innominate artery which passes towards the right shoulder. In this case, it shares a common origin with the left carotid artery. rca – right carotid artery, rsa – right subclavian artery, Inn A – innominate artery, lca – left carotid artery.

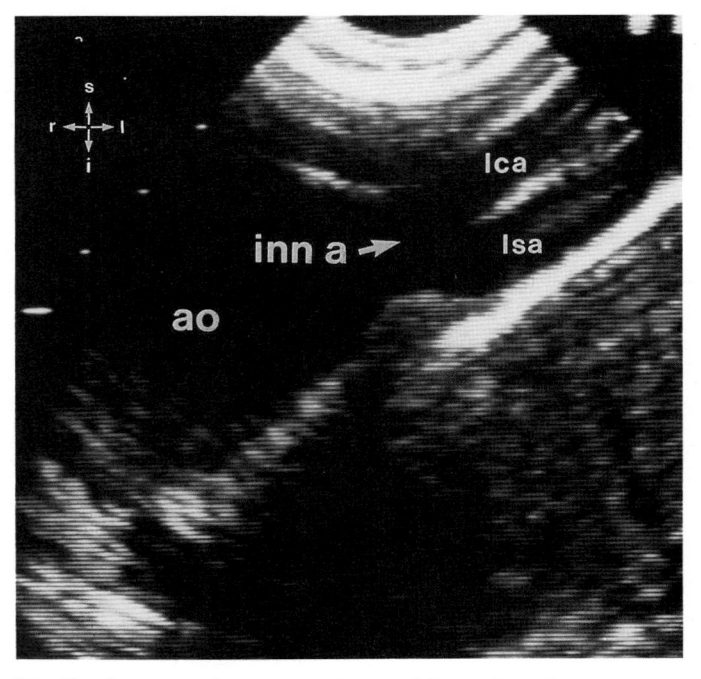

Fig. 57 Suprasternal paracoronal cut – right aortic arch demonstrating the innominate artery crossing to the left. lca – left carotid artery, lsa – left subclavian artery, inn a – innominate artery.

sion is retrograde flow via an arterial duct. Consequently, the ascending aorta is extremely hypoplastic while the pulmonary trunk is large (Fig. 55).

The side of the aortic arch in the mediastinum is determined by its relation to the trachea. While the orientation of the transducer and scanning plane may provide this information when the long axis of the arch is imaged from the suprasternal or high parasternal position, confusion may occur in situations where mediastinal shift has distorted the tracheal location from the midline. The branching pattern of the head and neck vessels is more reliable.[18] A left arch has the first aortic branch directed to the right, this being the innominate artery with its proximal bifurcation (Fig. 56). Conversely, the first branch from a right aortic arch passes towards the left shoulder (Fig. 57). A right arch typically has a tighter arc than a left arch (Fig. 58), whereas there is a broader arc than usual when the ascending aorta is anterior, as occurs with complete transposition of the great arteries (Fig. 59). A normal left sided aortic arch does not describe a simple arc, and it is unusual to be able to image the entire arch in one plane. Coarctation of the aorta is sometimes difficult to image, because of its posterior mediastinal location and variable morphology (Fig. 60). Reduced or absent pulsation of the descending aorta in the upper abdomen compared to the pulsation of the ascending aorta is useful supportive evidence for thoracic coarctation which might be mistakenly diagnosed instead of the rare 'abdominal coarctation' in patients with absent leg pulses.[19] Interruption of the aortic arch, which most commonly occurs between the left carotid

330 CARDIAC ULTRASOUND

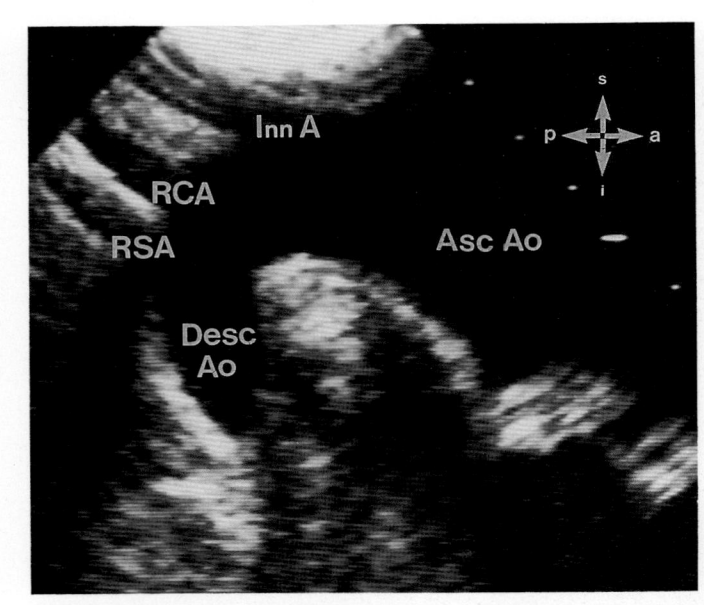

Fig. 58 Suprasternal long axis view – right aortic arch obtained by rotating the transducer clockwise from the coronal imaging position. Asc Ao – ascending aorta, Desc Ao – descending aorta, Inn A – innominate artery, RCA – right carotid artery, RSA – right subclavian artery.

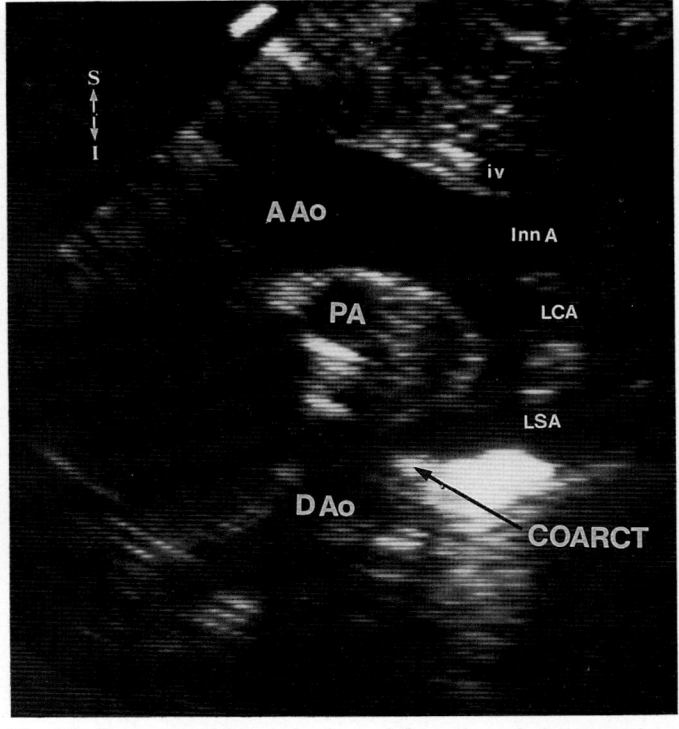

Fig. 60 Suprasternal long axis view – left aortic arch demonstrating discrete coarctation distal to the origin of the left subclavian artery. A Ao – ascending aorta, D Ao – descending aorta, iv – innominate vein, Inn A – innominate artery, LCA – left carotid artery, LSA – left subclavian artery, COARCT – coarctation.

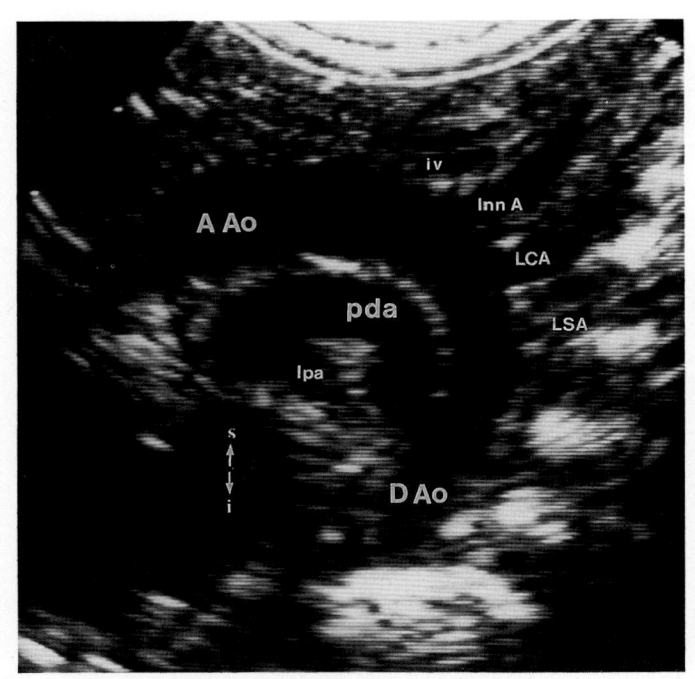

Fig. 59 Suprasternal long axis view – left aortic arch in a patient with transposition of the great arteries. A Ao – ascending aorta, D Ao – descending aorta, pda – patent ductus arteriosus, lpa – left pulmonary artery, iv – innominate vein, Inn A – innominate artery, LCA – left carotid artery, LSA – left subclavian artery.

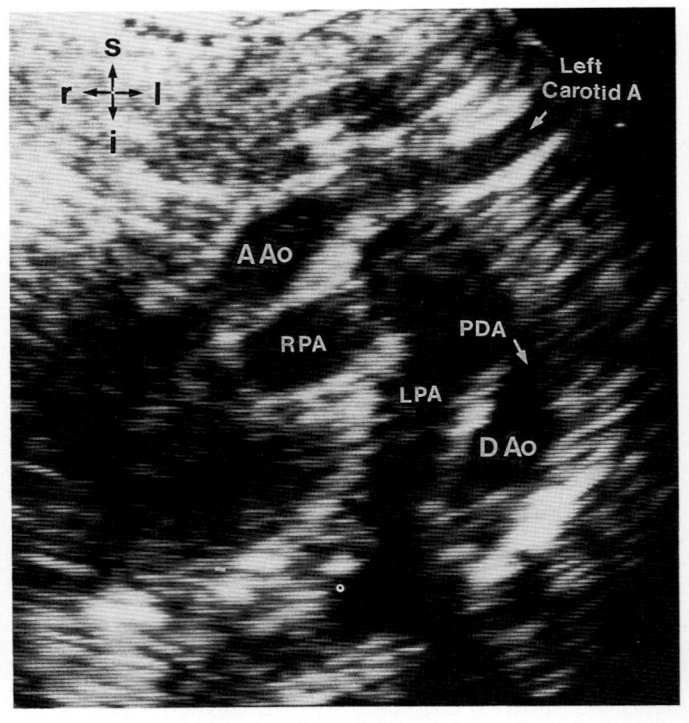

Fig. 61 Suprasternal view – interruption of the aortic arch distal to the left carotid artery. A Ao – Ascending aorta, D Ao – descending aorta, RPA – right pulmonary artery, LPA – left pulmonary artery, PDA – patent ductus arteriosus, Left Carotid A – left carotid artery.

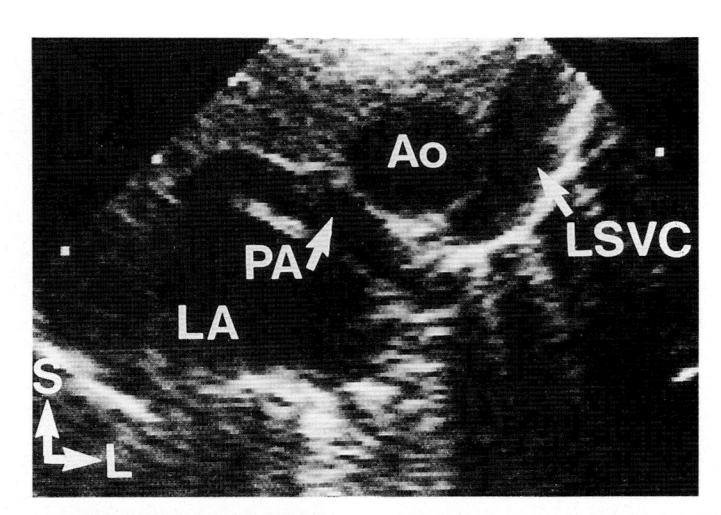

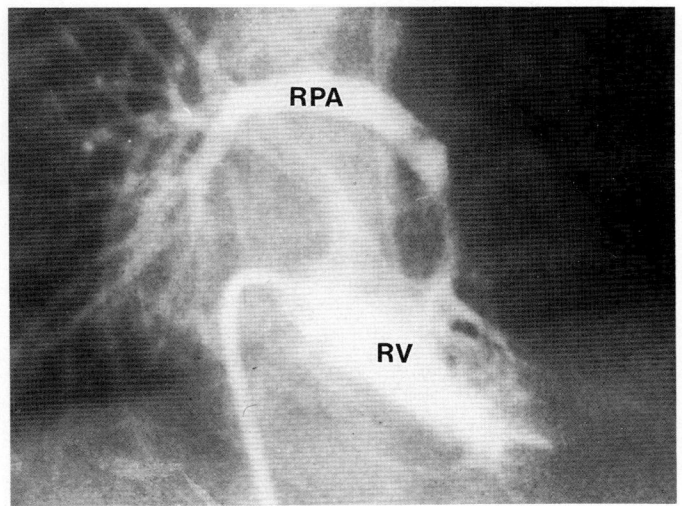

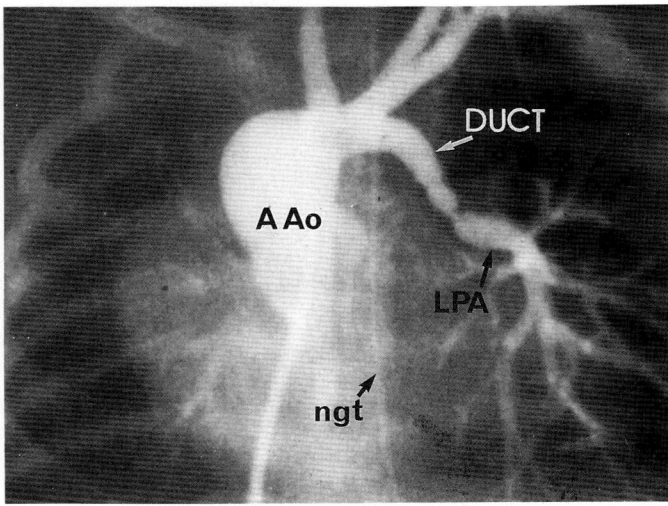

Fig. 62. **Tetralogy of Fallot.** On suprasternal imaging from a neonate with tetralogy of Fallot there is potential confusion as to whether the hypoplastic pulmonary arteries are confluent or not (top). Angiography demonstrates the right pulmonary artery is connected to the right ventricular outflow tract and pulmonary trunk (lower left), whereas the left pulmonary artery is disconnected, and perfused by an arterial duct which arises from the innominate artery. There is a right sided aortic arch (lower right). LSVC – left sided superior caval vein, ngt – nasogastric tube, RPA – right pulmonary artery, A Ao – ascending aorta, LPA – left pulmonary artery.

and left subclavian arteries, is characterised by a smooth sweep of the ascending aorta into its terminal branches, while the descending aortic blood flow arises from a large 'straight through' arterial duct (Fig. 61).

Size, confluence and evidence for obstruction to flow are features sought from images of the central pulmonary arteries. The normal pulmonary trunk is usually best seen from the precordium (Fig. 27), the proximal right pulmonary artery from a coronal suprasternal cut (Fig. 9), and the proximal left pulmonary artery from the same site by rotating the scanhead counter clockwise from the midline (Fig. 61). When pulmonary blood flow is duct dependent it is important to establish the site of ductal entry (Fig. 33), and the confluence or otherwise of hypoplastic central pulmonary arteries prior to construction of a palliative systemic to pulmonary artery shunt. Clamping of the contralateral pulmonary artery to construct the shunt will not result in cessation of pulmonary blood flow if the pulmonary arteries are centrally confluent. Non-confluent pulmonary arteries typically occur in pulmonary atresia with ventricular septal defect or tetralogy of Fallot (Fig. 62). Rarely, one pulmonary artery may arise from the ascending aorta (Fig. 63). The central pulmonary arteries cannot be imaged beyond the hila of the lungs, so that while proximal pulmonary artery stenosis will be evident, more distal branch stenoses will not be imaged. Indirect evidence for the presence of bilateral branch stenoses is obtained from the observation of excessive pulsatility of the pulmonary trunk.

The arterial duct is usually imaged parallel and just superior to the left pulmonary artery from the suprasternal or high left parasternal position (Fig. 59). It is a normal

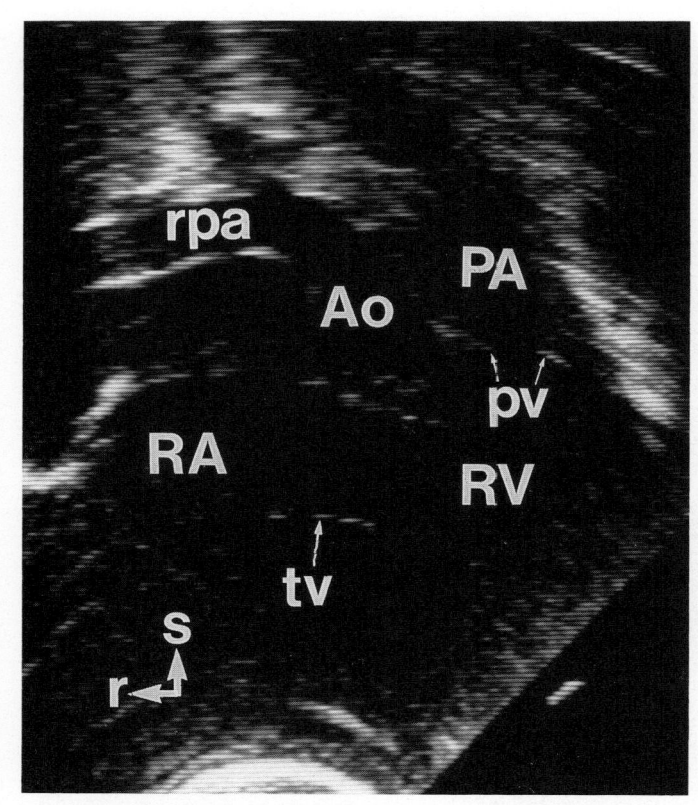

Fig. 63 Subcostal paracoronal view – **right pulmonary artery arising from ascending aorta** as an isolated abnormality. rpa – right pulmonary artery, pv – pulmonary valve.

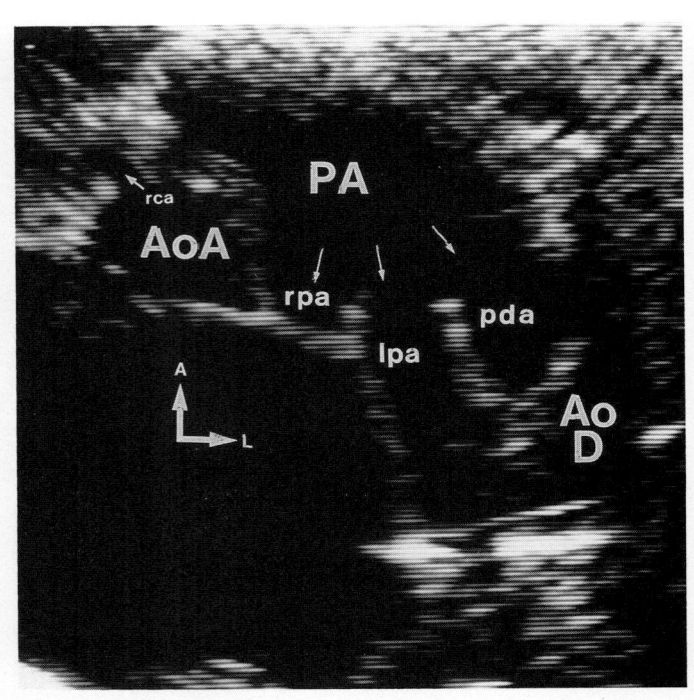

Fig. 64 Patent arterial duct. Modified parasternal short axis in a newborn demonstrating a widely patent arterial duct. The pulmonary trunk appears to trifurcate. AoA – ascending aorta, rca – right coronary artery, rpa – right pulmonary artery, lpa – left pulmonary artery, pda – patent ductus arteriosus, AoD – descending aorta.

structure in prenatal and immediate post-natal life (Fig. 64). After the duct has closed, the ductal ligament is usually evident in infants as a bright linear echo in the same location. The aortic end of the duct often has a vertical origin, and the duct a tortuous course when there is duct dependent pulmonary blood flow (Fig. 33). The ductal course may be difficult to image in the presence of a right sided aortic arch. The possibility of an innominate artery origin for the duct (Fig. 62) must be borne in mind. An aortopulmonary window is a communication between ascending aorta and pulmonary trunk which occurs just above the normal origin of the left coronary artery, and is usually best visualised from a subcostal cut through the right ventricular outflow tract or from parasternal short axis (Fig. 65). This is a lesion easily overlooked unless specifically sought.

An abnormal course or position of the great arteries may result in a vascular ring which compresses central mediastinal structures. The most common vascular ring resulting in stridor in infancy is a double aortic arch where the trachea and oesophagus are compressed in a vascular vice between the two arches. A double barrelled appearance of the ascending aorta may be identified on a parasternal short axis sweep up the ascending aorta from the base of the

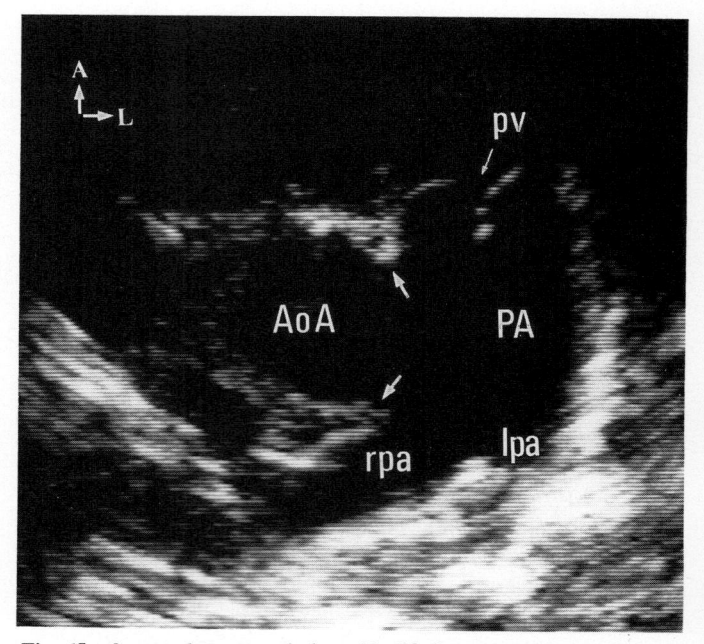

Fig. 65 Aortopulmonary window. Modified parasternal short axis view at the level of the great arteries demonstrating a large aortopulmonary window (margins delineated by arrows). AoA – ascending aorta, rpa – right pulmonary artery, lpa – left pulmonary artery.

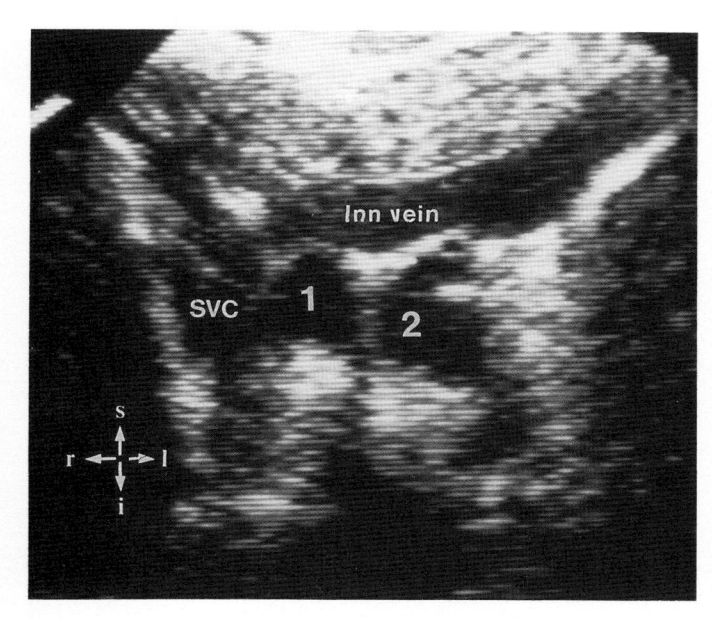

Fig. 66 Double aortic arch. Modified high parasternal short axis demonstrating a double aortic arch. 1 and 2 – separate aortic arches, SVC – superior vena cava, Inn vein – innominate vein.

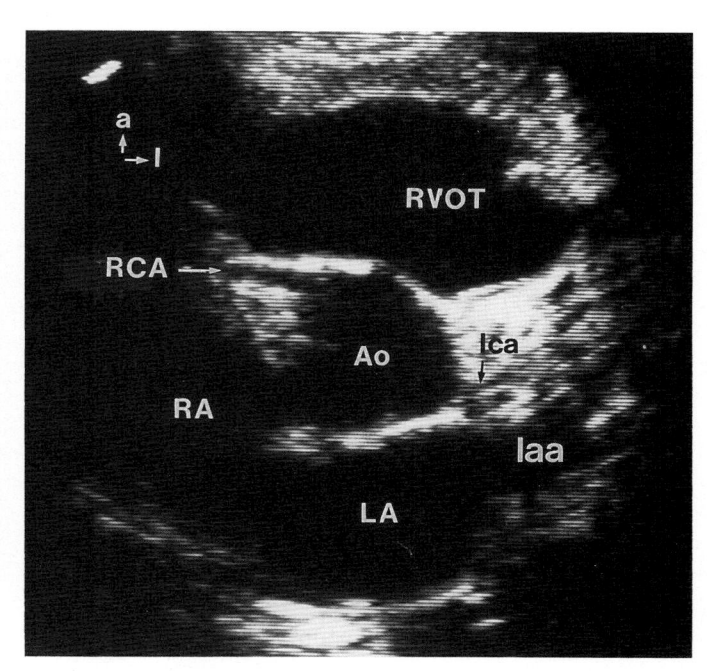

Fig. 68 Parasternal short axis view – normal proximal right coronary artery. RCA – right coronary artery, RVOT – right ventricular outflow tract, lca – left coronary artery, laa – left atrial appendage.

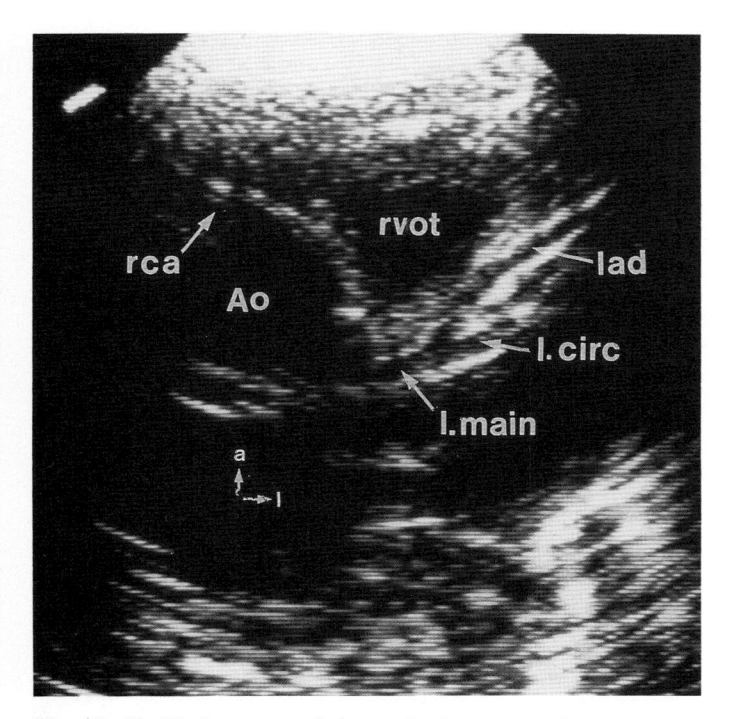

Fig. 67 Modified parasternal short axis view – normal proximal left coronary artery appearances. lad – left anterior descending branch, l.circ – left circumflex branch, l.main – left main coronary artery, rca – right coronary artery, rvot – right ventricular outflow tract.

heart (Fig. 66), or the two arches may be separately identified by gently rocking the scanhead from the long axis plane of one arch to that of the other from the suprasternal position. An anomalous right subclavian artery arising from the descending aorta is rarely symptomatic because it passes posterior to both trachea and oesophagus as it crosses the midline. It is difficult to image directly, but may be suspected if the 'innominate' artery appears smaller than expected and does not bifurcate in the usual way. A pulmonary artery sling is characterised by a more distal origin and more posterior course than usual of the left pulmonary artery as it arises from the right pulmonary artery, and then courses to the left between trachea and oesophagus. This may be a difficult echocardiographic diagnosis if there is associated mediastinal displacement but colour flow mapping may be helpful in identifying the abnormal left pulmonary artery origin.

The coronary arteries

The origins, course and size of the coronary arteries are important in a number of situations. Parasternal short axis views normally yield the best images of both proximal coronary arteries. The origin of the left coronary artery is seen when the ultrasound beam is angled just inferior to the pulmonary trunk and slight clockwise rotation of the transducer enables the bifurcation into the left anterior descending and left circumflex branches to be imaged (Fig. 67). In this view, the left anterior descending branch may be followed for 1 to 2 cm, and in some children, septal branches may also be demonstrated. The proximal right coronary artery is identified by slight cranial angulation

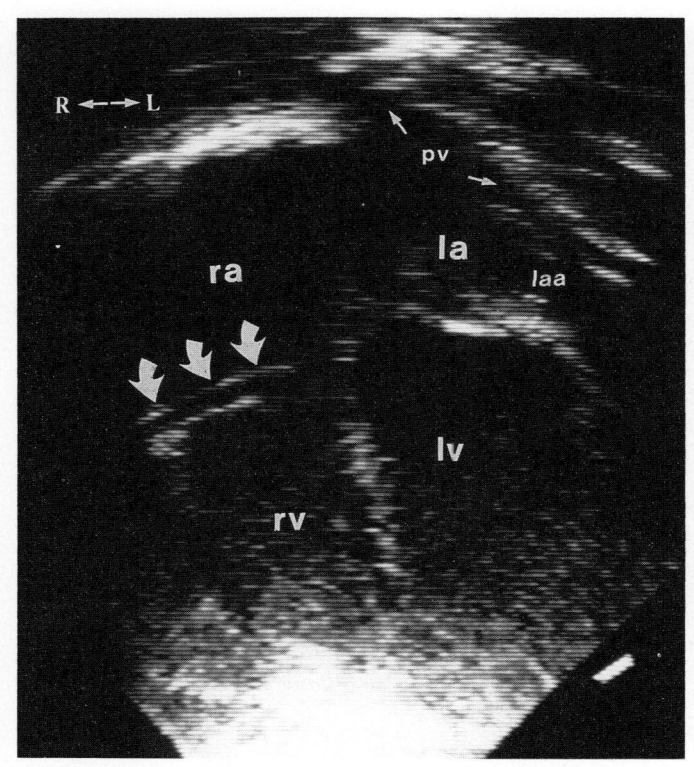

Fig. 69 Apical view with the transducer angled posteriorly to demonstrate the right coronary artery (arrows) as it passes posteriorly through the right atrioventricular groove. pv – pulmonary veins, laa – left atrial appendage.

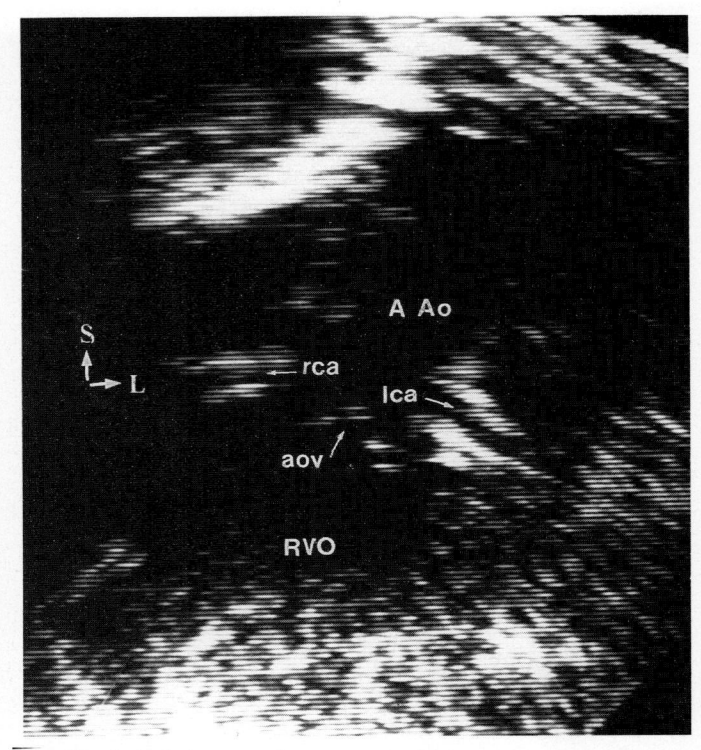

Fig. 70 Apical view showing separate origins of the coronary arteries in a neonate with transposition of the great arteries. rca – right coronary artery, lca – left coronary artery, A Ao – ascending aorta, aov – aortic valve, RVO – right ventricular outflow.

from this position, often also requiring slight clockwise rotation of the transducer (Fig. 68). The proximal right coronary artery swings in and out of the acoustic plane with each cardiac cycle. The more distal right coronary artery may be imaged as it passes posteriorly through the right atrioventricular groove from an apical view with the ultrasound beam angled posteriorly (Fig. 69). The proximal coronary arteries may be seen from the apex in neonates (Fig. 70) or in older children if the vessels are abnormally large (Fig. 71).

An anomalous origin of the left coronary artery from the pulmonary trunk must be distinguished from congestive cardiomyopathy in infancy. The anomalous origin can be imaged from a modified, high, left parasternal short axis cut (Fig. 72). A ratio of right coronary artery to ascending aortic diameter in excess of 0.20 also suggests the diagnosis (Fig. 72),[3] although this measurement requires equipment with high axial resolution and it may not be reliable in very young infants with poorly developed collateral flow from the right coronary artery. The transverse sinus of the pericardium can be mistaken for a normally arising left coronary artery[20] as it is an echo-free linear structure apparently arising from the ascending aorta.

Coronary-cameral fistulae (communications between a coronary artery and cardiac chamber) are also characterised

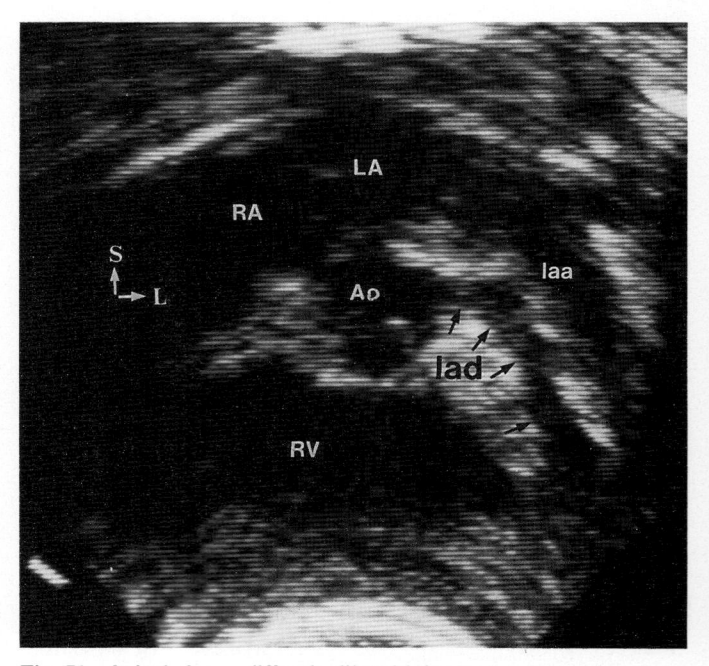

Fig. 71 Apical view – diffusely dilated left anterior descending coronary artery in a child with Kawasaki disease. lad – left anterior descending artery, laa – left atrial appendage.

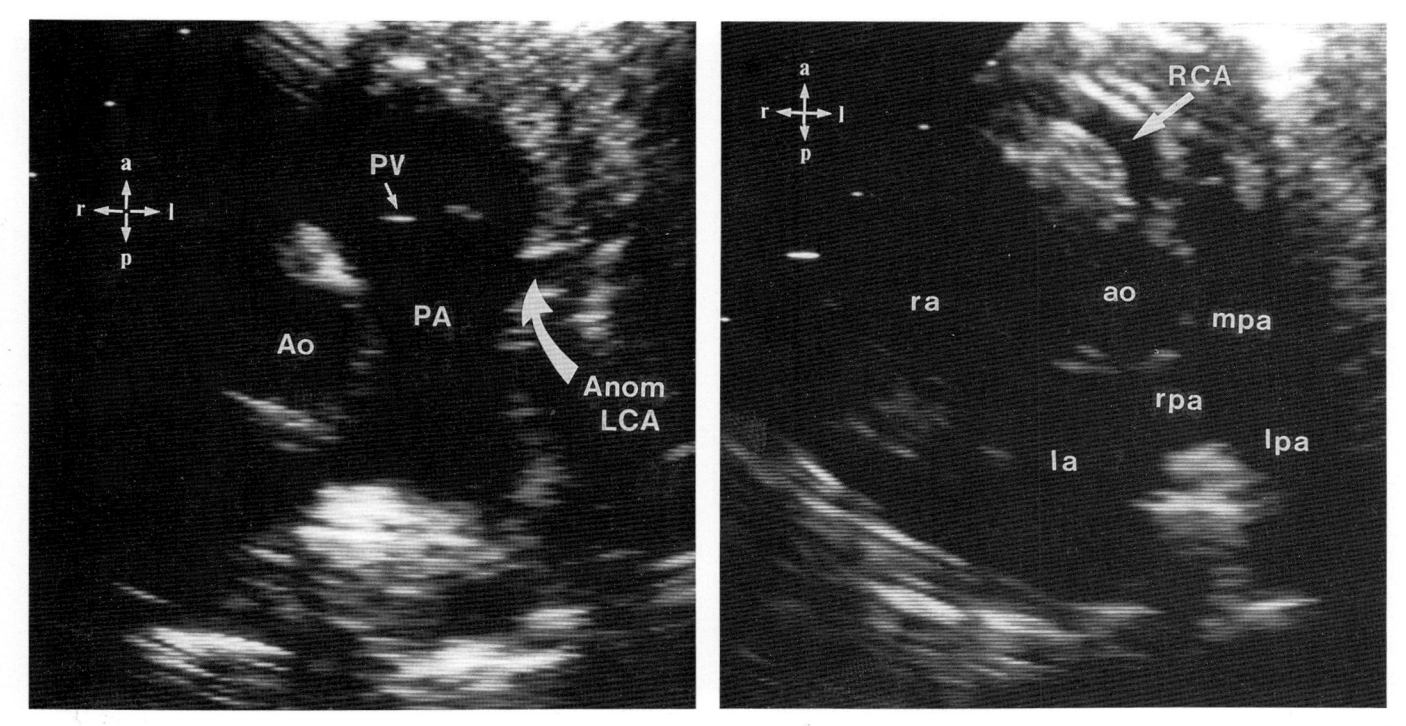

Fig. 72 Coronary artery anomalies. Left: modified high parasternal view in an infant demonstrating anomalous origin of the left coronary artery from the pulmonary trunk. Right: modified parasternal short axis view in the same patient demonstrates a dilated right coronary artery arising from the aorta. PA (mpa) – main pulmonary artery, Anom LCA – anomalous left coronary artery, RCA – right coronary artery, rpa – right pulmonary artery, lpa – left pulmonary artery.

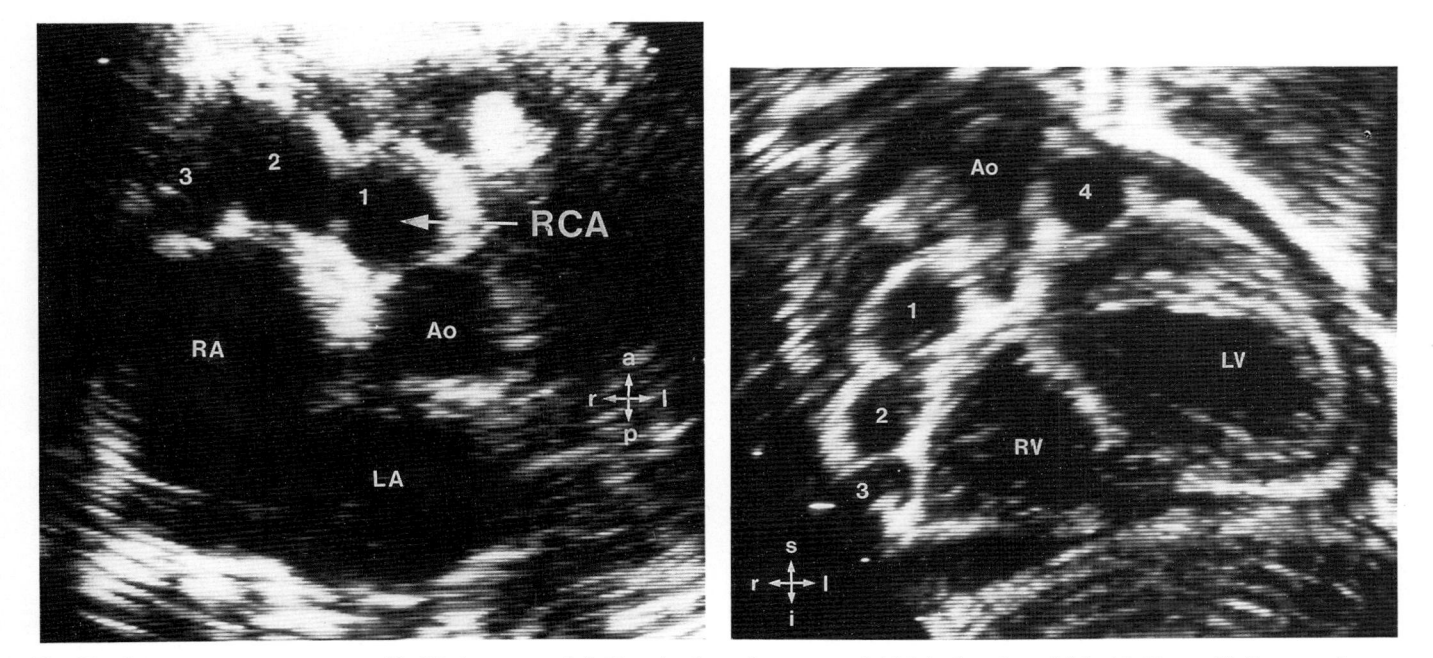

Fig. 73 Coronary artery aneurysm. Modified parasternal (left) and subcostal paracoronal (right) views in a child with Kawasaki disease and coronary aneurysm formation in the proximal right coronary artery (1, 2, 3), and proximal left (4) coronary arteries. RCA – right coronary artery.

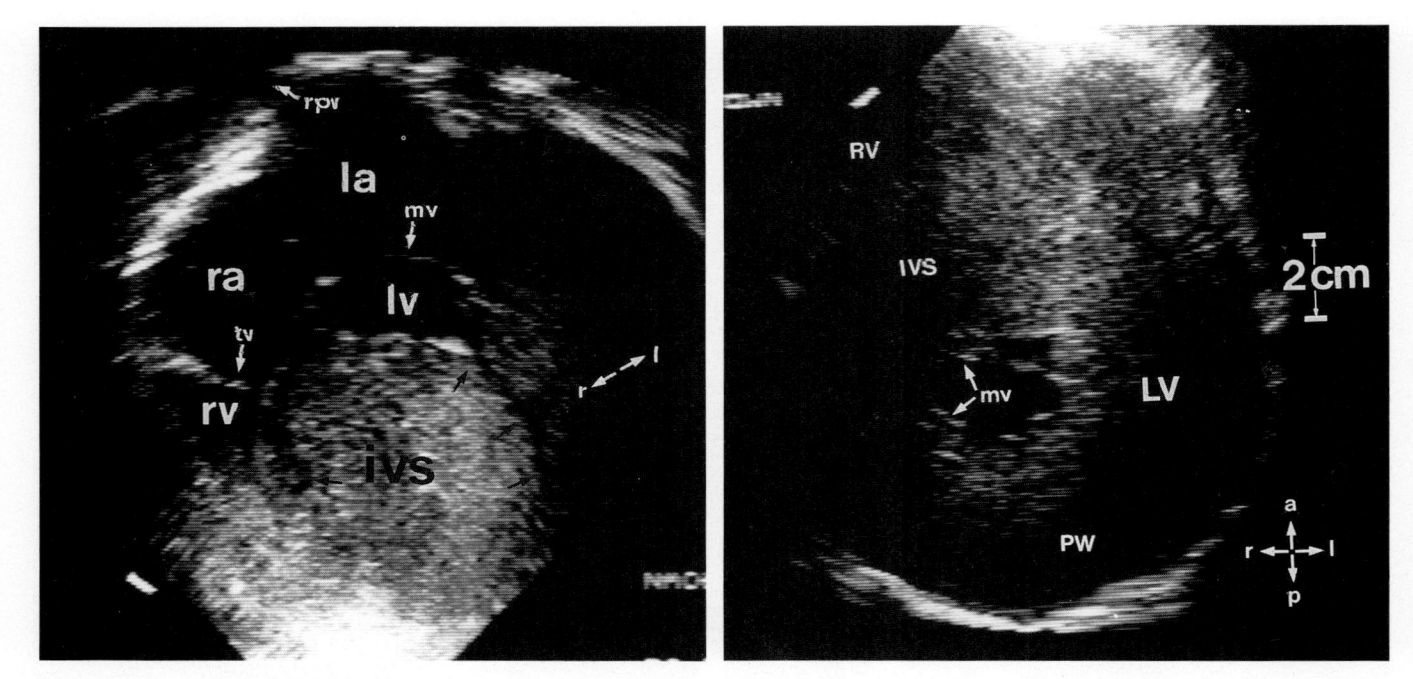

Fig. 74 Glycogen storage disease. Apical (left) and parasternal short axis (right) views in a child with gross myocardial thickening secondary to a glycogen storage disorder. ivs – inter-ventricular septum, rpv – right pulmonary vein, PW – left ventricular posterior wall.

by dilatation of the coronary artery which has the abnormal communication. The sites of origin of the coronary arteries from the aorta are important in the assessment for an arterial switch operation in cases of transposition of the great arteries. The coronary artery origins are usually from the aortic sinuses which face the pulmonary trunk (Fig. 70). Where there is a single coronary artery origin or the origins are immediately adjacent, the surgical transfer of the coronary arteries may be far more difficult. Coronary artery anatomy may also modify surgical strategy in other situations. In the tetralogy of Fallot,[21] demonstration that a major coronary artery passes across the right ventricular outflow tract is a relative contra-indication to complete repair in infancy, as a right ventricle to pulmonary artery conduit may be required to avoid division of the abnormally located coronary artery.

Acquired coronary artery dilatation and aneurysm formation is characteristic of Kawasaki disease (Figs 71 and 73) and may result in myocardial infarction. Echocardiographic diagnosis and serial monitoring of these lesions is now standard practice to provide a guide for therapy.

Acquired abnormalities

Acquired abnormalities may be apparent at any stage of the structured examination. Heart muscle abnormalities in childhood are uncommon. As in adults, dilated cardiomyopathy may be the result of viral myocarditis or drug toxicity, such as occurs with Adriamycin, but it is usually

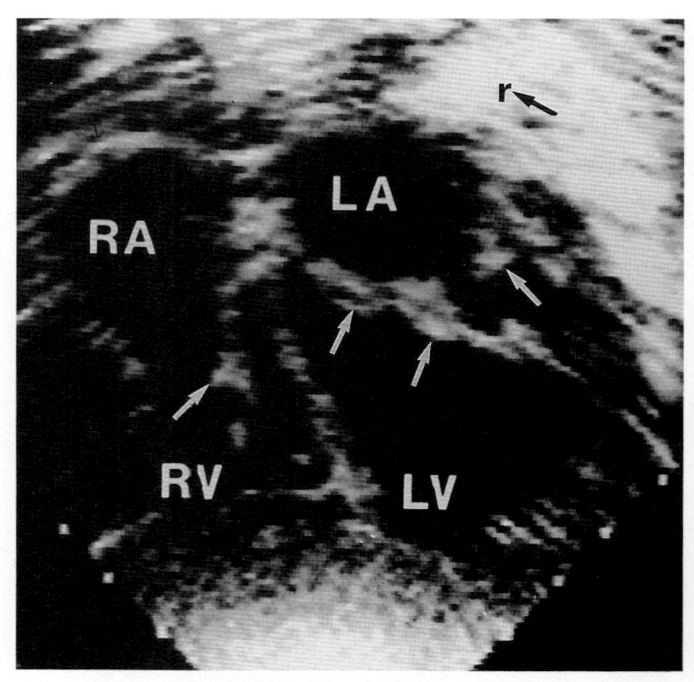

Fig. 75 Mucopolysaccharidosis. Apical view demonstrating nodular thickening (arrows) of the mitral and tricuspid valves in a child with a mucopolysaccharidosis.

idiopathic. However, 'thick walled' myocardium, with or without cavity enlargement, has a very wide range of possible causes more specific to infancy and childhood. Many

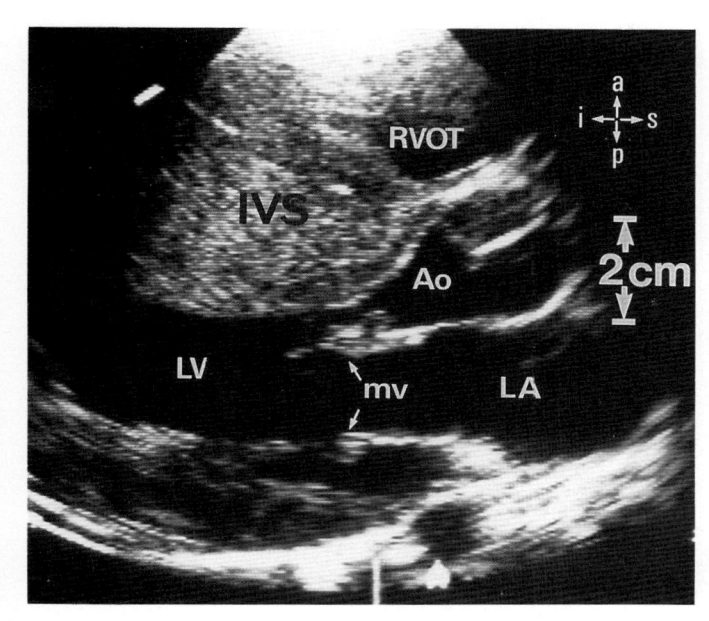

Fig. 76 Parasternal long axis view – child with hypertrophic cardiomyopathy. The septum (IVS) is more affected than the posterior wall. RVOT – right ventricular outflow tract.

of these have not been completely characterised. Storage disorders such as the mucopolysaccharidoses or glycogen storage disorders may result in myocardial deposition (Fig. 74), as may various abnormalities of energy utilisation such as 'carnitine deficiency'. Mucopolysaccharidoses may also result in nodular valvular thickening (Fig. 75). Infants of diabetic mothers typically have myocardial hypertrophy at birth with subsequent regression of the abnormal appearance. Noonan's syndrome may also result in myocardial hypertrophy (Fig. 76). Multiple intramyocardial tumours (rhabdomyomata) are typically associated with tuberous sclerosis (Fig. 77) and may be the only sign of the disorder.[22] Diffuse infiltration of the myocardium may result from malignant neoplasia (Fig. 78). Rarely, tumours at distant sites may present with cardiac manifestations in children. Intravascular extension of Wilms' tumour within the inferior caval vein into the cavity of the heart can cause obstruction to tricuspid valve flow (Fig. 79). Extrinsic compression of the heart may occur (Fig. 80). Arteriovenous malformations may result in high cardiac output with consequent enlargement of all cardiac chambers and features of 'heart failure'.

Vegetations (Fig. 81) or abscess formation (Fig. 82) may confirm infective endocarditis which is increasingly recognised in 'native' or surgically modified congenital heart disease. Intracardiac thrombus can occur at the tip of a central venous catheter or ventriculo-atrial shunt (inserted to relieve hydrocephalus) or on the endocardium of a dilated hypokinetic ventricle. Both vegetations and

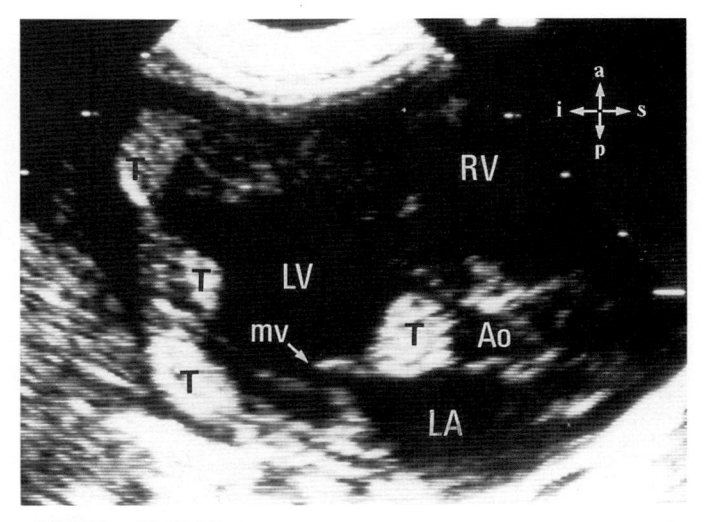

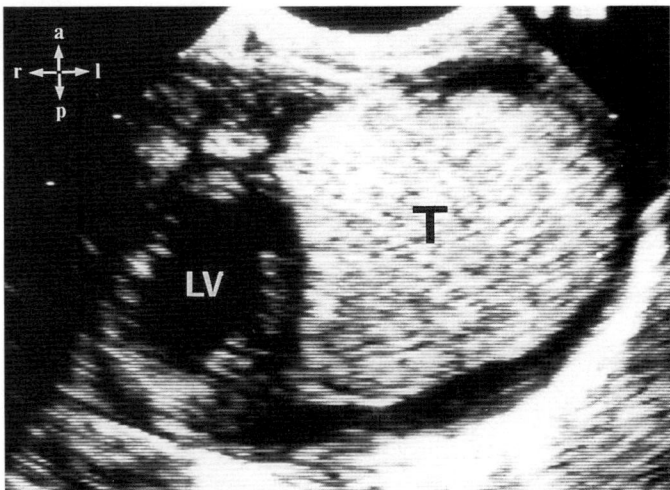

Fig. 77 Myocardial tumours. Apical long axis (top) and parasternal short axis (lower) in a neonate with multiple intramyocardial tumours (T), including a massive tumour mass arising in the left ventricular lateral wall.

thrombus are potential sources of emboli and this may determine their clinical presentation.

Extracardiac abnormalities may be apparent during systematic echocardiographic scanning. Renal abnormalities or abdominal cysts may be diagnosed (Fig. 83), while imaging the great vessels in the abdomen. Ascites may also be apparent. The visualisation of pleural fluid (Fig. 84) and assessment of suspected diaphragmatic palsy can be performed from a subcostal position. In both instances this information is often relevant early after cardiac surgery. Pericardial fluid is readily recognised (Fig. 85). Effusions with an infective or malignant aetiology often have tissue debris within the pericardial cavity. Purulent pericarditis may result in an organised effusion. This should not be

CARDIAC ULTRASOUND

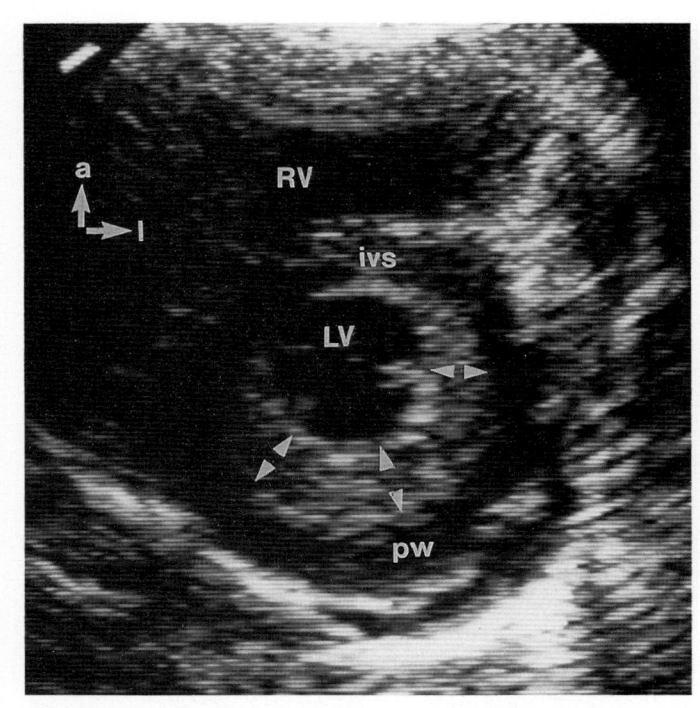

Fig. 78 Parasternal short axis view – eosinophilic infiltration in a crescentic fashion (delineated by arrowheads) which resulted in mitral regurgitation. ivs – inter-ventricular septum, pw – posterior left ventricular wall.

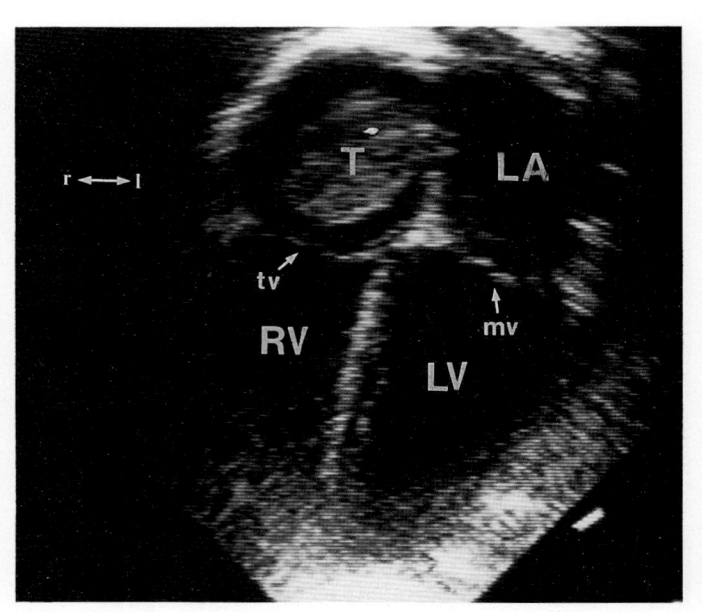

Fig. 79 Apical four chamber view – intravascular extension of Wilms' tumour (T) occupying the right atrium.

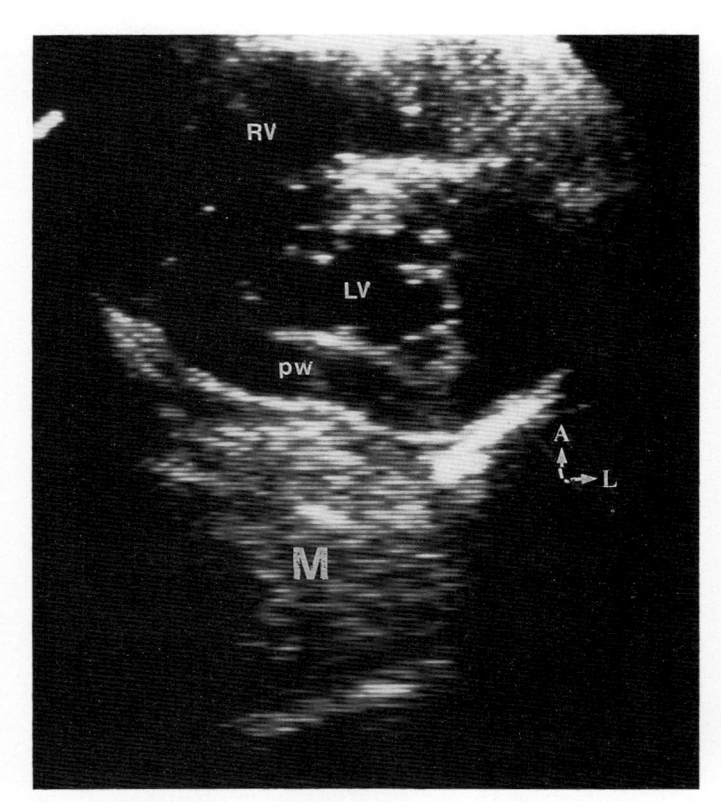

Fig. 80 Modified parasternal short axis view – mediastinal tumour (M) causing extrinsic compression of the heart. pw – posterior left ventricular wall.

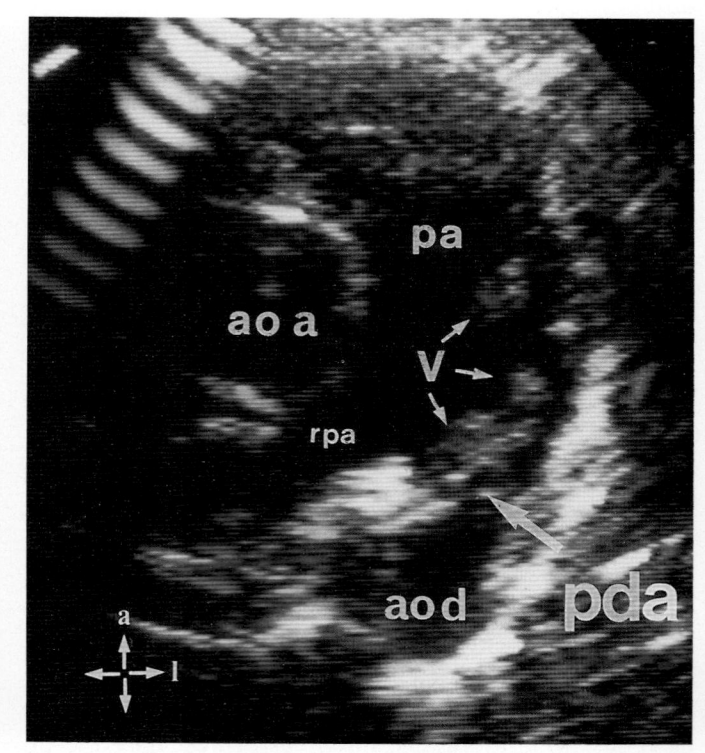

Fig. 81 Modified parasternal short axis view – vegetations (V) in the pulmonary trunk of a patient with a persistent arterial duct and a left to right shunt. aoa – ascending aorta, aod – descending aorta, rpa – right pulmonary artery, pda – arterial duct.

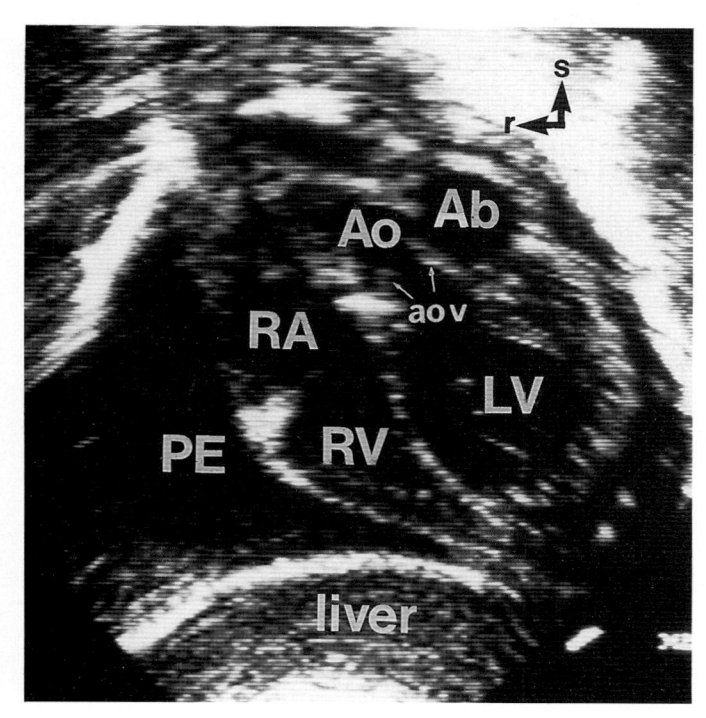

Fig. 82 Subcostal paracoronal view – **aortic root abscess** (Ab) in a patient with congenital aortic stenosis. Ao – aorta, aov – aortic valve, PE – pericardial effusion.

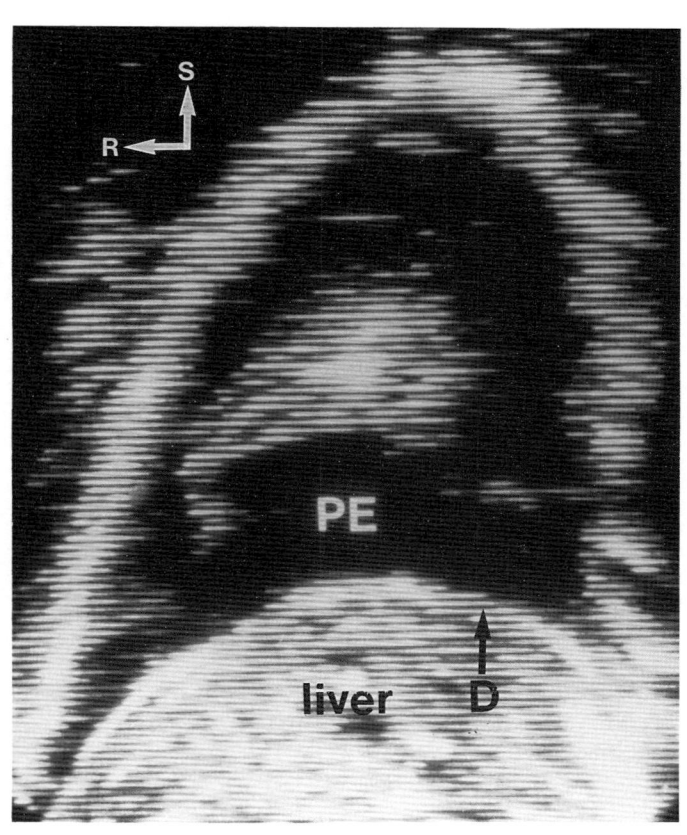

Fig. 84 **Pleural effusion**. Subcostal paracoronal view demonstrating a large right pleural effusion (PE) in an infant. D – diaphragm.

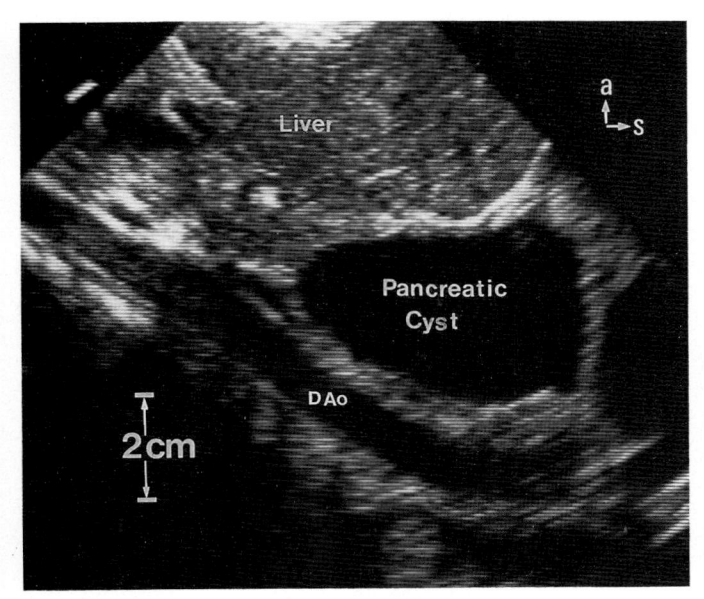

Fig. 83 **Pancreatic cyst**. Abdominal long axis view in a child who presented with pericardial effusion, demonstrating a large pancreatic cyst. DAo – descending aorta.

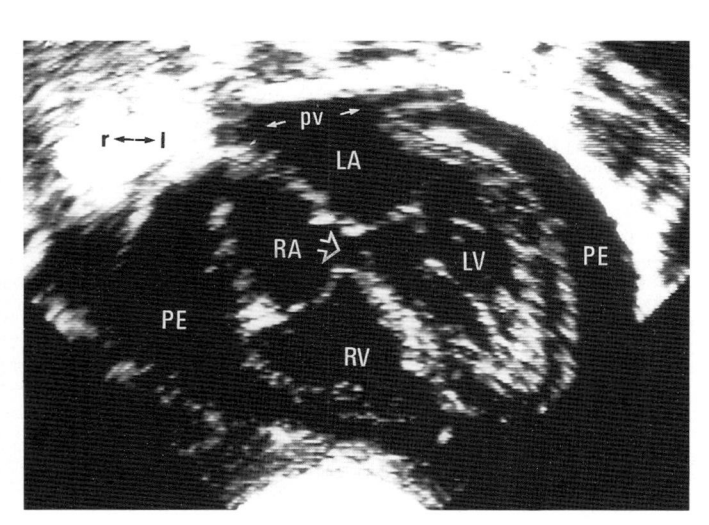

Fig. 85 Subcostal oblique four chamber view – **pericardial effusion** (PE). The muscular atrioventricular septum (open arrow) is well-demonstrated in this heart. pv – pulmonary veins.

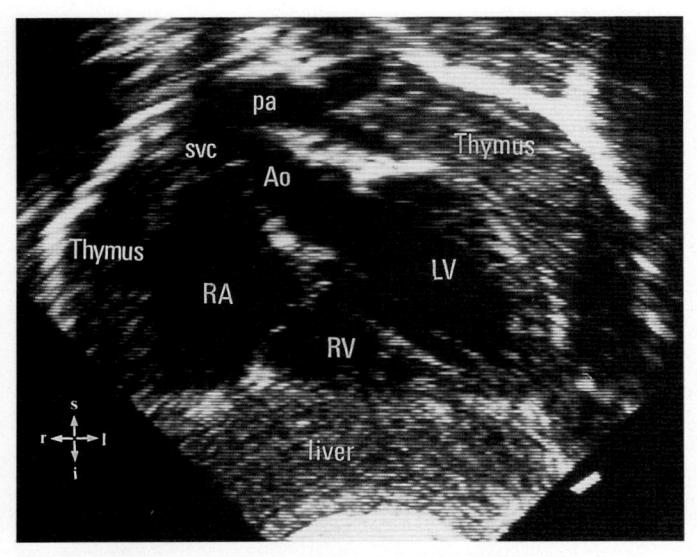

Fig. 86 Thymus. Subcostal paracoronal view with the transducer angled anteriorly shows thymic tissue extending unusually inferiorly.

confused with an unusually inferior extension of the thymus gland (Fig. 86).

Conclusion

The sequential segmental approach to the anatomic description of the heart provides a convenient framework for the description of congenital abnormalities.

While haemodynamic information may often be inferred from the structural images, associated developments in Doppler echocardiography have allowed accurate quantification of volumetric flow and pressure drops using pulsed and continuous wave Doppler velocimetry and colour flow mapping provides a valuable, largely qualitative, adjunct to flow assessment. The combination of detailed cross-sectional and Doppler echocardiographic assessment, with complementary diagnostic or interventional catheterisation procedures, provides an integrated approach to management throughout childhood.

REFERENCES

1 Anderson R H, Macartney F J, Shinebourne E A, Tynan M. eds. Terminology. In: Paediatric cardiology. Edinburgh: Churchill Livingstone. 1987: p 65–82
2 Smallhorn J, Rigby M L, Deanfield J E. Echocardiography. In: Anderson R H, Macartney F J, Shinebourne E A, Tynan M. eds. Paediatric cardiology. Edinburgh: Churchill Livingstone. 1987: p 319–349
3 Koike K, Musewe N N, Smallhorn J F, Freedom R M. Distinguishing between anomalous origin of the left coronary artery from the pulmonary trunk and dilated cardiomyopathy: role of echocardiographic measurement of the right coronary artery diameter. Br Heart J 1989; 61: 192–197
4 Henry W L, DeMaria A, Gramiak R, et al. Report of the American Society of Echocardiography Committee on nomenclature and standards in two-dimensional echocardiography. Circulation 1980; 62: 212–217
5 Gutgesell H P. Cardiac imaging with ultrasound: rightside up or upside down? Am J Cardiol 1985; 56: 479–480
6 Allen H D, Goldberg S J, Donnerstein R L, Marx G R. The normal cardiac ultrasonic examination. In: Moller J H, Neal W A. eds. Fetal, neonatal and infant cardiac disease. Norwalk: Appleton and Lange. 1990: p 261–291
7 Huhta J C, Smallhorn J F, Macartney F J. Two dimensional echocardiographic diagnosis of situs. Br Heart J 1982; 48: 97–108
8 Sapire D W, Ho S Y, Anderson R H, Rigby M L. Diagnosis and significance of atrial isomerism. Am J Cardiol 1986; 58: 342–346
9 Sapire D W. Atrial Isomerism. In: Anderson R H, Macartney F J, Shinebourne E A, Tynan M. eds. Paediatric cardiology. Edinburgh: Churchill Livingstone. 1987: p 473–496
10 de Leval M R, Kilner P, Gewillig M, Bull C. Total cavopulmonary connection: a logical alternative to atriopulmonary connection for complex Fontan operations. J Thorac Cardiovasc Surg 1988; 96: 682–695
11 Humes R A, Feldt R H, Porter C J, Julsrud P R, Puga F J, Danielson G K. The modified Fontan operation for asplenia and polysplenia syndromes. J Thorac Cardiovasc Surg 1988; 96: 212–218
12 Van Praagh R, Takao A. eds. Etiology and morphogenesis of congenital heart disease. Mount Kisco, New York: Futura Publishing. 1980
13 Griffin M L, Sullivan I D, Anderson R H, Macartney F J. Doubly committed subarterial ventricular septal defect: new morphological criteria with echocardiographic and angiographic correlation. Br Heart J 1988; 59: 474–479
14 Macartney F J, Rigby M L, Anderson R H, Stark J, Silverman N H. Double outlet right ventricle. Cross sectional echocardiographic findings, their anatomic explanation, and surgical relevance. Br Heart J 1984; 52: 167–177
15 Mortera C, Rissech M, Payola M, Miro C, Perich R. Cross sectional subcostal echocardiography: atrioventricular septal defects and the short axis cut. Br Heart J 1987; 58: 267–273
16 Baker E J, Leung M P, Anderson R H, Fischer D R, Zuberbuhler J R. The cross sectional anatomy of ventricular septal defects; a reappraisal. Br Heart J 1988; 59: 339–351
17 Ramaciotti C, Keren A, Silverman N H. Importance of (perimembranous) ventricular septal aneurysm in the natural history of isolated perimembranous ventricular septal defect. Am J Cardiol 1986; 57: 268–272
18 Huhta J C, Gutgesell H P, Latson L A, Huffines F D. Two-dimensional echocardiographic assessment of the aorta in infants and children with congenital heart disease. Circulation 1984; 70: 417–424
19 Smallhorn J F, Huhta J C, Adams P A, Anderson R H, Wilkinson J L, Macartney F J. Cross-sectional echocardiographic assessment of coarctation in the sick neonate and infant. Br Heart J 1983; 50: 349–361
20 Robinson P J, Sullivan I D, Kumpeng V, Anderson R H, Macartney F J. Anomalous origin of the left coronary artery from the pulmonary trunk. Br Heart J 1984; 52: 272–277
21 Jureidini S B, Appleton R S, Nouri S, Crawford C. Detection of coronary artery abnormalities in tetralogy of Fallot by two-dimensional echocardiography. JACC 1989; 14: 960–967
22 Smith H C, Watson G H, Patel R G, Super M. Cardiac rhabdomyomata in tuberous sclerosis: their course and diagnostic value. Arch Dis Child 1989; 69: 196–200

20

Left to right shunts

The atrial septum
The normal atrial septum
Atrial septal defect
Volume overload of the right heart and its differential diagnosis
Foramen ovale defect (secundum atrial septal defect)
Sinus venosus defect
Coronary sinus defect
Iatrogenic defects in the atrial septum
Transoesophageal echocardiography
Associated abnormalities
Postoperative appearances
Assessing shunt size
Atrioventricular septal defect
Atrioventricular junction abnormalities
Ventricular abnormalities
Haemodynamics
Associated abnormalities
Postoperative echocardiography
Estimation of shunt size and pulmonary artery pressure

Ventricular septal defect
Perimembranous defects
Muscular defects
Inlet muscular defects
Muscular defects in the midportion and apical region of the septum
Muscular outlet defects
Subaortic defects
Subpulmonary and doubly committed defects
Use of colour flow mapping in ventricular septal defect
Quantitative aspects of ventricular septal defects
Measurement of left to right shunt
Estimation of pulmonary artery pressure

Patent ductus arteriosus
Suprasternal long axis imaging
Left parasternal short axis imaging
Subcostal imaging
Doppler examination in patent ductus arteriosus
Quantifying the left to right shunt
Estimation of pulmonary artery pressure
Truncus arteriosus (common arterial truck)
Associated abnormalities
Differential diagnosis
Postoperative findings
Aortopulmonary window

John L. Gibbs and Neil Wilson

INTRODUCTION

The ultrasound findings of shunting at atrial, ventricular and arterial levels will be discussed in this chapter. It is useful to also consider echocardiographic abnormalities which may occur secondary to abnormal haemodynamics produced by shunts at various levels as these abnormalities will often provide the first clues to detailed ultrasound diagnosis. Individual abnormalities will be discussed separately in detail, but it must be emphasised that the ultrasound assessment of these defects should form just part of the overall process of sequential segmental analysis of congenital heart disease (see Ch. 19).[1-3]

THE ATRIAL SEPTUM

The atrial septum, because of the plane in which it lies, may not be seen clearly in standard precordial views.[4] The subcostal window, however, allows the septum to be imaged in its entirety in the majority of children and adults[5] (Fig. 1) and in rare cases where difficulties persist, imaging from the right sternal edge is useful.[6] Precordial views may be of some value in imaging the septum, but their real value lies in detecting abnormalities which occur secondary to left to right shunting.

A basic understanding of the anatomy of the various defects generally thought of as atrial septal defects is essential for the understanding of the ultrasound investigation of the defects. Defects may occur in any part of the atrial septum, they may be single or multiple or the septum may be absent. The commonest defect in the atrial septum (the 'secundum' defect) occurs within the oval foramen and is nowadays usually referred to as an oval foramen defect. Sinus venosus defects, commonly referred to as atrial septal defects, are not true defects of the atrial septum as they arise from developmental abnormalities of the venous sinus rather than the septum itself. Rarely, defects may occur in the coronary sinus roof (separating the lumen of the coronary sinus from the left atrium), resulting in interatrial shunting through the ostium of the coronary sinus. These defects are also usually included under the heading of atrial septal defects despite the lack of an actual defect in the septum. The so-called 'primum' atrial septal defect is a defect in the atrioventricular septum rather than the atrial septum and will be discussed with atrioventricular defects.

Thorough examination of the atrial septum including its surrounding structures is thus essential if accurate anatomical diagnosis is to be achieved and this is particularly important if surgical treatment is to be planned on the results of investigation by ultrasound alone.

The normal atrial septum

The oval foramen, situated in the central part of the atrial septum, is a thin structure which may remain anatomically patent for many years. The haemodynamic competence of the normal flap valve of the foramen, particularly in neonatal life, depends upon the relationship between right and left atrial pressure. Shunting may therefore occur in either direction across the septum in the absence of an actual anatomical defect in it. The shape of the atrial septum may provide useful clues to atrial pressure changes occurring in the newborn.[7]

The normal atrial septum in the neonate may show slight bulging from left to right in the first hours after birth when right heart pressures have yet to fall. When markedly elevated right atrial pressure is present (for instance in persistent pulmonary hypertension of the newborn) the septum, particularly in its central part, is seen to bulge from right to left (Fig. 2), usually reflecting the presence of right to left shunting across the foramen. Serial echocardiographic assessment of the shape of the septum may thus be useful in assessing the fall in right heart pressures associated with recovery from persistent fetal circulation.

The oval foramen remains very thin even into adult life. It is therefore less reflective of ultrasound than the remainder of the atrial septum and is difficult to image, sometimes appearing absent when it is not.[4,8] Such false positive diagnosis of a defect in this part of the septum is most likely to occur when the septum is imaged parallel to its long axis, for instance in an apical four chamber view. This error is least likely to occur when the ultrasound beam is at right angles to the septum, for instance in a subcostal view.[5] The delicate nature of the normal foramen is particularly well appreciated when it is imaged using transoesophageal echocardiography.

Doppler ultrasound is invaluable in the assessment of atrial shunting[9,10] and is of particular help in cases where

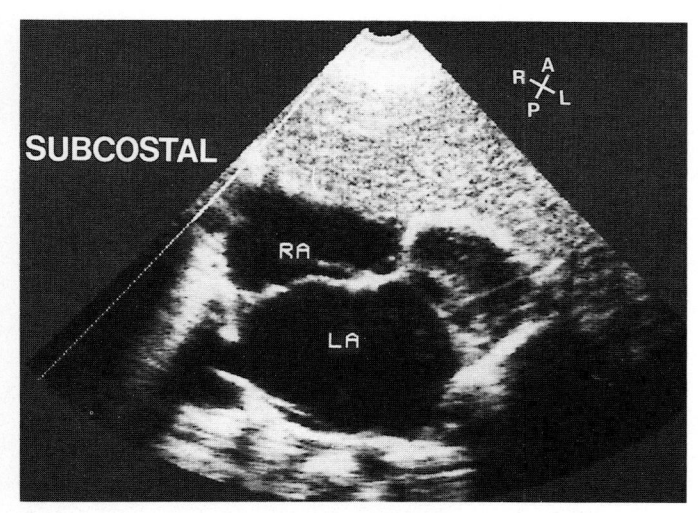

Fig. 1 The atrial septum is best imaged from the subcostal approach, when it may usually be seen in its full length and the anatomy of both atria and venous connections may also be appreciated. The central part of the normal atrial septum (the oval fossa) appears thinner than the remainder of the septum.

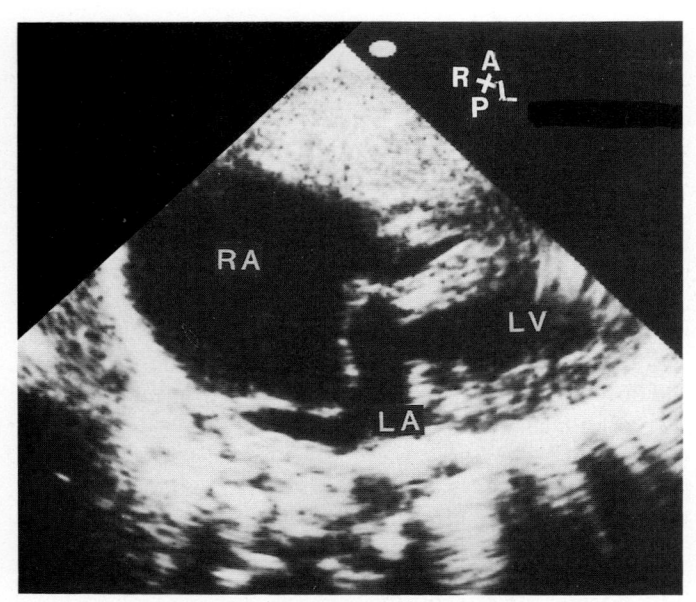

Fig. 2 The shape of the intact atrial septum may often give useful indirect evidence of the relationship between right and left atrial pressures. In this case the right atrial pressure is high and on this subcostal view there is marked bowing of the oval fossa into the left atrium. This finding will often be associated with right to left atrial shunting and is commonly seen in severe forms of persistent fetal circulation in the neonate.

the integrity of the septum cannot be confirmed by imaging alone. The sensitivity of Doppler ultrasound may, however, cause some confusion as a minor degree of left to right shunting across the oval foramen may be detected in a substantial number of babies who do not have defects in the foramen[11] (Plates 1A and 1B).

This is particularly common in premature babies with a patent arterial duct.[12] Furthermore, the velocity waveforms detectable in such cases may be indistinguishable from those seen in the presence of an atrial septal defect.[11,12] It may therefore be extremely difficult at times to differentiate between a small defect in the septum and normal neonatal atrial shunting across the foramen.[11] Colour flow Doppler mapping is often of considerable help in these circumstances,[13] when only a very small volume jet with a very narrow origin at the foramen is identifiable and there is no apparent defect in the septum. Single gate pulsed Doppler interrogation of the atrial septum must be performed alongside very careful cross-sectional imaging, as flow patterns very similar to those seen with atrial shunting may be due to normal coronary sinus or superior caval vein flow (Fig. 3). Again, colour flow imaging will usually allow the exact origin of flow to be determined,[14,15] thus avoiding false positive diagnosis of atrial shunting.

ATRIAL SEPTAL DEFECT

Volume overload of the right heart and its differential diagnosis

The first clue on cross-sectional echocardiography to the presence of left to right atrial shunting is the detection of abnormalities which arise as a result of volume overload of the right side of the heart, namely dilatation of the right ventricle and pulmonary artery[16–19] (Fig. 4) and paradoxical or reversed motion of the ventricular septum[17,20] (Fig. 5). The degree of right ventricular dilatation is related to the degree of volume loading of the ventricle and therefore to the size of the shunt,[19,20] but this serves as only a very crude means of assessing shunt size.

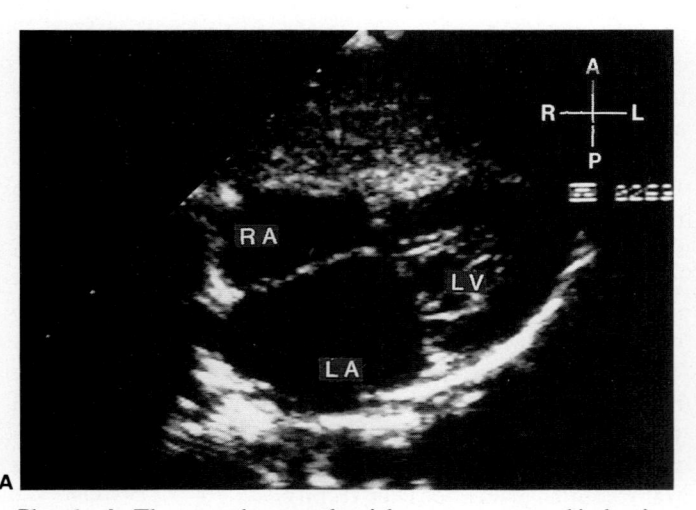

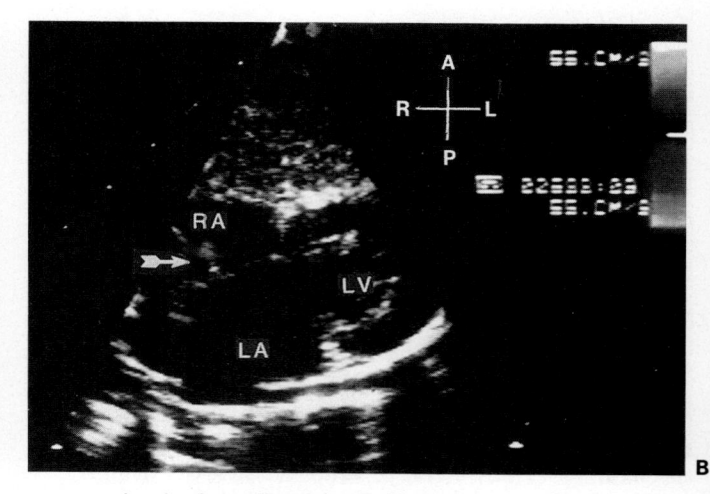

Plate 1 A: The normal neonatal atrial septum appears thin but intact on cross-sectional echocardiography. B: However, colour flow mapping will show a small left to right shunt (arrowed) across the foramen in a high percentage of normal babies and should be regarded as a normal finding. This figure is reproduced in colour in the colour plate section at the front of this volume.

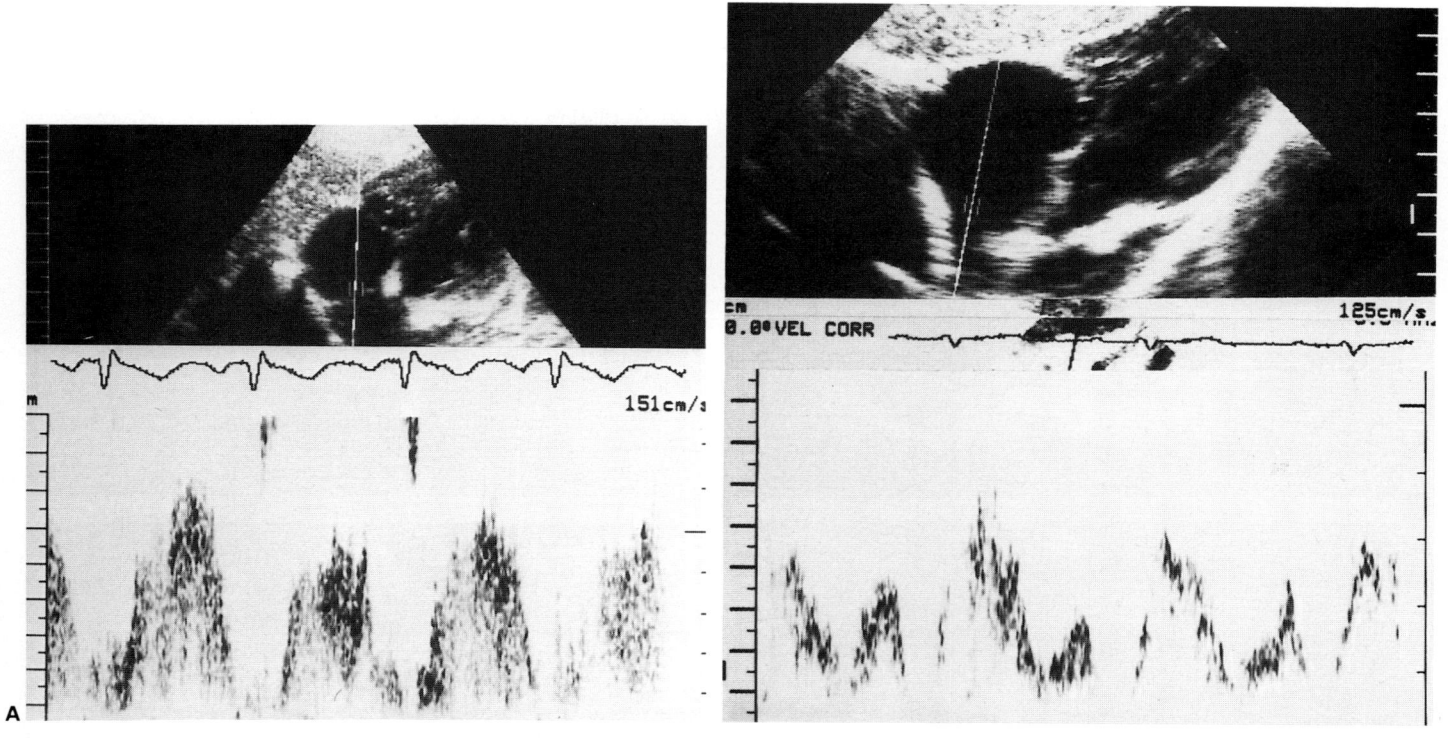

Fig. 3 A: Pulsed Doppler recording of left to right atrial shunting from a subcostal transducer position with the sample volume sited on the right side of the oval fossa. This appearance is commonly seen in the normal neonate without a true defect in the atrial septum. B: With only slight angulation of the transducer, superior caval vein flow into the right atrium is detected. These waveforms may be very easily confused with left to right atrial shunting and care has to be taken in older children and adults not to misinterpret normal superior caval vein flow as an atrial shunt.

Similarly, flow velocities across the tricuspid and pulmonary valves are usually elevated due to the increased flow across these valves (Fig. 6),[21] corresponding to the well known auscultatory findings of tricuspid and pulmonary flow murmurs. Flow velocities across the tricuspid valve may be elevated to as much as two or three times the normal, and flow velocities across the pulmonary valve may be as high as 3 m/s or more, mimicking the Doppler findings in mild pulmonary valve stenosis. The exclusion of pulmonary stenosis may sometimes be difficult in these circumstances, but it is usually possible by careful cross-sectional echocardiography of the pulmonary valve and by measuring right ventricular outflow tract velocities. The latter will be elevated in the presence of an atrial septal shunt but will be normal with pulmonary valve stenosis.

The echocardiographic abnormalities associated with right ventricular volume overload are, of course, not specific to left to right shunting at atrial level. The differential diagnosis of right ventricular dilatation includes volume loading due to other defects such as anomalous pulmonary venous drainage,[16,22] tricuspid regurgitation,[16] pulmonary regurgitation, coronary artery fistula to the right atrium, and peripheral or intracranial arteriovenous malformation.[23,24] The clinical and echocardiographic findings associated with a large left to right shunt through an arteriovenous malformation may so closely mimic those of atrial septal defect that the true diagnosis may only be suspected after atrial septal defect has been firmly excluded. Moving the transducer from the precordium to the anterior fontanelle may reveal the cause of the shunt.[24] Right ventricular dilatation may also be seen with left ventricular outflow obstruction (particularly aortic arch obstruction) in the neonate, with right ventricular cardiomyopathy[25] or with congenital parchment right ventricle (Uhl's anomaly).[26]

Paradoxical septal motion is best recorded using M-mode echocardiography from the left parasternal position. Although most commonly seen with right ventricular volume overload, it may be due to other causes. It is frequently seen transiently after cardiopulmonary bypass operations in adults,[27–29] with bundle branch block (usually left)[30] or with right ventricular pacing,[30–32] and after nonsurgical closure of the arterial duct.[33] Abnormal but not reversed motion may be seen after myocardial infarction[34] or with dilated cardiomyopathy[35] in adults. Conversely, ventricular septal motion will occasionally be normal even in the presence of a large atrial septal defect.[16,17,36] The term paradoxical is probably a misnomer for this pheno-

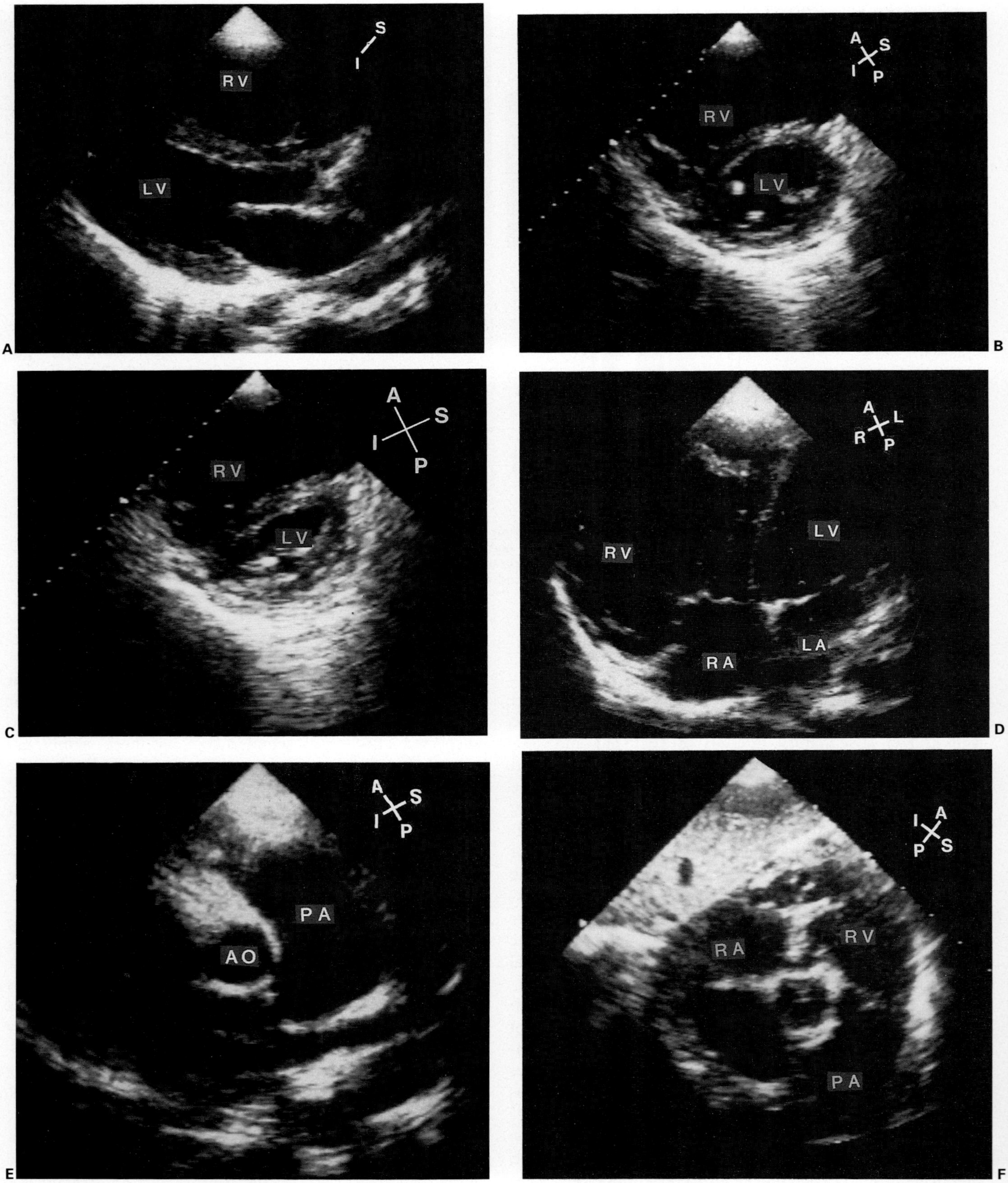
S
I
RV
LV
A
A
S
I
P
RV
LV
B
A
S
I
P
RV
LV
C
A
L
R
P
LV
RV
LA
RA
D
A
S
I
P
PA
AO
E
I
A
P
S
RA
RV
PA
F

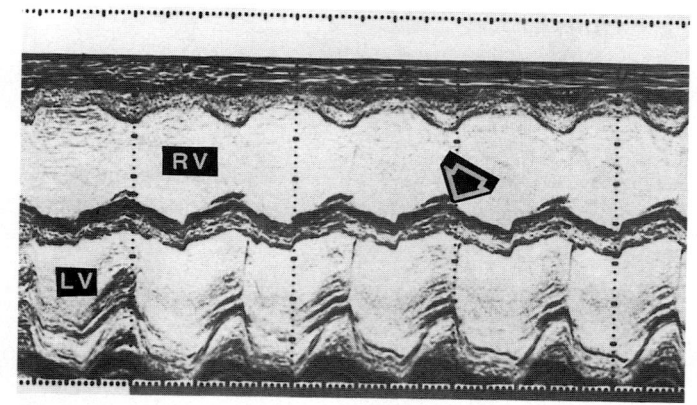

Fig. 5 Paradoxical septal motion. This M-mode appearance, recorded from a left parasternal transducer position, is a misnomer. The ventricular septum appears to move anteriorly in systole (arrowed). It is due to the change in shape of the left ventricle from diastole to systole (shown in Fig. 4B and 4C). It is not a specific indicator of right ventricular volume overload in itself.

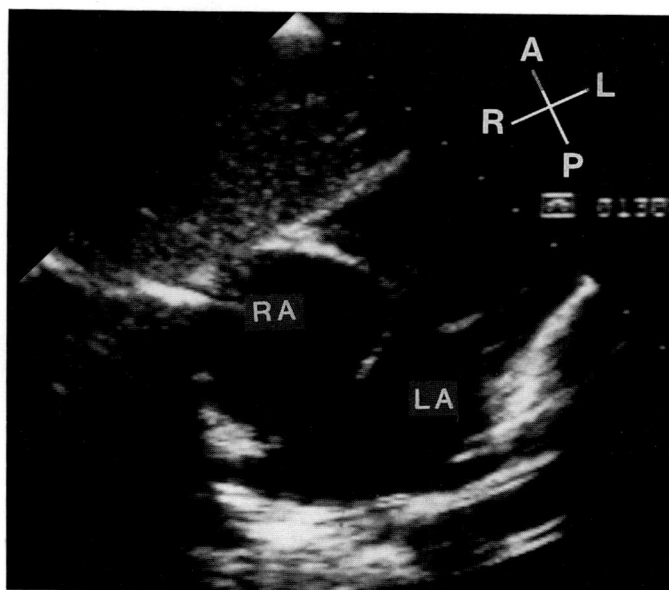

Fig. 7 A large oval fossa defect (secundum atrial septal defect) seen from the subcostal approach. Large single defects such as this are usually easily seen.

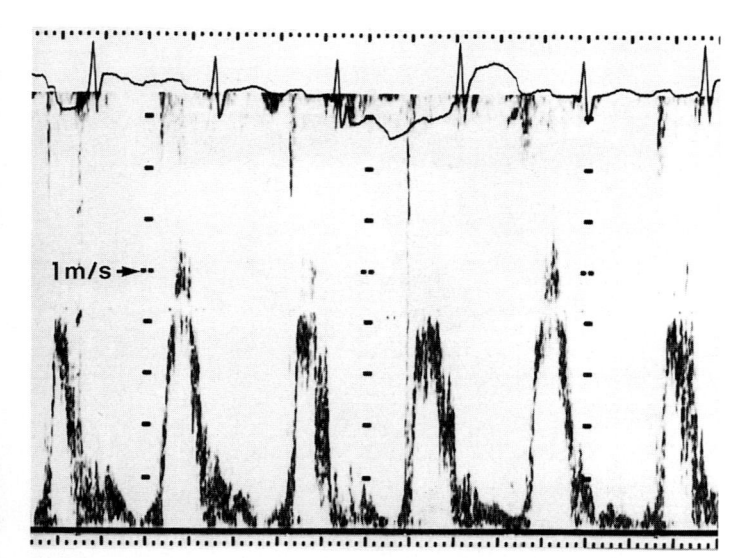

Fig. 6 High flow velocities across the tricuspid valve occur in the presence of significant left to right atrial shunting. In this example peak flow velocity across the tricuspid valve exceeds 1 m/s, well above the upper limit of normal.

Fig. 4 (opposite) Volume loading of the right side of the heart. A: In long axis parasternal view the right ventricle is seen to be dilated. In short axis parasternal view the right ventricular dilatation is again appreciated both **B:** during systole and **C:** diastole. In diastole the left ventricle appears oval in shape, returning to its normal circular cross-sectional appearance in systole. These changes in shape are largely responsible for the M-mode echo appearance of paradoxical motion of the ventricular septum associated with volume loading of the right ventricle. **D:** In the apical four chamber view, the right ventricular dilatation may distort the usual appearance of the left side of the heart and in particular may make the left ventricular shape appear abnormal. Views of the pulmonary artery from either **E:** the short axis parasternal view or **F:** the subcostal view will reveal dilatation of the pulmonary trunk which is best appreciated by comparison of the diameter of the pulmonary trunk with that of the aortic root seen in the same view.

menon; when it is seen postoperatively, detailed study has shown that ventricular septal motion is actually normal in relation to the posterior left ventricular wall, the apparent systolic anterior motion of the ventricular septum being due to exaggerated anterior motion of the whole left ventricle made possible by the loss of integrity of the pericardial sac.[27–29,37] It seems likely that a similar exaggerated movement of the left ventricle might also be made possible by right ventricular dilatation due to volume overload,[38] but it appears that changes in ventricular geometry play a major role in this group of patients, with the left ventricle losing its normal circular shape in diastole (and becoming oval in cross section), regaining its circular shape in systole[39–42] (see Fig. 4B and C).

Foramen ovale defect (secundum atrial septal defect)

Single, large defects in the oval foramen are usually easily detectable by cross-sectional echocardiography alone[4,5,43] (Fig. 7). However, small defects or multiple perforations[43] may be more difficult to detect (Plate 2). Particular difficulties arise in the presence of an aneurysm of the atrial septum (Fig. 8A, B, C, and Plate 3), which may or may not be fenestrated.[44,45] Signs of right heart volume overload on both M-mode and cross-sectional echocardiography will provide a useful pointer to the presence of a significant left to right shunt if present.[45] Aneurysms of the atrial septum usually involve the oval foramen. They may sometimes appear as large saccular structures within the right atrium and should not be mistaken for remnants of the venous

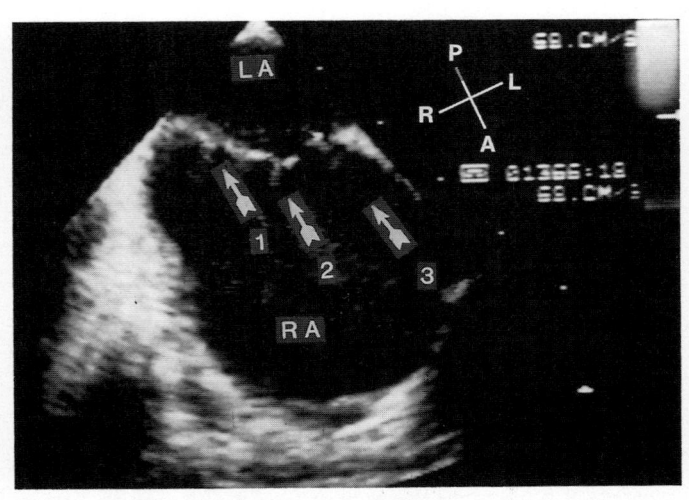

Plate 2 Multiple tiny holes are present in the oval fossa. The septum appears to be intact even with transoesophageal imaging, colour flow Doppler mapping is required to demonstrate the multiple jets across the septum (arrowed). This figure is reproduced in colour in the colour plate section at the front of this volume.

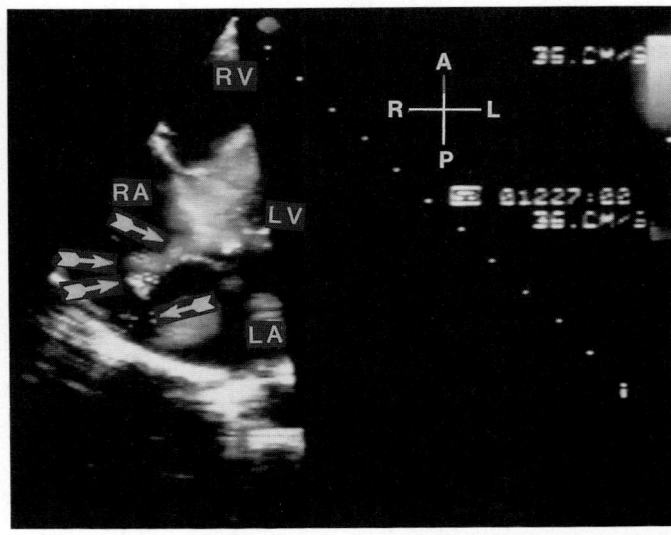

Plate 3 The same case as shown in Fig. 8. Colour flow Doppler mapping clearly reveals the presence of multiple fenestrations with left to right shunting in multiple jets (arrowed). This figure is reproduced in colour in the colour plate section at the front of this volume.

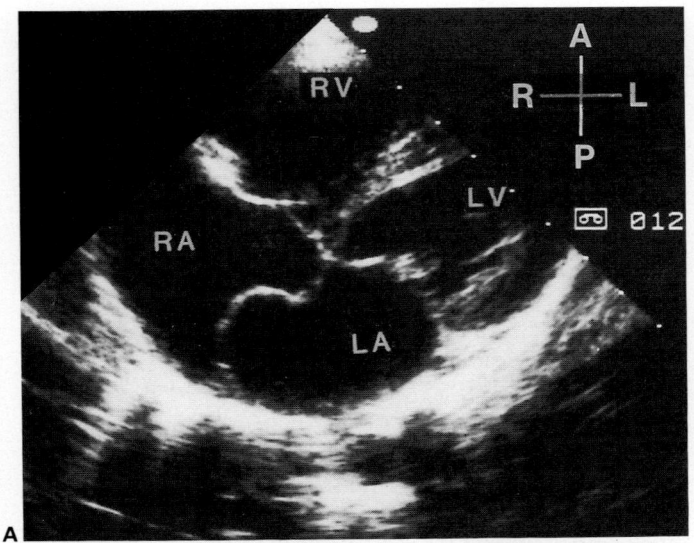

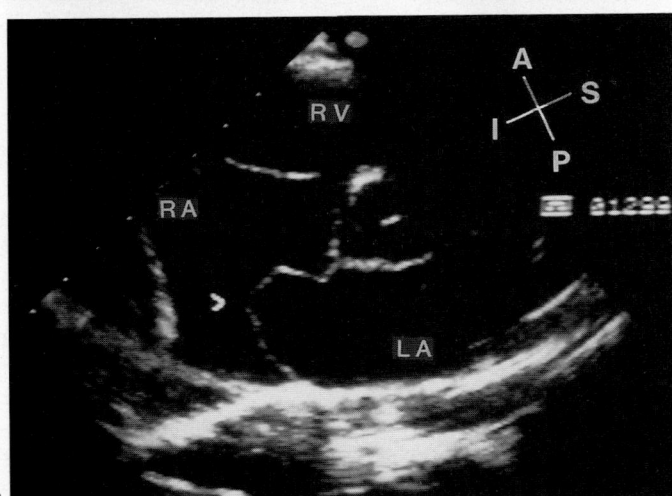

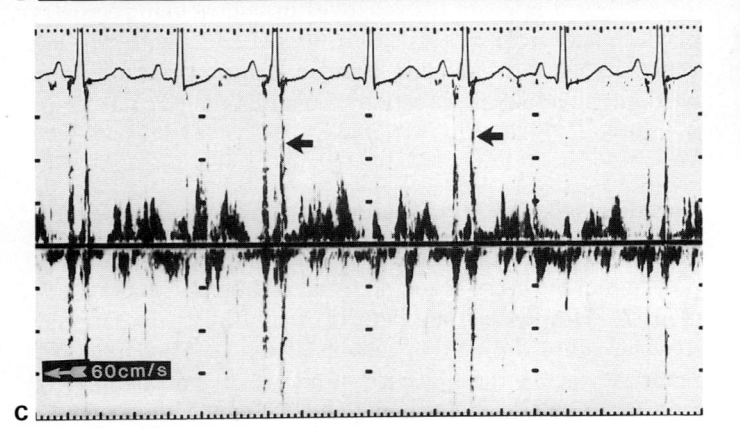

Fig. 8 Aneurysm of the atrial septum. A: Subcostal view showing the aneurysm bulging into the right atrium. **B:** In the short axis parasternal view the aneurysm is again clearly seen. In this view the appearances suggest the possibility of fenestration of the aneurysm (arrowed). The aneurysmal septum is very mobile and its motion throughout the cardiac cycle makes it very difficult to position a pulsed wave Doppler sample volume at the suspected site of shunting. **C:** The movement of the aneurysm produces motion artefact on the pulsed wave recording.

sinus (or Eustachian) valve or the Chiari network. Some remnants of these structures may be detectable in a high proportion of children and are only very rarely of any diagnostic importance.[46–48] It has been suggested that aneurysm formation around a defect in the oval foramen may contribute to spontaneous closure of atrial septal defect.[49] Spontaneous closure of secundum atrial septal defects diagnosed by both echocardiography[50] and by cardiac catheterisation[51] has been reported to occur in a surprising percentage of patients. In our experience spontaneous closure of atrial septal defects diagnosed by ultrasound and associated with signs of right heart volume overload is an exceedingly rare occurrence.

Contrast echocardiography may be useful in cases where an anatomical defect in the septum cannot be imaged but right heart volume overload is present.[52-55] When imaging quality is satisfactory, contrast studies add little if any useful information[43] and with recent improvements in imaging technology contrast injections are rarely required. The contrast used for injection does not appear to be important; blood, saline,[56] indocyanine green,[55] 5% dextrose[54] or even pure carbon dioxide[53] have all been successfully employed. The contrast effect seen after peripheral injection of these substances is due to reflection of ultrasound from microbubbles present in solution. In the presence of an atrial septal defect contrast is seen to enter the left atrium almost immediately after it reaches the right atrium, reflecting the fact that interatrial shunting is almost always bidirectional to some extent. However, contrast may be seen in the left atrium even in the presence of a very small defect and sometimes passage of contrast from right to left may even be seen with only a patent foramen.[57]

Doppler ultrasound has largely superseded contrast echocardiography in the diagnosis of interatrial shunting. Pulsed Doppler examination may confirm the site of the communication if used carefully and provides valuable information on the patterns of interatrial flow (Fig. 9). There can be no doubt however that colour flow imaging provides the quickest and most accurate means of assessing the integrity of the atrial septum[15,58] (Plate 4). It has substantial advantages because it is far less time consuming than searching for flow with single gate pulsed Doppler and because erroneous interpretation of superior caval vein or coronary sinus flow as left to right shunting is easily avoided. Colour flow imaging even allows rapid detection of small atrial shunts whose presence may not be suspected in the absence of right heart volume overload.

Sinus venosus defect

Venous sinus defects usually result in substantial left to right shunting at atrial level and are therefore almost always associated with clear echocardiographic signs of right ventricular volume overload.[59] The embryological development of these defects dictates, in the majority of cases, that one or more of the right pulmonary veins will drain anomalously to the right atrium or to the superior caval vein at its junction with the right atrium. Venous sinus defects occur at the uppermost margin of the atrial septum and may be best imaged, like atrial septal defects, using a subcostal transducer position[59,60] (Fig. 10). Care must always be taken to identify the right pulmonary veins and their site of drainage. When precordial imaging fails to demonstrate the anatomy clearly, transoesophageal imaging will usually allow clear visualisation of the defect itself, although identification of pulmonary venous drainage is rarely possible with confidence using this technique.[61]

Coronary sinus defect

Coronary sinus defect is a rare cause of interatrial shunting. Signs of right ventricular volume overload are, as might be expected, usually evident and cross-sectional echocardiography of the oval foramen will be normal unless there is a coincident defect. The clue to the site of the defect usually lies in the demonstration of a dilated coronary sinus orifice (Fig. 11) and the 'unroofing' of the coronary sinus which produces the communication between the coronary sinus and the left atrium may be directly visualised in some cases (Plate 5A, B, C, D, E).

On very rare occasions a left to right shunt through the coronary sinus may be due to a fistula between the left ventricle and the coronary sinus, when colour flow imaging is particularly useful in differentiating the high velocity jet into the coronary sinus from a mitral regurgitant jet.[62] If a shunt at atrial level is suspected and the coronary sinus is dilated but no defect in it is visible, care must be taken to exclude other causes of dilatation of the coronary sinus such as anomalous pulmonary venous drainage to the coronary sinus.[63] Persistence of the left superior caval vein or anomalous systemic venous drainage to the coronary sinus will also cause the sinus to be dilated but these abnormalities alone will not cause dilatation of the right heart.

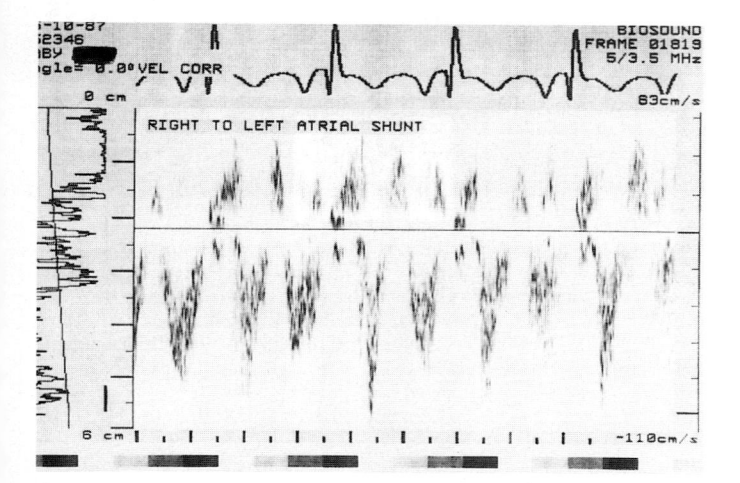

Fig. 9 Pulsed wave Doppler recording from the subcostal position showing predominant right to left atrial shunting across an atrial septal defect recorded below the zero flow baseline. The presence of a defect in the atrial septum does not necessarily imply that left to right shunting is taking place and Doppler ultrasound has an important role in establishing the haemodynamic consequences of the defect.

350 CARDIAC ULTRASOUND

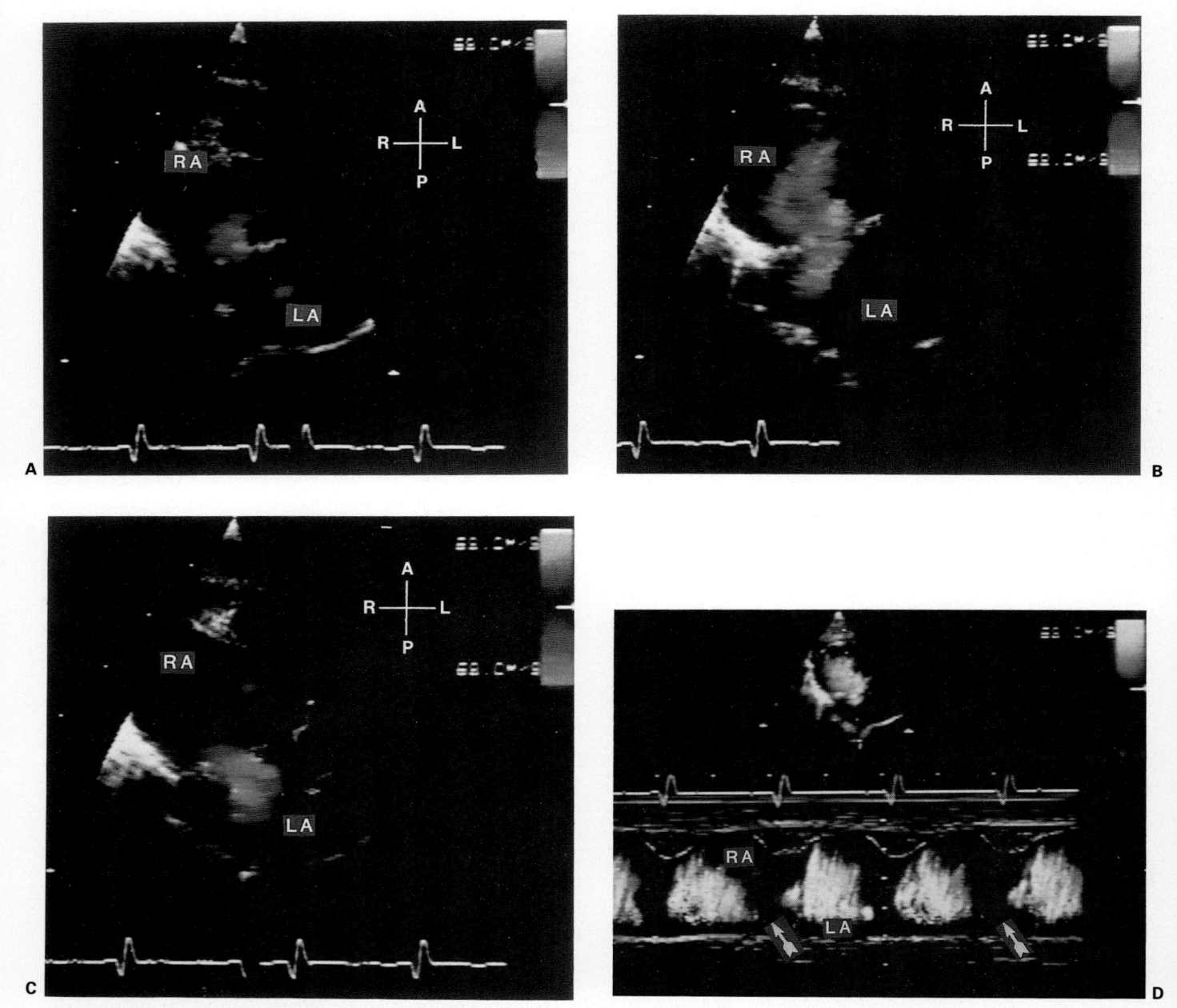

Plate 4 Frame by frame analysis of colour flow Doppler mapping reveals that patterns of interatrial shunting may be complex even in the presence of a straightforward oval fossa defect, when shunting is often bidirectional but predominantly from left to right. The shunt haemodynamics vary with both the stage of the cardiac cycle and the stage of respiration. In early diastole (on the T wave of the electrocardiogram) there is usually a small left to right shunt **A**, which increases during the phases of ventricular filling **B. C:** At the onset of systole, however, the shunt direction in this patient can be seen to change from left to right to right to left. The timing of the changes in flow direction is best appreciated using colour flow M-mode Doppler examination **D**. Shunt reversal is shown by a change in colour of the trans septal flow from orange to blue (arrowed). This figure is reproduced in colour in the colour plate section at the front of this volume.

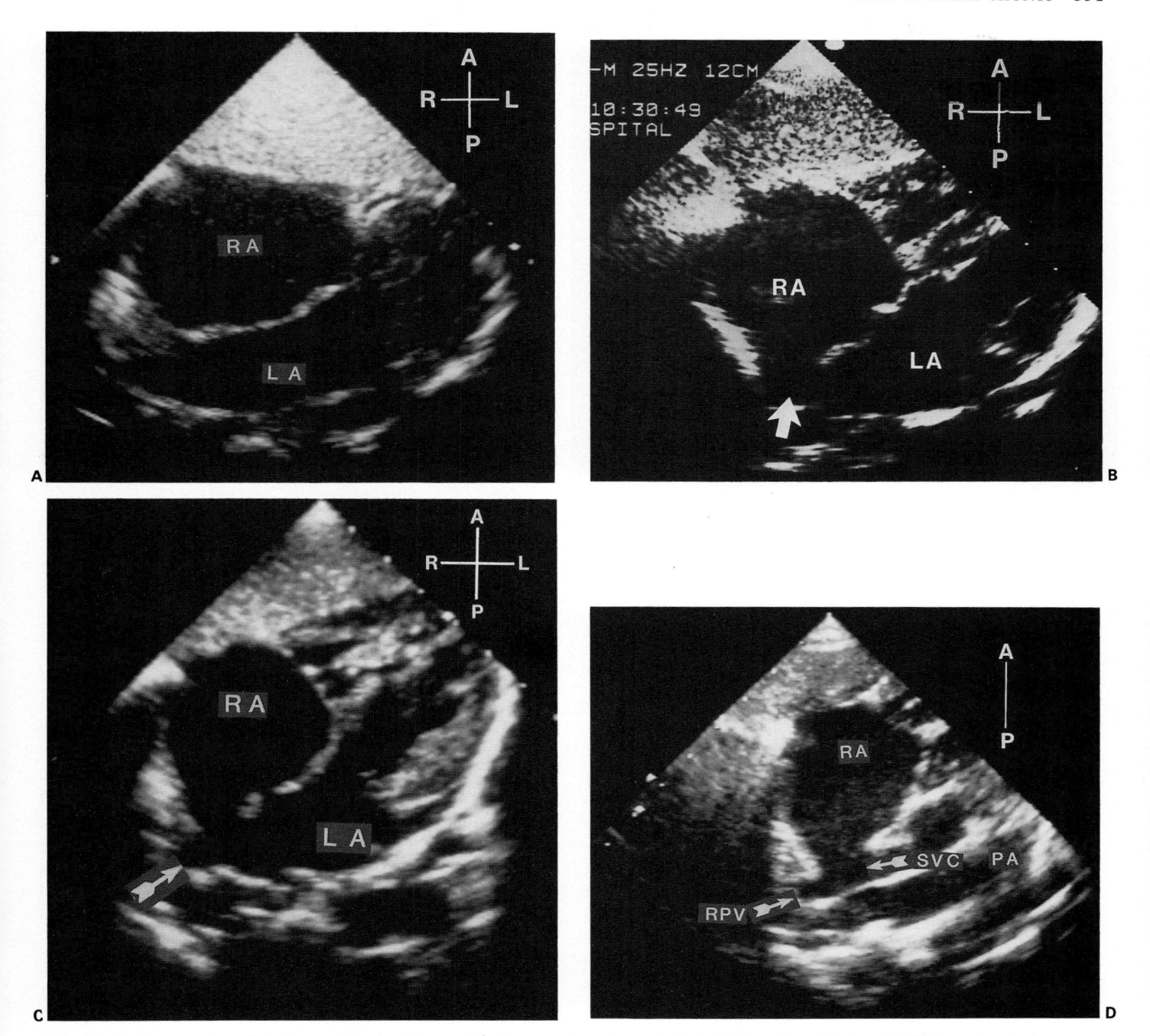

Fig. 10 **A: Sinus venosus defects may be missed by angling the transducer too anteriorly in the subcostal view. B:** With more posterior angulation the defect may usually be clearly seen. **C:** With still further angulation posteriorly the abnormal site of drainage of the right lower lobe (but sometimes a separate middle lobe vein) may be seen (arrowed). **D:** Anterior angulation of the transducer with some clockwise rotation to bring the superior caval vein into view may reveal abnormal drainage of the right upper lobe pulmonary vein (RPV) into the superior caval vein (SVC) at its junction with the right atrium.

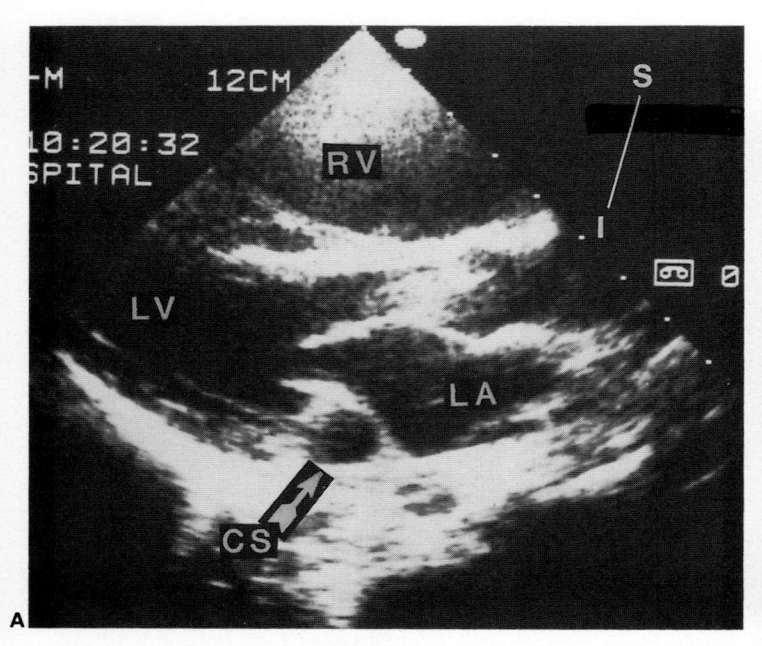

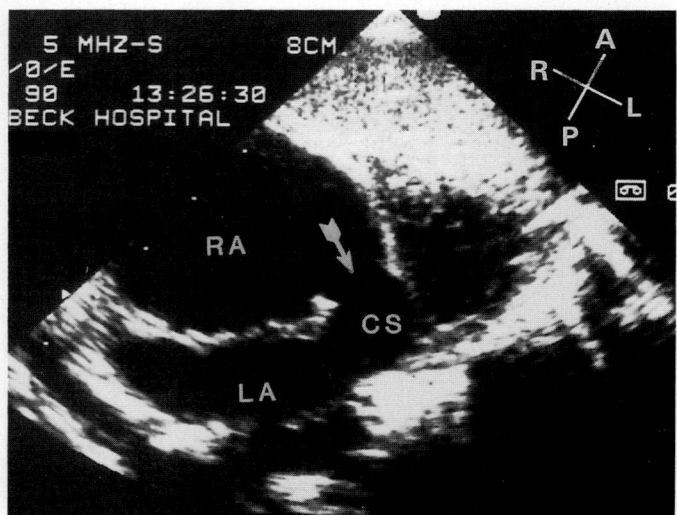

Fig. 11 A: Long axis parasternal and B: subcostal views of a dilated coronary sinus, one of the first clues to the presence of a coronary sinus defect. When gross dilatation as in B is present, care must be taken not to confuse the appearance with that of a partial atrioventricular septal defect (a primum atrial septal defect).

Iatrogenic defects in the atrial septum

The creation of an atrial septal defect may be beneficial in some forms of congenital heart disease and, just as for naturally occurring defects, echocardiography is valuable in their assessment. Varying appearances may be seen, depending on the technique used to create the defect. A closed surgical septectomy (Blalock Hanlon procedure) produces a defect in the superior part of the septum, producing an appearance somewhat similar to that of a venous sinus defect, whilst septectomy performed on cardiopulmonary bypass usually produces a large central defect in the septum. When the defect is produced by balloon septostomy (Rashkind procedure) the defect is usually restricted to the confines of the oval foramen. Traditionally balloon septostomy has been performed in the catheter laboratory using an X-ray image intensifier, but it is now clear that the procedure may be performed easily and more quickly purely under echocardiographic control[64,65] (Fig. 12).

This technique has considerable advantages as it avoids the need to transfer ill neonates to the catheter laboratory, it allows direct visualisation of the catheter tip position (which may be difficult with X-ray control, particularly in the presence of juxtaposition of the atrial appendages[66] or a large coronary sinus). Additionally, echocardiography allows the result of the septostomy to be assessed immediately.

Transoesophageal echocardiography

In rare cases where the anatomy of the atrial septum is in doubt after traditional cross-sectional and Doppler echocardiography transoesophageal imaging and Doppler may prove invaluable[67,61] (see Plate 2). Imaging the heart from the oesophagus, which lies immediately behind the left atrium, enables extremely high quality images to be obtained. The technique is particularly well suited to the assessment of atrial morphology and pathology in patients who have respiratory disease or chest deformity. A detailed account of the technique and its applications is given in Chapter 9.

Associated abnormalities

Defects in the atrial septum may occur in combination with any other congenital heart defect. A defect in the oval foramen most commonly occurs in isolation, but prolapse of the mitral valve has been reported to be a particular association,[68,69,38] some studies suggesting that mitral valve abnormalities may occur in over 50% of cases.[70] Such findings have been reported in angiographic studies[68,71] as well as on echocardiography, but reassuringly there is some evidence that these appearances have been misinterpreted and that true mitral prolapse is a much less common association than had initially been suggested.[72]

Indeed, histological study of the mitral valve in such cases has failed to show the usual characteristics of mitral

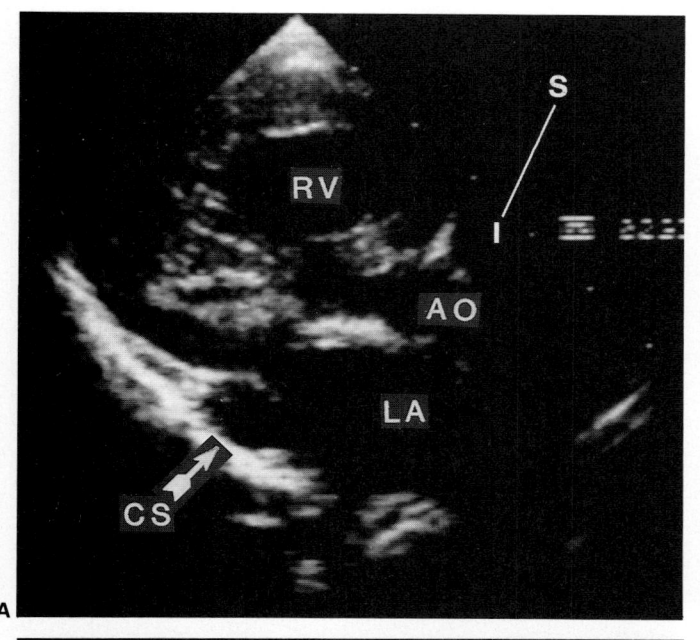

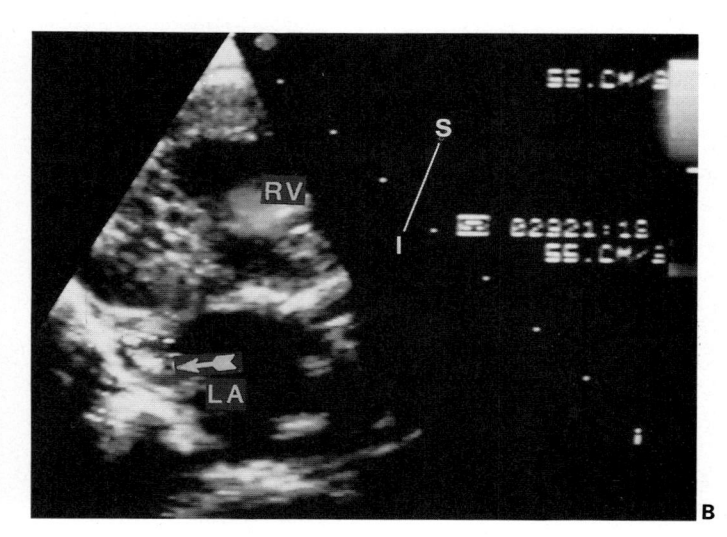

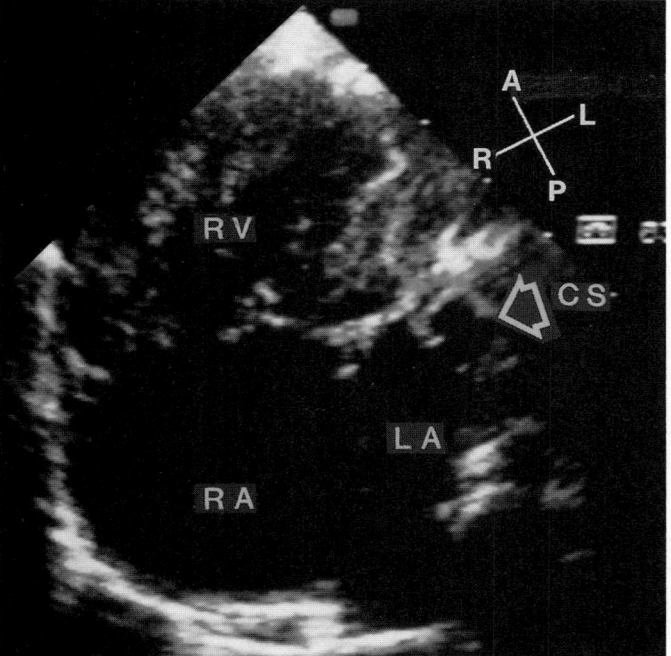

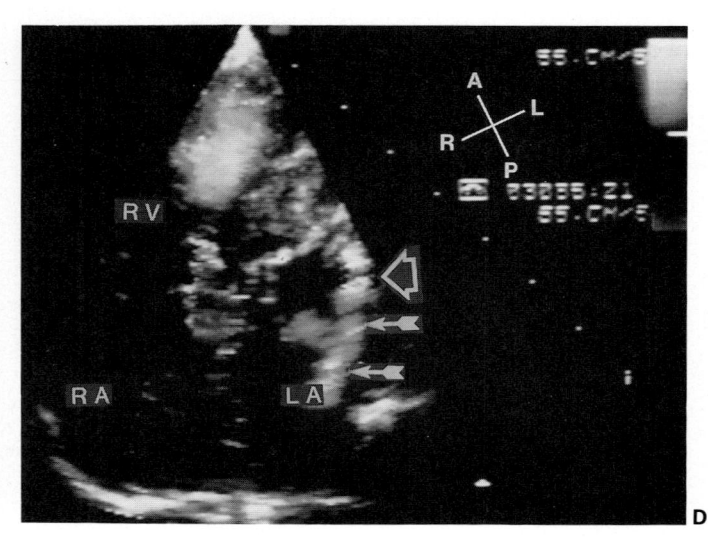

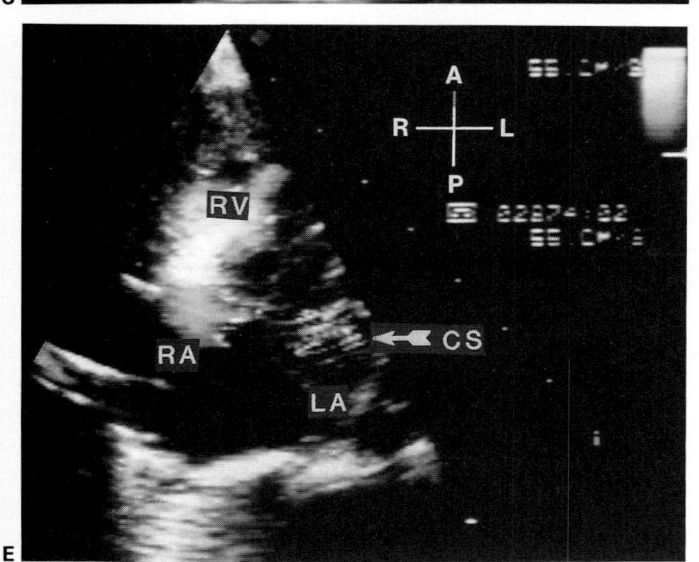

Plate 5 **A: Parasternal long axis view of a coronary sinus defect.** The dilated coronary sinus (arrowed) is seen to communicate with the left atrium. **B:** Colour flow mapping shows turbulent flow (arrowed) within the coronary sinus (the patient also has mitral atresia, the coronary sinus defect being the only escape route from the left atrium). **C:** The dilated coronary sinus (arrowed) and its communication with the left atrium is also seen in an apical four chamber view. **D:** In this view colour flow mapping shows blood streaming (small arrows) from the left atrium into the coronary sinus, where the flow becomes turbulent (large arrow). There is also a jet of tricuspid regurgitation. **E:** Posterior angulation of the transducer allows visualisation of the coronary sinus draining into the right atrium (flow in blue) and thence through the tricuspid valve to the right ventricle (flow in orange). This figure is reproduced in colour in the colour plate section at the front of this volume.

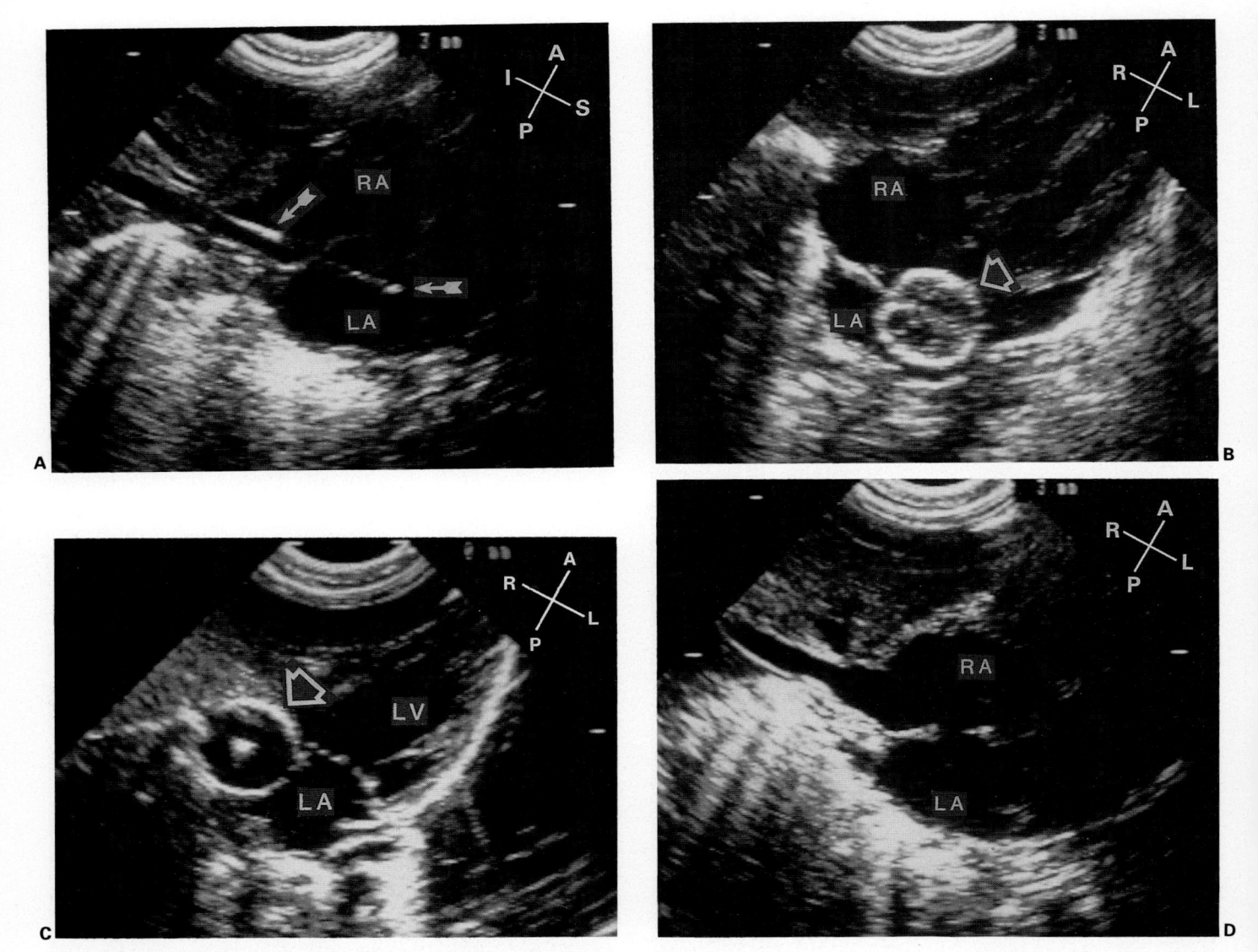

Fig. 12 Balloon atrial septostomy under echocardiographic guidance. **A:** The balloon catheter (arrowed) can be seen emerging from the inferior caval vein to enter the right atrium and pass through the oval foramen to lie in the left atrium. **B:** The balloon (arrowed) is inflated with saline in the left atrium. **C:** The balloon is pulled sharply back across the septum into the right atrium. **D:** The balloon is deflated and the defect in the septum is clearly visible.

valve prolapse.[73] It seems therefore that, whilst mitral prolapse may occur in some patients with atrial septal defect, it has almost certainly been overdiagnosed in the past. This illustrates the important general rule that it is rarely wise to interpret echocardiographic appearances in isolation without taking clinical signs into account. Mitral stenosis may also very rarely occur alongside atrial septal defect (Lutembacher's syndrome), but the association is sufficiently rare to be an incidental finding.

Defects in the oval foramen should be sought in the presence of subdivision of the left atrium (cor triatriatum) as atrial shunting occurs in up to half such cases. The defect may be either proximal or distal to the obstructing membrane.

A coronary sinus defect rarely occurs as an isolated abnormality and is most commonly seen in the presence of complex congenital heart disease. Venous sinus defects are almost invariably associated with abnormal connection of the superior caval vein (overriding the crest of the atrial septum) as well as anomalous drainage of one or more of the right pulmonary veins.[60]

Postoperative appearances

If repair of a defect in the oval foramen has been carried out by direct suturing alone, the site of repair may not be apparent on postoperative cross-sectional echocardiography, but if a patch of synthetic material or pericardium has been used it may usually be identified.

After surgical repair the echocardiographic changes due

to right heart volume overload will usually improve rapidly. Obvious right ventricular dilatation on cross-sectional imaging and frankly paradoxical septal motion both usually appear to resolve within a few months of surgery. However, critical analysis shows that right ventricular dimensions and ventricular septal motion remain subtly abnormal in the majority of patients[74,75] and that these abnormalities may persist for at least 5 years after operation.[76] There is some degree of correlation between the persistence of these abnormalities and age at surgical treatment, leading to the hypothesis that failure of the echocardiogram to return to normal is a result of chronic right ventricular volume overload. This in turn implies that early surgical intervention in children with marked signs of volume overload may increase the likelihood of a return to echocardiographic normality.[76] Further study of children who have early surgical treatment will be necessary to determine whether the avoidance of persistent echocardiographic abnormalities is possible or, indeed, necessarily desirable.

A surprising finding in long-term echocardiographic follow up after surgical closure of oval foramen defects is that left ventricular fractional shortening is unusually high in almost 50% of cases. The reason for this is not clear, but a variation from normal left ventricular geometry as a result of preoperative right ventricular dilatation may be responsible.[76] Very little long-term follow-up data is available in patients who have undergone closure of sinus venosus or coronary sinus defects, but it seems likely that some late postoperative echocardiographic evidence of right heart volume overload would also be present in these patients.

Interatrial shunting may also occur after venous redirection operations for transposition of the great arteries. Although atrial anatomy is complex in such patients, the same basic rules used in the investigation of atrial septal defects apply, bearing in mind that shunt direction may often be right to left in such cases (see Ch. 22).

Both M-mode and cross-sectional contrast echocardiography may also show persistent abnormalities after surgical closure of atrial septal defect, with clear evidence of a small, haemodynamically insignificant left to right atrial shunt being detectable in about one third of cases who have had otherwise apparently completely successful repair.[77] Our own experience is that trivial very small residual postoperative left to right jets across the septum are not infrequently detectable by colour flow imaging. A small persistent atrial shunt does not necessarily imply inadequate repair and such findings must be interpreted with caution and diplomacy!

Assessing shunt size

Many different methods for crude indirect assessment of shunt size in atrial septal defect have been proposed. These include estimation of the severity of right heart volume overload by the measurement of right ventricular dimensions[78] or their variation with respiration,[20] measurement of the size of the pulmonary arteries,[18,79] or even by comparing the diameters of the tricuspid and mitral valve orifices on M-mode echocardiography.[80] Systolic and diastolic time intervals have also been used to assess shunt size indirectly with limited success.[81] Direct cross-sectional echocardiographic measurement of the size of the defect in the septum may be helpful in some cases,[19,43] but this may be misleading in the presence of multiple fenestrations of the foramen.[43]

The integral of the transatrial flow velocity pulsed Doppler waveform bears some relationship to shunt magnitude,[82] as does the area of flow across the septum seen on colour flow imaging.[13,83]

None of the above indirect methods provide accurate estimates of shunt size in individual patients and they can only give a crude indication of pulmonary to systemic flow ratio. Quantitative estimation of systemic and pulmonary blood flow using Doppler echocardiography offers the most promising approach to ultrasound assessment of shunt size. The different approaches to these measurements and their limitations are discussed separately in Chapter 8 on flow measurement.

ATRIOVENTRICULAR SEPTAL DEFECT

Introduction

The atrioventricular septum separates the right atrium from the left ventricle. It exists because the septal leaflet of the tricuspid valve is inserted more apically than the septal leaflet of the mitral valve (Fig. 13). An echocardiographic hallmark of atrioventricular septal defects is

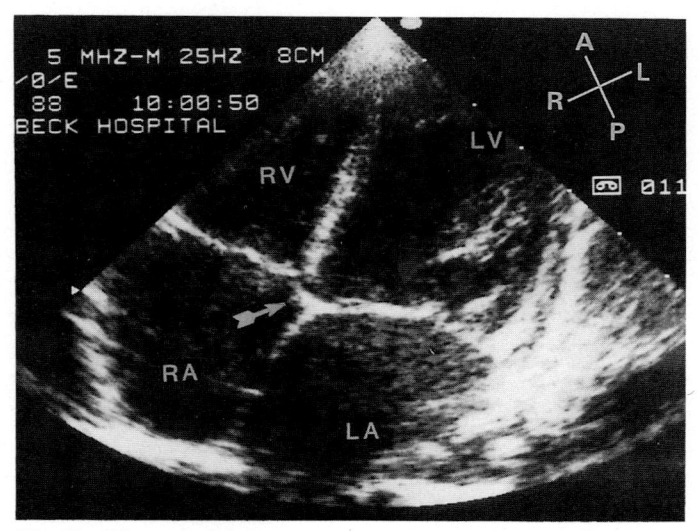

Fig. 13 The atrioventricular septum (arrowed) seen in an apical four chamber view. In the normal heart the septal leaflet of the tricuspid valve can be seen to be attached more apically than the septal attachment of the mitral valve. The atrioventricular septum thus separates the left ventricle from the right atrium.

the absence of this normal 'offsetting' of the septal insertions of the atrioventricular valves.[84-86] The structural abnormalities of the atrioventricular valves present in atrioventricular defects are best explained by the presence of a common atrioventricular valve rather than two separate valves; the common valve may or may not be divided into left and right components, but it is always abnormal.[87,88] The abnormalities present in atrioventricular septal defects are not restricted to the atrioventricular junction, but are associated with variable degrees of abnormality of ventricular morphology. In addition, both the practice and interpretation of cross-sectional echocardiography may be complicated by abnormalities of visceroatrial situs.[87,89,90] Although early reports suggested that M-mode echocardiography might be useful in the anatomical assessment of atrioventricular defects,[91-93] this has been superseded by cross-sectional imaging.

Atrioventricular junction abnormalities

Defects in the atrioventricular septum may be partial or complete and of variable size. Each type of atrioventricular septal defect may be best understood morphologically and echocardiographically by consideration of the central attachment of the common valve.

This attachment may be to the crest of the ventricular septum, forming what is commonly referred to as a 'primum' atrial septal defect (Fig. 14), on rare occasions to the atrial septum, forming an inlet ventricular septal defect otherwise known as a 'ventricular septal defect of canal type'; or there may be no central attachment, forming a complete atrioventricular septal defect (otherwise known as a complete atrioventricular canal defect or endocardial cushion defect)[88,94] (Fig. 15).

There is some controversy over the question of whether an inlet ventricular septal defect with separate atrioventricular valves which arise at the same level represents a form of atrioventricular septal defect or a form of ventricular septal defect. Whilst there is clearly an absence of the atrioventricular septum when both atrioventricular

Fig. 14 A partial atrioventricular septal defect (previously known as an ostium primum atrial septal defect) seen in an apical four chamber view. There is a large communication between the left atrium and the right atrium at the lower end of the septum and the atrioventricular valves arise at the same level, so there is no atrioventricular septum. There is no ventricular component to the defect as the leaflets of the atrioventricular valve are inserted into the crest of the ventricular septum.

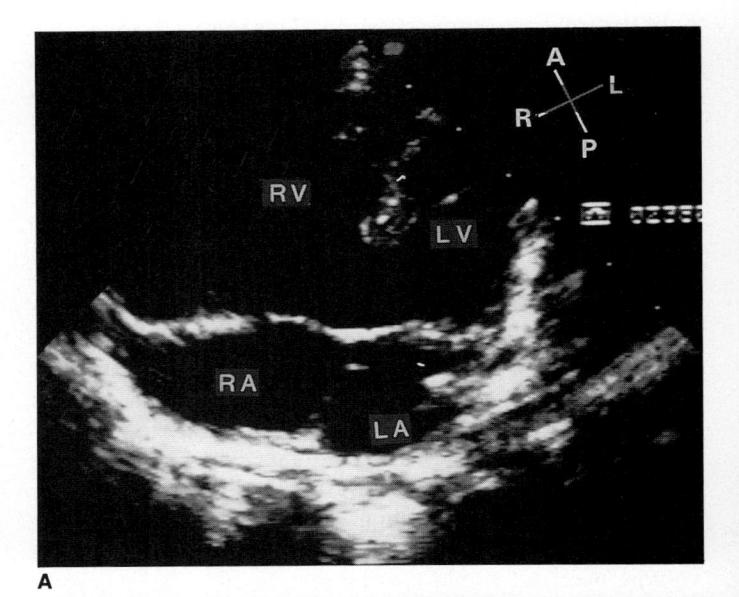

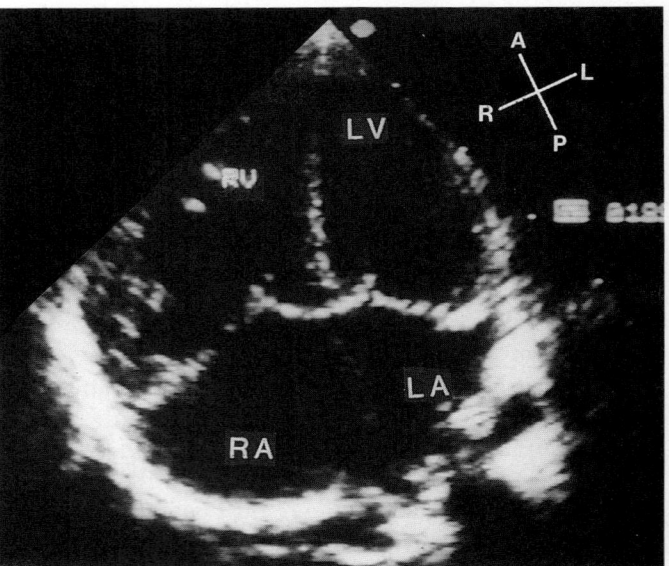

Fig. 15 A: A complete atrioventricular septal defect seen in an apical four chamber view. In this example the atrial component to the defect is relatively small, but there is a large ventricular component. **B:** In this patient with a smaller ventricular component slight anterior angulation of the transducer clearly shows the common bridging anterior leaflet of the atrioventricular valve.

valves arise at the same level, an inlet ventricular septal defect is frequently accompanied by separate atrioventricular valves which have the morphologic appearance of normal tricuspid and mitral valves[86,95] and is anatomically and functionally distinct from an atrioventricular defect without an atrial communication.[85,86,95,96] The problem is largely semantic, the importance in practical terms being careful assessment of atrioventricular valve morphology in all cases where the atrioventricular septum is absent. If, in these cases, the atrioventricular valves appear normal it is convenient to term the defect an inlet ventricular septal defect. This in turn should lead to a careful search for either atrioventricular valve overriding or straddling of the ventricular septum.[86,97] Similar difficulties may arise in some forms of single ventricle when the atrioventricular valves arise at the same level.

In these complex cases cross-sectional echocardiography is equally effective at establishing valve morphology.[98–100] and it is usually best simply to describe the echocardiographic findings rather than to attempt to fit the abnormalities into a distinct single category.

Although, as already stated, the normal atrioventricular septum separates the right atrium from the left ventricle it may be appreciated that, because the normal atrioventricular valve offsetting is absent in these defects, atrioventricular septal defects do not result in isolated communications between the right atrium and the left ventricle (the 'Gerbode defect'). Left to right shunting from the left ventricle to the right atrium may however occur. In the authors' experience when these shunts occur with atrioventricular septal defect they may usually be shown by colour flow imaging to be due to regurgitation through the left component of the atrioventricular valve with the regurgitant jet directed towards the right atrium. Left ventricular to right atrial shunting may also occur in the absence of an atrioventricular septal defect but in the presence of a ventricular septal defect and coincident tricuspid regurgitation,[101–105] the jet across the ventricular septum being directed towards the tricuspid valve orifice. In the very few reported cases of genuinely isolated left ventricular to right atrial communication there is normal offsetting of the atrioventricular valves and it has been suggested that this is due to a defect in the central fibrous body rather than in the atrioventricular septum.[106]

In the presence of a common atrioventricular valve it is not surprising that the left component of the valve, even in a partial atrioventricular septal defect, is structurally different to the normal mitral valve and that therefore its function is usually abnormal too. The most obvious abnormality of the left component of the valve on echocardiography is an apparent cleft,[94,107,108] although further study has shown this to be a commissure of the common valve.[85,87] This apparent cleft is a separate entity from isolated clefts which may occur in the anterior leaflet of the mitral valve.[107,108] Other abnormalities of the atrioventricular valves such as stenosis[109] or even double orifice[110] may occur. Subcostal short axis imaging is particularly useful in assessing valve morphology in these cases.[111] The valve abnormalities in atrioventricular defects are not restricted to the cusps and short axis parasternal or subcostal imaging will usually show abnormally situated papillary muscles in the left ventricle.[112] Careful echocardiographic assessment of atrioventricular valve structure and function is thus extremely important even in patients with a partial atrioventricular septal defect.

Ventricular abnormalities

Ventricular morphology as well as the atrioventricular junction is abnormal in these defects; left ventricular geometry is altered and the left ventricular outflow tract is narrower than in the normal heart[87] (Fig. 16). These relatively subtle morphological abnormalities are not always obvious on cross-sectional echocardiography. However, important abnormalities of ventricular anatomy are usually immediately apparent and may occur in patients with either partial or complete defects.

One of the most important of these abnormalities from the viewpoint of surgical correction is that known as ventricular dominance, where there is marked inequality in the size of the two ventricles.[87,88,113] This appears to be related to the balance between flow through the right and left components of the atrioventricular valve into the respective ventricular chambers. If the orifice of the left sided component of the valve is small or the common valve is predominantly committed to (i.e. preferentially fills) the

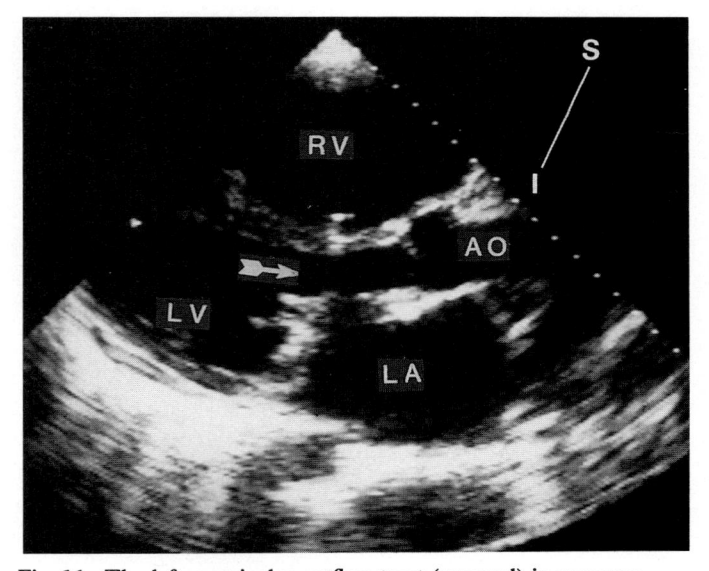

Fig. 16 The left ventricular outflow tract (arrowed) is narrower than normal in the presence of either partial or complete atrioventricular septal defect. In this example the right ventricle is dilated due to volume loading and the left ventricular outflow tract is strikingly narrower than normal although no obstruction to flow was detectable by Doppler examination.

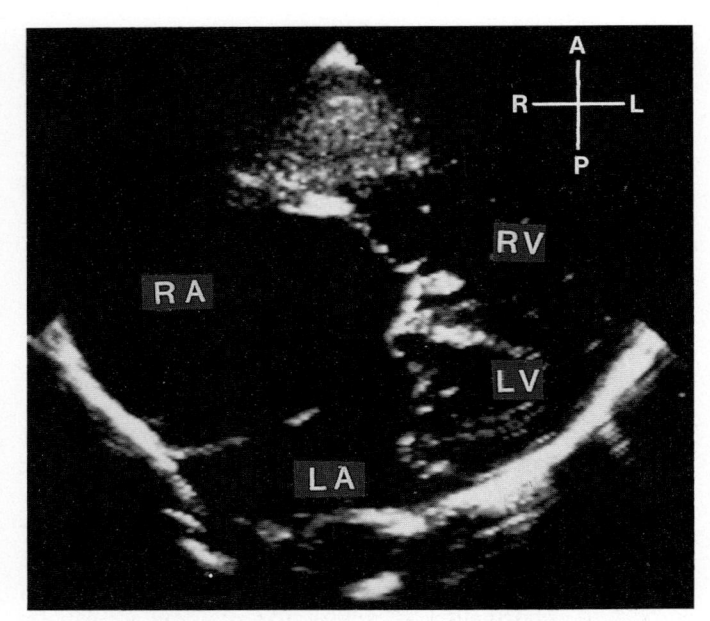

Fig. 17 A subcostal view of a partial atrioventricular septal defect with right dominance. The left atrium and left ventricle are small. The right atrium and the right ventricle are markedly dilated and the free lower edge of the atrial septum appears to override the orifice of the left component of the atrioventricular valve.

right ventricle, the right ventricle and the pulmonary artery will be seen to be dilated and the left ventricle (and sometimes the aortic root and aortic arch) will be hypoplastic to some degree (Fig. 17). Conversely, right heart hypoplasia with left ventricular dominance may occur.[88] On rare occasions atrial rather than ventricular dominance may be seen with complete defects, where the common atrioventricular valve predominantly arises from either the right or the left atrium, an arrangement sometimes referred to as double outlet atrium.[114] Right atrial dominance with an atrioventricular septal defect may sometimes be very difficult to distinguish from mitral atresia with ventricular septal defect and left atrial dominance may be difficult to distinguish from tricuspid atresia.[115,116]

The narrowing of the left ventricular outflow tract in atrioventricular septal defects is not often of haemodynamic significance, but important subaortic stenosis may occur and is usually readily detectable by echocardiography.[117] The inherent narrowing of the outflow tract may be partially responsible for this, but protrusion of abnormal atrioventricular valve tissue into the outflow tract appears to be a major contributing factor.[117]

Abnormal motion of the left atrioventricular valve in diastole rather than systole causing narrowing of the left ventricular outflow tract (the 'goose neck or swan neck appearance') is detectable in most patients with atrioventricular septal defect (Fig. 18).[118]

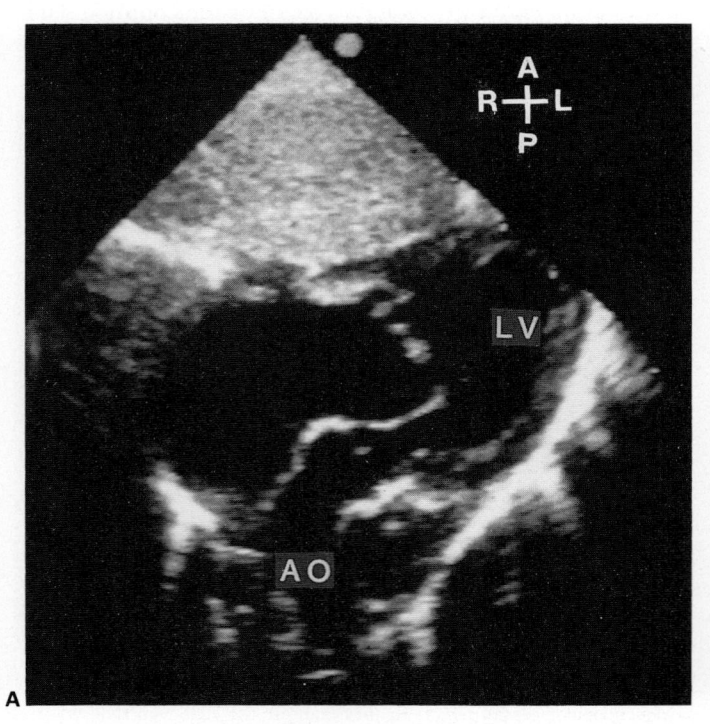

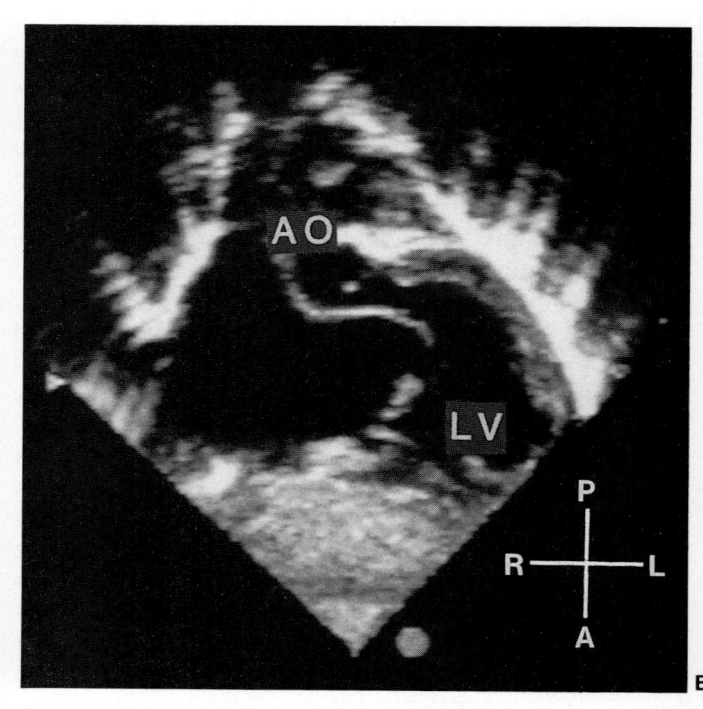

Fig. 18 A: The swan neck (or goose neck) deformity of the left ventricular outflow tract can be seen from the subcostal position in conventional orientation. B: It may be better appreciated in anatomical orientation. This appearance is seen in diastole and is due to the abnormal anterior atrioventricular valve leaflet bowing into the inherently narrow left ventricular outflow tract.

The presence of ventricular dominance or of subaortic obstruction are of extreme importance when considering surgical repair. These, as well as the complexities of the anatomy of the atrioventricular junction, are usually far better appreciated using ultrasound than by invasive investigation, and careful and complete sequential segmental analysis of the cardiac and great artery anatomy should provide sufficient information to allow surgical treatment to take place without cardiac catheterisation in the majority of patients.

Haemodynamics

Single gate pulsed Doppler has little to offer in atrioventricular septal defect as blood flow patterns may be extremely complex with variable mixtures of mitral and tricuspid regurgitation, interatrial and interventricular shunting and shunting between the left ventricle and the right atrium. However, colour flow imaging may allow some qualitative analysis of flow patterns and jet directions as well as allowing semiquantitative assessment of atrioventricular valve regurgitation by evaluation of the spatial extent of the regurgitant jet (Plate 6A and B). Continuous wave examination, like single gate pulsed wave Doppler examination, may also prove very difficult to interpret unless guided by colour flow imaging.

Although it is widely accepted that ultrasound provides detailed anatomical information some authorities still recommend routine cardiac catheterisation for preoperative haemodynamic assessment of infants with atrioventricular defects,[119] in particular for the calculation of pulmonary vascular resistance.

Associated abnormalities

Abnormalities such as volume loading of the right ventricle and pulmonary arterial dilatation will be seen in patients who have predominance of shunting at atrial level. Right ventricular hypertrophy, often best evaluated by assessment of the thickness of the right ventricular free wall on a subcostal view, will be seen in patients with elevated right ventricular pressure, and this is a most useful indicator of pulmonary hypertension.

Other structural abnormalities may occur in the presence of atrioventricular septal defects, the commonest being atrial isomerism,[89,90] when it is important to assess the spatial orientation of the ventricular chambers as part of the process of sequential analysis.[120] There is also an infrequent association of atrioventricular defect with tetralogy of Fallot.[87]

Postoperative echocardiography

Ultrasound is invaluable after surgery for atrioventricular septal defects. It allows visualisation of the patch used to

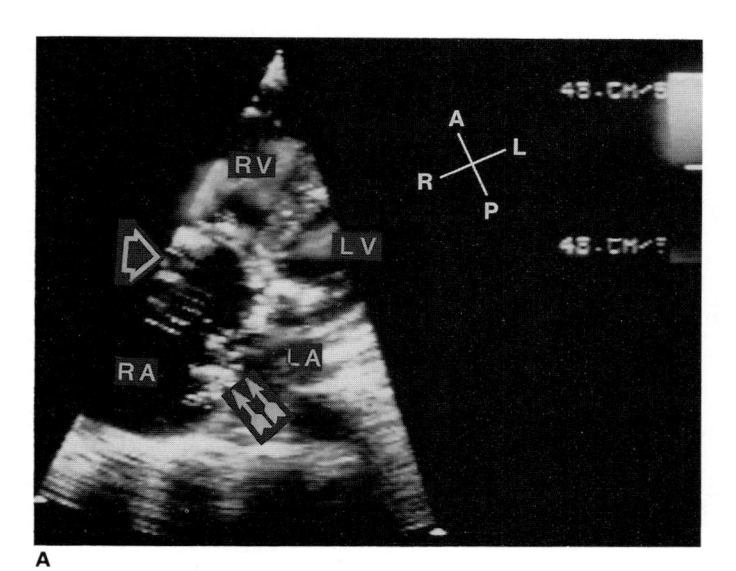

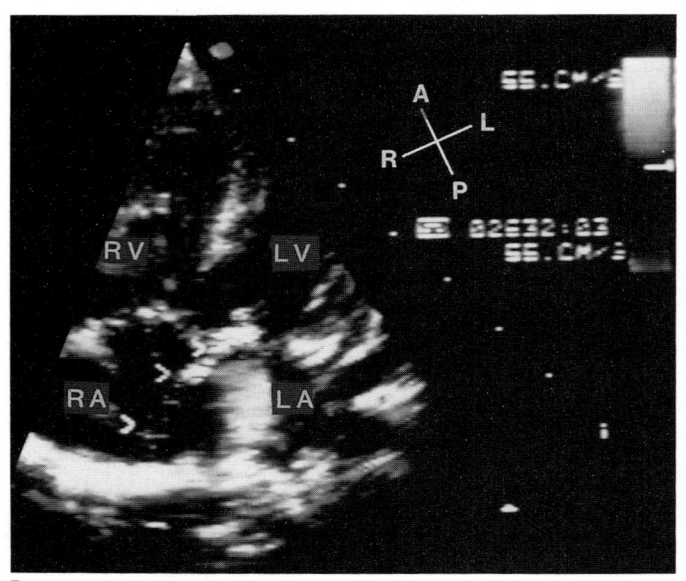

Plate 6 Both left and right sided atrioventricular valve regurgitation are common with atrioventricular septal defects. **A:** In colour flow Doppler mapping, an apical view shows jets of regurgitation into both the left atrium (small arrows) and the right atrium (large arrow). **B:** There is a left sided regurgitant jet which is directed across the atrial septum into the right atrium. This finding is often associated with a very large atrial shunt (effectively a left ventricular to right atrial shunt), along with particularly marked echocardiographic changes of right ventricular volume overload. This figure is reproduced in colour in the colour plate section at the front of this volume.

close the defect, assessment of ventricular function, assessment of pulmonary arterial systolic pressure and serial follow up of atrioventricular valve function, the latter being of particular importance as many patients will be left with some degree of mitral regurgitation.[121]

It has been suggested that intraoperative echocardiography may be of value in assessing the immediate results of mitral valve repair[122] and colour flow imaging will no doubt prove a valuable intraoperative asset in the future. Although there are reports of the value of pulsed Doppler mapping in the assessment of severity of atrioventricular regurgitation,[123,124] the spatial extent of a regurgitant jet is affected by many factors other than the degree of regurgitation and cannot therefore be used to provide a quantitative estimate of severity.[125-128]

Long-term echocardiographic follow up of patients who have undergone surgical repair may show persistent abnormalities of ventricular septal motion and right ventricular dimensions as frequently seen after surgical repair of atrial septal defect. Progressive subaortic stenosis may appear late after surgical repair even in patients who have no obvious narrowing of the left ventricular outflow tract at the time of operation.[129] This is readily detectable by cross-sectional echocardiography. It appears to be related to the inherent narrowing of the outflow tract that is present in these patients rather than being related to the patch used to close the defect. Those patients who go on to develop such outflow stenosis have, however, often had a particularly marked gooseneck appearance on cross-sectional echocardiography prior to surgical correction.[129] Continuous wave Doppler examination allows serial postoperative evaluation of changing left ventricular outflow velocities and estimation of pressure drop using the modified Bernoulli equation.

Estimation of shunt size and pulmonary artery pressure

The same indirect methods of crudely assessing shunt size in atrial septal defects may be applied to atrioventricular septal defects but in practice these methods are too inaccurate in individual patients to be of great clinical value. Quantitative calculation of pulmonary and systemic blood flow using Doppler echocardiography is possible in some patients and is discussed separately in Chapter 8 on flow measurement.

Estimation of pulmonary artery systolic pressure may be attempted using several different methods including measurement of the velocity of flow across the ventricular septum or the velocity of tricuspid regurgitation. These methods are discussed in detail in Chapter 7 on quantitative pressure calculations.

VENTRICULAR SEPTAL DEFECT

Introduction

Ventricular septal defect is the commonest congenital abnormality of the heart and it accounts for up to 34% of all lesions.[130] Although this section refers to ventricular septal defect as an isolated lesion, such defects may be a composite part of more complex congenital heart lesions such as tetralogy of Fallot, atrioventricular septal defect, truncus arteriosus, double outlet ventricle and some forms of pulmonary atresia. These complex lesions are discussed elsewhere in this book. Even in the so-called isolated cases of ventricular septal defect, acquired right ventricular outflow tract obstruction may develop. Aortic regurgitation due to prolapse of one or more of the cusps of the aortic valve is also well recognised. There are many different types of ventricular septal defect, and classification is best made according to the strict anatomical position of the defect in the ventricular septum. By convention the septum is described as viewed from the right ventricle. The anatomical regions of the septum can be divided approximately into inlet, trabecular, or outlet regions. In addition to classification according to inlet, trabecular and outlet there is further subdivision according to the morphology of the ventricular septum in that area (Fig. 19). The two morphological areas of the septum are perimembranous (or membranous) and muscular (sometimes also referred to as trabecular when referring to defects at the apex of the septum). Additionally, defects may be single or multiple and be present in different parts of the septum. It can be seen from Figure 19 that large defects may involve both the perimembranous and muscular regions of the septum and may extend from inlet to outlet. Such defects are termed confluent.

Although there have been several methods of classification suggested, the approach suggested by Soto[131] avoids ambiguity and perhaps has more international application than its alternatives or modifications.[132-135] Capelli[135] has supplied a classification of site of the ventricular septal defect based on the proximity to the atrioventricular and semilunar valves. A useful goal which has emerged from the debate is to consider simple description of a defect rather than its classification into a specific category at all costs.[136] The accuracy of identification of ventricular septal defects using ultrasound is well recognised[137] and anatomical classification is essential for reasons of referral for surgical treatment which is often possible without invasive investigation[138] and the obvious influence this will have on the surgeon's approach to the defect, including the avoidance of atrioventricular conduction tissue.[139] The site of a defect in the septum is also important as some defects, depending on their site and appearance, may diminish in size with the growth of the child.[140-142] Postoperative study of the ventricular septum is also important in patients having undergone ventricular septal defect closure in order to monitor haemodynamic progress.[143] Ventricular septal defects may be single or multiple and the multiple defects may be in entirely different anatomical sites. The size of a ventricular septal defect is conventionally expressed as small, medium or large. This is based on the size of the defect in relation to the size of the aortic root. Ventricular septal defects less than one third the diameter of the aortic root are said to be small. Those up to one half the diameter of the aortic root are medium sized, and those more than half the aortic root diameter, large.

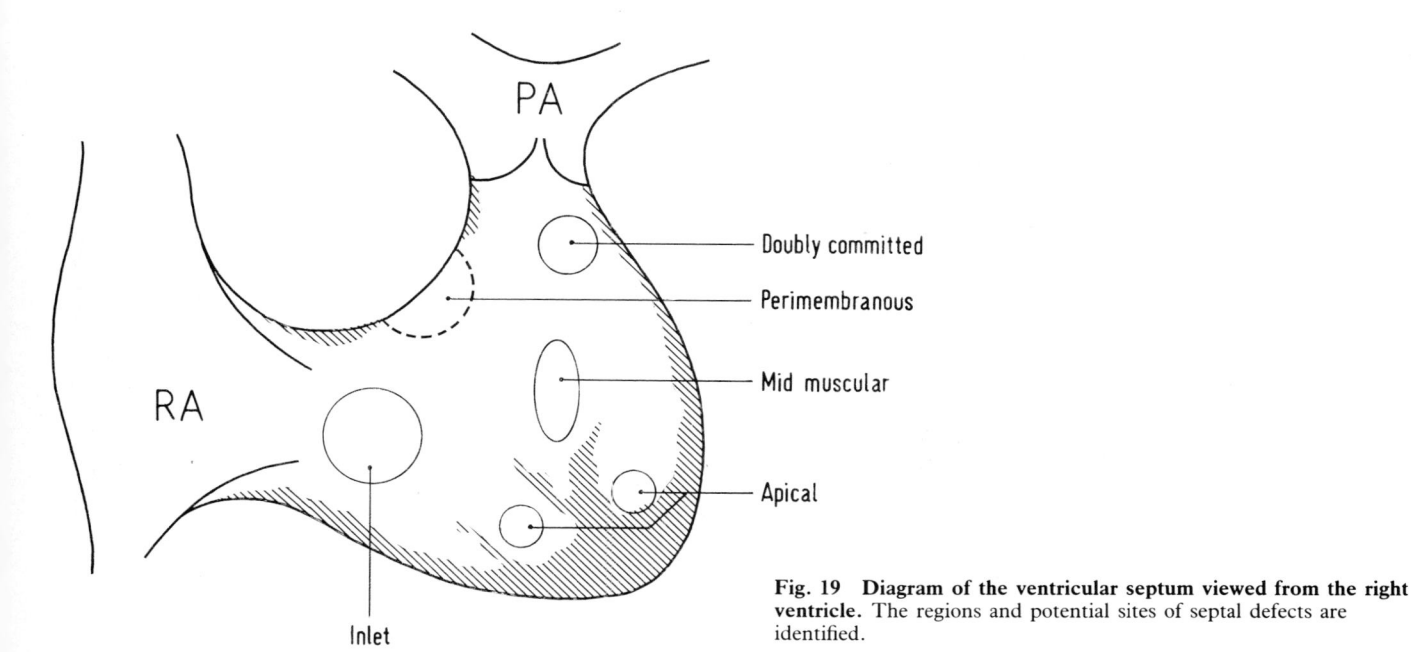

Fig. 19 Diagram of the ventricular septum viewed from the right ventricle. The regions and potential sites of septal defects are identified.

The examination

M-mode echocardiography has little part to play in the direct assessment of ventricular septal defects, although it may be useful to assess left atrial dilatation, a consequence of left to right shunting across the ventricular septum. The ratio of the left atrial:aortic root diameters has been used as a crude indicator of the magnitude of the left to right shunt.[144] This topic will be discussed in greater detail in the section dealing with quantitative assessment of ventricular septal defects.

Ventricular septal defects may be imaged using cross-sectional echocardiography from any of the standard precordial[145] or subcostal[146] planes. The conventional cross-sectional 'cuts' may be adapted slightly, depending on the site of the defect and the individual patient characteristics, notably the availability of a good echocardiographic window. As with ultrasound examination of any organ, there are potential problems of artefact. In particular there may be areas of echo 'drop out' in the ventricular septum with the attendant risk of false positive diagnosis. It is important therefore to attempt identification of a suspected defect in several different views, a practice which should limit false positive errors.[147] The usual physical limitations of ultrasound apply in the thorax, particularly poor ultrasonic penetration due to interposition of air in the lungs between the transducer and the heart.

When a defect cannot be identified by imaging alone, Doppler studies are of great value in pulsed,[148] continuous[149] and colour flow modes.[150,151] Similarly, Doppler examination may be used to differentiate between mitral regurgitation and ventricular septal defect, where the clinical distinction may sometimes be difficult.[152] It has also been postulated that colour flow mapping may be of value in the prediction of the natural history of ventricular septal defects, identifying those which may get smaller or close spontaneously.[142] In addition Doppler studies may also be used to give some quantitative information about the haemodynamics of the defect including an estimate of right ventricular pressure by obtaining a septal pressure gradient using continuous wave Doppler measurement.[153,154] It is technically feasible (but in practice extremely difficult) to estimate the pulmonary to systemic flow ratio by using a combination of pulsed Doppler flow measurement and imaging.[155,156] The potential errors inherent in these measurements probably exclude them from widespread clinical use; they are discussed in more detail in Chapter 8 on quantitative flow measurements.

Perimembranous defects

This is the commonest type of ventricular septal defect. They may be small, medium or large in size but are almost invariably single. They are frequently associated with aneurysmal tissue formed around the edges of the defect. They can be imaged from an apical four chamber view, when the defect is usually seen directly adjacent to the septal leaflet of the tricuspid valve (Fig. 20). Indeed parts of the tricuspid valve apparatus may be indistinguishable from the aneurysm around the defect. Anterior angulation of the transducer will bring the left ventricular outflow tract into view, producing the so called 'five chamber view' and this manoeuvre should be performed to assess extension of the defect into the outlet region.

At times the aneurysm around the defect may appear

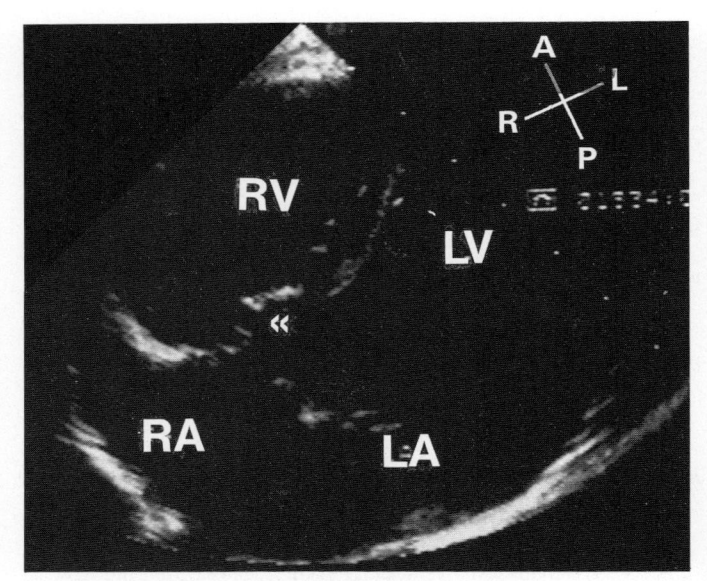

Fig. 20 A perimembranous ventricular septal defect (arrowed) seen from an apical four chamber view, demonstrating the proximity of the defect to the septal leaflet of the tricuspid valve.

complete and a defect on imaging alone may not be apparent (Plate 7A). Under these circumstances either pulsed or colour flow Doppler studies can be used to confirm that there is blood flow from left to right ventricle (Plate 7B). Perimembranous defects may also be imaged from the subcostal four chamber position.[146] The proximity of the defect to the leaflets and chordae of the tricuspid valve can easily be appreciated from this view. It is tricuspid valve tissue which usually forms the basis of the closure mechanism of these defects.[157,158] Large perimembranous defects may be imaged from a short axis left parasternal view, with the aorta in cross section and the right ventricular outflow tract wrapping around it. In this imaging position the defect appears as an aneurysmal deficiency in the aortic root.[159] These defects are by definition in the perimembranous region of the septum but frequently extend into the body of the ventricle where they will encroach on to the muscular part of the septum (Fig. 21). Likewise extension may occur into the outlet portion of the septum where again a muscular rim will be visible. This latter type of perimembranous defect may extend into the muscular outlet septum. The confluent defect thus formed may be associated with the additional complication of prolapse of the right coronary cusp of the aortic valve,[160] leading to aortic regurgitation (see below). Prolapse of the right coronary cusp is most easily identified in a long axis left parasternal view where one would normally expect to image the ventricular septum and the aortic root in continuity. In the presence of a ventricular septal defect the right coronary cusp may be seen to prolapse into the cavity of the right ventricle in diastole. The size of the defect and the degree of prolapse varies from patient to patient. It is

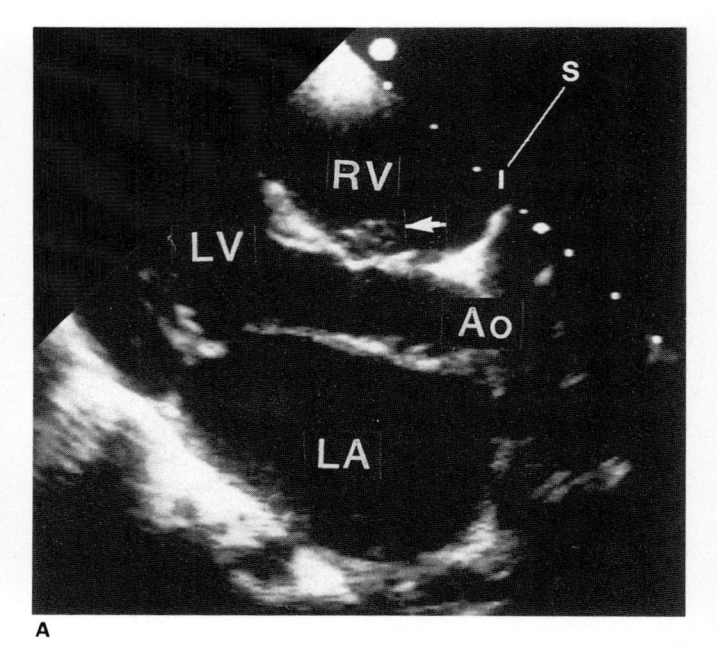

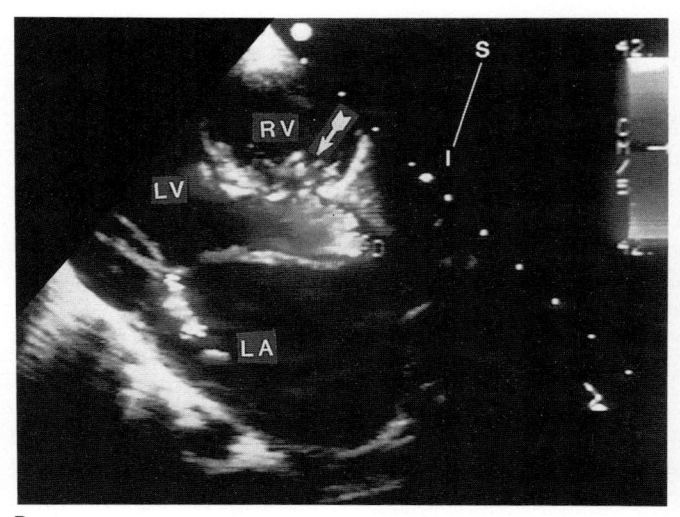

Plate 7 A: A perimembranous defect seen in long axis left parasternal view. The defect appears to be completely closed by aneurysm formation. **B:** Colour flow Doppler mapping however shows a persistent left to right shunt across the defect (arrowed) as well as a jet of mitral regurgitation into the left atrium. This figure is reproduced in colour in the colour plate section at the front of this volume.

quite possible to have a patient with a ventricular septal defect in which prolapse of the aortic valve cusp virtually occludes the defect.

Indeed this is stated as one of the possible mechanisms of closure of this type of defect. It is important therefore to scan the membranous septum from all of the above mentioned sites to assess the full extent of the defect. Likewise in the case of membranous defects extending into the outlet septum, a good case is made for looking for aortic regurgitation using Doppler techniques. This is perhaps easiest

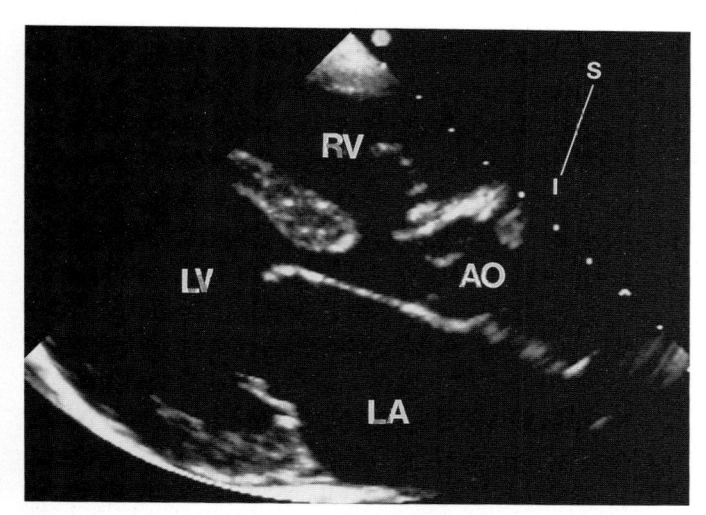

Fig. 21 A perimembranous defect from a left parasternal view, demonstrating the defect extending into the muscular septum towards the aorta.

using colour flow mapping, but pulsed and continuous wave examination should be used to confirm or refute the presence of aortic regurgitation in this situation.

Muscular defects

These defects may exist in the inlet, outlet or apical regions of the septum. They may be single, but not uncommonly may be multiple, in which case they are likely to be found in the apical septum. In these circumstances Doppler colour flow mapping is extremely helpful.[161,150] It is of course possible to have one defect in the perimembranous region and another in the apical region.

Inlet muscular defects

The inlet defect is characterised by having its roof formed by the tricuspid and mitral valves. This area of the septum may be imaged best either from the apical four chamber view or the subcostal four chamber view. In the apical four chamber view it is slightly easier to expose fully the leaflets of both the mitral and tricuspid valves. Larger defects will also be partly identified in a long axis left parasternal view. Whilst exposure of both atrioventricular valves is possible from the subcostal approach also, the mitral valve may be foreshortened depending on rotation of the transducer, and it is possible that a smaller inlet defect could be classified mistakenly as being perimembranous.

In these circumstances care must be taken to image the mitral valve and tricuspid valve together in relation to the defect. Figure 22A, an apical four chamber view, demonstrates a large inlet muscular defect, the mitral and tricuspid valves are clearly seen forming the roof of the defect. The defect is also visible in the parasternal long axis view (Fig. 22B).

Inlet muscular defects may be associated with malalignment of the atrioventricular valves. This is a situation in which either the tricuspid or mitral valve appears to override the ventricular septum. Extremes of overriding may result in a situation in which both atrioventricular valves or all of one atrioventricular valve and a majority of the other atrioventricular valve may appear to be committed to only one of the ventricles.[100,162] This may be termed 'double inlet ventricle'. In addition, with large inlet defects it is possible that atrioventricular valve apparatus will attach to the contralateral side of the septum. This is described as a straddling atrioventricular valve.

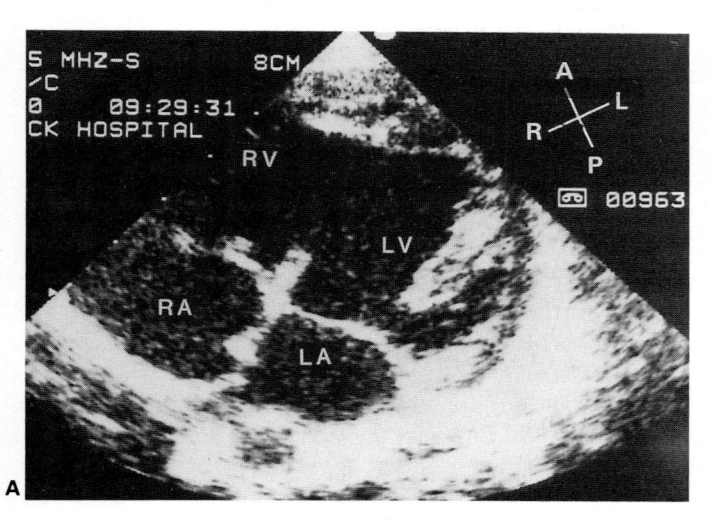

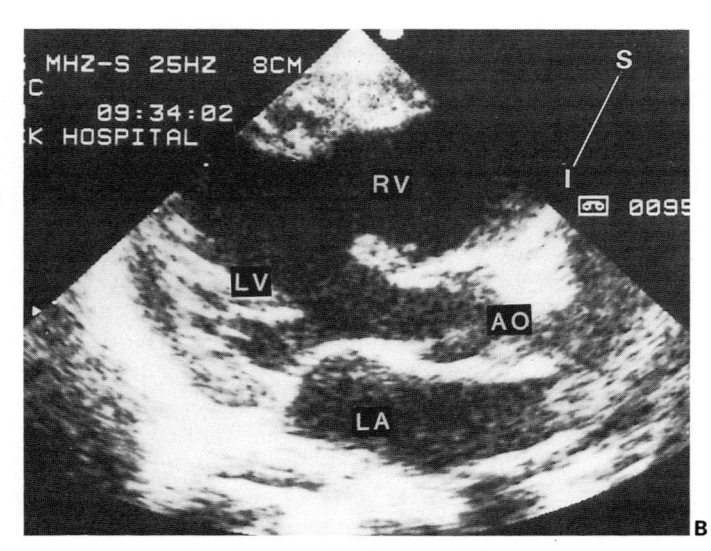

Fig. 22 A: A large inlet muscular defect. Note that the defect is roofed by the mitral and tricuspid valves. B: The same defect in the parasternal long axis view.

Muscular defects in the midportion and apical region of the septum

These defects which are often referred to as trabecular defects can be very difficult to image owing to the potentially obscuring effects of the coarse trabeculations and moderator band of the right ventricle which are to be found in this portion of the septum, and defects in this area are more likely to be missed than elsewhere in the septum.[151] In these circumstances the defects may only be suspected due to an imaged area of thinning of the septum. A complete defect may not be apparent. They may also be rather tortuous, passing through the septum obliquely, and thus imaging the defect in its entirety through the septum may be very difficult, necessitating sections of the septum from different angles.

They may be seen from all of the standard sections of the heart, perhaps most commonly four chamber apical and subcostal views. The short axis left parasternal view, which is more commonly used to image the body of the left ventricle inferior to the mitral valve, is also helpful when looking at the midportion of the septum. In addition, Doppler colour flow mapping studies probably contribute more to the diagnosis of defects in these areas than any other.[150,151,163,164] Plate 8A demonstrates an oblique apical ventricular septal defect, with left to right shunting across it clearly demonstrated by colour flow Doppler (Plate 8B). Plate 9A demonstrates a mid-muscular defect obscured by trabeculations which appears as an area of thinning of the septum. It is only fully identified using Doppler colour flow mapping (Plate 9B). The usefulness of the short axis section of the ventricular septum is demonstrated in Figure 23 which identifies two small mid muscular defects. In the case of multiple small defects the overall left to right shunt may be substantial despite the apparently unimpressive size of the individual defects seen on imaging. In patients with volume overload of the left heart but with only a small ventricular septal defect visible, the possibility of multiple small muscular defects should be considered.

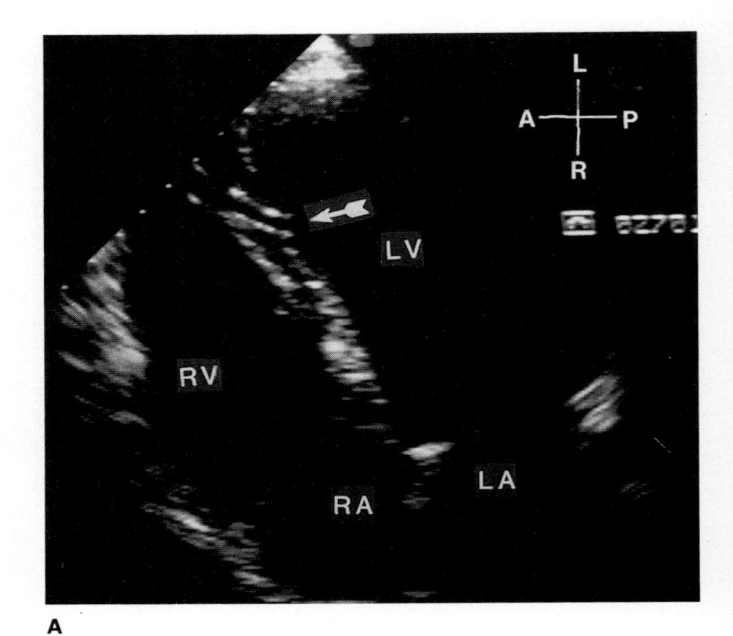

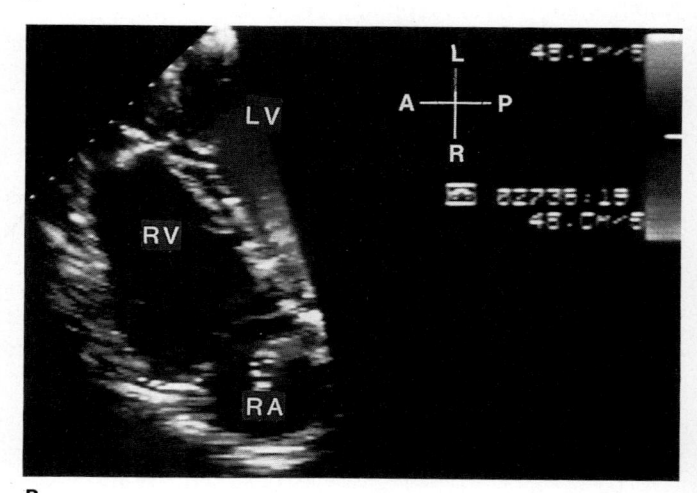

Plate 8 A: An oblique muscular apical defect seen from an apical four chamber view. B: Left to right shunting across the defect is confirmed by colour flow Doppler mapping. This figure is reproduced in colour in the colour plate section at the front of this volume.

Muscular outlet defects

These defects in the outlet part of the septum are generally described as being subaortic, subpulmonary or doubly committed. Subaortic defects have the leaflets of the aortic valve as their roof. Subpulmonary defects have the pulmonary valve leaflets forming the roof of the defect, whilst doubly committed ventricular septal defects have both aortic and pulmonary valves in fibrous continuity forming their roof.[165] The distinction between subpulmonary and doubly committed defects may be difficult to make. They are often difficult to image, lying anteriorly in the heart and therefore more than other defects tend to be obscured in those patients with a poor parasternal window.

Subaortic defects

Muscular subaortic defects may be isolated but are most often seen as part of complex malformations, notably tetralogy of Fallot, truncus arteriosus and pulmonary atresia. In these circumstances the defect is often large and appears to be overridden by the aorta or arterial trunk. They are usually easily imaged in the parasternal long axis view or in a four chamber apical view with the transducer tilted anteriorly to reveal the left ventricular outflow tract. This is sometimes referred to as the five chamber view. Figures 24A and 24B demonstrate images of a large subaortic defect seen from parasternal long axis and five chamber views respectively. It is common with such sub-

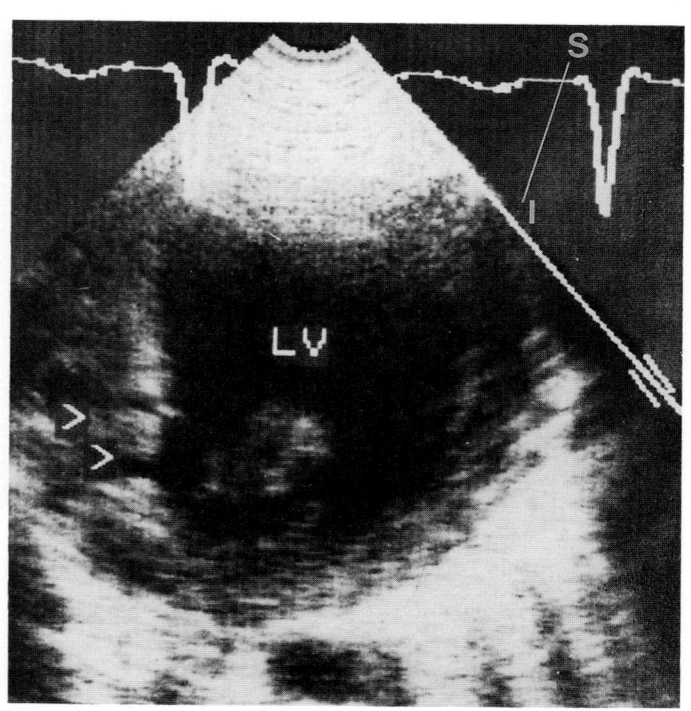

Fig. 23 Short axis apical view of two muscular defects.

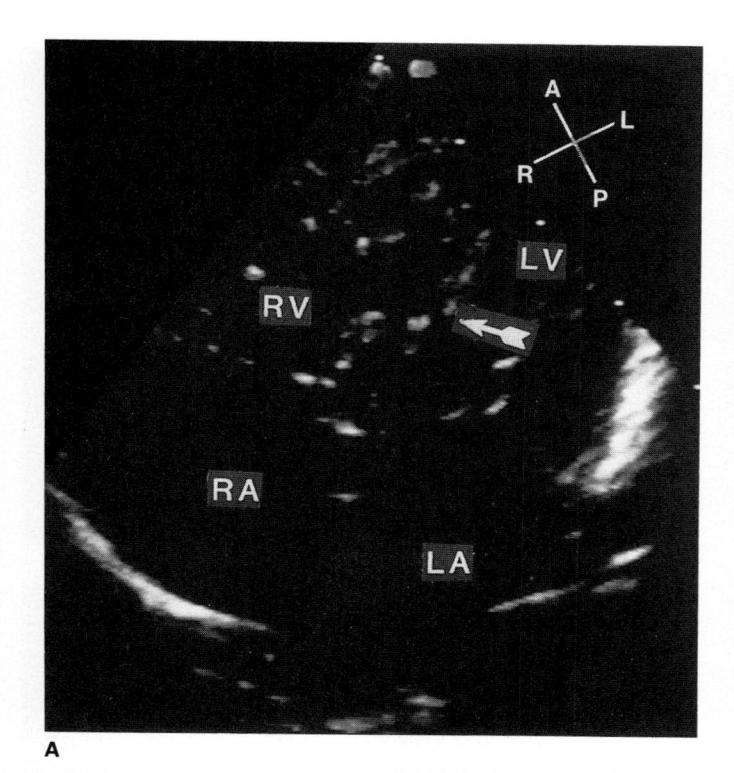

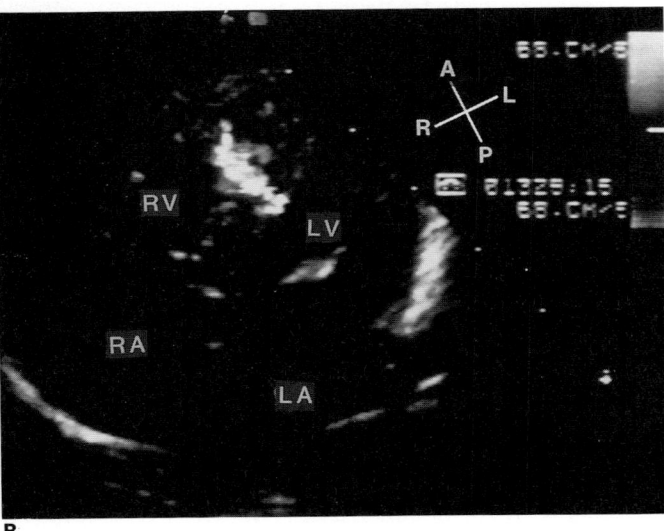

Plate 9 A: A mid muscular defect. There is thinning of the ventricular septum, but an actual defect is not appreciated using imaging alone. **B:** Left to right shunting across the defect is clearly present on colour flow Doppler mapping. This figure is reproduced in colour in the colour plate section at the front of this volume.

aortic defects for the aorta to override the ventricular septum, as is seen in the figures illustrated. The degree of aortic override is generally expressed as a percentage of the diameter of the aortic root, as explained in the legend. When the percentage of override as judged from the long axis and five chamber views is greater than 50%, the right ventricle is said to be 'double outlet'.

This lesion is most commonly associated with other abnormalities of the heart such as right ventricular outflow tract obstruction and malposition of the great arteries.

Subpulmonary and doubly committed defects

Subpulmonary defects are best imaged in the short axis left parasternal view, which one would normally choose to image the right ventricular outflow tract with the main and branch pulmonary arteries in view. Alternatively, a subcostal 'paracoronal' view has been used with the transducer directed towards the left shoulder, this being particularly useful when the parasternal window is poor. A doubly committed ventricular septal defect is illustrated in Figure 25 in the left parasternal short axis view (A) and in subcostal paracoronal view (B). It is worth appreciating that with subpulmonary or doubly committed defects the jet of blood passing through the septum travels virtually directly into the pulmonary artery. This has the effect of producing dilatation of the pulmonary artery which is disproportionate to the size of the imaged defect. It may also lead to the erroneous diagnosis of associated pulmonary stenosis as blood flow in the pulmonary artery distal to the pulmonary valve will be turbulent and at high velocity.[149] In such circumstances colour flow mapping or pulsed Doppler sampling will demonstrate that the turbulence starts in the right ventricular outflow tract proximal to the pulmonary valve. Despite this however it is easy to make

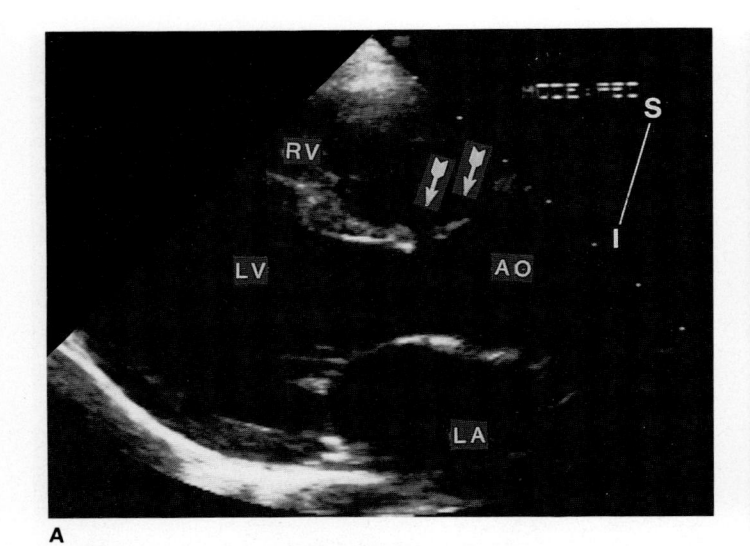

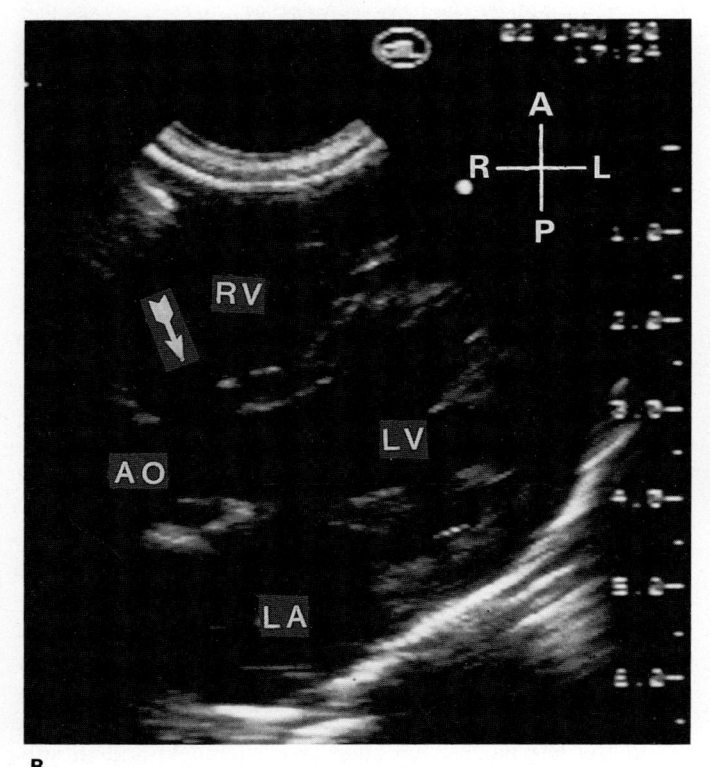

Fig. 24 A: A subaortic defect seen in a long axis parasternal view demonstrating override of the aorta of approximately 30% and in a subcostal five chamber view (B).

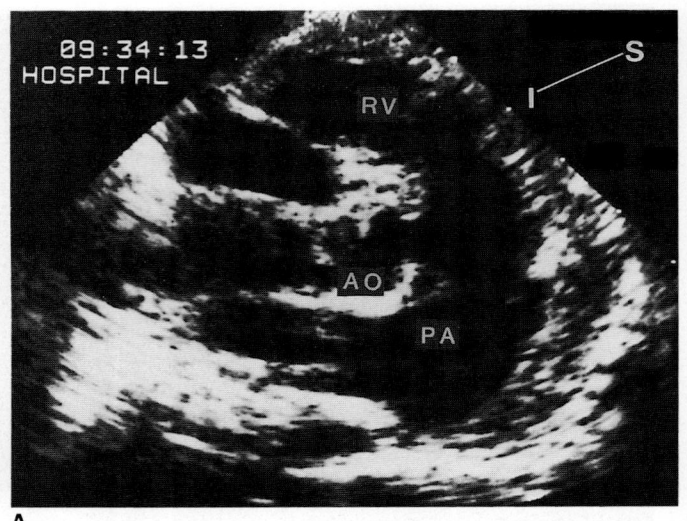

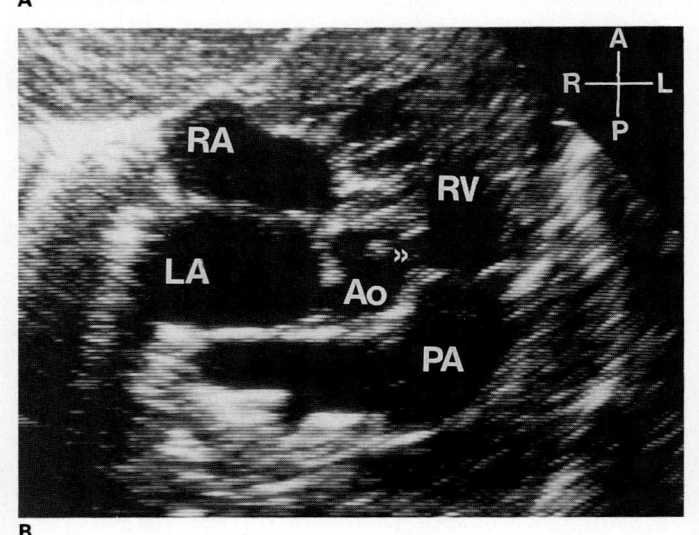

Fig. 25 A: A doubly committed subarterial defect seen in the left parasternal short axis view and in the subcostal view (B).

a false positive diagnosis of pulmonary stenosis in these circumstances.

Use of colour flow mapping in ventricular septal defect

Colour flow mapping is most useful for detecting small ventricular septal defects whose size is below imaging resolution.[150,166] In practice these defects are usually situated in the apical part of the septum, being obscured by the muscular trabeculations in this region, and occasionally by the oblique passage they may take. They may also be multiple. Apical defects are best identified in either apical four chamber or subcostal four chamber views, the parasternal long axis view being more useful for midmuscular defects. The defects are seen as tiny jets of mosaic colour on the right side of the ventricular septum. Plate 10 demonstrates two very small apical muscular defects identified on colour flow Doppler mapping which were not imaged on cross-sectional echocardiography. As mentioned above in relation to subpulmonary and doubly committed defects, colour flow mapping helps to identify high velocity flow in the right ventricular outflow tract proximal to the pulmonary valve. This may help discrimination between true and apparent right ventricular outflow tract obstruction.

LEFT TO RIGHT SHUNTS 367

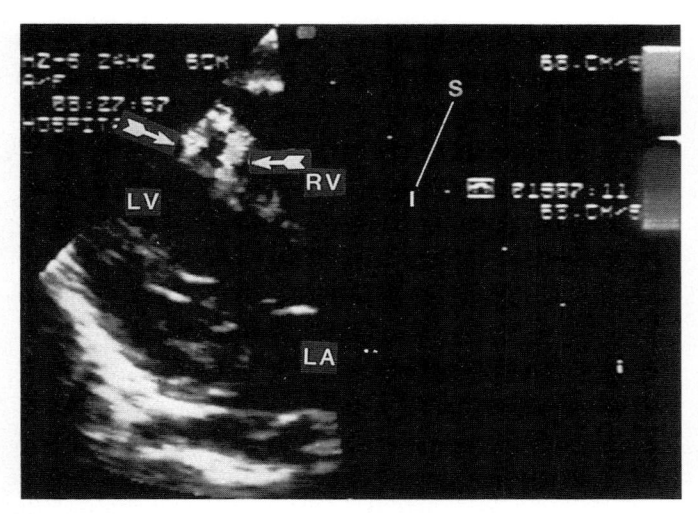

Plate 10 Colour flow mapping study of multiple apical defects (arrowed) in the long axis left parasternal view. This figure is reproduced in colour in the colour plate section at the front of this volume.

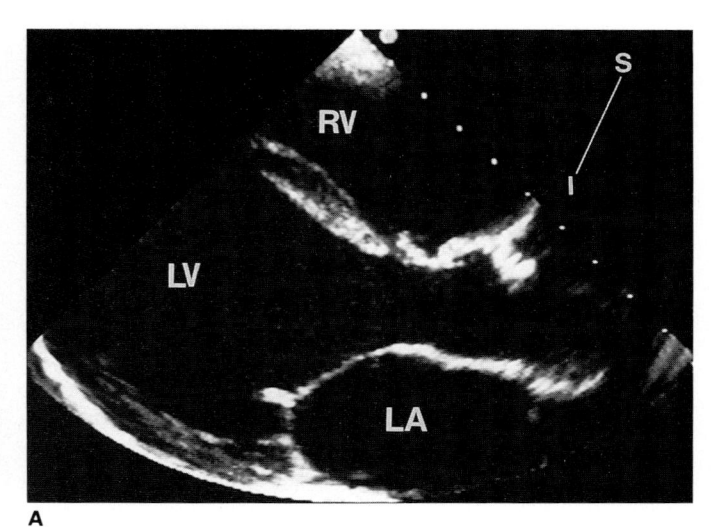

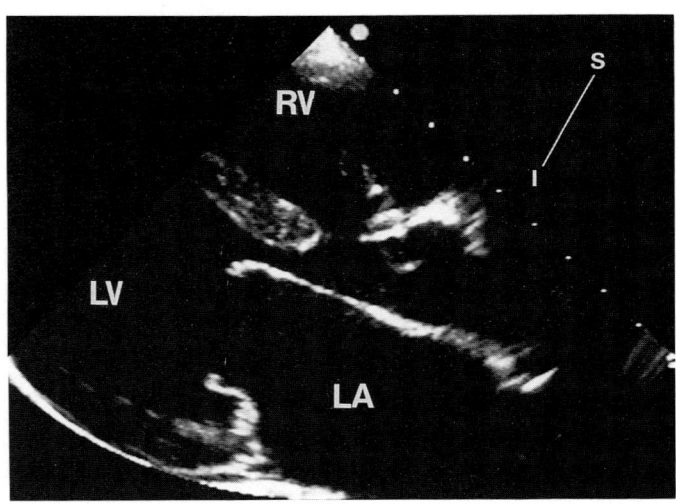

Fig. 26 A muscular subaortic defect seen in systole (**A**) and in diastole (**B**). Note the marked difference in the diameter of the defect at these different stages of the cardiac cycle.

Quantitative aspects of ventricular septal defects

It will be immediately apparent that much of the clinical management of ventricular septal defects depends on their size. Quantitation may be divided into assessment of the anatomical size of the defect by direct imaging, the magnitude of the left to right shunt by inferred or direct volume flow calculations and estimation of pulmonary artery pressure. At the present time there is no ultrasonic method available for the calculation of pulmonary vascular resistance.

There have been several studies on the accuracy of cross-sectional imaging in assessing the size of a ventricular septal defect compared to measured size at cardiac catheterisation or operation and *in vitro* experiments.[167,168] This is reasonably accurate within the caveats of measurement of any ultrasonic image, providing that the defects are imaged from at least two different planes and the operator is aware that they are rarely circular. There are obvious pitfalls; it is possible that a defect is imaged not at its widest part, but tangentially, producing a chord-like section in which case the ultrasonic measurement is likely to underestimate the actual size of the defect.[168] In early cardiac ultrasound machines the limits in beam shape and transducer penetration were particularly important in the identification of defects[169] though even in these early systems resolution of defects as small as 3 mm was described. The quality of modern instruments is such that penetration and beam focus are unlikely to be a problem in children.

There may be considerable change in the size of a defect between systole and diastole. This change appears greatest with muscular defects when they may appear to close completely, with only colour flow mapping revealing that there is in fact still a defect present. There may be similar but usually less marked appearances with perimembranous defects. Figure 26 demonstrates the considerable change in dimensions of a ventricular septal defect which may be seen between systole and diastole.

Measurement of left to right shunt

Indirect estimation of the size of the left to right shunt through a ventricular septal defect was first made by measuring the diameter of the aortic root and left atrium in the same plane and expressing them as a ratio.[144] This measurement is made using the M-mode cursor across the aortic root and left atrium in a long axis left parasternal view. There is some debate as to what constitutes a normal left atrium:aortic root ratio. Lewis and workers[144] reported a ratio greater than 1.1 correlating well with a pulmonary to systemic flow ratio of 2:1. In premature babies a left atrium:aortic root ratio of greater than 1.4 has been suggested to indicate a significant left to right shunt.[170] Figure 27 demonstrates a dilated left atrium in a patient with a large left to right shunt through a ventricular septal defect. Note the left atrium:aortic root ratio of more than 2:1.

A more direct method of estimating the size of the left to right shunt resulting from a ventricular septal defect employs the principles of volumetric flow calculation. This principle states that blood flow in a particular site can be calculated as the product of the cross-sectional area of that site and the mean velocity of blood flowing across it. With area in cm^2 and mean velocity in cm/s the product is further multiplied by 60 to give flow in cm^3/min. The method is covered in detail elsewhere but briefly involves an M-mode or cross-sectional study to calculate the cross-sectional areas of both the aorta and the pulmonary artery. The mean flow velocity at these sites is then calculated using pulsed or continuous wave Doppler traces by digitising the Doppler waveforms produced. The ratio of the two calculated flows equates with the pulmonary to systemic flow ratio.

Linear correlation with invasive methods of calculating the size of the left to right shunt through a ventricular septal defect is reported as very good in experimental[171] and clinical[172-174] studies. There is however a very large standard error with this method. This error is consequent mainly on the measurement of the cross-sectional area of the interrogated vessel. In this calculation the diameter measurement is squared, compounding even small errors in its estimation. Another potential pitfall is the calculation of mean velocity in the pulmonary artery. In many patients with a ventricular septal defect the blood flow in the pulmonary artery is too turbulent to allow accurate digitisation of the velocity envelope. Under these circumstances however it is possible to use the mitral valve orifice and mitral flow velocity to calculate the pulmonary blood flow.[175,176] This modification of calculating pulmonary flow also gives good linear correlation but has a wide standard error.

Estimation of pulmonary artery pressure

There have been many attempts to estimate pulmonary artery pressure non-invasively with echocardiography. The early attempts were modifications of the principles of the Burstin nomogram[177] which equated pulmonary artery pressure measured invasively with external graphic measurements of the time between pulmonary valve closure and tricuspid valve opening. Hatle[149] used Doppler flow signals to measure the pulmonary valve closure to tricuspid valve opening time, and found good correlation of systolic pulmonary artery pressure using the Burstin nomogram. In the light of subsequent related work, the original Burstin paper must be viewed as reasonably sound theoretically, but extraordinary in terms of the high level of correlation and narrow confidence limits achieved.

Doppler examination has been used to attempt supposedly accurate estimations of flow times in the pulmonary artery[178] by correlating the time taken to achieve peak systolic velocity in the pulmonary artery with invasive measurements of pulmonary artery pressure. Once again whilst achieving reasonable linear correlation, wide confidence limits restrict the use of this method to anything but a very crude screening test in adults, in which a time to peak velocity of less than 80 milliseconds may indicate some elevation of pulmonary artery pressure.[179,180]

There are also cross-sectional echocardiographic appearances which are suggestive of pulmonary hypertension. In the presence of a ventricular septal defect hypertrophy and dilatation of the right ventricle and pulmonary artery are reasonable non-quantitative indicators of elevated pulmonary artery pressure. Prolapse of the pulmonary valve cusps in diastole gives a rather subjective suggestion of elevated pulmonary artery pressure. Despite the work of Robinson[181] in a group of children with ventricular septal defects, this method is not sufficiently reliable to be widely applicable. Colour flow Doppler mapping may identify right ventricular hypertension by demonstrating bidirectional or even right to left flow across a ventricular septal defect.[182] The method is not at all quantitative and cannot exclusively be relied upon to reflect accurately the pulmonary artery pressure, as bidirectional and right to left shunting may occur across a defect when there is severe right ventricular outflow tract obstruction. Nevertheless if

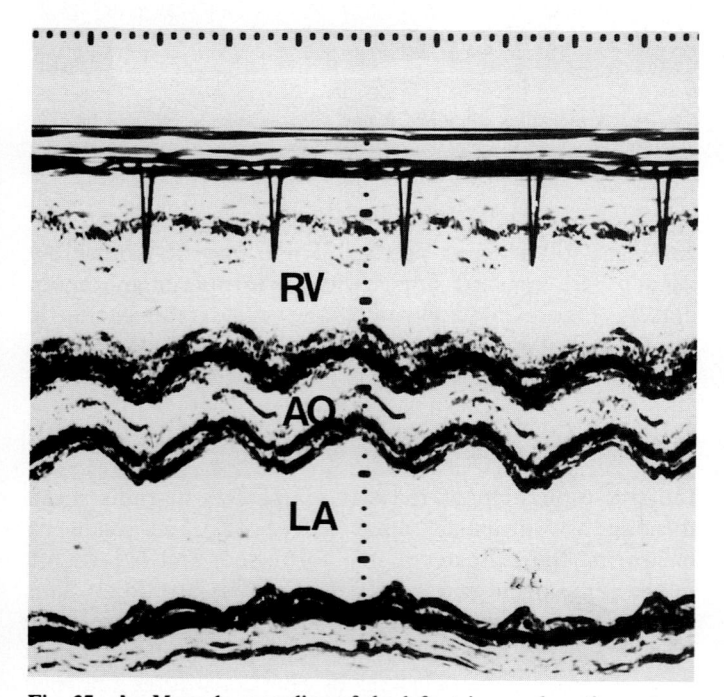

Fig. 27 An M-mode recording of the left atrium and aortic root. Note the marked dilatation of the left atrium and an LA:AO ratio of 1.8 indicating a large left to right shunt.

this latter association is excluded, the operator has yet another qualitative tool with which to screen for elevated pulmonary artery pressure.

The most accurate method of estimating pulmonary artery pressure in patients with a ventricular septal defect is to use the continuous wave Doppler technique to measure the peak blood flow velocity across the defect, and apply the modified Bernoulli equation to it to obtain a pressure difference between the left ventricle and right ventricle. This is sometimes termed the septal gradient. A reasonably accurate estimate of right ventricular, and in the absence of right ventricular outflow tract obstruction, pulmonary artery pressure is made by subtracting this pressure difference from the systolic blood pressure measured in the arm.[153,154,183] Underestimation of the pressure difference across the ventricular septal defect in some patients with normal or only mildly elevated pulmonary artery pressure has been reported by some workers,[184] tending therefore to overestimate the pulmonary artery pressure. Generally however patients with normal or only mild elevation of pulmonary artery pressure will have high velocity flow across the septum and therefore a large septal gradient, and those with severe pulmonary hypertension will have a relatively low velocity and a small septal gradient. Figure 28 demonstrates velocity recordings across ventricular septal defects in two patients, one with normal pulmonary artery pressure (A), and one with significant pulmonary hypertension (B). In the presence of a very large ventricular septal defect, or a defect associated with pulmonary vascular disease and severe pulmonary hypertension there will not of course be any difference in pressure between the left and right ventricles. In these circumstances there is no septal gradient, the velocity of blood passing through the defect in either direction being in the region of 1–2 m/s. The technique of eliciting a septal gradient involves locating the direction of the jet of blood passing through the defect with the continuous wave transducer placed at the mid left parasternal edge. If there is a palpable thrill it is logical to start interrogating the jet at this site. Once in the vicinity of the jet small movements of the transducer should be made to ensure full alignment with flow. This is confirmed by a pure tone audio signal and a well-defined envelope of spectral analysis with minimal gain settings. Understandably this method is not applicable to all defects. Some for example will have rather eccentrically directed jets, particularly those associated with an aneurysm of the ventricular septum. In addition blood passing through very small defects may do so in a spray fashion and thus accurate flow alignment is impossible.

The modified Bernoulli equation applied to the tricuspid regurgitation jet can be used to estimate right ventricular pressure in those patients in whom it is possible to obtain a high quality Doppler signal.[185,186] A right ventricle to right atrium pressure difference is obtained in millimetres of mercury and an estimate of mean right atrial pressure is added to this value. This sum is a reasonable estimate of right ventricular systolic pressure and, in the absence of right ventricular outflow tract obstruction, of pulmonary artery systolic pressure.

Thus the commonest of congenital heart lesions may be fully assessed using the medium of ultrasound in all modes applied to the heart. Whilst M-mode studies perhaps offer least information, modern colour flow mapping studies may aid rapid diagnosis even for the novice. Transoesophageal studies in children are very much in their early stages, but there is little doubt that this mode of car-

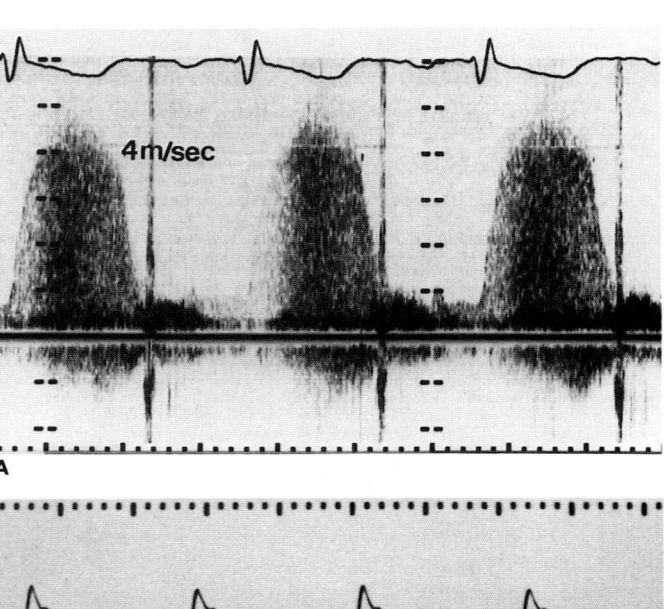

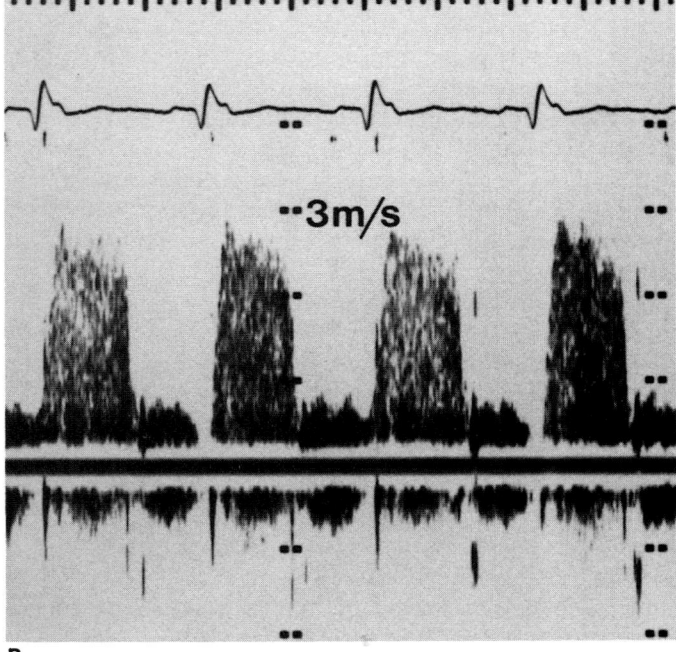

Fig. 28 Continuous wave Doppler recordings. A: A Septal jet with peak velocity of almost 5 m/s in a patient with normal pulmonary artery pressure and B: with a peak velocity of less than 3 m/s in a patient with elevated pulmonary artery pressure.

diac ultrasound will find its place.[187] It seems likely that in the first instance this will be of most benefit to those children with a poor precordial ultrasound window, particularly those having just undergone cardiac surgery.

Anatomical and haemodynamic information may be obtained using cardiac ultrasound and it is a great tribute to the technique that experienced operators in many centres refer patients for surgery on the basis of ultrasound diagnosis alone.

PATENT DUCTUS ARTERIOSUS

Introduction

The ductus arteriosus is a communication between the descending aorta and the pulmonary artery. Constriction of the ductus arteriosus begins in the early hours of life; functional closure in term babies is usually complete in the first 24 hours of life and complete anatomical obliteration is usually achieved by the age of 21 days.[188] Isolated patency of the ductus arteriosus in term infants is the second commonest congenital heart abnormality, and constitutes between 5 and 10% of all congenital abnormalities of the heart.[189]

Under normal circumstances patency of the ductus arteriosus beyond the early days of life is associated with flow of blood from aorta to pulmonary artery. Nomenclature of this lesion has varied over the years. Whilst patent ductus arteriosus is probably the most widely understood name for this lesion internationally, some authors have advocated ductus arteriosus, persistent ductus arteriosus, and most recently arterial duct, as alternatives. Abbreviation of patent ductus arteriosus to PDA is widely used and understood.

As with any of the congenital heart lesions, a ductus arteriosus may exist as an isolated lesion, or as part of a combination with virtually any congenital heart abnormality. Common complex lesions associated with a ductus arteriosus include pulmonary atresia, critical left heart obstructive lesions such as coarctation of the aorta, interruption of the aortic arch, hypoplastic left heart syndrome and critical aortic stenosis.

In this situation the co-existence of a ductus arteriosus may be beneficial to the patient in providing temporary perfusion of the systemic or pulmonary circulation in the newborn period. This chapter will deal only with isolated ductus arteriosus, and will concentrate on those shunting from left to right shunt.

Cross-sectional echocardiography is the most useful mode of ultrasound for qualitative and quantitative assessment of the ductus arteriosus. M-mode echocardiography has very little place in the diagnosis of ductus arteriosus but it may detect left atrial dilatation, indirectly supporting a clinical suspicion of a left to right shunt,[190] albeit with poor sensitivity and specificity.[191] Doppler ultrasound has improved the diagnostic yield of ultrasound in making the diagnosis of a ductus arteriosus.[192–194] In some cases a practical estimate of pulmonary artery pressure may be made[195] and within limitations, quantification of the left to right shunt may also be possible.[155,196] Much of our knowledge of the anatomy of the ductus arteriosus has come from studies of premature newborns by virtue of the increased incidence in this group.

The examination

Imaging the ductus arteriosus may be achieved from either the suprasternal long axis, left parasternal short axis, or subcostal imaging planes.

Suprasternal long axis imaging

This plane of imaging was initially validated by Smallhorn[197] who predicted ductal patency in 87 out of a group of 94 patients ranging from premature neonates to those aged more than 1 year.

The transducer is placed either directly in the suprasternal notch, or just to the right of it, virtually overlying the head of the right clavicle. It is held almost midway between a coronal and sagittal section. In addition it may be possible to obtain this section with the transducer overlying the left sternoclavicular joint. The plane of imaging is thus directed to the left and posterior in the plane of the aortic arch. A standard view of the aortic arch is obtained which displays the three main head and neck branches. With fine manipulation, occasionally necessitating moving the transducer down an intercostal space, the ductus may be brought into view between the proximal descending aorta and the main pulmonary artery (Fig. 29). Care must be taken to identify the left pulmonary artery and the ductus arteriosus separately. The left pulmonary artery lies inferior and anterior to the ductus arteriosus but can so convincingly appear to communicate with the lumen of the descending aorta that a false positive diagnosis can easily be made. It is unusual to be able to identify both the left pulmonary artery and the ductus arteriosus in their entirety in the same echocardiographic section, particularly if the ductus is small. However, portions of both may be imaged together which further avoids the pitfall of false positive diagnosis. If there is any doubt, attempts to image the ductus from the left parasternal short axis plane or the subcostal plane should be made. If Doppler ultrasound is available this is likely to resolve any uncertainty as to the diagnosis.

False negative diagnosis may occur with imaging alone in the case of very small ducts approaching 2 mm diameter[198] which are likely to be close to the limits of lateral resolution of the transducer.[199]

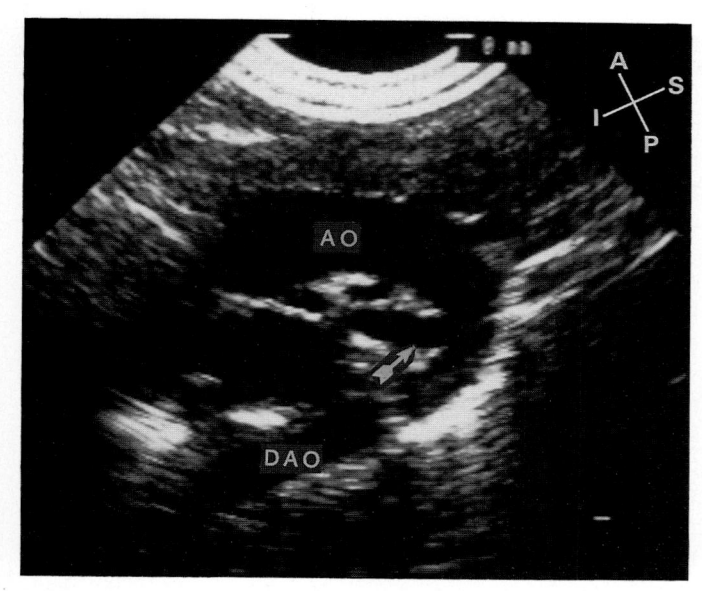

Fig. 29 A long axis suprasternal view of the aortic arch showing a patent ductus arteriosus.

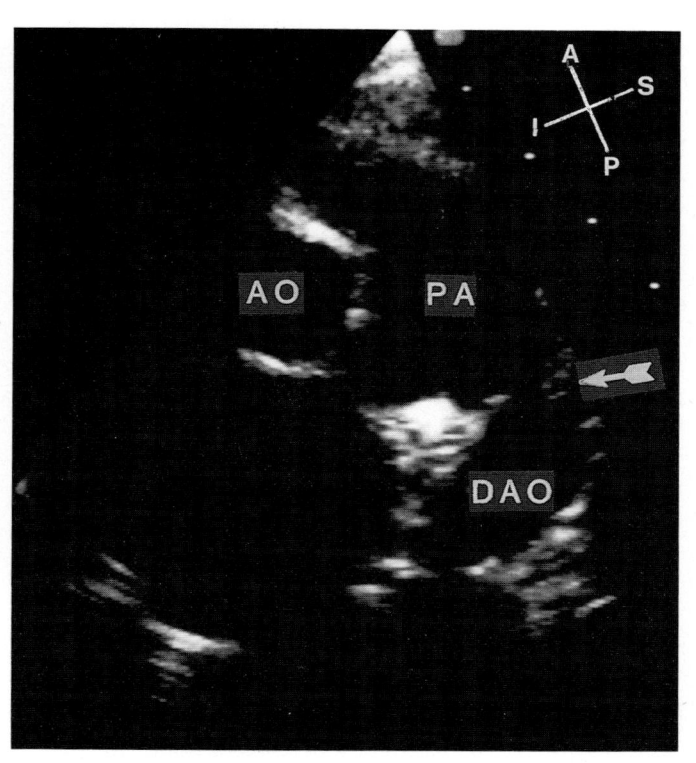

Fig. 30 A left parasternal short axis view showing a patent ductus arteriosus.

Left parasternal short axis imaging

This plane of imaging for identifying the ductus arteriosus was popularised by Sahn.[200] It relies on a cross-sectional cut which sections the main pulmonary artery, the ductus arteriosus and the descending aorta in continuity. The transducer is placed to the left of the sternum in the second or third intercostal space and directed posteriorly. The pulmonary artery is easily identified and if the transducer is rotated anticlockwise the communication between it and the descending aorta via the ductus arteriosus may be seen (Fig. 30). In this view the ductus may appear as a very short structure and if care is not taken the diagnosis may be missed. Stenosis at the pulmonary artery end of the ductus is relatively common. It is seen as a 'tear drop' appearance of the communication between the aorta and pulmonary artery. Some authors[201-203] claim that serial echocardiographic studies can document gradual stenosis and closure of the ductus arteriosus in premature babies, and can thus be used to monitor the therapeutic response to pharmacological manipulation, or in assessment for surgical closure. Once again lack of imaging resolution may result in the potential for false negative diagnosis for very small ductuses. Doppler ultrasound and particularly colour flow mapping increase the diagnostic accuracy.

The main pitfall of the left parasternal technique is the availability of a good echocardiographic window. In many patients, particularly premature neonates with their common problem of lung disease, good images cannot be obtained from this position because of the interposition of air between the heart and the transducer. This latter problem may be overcome by using the subcostal approach.

Subcostal imaging

This echocardiographic section necessitates placing the transducer at the xiphisternum and directing the ultrasound beam upwards and to the left. In this section the distal aortic arch and proximal descending aorta may be imaged and the ductus identified in the similar but reciprocal view to that seen from the suprasternal notch. The drawback of this method of imaging the ductus is that as the aortic arch and ductus are relatively far away from the transducer, it tends to be limited to babies and infants. In addition, hepatomegaly or abdominal distension may preclude obtaining a good transducer position. A transducer with a relatively narrow radius convex head is more suited to imaging from the subcostal position. As mentioned above, this approach does have the advantage of being useful in those patients with a limited parasternal window secondary to lung disease or chest deformity. Premature neonates come into this category and this view can be particularly useful in these patients who will tend to have hyperinflated lung overlying much of the heart. Using a combination of the above imaging techniques it is possible to determine ductal patency with great sensitivity and specificity. Most paediatric cardiologists throughout the world are confident to refer patients for surgical or interventional treatment of a ductus arteriosus on the basis of imaging confirmation by echocardiography.

Doppler examination in patent ductus arteriosus

The most useful application of Doppler ultrasound to the patent ductus arteriosus is in qualitative diagnosis. It may be used to support an imaging diagnosis, or confirm the diagnosis when the imaging study is equivocal. Pulsed wave,[192,196] continuous wave[204] or colour flow mapping[194] Doppler examinations in particular afford rapid confirmation of flow in the pulmonary artery from a ductus arteriosus.

Quantitative information such as an estimate of pulmonary artery pressure or the size of the left to right shunt may also be obtained using Doppler studies as discussed below.

Doppler ultrasound was initially used to confirm the presence of a ductus arteriosus by demonstrating flow reversal in the descending aorta[205] or brachial artery[206] using analogue displays of the Doppler waveforms. If the lumen of the descending aorta is interrogated from the suprasternal notch the Doppler signal obtained consists of a systolic peak directed away from the transducer followed by an early diastolic peak directed back towards the transducer. This is an accentuation of the normal diastolic Doppler waveform seen as a consequence of flow reversal filling the aortic sinuses and coronary arteries. The appearance is not specific to ductus arteriosus however and may be found in other pathological conditions with diastolic run off from the aorta, notably aortic regurgitation, aortopulmonary window, and in patients with a systemic to pulmonary artery shunt.

Pulsed Doppler sampling of blood flow in the pulmonary artery produces characteristic waveforms depending on the site of sampling within the pulmonary artery.[192,207] There is a systolic waveform directed away from the transducer followed by a diastolic peak of disturbed flow in the same direction with the Doppler sample volume placed in the centre of the pulmonary artery as viewed in the standard left parasternal short axis view (Fig. 31). This diastolic peak represents blood which has flowed from aorta to pulmonary artery, met a closed pulmonary valve and has subsequently turned antegradely down the pulmonary artery.

High velocity disturbed flow directed towards the transducer is seen with the sample volume placed a little more laterally and thus lying close to the pulmonary artery end of the ductus orifice. When this same orifice is interrogated with a continuous wave Doppler beam a characteristic 'saw tooth' Doppler waveform of high velocity throughout systole and diastole is seen (Fig. 32). This interrogation of the ductus may be obtained by placing the continuous wave transducer in the suprasternal notch and directing it posteriorly and to the left. Alternatively, the waveform may be recorded from the left parasternal position with the transducer directed posteriorly and to the left. The characteristic continuous audio signal is heard and with fine manipulation the complete waveform is obtained. The typical waveform is of continuous flow with the maximum velocity in systole and a lower velocity in diastole.[208] This type of Doppler signal may also be used to estimate pulmonary artery pressure (see below). As most patients will have normal pulmonary artery pressure the velocities measured both in systole and diastole will be high and the audio signal when fully aligned can be described as a continuous hissing sound.

Colour flow Doppler mapping applied to the image obtained in the left parasternal short axis section of the pulmonary artery–ductus–descending aorta section gives rapid confirmation of flow through the ductus to pulmonary artery with high velocity flow seen as a mosaic pattern directed towards the transducer (Plate 11). Flow is

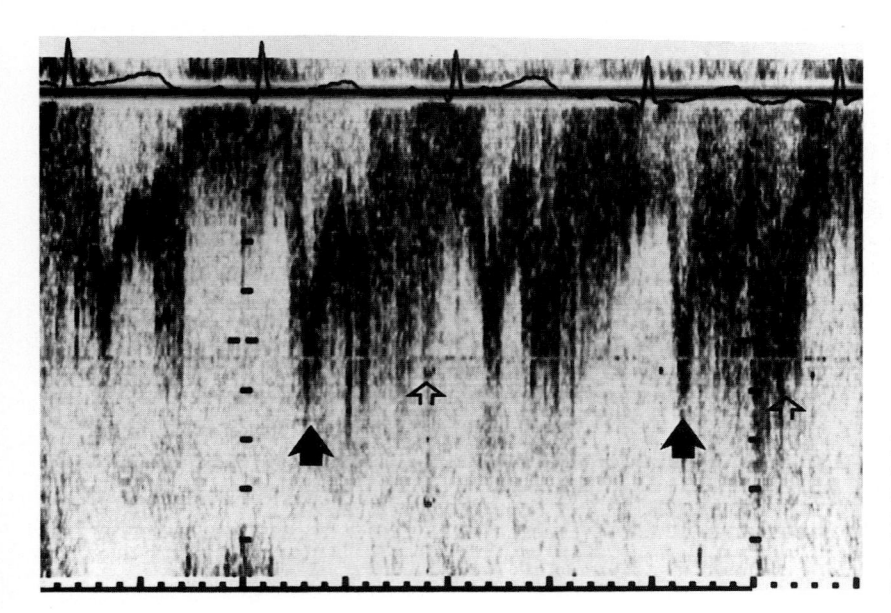

Fig. 31 A pulsed Doppler recording of pulmonary artery flow, taken using a parasternal short axis approach. The sample volume is placed in the main pulmonary artery approximately half way between the valve and the bifurcation. There are both systolic (closed arrow) and diastolic (open arrow) signals directed away from the transducer.

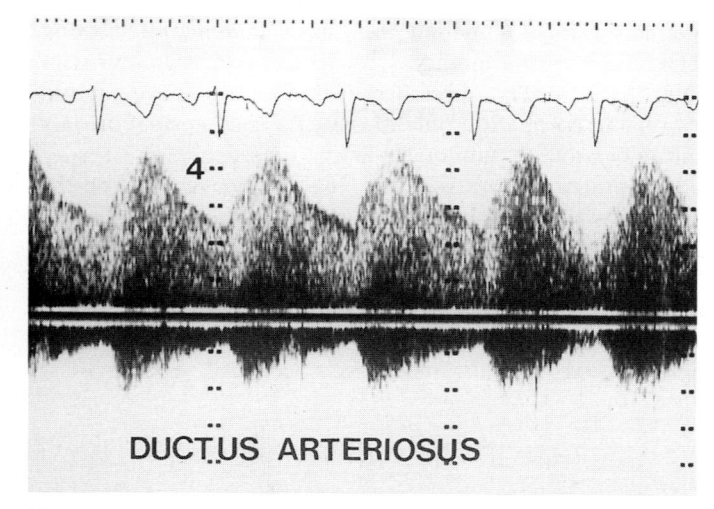

Fig. 32 A continuous wave Doppler recording from the suprasternal notch showing the typical high velocity sawtooth pattern. High velocity flow from aorta to pulmonary artery throughout the cardiac cycle indicates low pulmonary artery pressure.

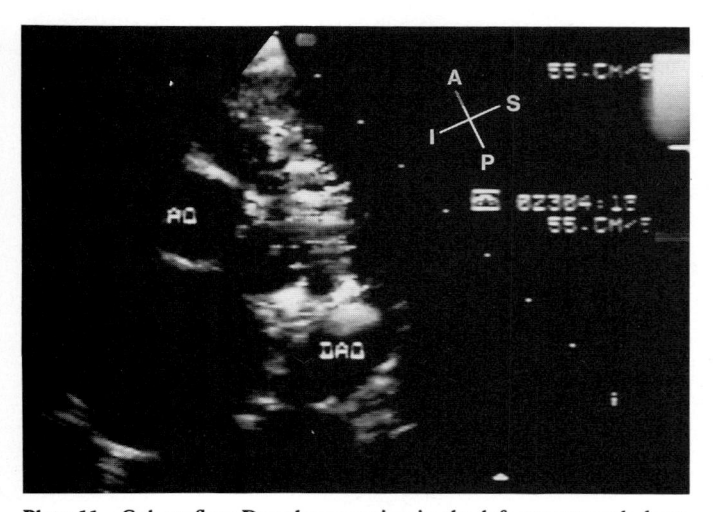

Plate 11 Colour flow Doppler mapping in the left parasternal short axis view demonstrating a broad, centrally placed mosaic jet from aorta into the pulmonary artery (anatomy as in Fig. 30). This figure is reproduced in colour in the colour plate section at the front of this volume.

seen as a narrow turbulent jet applied along the lateral wall of the pulmonary artery when the ductus orifice is small and not directly interrogated.[194]

Colour flow mapping applied to the imaging obtained from the suprasternal notch is not so reliably helpful due to the relatively large distance between the ductus and the transducer, as at such distances the lateral resolution of the transducer is compromised. It may be possible to observe a continuous mosaic pattern of colour in the pulmonary artery from this approach but care must be taken not to mistake this for aliasing of a normal pulmonary artery velocity signal.

Quantifying the left to right shunt

The consequence of a large left to right shunt through a ductus arteriosus is volume loading of the left heart. This results in dilatation of both the left atrium and left ventricle, the latter of which is usually hypercontractile.[209] In addition, the pulmonary veins entering the back of the left atrium may also appear dilated. These appearances may be appreciated using cross-sectional echocardiography, but of course are not specific to ductus arteriosus as they are also seen in patients with any large left to right shunt at ventricular or arterial level. The subsequent increased flow across the mitral valve can be documented using pulsed Doppler interrogation,[21] when peak velocities outside the normal range are to be found in the presence of a significant left to right shunt. In addition mitral velocity may be used in the calculation of pulmonary blood flow (see below). The left atrium is more distensible than the aortic root so the size of the left atrium in comparison to that of the aortic root increases in patients with a significant left to right shunt. Authors have tried to quantitate the size of the left to right shunt in terms of the dimensions of the left atrium and aortic root expressed as a ratio (LA/AO).[207,210] The dimensions are usually taken from the precordial position and are usually measured using the leading edge method.[211]

There is some evidence[212] to suggest that the flattening of the chest in babies with pronounced sternal retraction produces left atrial flattening and the precordial anteroposterior measurement may not reflect atrial distension which has been forced to occur in a superior–inferior direction. This results[213] in the potential for false negative diagnosis. As a serial measurement in the same patient by the same operator this ratio is probably a reasonable indicator of changes in the size of the left to right shunt,[214] with a ratio in excess of 1:2 being considered abnormal,[215] though some authors[210] would recommend 1.4 as a more reliable figure. This debate would seem to be further evidence that individual isolated measurements may not be sensitive or specific[191] particularly in fluid-restricted infants. The measurement is made from a long axis left parasternal section of the heart with the M-mode cursor line placed vertical to the aortic root and transecting the left atrium. The inference is that the larger the shunt the higher the ratio. Figure 33 demonstrates a dilated left atrium in a patient with a large ductus arteriosus.

Calculation of the left to right shunt through a ductus arteriosus is performed using principles of volumetric flow calculation covered in detail elsewhere in this book. In short this consists of estimating the pulmonary blood flow using the product of mean velocity across the mitral valve and an estimate of cross-sectional area of the mitral valve orifice. There are in vitro and clinical validations of this technique.[155,216] Systemic blood flow is calculated as the product of the mean velocity of blood in the aorta (usually

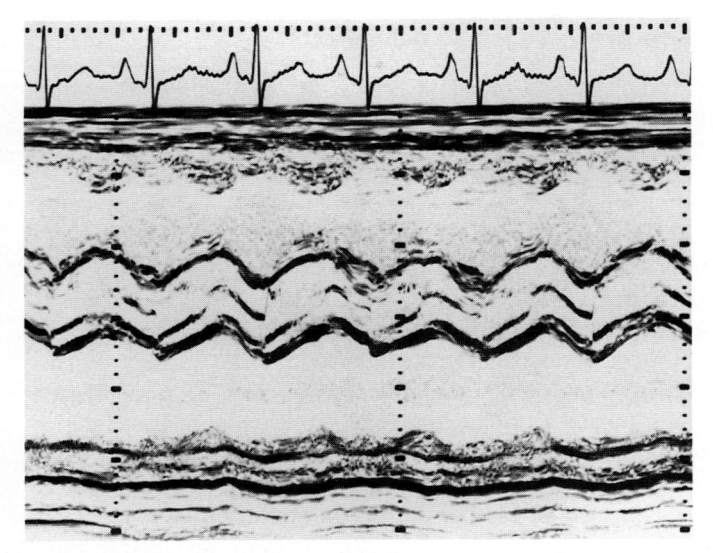

Fig. 33 An M-mode recording of the aortic root and the left atrium from a patient with a large left to right ductal shunt. The ratio of aortic root diameter to left atrial diameter is 1.6, indicating left atrial dilatation due to the large shunt.

just above the sinuses of Valsalva) and the cross-sectional area of the aorta at this point.[217] Mean velocity is best calculated using pulsed Doppler traces and digitised hard copy or on screen software.

Cross-sectional area is calculated from measurements made using M-mode or cross-sectional images. Whilst this method correlates acceptably with simultaneous invasive methods the standard error of the estimate is large, in the region of 25%[174] and precludes it as a useful single measurement in an individual. Repeated calculations in the same patient may be more valid as errors in calculation of cross-sectional area are likely to be constant.

Estimation of pulmonary artery pressure

In the past pulsed Doppler recordings[218] have been used to correlate the duration of diastolic flow from the ductus to the pulmonary artery with pulmonary artery pressure. Abbreviation of the duration of flow into the pulmonary artery in diastole would appear to be a reliable indicator of elevated pulmonary artery pressure, though the method is not accurate enough for use as an individual measurement.

For the purposes of more accurate estimation of pulmonary artery pressure the ductus arteriosus is seen as a stenotic lesion between the systemic and pulmonary artery circulations. Thus the peak velocity of the waveform in metres per second in either systole or diastole may be applied to the modified Bernoulli equation. The resulting pressure drop calculated in millimetres of mercury is subtracted from the systolic or diastolic blood pressure measured in the arm with a sphygmomanometer and thus pulmonary artery systolic or diastolic pressure can be calculated. Whilst some authors have demonstrated good correlation of this method with invasive measurements of pulmonary artery pressure,[219] others[195] have found reasonable correlation only in patients with normal or only mild elevation of pulmonary artery pressure.

For practical purposes, the higher the velocity of the blood flow through the ductus arteriosus the lower the pulmonary artery pressure. Figure 34 shows recordings from two patients, one with normal pulmonary artery pressure and one with pulmonary hypertension. At the extremes of pulmonary hypertension blood may only flow from left to right during diastole and at low velocity. Under these

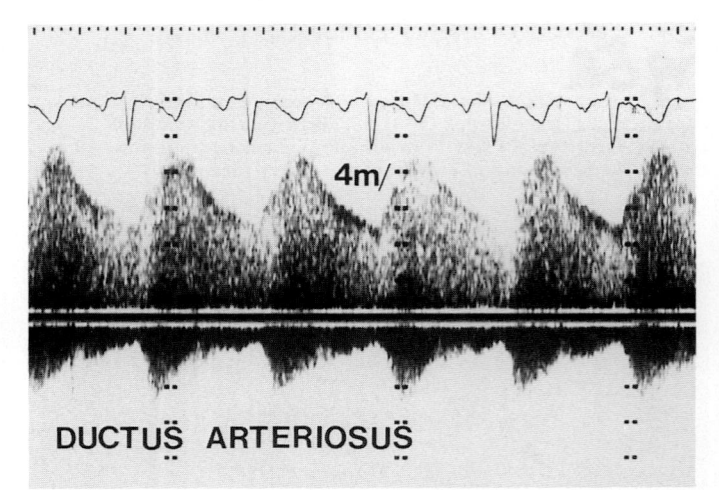

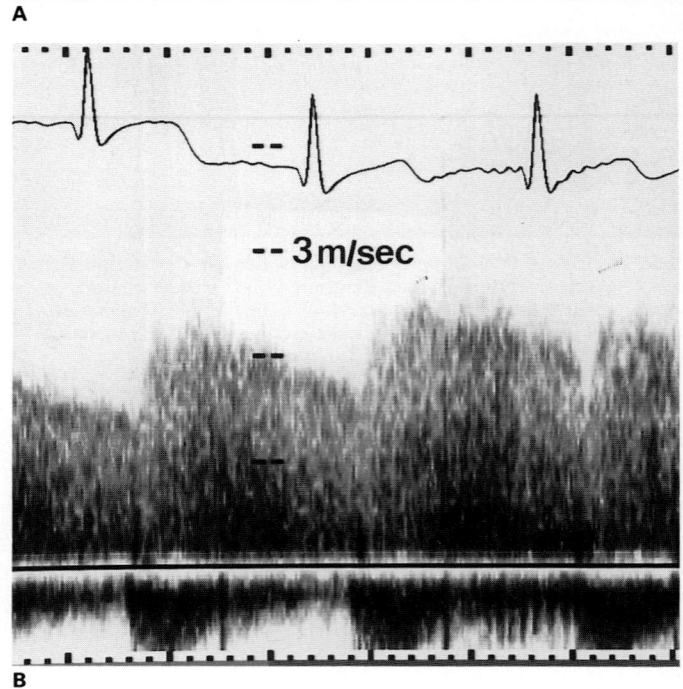

Fig. 34 Continuous wave Doppler recordings. A: Ductal flow velocities with a peak velocity of over 4 m/s in a patient with normal pulmonary artery pressure and **B:** with a peak velocity of just over 2 m/s in a patient with pulmonary systolic and diastolic hypertension.

circumstances there may also be bidirectional shunting through the ductus at low velocity. It has also been postulated that colour flow mapping can help to identify patients with pulmonary hypertension as it shows loss of the usual mosaic pattern of high velocity flow through the ductus in patients with severe elevation of pulmonary artery pressure.[220]

Diagnostic information of a qualitative and quantitative nature is available using all forms of echocardiography. The new technique of transoesophageal echocardiography is becoming more feasible in children.[187] Its role in ductus arteriosus is not yet defined, though this may be a useful tool in interventional procedures on the ductus arteriosus such as occlusion using the Rashkind double umbrella technique.

TRUNCUS ARTERIOSUS (COMMON ARTERIAL TRUNK)

The echocardiographic diagnosis of common arterial trunk rests upon the demonstration of a single great artery arising from the heart with the aorta and the main pulmonary artery or the branch pulmonary arteries arising from it.

Common arterial trunk is most frequently associated with an outlet ventricular septal defect with the trunk overriding the crest of the ventricular septum. Varying degrees of override may be seen; the majority will show approximately 50% override but more or less than this may occur, resulting in the trunk arising predominantly from one ventricular chamber.[221] The degree of override is usually clearly seen on parasternal long axis imaging (Fig. 35) and may be confirmed and better appreciated in three dimensions by additional use of subcostal and apical views.[221-224] Short axis parasternal imaging will reveal the absence of a right ventricular infundibulum and is important in the exclusion of tetralogy of Fallot or pulmonary atresia with ventricular septal defect, both of which are also associated with a large great artery overriding the ventricular septum.[225] As with other left to right shunts at ventricular or arterial level, high pulmonary blood flow will be reflected by left atrial dilatation and high mitral flow velocities.

The echocardiographic technique best suited to demonstration of the origin of the pulmonary arteries will depend to a certain extent on the site of their origin from the trunk. In the commonest anatomical arrangement, when the main pulmonary artery arises from the posterior aspect of the trunk above the sinuses of Valsalva, the origin of the main pulmonary artery may usually be seen in parasternal long axis, suprasternal and subcostal views (Fig. 36). Identification of the pulmonary artery bifurcation and its branches usually requires some modification of this view, with clockwise rotation of the transducer halfway towards a short axis view (either from the parasternal or subcostal approaches) often allowing visualisation of the proximal branches[223,224,226-228] (Fig. 37).

Stenosis of the proximal branch pulmonary arteries may occur with a common arterial trunk and may, at least in theory, be detectable by cross-sectional echocardiography. The suprasternal approach is particularly useful for imaging the proximal pulmonary artery branches and their origins; the right pulmonary artery may be imaged in its long axis to include its origin, and rotation of the transducer through 90° to image the ascending aorta in its long axis usually allows visualisation of the origin of the left pulmonary artery.[222] When the main pulmonary artery is absent and the right and left pulmonary arteries arise separately from the posterior aspect of the trunk (or more rarely from its lateral aspects), a combination of transducer positions will still usually allow detection of their sites of origin.[227,228] Common arterial trunk has been subdivided into different types or categories based upon the origin of the pulmonary arteries, but unfortunately more than one system of classification has been suggested.[229] Confusion may be avoided by simply stating the anatomical arrangement detected at echocardiography, with particular reference to the site(s) of origin of the pulmonary arteries.

The valve of the common trunk is abnormal; it may have 2, 3 or 4 cusps which may be thickened and dysplastic and the valve may be stenosed or incompetent. Dysplasia and stenosis will usually be apparent on cross-sectional imaging of the truncal valve in its long axis (Fig. 38) and short axis views may allow determination of the number of valve cusps.[230]

M-mode echocardiography is of little value in the anatomical diagnosis of common arterial trunk, but prior to the advent of cross-sectional echocardiography it allowed detection of a single, large, overriding great artery and

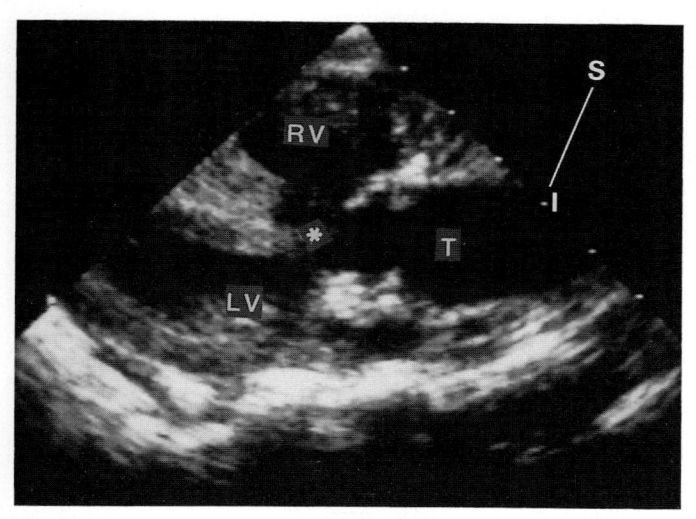

Fig. 35 A common arterial trunk (T) overriding the ventricular septum by about 50%, with the usual single outlet ventricular septal defect (*) seen in long axis parasternal view. The origin of the pulmonary artery is not seen in this view.

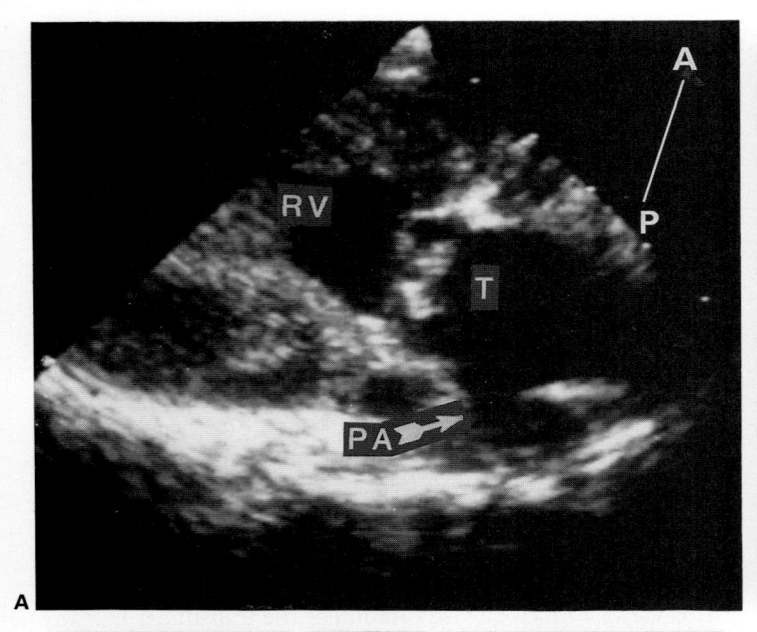

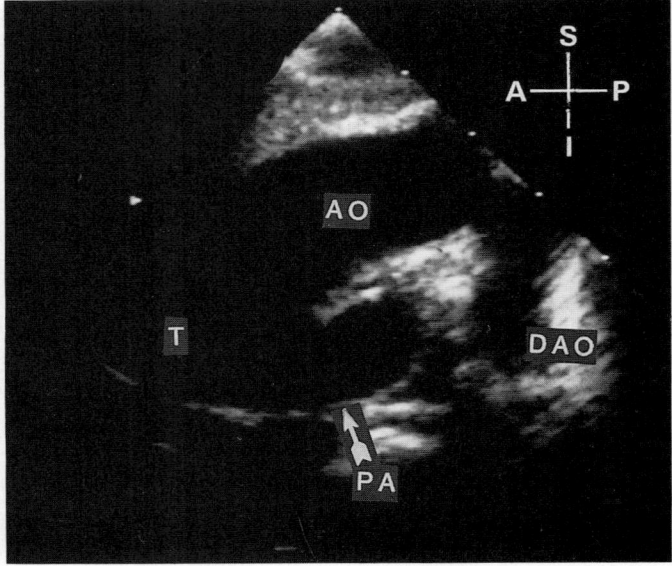

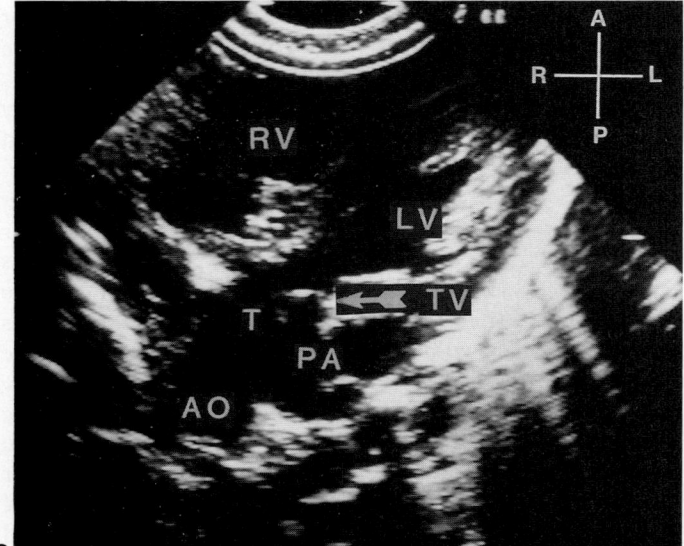

Fig. 36 Common arterial trunk (**T**). The origin of the main pulmonary artery may be seen using **A**: a modified parasternal long axis approach (the trunk is largely arising from the right ventricle in this example), **B**: using a suprasternal approach, or **C**: from the subcostal approach. T – truncal valve.

truncal valve dysplasia when present.[231,232,225]

Doppler ultrasound allows quantitative estimation of pressure drop across the truncal valve, but this information can be difficult to interpret in the inevitable presence of high flow across the valve prior to surgery. Colour flow imaging allows semiquantitative assessment of truncal valve incompetence.

Associated abnormalities

Full sequential segmental echocardiographic analysis of cardiac anatomy is an essential part of the ultrasound diagnosis of common arterial trunk, with particular attention being paid to aortic arch abnormalities. Right aortic arch

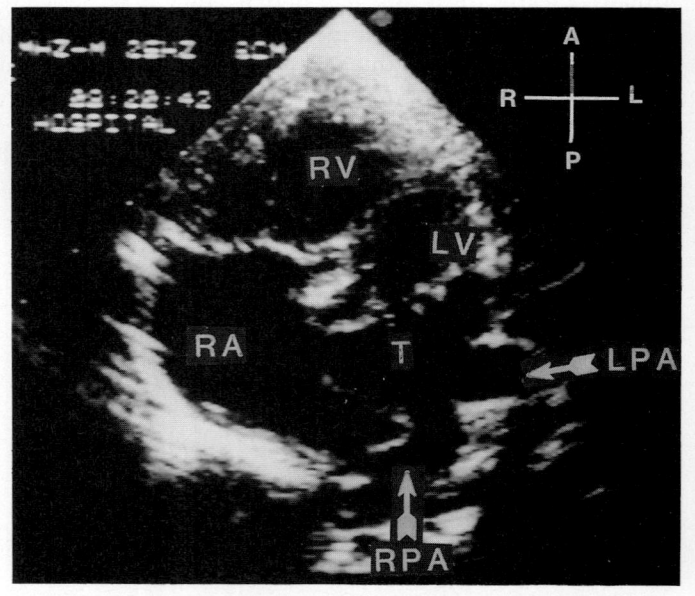

Fig. 37 Modification of the views in Fig. 36 will usually allow visualisation of the pulmonary artery bifurcation. In this example of a modified subcostal view, the right and left pulmonary arteries are clearly identified (RPA, LPA). The main pulmonary artery is very short in this patient, with the pulmonary artery bifurcating almost immediately after it arises from the common arterial trunk.

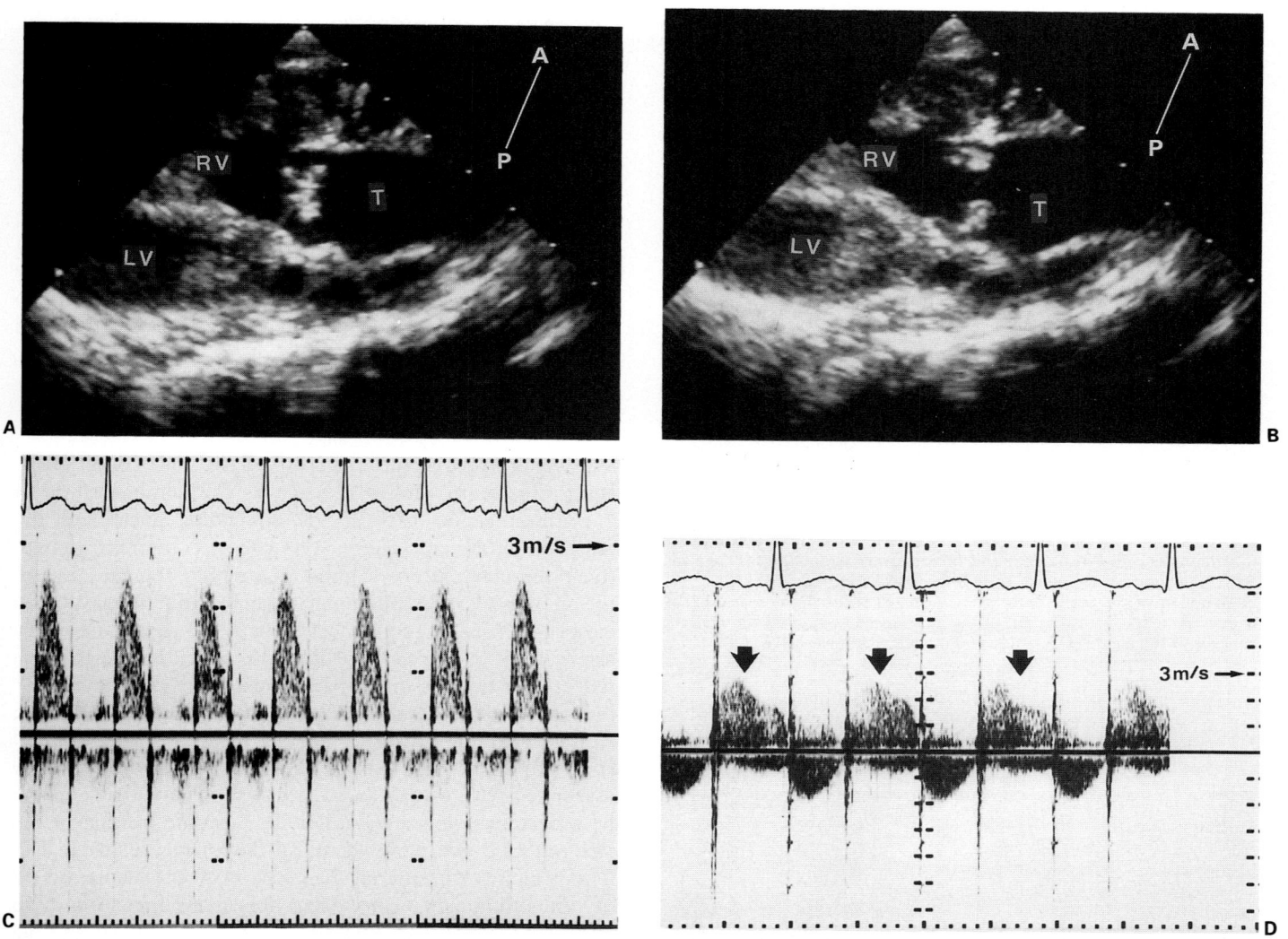

Fig. 38 Truncal valves are frequently functionally abnormal and often appear dysplastic and stenosed as in this example. In long axis parasternal view the truncal valve leaflets are clearly grossly thickened when seen **A**: in diastole and **B**: the cusp excursion is limited in systole. **C**: A continuous wave Doppler recording of truncal flow velocities taken from the suprasternal notch shows a peak velocity of about 2.5 m/s (a pressure drop of about 25 mmHg), representing mild truncal valve stenosis. **D**: A continuous wave recording of truncal valve flow using an apical approach demonstrates truncal valve regurgitation (arrowed).

(Fig. 39), coarctation of the aorta and interruption of the aortic arch are notable associations. Common arterial trunk may also be associated with thymic aplasia as part of the DiGeorge syndrome.[233] In the neonate the thymus may usually be detected by parasternal and suprasternal imaging and a brief search for thymic tissue may occasionally be helpful, but unfortunately ultrasound cannot reliably exclude the presence of thymic tissue.

Differential diagnosis

The diagnosis of common arterial trunk is usually clear on cross-sectional echocardiography. However, care must be taken to avoid erroneous diagnosis of other conditions associated with a large great artery which overrides the ventricular septum. Such conditions include tetralogy of Fallot, pulmonary atresia with ventricular septal defect, and aortic atresia with ventricular septal defect. Rarely one pulmonary artery may arise directly from the ascending aorta with the other pulmonary artery arising normally from the main pulmonary artery (sometimes referred to as a hemitruncus). This may give a similar appearance in long axis parasternal view to that seen with common arterial trunk, but more detailed examination will reveal the normal origin of the main pulmonary artery from the right ventricle.[234–237] Even more rarely, both branch pulmonary arteries may arise from the ascending aorta with the main

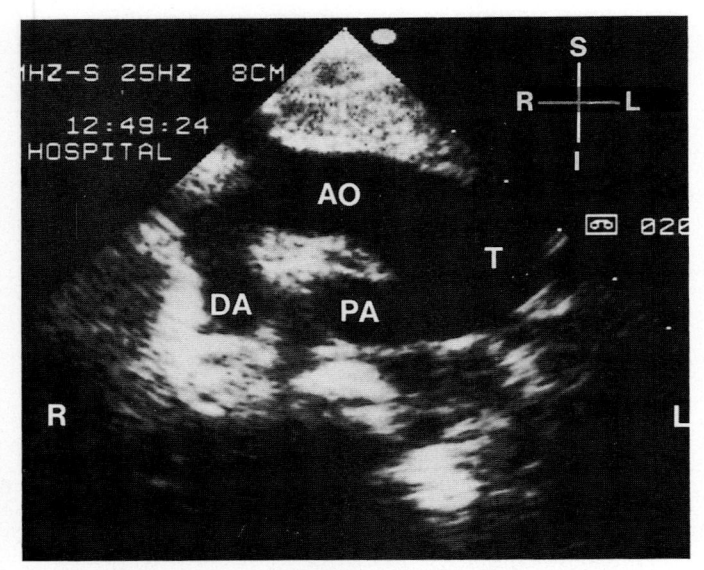

Fig. 39 Right sided aortic arch with a common arterial trunk. This is a relatively common association. A standard left arch view will fail to demonstrate the aortic arch and proximal descending aorta. Care must be taken not to interpret such findings as indicative of interruption of the aortic arch (also associated with common arterial trunk). Anticlockwise rotation of the transducer will reveal the arch curving to the right. (DA – descending aorta, truncal valve – T).

pulmonary artery arising normally but leading only to the arterial duct.[238]

Postoperative findings

Postoperative echocardiography allows assessment of right and left ventricular function, evaluation of aortic valve function, confirmation of successful closure of the ventricular septum and evaluation of blood flow velocity in the conduit between the right ventricle and the pulmonary arteries. Colour flow imaging is particularly useful in the detection of residual left to right ventricular shunting and aortic regurgitation.

AORTOPULMONARY WINDOW

The echocardiographic diagnosis of the rare condition of aortopulmonary window is made by the demonstration of a communication between the ascending aorta and the adjacent pulmonary artery. The site of communication to the pulmonary artery is most commonly the junction of the main and right pulmonary arteries, but it may be to either the main pulmonary artery or to the right pulmonary artery itself as it passes behind the ascending aorta. The defect may be seen in the parasternal short axis view,[239,240] but in breathless children this may be difficult, when suprasternal or subcostal imaging are most useful[222,241] (Fig. 40, Plate 12). Aortopulmonary window is usually associated with a substantial left to right shunt which will be reflected by left atrial dilatation, volume loading of the left ventricle and elevated mitral flow velocities (Fig. 41). The principal differential diagnosis is of anomalous origin of one pulmonary artery from the ascending aorta with the other pulmonary artery arising normally from the

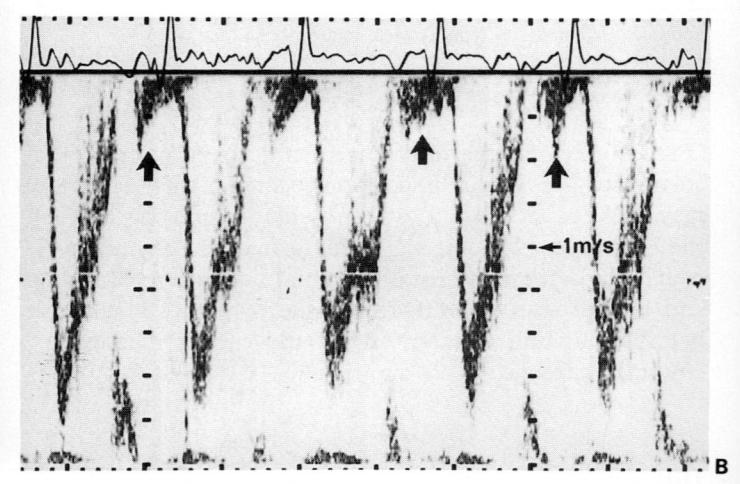

Fig. 40 Aortopulmonary window in its most common form. A: In the suprasternal view there is a wide communication (arrowed) between the posterior wall of the ascending aorta (AAO) and the proximal right pulmonary artery. **B:** The subcostal approach is well suited to pulsed Doppler assessment of pulmonary artery flow velocities, which have a similar appearance to that seen in the presence of a large arterial duct, with forward flow occurring down the main pulmonary artery in both systole and diastole (arrowed).

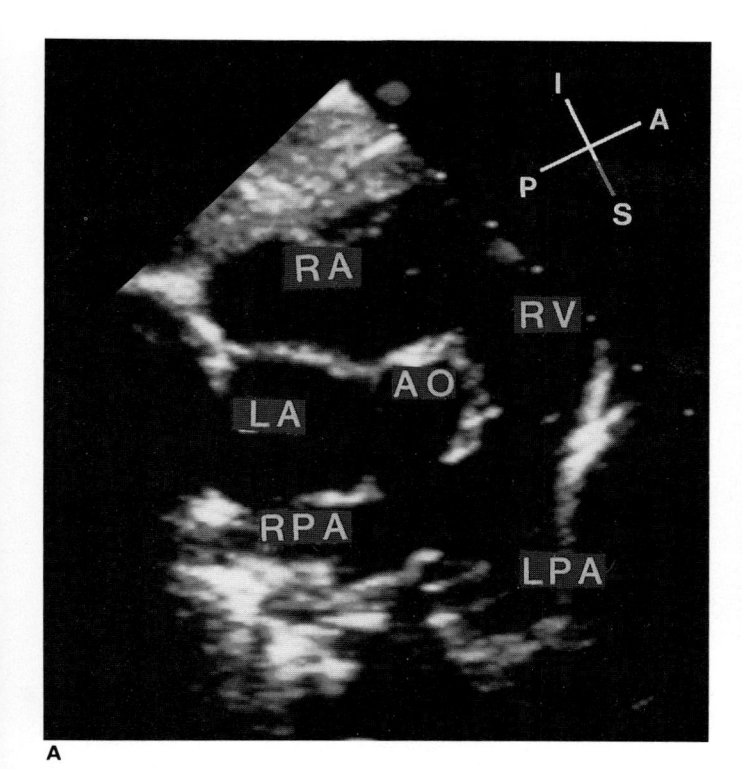

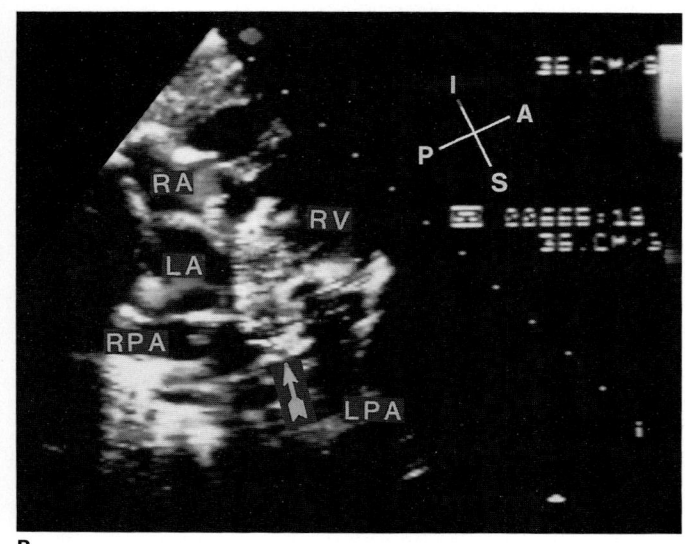

Plate 12 In breathless children with aortopulmonary window the subcostal approach may prove to be useful. **A:** This example shows a large window between the posterior aspect of the ascending aorta and the origin of the right pulmonary artery **B:** Colour flow Doppler mapping shows a wide, turbulent jet (arrowed) directed from the aorta into the pulmonary artery. This figure is reproduced in colour in the colour plate section at the front of this volume.

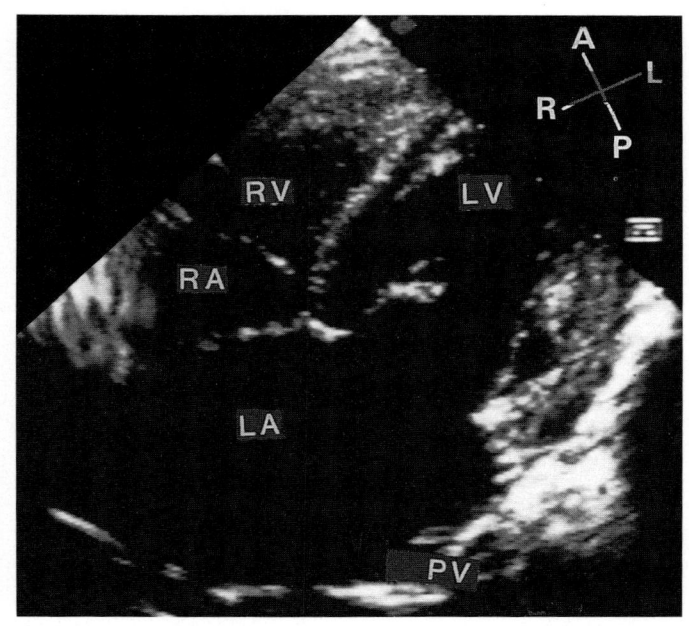

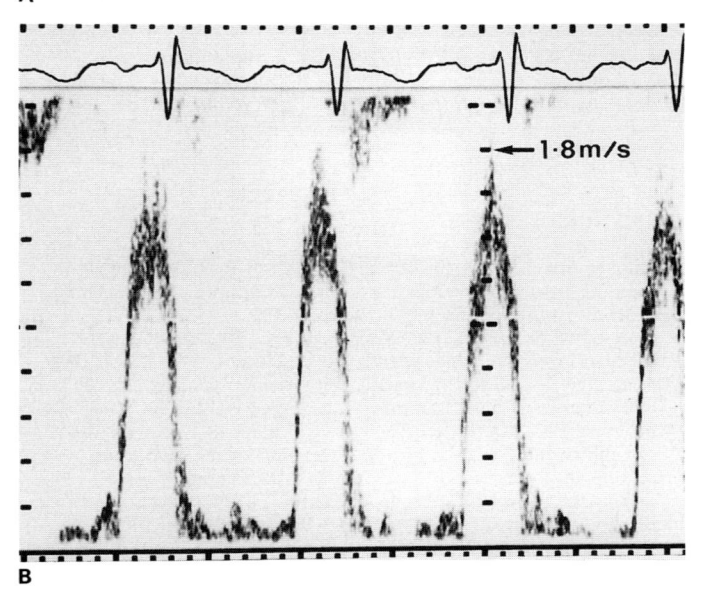

Fig. 41 A: Marked left atrial dilatation seen in the subcostal view. The pulmonary veins are also dilated (PV – pulmonary vein). Volume loading of the left heart is an almost invariable finding in aortopulmonary window. **B:** The large left to right shunt causes high pulmonary blood flow with consequent high mitral blood flow reflected by high mitral flow velocities, in this case reaching a peak velocity of 1.7 m/s.

right ventricle.[242,237] Echocardiography is also valuable in the postoperative period to confirm satisfactory repair (Plate 13).

Aortopulmonary window may occur in isolation but additional abnormalities are present in about 50% of cases. Associations which should be sought by the echocardiographer include an arterial duct, interruption of the aortic arch, tetralogy of Fallot, ventricular septal defect, atrial septal defect, right aortic arch and aortic origin of the right pulmonary artery.[235,243,244]

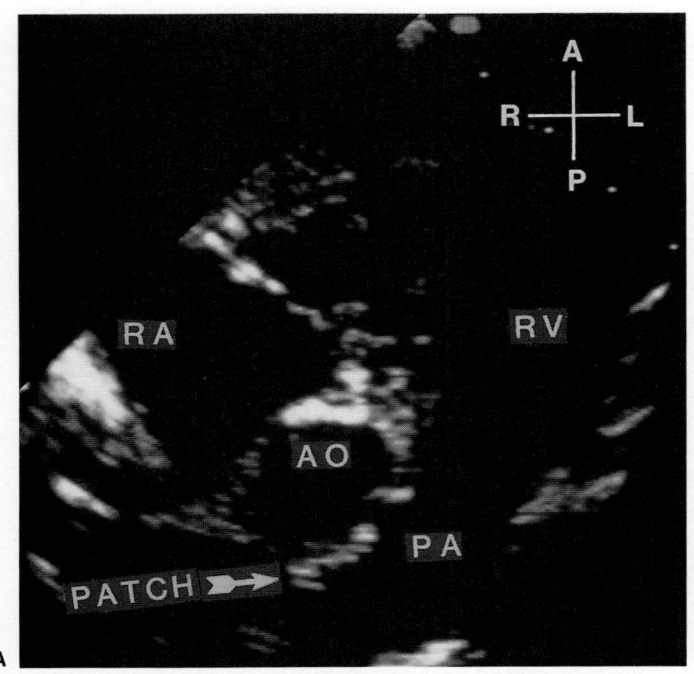

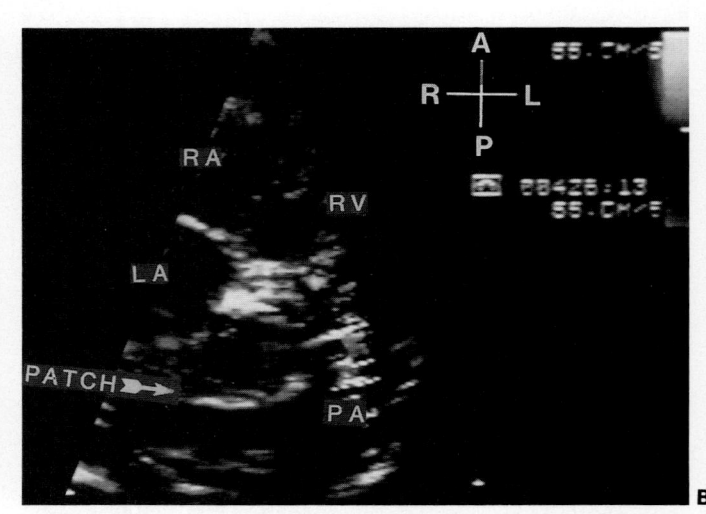

Plate 13 A: After surgical repair of the aortopulmonary window the patch closure of the defect is clearly visible on subcostal imaging. **B:** Colour flow Doppler mapping shows normal flow patterns in the pulmonary artery, with no residual aortopulmonary shunt, in marked contrast to Plate 12. This figure is reproduced in colour in the colour plate section at the front of this volume.

REFERENCES

1. Shinebourne E A, Macartney F J, Anderson R H. Sequential chamber localisation – logical approach to diagnosis in congenital heart disease. Br Heart J 1976; 38: 327–340
2. Huhta J C, Smallhorn J F, Macartney F J. Two dimensional echocardiographic diagnosis of situs. Br Heart J 1982; 48: 97–108
3. Macartney F J. Cross sectional echocardiographic diagnosis of congenital heart disease in infants. Br Heart J 1983; 50: 501–505
4. Schapira J N, Martin R P, Fowles R E, Popp R L. Single and two-dimensional echocardiographic features of the interatrial septum in normal subjects and patients with an atrial septal defect. Am J Cardiol 1979; 43: 816–819
5. Shub C, Dimopoulos I N, Seward J B, Callahan J A, Tancredi R G, Schattenberg T T, Reeder G S, Hagler D J, Tajik A J. Sensitivity of two-dimensional echocardiography in the direct visualization of atrial septal defect utilizing the subcostal approach: experience with 154 patients. J Am Coll Cardiol 1983; 2: 127–135
6. Iliceto S, Antonelli G, Sorino M, Ricci A. Detection of atrial septal defect by right sternal border echocardiography. Am J Cardiol 1984; 54: 376–378
7. Kupferschmid C, Lang D. The valve of the foramen ovale in interatrial right-to-left shunt: echocardiographic cineangiographic and hemodynamic observations. Am J Cardiol 1983; 51: 1489–1494
8. Dillon J C, Weyman A E, Feigenbaum H, Eggleton R C, Johnston K. Cross-sectional echocardiographic examination of the interatrial septum. Circulation 1977; 55: 115–120
9. Goldberg S J, Areias J C, Spitaels S E C, de Villeneuve V H. Use of time interval histographic output from echo-Doppler to detect left-to-right atrial shunts. Circulation 1978; 58: 147–152
10. Minagoe S, Tei C, Kisanuki A, Arikawa K, Nakazono Y, Yoshimura H, Kashima T, Tanaka H. Non invasive pulsed Doppler echocardiographic detection of the direction of shunt flow in patients with atrial septal defect: usefulness of the right parasternal approach. Circulation 1985; 71: 745–753
11. Oberhoffer R, Lang D. Diagnostic criteria of interatrial defects: a single gate pulsed Doppler echocardiographic study. Int J Cardiol 1989; 25: 167–171
12. Zhou T-F, Guntheroth W G. Valve incompetent foramen ovale in premature infants with ductus arteriosus: a Doppler echocardiographic study. J Am Coll Cardiol 1987; 10: 193–199
13. Sherman F S, Sahn D J, Valdez-Cruz L M, Chung K G, Elias C W. Two-dimensional Doppler colour flow mapping for detecting atrial and ventricular septal defects. Herz 1987; 12: 212–216
14. Miyatake K, Okamoto M, Kinoshita N, Izumi S, Owa M, Takao S, Sakakibara H, Nimura Y. Clinical applications of a new type of real-time two-dimensional Doppler flow imaging system. Am J Cardiol 1984; 54: 857–868
15. Suzuki Y, Kambara H, Kadota K, Tamaki S, Yamazato A, Nohara R, Osakada G, Kawai C. Detection of intracardiac shunt flow in atrial septal defect using a real-time two-dimensional colour-coded Doppler flow imaging system and comparison with contrast two-dimensional echocardiography. Am J Cardiol 1985; 56: 347–350
16. McCann W D, Harbold N B, Giuliani E R. The echocardiogram in right ventricular volume overload. JAMA 1972; 221: 1243–1245
17. Radtke W E, Tajik A J, Gau G T, Schattenberg T T, Giuliani E R, Tancredi R G. Atrial septal defect: echocardiographic observations. Studies in 120 patients. Ann Int Med 1976; 84: 246–253
18. Kasper W, Treese N, Pop T, Meinertz T. Diagnosis of increased pulmonary blood flow by suprasternal M-mode echocardiography in atrial septal defect. Am J Cardiol 1983; 52: 1272–1274
19. Chen C, Kremer P, Schroeder E, Rodewald G, Bleifeld W. Usefulness of anatomic parameters derived from two-dimensional echocardiography for estimating magnitude of left to right shunt in patients with atrial septal defect. Clin Cardiol 1987; 10: 316–321.
20. Mauran P, Fouron J-C, Carceller A-M, Douste-Blazy M-Y, van Doesburg N H, Guerin R, Ducharme G, Davignon A. Value of

respiratory variations of right ventricular dimension in the identification of small atrial septal defects (secundum type) not requiring surgery: an echocardiographic study. Am Heart J 1986; 112: 548–553
21 Goldberg S J, Wilson N, Dickinson D F. Increased blood velocities in the heart and great vessels of patients with congenital heart disease. An assessment of their significance in the absence of valvar stenosis. Br Heart J 1985; 53: 640–644
22 Paquet M, Gutgesell H. Echocardiographic features of total anomalous pulmonary venous connection. Circulation 1975; 51: 599–605
23 Stanbridge R de L, Westaby S, Smallhorn J F, Taylor J F N. Intracranial arteriovenous malformation with aneurysm of the vein of Galen as cause of heart failure in infancy. Echocardiographic diagnosis and results of treatment. Br Heart J 1983; 49: 157–162
24 Snider A R, Soifer S J, Silverman N H. Detection of intracranial arteriovenous fistula by two-dimensional ultrasonography. Circulation 1981; 63: 1179–1185
25 Bahler A S, Meller J, Brik H, Herman M V, Teichholz L E. Paradoxical motion of the interventricular septum with right ventricular dilatation in the absence of shunting. Am J Cardiol 1976; 38: 654–657
26 Ribeiro P A, Shapiro L M, Foale R A, Crean P, Oakley C M. Echocardiographic features of right ventricular dilated cardiomyopathy and Uhl's anomaly. Eur Heart J 1987; 8: 65–71
27 Righetti A, Crawford M H, O'Rourke R A, Schelbert H, Daily P O, Ross J. Interventricular septal motion and left ventricular function after coronary bypass surgery. Evaluation with echocardiography and radionuclide angiography. Am J Cardiol 1977; 39: 372–377
28 Waggoner A D, Shah A A, Schuessler J S, Crawford E S, Nelson J G, Miller R R, Quinones M A. Effect of cardiac surgery on ventricular septal motion: assessment by intraoperative echocardiography and cross-sectional echocardiography. Am Heart J 1982; 104: 1271–1278
29 Kerber R E, Litchfield R. Postoperative abnormalities of interventricular septal motion: two-dimensional and M-mode echocardiographic correlations. Am Heart J 1982; 104: 263–268
30 Fujii J J, Watanabe H, Watanabe T, Takahashi N, Ohta A, Kato K. M-mode and cross-sectional echocardiographic study of the left ventricular wall motions in complete left bundle branch block. Br Heart J 1979; 42: 255–260
31 Zoneraich S, Zoneraich O, Rhee J J. Echocardiographic evaluation of septal motion in patients with artificial pacemakers: vectorcardiographic correlations. Am Heart J 1977; 93: 596–602
32 Little W C, Reeves R C, Arciniegas J, Katholi R E, Rogers E W. Mechanism of abnormal interventricular septal motion during delayed left ventricular activation. Circulation 1982; 65: 1486–1491
33 Beppu S, Masuda Y, Sakakibara H, Izumi S, Park Y-D, Nagata S, Miyatake K, Nimura Y. Transient abnormal septal motion after non-surgical closure of the ductus arteriosus. Br Heart J 1988; 59: 706–711
34 Corya B C, Rasmussen S, Knoebel S B, Feigenbaum H. Echocardiography in acute myocardial infarction. Am J Cardiol 1975; 36: 1–10
35 Burch G E, Giles T D, Martinez E C. Echocardiographic abnormalities of interventricular septum associated with 'absent Q' syndrome. JAMA 1974; 228: 1665–1666
36 Tajik A J, Gau G T, Schattenberg T T, Ritter D G. Normal ventricular septal motion in atrial septal defect. An echocardiographic observation. Mayo Clin Proc 1972; 47: 635–638
37 Payvandi M, Kerber R E. Echocardiography in congenital and acquired absence of the pericardium. An echocardiographic mimic of right ventricular volume overload. Circulation 1976; 53: 86–92
38 Lieppe W, Scallion R, Behar V S, Kisslo J A. Two-dimensional echocardiographic findings in atrial septal defect. Circulation 1977; 56: 447–456
39 Hung J, Uren R F, Richmond D R, Kelly D T. The mechanism of abnormal septal motion in atrial septal defect: pre- and post-operative study by radionuclide ventriculography in adults. Circulation 1981; 63: 142–148
40 Weyman A E, Wann S, Feigenbaum H, Dillon J C. Mechanism of abnormal septal motion in patients with right ventricular volume overload. Circulation 1976; 54: 179–186
41 Mueller T M, Kerber R E, Marcus M L. Comparison of interventricular septal motion studied by ventriculography and echocardiography in patients with atrial septal defect. Br Heart J 1978; 40: 984–991
42 Popio K A, Gorlin R, Teichholz L E, Cohn P F, Bechtel D, Herman M V. Abnormalities of left ventricular function and geometry in adults with an atrial septal defect. Ventriculographic, hemodynamic and echocardiographic studies. Am J Cardiol 1975; 36: 302–308
43 Forfar J C, Godman M J. Functional and anatomic correlates in atrial septal defect. An echocardiographic study. Br Heart J 1985; 54: 193–200
44 Gondi B, Nanda N C. Two-dimensional echocardiographic features of atrial septal aneurysms. Circulation 1981; 63: 452–457
45 Belkin R N, Waugh R A, Kisslo J. Interatrial shunting in atrial septal aneurysm. Am J Cardiol 1986; 57: 310–312
46 Limacher M C, Gutgesell H P, Vick G W, Cohen M H, Huhta J H. Echocardiographic anatomy of the Eustachian valve. Am J Cardiol 1986; 57: 363–365
47 Battle-Diaz J, Stanley P, Kratz C, Fouron J-C, Guerin R, Davignon A. Echocardiographic manifestations of persistence of the right sinus venosus valve. Am J Cardiol 1979; 43: 850–853
48 Werner J A, Cheitlin M D, Gross B W, Speck S M, Ivey T D. Echocardiographic appearance of the Chiari network: differentiation from right heart pathology. Circulation 1981; 63: 1104–1109
49 Awan I H, Rice R, Moodie D S. Spontaneous closure of atrial septal defect with interatrial aneurysm formation. Pediatr Cardiol 1982; 3: 143–145
50 Gishla R P, Hannon D W, Meyer R A, Kaplan S. Spontaneous closure of isolated secundum atrial septal defects in infants: an echocardiographic study. Am Heart J 1985; 109: 1327–1333
51 Cockerham J T, Martin T C, Gutierrez F R, Hartmann A F, Goldring D, Strauss A W. Spontaneous closure of secundum atrial septal defect in infants and young children. Am J Cardiol 1983; 52: 1267–1271
52 Seward J B, Tajik A J, Hagler D J, Ritter D G. Peripheral venous contrast echocardiography. Am J Cardiol 1977; 39: 202–212
53 Munoz S, Berti C, Pulido C, Blanco P. Two-dimensional echocardiography with carbon dioxide in the detection of congenital cardiac shunts. Am J Cardiol 1984; 53: 206–210
54 Serruys P W, Van den Brand M, Hugenholtz P G, Roelandt J. Intracardiac right-to-left shunts demonstrated by two-dimensional echocardiography after peripheral vein injection. Br Heart J 1979; 42: 429–437
55 Bourdillon P D V, Foale R A, Rickards A F. Identification of atrial septal defects by cross-sectional contrast echocardiography. Br Heart J 1980; 44: 401–405
56 Duff D F, Gutgesell H P. The use of saline or blood for ultrasonic detection of a right to left shunt in the early postoperative patient. Am Heart J 1977; 94: 402–406
57 Kronik G, Mosslacher H. Positive contrast echocardiography in patients with patent foramen ovale and normal right heart hemodynamics. Am J Cardiol 1982; 49: 1806–1809
58 Khandheria B K, Shub C, Tajik A J, Taylor C L, Hagler D J, Seward J B. Utility of color flow imaging for visualizing shunt flow in atrial septal defect. Int J Cardiol 1989; 23: 91–98
59 Nasser F N, Tajik A J, Seward J B, Hagler D J. Diagnosis of sinus venosus atrial septal defect by two-dimensional echocardiography. Mayo Clin Proc 1981; 56: 568–572
60 Ettedgui J A, Siewers R D, Anderson R H, Park S C, Pahl E, Zuberbuhler J R. The diagnostic echocardiographic features of the superior caval ('sinus venosus') interatrial communication. Br Heart J 1990, 64: 329–331
61 Oh J K, Seward J B, Khandheria B K, Danielson G K, Tajik A J. Visualization of sinus venosus atrial septal defect by transesophageal echocardiography. J Am Soc Echocardiog 1988; 1: 275–277
62 Gnanapragasam J P, Houston A B, Lilley S. Congenital fistula

between the left ventricle and coronary sinus: elucidation by colour Doppler flow mapping. Br Heart J 1989; 62: 406–408
63 Snider A R, Ports T A, Silverman N H. Venous anomalies of the coronary sinus: detection by M-mode, two-dimensional and contrast echocardiography. Circulation 1979; 60: 721–727
64 Allan L D, Leanage R, Wainwright R, Joseph M, Tynan M. Balloon atrial septostomy under two-dimensional echocardiographic control. Br Heart J 1982; 47: 41–43
65 Lau K-C, Mok C-K, Lo R N S, Leung M P, Yeung C-Y. Balloon atrial septostomy under two-dimensional echocardiographic control. Pediatr Cardiol 1987; 8: 35–37
66 Rice M J, Seward J B, Hagler D J, Edwards W D, Julsrud P R, Tajik A J. Left juxtaposed atrial appendages: diagnostic two-dimensional echocardiographic features. J Am Coll Cardiol 1983; 1: 1330–1336
67 Hanrath P, Schluter M, Langenstein B A, Polster J, Engel S, Kremer P, Krebber H-J. Detection of ostium secundum atrial septal defects by transoesophageal echocardiography. Br Heart J 1983; 49: 350–358
68 Betriu A, Wigle E D, Felderhof C H, McLoughlin M J. Prolapse of the posterior leaflet of the mitral valve associated with secundum atrial septal defect. Am J Cardiol 1975; 35: 363–369
69 Nagata S, Nimura Y, Sakakibara H, Beppu S, Park Y-D, Kawazoe K, Fujita T. Mitral valve lesion associated with secundum atrial septal defect. Analysis by real time two dimensional echocardiography. Br Heart J 1983; 49: 51–58
70 Kambe T, Ichimiya S, Toguchi M, Hibi N, Fukui Y, Nishimura K. Cross-sectional echocardiographic study on the mitral valve prolapse associated with secundum atrial septal defect. Pre- and post-operative comparison. Jpn Circ J 1981; 45: 260–267
71 Leachman R D, Cokkinos D V, Cooley D A. Association of ostium secundum atrial septal defects with mitral valve prolapse. Am J Cardiol 1976; 38: 167–169
72 Somerville J, Kaku S, Saravalli O. Prolapsed mitral cusps in atrial septal defect. An erroneous radiological interpretation. Br Heart J 1978; 40: 58–63
73 Davies M J. Mitral valve anomalies in secundum atrial septal defects. Br Heart J 1981; 46: 126–128
74 Pearlman A S, Borer J S, Clark C E, Henry W L, Redwood D R, Morrow A G, Epstein S E. Abnormal right ventricular size and ventricular septal motion after atrial septal defect closure. Am J Cardiol 1978; 41: 295–301
75 Hanseus K, Bjorkhem G, Lundstrom N-R, Soeroso S. Cross-sectional echocardiographic measurement of right atrial and right ventricular size in children with atrial septal defect before and after surgery. Pediatr Cardiol 1988; 9: 231–236
76 Meyer R A, Korfhagen J C, Covitz W, Kaplan S. Long-term follow-up study after closure of secundum atrial septal defect in children: an echocardiographic study. Am J Cardiol 1982; 50: 143–148
77 Santoso T, Meltzer R S, Castellanos S, Serruys P W, Roelandt J. Contrast echocardiographic shunts may persist after atrial septal defect repair. Eur Heart J 1983; 4: 129–136
78 Hiraishi S, DiSessa T G, Jarmakani J M, Nakanishi T, Isabel-Jones J B, Friedman W F. Two-dimensional echocardiographic assessment of right ventricular volume in children with congenital heart disease. Am J Cardiol 1982; 50: 1368–1375
79 Snider A R, Silverman N H. Suprasternal notch echocardiography: a two-dimensional technique for evaluating congenital heart disease. Circulation 1981; 63: 165–173
80 Walker J K, Jones P R M, Dighton G P. Non-invasive assessment of isolated atrial defects. Br Heart J 1983; 49: 163–166
81 Veyrat C, Gourtchiglouian C, Bas S, Abitbol G, Kalmanson D. Quantification of left to right shunt in atrial septal defect using systolic time intervals derived from pulsed Doppler velocimetry. Br Heart J 1984; 52: 633–640
82 Marx G R, Allen H D, Goldberg S J, Flinn C J. Transatrial septal velocity measurement by Doppler echocardiography in atrial septal defect: correlation with Qp:Qs ratio. Am J Cardiol 1985; 55: 1162–1167
83 Pollick C, Sullivan H, Cujec B, Wilansky S. Doppler colour-flow imaging assessment of shunt size in atrial septal defect. Circulation 1988; 78: 522–528

84 Beppu S, Nimura Y, Nagata S, Tamai M, Matsuo H, Matsumoto M, Kawashima Y, Sakakibara H, Abe H. Diagnosis of endocardial cushion defect with cross-sectional and M-mode scanning echocardiography. Differentiation from secundum atrial septal defect. Br Heart J 1976; 38: 911–920
85 Smallhorn J F, Tommasini G, Anderson R H, Macartney F J. Assessment of atrioventricular defects by two dimensional echocardiography. Br Heart J 1982; 47: 109–121
86 Smallhorn J F, Sutherland G R, Anderson R H, Macartney F J. Cross-sectional echocardiographic assessment of conditions with atrioventricular valve leaflets attached to the atrial septum at the same level. Br Heart J 1982; 48: 331–341
87 Anderson R H, Ho S Y. The clinical anatomy of congenital heart disease. Cardiology in Practice 1989; 7: 128–139
88 Silverman N H, Zuberbuhler J R, Anderson R H. Atrioventricular septal defects: cross-sectional echocardiographic and morphologic comparisons. Int J Cardiol 1986; 13: 1289–1331
89 Arisawa J, Morimoto S, Ikezoe J, Hamada S, Kozuka T, Sano T, Ogawa M, Matsuda H, Kawashima Y. Cross sectional echocardiographic anatomy of common atrioventricular valve in atrial isomerism. Br Heart J 1989; 62: 291–297
90 De Tommasi S M, Daliento L, Ho S Y, Macartney F J, Anderson R H. Analysis of atrioventricular junction, ventricular mass, and ventriculoarterial junction in 43 specimens with atrial isomerism. Br Heart J 1981; 45: 236–247
91 Komatsu Y, Nagai Y, Shibuya M, Takao A, Hirosawa K. Echocardiographic analysis of intracardiac anatomy in endocardial cushion defect. Am Heart J 1976; 91: 210–218
92 Aceytuno A M F, Gonzalez A B, Miguel C M, Tynan M, Anderson R H. Subxiphoid M-mode echocardiography in atrioventricular defects. Pediatr Cardiol 1982; 3: 119–125
93 Sutherland G R, Van Mill G J, Anderson R H, Hunter S. Sub-xiphoid echocardiography – a new approach to the diagnosis and differentiation of atrioventricular defects. Eur Heart J 1980; 1: 45–54
94 Hagler D J, Tajik A J, Seward J B, Mair D D, Ritter D G. Real-time wide-angle sector echocardiography: atrioventricular canal defects. Circulation 1979; 59: 140–150
95 Penkoske P A, Neches W H, Anderson R H, Zuberbuhler J R. Further observations on the morphology of atrioventricular defects. J Thorac Cardiovasc Surg 1985; 90: 611–622
96 LaCorte M A, Cooper R S, Kauffman S L, Schiller M S, Golinko R J, Griepp R B. Atrioventricular canal ventricular septal defect with cleft mitral valve. Angiographic and echocardiographic features. Pediatr Cardiol 1982; 2: 289–295
97 LaCorte M A, Fellows K E, Williams R G. Overriding tricuspid valve: echocardiographic and angiocardiographic features. Am J Cardiol 1976; 37: 911–919
98 Smallhorn J F, Tommasini G, Macartney F J. Two-dimensional echocardiographic assessment of common atrioventricular valves in univentricular hearts. Br Heart J 1981; 46: 128–134
99 Freedom R M, Picchio F, Duncan W J, Harder J R, Moes C A F, Rowe R D. The atrioventricular junction in the univentricular heart: a two-dimensional echocardiographic analysis. Pediatr Cardiol 1982; 3: 105–117
100 Rigby M L, Anderson R H, Gibson D, Jones O D H, Joseph M C, Shinebourne E A. Two dimensional echocardiographic categorisation of the univentricular heart. Ventricular morphology, type and mode of atrioventricular connection. Br Heart J 1981; 46: 603–612
101 Grenadier E, Keidar S, Palant A. Contrast echocardiographic right-to-left flow in left ventricular-to-right-atrial shunt. Am Heart J 1983; 106: 1157–1159
102 Shanes J G, Levitsky S, Seyal M S, Welch W, Kondos G, Silverman N, Rich S, Pietras R J. Diagnosis of left ventricular to right atrial shunt using contrast echocardiography. Am J Cardiol 1983; 52: 650
103 Grenadier E, Shem-Tov A, Motro M, Palant A. Echocardiographic diagnosis of left ventricular-right atrial communication. Am Heart J 1983; 106: 407–409
104 Mills P, McLaurin L, Smith C, Murray G, Craige E. Echocardiographic findings in left ventricular to right atrial shunts. Br Heart J 1977; 39: 594–597
105 Grenadier E, Keidar S, Palant A. Contrast echocardiographic

105 right-to-left flow in left ventricular-to-right atrial shunt. Am Heart J 1983; 106: 1157–1159
106 McKay R, Battistessa S A, Wilkinson J L, Wright J P. A communication from the left ventricle to the right atrium: a defect in the central fibrous body. Int J Cardiol 1989; 23: 117–123
107 Beppu S, Nimura Y, Sakakibara H, Nagata S, Park Y-D, Baba K, Naito Y, Ohta M, Kamiya T, Koyanagi H, Fujita T. Mitral cleft in ostium primum atrial septal defect assessed by cross-sectional echocardiography. Circulation 1980; 62: 1099–1107
108 Smallhorn J F, de Leval M, Stark J, Somerville J, Taylor J F N, Anderson R H, Macartney F J. Isolated anterior mitral cleft. Two dimensional echocardiographic assessment and differentiation from 'clefts' associated with atrioventricular septal defect. Br Heart J 1982; 48: 109–116
109 Bloom K R, Freedom R M, Williams C M, Trusler G A, Rowe R D. Echocardiographic recognition of atrioventricular valve stenosis associated with endocardial cushion defect: pathologic and surgical correlates. Pediatr Cardiol 1979; 44: 1326–1331
110 Warnes C, Somerville J. Double mitral valve orifice in atrioventricular defects. Br Heart J 1983; 49: 59–64
111 Mortera C, Rissech M, Payola M, Miro C, Perich R. Cross sectional subcostal echocardiography: atrioventricular septal defects and the short axis cut. Br Heart J 1987; 58: 267–273
112 Chin A J, Bierman F Z, Sanders S P, Williams R G, Norwood W I, Castaneda A R. Subxiphoid 2-dimensional echocardiographic identification of left papillary muscle abnormalities in complete common atrioventricular canal. Am J Cardiol 1983; 51: 1695–1699
113 Mehta S, Hirschfield S, Riggs T, Liebamn J. Echocardiographic estimation of ventricular hypoplasia in complete atrioventricular canal. Circulation 1979; 59: 888–893
114 Corwin R D, Singh A K, Karlson K E. Double-outlet right atrium: a rare endocardial cushion defect. Am Heart J 1983; 106: 1156–1157
115 Rao P S. Atrioventricular canal mimicking tricuspid atresia: echocardiographic and angiographic features. Br Heart J 1987; 58: 409–412
116 Beppu S, Nimura Y, Tamai M, Nagata S, Matsuo H, Kawashima Y, Kozuka T, Sakakibara H. Two-dimensional echocardiography in diagnosing tricuspid atresia. Differentiation from other hypoplastic right heart syndromes and common atrioventricular canal. Br Heart J 1978; 40: 1174–1183
117 Lappen R S, Muster A J, Idriss F S, Riggs T W, Ilbawi M, Paul M H, Bharati S, Lev M. Masked subaortic stenosis in ostium primum atrial septal defect: recognition and treatment. Am J Cardiol 1983; 52: 336–340
118 Yoshida H, Funabashi T, Nakaya S, Maeda T, Taniguchi N. Subxiphoid cross-sectional echocardiographic imaging of the 'goose neck' deformity in endocardial cushion defect. Circulation 1980; 62: 1319–1323
119 Ebels T. Echocardiography and surgery for atrioventricular septal defect. Int J Cardiol 1986; 13: 353–360
120 Carvalho J S, Rigby M L, Shinebourne E A, Anderson R H. Cross sectional echocardiography for recognition of ventricular topology in atrioventricular septal defect. Br Heart J 1989; 61: 285–288
121 Meijboom E J, Ebels T, Anderson R H, Schasfoort van Leeuwen M J M, Deanfield J E, Eijgelaar A, van der Heide H. Left atrioventricular valve after surgical repair in atrioventricular septal defect with separate valve orifices (ostium primum atrial septal defect): an echo-Doppler study. Am J Cardiol 1986; 57: 433–436
122 Goldman M E, Fuster V, Guarino T, Mindich B P. Intraoperative echocardiography for the evaluation of valvar regurgitation: experience in 263 patients. Circulation 1986; 74(suppl I): 143–149
123 Meijboom E J, Wyse R K H, Ebels T, Deanfield J E, Quagebeur J M, Anderson R H, Brenner J I. Doppler mapping of postoperative left atrioventricular valve regurgitation. Circulation 1988; 77: 311–315
124 Miyatake K, Izumi S, Okamoto M, Kinoshita N, Asonuma H, Nakagawa H, Yamamoto K, Takamiya M, Sakakibara H, Nimura Y. Semiquantitative grading of severity of mitral regurgitation by real-time two-dimensional Doppler flow imaging technique. J Am Coll Cardiol 1986; 7: 82–88
125 Monaghan M, Mills P. Doppler colour flow mapping: technology in search of an application? Br Heart J 1989; 61: 133–138

126 Bolger A F, Eigler N L, Maurer G. Quantifying valvular regurgitation. Limitations and inherent assumptions of Doppler techniques. Circulation 1988; 78: 1316–1318
127 Goldman M E. Real-time two-dimensional Doppler flow imaging: a word of caution. J Am Coll Cardiol 1986; 7: 89–90
128 Roelandt J. Colour-coded Doppler flow imaging: what are the prospects? Eur Heart J 1986; 7: 184–189
129 Taylor N C, Somerville J. Fixed subaortic stenosis after repair of ostium primum defects. Br Heart J 1981; 45: 689–697
130 Dickinson D F, Arnold R, Wilkinson J L. Ventricular septal defect in children born in Liverpool 1960–1969. Evaluation of natural course and surgical implications in an unselected population. Br Heart J 1981; 46: 47–54
131 Soto B, Becker A, Moulaert A J, Lie J T, Anderson R H. Classification of ventricular septal defects. Br Heart J 1980; 43: 332–343
132 Sutherland G R, Godman M J, Smallhorn J F, Guiterras P, Anderson R H, Hunter S. Ventricular septal defects. Two dimensional echocardiographic and morphological correlations. Br Heart J 1982; 47: 316–328
133 Baker E J, Leung M P, Anderson R H, Fischer D R, Zuberbuhler J R. The cross sectional anatomy of ventricular septal defects: a reappraisal. Br Heart J 1988; 59: 339–351
134 Hagler D J, Edwards W D, Seward J B, Tajik A J. Standardised nomenclature of the ventricular septum and ventricular septal defects, with applications for two dimensional echocardiography. Mayo Clin Proc 1985; 60: 741–752
135 Capelli H, Andrade J L, Somerville J. Classification of the site of ventricular septal defect by 2-dimensional echocardiography. Am J Cardiol 1983; 51: 1474–1480
136 Anderson R H. Description of ventricular septal defects – or how long is a piece of string? Int J Cardiol 1986; 13: 267–278
137 Piot J D, Lucet P, Losay J et al. Diagnostic et localisation des communications interventriculaires par l'echocardiographie bidimensionelle. Arch Mal Coeur 1981; 9: 1001–1009
138 Shore D F, Rigby M L, Anderson R H, Lincoln C. Surgical closure of ventricular septal defects without cardiac catheterisation and angiography. Proceedings 1st World congress paediatric cardiac surgery. Ghedini Editore, Milano 1988; p 22
139 Milo S, Ho S Y, Macartney F J, Wilkinson J L, Anderson R H. The surgical anatomy and atrioventricular conduction tissues of hearts with ventricular septal defects. J Thorac Cardiovasc Surgery 1980; 79: 244–255
140 Ramaciotti C, Keren A, Silverman N. Importance of (perimembranous) ventricular septal aneurysm in the natural history of isolated perimembranous ventricular septal defect. Am J Cardiol 1986; 57: 268–272
141 Alpert B S, Mellitis E D, Rowe R D. Spontaneous closure of small ventricular septal defects. Probability rates in the first five years of life. Am J Dis Child 1973; 125: 194–196
142 Hornberger L K, Sahn D J, Krabill K A et al. Elucidation of the natural history of ventricular septal defects by serial Doppler colour flow mapping studies. J Am Coll Cardiol 1989; 13: 1111–1118
143 Stevenson J G, Kawabori I, Stamm S J et al. Pulsed Doppler evaluation of ventricular septal defect patches. Circulation 1984; 70(suppl 1): 38–45
144 Lewis A B, Takahashi M. Echocardiographic assessment of left to right shunt volume in children with ventricular septal defect. Circulation 1976; 54: 78–82
145 Silverman N, Hunter S, Anderson R H, Ho S Y, Sutherland G R, Davies M J. Anatomical basis of cross sectional echocardiography. Br Heart J 1983; 50: 421–431
146 Bierman F Z, Fellows K, Williams R G. Prospective identification of ventricular septal defects in infancy using subxiphoid two dimensional echocardiography. Circulation 1980; 62: 807–817
147 Canale J M, Sahn D J, Allen H D et al. Factors affecting real time cross sectional imaging of perimembranous ventricular septal defects. Circulation 1981; 63: 689–697
148 Stevenson J G, Kawabori I, Dooley T, Guntheroth W G. Diagnosis of ventricular septal defect by pulsed Doppler echocardiography. Sensitivity, specificity and limitations. Am J Cardiol 1978; 58: 322–326
149 Hatle L, Rokseth R. Noninvasive diagnosis and assessment of

ventricular septal defect by Doppler ultrasound. Acta Med Scand 1981; 645: 47-56
150 Ortiz E, Robinson P J, Deanfield J E, Franklin R, Macartney F J, Wyse R K H. Localisation of ventricular septal defects by simultaneous display of superimposed colour Doppler and cross sectional echocardiographic images. Br Heart J 1985; 54: 53-60
151 Sutherland G R, Smyllie J H, Ogilvie B C, Keeton B R. Colour flow imaging in the diagnosis of multiple ventricular septal defects. Br Heart J 1989; 62: 43-49
152 Stevenson J G, Kawabori I, Guntheroth W G. Differentiation of ventricular septal defects from mitral regurgitation by pulsed Doppler echocardiography. Circulation 1977; 56: 14-18
153 Murphy D J, Ludomirsky A, Huhta J C. Continuous wave Doppler in children with ventricular septal defect: noninvasive estimation of interventricular pressure gradient. Am J Cardiol 1986; 57: 428-432
154 Silbert D R, Brunson S C, Schiff R, Diamant S. Determination of right ventricular pressure in the presence of a ventricular septal defect using continuous wave Doppler ultrasound. J Am Coll Cardiol 1986; 8: 379-384
155 Dickinson D F, Goldberg S J, Wilson N. A comparison of information obtained by ultrasound examination and cardiac catheterisation in paediatric patients with congenital heart disease. Int J Cardiol 1985; 9: 275-285
156 Valdes-Cruz L M, Horowitz S, Mesel E et al. A pulsed Doppler echocardiographic method for calculation of pulmonary and systemic flow: accuracy in a canine model with ventricular septal defect. Circulation 1983; 68: 597-602
157 Anderson R H, Lenox C C, Zuberbuhler J R. Mechanisms of closure of perimembranous ventricular septal defect. Am J Cardiol 1983; 52: 341-345
158 Sutherland G R, Godman M J. Natural history of ventricular septal defects. In: Hunter S, Hall R. eds. Clinical echocardiography; Castle House Publications, pp 129-138
159 Snider R, Silverman N H, Schiller N B, Ports T A. Echocardiographic evaluation of ventricular septal aneurysms. Circulation 1979; 59: 920-926
160 Craig B G, Smallhorn J F, Burrows P, Trusler G A, Rowe R D. Cross sectional echocardiography in the evaluation of aortic valve prolapse associated with ventricular septal defect. Am Heart J 1986; 112: 800-807
161 Ludomirsky A, Huhta J C, Vick G W, Murphy D J, Danford D A, Morrow W R. Colour Doppler detection of multiple ventricular septal defects. Circulation 1986; 74: 1317-1322
162 Shiraishi H, Silverman N. Echocardiographic spectrum of double inlet ventricle: evaluation of the interventricular communication. J Am Coll Cardiol 1990; 15: 1401-1408
163 Sahn D J, Swensson R E, Valdes-Cruz L M, Scagnelli S, Main J. Two dimensional colour flow mapping for evaluation of ventricular septal defect shunts: a new diagnostic modality. Circulation 1984; 70: II 364
164 Kapusta L, Hopman J C W, Daniels O. The usefulness of cross sectional Doppler flow imaging in the detection of small ventricular septal defects with left to right shunt. Eur Heart J 1987; 8: 1002-1006
165 Griffin M L, Sullivan I, Anderson R H, Macartney F J. Doubly committed subarterial ventricular septal defect: new morphologic criteria with echocardiographic and angiographic correlation. Br Heart J 1988; 59: 474-479
166 Swennson R E, Sahn D J, Valdes-Cruz L M. Colour flow Doppler mapping in congenital heart disease. Echocardiography 1985; 2: 545-549
167 Cheatham J P, Latson L A, Gutgesell H P. Ventricular septal defect in infancy: detection with two dimensional echocardiography. Am J Cardiol 1981; 47: 85-89
168 Kececioglu-Draelos Z, Goldberg S J, Sahn D J. How accurate is the ultrasonic estimation of ventricular septal defect size? Pediatr Cardiol 1982; 3: 189-195
169 Jaffe C C, Atkinson P, Taylor K J W. Physical parameters affecting the visibility of small ventricular septal defects using two dimensional echocardiography. Invest Radiol 1979; 14: 149-155
170 Kupferschmid C, Land D, Pohlandt F. Sensitivity, specificity and predictive value of clinical findings, M-mode echocardiography and continuous wave Doppler sonography in the diagnosis of symptomatic patent ductus in preterm infants. Eur J Pediatr 1988; 147: 279-282
171 Meijboom E J, Valdes-Cruz L M, Horowitz S et al. A two dimensional Doppler echocardiographic method for calculation of pulmonary and systemic blood flow in a canine model with a variable sized left to right extracardiac shunt. Circulation 1983; 68: 437-445
172 Goldberg S J, Sahn D J, Allen H D, Valdes-Cruz L M, Hoenecke H, Carnahan Y. Evaluation of pulmonary and systemic blood flow by 2 dimensional Doppler echocardiography using fast Fourier transform spectral analysis. Am J Cardiol 1982; 50: 1394-1400
173 Sanders S P, Yeager S, Williams R G. Measurements of systemic and pulmonary blood flow and QP/QS ratio using Doppler and two dimensional echocardiography. Am J Cardiol 1983; 51: 952-956
174 Barron J V, Sahn D J, Valdes-Cruz L M et al. Clinical utility of two dimensional Doppler echocardiographic techniques for estimating pulmonary to systemic blood flow ratios in children with left to right shunting atrial septal defect, ventricular septal defect or patent ductus arteriosus. J Am Coll Cardiol 1984; 3: 169-178
175 Fisher D C, Sahn D J, Friedman M J, et al. The mitral valve method for noninvasive two dimensional echo Doppler determinations of cardiac output. Circulation 1983; 67: 872-877
176 Goldberg S J, Dickinson D F, Wilson N. Evaluation of an elliptical area technique for calculating mitral blood flow by Doppler echocardiography. Br Heart J 1985; 54: 68-75
177 Burstin L. Determination of pressure in the pulmonary artery by external graphic recordings. Br Heart J 1967; 29: 396-404
178 Kosturakis D, Goldberg S J, Allen H D, Loeber C. Doppler echocardiographic prediction of pulmonary arterial hypertension in congenital heart disease. Am J Cardiol 1984; 53: 1110-1115
179 Mahan G, Dabestani A, Gardin J, Allfie A, Burn C, Henry W. Estimation of pulmonary artery pressure by pulsed Doppler echocardiography (abstract). Circulation 1983; 68 (suppl 2) 367
180 Kitabatake A, Inoue M, Asao M et al. Noninvasive evaluation of pulmonary hypertension by a pulsed Doppler technique. Circulation 1983; 68: 302-309
181 Robinson P J, Wyse R K H, Macartney F J. Significance of pulmonary valve prolapse: a cross sectional echocardiographic study. Br Heart J 1984; 52: 266-271
182 Zeevi B, Keren G, Sherez J, Berant M, Blieden L C, Laniado S. Bidirectional flow in congenital ventricular septal defect: a Doppler echocardiographic study. Clin Cardiol 1987; 10: 143-146
183 Hatle L, Angelsen B. Doppler ultrasound in cardiology; physical principles and clinical applications. 2nd edition. Philadelphia: Lea and Febiger. 1985, p 236
184 Houston A B. In: Houston A B, Simpson I A eds. Cardiac Doppler ultrasound: a clinical perspective. Cambridge: Butterworths. 1988
185 Currie P J, Seward J B, Chan K L et al. Continuous wave Doppler determination of right ventricular pressure: a simultaneous Doppler catheterisation study in 127 patients. J Am Coll Cardiol 1985; 6: 75-76
186 Yock P, Popp R. Noninvasive measurement of right ventricular systolic pressure by Doppler ultrasound in patients with tricuspid regurgitation. Circulation 1984; 70: 657-662
187 Cyran S E, Kimball T R, Meyer R A et al. Efficacy of intraoperative transoesophageal echocardiography in children with congenital heart disease. Am J Cardiol 1989; 63: 594-598
188 Rudolph A M. In: Congenital diseases of the heart. Clinical and physiologic considerations in diagnosis and management. Chicago: Year Book Medical Publishers Inc. pp 171-172
189 Mitchell S C, Korones S B, Berendes H W. Congenital heart disease in 56109 births: incidence and natural history. Circulation 1971; 43: 323-332
190 Silverman N H, Lewis A B, Heymann M A, Rudolph A M. Echocardiographic assessment of ductus arteriosus shunt in premature infants. Circulation 1974; 50: 821-825
191 Valdes-Cruz L M, Dudell G G. Specificity and accuracy of echocardiographic and clinical criteria for diagnosis of patent ductus arteriosus in fluid restricted infants. J Pediatrics 1981; 98: 298-305

192 Wilson N, Dickinson D F, Goldberg S J, Scott O. Pulmonary artery velocity patterns in ductus arteriosus. Br Heart J 1984; 52: 462–464
193 Huhta J C, Cohen M, Gutgesell H P. Patency of the ductus arteriosus in normal neonates: two dimensional echocardiography versus Doppler assessment. J Am Coll Cardiol 1984; 4: 561–564
194 Swensson R E, Valdes Cruz L M, Sahn D J, et al. Real time Doppler color flow mapping for detection of patent arterial ductus. J Am Coll Cardiol 1986; 8: 1105–1112
195 Houston A B, Lim M K, Doig W B et al. Doppler flow characteristics in the assessment of pulmonary artery pressure in ductus arteriosus. Br Heart J 1989; 62: 284–290
196 Stevenson J G. The use of Doppler for detection and estimation of severity of patent ductus arteriosus, ventricular septal defect, and atrial septal defect. Echocardiography 1987; 4: 321–346
197 Smallhorn J F, Huhta J C, Anderson R H, Macartney F J. Suprasternal echocardiography in assessment of patent ductus arteriosus. Br Heart J 1982; 48: 321–330
198 Allen H D, Goldberg S J, Valdes-Cruz L M, Sahn D J. Use of echocardiography in newborns with patent ductus arteriosus: a review. Pediatr Cardiol 1982; 3: 65–70
199 Smallhorn J F. Patent ductus arteriosus – evaluation by echocardiography. Echocardiography 1987; 4: 101–118
200 Sahn D J, Allen H D. Real time cross sectional echocardiographic imaging and measurement of the patent ductus arteriosus in infants and children. Circulation 1978; 58: 343–354
201 Rigby M L, Pickering D, Wilkinson A. Cross sectional echocardiography in determining persistent patency of the ductus arteriosus in preterm infants. Arch Dis Child 1984; 59: 341–345
202 Huhta J C. In: Pediatric imaging/Doppler ultrasound of the chest: extracardiac diagnosis. Philadelphia: Lea and Febiger. pp 104–106
203 Vick W G, Huhta J C, Gutgesell H P. Assessment of the ductus arteriosus in preterm infants utilising suprasternal two dimensional Doppler echocardiography. J Am Coll Cardiol 1985; 5: 973–977
204 Murphy D J Jr, Vick G W III, Ramsay J M, Danford D A, Huhta J C. Continuous wave Doppler echocardiography in patent ductus arteriosus. J Cardiovasc Ultrasonogr 1987; 6: 273–278
205 Serwer G A, Armstrong B E, Anderson P A W. Noninvasive detection of retrograde descending aortic flow in infants using continuous wave Doppler ultrasonography. Implications for aortic run off lesions. J Pediatr 1980; 97: 394–400
206 Feldtman R W, Andrassy R J, Alexander J A, Stanford W. Doppler ultrasonic flow detection as an adjunct in the diagnosis of patent ductus arteriosus in premature infants. J Thorac Cardiovasc Surg 1976; 72: 288–290
207 Daniels O, Hopman J C W, Stoelinga G B A, Busch H J, Peer P G M. Doppler flow characteristics in the main pulmonary artery and the LA/Ao ratio before and after ductal closure in healthy newborns. Ped Cardiol 1982; 3: 99–104
208 Hatle L, Angelsen B. Doppler ultrasound in cardiology: physical principles and clinical applications. 2nd edition: Philadelphia: Lea and Febiger. 1985; pp 222–223
209 Baylen B G, Meyer R A, Korfhagen J, Benzing G, Bubb M E, Kaplan S. Left ventricular performance in the critically ill premature infant with patent ductus arteriosus and pulmonary disease. Circulation 1977; 55: 182–188
210 Kupferschmid C, Lang D, Pohlandt F. Sensitivity, specificity and predictive value of clinical findings, M mode echocardiography and continuous wave Doppler sonography in the diagnosis of symptomatic patent ductus arteriosus in preterm infants. Eur J Pediatr 1988; 147: 279–282
211 Recommendation of the American Society of Echocardiography regarding quantitation in M mode echocardiography. March 1978
212 Allen H D, Goldberg S J, Sahn D J, Ovitt T W, Goldberg B B. Suprasternal notch echocardiography. Assessment of its clinical utility in pediatric cardiology. Circulation 1977; 55: 605–613
213 Hirshklau M J, DiSessa T G, Higgins C B, Friedman W F. Echocardiographic diagnosis: pitfalls in the premature infant with a large patent ductus arteriosus. J Pediatr 1978; 92: 474–477
214 Halliday H L, Hirata T, Brady J P. Echocardiographic findings of large patent ductus arteriosus in the very low birthweight infant before and after treatment with indomethacin. Arch Dis Child 1979; 54: 744–749
215 Heymann M A. In: Adams F H, Emmanouilides G C. eds. Moss' heart disease in children and adolescents. Baltimore/London: Williams & Wilkins p. 162
216 Meijboom E J, Valdes Cruz L M, Horowitz S et al. A two dimensional echocardiographic method for calculation of pulmonary and systemic blood flow in a canine model with a variable sized left to right extracardiac shunt. Circulation 1983; 68: 437–445
217 Alverson D C, Eldridge M, Dillon T, Yabek S M, Berman W. Noninvasive pulsed Doppler determination of cardiac output in neonates and children. J Pediatrics 1982; 101: 46–50
218 Stevenson J G, Kawabori I, Guntheroth W G. Noninvasive detection of pulmonary hypertension in patent ductus arteriosus by pulsed Doppler echocardiography. Circulation 1979; 60: 355–359
219 Musewe N N, Smallhorn J F, Benson L N, Burrows P E, Freedom R M. Validation of Doppler derived pulmonary arterial pressure in patients with ductus arteriosus under different hemodynamic states. Circulation 1987; 76: 1081–1091
220 Aziz K, Tasneem H. Evaluation of pulmonary artery pressure by Doppler colour flow mapping in patients with a ductus arteriosus. Br Heart J 1990; 63: 295–299
221 Houston A B, Gregory N L, Murtagh E, Coleman E N. Two-dimensional echocardiography in infants with persistent truncus arteriosus. Br Heart J 1981; 46: 492–497
222 Smallhorn J F, Anderson R H, Macartney F J. Two dimensional echocardiographic assessment of communications between ascending aorta and pulmonary trunk or individual pulmonary arteries. Br Heart J 1982; 47: 563–572
223 Hagler D J, Tajik A J, Seward J B, Mair D D, Ritter D G. Wide-angle two-dimensional echocardiographic profiles of conotruncal abnormalities. Mayo Clin Proc 1980; 55: 73–82
224 Sanders S P, Bierman F Z, Williams R G. Conotruncal malformations: diagnosis in infancy using subxiphoid 2-dimensional echocardiography. Am J Cardiol 1982; 50: 1361–1367
225 Assad-Morell J L, Seward J B, Tajik A J, Hagler D J, Giuliani E R, Ritter D G. Echo-phonocardiographic and contrast studies in conditions associated with systemic arterial trunk overriding the ventricular septum. Truncus arteriosus, tetralogy of Fallot, and pulmonary atresia with ventricular septal defect. Circulation 1976; 53: 663–673
226 Rice M J, Seward J B, Hagler D J, Mair D D, Tajik A J. Definitive diagnosis of truncus arteriosus by two-dimensional echocardiography. Mayo Clin Proc 1982; 57: 476–481
227 Marin-Garcia J, Tonkin I L D. Two-dimensional echocardiographic evaluation of persistent truncus arteriosus. Am J Cardiol 1982; 50: 1376–1379
228 Riggs T W, Paul M H. Two-dimensional echocardiographic prospective diagnosis of common truncus arteriosus in infants. Am J Cardiol 1982; 50: 1380–1384
229 Yoshizato T, Julsrud P R. Truncus arteriosus revisited: an angiographic demonstration. Pediatr Cardiol 1990; 11: 36–40
230 Gerlis L M, Wilson N, Dickinson D F, Scott O. Valvar stenosis in truncus arteriosus. Br Heart J 1984; 52: 440–445
231 Patel R G, Freedom R M, Bloom K R, Rowe R D. Truncal or aortic valve stenosis in functionally single arterial trunk. A clinical, hemodynamic and pathological study of six cases. Am J Cardiol 1978; 42: 800–809
232 Chandraratna P A N, Bhaduri U, Littman B B, Hildner F J. Echocardiographic findings in persistent truncus arteriosus in a young adult. Br Heart J 1974; 36: 732–736
233 Moerman P, Godeeris P, Lauwerijns J, Van der Hauwert L G. Cardiovascular malformations in DiGeorge syndrome (congenital absence or hypoplasia of the thymus). Br Heart J 1980; 44: 452–459
234 Lo R N S, Mok C, Leung M P, Lau K, Cheung D L C. Cross-sectional and pulsed Doppler echocardiographic features of anomalous origin of the right pulmonary artery from the ascending aorta. Am J Cardiol 1987; 60: 921–924
235 Mendoza D A, Ueda T, Nishioka K, Yokota Y, Mikawa H, Nomoto S, Yamazoto A, Fukumasu H, Ban T. Aortopulmonary window, aortic origin of the pulmonary artery, and interrupted aortic arch: detection by two-dimensional and colour Doppler echocardiography in an infant. Pediatr Cardiol 1986; 7: 49–52

236 Fong L V, Anderson R H, Siewers R D, Trento A, Park S C. Anomalous origin of one pulmonary artery from the ascending aorta: a review of echocardiographic, catheter and morphological features. Br Heart J 1989; 62: 389–395
237 Duncan W J, Freedom R M, Olley P M, Rowe R D. Two-dimensional echocardiographic identification of hemitruncus: anomalous origin of one pulmonary artery from ascending aorta with the other pulmonary artery arising normally from the right ventricle. Am Heart J 1981; 102: 892–896
238 Beitzke A, Shinebourne E A. Single origin of right and left pulmonary arteries from ascending aorta, with main pulmonary artery from right ventricle. Br Heart J 1980; 43: 363–365
239 Satomi G, Nakamura K, Imai Y, Takao A. Two-dimensional echocardiographic diagnosis of aortopulmonary window. Br Heart J 1980; 43: 351–356
240 Donaldson R M, Ballester M, Rickards A F. Diagnosis of aortico-pulmonary window by two-dimensional echocardiography. Cathet Cardiovasc Diagn 1982; 8: 185–189
241 Rice M J, Seward J B, Hagler D J, Mair D D, Tajik A J. Visualization of aortopulmonary window by two-dimensional echocardiography. Mayo Clin Proc 1982; 57: 482–487
242 King O H, Huhta J C, Gutgesell H P, Ott D A. Two-dimensional echocardiographic diagnosis of anomalous origin of the right pulmonary artery from the aorta: differentiation from aortopulmonary window. J Am Coll Cardiol 1984; 4: 351–355
243 Blieden L C, Moller J H. Aorticopulmonary septal defect: an experience with 17 patients. Br Heart J 1974; 36: 630–635
244 Carminatti M, Borghi A, Valsecchi O, Quattrociocchi M, Balduzzi A, Rusconi P, Russo M G, Festa P, Preda L, Tiraboschi R. Aortopulmonary window coexisting with tetralogy of Fallot: echocardiographic diagnosis. Pediatr Cardiol 1990; 11: 41–43

21

Left sided obstruction

Aortic stenosis
Bicuspid aortic valve
Aortic valve stenosis
M-mode echocardiography
Cross-sectional echocardiography
Doppler ultrasound
Fixed subaortic stenosis
Supravalve aortic stenosis

Hypoplastic left heart syndrome
Coarctation of the aorta
Imaging of coarctation of the aorta
Doppler examination in coarctation of the aorta
Interrupted aortic arch

Alan Houston

AORTIC STENOSIS

Congenital aortic stenosis can be situated at subvalve, valve or supravalve level and it is occasionally present at more than one site. Approximately three quarters of cases of congenital aortic stenosis are of valve stenosis, one quarter have subvalve stenosis and only 1–2% have supravalve stenosis. Any of the forms of left ventricular outflow tract obstruction may be associated with secondary left ventricular hypertrophy which is usually concentric but in a minority of cases the interventricular septum is thicker than the posterior wall. The assessment of the nature and severity of the obstruction has been greatly simplified by ultrasound, with cross-sectional echocardiography accurately localising the level of obstruction and Doppler ultrasound providing an accurate assessment of the gradient across it. The echocardiographic features for the different types of aortic stenosis will be considered individually. A bicuspid aortic valve may be associated with stenosis and this condition will be considered first.

Bicuspid aortic valve

The bicuspid aortic valve is a very common congenital cardiac defect, occurring in 1–2% of normal subjects and more commonly with certain lesions, particularly coarctation of the aorta. It may be suspected clinically by the presence of an ejection click or it may first be recognised from an echocardiographic study. In most cases the valve does not have two simple leaflets but rather has two functional leaflets, one being formed from two fused segments with a raphe between them.

The bicuspid aortic valve can often be recognised on M-mode echocardiography from the diastolic pattern of eccentric closure of the valve cusps (Fig. 1). It has been suggested that this can be quantified with an eccentricity index which is the ratio of half the aortic diameter to the distance from the nearest aortic wall to the closure echo. A ratio of greater than 1.3 has been considered abnormal using the leading edge method at the onset of diastole.[1] This is not, however, a completely reliable sign and the degree of eccentricity can be altered by modifying the transducer angulation to traverse the cusp closure line in different positions and it may even appear to be abnormal in up to 20% of normal subjects.[1,2]

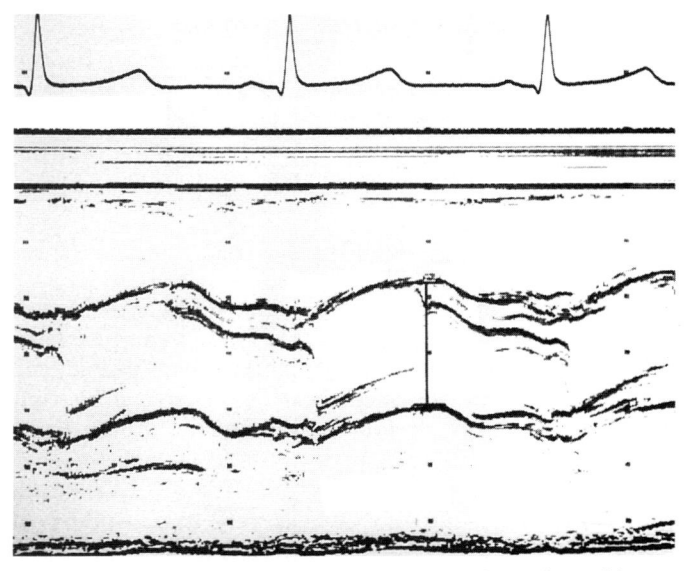

Fig. 1 **M-mode study through the aortic root of a patient with a bicuspid aortic valve.** In diastole the echo from the closed cusps is eccentric, lying much nearer to the anterior than the posterior wall.

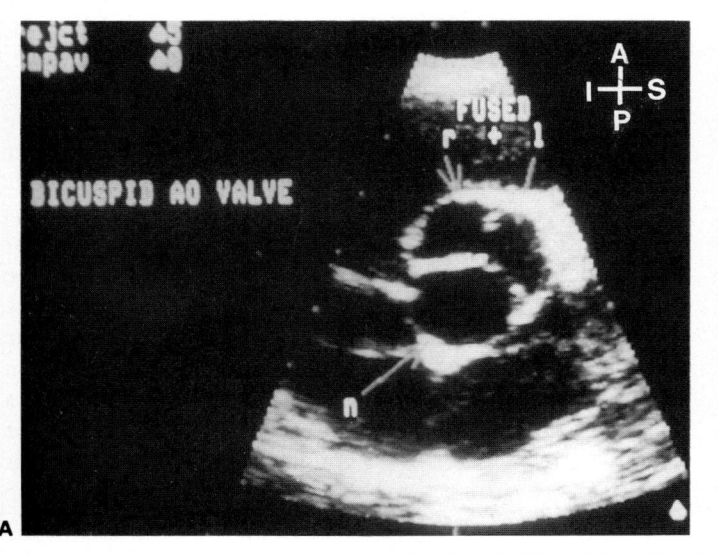

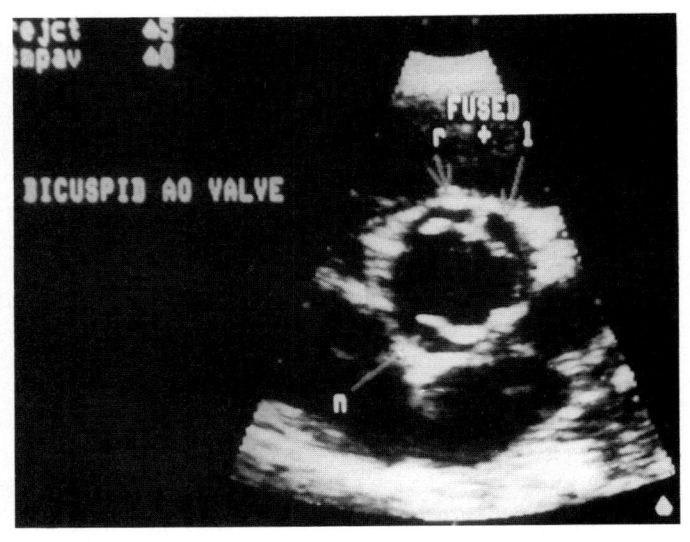

Fig. 2 **Short axis systolic images of a functionally bicuspid aortic valve.** In diastole (**A**) there appear to be 3 cusps but in systole (**B**) it is apparent that there is a functionally single anterior cusp formed from right (r) and left (l) segments which is slightly larger than the posterior non-coronary (n) cusps.

Cross-sectional echocardiography is a much more reliable method of making the diagnosis.[3] A short axis view of the aortic root and valve is used for direct visualisation of the cusps. In the relatively uncommon situation where there are clearly two separate cusps (14% of cases) this may be apparent in diastole. More commonly one cusp is formed of two segments joined by a raphe and in diastole the valve may appear to have three cusps although they can be of different sizes. The diagnosis is made in systolic frames when the commissures between the individual cusps and the opening pattern of two or three cusps can be seen (Fig. 2). Although definite assessment of the aortic valve morphology is not possible in some older patients[4] it is usually possible in younger subjects. Long axis views will show that the valve opens well. In most cases a bicuspid valve is not stenotic in childhood but in some patients the flow velocity can be slightly increased. Although this velocity is usually less than 2.5m/s it may indicate mild obstruction.

Aortic valve stenosis

In congenital aortic stenosis in young subjects the valve is morphologically different from that found in aortic stenosis in later life. In the majority of patients it is pliable, relatively mobile and not calcified. Most often it is bicuspid, either anatomically or functionally, with a central raphe and fused lateral commissures. Systolic movement results in doming of the valve leaflets since the orifice is restrictive. Less frequently the valve is very thick, lumpy and disorganised and has restricted systolic movement. This is more often seen in very young patients, particularly in those infants with severe obstruction.

M-mode echocardiography

The left ventricular appearance on M-mode echocardiography will be similar in all forms of aortic stenosis and depends on the severity of the obstruction. The left ventricular wall may be thickened. This hypertrophy is usually concentric but it is possible to have relatively greater septal thickening. This asymmetrical hypertrophy is not indicative of hypertrophic cardiomyopathy. Catheterisation studies have demonstrated that unlike adults, children with aortic stenosis often have reduced systolic wall stress with supernormal indices of left ventricular pump function.[5] The ejection fraction and velocity of circumferential fibre shortening will be increased in these cases. It is important to ensure that left ventricular function is normal when Doppler examination is used to assess severity of stenosis since a low gradient or pressure drop will be found with severe stenosis in the presence of poor left ventricular function. Poor function can occur with severe obstruction and secondary cardiac failure, this most often being associated with symptomatic critical aortic stenosis in the newborn.[6]

It is possible to obtain an estimate of the left ventricular pressure in aortic stenosis in children by using a modification of the wall stress formula. Left ventricular systolic wall thickness (LVWT) and internal dimension (LVID) are measured and the pressure (LVP) calculated from

$$LVP = LVWT/LVID \times K.$$

K represents a constant which has been calculated to be from 220^7 to $245.^8$ The main difficulty with this technique is in ensuring that the posterior wall has been accurately measured and that other echoes, such as those from the chordae tendineae, are not included. No matter which constant is used this formula gives a useful prediction of the severity of stenosis when left ventricular function is normal. It is important to be aware that this is not the actual left ventricular pressure and the gradient calculated from this is not comparable to that obtained with Doppler examination. If Doppler equipment is not available this formula can be of value in detecting those patients with a low gradient who do not need further investigation.

It is inappropriate to attempt to measure the cusp separation with M-mode echocardiography since it is impossible to be sure that the recorded echoes represent the cusps at the true orifice and not an area of doming below it.

Cross-sectional echocardiography

Cross-sectional echocardiography shows the morphology of the aortic valve and better defines its orifice. In systole there will be the characteristic domed appearance[9] of the pliable valve (Fig. 3B). The long axis view in aortic valve stenosis in diastole may show the leaflets to be thickened (Fig. 3A). The anterior and posterior cusps are usually apparent with the valve orifice being delineated by the tips of the valve leaflets. In some cases it is difficult to show the anterior and posterior cusps equally well and the appearance may be of doming of just one margin of the valve, usually the anterior, and the orifice will not then be shown. The apical four chamber view may show the doming more clearly but in older subjects the distance of the transducer from the valve limits the image quality obtained in this view. An estimation of the severity of the valve stenosis can be made from the long axis view by the measurement of the maximum aortic cusp separation at the orifice.[9] The orifice should be located at the apex of the domed valve and the scanning plane moved across this to determine the greatest separation of the leaflet tips. The inner dimension is measured at that point. In adults this distance bears a relation to the severity of stenosis and can be corrected for body surface area[10] but in children this correction is not valid since the aortic cusp separation increases relative to body surface area as size increases. The ratio of the maximum aortic cusp separation to aortic root dimension can be used instead. In normal subjects this should be between 0.6 and 0.9, in patients with mild stenosis (gradient less

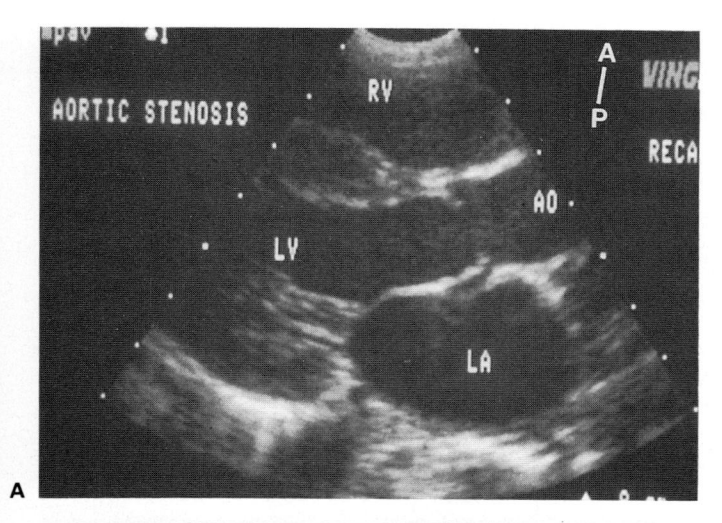

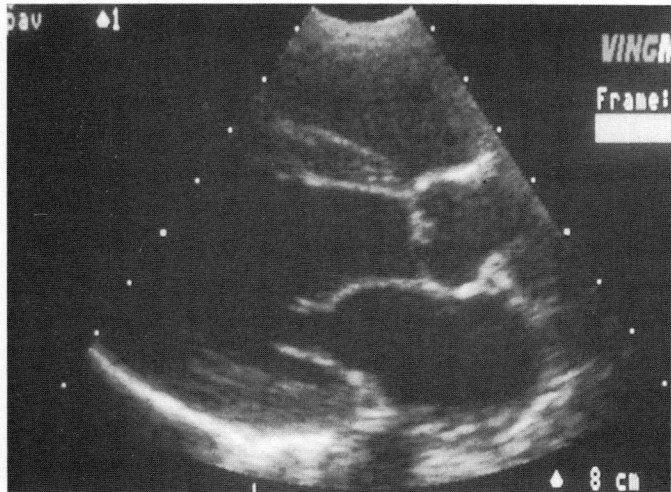

Fig. 3 Long axis views in a patient with moderate aortic valve stenosis. **A:** In systole there is doming of the valve though the posterior margin of the orifice is not as clearly shown as the anterior one in this frame. **B:** In diastole multiple echoes are apparent at the point of apposition of the leaflets, indicating thickening of the valve.

than 50 mmHg) the ratio is from 0.4 to 0.6, and in patients with more severe obstruction (over 50 mmHg) the ratio is from 0.2 to 0.4.[9] Since Doppler examination gives a more accurate measurement of gradient this measurement is now of limited practical value in deciding on appropriate patient management.

Short axis views of the valve may show an abnormal cusp pattern in diastole and the restricted movement of the cusps in systole. It is not, however, possible to obtain a sufficiently clear image showing the exact valve orifice to allow reliable area measurement. There is potential for error in that the apparent orifice shown may be below the valve tips with resultant overestimation of the true area.

In the less common situation of the symptomatic infant with critical stenosis the valve is thickened and distorted. Doming may be minimal with the cusps being relatively immobile and thick in both systole and diastole. In addition there is usually post stenotic dilatation of the aorta and there may be increased echogenicity of the papillary muscles and enlargement of the right ventricle.[6]

Doppler ultrasound

Doppler ultrasound provides an accurate non-invasive means of determining the valve gradient in aortic valve stenosis in children.[11] The technique is similar to that used in adults with aortic stenosis for the measurement of the instantaneous maximum gradient with the modified Bernoulli formula[12] and, if considered appropriate, for estimating the aortic valve area with the continuity equation.[13] In infants and young children it is commonly possible to obtain satisfactory continuous wave Doppler signals from all positions, namely suprasternal, right supraclavicular, right upper sternal edge, left sternal edge, subxiphoid and apical. All sites must be used since the one from which the maximum velocity will be obtained cannot be predicted and there may be a significant difference between them. If all are explored it is unlikely that the angle of incidence of the beam to the jet will be high in every case and there should consequently be little underestimation of the instantaneous maximum gradient calculated from the maximum velocity recorded. The difference between the peak-to-peak and instantaneous maximum gradient[14] should be borne in mind in interpreting the clinical significance of this value and as with adults[15] all clinical and non-invasive findings should be considered together. Children are more likely than adults to be active before the study or be excited or worried by it and the state of activity will affect the maximum velocity obtained. If the flow velocity proximal to the aortic valve is greater than 1.0 m/s it will be necessary to consider it in the calculation.[16] A higher value may be obtained from a patient who is sedated or anaesthetised for cardiac catheterisation, as has been shown in children with pulmonary stenosis.[17] The catheter derived peak-to-peak gradient has traditionally been measured and used for deciding on management and it may well be that the higher Doppler gradient obtained from the active child more accurately indicates the need for restriction of activity or surgical or balloon intervention. In the infant with cardiac failure and critical aortic stenosis the gradient is often low but the echocardiographic appearance of severely decreased left ventricular function indicates that there is marked reduction of the aortic valve area and thus critical aortic stenosis can be inferred. The Doppler gradient must not be considered on its own and all clinical and echocardiographic findings must be considered.

Colour Doppler flow mapping is of little practical value in aortic valve stenosis. It seldom shows a clear jet through the valve, in most cases there being a relatively wide region of turbulence or variance immediately distal to it. Under no circumstances should an attempt be made to measure the angle of incidence of the ultrasound beam to the jet and use this to correct for the angle of incidence of the spectral beam as many misinterpretations can occur (see Quantitative Doppler Techniques — Ch. 6).

Fixed subaortic stenosis

This defect can occur in isolation or with other congenital malformations such as coarctation of the aorta, ventricular septal defect, atrio-ventricular septal defect, arterial duct, or aortic valve disease. The lesion most often takes the form of a complete or partial ring of fibromuscular tissue about 5 to 10 mm below the aortic valve. Although the lesion is almost always a fibromuscular ridge, echocardiography shows what appear to be two different types of discrete obstruction, either a membranous diaphragm quite close to the aortic valve or a fibrous ridge further below it. The difference between these types is, to a degree, a qualitative one which is related to the thickness of the ridge. In many cases this abnormality cannot be recognised in early life and it only becomes apparent after infancy. Less commonly the obstruction is a tunnel-like narrowing involving a length of the left ventricular outflow tract rather than a discrete part of it.

M-mode echocardiography will suggest the presence of the abnormality but definitive diagnosis requires the use of cross-sectional imaging. The M-mode study through the left ventricle may show thickening of its wall as in aortic valve stenosis. A sweep up through the left ventricular outflow tract can demonstrate prolonged narrowing with tunnel obstruction but the linear echo of a discrete diaphragm in the immediate subvalve region is difficult to show and M-mode studies are not a reliable means of reaching the diagnosis. The M-mode record through the aortic valve is extremely useful and may point to the need for a more assiduous study of the subvalve area. In subaortic stenosis the aortic valve cusps classically show coarse systolic fluttering with a prominent notch due to early and abrupt systolic closure of the valve after which the valve again opens partially and closes slowly throughout the rest of systole[18,19] (Fig. 4). This is, however, an indirect and non-specific finding and a similar appearance can occur in other situations such as ventricular septal defect or hypertrophic obstructive cardiomyopathy where there is interference with left ventricular outlet tract flow. Occasionally there may be flutter of the mitral valve due to aortic regurgitation which is an almost universal accompaniment of subaortic stenosis.

Cross-sectional echocardiography will usually allow the diagnosis to be reached and this modality can provide a distinction between the different forms of obstruction. Where there is a discrete obstruction the narrowing may be apparent in a parasternal long axis view.[20,21] There may

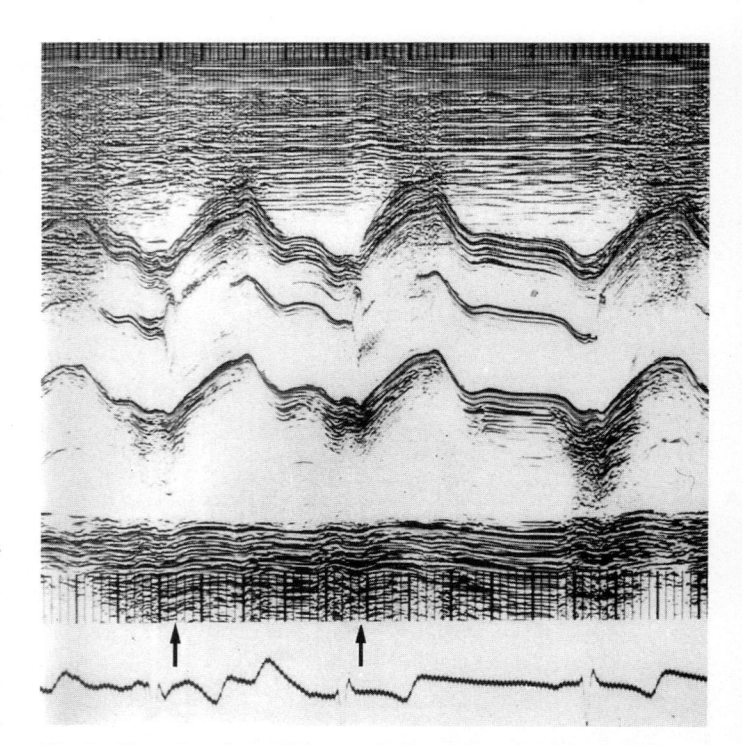

Fig. 4 M-mode echocardiogram of the aortic valve in a patient with subaortic stenosis. The early systolic closure (arrowed) and systolic flutter of the leaflets is best seen in the first period of systole in the anterior cusp.

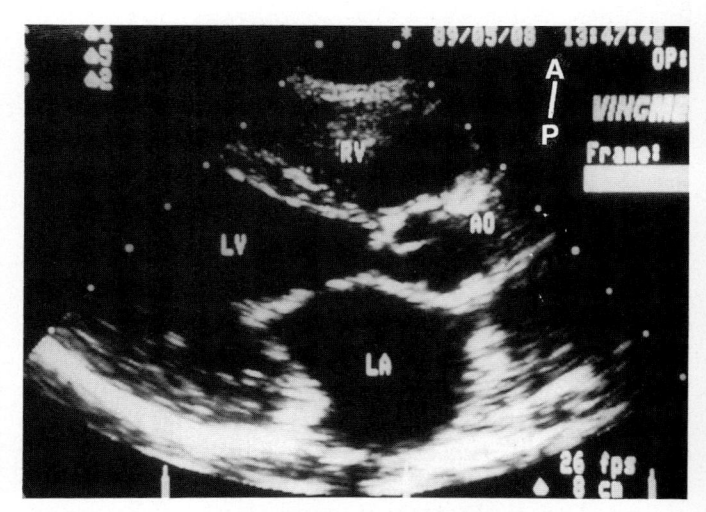

Fig. 5 A long axis view in a patient with subaortic stenosis showing a relatively narrow left ventricular outflow tract and a subaortic membrane.

be associated narrowing of the left ventricular outflow tract (Fig. 5) or the obstruction may be seen as a relatively thin bright echogenic membrane-like structure immediately below the aortic valve, protruding from the posterior aspect of the upper ventricular septum into the left ventricular outflow tract (Fig. 6). In some cases a thicker fibrous ridge

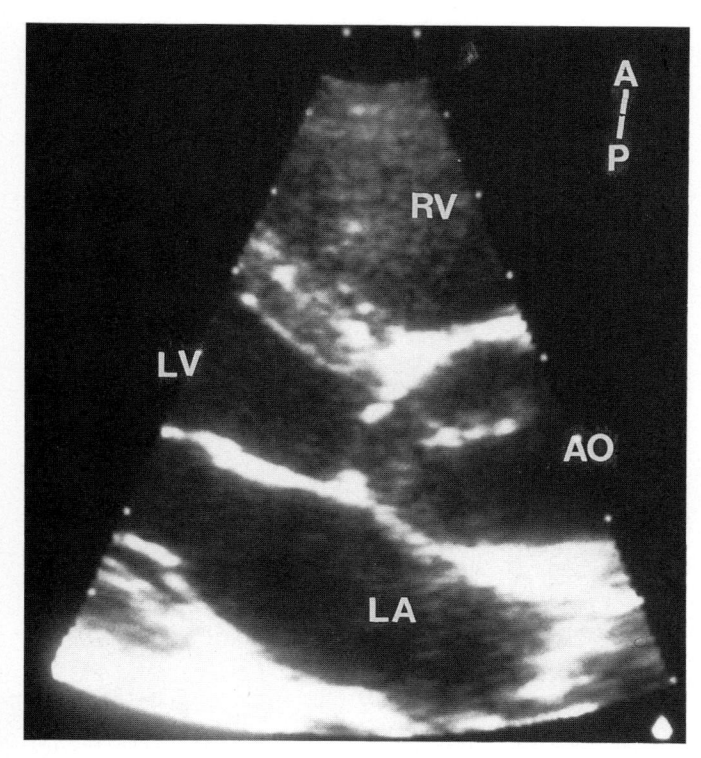

Fig. 6 Modified long axis view in a patient with subaortic stenosis showing a relatively thin subaortic membrane below the aortic cusp.

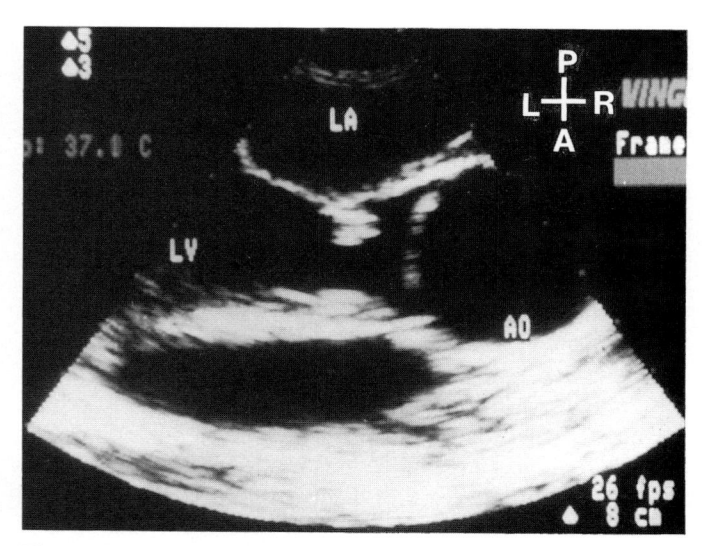

Fig. 7 Transoesophageal image from a child with subaortic stenosis in whom the membrane was not clearly shown with transthoracic ultrasound. The posterior margin related to the mitral valve is particularly clearly shown.

is apparent in the outflow tract a little more proximally (at a slightly greater distance from the aortic valve). It is not always possible to show the posterior margin of this ridge in relation to the anterior leaflet of the mitral valve but adjustment of the scanning plane may improve its demonstration.[21] Since a ring or membrane is parallel to the ultrasound beam in the parasternal view it may be poorly shown when it is thin and membrane-like. An apical long axis view will then bring it into a more suitable position for imaging and can improve its recognition[22] and in particular will demonstrate its adherence to the mitral valve. A similar lesion can occur with subpulmonary obstruction in transposition of the great arteries.[23] It has been reported that it is possible to miss a thin membrane with echocardiography[21] and it is thus important to use multiple transducer positions when the diagnosis is suspected but a membrane or ridge is not clearly shown. Difficulty can arise in some cases where there appears to be a ridge arising from the ventricular septum but no obstruction is demonstrated. The use of multiple views and, more importantly, Doppler examination to determine whether there is a clinically significant left ventricular outflow tract gradient will then indicate its clinical significance.

The fibrous ridge can almost always be shown with echocardiography in a sufficiently clear manner for the surgeon to undertake operation without catheterisation.

Indeed it is often difficult to show this ridge with angiocardiography and echocardiography is generally superior in the detection and demonstration of subvalve left ventricular outflow tract obstruction.[24] In cases of doubt an exceptionally clear image of the subaortic area is provided by transoesophageal echocardiography using the standard view showing the mitral and aortic valves. Even when the lesion has been shown from a transthoracic position this technique will greatly improve the detail of the lesion (Fig. 7) and is undoubtedly superior to angiography.[25]

Tunnel obstruction is characterised by widespread narrowing in the subaortic region, often with irregular borders. On some occasions the obstruction can be the result of accessory tissue on the anterior mitral leaflet and this can be shown in an apical view as a mass of echoes attached to the mitral valve and prolapsing into the left ventricular outflow tract. Accurate measurement of the area of obstruction is difficult and imaging echocardiography has little part to play in the assessment of the severity of subaortic stenosis, but, as with aortic valve stenosis, an estimation of the left ventricular pressure and thence gradient (or pressure drop) may be reached by the application of wall stress calculations.

Colour Doppler flow mapping can be helpful in localising the exact site of narrowing when this is not clear on imaging. Proximal flow acceleration and turbulence at the site of the obstruction will usually be apparent. Spectral Doppler echocardiography allows the gradient across the narrowing to be assessed. It is used in the same way as in aortic valve stenosis in adults or children. The angle of the jet cannot be predicted and it is particularly important to search all sites for the maximal velocity. There is no clear evidence that there are any particular problems in applying the technique in subvalve rather than valve stenosis. There are, however, theoretical considerations that may result in differences between the Doppler and catheter measured gradient if the obstruction is elongated or at different levels[26,27] and there may be more difficulty in obtaining adequate alignment with the jet flow. Thus the study must be meticulously performed from every possible site. All the non-invasive results must be taken into consideration in interpreting the findings. Some authorities would argue that the gradient is unimportant and that subaortic stenosis is a progressive lesion and should be operated upon even if the gradient is low. There is no practical means to obtain the area of the obstruction in subaortic stenosis since the continuity equation cannot be applied. This is because there is no suitable region for measurement lying proximal to the stenosis. In virtually all subjects there will also be aortic regurgitation and the diagnosis of subaortic stenosis in the absence of this should be reconsidered.

Supravalve aortic stenosis

Supravalve aortic stenosis usually occurs above the aortic sinuses which appear to bulge out below the narrowed area which may be discrete, diffuse or tubular. On occasions the stenosis may be at the level of the sinuses (Fig. 8). The

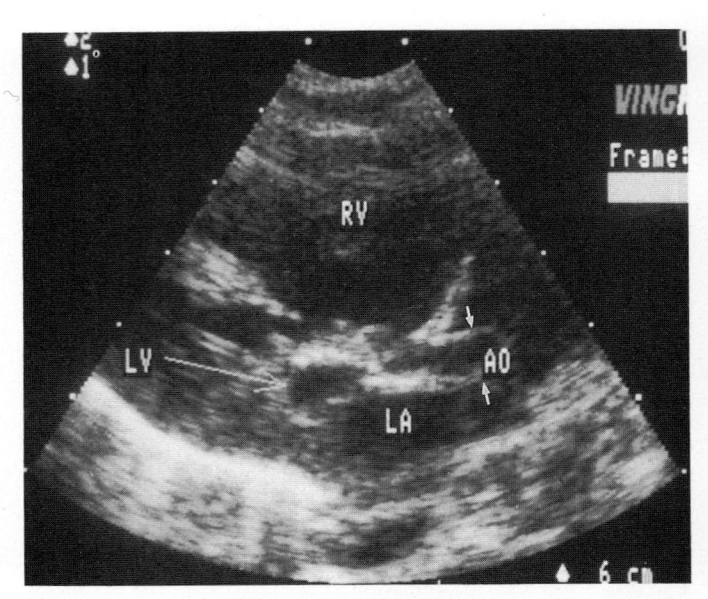

Fig. 9 Long axis view in a patient with supravalve aortic stenosis and hypoplasia of the ascending aorta (arrowed). The right ventricle is large.

ultrasound appearances will depend on the basic malformation. M-mode echocardiography can show thickened left ventricular walls and a somewhat smaller than normal aortic root. It is theoretically possible to continue a sweep upwards to demonstrate that the ascending aorta is small[28] but this is subject to error and cross-sectional echocardiography should be used to show the area of abnormality. The aortic root may be smaller than normal and the coronary arteries may be dilated. In the normal subject the diameter of the aorta just above the valve sinuses is approximately equal to or slightly larger than that at the valve ring and an area of greater narrowing is in keeping with a diagnosis of supravalve aortic stenosis.[29,30] A parasternal long axis view is more useful for these assessments (Fig. 9), often with the transducer moved to a higher interspace than that normally used to show the left ventricular outflow tract and the aortic valve. The right parasternal window may sometimes be useful in this condition also. Colour Doppler flow mapping will confirm the site of narrowing but it is of little additional practical value. Spectral Doppler examination can provide a measurement of the gradient but in this situation it is sometimes less easy than in valve or subvalve stenosis to obtain the maximum velocity signal.

HYPOPLASTIC LEFT HEART SYNDROME

The hypoplastic left heart syndrome is a relatively common defect which, if untreated, usually results in death in the neonatal period. It was long considered to be inoperable but in the last decade treatment by palliative surgery or cardiac transplantation has become available. There is no universal agreement that surgical treatment should be

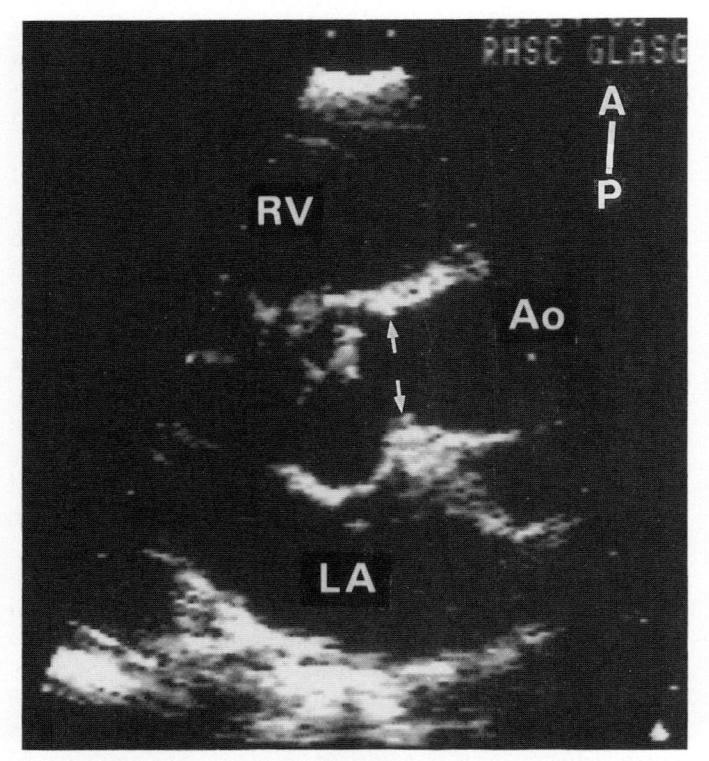

Fig. 8 Long axis view in a patient with supravalve aortic stenosis (arrowed) with hypoplasia of the aortic root and proximal ascending aorta.

offered and which form it might take, but the necessity of making a detailed anatomical diagnosis has become of more clinical relevance and echocardiography has become accepted as the definitive means of doing this. The condition can occasionally be diagnosed antenatally during fetal echocardiography.

The syndrome consists of a spectrum of differing degrees of hypoplasia of the left atrium, the left ventricle and the aorta, with stenosis or atresia of the aortic and mitral valves. Ultrasound examination should include assessment of all these structures. The capability of echocardiography to make the basic diagnosis of hypoplastic left heart syndrome was recognised with M-mode echocardiography before the routine use of cross-sectional imaging.[31,32] The diagnosis is based on the presence of a small left ventricular cavity and ascending aorta, but the small size of these structures makes demonstration and exact measurement with M-mode echocardiography difficult. Different criteria for making the diagnosis[33,34] have been suggested with M-mode echocardiography. There are differences between the measurements obtained in different studies, probably because of inaccuracies in beam alignment, and in this situation accurate measurement with M-mode echocardiography requires the use of cross-sectional imaging to guide the beam. Furthermore M-mode echocardiography alone can sometimes give an incorrect impression of the size of the left ventricle if echoes from prominent right ventricular trabeculations or papillary muscles are mistaken as representing the ventricular septum and the true chamber is not seen.[35] More recently the group which has pioneered the palliative surgical approach has used the following echocardiographic criteria for the definition of hypoplastic left heart syndrome.[36] The mitral valve annulus diameter is 6 mm or less, the left ventricular cavity end diastolic dimension is less than 10 mm and the ascending aorta external diameter is less than 7 mm with aortic valve atresia, hypoplasia, or stenosis. Cross-sectional echocardiography, by facilitating M-mode alignment and showing other features of the syndrome, is the ideal means for assessing the anatomy in hypoplastic left heart syndrome.[37] There are few reports on the simple cross-sectional diagnosis,[38] perhaps because the assessment is relatively straightforward and studies concentrate on the relevance of different findings to palliative surgery.[34,36,39]

The diagnosis is made using standard views but because of the small size of the left-sided structures the transducer angulation has to be modified as necessary to show each feature optimally. Since the syndrome comprises a variety of different features the appearances will vary from one patient to another. A standard parasternal long axis view will show the small aorta, the left atrium and the left ventricle but it may not be possible to show all these structures and the ascending aorta optimally in a single view. When the left ventricle is very small it is difficult or impossible to demonstrate the cavity, and the distinction of hypoplastic left heart syndrome from a univentricular heart may require the use of a variety of other views. The left ventricular diastolic dimension will usually be less than 10 mm but in some atypical forms of the syndrome this may be greater. The mitral valve leaflets show very limited motion and imaging does not usually allow a clear distinction to be made between atresia or severe stenosis. When individual cusps are seen to open, particularly if their movement can be recorded with M-mode echocardiography, the mitral valve is not considered to be atretic and the orifice is likely to be greater than 3 mm diameter.[34] The mitral valve ring can be measured directly[40] but its size is of no surgical or prognostic significance.

The transducer may have to be moved to a high position with rightward tilt to show the aortic root. The ascending aorta is best seen from a suprasternal site from where the aortic arch can also be imaged (Plate 1). The aortic annulus is imaged from a mid or high parasternal position and the valve motion and morphology are best seen in a long axis view. In cases where the aorta is very small the aortic cusps can appear as relatively immobile and thick, representing probable atresia. Even when the aortic root is larger than usual it is not commonly possible to show the mobile doming valve cusps in systole.

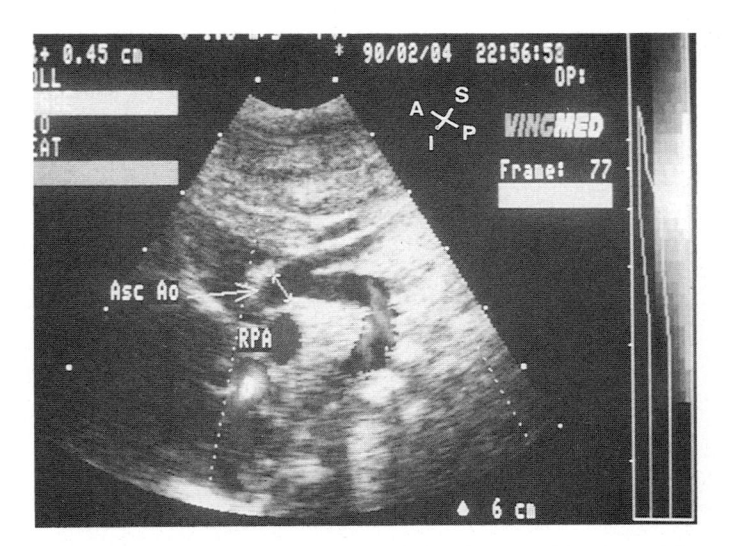

Plate 1 **Suprasternal view of the ascending aorta and aortic arch** in hypoplastic left heart syndrome. The red/orange colour indicates retrograde flow in the arch from the descending aorta to the arch and thence to the ascending aorta. This figure is reproduced in colour in the colour plate section at the front of this volume.

Short axis views are often more suitable for showing the left ventricle (Fig. 10) and ascending aorta (Fig. 11) and measuring their dimensions. A four chamber view (Fig. 12) may show the left ventricular cavity when it is not apparent from long and short axis views. Even with the use of all these cross-sectional views, the left

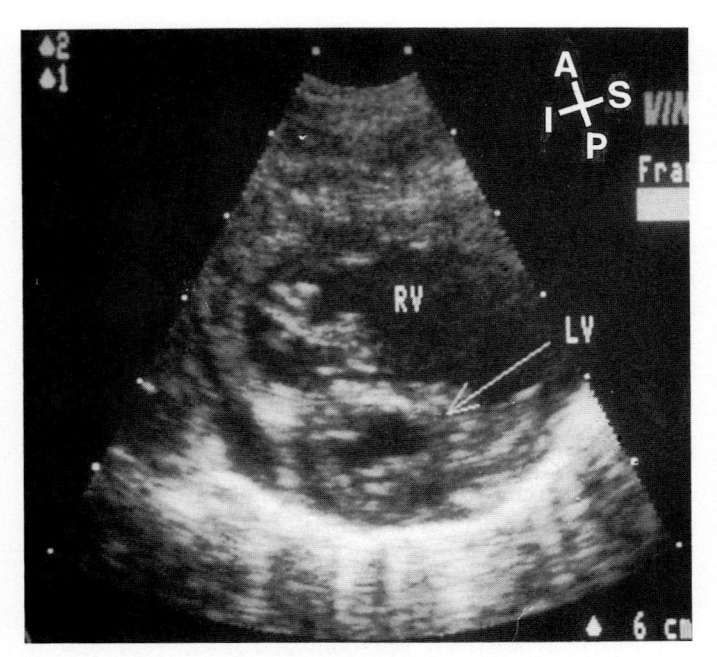

Fig. 10 Short axis view of the ventricles in a patient with left heart hypoplasia. There is a very small left ventricular cavity and large right ventricle, the walls of which are clearly shown.

ventricular cavity can sometimes be impossible to show and indeed no cavity may be found at autopsy.

Abnormalities of right ventricular regional wall motion can occur at the time of initial presentation and these are best shown on a short axis sweep. The exact quantitation of this abnormality is difficult but a qualitative assessment can be made from short axis views through the ventricles (Fig. 10). The atrial septal anatomy can show some variation with the septum primum often having an abnormal orientation, its superior aspect being displaced leftward and attached directly on to the atrial wall, distant from its normal position on the superior limbus of the septum secundum near the entrance of the superior caval vein. The unusual curvature of the thin superior part of the septum primum can result in echocardiographic drop out in short and long axis views, incorrectly suggesting the presence of a large atrial septal defect. It is then appropriate to use a subcostal position with four chamber and long axial views,[41] the latter providing the best angle for optimal demonstration of any leftward deviation of the superior attachment of the septum primum.[39] These views will also demonstrate the size of the foramen ovale and any atrial septal defect (Fig. 12).

The ascending aorta, arch and periductal region are shown from a high parasternal or suprasternal site (Plate 1). The ascending aorta will have an internal diameter from 2 to 7 mm and may be seen to widen at the proximal arch just before the innominate artery origin and again in the post ductal region. Coarctation of the aorta is a common accompaniment, its incidence depending on the exact definition used.[36] A posterior juxtaductal ridge can occur in patients with hypoplastic left heart syndrome and it has been suggested that coarctation of the aorta should

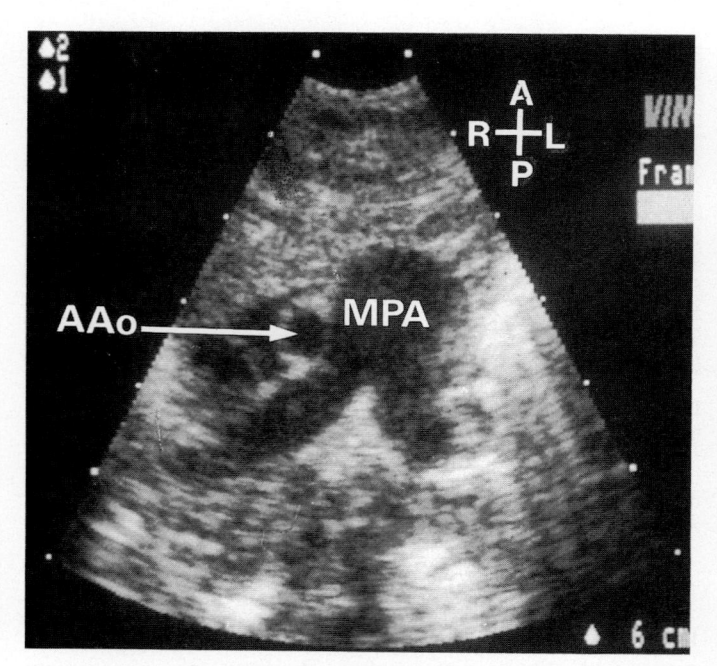

Fig. 11 Short axis view of the great arteries above the level of the aortic valve in a patient with left heart hypoplasia showing the very small ascending aorta (AAo) to the right of the large main right pulmonary artery (MPA). The proximal pulmonary arteries are shown to be of good size.

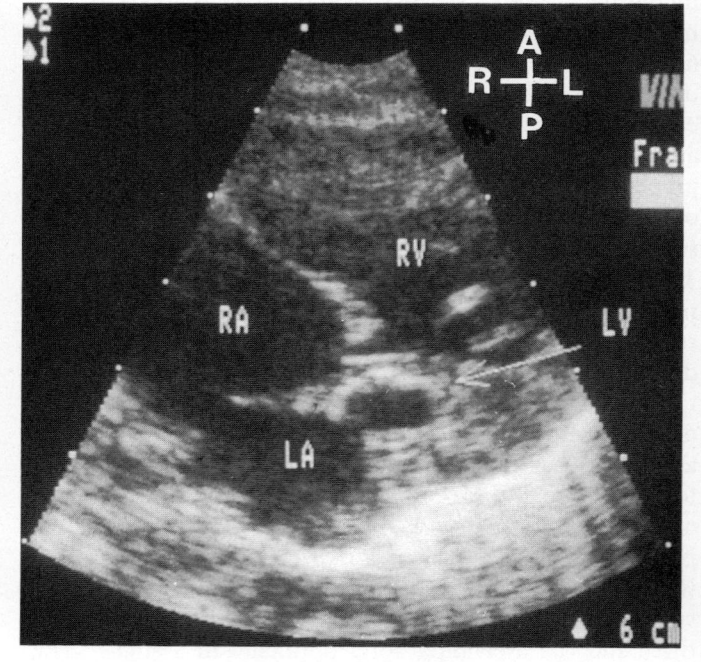

Fig. 12 Subxyphoid 4 chamber view in hypoplastic left heart syndrome. The atrial septum and atrial septal defect are shown optimally and the septum primum is inserted normally.

not be diagnosed unless this ridge reduces the internal diameter of the distal isthmus by at least 50%. Standard views of the arterial duct will show its continuity with the descending aorta.

The usual surgical approach necessitates atrial septectomy and augmentation of the ascending, transverse and descending aorta and it might be expected that certain individual features of the hypoplastic left heart syndrome might be of prognostic relevance in relation to palliative surgery. However, echocardiographic assessment has shown that the anatomy of the atrial septum, the aortic root size and distal arch anatomy, the right ventricular wall thickness and function, and the severity of tricuspid regurgitation are of no prognostic significance.[36] Thus, whilst it is appropriate to assess all these features, any difficulty in defining exactly the atrial anatomy or the presence of coarctation should not preclude surgical treatment on the basis of echocardiography alone.

In a study of the accuracy of echocardiography in hypoplastic left heart syndrome it was reported that a hypoplastic branch pulmonary artery and left superior vena cava were not shown with echocardiograph.[37] Such information would undoubtedly be of value to the surgeon and thus although these and other abnormalities are rare it is appropriate to attempt to define as far as possible the pulmonary artery branches and the venous connections. Colour Doppler flow mapping can be of help in this assessment by showing increased velocity where there is a stenotic lesion. It will also improve definition of venous channels and their site of entry into the heart.

Doppler ultrasound is of limited practical value in the diagnosis and assessment of hypoplastic left heart syndrome. Flow through the mitral and aortic valves may be shown with spectral Doppler examination or colour flow mapping but the size of the left ventricle, rather than valve function, is the important determinant of the surgical approach. Tricuspid regurgitation can be demonstrated in the majority of patients. An estimate of the severity of tricuspid regurgitation can be obtained with colour Doppler flow mapping but interpretation is subject to the potential difficulties of the technique,[42] and it appears to be of no clinical significance unless it is very severe. Spectral or colour Doppler interrogation of the arterial duct will show the typical pattern of flow, mainly from the pulmonary artery to the aorta with a short period of reverse flow in late diastole (Fig. 13). The flow from aorta to pulmonary artery occurring in diastole is simply a reflection of the difference in the diastolic resistance between the pulmonary and systemic circulations. It does not indicate that flow has occurred through the ascending aorta and arch and thence into the duct and pulmonary artery. Colour Doppler studies will also show that flow in the isthmus and ascending aorta is retrograde when aortic atresia is present (Plate 1).

Echocardiography will be applied increasingly in the assessment of palliative surgery for the left heart hypoplasia syndrome and the echocardiographic appearances have been confirmed from a study of fixed autopsy specimens of hearts which have undergone this procedure.[39] Ultrasound imaging has shown differential growth patterns in the pulmonary arteries in those who have had a Blalock shunt as opposed to a central one,[43] and Doppler examination has shown mild to moderate semilunar valve regurgitation in about 25% of these patients.[44]

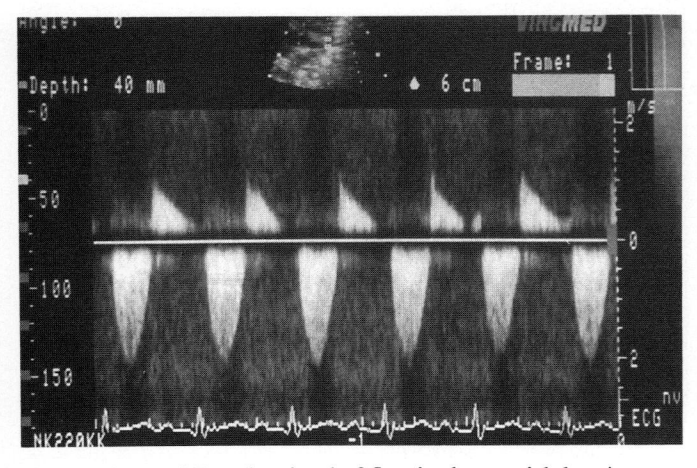

Fig. 13 Spectral Doppler signal of flow in the arterial duct in a patient with hypoplastic left heart syndrome recorded from the parasternal position. Flow in systole is from the pulmonary artery to the aorta but in diastole is reversed.

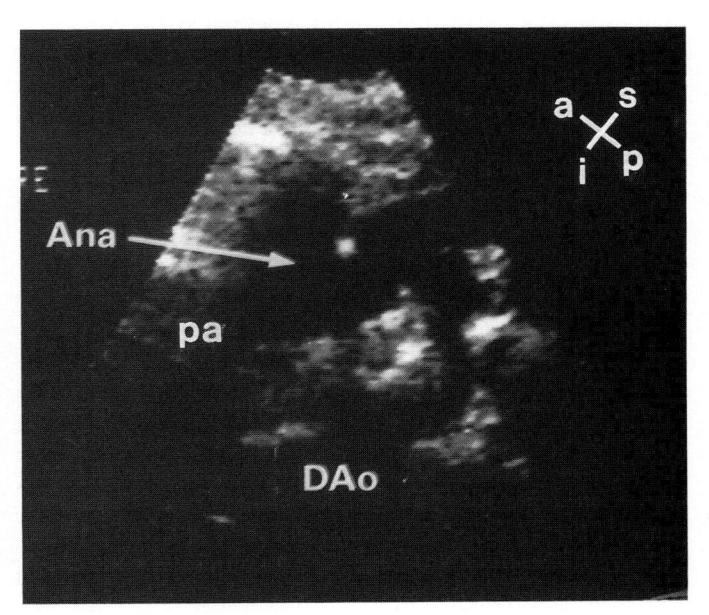

Fig. 14 High parasternal view in an infant who has undergone palliative surgery for hypoplastic left heart syndrome. The anastomosis between the pulmonary artery and aorta is shown and the distal arch though relatively narrow shows no discrete obstruction. Ana = anastomosis; DA = descending aorta.

Echocardiography can demonstrate the anastomosis of the pulmonary artery to the aorta, presence or absence of aortic coarctation (Fig. 14), and atrial septal and shunt flow but detailed evaluation of its practical value in the individual patient following surgery is awaited.

COARCTATION OF THE AORTA

Patients with coarctation of the aorta commonly present with congestive cardiac failure in the neonatal period or with diminished femoral pulses in later infancy or childhood. There has been some difference of opinion as to the morphology and terminology of aortic coarctation. A practical classification which, in the newborn, can be recognised by echocardiography is that of preductal, paraductal and postductal coarctation. The most common is preductal coarctation where there is a shelf at the junction of the aortic isthmus and duct. In infants this shelf is composed of an extension of ductal tissue, usually with hypoplasia of the isthmus which tapers down towards the waist. Less commonly the coarctation is paraductal, lying directly opposite the mouth of the arterial duct or ligamentum, or in a postductal position, usually immediately beyond the arterial duct. Paraductal coarctation is most often found in the left heart hypoplasia syndrome.

In most cases of coarctation there is a discrete shelf-like lesion with gradual tapering in the aortic arch proximal to it. Variations in the anatomical nature of the coarctation will determine the echocardiographic findings but in the older subject these different sites are less apparent. Early ultrasonic descriptions were of a discrete membrane, an hourglass type narrowing, a long segment narrowing, or a generalised hypoplasia of the isthmus.[45] The diagnosis is usually reached on the basis of clinical examination and further investigations are directed to defining its site and nature to permit the correct surgical approach. The main exception to this occurs in the newborn infant where clinical signs can be difficult to elucidate, particularly if prostaglandin therapy has been started and the arterial duct is open.

Imaging of coarctation of the aorta

The initial parasternal echocardiographic study will often demonstrate ventricular abnormality. In older subjects the left ventricular cavity is usually normal in size and function though its walls may be somewhat thickened. In infants the right ventricle is often enlarged and the left ventricle is smaller than normal with decreased function.[46] In some patients, generally presenting later in infancy, the left ventricle can be dilated with diminished function and mitral regurgitation. Abnormalities of the aortic valve are associated with coarctation, the most common being a bicuspid valve, though valve or subvalve stenosis also

occur. Ventricular septal defect frequently occurs with symptomatic coarctation in the newborn.

Imaging of coarctation is undertaken from the suprasternal notch[45,47,48] or high parasternal sites[49] using the standard views for demonstrating the aortic arch and arterial duct. The transducer should first be placed in the suprasternal notch and (for a left arch) rotated clockwise from an antero-posterior plane with minor modifications of the angulation being undertaken to show the ascending aorta, arch, and proximal descending aorta as an arcuate echo free structure. In some younger patients this view may be better obtained from a high parasternal position, either right or left. These are the optimal views for demonstrating the origin of the head and neck vessels from the superior margin of the aortic arch[50] and they should be used to establish the size and relationship of the left subclavian artery to the coarctation site (Fig. 15) and ascertain that the right subclavian artery does not have an anomalous origin distal to the coarctation. The normal bifurcation of the brachiocephalic artery into the right carotid and subclavian arteries may be shown by turning the transducer towards the right shoulder to follow the most proximal vessel from the arch. If the normal right brachiocephalic artery bifurcation is not seen it is appropriate to attempt to image the origin and course of each vessel to try to confirm or exclude an anomalous origin of the right subclavian

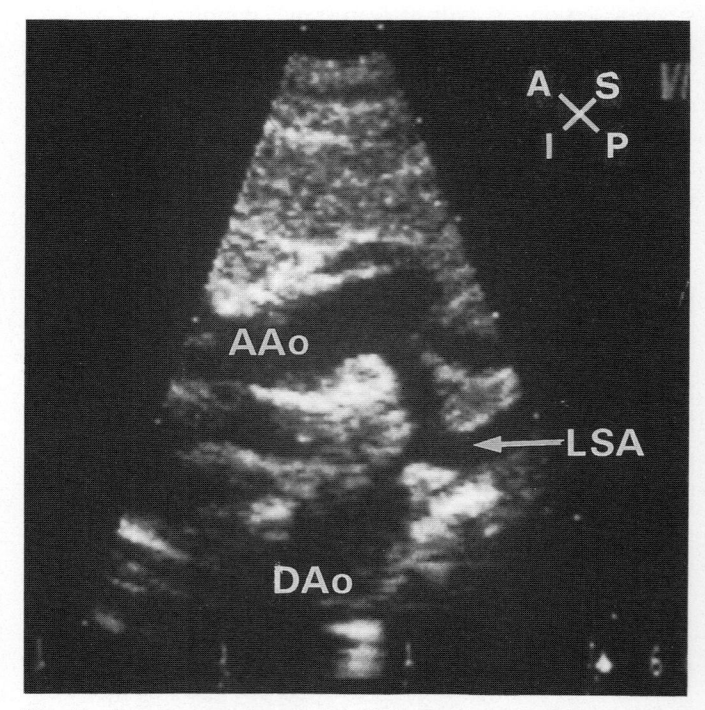

Fig. 15 Suprasternal view from an infant with preductal coarctation of the aorta. The left carotid and subclavian arteries are apparent with coarctation immediately distal to the subclavian artery. There is also poststenotic dilatation of the descending aorta. AAo = ascending aorta; DAo = descending aorta; LSA = left subclavian artery.

artery. Where there is difficulty or doubt as to whether a vessel being studied is an artery or vein, the use of Doppler examination to determine the direction of flow will prevent any confusion.

In older patients in whom coarctation can be recognised it will usually be apparent in the suprasternal view. There is no standard appearance of a coarctation on echocardiography and this will vary depending on the nature of the lesion and the aorta immediately proximal and distal to it. In some cases there will be evidence of discrete narrowing, often with post-stenotic dilatation (Fig. 15). This dilatation is more apparent in older subjects and its demonstration can help to pin-point the site of the coarctation in cases where a clear narrowing or transverse membrane is not shown but this is not completely reliable as post-stenotic dilatation does not always occur. Rarely there may be the appearance of more than one membrane (Fig. 16) due to a coarctation with a 'fold' in the aorta at the site. In a considerable number of older children and adults it is not possible to show the coarctation site with imaging echocardiography alone[51] because it is relatively far round the arch and is often shadowed by a mass of echoes from structures under the aortic arch. In this situation colour Doppler flow mapping may be of value in highlighting the narrow area.

The arch examination is technically easier in infants than older subjects and the coarctation can be shown with echocardiography in most infants, particularly the newborn. In this age group the coarctation may be better shown if the transducer is adjusted to view the area adjacent to and below the arterial duct by rotating the probe anti-clockwise and tilting it to the left. This is often better shown with the transducer in the left subclavicular area. This manoeuvre is designed to show the distal aortic arch and descending aorta in relation to the main and left pulmonary arteries and arterial duct and is usually out of the plane of the ascending aorta and arch branches.[52] In the newborn the relationship of the narrowing to the arterial duct will be apparent using this approach.[49] In most cases the narrowing is preductal (Fig. 17) with a shelf protruding into the lumen, often with some degree of hypoplasia of the isthmus. With coarctation of the aorta this shelf will also involve the posterior part of the aorta and care should be taken to ensure that an apparent anterior ridge due to normal ductal insertion into the aorta (Fig. 18) is not mistaken for coarctation in a normal infant.

Difficulties in interpretation may occur when the isthmus is narrow but a shelf is not clearly shown. The question as to whether this is a normal variant may then arise and clinical findings are then important in considering the requirement for operation. In infants with preductal coarctation the internal diameter of the isthmus is generally 3 mm or less but it is greater than 3.3 mm in 80% of normal subjects.[49] In cases where narrowing in the thoracic aorta cannot be demonstrated despite clinical findings of coarctation, the abdominal aorta should be examined. Coarctation in this site is rare and usually takes the form of diffuse hypoplasia rather than a discrete shelf. This can sometimes be imaged from the epigastrium but the distal

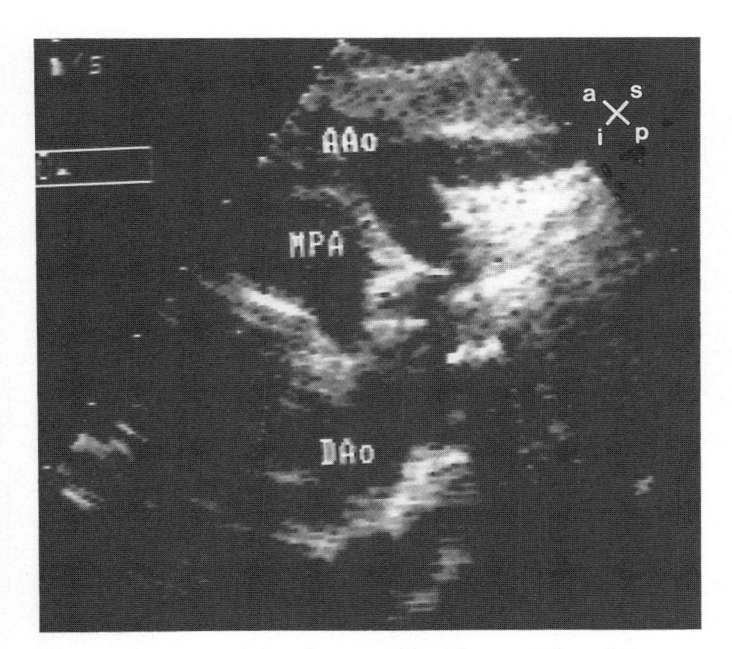

Fig. 16 Suprasternal view from a child with coarctation of the aorta in whom an appearance of more than one membrane is produced by the serpiginous course of the aorta. A discrete coarctation was found at surgery. AAo = ascending aorta; DAo = descending aorta.

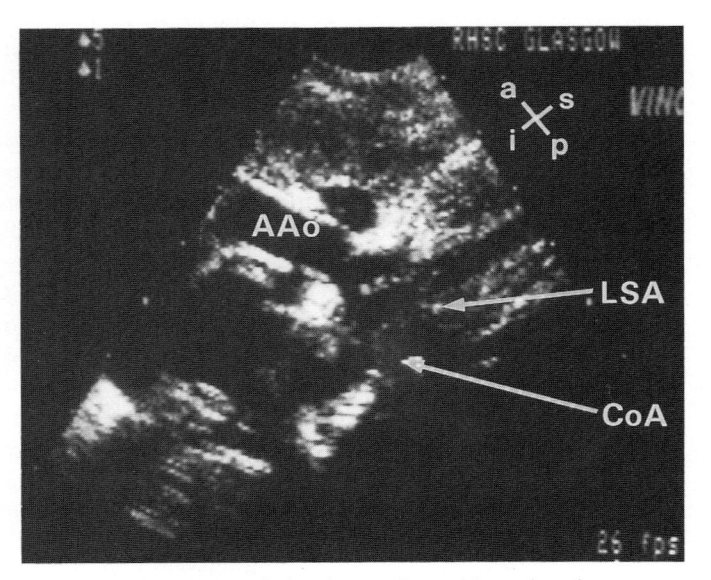

Fig. 17 High parasternal view in a patient with preductal coarctation of the aorta and a widely patent arterial duct. The arrow indicates the site of obstruction just distal to the left subclavian artery. LSA = left subclavian artery; CoA = coarctation.

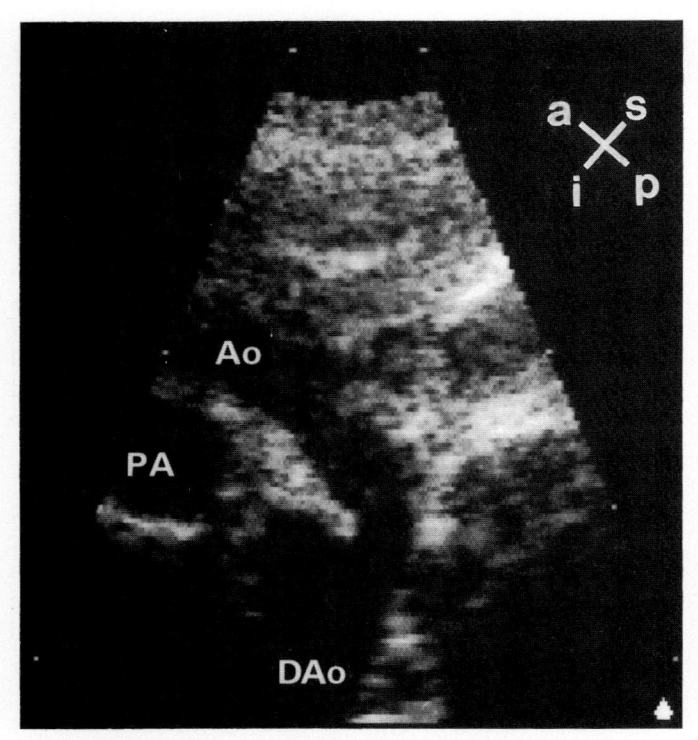

Fig. 18 High parasternal view from a newborn infant with no coarctation but an open arterial duct. The shelf at the superior margin of the arterial duct could be mistaken for a coarctation but there is no posterior extension of this. DAo = descending aorta.

abdominal aorta and bifurcation in infants is generally more easily seen from the lumbar site.[53] The descending thoracic aorta can be shown in a long axis plane from a subxiphoid position and with coarctation of the aorta it will usually exhibit diminished pulsation, but this sign, though helpful in some situations, is non-specific.

Assessment of the severity of the obstruction in coarctation is not practical with imaging ultrasound, and echocardiographic and angiocardiographic measurements of the diameter of the narrow area show a relatively poor correlation.[54] If coarctation is recognised clinically it will require surgery or balloon angioplasty treatment and the severity of the obstruction or gradient across it is of limited clinical significance. It is more important that the surgeon knows the exact site of the coarctation and the anatomy of the adjacent aorta and head and neck vessels.

Although imaging echocardiography often provides sufficient information to allow surgery to be undertaken safely without catheterisation in infants, it can be difficult to demonstrate the coarctation site in older subjects.[51] Indeed it has been commented upon that coarctation of the aorta is 'one of the most difficult lesions to diagnose confidently with two-dimensional echocardiography'.[55] Where a clear echocardiographic image of the coarctation site is not obtained, Doppler ultrasound can be useful in demonstrating its site. In addition Doppler examination has the potential ability to give information on the pressure gradient across the obstruction.

Doppler examination in coarctation of the aorta

In the normal individual, forward flow in both the ascending and descending aorta is of approximately the same velocity, less than 2 m/s, and is usually confined to systole. Flow in the descending aorta can be recorded from the suprasternal or high parasternal positions with a 'stand alone' or duplex transducer. In older subjects with coarctation, the flow velocity in the descending aorta will be increased, usually with a maximum velocity greater than 3 m/s. The classical spectral signal shows flow reaching its maximum velocity in mid systole, falling to a relatively low level at end systole and continuing with decreasing velocity for a variable time into diastolic (Fig. 19).[56] The velocity of the diastolic flow is variable and its recognition may require reduction of the high pass filter to the lowest possible level. The flow may continue through all or only part of diastole and in some patients no diastolic flow can be recognised. Diastolic flow reflects the pressure difference across the coarctation in diastole and has no relationship to the maximum velocity or gradient. It has been suggested that this flow pattern may be related to the collateral flow but there is no good evidence for this. If continuous wave Doppler examination or high pulse repetition frequency Doppler examination with a large sample volume is used, the systolic signal frequently demonstrates superimposed lower velocity flow from the aorta proximal to the obstruction (Fig. 19). If an attempt is made to calculate the pressure gradient across the coarctation this proximal velocity should be taken into account, using the equation $p = 4(v_2^2 - v_1^2)$, where p is the pressure difference in

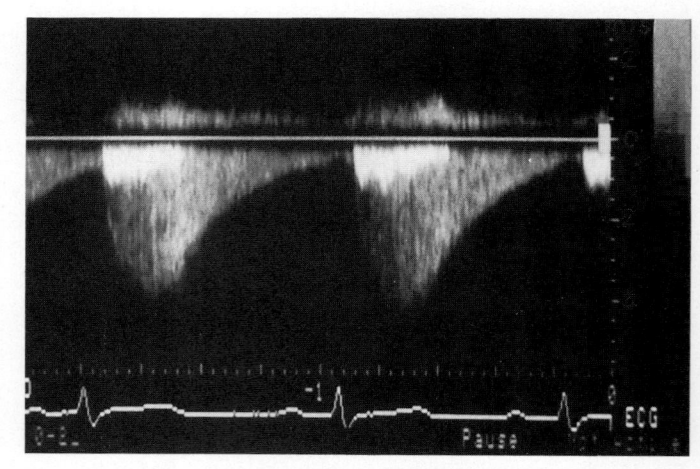

Fig. 19 Continuous wave spectral Doppler signal from a patient with coarctation of the aorta. The flow signal indicates continuous flow throughout diastole. Note that superimposed on the high velocity signal is a relatively low velocity one (less than 1 m/s) due to flow proximal to the obstruction.

mmHg, v_2 is the maximum velocity in the coarctation in m/s and v_1 is the velocity before the coarctation in m/s. Increased flow velocity in the aortic arch also occurs with a large shunt through an arterial duct but in this situation the increased velocity will occur through the whole arch.

Doppler examination has proved to be less reliable in estimating the gradient in coarctation of the aorta than with semilunar valve stenosis.[57,58] The reasons for this are uncertain. While differences between instantaneous and peak-to-peak pressure differences do not seem to account for overestimations, underestimation may be due to poor beam alignment or may result from the tendency for Doppler studies to give lower values where the orifice is small.[59] Attempts have been made to improve the Doppler assessment of pressure drop by developing a formula taking into account acceleration time and antegrade flow time from the distal flow signa.[58] This is relatively complicated, however, and cannot be considered to provide a measurement of gradient comparable to that obtained in semilunar valve stenosis. In the majority of patients, however, the decision to operate in coarctation is based on clinical findings and thus the exact gradient is of little practical importance.

A difficulty can occur in a normotensive patient with no clinical evidence of coarctation or arterial duct in whom the ultrasound study, performed for another reason, demonstrates increased velocity in the descending aorta, typically between 2.3 and 2.7 m/s. Furthermore in those patients who have undergone apparently successful surgical repair of coarctation a similar increase in velocity of up to 2.7 m/s (equivalent to 30 mmHg pressure drop) can be found. It is likely that both these situations represent mild narrowing of the aorta and there is little information on the natural history of such a mild abnormality. The author's present practice is to review these patients every two or three years. In some patients with severe obstruction in whom the narrowing cannot be demonstrated it is not possible to show an increased flow velocity from a transthoracic position, either due to the angle at which blood flows through the coarctation segment or because the lumen is occluded. The transoesophageal approach will then be the only means of demonstrating the coarctation with ultrasound. Other flow signals from collateral arteries may be obtained when the flow signal through the obstruction is not found. These are generally continuous flow signals with a maximum systolic velocity of less than 2.5 m/s.[57]

In infants there can be difficulties in ascertaining that recorded flow is from the coarctation site and not the arterial duct, even if colour Doppler flow mapping is used. The signal of increased flow velocity through the coarctation can generally be obtained but if the arterial duct is open and pulmonary artery and aortic pressures are similar, the velocity of flow across the coarctation may be lower than 2.5 m/s. Even with arch interruption a flow signal away from the transducer can be shown,[57] which represents flow through the arterial duct from the pulmonary artery to the descending aorta. In virtually all cases, however, this flow will be bidirectional, similar to that in the hypoplastic left heart syndrome illustrated in Figure 13. The relative pulmonary artery and aortic pressures will be reflected in the flow patterns in the arterial duct[60] and the right ventricular pressure will be reflected in the velocity of any tricuspid regurgitation jet. The information on pulmonary pressure and ductal flow provided by these signals should be taken into account when interpreting the flow velocity and pattern through a suspected coarctation.

It is important to emphasise that the maximum flow velocity through the coarctation, and thus the pressure gradient across it, has only a limited relationship to the severity of the obstruction and clinical factors remain the ideal means of deciding whether or not surgery is appropriate. The Doppler signal in the descending aorta beyond the coarctation can be significantly different from that in the ascending aorta and also from that in the descending aorta in normal subjects. The forward flow time is prolonged with diminished maximum velocity and the signal looks wider and flatter. Attempts have been made to use these changes in the Doppler flow pattern in the descending aorta as a more definite indicator of coarctation.[61] These studies found that acceleration time and antegrade flow time in the descending aorta are similar to those in the ascending aorta in normal subjects but are prolonged in coarctation. Values for acceleration and deceleration slope and peak velocity are lower in the descending than the ascending aorta in normal subjects but this difference becomes more marked in coarctation. The greatest difference between those with coarctation and normal subjects was with the corrected acceleration time and the acceleration slope. Corrected acceleration time is obtained by dividing acceleration time by the R–R internal from the electrocardiogram. Normal corrected acceleration time is 90+/−20 ms. This value rises to 190+/−67 ms in cases of coarctation. The acceleration slope is 58+/−22 m/s^2 normals but drops to 14+/−13 m/s^2 in patients with coarctation. Whilst it is unlikely that a normal subject would be considered to have coarctation on the basis of these criteria, they do not allow a clear distinction between normal and abnormal and the diagnosis can be missed using these criteria alone. In infants with coarctation and an arterial duct, for example, an antegrade flow time is not prolonged though other parameters are abnormal. In addition these techniques do not pin-point the site of obstruction.

Spectral Doppler examination is an important adjunct to imaging in those patients in whom the coarctation site cannot be shown clearly. It adds to the certainty of the ultrasound diagnosis by confirming the presence of an obstructive lesion in doubtful cases. It adds to the certainty of the ultrasound diagnosis and allows surgical treatment without catheterisation in many infants[62] and children.

Spectral Doppler examination, usually with continuous wave techniques, simply indicates that there must be obstruction and does not help to outline or highlight the exact site of obstruction when this is unclear from images. Colour Doppler flow mapping can be of particular value in this situation. Colour Doppler flow mapping will show flow acceleration proximal to the obstruction as aliasing from blue to red and again to blue.[54] The lumen of the narrowed area is usually delineated exactly with the colour mapping and the aorta immediately distal to the narrowing is filled in with a mosaic of colour or variance due to the poststenotic turbulence. Thus when the site of the coarctation is not clearly shown, colour Doppler flow mapping becomes of particular value in highlighting the area of coarctation with the flow disturbance pattern, thus permitting its exact localisation (Plate 2). The addition of colour will provide absolute confirmation that this is the site of obstruction and will add to the diagnostic certainty of the study, even when it is thought that the coarctation site has been correctly identified. In some situations where the coarctation is relatively distal it can be difficult to demonstrate from the suprasternal or high parasternal sites with either imaging or colour Doppler examination and a lower position can be useful. Colour Doppler flow mapping has an additional advantage over spectral Doppler in that it can occasionally be difficult with duplex spectral imaging to be certain that the increased velocity signal does not come from flow in a stenotic left pulmonary artery. Colour Doppler mapping provides a more convincing and definite demonstration of the obstruction site which is acceptable to the surgeon by demonstrating the exact site of the flow disturbance in relation to the echocardiographic image. Colour Doppler flow mapping can give some information on the anatomical severity of narrowing. The diameter of the narrow area filled in by colour gives a more accurate correlation with the angiocardiographic diameter than the two dimensional image.[54] It is probable that this is because the lateral resolution of the colour Doppler is improved by the high signal to noise ratio while two-dimensional echocardiography is still subject to lateral resolution artefacts. The anatomical severity rather than pressure gradient is also related to the width of the accelerating stream[54] but the clinical significance of this is as yet uncertain.

On rare occasions the coarctation may not be shown from a transthoracic position, even with colour Doppler examination. Transoesophageal echocardiography has the advantage of positioning the transducer very close to the thoracic aorta and distal aortic arch. The technique thus has the ability to show the presence of coarctation of the aorta even in patients in whom this is not possible with transthoracic imaging or Doppler. The usual transoesophageal transducer provides a transverse section of the normal aortic arch which can be seen as an elongated sausage shaped structure which becomes the circular descending thoracic aorta as the transducer is inserted further. In cases of coarctation the descending aorta narrows abruptly and then widens beyond the obstruction. Biplane transoesophageal transducers are now being introduced. The additional vertically orientated plane may facilitate visualisation of coarctations. The normal pulsations in the arch and thoracic aorta decrease as the transducer moves downwards beyond the obstruction. Colour Doppler flow mapping will show turbulence at the coarctation site and will outline its boundaries. Spectral Doppler examination may show a typical coarctation signal, the maximal velocity usually being lower than that from a transthoracic position since it is dependent on the angle between the flow direction and ultrasound beam which will be large in the case of transoesophageal examination. Colour Doppler examination shows the boundaries of the narrowed area and the flow from collateral arteries into the distal aorta. At present it is uncertain whether recognition of this collateral flow is of any value in monitoring the possible effects of cross-clamping the aorta during surgical repair of coarctation.

Ultrasound will allow the site of coarctation of the aorta to be shown in most subjects. In older patients where the arch and coarctation are not well seen with imaging and the coarctation is only shown with Doppler or transoesophageal imaging, the question arises whether catheterisation is necessary to show the exact site of coarctation, the anatomy of the head and neck vessels, and the collateral flow. Although angiography will give a more detailed demonstration of these features it is not necessary in most cases but the need for this investigation will depend on the preference of the surgeon undertaking the operative pro-

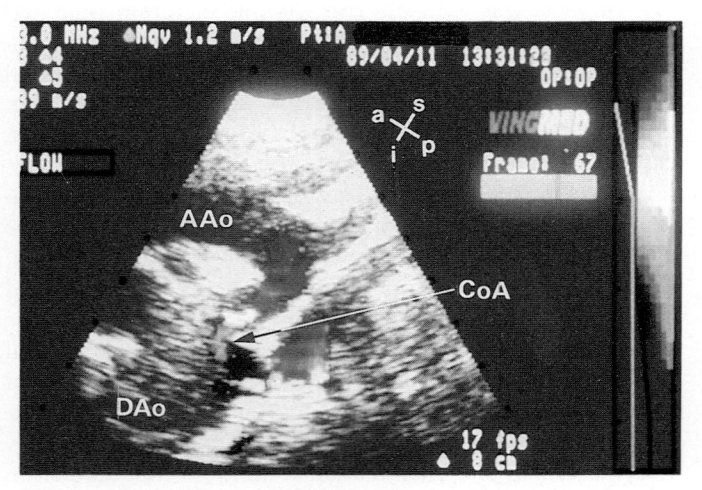

Plate 2 Suprasternal view from a patient with coarctation of the aorta in whom the site of obstruction was not clearly shown with imaging. The colour signal shows acceleration towards the site of the coarctation which is outlined with the posterior aspect of the poststenotic area clearly seen outlined in red. AAo = ascending aorta; DAo = descending aorta; CoA = coarctation. This figure is reproduced in colour in the colour plate section at the front of this volume.

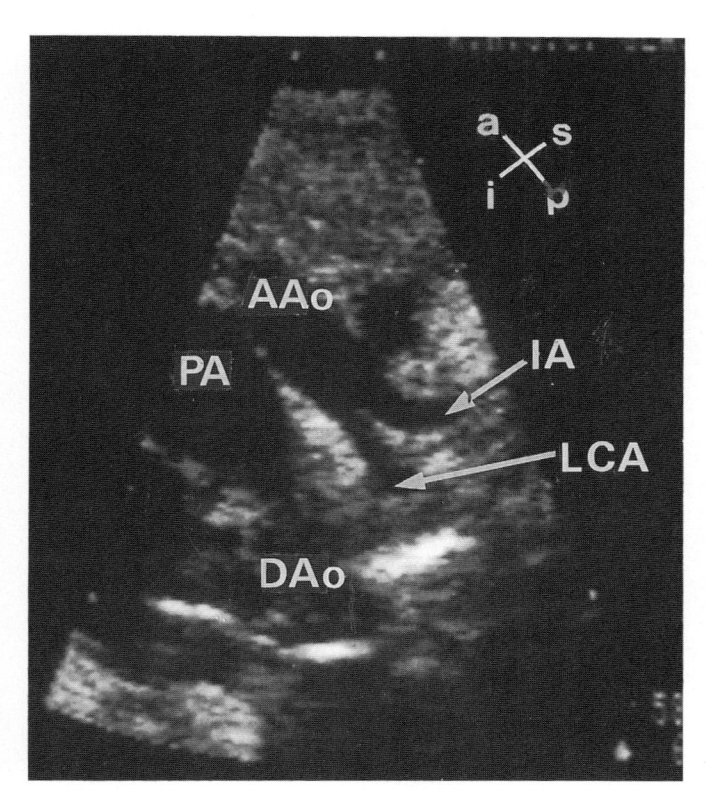

Fig. 20 Two-dimensional image from a patient with type B interruption of the aortic arch showing the aorta dividing into the innominate artery and left carotid artery. AAo = ascending aorta; DAo = descending aorta; IA = innominate artery.

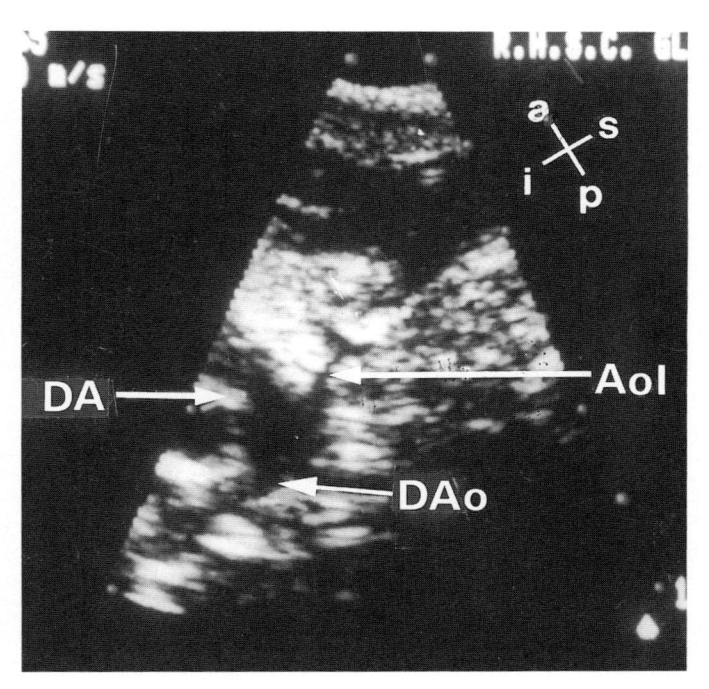

Fig. 21 Parasternal view from an infant with extreme hypoplasia of the isthmus. In this view a thread representing the distal arch can be seen to join the descending aorta at the site of the arterial duct. DA = arterial duct; AoI = aortic isthmus; DAo = descending aorta.

cedure. Magnetic resonance imaging will have an increasing role in the assessment of this anatomy.

Interrupted aortic arch

Interrupted aortic arch has been classified on the basis of its site in relation to the head and neck vessels. Most commonly it is type A in which the interruption is beyond the left subclavian artery. Less frequently it is of type B in which the obstruction lies between the left carotid and left subclavian arteries. Rarely, the interruption is of type C where the lesion lies between the innominate and left carotid arteries. Interrupted aortic arch is often associated with another abnormality, most commonly a ventricular septal defect with leftward deviation of the conus septum and malalignment. A search should be made for an unrecognised feature such as an aortopulmonary window when there appears to be an interrupted aortic arch with no other abnormality.

The ascending aorta is almost invariably small in this condition and in classical cases the differentiation of interrupted aortic arch from coarctation is relatively simple. Typically the aorta is shown to terminate in one of the head and neck vessels and there is a clear gap between this and the descending aorta. In type A aortic interruption, the ascending aorta and the left subclavian artery are separated from the descending aorta which can be shown to arise from the arterial duct with no arch joining the ascending and descending segments. With type B interruption there is classically a Y sign (Fig. 20) with the ascending aorta being shown to bifurcate and continue upwards into the neck with no posterior arching.[63] Adjustment of the transducer angle to the ductal view can then show the left subclavian artery in relation to the descending aorta and arterial duct. Difficulty may be experienced in confirming that there is no continuity between the arch and the descending aorta because a hypoplastic isthmus can be difficult to recognise. In cases where there is a thread-like communication between the ascending and descending aorta, the lesion is morphologically severe hypoplasia although it may be functionally interrupted (Fig. 21). In this context colour Doppler studies can confirm whether or not there is flow in the segment.

On occasions there can be difficulty in being completely sure of the identity of the head and neck vessels and this requires careful tracing of their course. It can be easy to confuse the two branches from the ascending aorta in type B interruption with the bifurcation of the innominate artery in a type C lesion.

REFERENCES

1. Radford D, Bloom K R, Izukawa T et al. Echocardiographic assessment of bicuspid aortic valves. Circulation 1976; 53: 80–85.
2. Kececiolgu-Draelos Z, Goldberg S J. Role of M-mode echocardiography in congenital aortic stenosis. Am J Cardiol 1981; 47: 1267–1272.
3. Fowles R E, Martin R P, Abrams J M et al. Two-dimensional echocardiographic features of bicuspid aortic valve. Chest 1979; 75: 434–440.
4. Zema M J, Caccuvano M. Two-dimensional echocardiographic assessment of aortic valve morphology: feasibility of bicuspid valve detection. Br Heart J 1982; 48: 428–433.
5. Assey M A, Wisenbaugh T, Spann J F et al. Unexpected persistence into adulthood of low wall stress in patients with congenital aortic stenosis: is there a fundamental difference in the hypertrophic response to a pressure overload present from birth? Circulation 1987; 75: 973–979.
6. Huhta J C, Latson L A, Gutgessell H P et al. Echocardiography in the diagnosis and management of symptomatic aortic valve stenosis in infants. Circulation 1984; 70: 438–444.
7. Brenner J I, Baker K R, Berman M A. Prediction of left ventricular pressure in infants with aortic stenosis. Br Heart J 1978; 44: 406–410.
8. Blackwood R A, Bloom K R, Williams C M. Aortic stenosis in children. Experience with echocardiographic prediction of severity. Circulation 1978; 57: 263–268.
9. Weyman A E, Feigenbaum H, Hurwitz R A et al. Cross-sectional echocardiographic assessment of the severity of aortic stenosis in children. Circulation 1977; 55: 773–778.
10. De Maria A N, Bommer W, Joye J et al. Value and limitations of cross-sectional echocardiography of the aortic valve in the diagnosis and quantification of valvular aortic stenosis. Circulation 1980; 62: 304–312.
11. Lima C O, Sahn D J, Valdes-Cruz L M et al. Prediction of the severity of left ventricular outflow tract obstruction by quantitative two-dimensional echocardiographic Doppler studies. Circulation 1983; 68: 348–354.
12. Currie P J, Seward J B, Reeder G S et al. Continuous-wave Doppler echocardiographic assessment of severity of calcific aortic stenosis: a simultaneous Doppler catheter correlative study in 100 adult patients. Circulation 1985; 71: 1162–1169.
13. Skjaerpe T J, Hegrenaes L, Hatle L. Noninvasive estimation of valve area in patients with aortic stenosis by Doppler ultrasound and two-dimensional echocardiography. Circulation 1985; 72: 1106–1118.
14. Currie P J, Hagler D J, Seward J B et al. Instantaneous pressure gradient: a simultaneous Doppler and dual catheter study. J M Coll Cardiol 1986; 7: 800–806.
15. Simpson I A, Houston A B, Sheldon C S et al. Clinical value of Doppler echocardiography in the assessment of adults with aortic stenosis. Br Heart J 1985; 53: 636–639.
16. Martin G R, Soifer S J, Silverman N H. Effects of activity on ascending aorta velocity in children with valvar aortic stenosis. Am J Cardiol 1987; 59: 1386–1390.
17. Lim M K, Houston A B, Doig W B et al. The variability in the Doppler gradient in pulmonary stenosis before and after balloon valvoplasty. Br Heart J 1989; 62: 212–216.
18. Davis R H, Feigenbaum H, Chang S et al. Echocardiographic manifestations of discrete subaortic stenosis. Am J Cardiol 1974; 33: 277–280.
19. Krueger S K, French J W, Forker A D et al. Echocardiography in discrete subaortic stenosis. Circulation 1979; 59: 506–513.
20. Weyman A E, Feigenbaum H, Hurwitz R A et al. Cross-sectional echocardiography in evaluating patients with discrete subaortic stenosis. Am J Cardiol 1976; 37: 358–365.
21. Motro M, Schneeweiss A, Shem-Tov A et al. Two-dimensional echocardiography in discrete subaortic stenosis. Am J Cardiol 1984; 53: 896–907.
22. Di Sessa T G, Hagan A D, Isobel-Jones J B et al. Two-dimensional echocardiographic evaluation of discrete subaortic stenosis from the apical long axis view. Am Heart J 1981; 101: 774–782.
23. Chin A J, Yeager S B, Sanders S P et al. Accuracy of prospective two-dimensional echocardiographic evaluation of left ventricular outflow tract in complete transposition of the great arteries. Am J Cardiol 1985; 55: 759–764.
24. Wilcox W D, Seward J B, Hagler D J et al. Discrete subaortic stenosis. Two-dimensional echocardiographic features with angiocardiographic and surgical correlation. Mayo Clin Proc 1980; 55: 425–433.
25. Mugge A, Daniel W G, Wolpers H G et al. Improved visualisation of discrete subvalvar aortic stenosis by transesophageal color coded Doppler echocardiography. Am Heart J 1989; 117: 474–475.
26. Yoganathan A P, Valdes-Cruz L M, Schmidt-Dohna M S et al. Continuous-wave Doppler velocities and gradients across fixed tunnel obstruction: studies in vitro and in vivo. Circulation 1987; 76: 657–666.
27. Simpson I A, Valdes-Cruz L M, Yoganathan A P et al. Spatial 17 velocity distribution and acceleration in serial subvalve tunnel and valvular obstructions: an in vitro study using Doppler color flow mapping. J Am Coll Cardiol 1989; 13: 241–248.
28. Bolen J L, Popp R L, French J W. Echocardiographic features of subvalve aortic stenosis. Circulation 1975; 52: 817–822.
29. Weyman A E, Caldwell R L, Hurwitz R A et al. Cross-sectional echocardiographic characterisation of aortic obstruction. 1. Supravalvar aortic stenosis and hypoplasia. Circulation 1978; 57: 491–497.
30. Vogt J, Rupprath G, Grimm T, Beuren A J. Qualitative and quantitative evaluation of supravalve aortic stenosis by cross-sectional echocardiography. A report of 80 patients. Pediatr Cardiol 1982; 3: 13–17.
31. Lundstrom N R. Ultrasound cardiographic studies of the mitral valve region in young infants with mitral atresia, mitral stenosis, hypoplasia of the left ventricle and cor triatriatum. Circulation 1971; 45: 324–334.
32. Meyer R A, Kaplan S. Echocardiography in the diagnosis of hypoplasia of the left or right ventricles in the neonate. Circulation 1971; 46: 55–64.
33. Farroki Z Q, Henry J G, Green E W. Echocardiographic spectrum of the hypoplastic left heart syndrome. Am J Cardiol 1976; 38: 337–343.
34. Bass J L, Ben-Shachar G, Edwards J E. Comparison of M-mode echocardiography and pathologic findings in the left heart hypoplasia syndrome. Am J Cardiol 1980; 45: 79–86.
35. Rushaupt D J, Moshiree M, Lev M et al. Echocardiogram in mitral-aortic atresia: false identification of the ventricular septum and left ventricle. Pediatr Cardiol 1980; 1: 281–285.
36. Helton J G, Aglira B A, Chin A J et al. Analysis of potential anatomic or physiologic determinants of outcome of palliative surgery for hypoplastic left heart syndrome. Circulation 1986; 74 (Suppl 1): I 70–77.
37. Bash S E, Huhta J C, Vick G W et al. Hypoplastic left heart syndrome: is echocardiography accurate enough to guide surgical palliation. J Am Coll Cardiol 1986; 7: 601–606.
38. Lange L W, Sahn D J, Allen H D et al. Cross-sectional echocardiography in hypoplastic left ventricle: echocardiographic-angiographic-anatomic correlations. Pediatr Cardiol 1980; 1: 287–299.
39. Weinberg P M, Chin A J, Murphy J D et al. Postmortem echocardiography and tomographic anatomy of hypoplastic left heart syndrome after palliative surgery. Am J Cardiol 1986; 58: 1228–1232.
40. Smallhorn J, Tommasini G, Deanfield J et al. Congenital mitral stenosis. Anatomical and functional assessment by echocardiography. Br Heart J 1981; 45: 527–534.
41. Chin A J, Yeager S B, Sanders S P et al. Accuracy of prospective two-dimensional echocardiographic evaluation of left ventricular outflow tract in complete transposition of the great arteries. Am J Cardiol 1985; 55: 759–764.

42 Simpson I A, Valdes-Cruz L M, Sahn D J et al. Color Doppler flow mapping of simulated in vitro regurgitant jets: evaluation of the effects of orifice size and hemodynamic variables. J Am Coll Cardiol 1989; 13: 1195–1207.
43 Alboliras E T, Chin A J, Barber G et al. Pulmonary artery configuration after palliative operations for hypoplastic left heart syndrome. J Thorac Cardiovasc Surg 1989; 97: 878–885.
44 Chin A J, Barber G, Helton J G et al. Fate of the pulmonic valve after proximal pulmonary artery-to-ascending aorta anastomosis for aortic outflow obstruction. Am J Cardiol 1988; 62: 435–438.
45 Sahn D J, Allen H D, McDonald G et al. Real-time cross-sectional echocardiographic diagnosis of coarctation of the aorta: a prospective study of echocardiographic-angiographic correlations. Circulation 1977; 56: 762–769.
46 Wing J P, Findlay W A, Sahn D J et al. Serial echocardiographic profiles in infants and children with coarctation of the aorta. Am J Cardiol 1978; 41: 1270–1277.
47 Weyman A E, Caldwell R L, Hurwitz R A et al. Cross-sectional echocardiographic detection of aortic obstruction. 2. Coarctation of the aorta. Circulation 1978; 57: 498–502.
48 Duncan W J, Ninomiya K, Cook D H et al. Noninvasive diagnosis of neonatal coarctation and associated anomalies using two-dimensional echocardiography. Am Heart J 1983; 106: 63–69.
49 Smallhorn J F, Huhta J C, Adams P A et al. Cross-sectional echocardiographic assessment of coarctation in the sick neonate and infant. Br Heart J 1983; 50: 349–361.
50 Huhta J C, Gutgessel H P, Latson L A et al. Two-dimensional echocardiographic assessment of the aorta in infants and children with congenital heart disease. Circulation 1984; 70: 417–424.
51 Modena M G, Benassi A, Mattioli G et al. Computerised tomography and ultrasound in the noninvasive evaluation of coarctation of the aorta. Am J Cardiol 1985; 56: 822–824.
52 Smallhorn J F, Huhta J C, Anderson R H et al. Suprasternal cross-sectional echocardiography in assessment of patent ductus arteriosus. Br Heart J 1982; 48: 321–330.
53 Garg A K, Houston A B, Laing J M et al. Positioning of umbilical arterial catheters with ultrasound. Arch Dis Child 1983; 58: 1017–1018.
54 Simpson I A, Sahn D J, Valdes-Cruz et al. Color Doppler flow mapping in patients with coarctation of the aorta: new observations and improved evaluation with color flow diameter and proximal acceleration as predictors of severity. Circulation 1988; 77: 736–744.
55 Hagler D T, Tajik A J, Seward J B et al. Noninvasive assessment of pulmonary valve stenosis, aortic valve stenosis and coarctation of the aorta in critically ill neonates. Am J Cardiol 1986; 57: 369–372.
56 Hatle L, Angelson B. Doppler ultrasound in cardiology: physical principles and clinical applications. Philadelphia: Lea and Febiger, 1985; 217–220.
57 Houston A B, Simpson I A, Pollock et al. Doppler ultrasound in the assessment of severity of coarctation of the aorta and interruption of the aortic arch. Br Heart J 1987; 57: 38–43.
58 Rao P S, Carey P. Doppler ultrasound in the prediction of pressure gradients across aortic coarctation. Am Heart J 1989; 118: 299–307.
59 Teirstein P S, Yock P G, Popp R L. The accuracy of Doppler ultrasound measurement of pressure gradients across irregular, dual and tunnel-like obstructions to blood flow. Circulation 1985; 72: 577–584.
60 Houston A B, Lim M K, Doig W B et al. Doppler flow characteristics in the assessment of pulmonary artery pressure in ductus arteriosus. Br Heart J 1989; 62: 285–290.
61 Shaddy R E, Snider A R, Silverman N H et al. Pulsed Doppler findings in patients with coarctation of the aorta. Circulation 1986; 73: 82–88.
62 George B, Di Sessa T G, Williams R et al. Coarctation repair without cardiac catheterisation in infants. Am Heart J 1987; 114: 1421–1425.
63 Smallhorn J F, Anderson R H, Macartney F J. Cross-sectional echocardiographic recognition of interruption of aortic arch between left carotid and subclavian arteries. Br Heart J 1982; 48: 229–235.

22

Abnormalities of ventriculo-arterial connection

Complete transposition with intact ventricular septum
Balloon atrial septostomy
Complete transposition with ventricular septal defect
Straddling atrioventricular valves
Other abnormalities of the chordal attachments
Complete transposition with left ventricular outflow obstruction
Complete transposition with aortic arch abnormalities and subaortic stenosis
Rare associated abnormalities

Evaluation after corrective surgery for complete transposition
Atrial redirection operations
Arterial switch operations
Rastelli operations
Double outlet right ventricle
Subaortic ventricular septal defect
Subpulmonary ventricular septal defect
Doubly committed ventricular septal defect
Non-committed ventricular septal defect
Associated lesions
Double outlet left ventricle

Congenitally corrected transposition of the great arteries
Corrected transposition with ventricular septal defect
Corrected transposition with left ventricular outflow obstruction
Corrected transposition with abnormalities of the left atrioventricular valve
Corrected transposition with right ventricular outflow obstruction
Double outlet right ventricle with atrioventricular discordance
Criss-cross atrioventricular connection and superior-inferior ventricles
Atrioventricular discordance with a concordant ventriculo-arterial connection

Robin P. Martin

COMPLETE TRANSPOSITION WITH INTACT VENTRICULAR SEPTUM

Introduction

Transposition of the great arteries is present in approximately 5% of children with congenital heart disease[1] and it is the commonest cyanotic lesion to present in the neonatal period.

There has been much debate regarding the appropriate definition and terminology of this condition.[2] The term complete transposition is used to describe the presence of a normal (concordant) atrioventricular connection with a discordant ventriculo-arterial connection, i.e. the morphological right ventricle dominantly connecting to the aorta and the morphological left ventricle to the pulmonary artery. This chapter does not include abnormalities of atrioventricular connection where there are double inlet, ambiguous or absent connections. A later section describes 'congenitally corrected transposition of the great arteries' where ventriculo-arterial discordance is combined with atrioventricular discordance.

M-mode echocardiography may demonstrate the abnormal spatial relationship of the two great arteries but this technique is not specific for complete transposition. Cross-sectional echocardiography has supplanted M-mode examination with its ability to examine the cardiac connections sequentially.

Cross-sectional examination will reveal normal atrial situs and systemic and pulmonary venous connections from the subcostal approach. A standard four chamber view will demonstrate the normal atrioventricular connection, the right atrium connecting to the heavily trabeculated right ventricle with its coarse septal surface and the left atrium connecting to the left ventricle with its relatively smooth septal surface. Superior angulation of the transducer will show the pulmonary artery originating from the left ventricle (Fig. 1). The bifurcation of the pulmonary artery should be identified and this may require a minor degree of anticlockwise rotation of the transducer. Further superior angulation will reveal the aorta originating from the right ventricle, this vessel usually lying anterior and to the right of the pulmonary trunk. The aorta will always be recognised as the artery giving rise to the head and neck vessels. Alternatively, it may be possible to demonstrate both great arteries and their origins from their respective ventricles by superior angulation combined with a moderate degree of clockwise rotation of the transducer (Fig. 2).

The spatial relationship of the great arteries is variable and can be established from the parasternal views. A parasternal long axis view will often show the aorta anterior to the pulmonary artery with the pulmonary artery characteristically 'dipping' posteriorly in contrast to the more anterior and superior course of the aorta when the arterial connection is normal (Fig. 3). This can be confirmed with

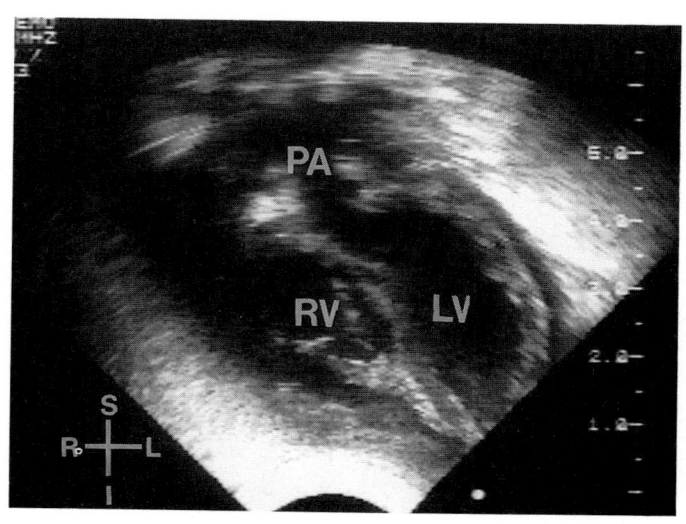

Fig. 1 Subcostal view of the left ventricular outflow in complete transposition with intact ventricular septum. Superior angulation and slight anticlockwise rotation shows the connection of the left ventricle to the pulmonary trunk.

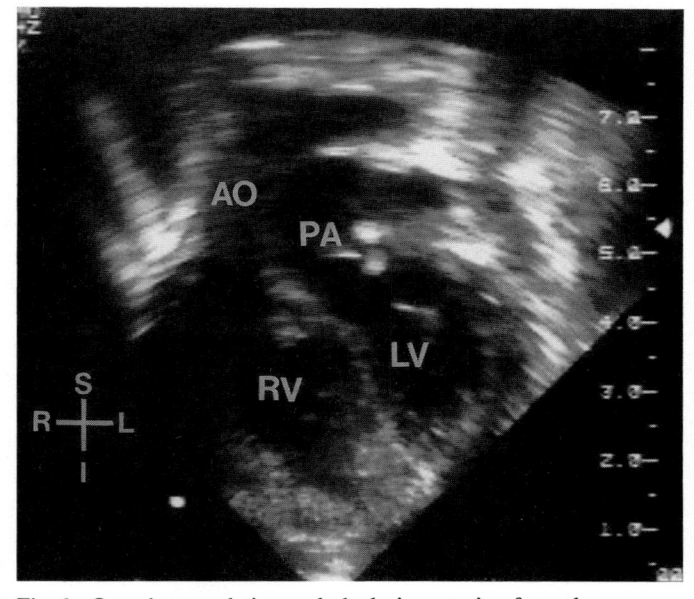

Fig. 2 Superior angulation and clockwise rotation from the standard subcostal four chamber view shows the aorta arising from the right ventricle in a child with transposition and intact ventricular septum.

the parasternal short axis views where the posterior great artery can be seen to bifurcate (Fig. 4). It should also be possible to appreciate that the great arteries have a parallel course unlike the usual crossing arrangement seen with a concordant ventriculo-arterial connection. The most frequently seen orientation of the great arteries is one where the aorta is anterior and slightly to the right of the pulmonary artery.[3] Other variations, such as the aorta directly

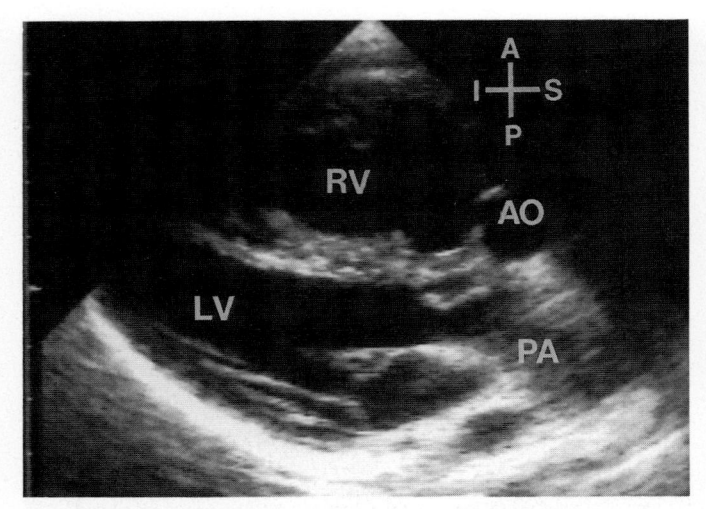

Fig. 3 Parasternal long axis view in complete transposition with intact ventricular septum. The posterior great artery (pulmonary artery) dips posteriorly. The aorta can also be seen anterior to the pulmonary artery.

anterior or in a left anterior position are also common. Rarely the aorta may be posterior and to the right of the pulmonary trunk, so-called 'posterior transposition'. A side by side arterial relationship is more commonly seen when there is an associated ventricular septal defect. Ventriculo-arterial connections should not be inferred from great arterial positions.

The ability to demonstrate the coronary artery anatomy has become important with the increased use of the arterial switch operation to repair the defect. The coronary anatomy is usually best seen from the parasternal short axis views, but angulated apical or subcostal views may sometimes be helpful.[4] The coronary artery arrangement is variable and has been the subject of a variety of classifications.[5,6] These have been based on the cardiac surgeon's viewpoint rather than that of the echocardiographer. Fortunately the coronary arteries usually originate from one or both of the aortic sinuses that face the pulmonary trunk. From the surgeon's viewpoint the usual arrangement is for the left anterior descending and circumflex branches of the left coronary artery to originate from his right-handed facing sinus and the right coronary artery from the left-handed facing sinus. In the parasternal short axis view this equates to the left coronary originating from the left-sided facing sinus and the right coronary from the right-sided facing sinus. A number of variations of the branching pattern may be seen which include origin of the circumflex branch from the right coronary artery and a single origin to the coronary arteries from either of the facing sinuses. Careful examination of the early branching of these arteries will usually identify the particular variation present.

The aortic arch can be visualised from standard high parasternal or suprasternal views. Coarctation is uncom-

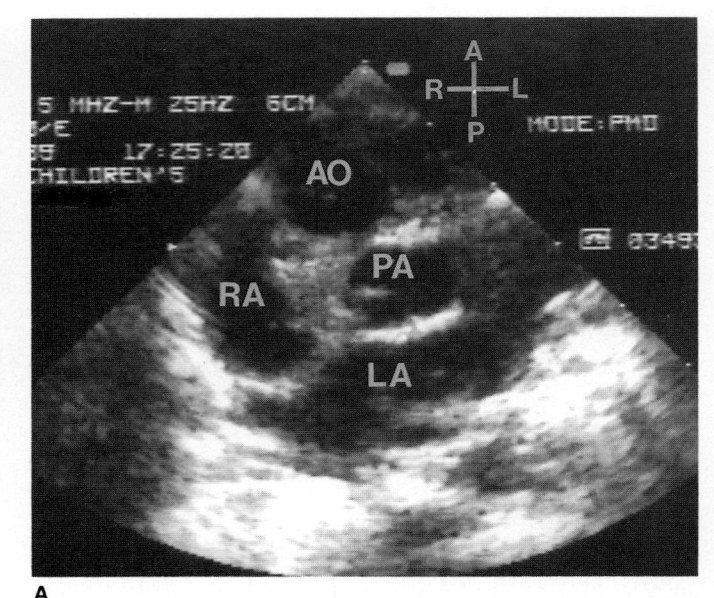

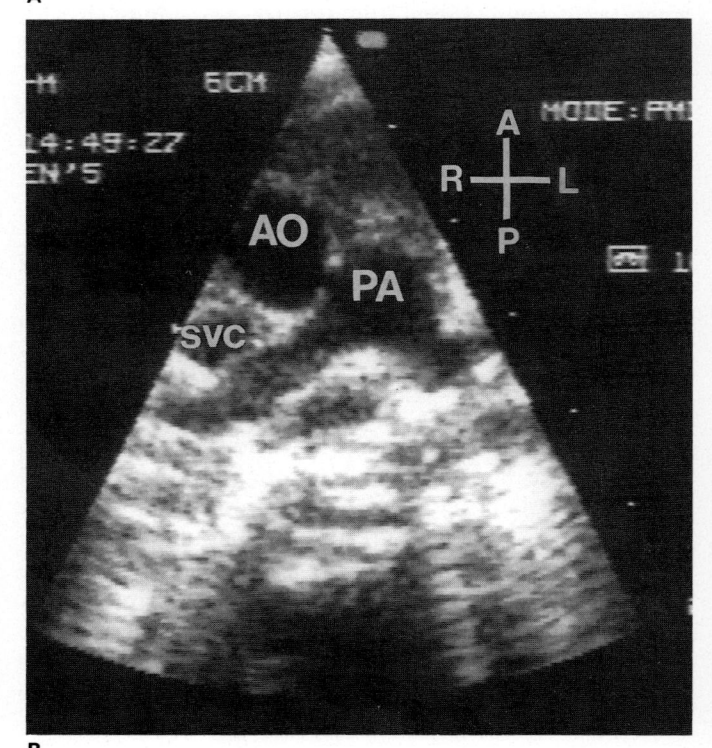

Fig. 4 A: Parasternal short axis view in complete transposition. The aortic valve is anterior and to the right of the pulmonary valve. **B:** Parasternal short axis view angulating slightly superior to **A** shows the posterior great artery bifurcating indicating it is the pulmonary trunk.

mon in complete transposition with intact ventricular septum and is more frequently seen in transposition with ventricular septal defect.

A patent arterial duct should be sought and persistent flow may be noted on Doppler examination (colour flow

ABNORMALITIES OF VENTRICULO-ARTERIAL CONNECTION 411

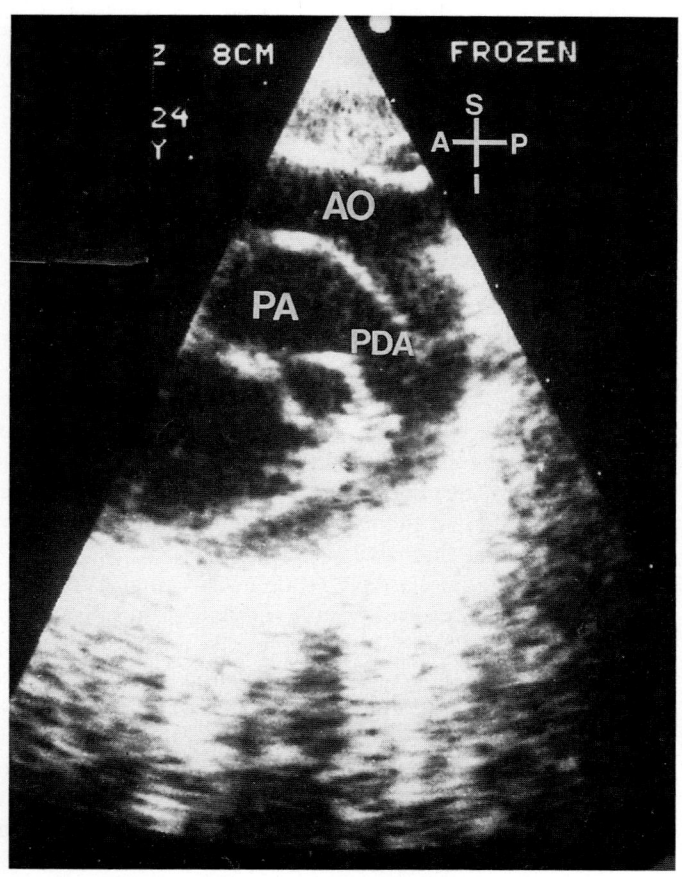

Fig. 5 High parasternal view of the aortic arch in an infant with transposition of the great arteries. The large persistent ductus arteriosus is orientated in the same plane as the aortic arch. PDA – Persistent ductus arteriosus.

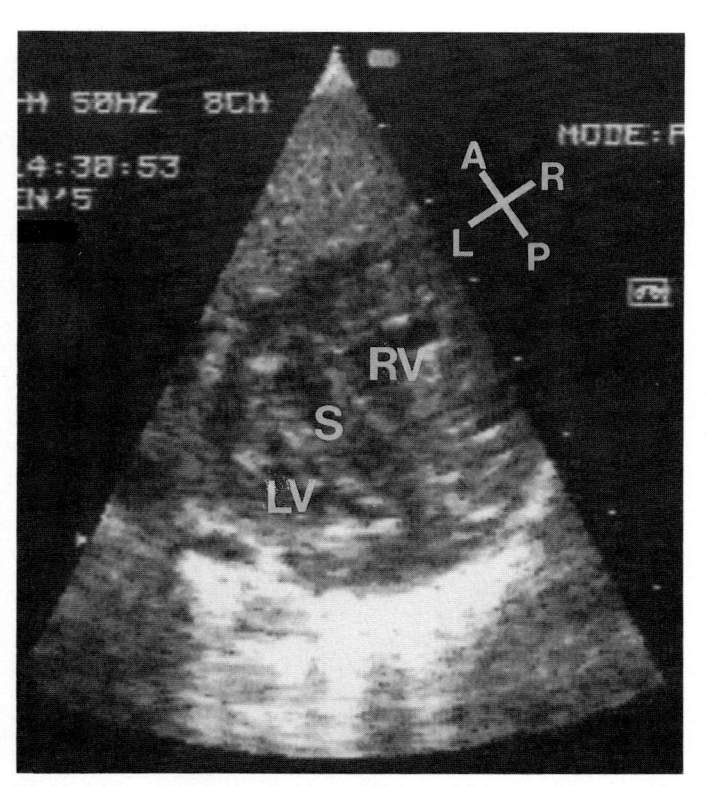

Fig. 6 Subcostal short axis view of right and left ventricles. In this child with complete transposition and severe left ventricular outflow obstruction, the interventricular septum is flat indicating that the left ventricular pressure is at systemic level. S – interventricular septum.

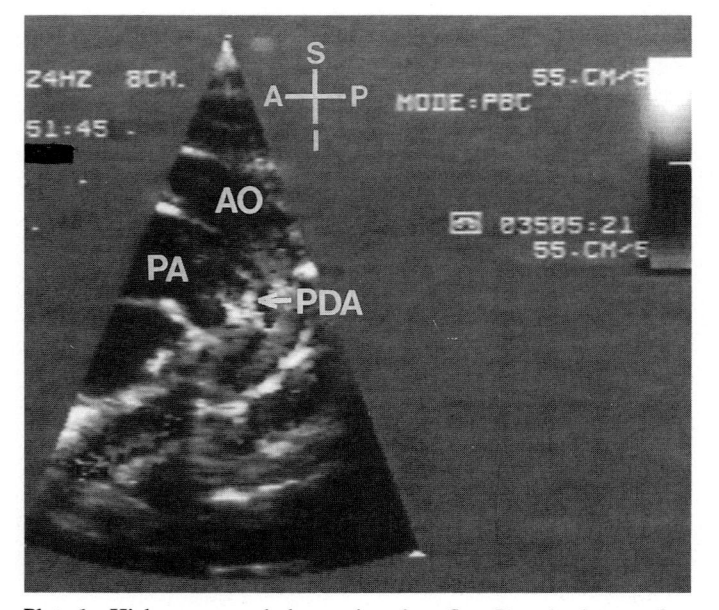

Plate 1 High parasternal short axis colour flow Doppler image of the great arteries in complete transposition. The systolic (blue) flow in the aorta and pulmonary trunk can be seen with flow in the persistent arterial duct showing as an orange jet passing from descending thoracic aorta anteriorly into the pulmonary artery. This figure is reproduced in colour in the colour plate section at the front of this volume.

mapping may be particularly useful for this). The arterial duct tends to be oriented in the same plane as the aortic arch and is usually seen in the standard aortic arch view (Fig. 5 and Plate 1).

A careful examination should include a search for associated abnormalities such as ventricular septal defect and obstruction to the left and right ventricular outflows. These will be discussed in later sections.

The left and right ventricles can be examined from parasternal and subcostal views in order to estimate their function and to assess the relative pressure difference between the two ventricles. Left ventricular function can be measured using standard M-mode indices of systolic function but it must be remembered that this is not the systemic ventricle and that in uncomplicated transposition with intact ventricular septum the left ventricular muscle mass will fall as the pulmonary artery pressures fall. Coinciding with the fall in muscle mass will be a change in the shape of the left ventricle due to alteration of the interventricular septal contour. This can be evaluated from a subcostal short axis cut of the left ventricle at the level of the papillary muscles (Fig. 6). This may be a useful noninvasive method of estimating left ventricular pressure.[7] As left ventricular pressure falls the interventricular septum bows into the left ventricular cavity, giving it a 'banana' shape. If left ventricular pressure rises as in the case of pulmonary hypertension or left ventricular outflow obstruction then the septal contour becomes increasingly flattened. If suprasystemic pressures develop in the left ventricle the septal contour becomes convex to the right as seen in the normal heart.

The assessment of right ventricular function by echocardiography is difficult because of its retrosternal location and irregular shape. In clinical practice, a subjective assessment of right ventricular dilatation and wall motion is often performed but this is unreliable. It is possible to calculate right ventricular volume and ejection fraction from cross-sectional images. Single plane measurements or a variety of biplane methods with the area length method or Simpson's rule have been described.[8-10] None of these are widely used and many centres rely on other methods, such as radionuclide angiography or invasive study by cardiac catheterisation.

Balloon atrial septostomy

The atrial septum can be examined for the presence of an atrial septal defect from the subcostal views. The flow across any defect and across the foramen ovale can be assessed by Doppler examination.[11] If there is not a large atrial septal defect, balloon atrial septostomy will need to be performed in a child with an intact interventricular septum. This can be performed under echocardiographic monitoring, either in the cardiac catheterisation laboratory or in the neonatal intensive care unit.[12-14]

The technique is relatively straightforward and requires placement of the septostomy catheter via the umbilical vein or femoral vein. The umbilical vein is particularly easy to use in the first 48 hours of life, when the ductus venosus is open. The passage of the catheter through the hepatic veins or the inferior vena cava (depending upon the site of entry), can be monitored using a subcostal sagittal view to show the junction of the inferior vena cava with the right atrium. It must be remembered that echocardiography is a cross-sectional technique and the tip of the catheter may not be in the plane of the examination at all times. Careful movements of the septostomy catheter and co-operation between the septostomy operator and the echocardiographer is required. When the catheter is in the right atrium, the echocardiographer should change to a four

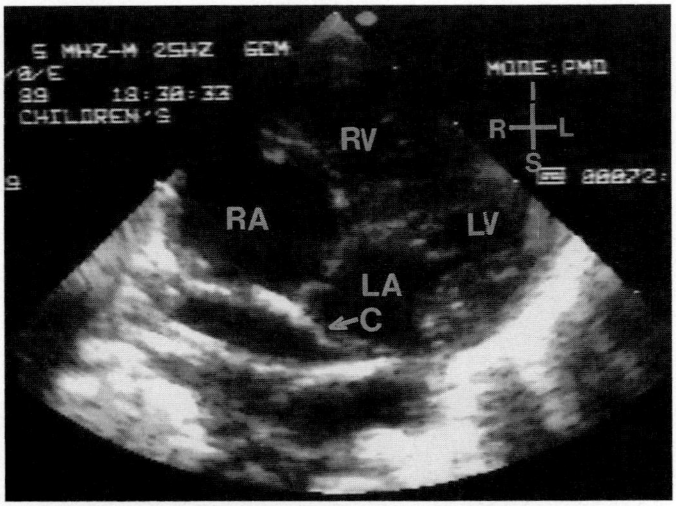

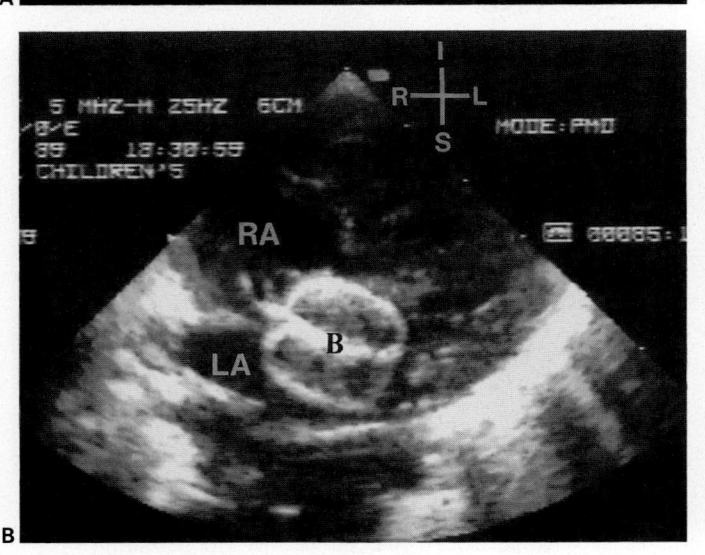

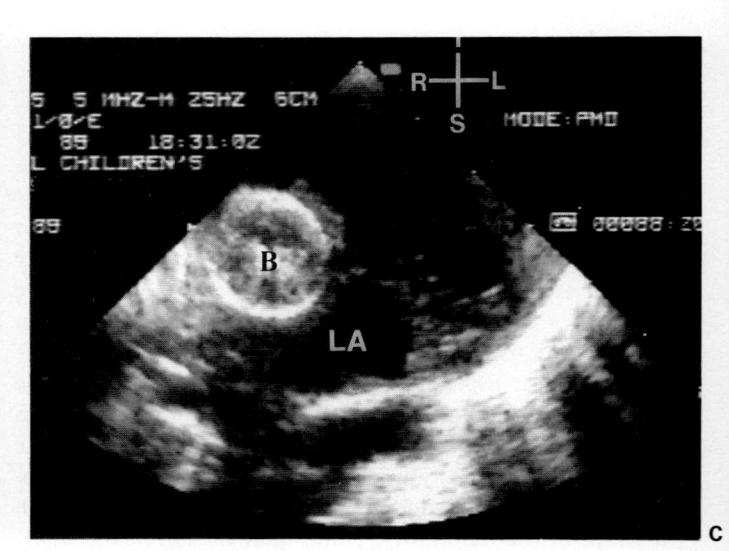

Fig. 7 Balloon atrial septostomy with echocardiographic guidance. A: Subcostal four chamber view showing the catheter after it has been passed via the foramen ovale into the left atrium. C – catheter. **B:** Subcostal four chamber view showing the balloon after it has been inflated in the left atrium. B – balloon. **C:** Subcostal four chamber view after the inflated balloon has been pulled back through the atrial septum into the right atrium.

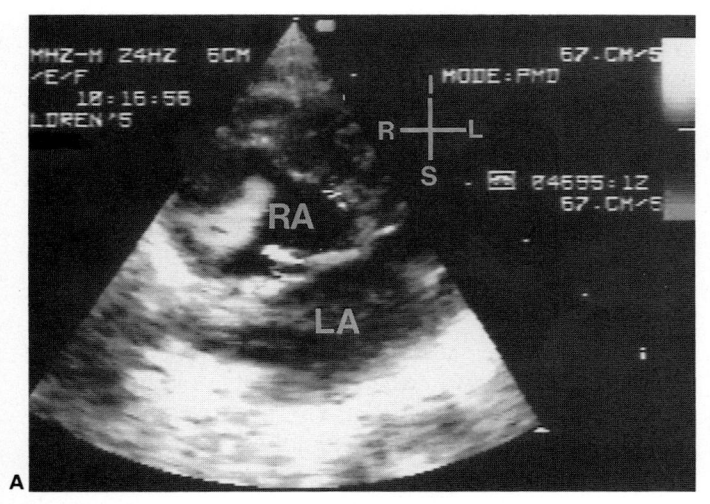

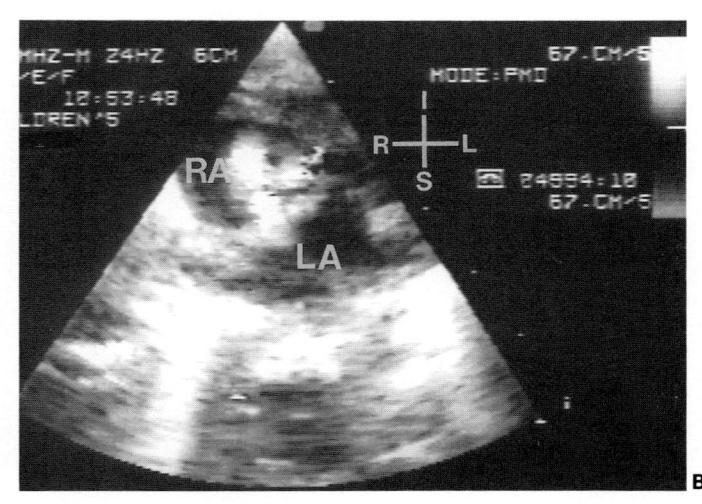

Plate 2 Colour flow images before and after balloon atrial septostomy. A: Subcostal four chamber view of atrial septum showing a narrow jet of left to right flow across the foramen ovale. **B:** Similar view in same patient after balloon atrial septostomy. There is now a moderate sized atrial septal defect with low velocity (orange) left to right flow. This figure is reproduced in colour in the colour plate section at the front of this volume.

chamber subcostal view that shows the foramen ovale. The catheter may then be passed into the left atrium and the balloon gently inflated to ascertain correct positioning. The balloon will be seen to inflate in the left atrium and the septostomy can then be performed in the standard manner (Fig. 7). This method does require certain modifications to technique compared to the standard method using biplane X-ray screening but there are a number of advantages. It is possible to be certain of correct positioning of the catheter in the left atrium and the atrial septal defect produced can be visualised so that further pull backs can be performed if the defect appears inadequate (Plate 2). In critically ill infants it can be performed on the intensive care unit thus avoiding the stress of moving a sick child. It is also possible to ensure that the septostomy balloon does not prolapse from the left atrium into the mitral valve orifice.

COMPLETE TRANSPOSITION WITH VENTRICULAR SEPTAL DEFECT

The most common associated lesion found with transposition of the great arteries is a ventricular septal defect. Such defects may occupy similar sites to those encountered when ventricular septal defects occur as isolated lesions. Perimembranous defect may extend into the inlet, trabecular or outlet portions of the septum. Conversely defects of the trabecular, inlet outlet septum or doubly committed subarterial defects may occur, muscular outlet defects being the most frequently encountered (Fig. 8 and Plate 3).

Malalignment of the outlet septum with the trabecular septum may be seen and this results in a variety of associated abnormalities. If the outlet septum is deviated

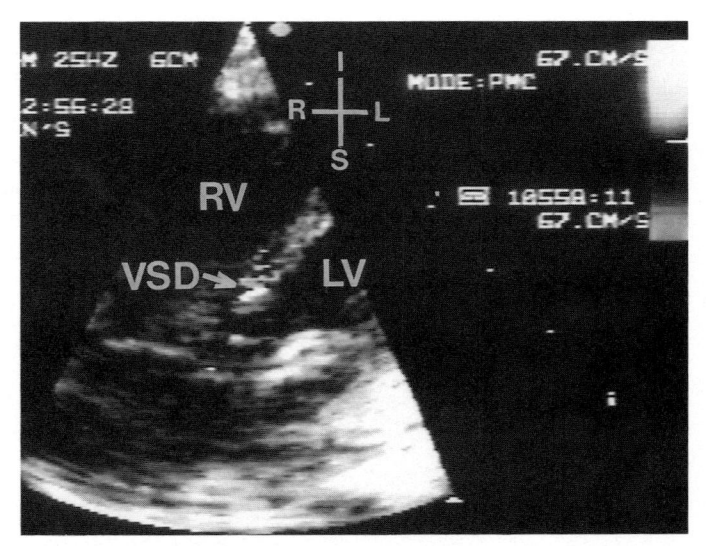

Plate 3 Colour flow Doppler image in an infant with transposition and a perimembranous ventricular septal defect. Note that the flow through the defect is blue indicating right to left flow. This is the normal direction of flow in transposition where the right ventricular pressure is likely to be higher than the left. This figure is reproduced in colour in the colour plate section at the front of this volume.

posteriorly it may result in subpulmonary narrowing and with anterior deviation there can be subaortic narrowing. This is often best appreciated from the parasternal long axis view or from a subcostal long axis view. These malalignment defects may have a muscular margin or they may extend into the perimembranous position where there is continuity with the central fibrous body. A combination of views may be required to be certain on this point, superior angulation from the subcostal four chamber view

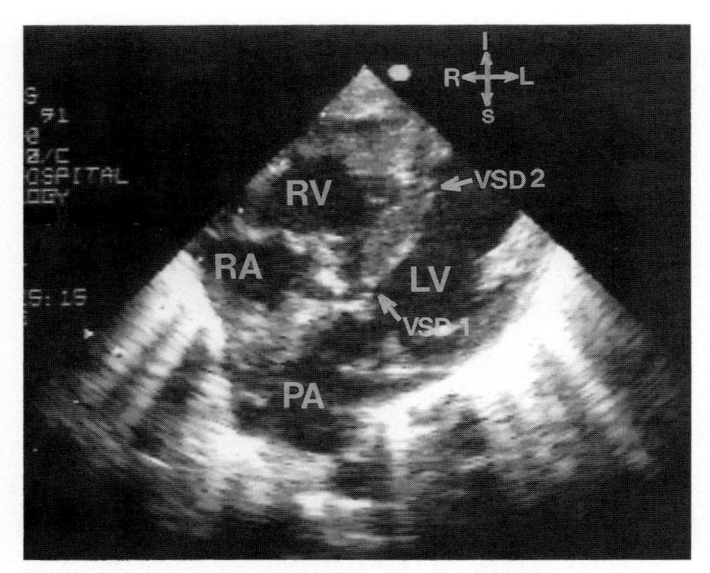

Fig. 8 Subcostal left ventricular outflow view with transposition and multiple ventricular septal defects. A small perimembranous defect is shown (VSD 1) with a second defect in the trabecular septum (VSD 2).

being particularly useful. Septal malalignment may result in the pulmonary artery overriding the septum (Fig. 9) and if the degree of override exceeds 50%, such defects are classified as double outlet right ventricle (Taussig-Bing anomaly) rather than complete transposition. In borderline cases it may not always be easy to make this distinction.

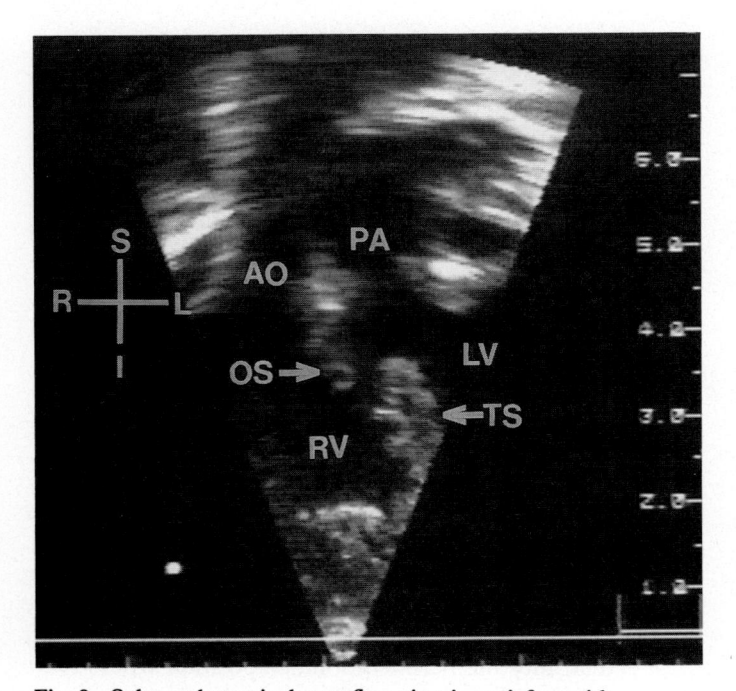

Fig. 9 Subcostal ventricular outflow view in an infant with transposition and a subpulmonary ventricular septal defect. There is malalignment of the outlet septum (OS) and trabecular septum (TS). This results in the pulmonary artery overriding the trabecular septum.

Straddling atrioventricular valves

A straddling valve is defined as one in which the tensor apparatus is shared between two ventricles. A straddling mitral valve for instance will have some of its tensor apparatus traversing the ventricular septal defect to insert into the right ventricle and a straddling tricuspid valve will have some of its tensor apparatus inserting into the left ventricle. This has important implications when the surgical closure of the ventricular septal defect is being considered.

This must be distinguished from an overriding atrioventricular valve where the valve overrides the ventricular septum but all of its chordal attachments are to the appropriate ventricle. A straddling valve usually but not always overrides the ventricular septum (Fig. 10).

Straddling of the mitral valve occurs with an anteriorly positioned ventricular septal defect, often a muscular outlet defect. This may be appreciated from careful review of the precordial long and short axis views where the tensor apparatus will be seen crossing the ventricular septal defect and inserting into the right side of the ventricular septum.

Straddling of the tricuspid valve occurs with a more posteriorly positioned ventricular septal defect involving the inlet portion of the ventricular septum. This is best appreciated from apical or subcostal four chamber views.

Other abnormalities of the chordal attachments

The tricuspid valve may have some of its chordal attachments inserting into the right ventricular aspect of the outlet septum. This is important to recognise as it complicates the closure of the ventricular septal defect to the aorta as part of a Rastelli operation.

Rarely some of the tricuspid valve and its chordae may herniate through the ventricular septal defect in systole, producing left ventricular outflow obstruction. Abnormal attachments of the mitral valve to the left ventricular outflow can occur which may also result in left ventricular outflow obstruction.

COMPLETE TRANSPOSITION WITH LEFT VENTRICULAR OUTFLOW OBSTRUCTION

The pulmonary valve and the subpulmonary region need careful evaluation in all patients with complete transposition. This area becomes of vital importance if an arterial switch operation is to be considered, as this then becomes the 'new' aortic valve and subaortic region. Even in the absence of a significant pressure gradient the left ventricular outflow may appear narrow, particularly in those patients with an intact ventricular septum where the septum bulges posteriorly just below the pulmonary valve. This region can best be assessed from parasternal long axis views or oblique subcostal views,[15] paying particular attention to diastolic views when fixed obstructive lesions may be best appreciated. It may be difficult to obtain good alignment with flow when performing Doppler studies because of the tortuous course of the left ventricular outflow in transposition, and this can make accurate estimation of pressure gradients difficult. Attention should also be paid to the contour of the interventricular septum on the subcostal short axis view, as this gives an indirect estimate of the left ventricular pressure.

Several types of left ventricular outflow obstruction are recognised. Isolated pulmonary valve stenosis is rare, more commonly coexisting with subpulmonary obstruction. The latter may be dynamic or fixed. Dynamic obstruction is commonly seen with an intact interventricular septum where the appearances may be similar to those seen in hypertrophic obstructive cardiomyopathy (Fig. 11). The higher right ventricular pressure is associated with the septum bulging posteriorly into the subpulmonary region and there may be associated systolic anterior motion of the mitral valve from the resulting 'Venturi' effect. This type of obstruction will usually resolve after an arterial switch operation, once the normal pressure relationships between the two ventricles is restored.[16] The absence of apposition of the anterior mitral valve leaflet to the ventricular septum during systole appears to exclude the presence of significant dynamic obstruction. However, systolic anterior motion of the mitral valve, apposition of the anterior mitral leaflet to the ventricular septum in systole and premature systolic closure of the pulmonary valve, have all been described in patients without significant outflow gradients.[17,18] These parameters should not be used in isolation and other features such as the ventricular septal contour, and the Doppler flow velocity in the left ventricular outflow should be evaluated (Plate 4).

Fixed obstruction may result from a discrete subpulmonary fibromuscular shelf extending from the septum around posteriorly to the anterior mitral leaflet (Fig. 12). Occasionally the fibrous narrowing may be of the 'tunnel' variety. Abnormal mitral attachments, and aneurysmal tissue tags, can also produce obstruction (Fig. 13). There may be obstruction resulting from posterior deviation of the outlet septum or from herniation of tricuspid valve tissue through a ventricular septal defect.

In patients with fixed severe left ventricular outflow obstruction and a ventricular septal defect, the preferred method of repair is a Rastelli operation.[19] It requires patching of the ventricular septal defect to the subaortic infundibulum. The pulmonary trunk is then ligated and divided and an extracardiac conduit is placed between the

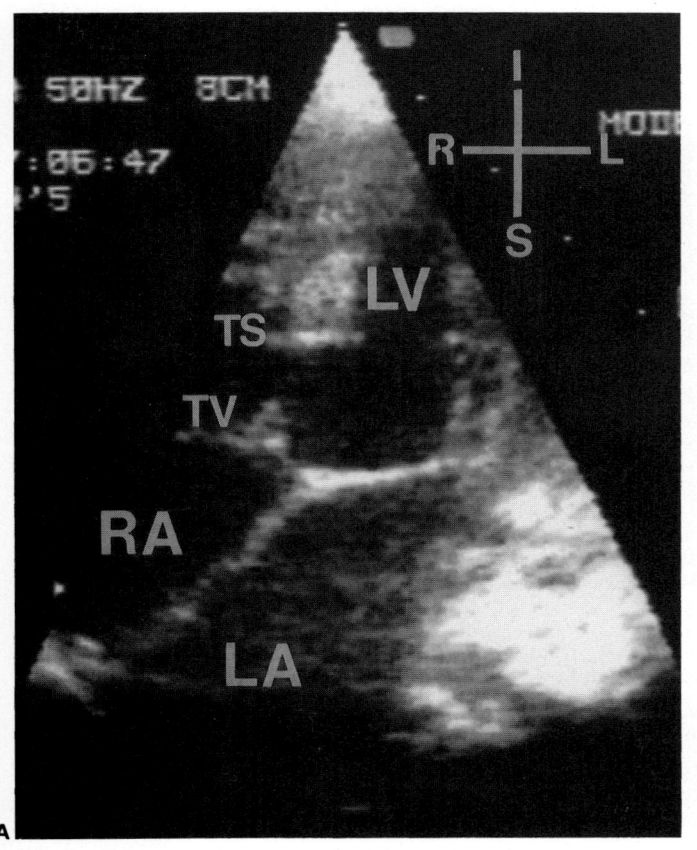

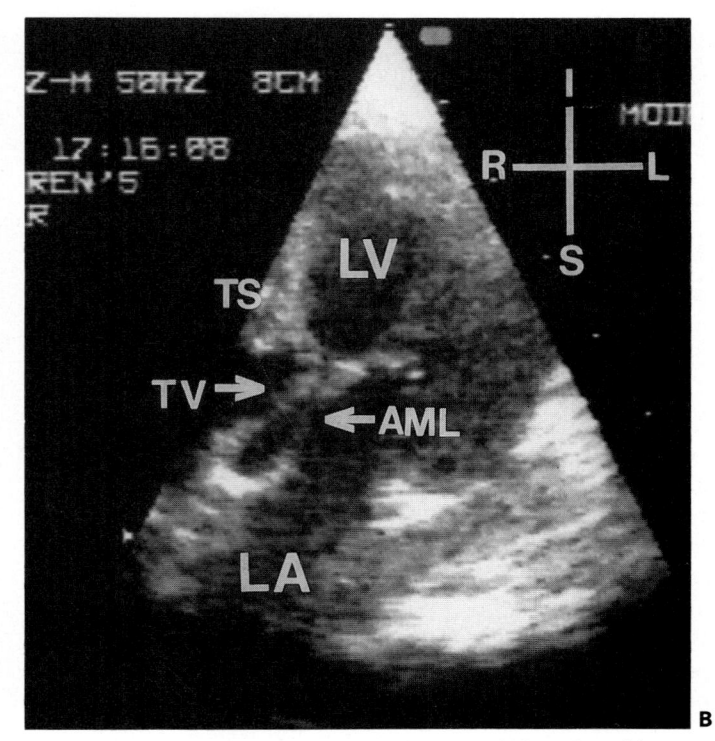

Fig. 10 Modified apical four chamber view in a child with transposition and an inlet ventricular septal defect with a straddling tricuspid valve. **A:** The tricuspid valve overrides the trabecular septum (TS). **B:** The septal leaflet of the tricuspid valve straddles the ventricular septal defect and has chordal attachments on the left side of the trabecular septum. AML – anterior mitral leaflet.

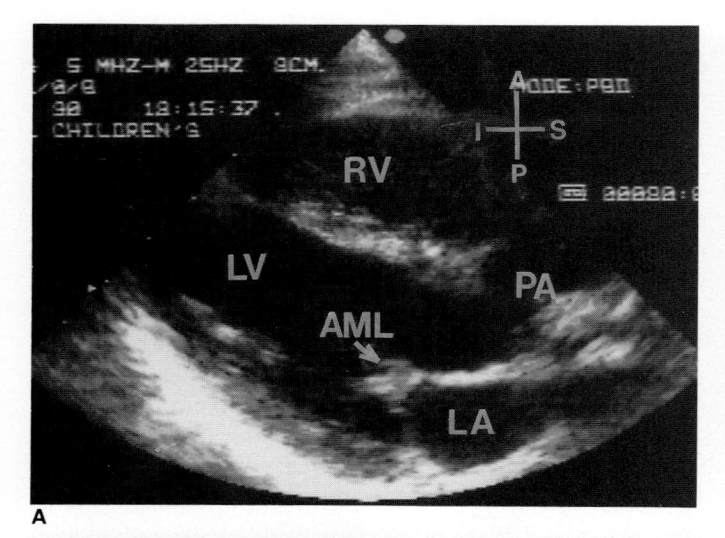

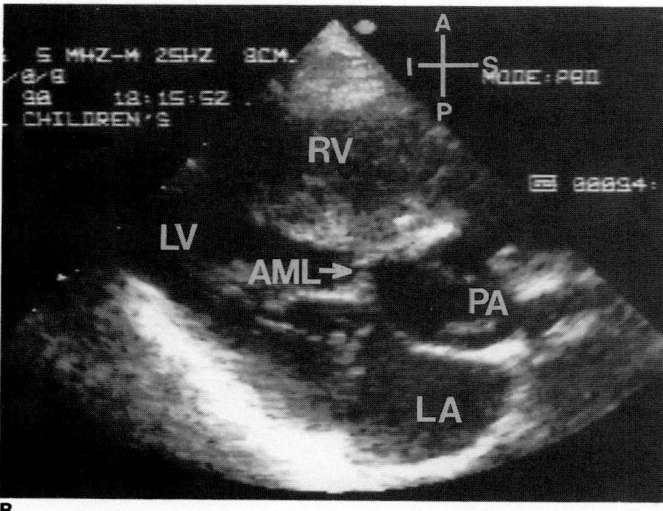

Fig. 11 Dynamic left ventricular outflow obstruction in transposition with intact ventricular septum. A: Parasternal long axis view in early systole. The anterior leaflet of the mitral valve (AML) is in a normal position. **B:** Later systolic frame in the same patient. There is systolic anterior motion of the anterior leaflet of the mitral valve and it is now in apposition to the ventricular septum.

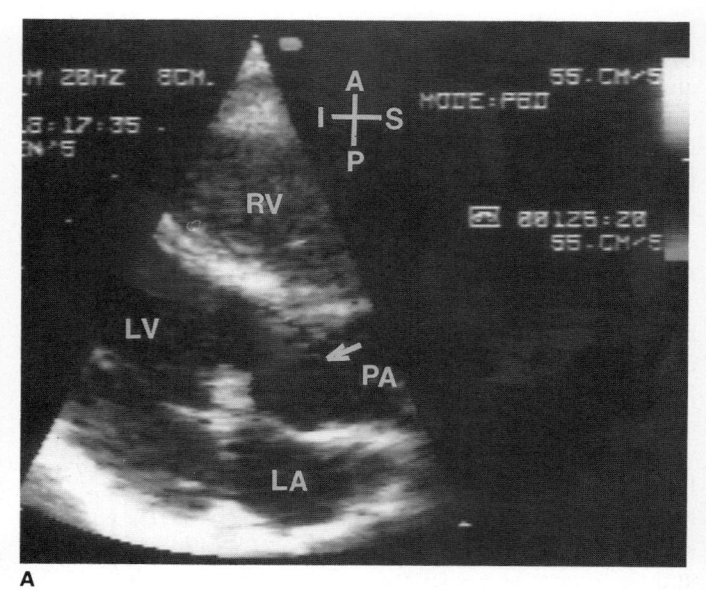

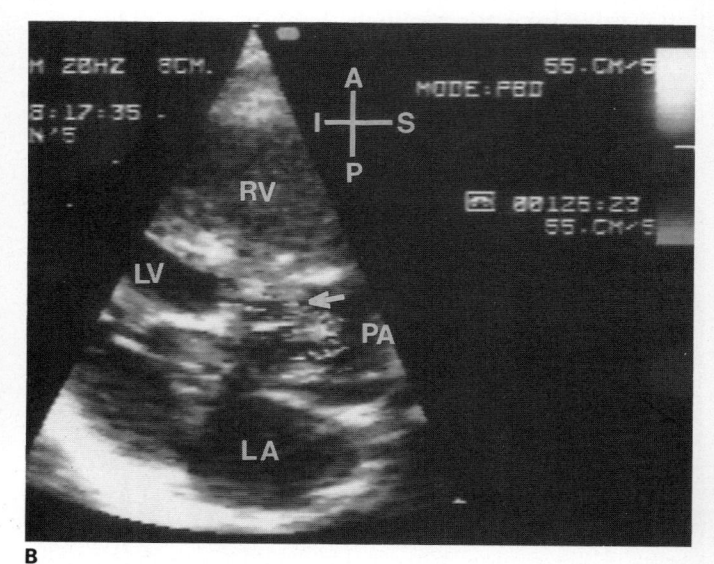

Plate 4 Colour flow Doppler images showing dynamic left ventricular outflow obstruction in transposition with intact ventricular septum. A: Parasternal long axis image in early systole shows low velocity blue flow in the left ventricular outflow (arrowed). **B:** Similar view in mid systole shows that the anterior mitral valve leaflet has moved anteriorly producing obstruction to the left ventricular outflow. There is high velocity turbulent flow just distal to the mitral leaflet (arrowed). This figure is reproduced in colour in the colour plate section at the front of this volume.

right ventricle and the distal pulmonary trunk. The left ventricle then becomes the systemic pump as it is connected via the ventricular septal defect to the aorta. The ventricular septal defect needs to be of adequate size and appropriately positioned for this to be successful so that the left ventricular to aortic outflow is unobstructed. This needs to be considered when such patients are examined. When the ventricular septal defect is associated with posterior deviation of the outlet septum there is rarely a problem. This is not so for inlet or trabecular defects and difficulties may be encountered if the tricuspid valve has abnormal chordal attachments in the right ventricular outflow.

COMPLETE TRANSPOSITION WITH AORTIC ARCH ABNORMALITIES AND SUBAORTIC STENOSIS

Abnormalities of the aortic arch occur in approximately 5% of children with complete transposition. Coarctation, tubular arch hypoplasia and interrupted aortic arch have all been described.[20] These can be diagnosed on cross-

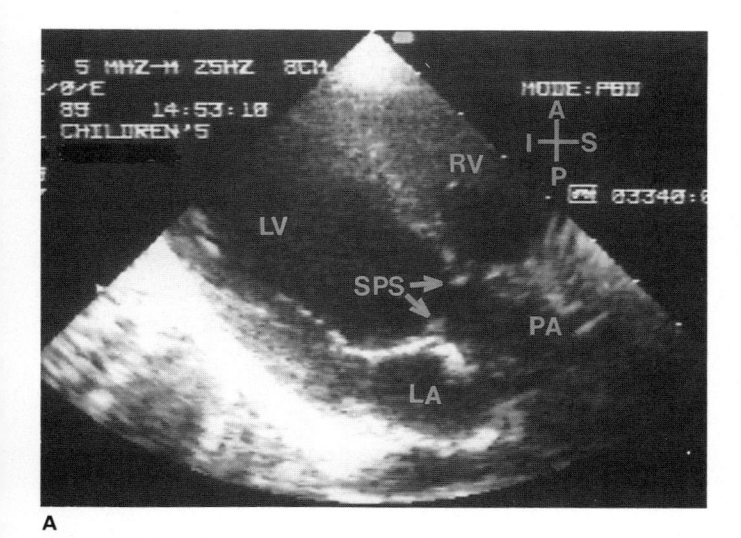

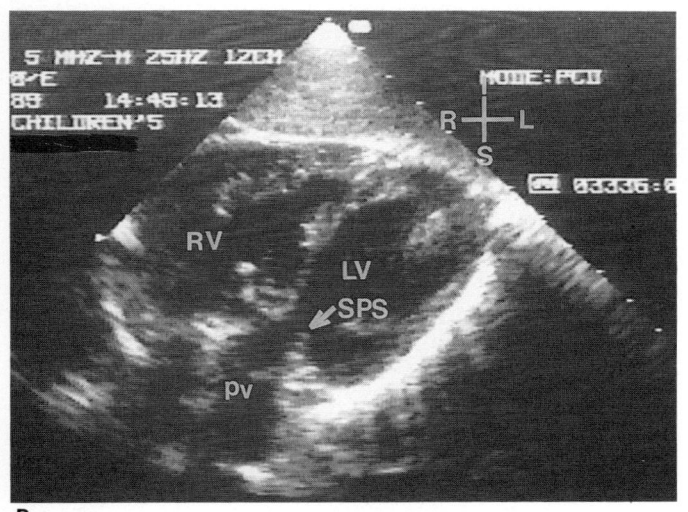

Fig. 12 Fixed membranous subpulmonary stenosis in transposition.
A: Parasternal long axis view in early systole. There is a discrete subpulmonary shelf arrowed (SPS). **B:** Subcostal left ventricular outflow view in the same patient. The stenotic membrane (SPS) is shown and is clearly separated from the pulmonary valve leaflets.

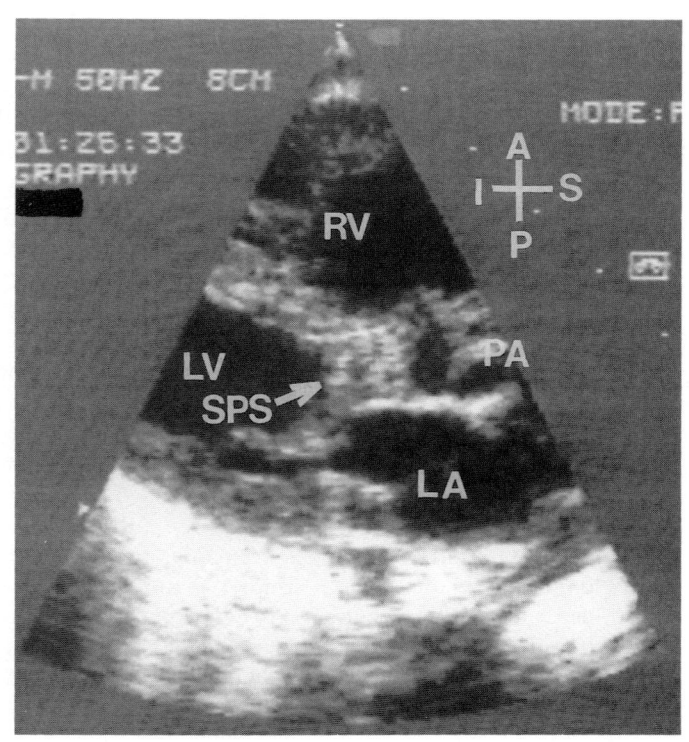

Fig. 13 Subpulmonary stenosis (SPS) in transposition secondary to anomalous attachment of the anterior leaflet of the mitral valve to the interventricular septum with a large tissue tag on the leaflet contributing to the stenosis.

sectional imaging from the suprasternal notch or from high parasternal sagittal cuts. Aortic arch obstruction is usually seen in association with a ventricular septal defect. Careful evaluation of the subaortic region should be performed because of the frequent coexistence of subaortic stenosis. This may be caused by anterior deviation of the outlet septum in a malalignment ventricular septal defect or from abnormal muscle bundles in the right ventricular outflow or a prominent ventriculo-infundibular fold. Parasternal long axis views and oblique subcostal views are the best for evaluating this problem. Subaortic obstruction and aortic arch anomalies may be associated with right ventricular hypoplasia. When present this would be a relative contraindication to a Mustard or Senning operation and an arterial switch operation would be the corrective procedure of choice.

Rare associated abnormalities

Atrioventricular septal defect may occur with complete transposition and the morphology of the defect is similar to that seen as an isolated lesion.

Abnormalities of the pulmonary and systemic venous connections are uncommon. These can be identified in the standard manner from a combination of subcostal and suprasternal views.

EVALUATION AFTER CORRECTIVE SURGERY FOR COMPLETE TRANSPOSITION

There are two approaches that can be used to 'correct' complete transposition of the great arteries, namely physiological correction by an atrial redirection procedure or anatomical correction by an arterial switch operation.

Atrial redirection operations

Mustard's and Senning's operations are the methods of atrial redirection that have been used widely. Both methods involve redirecting the systemic and pulmonary venous inflow to the heart. Prosthetic material is used in the Mustard operation and natural atrial tissue is used in the Senning operation. The systemic venous blood from the inferior and superior caval veins is redirected to the mitral valve and thence the left ventricle by constructing a baffle to redirect flow. Similarly, the pulmonary venous return is redirected to the tricuspid valve and right ventricle. This achieves a physiological correction but leaves the right ventricle as the systemic pump and the left ventricle on the pulmonary side of the circulation.

When performing echocardiography in these patients, a number of factors need to be considered. Firstly, the pressure relationships between the two ventricles is likely to be unchanged (unless a ventricular septal defect has been closed or subpulmonary stenosis relieved). The right ventricle will remain hypertrophied and the substrate for dynamic subpulmonary stenosis remains in the left ventricle. Secondly there are a number of potential complications of the surgery that should be sought.

It is important to evaluate right ventricular function, as symptomatic dysfunction occurs in approximately 10% of patients after operation.[21] Ventricular function may be measured using methods described previously. Dysfunction will be associated with an increased right ventricular end-diastolic volume and reduced ejection fraction. The application of normal values of right ventricular function obtained from individuals without transposition should be avoided as the loading characteristics of the ventricles are different. Most angiographic studies after Mustard and Senning operations have shown that the right ventricular volume is increased and the right ventricular ejection fraction is reduced compared to normal individuals. Whether this reflects true dysfunction in all cases is debatable, as it might result from adaptation to the different loading conditions.

Tricuspid regurgitation is frequently seen after corrective surgery. Usually this is mild but it may be more severe if there is right ventricular dysfunction or if abnormalities of the tricuspid valve result from closure of a ventricular septal defect with a straddling tricuspid valve.[22]

Much attention has been focused on the diagnosis of baffle obstruction after the Mustard and Senning operations. As might be expected, with growth of the patient the systemic and pulmonary venous pathways may become obstructed. This is predominantly a problem encountered after the Mustard operation, presumably because the prosthetic material does not have the potential for growth of the atrial tissue. Systemic venous pathway obstruction often occurs in the superior caval vein limb of the baffle. This may be diagnosed by a combination of cross-sectional imaging, contrast echocardiography and pulsed Doppler study.[23-25] The apical four chamber view allows the mid portion of the baffle to be seen, a common site of obstruction. Pulsed Doppler interrogation or colour flow mapping can also be used from this approach and as alignment with the direction of flow is possible this can be used for quantitative assessment of flow gradients (Plate 5). The systemic venous pathway can appear narrow from this view in the absence of obstruction because of its oblique nature. The superior and inferior caval limbs to the baffle can be further evaluated by short axis parasternal and subcostal views respectively. The junction of the superior caval vein and the baffle may be particularly difficult to visualise. Contrast echocardiography can be helpful in this situation. There is usually run-off via the azygos vein with partial or total

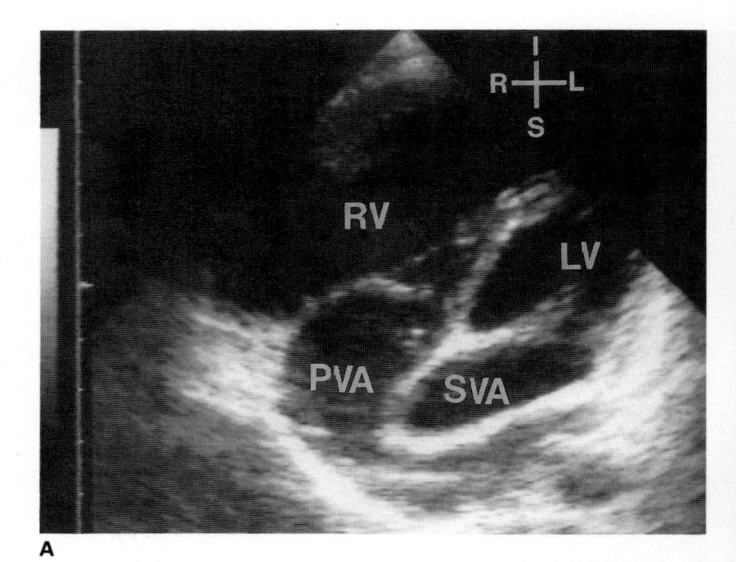

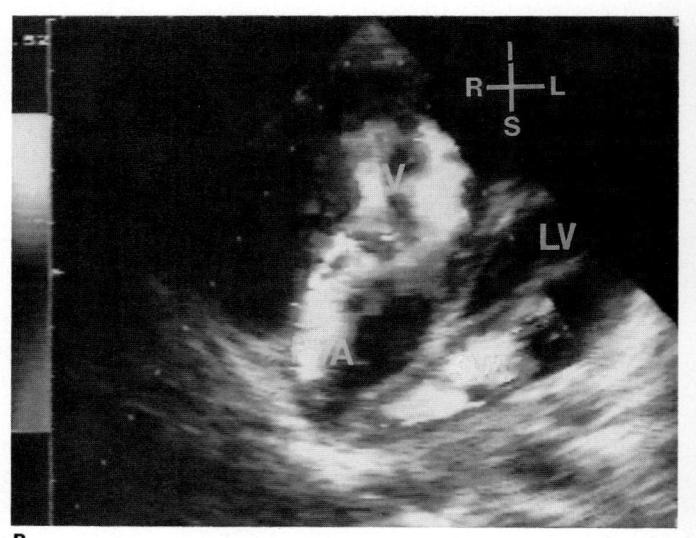

Plate 5 A: Apical four chamber view after the Senning operation for complete transposition with intact ventricular septum. The pulmonary veins connect to the pulmonary venous atrium (PVA) posterior and to the right of the systemic venous atrium (SVA). **B:** Colour flow Doppler image showing low velocity, non-turbulent (orange) flow in the pulmonary and systemic venous pathways. This figure is reproduced in colour in the colour plate section at the front of this volume.

obstruction to this pathway. Thus if obstruction is complete contrast medium that is injected into a right arm vein will pass down the azygos vein and then into the heart via the inferior caval vein. This may be appreciated by imaging the inferior caval vein from the subcostal approach. In lesser degrees of obstruction, contrast will be seen entering the heart from above and below.

Pulmonary venous pathway obstruction is less common but is clinically more important. The pathway may become obstructed in its mid portion or there may be selective obstruction to one or more of the pulmonary veins. This may best be visualised from posteriorly angulated apical four chamber views or subcostal views.[26] Doppler interrogation can be performed from the apical four chamber view and in the presence of obstruction there will be characteristic high velocity turbulent, continuous flow distal to the site of obstruction.[27] If pulmonary hypertension results from the obstruction then the left ventricle will appear more hypertrophied and the interventricular septal contour will become more flattened.

Residual atrial shunts due to a baffle leak are rarely large enough to require reoperation. Contrast echocardiography is very sensitive at detecting such shunts and they may be localised by cross-sectional imaging[28] and colour flow Doppler examination.

The development of pulmonary vascular disease should be suspected if there is evidence of left ventricular hypertension (i.e. left ventricular hypertrophy and change in the interventricular septal contour) in the absence of left ventricular outflow obstruction or pulmonary venous pathway obstruction.

Arterial switch operations

The arterial switch operation or anatomical correction has become increasingly used to treat complete transposition. Repair is achieved by transecting the great arteries above the aortic and pulmonary valves and then re-anastomosing them to the appropriate ventricle. This is combined with separate transfer of the coronary arteries to the new aortic root. This achieves an anatomical correction as the left ventricle reverts to its normal role of the systemic pump.

Studies of left ventricular function after the arterial switch operation have generally shown normal[29] or near-normal[30] function although the left ventricle may have a more globular shape.[31] The major abnormalities, that should be sought relate to the aortic and pulmonary anastomoses.[32,33] The pulmonary artery tends to be distorted or irregular at the anastomotic site and this may be associated with supravalvar pulmonary stenosis. Narrowing of the proximal branch pulmonary arteries may also occur. These abnormalities can be appreciated from the standard subcostal and precordial views. Doppler examination allows prediction of the severity of the stenosis. It should be remembered that the great artery positional relationships will remain abnormal, though their precise positions will vary depending on the preoperative anatomy and the method of pulmonary artery reconstruction that has been used.

The aortic anastomosis may also become narrowed, though this is relatively uncommon. Mild aortic regurgitation is often seen, particularly in those patients who have had previous banding of the pulmonary artery.[34] This may relate to a degree of dilatation of the aortic root, a feature that may be striking in some patients.

Rastelli operations

The principle of the operation has been described before. There are a number of factors that need to be considered when performing echocardiography in these patients. Left ventricular function may be impaired and can be assessed from the M-mode echocardiogram.[35] The presence of left ventricular outflow obstruction or residual ventricular septal defect should be determined. Colour flow imaging is likely to be helpful for both these diagnoses. The right ventricular to pulmonary artery conduit should also be examined as conduit stenosis is likely to develop as the patient grows. These conduits may be constructed of prosthetic or homograft material. Conduits may become obstructed at the level of the valve or at the distal insertion into the pulmonary trunk. Careful cross-sectional imaging and Doppler examination should reveal the site of any obstruction. The conduits are often best imaged from the precordium as subcostal imaging may be difficult due to the very anterior course of the conduit and the older age of the patient (generally Rastelli operations are not undertaken until 4 or more years of age).

DOUBLE OUTLET RIGHT VENTRICLE

In this condition both great arteries are connected entirely or predominantly to the right ventricle. In malformations where an arterial valve overrides the ventricular septum, double outlet ventricle is considered to be present when greater than 50% of the circumference of the aortic and pulmonary valves is connected to the right ventricle.[2] It is simply a description of ventriculo-arterial connection and may occur with a variety of atrial arrangements and atrioventricular connections. This account will not include double outlet ventricle when there are abnormalities of atrial situs, double inlet or absent atrioventricular connection. A later section will describe double outlet right ventricle in association with atrioventricular discordance.

Double outlet right ventricle is generally subdivided into different groups depending on the relationship of the ventricular septal defect to the great arteries. This crucial feature determines the likely surgical treatment that can be offered. Cross-sectional echocardiography allows the determination of the margins of the ventricular septal defect and its relationship to the aorta and pulmonary artery, something that may be difficult to determine by angiography. Thus double outlet right ventricle may occur with a subaortic, subpulmonary or doubly committed ventricular septal defect, depending on the size and orientation of the outlet septum. Alternatively the ventricular septal defect may be unrelated to the great arteries, because of its location in the trabecular septum or the inlet region; so called non-committed defects.[36-38]

The initial part of the examination is performed to determine the atrial arrangement and the atrioventricular connection as described previously. The great arteries can then be identified by their course and branching pattern. The ventriculo-arterial connection can then be evaluated from a combination of parasternal long and short axis views[39,40] and subcostal views.[38,41]

The parasternal long axis view will show both great arteries originating anterior to the ventricular septum and will show whether there is a left sided ventriculo-infundibular fold or mitral/great artery fibrous continuity (Fig. 14). The presence of bilateral infundibulae (and therefore a left-sided ventriculo-infundibular fold) is frequently seen in double outlet right ventricle but is not a prerequisite for the diagnosis. When the aorta or pulmonary artery override the ventricular septum, the semilunar valve closure lines and their relationship to the septum should be noted. If the degree of override of both valves on to the right ventricle exceeds 50% then the criteria for double outlet right ventricle are fulfilled.

The parasternal short axis views will identify the positional relationship of the two great arteries. In the majority of cases the aorta will be to the right of the pulmonary artery, either with a side to side relationship or with the aorta slightly anterior to the pulmonary artery.[36] The transducer can be angled down from the base to the apex to assess the relationship of the great arteries to the ventricular septal defect, the outlet septum and the right sided ventriculo-infundibular fold.

Subcostal views should begin with the standard four chamber view and any straddling or abnormal chordal attachments of the mitral or tricuspid valves can be assessed. Clockwise rotation of the transducer, to show the left ventricular outlet, will show the ventricular septal defect. Note should be taken of the site and size of this defect. The majority of defects will be perimembranous, having the region of mitral/tricuspid or tricuspid/aortic fibrous continuity as one of the margins of the defect. A muscular posterior rim to the defect, producing a muscular outlet defect is relatively common and double committed defects with absence of the outlet septum may also be seen. The transducer can be rotated clockwise to visualise the ventricular outlets, the size of the outlet septum and a two chamber long axis view of the right ventricle. Care should be taken with the subcostal views as changes in the angulation of the transducer may make an overriding great artery appear to be dominantly connected to the right ventricle or the left ventricle alternately. Whether or not this is a spurious finding can be determined from the parasternal views.

Subaortic ventricular septal defect

The features to be observed when the ventricular septal defect is subaortic are best appreciated from the subcostal long axis view and serial short axis views. It is important to look at the size and orientation of the outlet septum. If the outlet septum, descending from the junction of the aortic and pulmonary valves, curves leftwards to fuse with the ventriculo-infundibular fold, then the ventricular septal defect will be subaortic (Fig. 15).

This causes the pulmonary outflow tract to appear as an elliptical structure, clearly separated from the ventricular septal defect and thence the left ventricle. The leftwards orientation of the outlet septum may also be noted on the serial short axis parasternal views.

The anatomy of this defect may be similar to that seen in classical tetralogy of Fallot, as the leftwards and anterior deviation of the outlet septum may result in subpulmonary stenosis. In addition to the infundibular stenosis there may be additional stenosis of the pulmonary valve and branch pulmonary arteries. There has been much debate about whether such defects should be classified as double outlet right ventricle or whether it is simpler to classify them as the tetralogy of Fallot as their treatment is identical to that of the tetralogy of Fallot with a lesser degree of aortic override.

There is no such problem when there is no associated subpulmonary stenosis. These cases often, but not always,

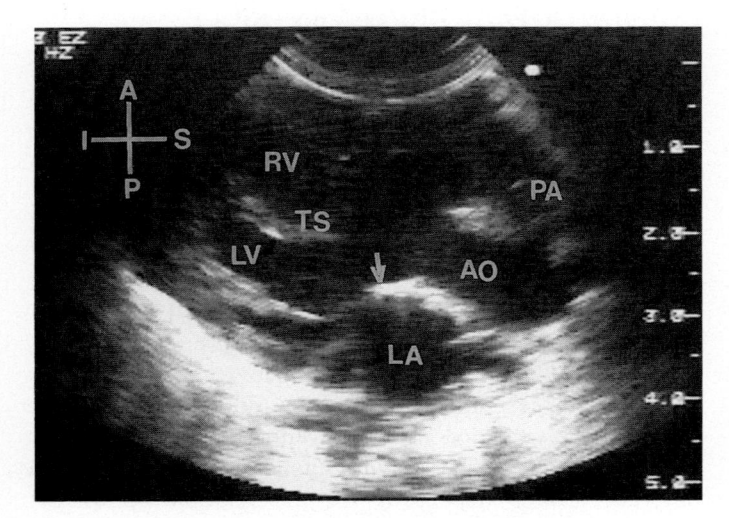

Fig. 14 **Parasternal long axis view in double outlet right ventricle with a subaortic ventricular septal defect.** There is fibrous continuity between mitral and aortic valves (arrowed). The aorta overrides the trabecular septum (TS) by over 50% fulfilling the definition of double outlet right ventricle.

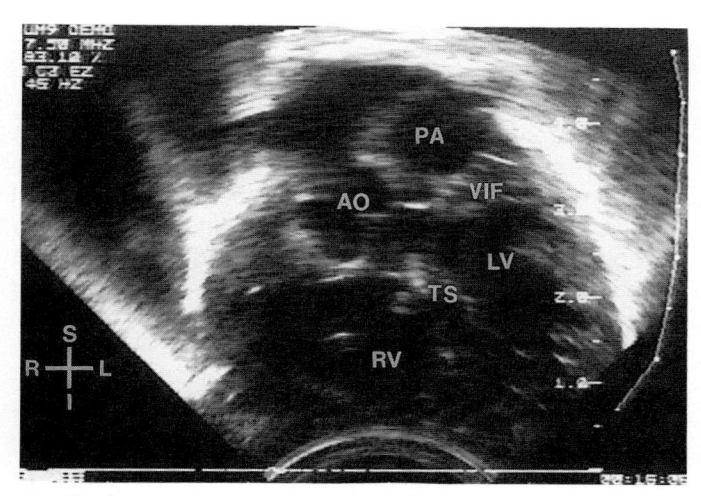

Fig. 15 Subcostal ventricular outflow view showing double outlet right ventricle with a subaortic ventricular septal defect. The aorta overrides the trabecular septum by over 50%. Note the fusion of the outlet septum with the ventriculo-infundibular fold (VIF) that results in the pulmonary outflow appearing as an elliptical structure.

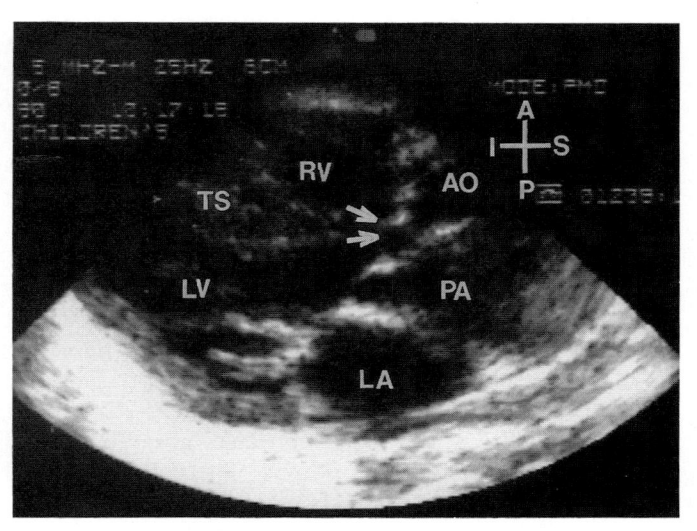

Fig. 16 Parasternal long axis view in double outlet right ventricle with a doubly committed ventricular septal defect. There is absence of the outlet septum with fibrous continuity between the pulmonary and aortic valve leaflets (arrowed). In this case the pulmonary artery overrides the trabecular septum.

have a subaortic infundibulum. Important associated lesions to look for are coarctation of the aorta and a restrictive ventricular septal defect resulting in left ventricular outflow obstruction.

Subpulmonary ventricular septal defect

This condition has similarity to complete transposition with ventricular septal defect but the pulmonary artery overrides the ventricular septal defect by greater than the required 50% thus rendering it double outlet right ventricle. It has been called the Taussig-Bing anomaly.[42] The aorta is likely to be to the right of the pulmonary trunk, either side by side or in a right anterior position. There may be fibrous continuity between the pulmonary and mitral valves or there may be bilateral infundibulae. The ventricular septal defect is perimembranous in 60% and muscular in the remainder.[36]

The key to diagnosis again relates to observing the orientation of the outlet septum from the subcostal or parasternal short axis views. With a subpulmonary defect the outlet septum will deviate to the right, or appear to travel straight downwards, to fuse with the right ventriculo-infundibular fold. This contrasts to a subaortic defect where the outlet septum deviates to the left. There is seldom pulmonary stenosis but coarctation of the aorta is a common finding.[43] Straddling of the mitral valve may be seen and a restrictive ventricular septal defect is very rare.

Doubly committed ventricular septal defect

In this kind of defect there is virtual or complete absence of the outlet septum, thus leaving both great arteries related to the ventricular septal defect. One of the great arteries, usually the pulmonary artery, may be closest to the ventricular septal defect or may override it (Fig. 16).

The aortic and pulmonary valves will be seen in fibrous continuity from the subcostal long axis view, with either absence of the outlet septum or a small rim of outlet septum lying underneath them.

Non-committed ventricular septal defect

The ventricular septal defect is remote from the great arteries, usually either a perimembranous defect extending into the inlet septum or a muscular inlet defect. Such defects are commonly associated with overriding or straddling of the atrioventricular valves and may best be observed from apical or subcostal four chamber views. Serial short axis scans from base to apex will show both great arteries originating from the right ventricle with the outlet septum deviating to left or right, and the posteriorly positioned ventricular septal defect remote from the great arteries.

Other types of non-committed defects that may be seen include complete atrioventricular septal defect and muscular defects in the trabecular septum. Non-committed defects are very important to examine carefully, as surgical closure of the defect to one of the great arteries may be difficult, particularly with a straddling atrioventricular valve.

Associated lesions

Multiple ventricular septal defects were found in 5 of the

84 cases reported by Wilkinson,[36] usually including a separate inlet muscular defect. Restrictive defects may occur with subaortic ventricular septal defects. This produces left ventricular outflow obstruction with consequent left ventricular hypertrophy. Doppler echocardiographic assessment from the parasternal region should allow quantification of the pressure difference between the two ventricles.

Subaortic stenosis may occur in subpulmonary defects as a consequence of the rightwards displacement of the outlet septum or there may be dynamic obstruction originating from the muscular subaortic infundibulum. In subaortic ventricular septal defects, subaortic stenosis may result from prominence of the right ventriculo-infundibular fold or there may be discrete fibrous obstruction. Careful examination of the aortic arch is required, because coarctation and interruption of the aortic arch, are frequent accompaniments.

Subpulmonary stenosis is frequently seen with a subaortic defect, as previously mentioned. It is rarely seen with subpulmonary or double committed defects.

Double outlet right ventricle with an intact ventricular septum has been described,[44] and is associated with severe left ventricular hypoplasia.

DOUBLE OUTLET LEFT VENTRICLE

This is a very rare condition characterised by both great arteries being committed to the left ventricle. The few descriptions in the literature show that it has variable morphology.[45,46] It normally occurs with usual atrial arrangement and concordant atrioventricular connection. The vast majority of the ventricular septal defects are subaortic, with a small number that are subpulmonary or doubly committed. The spatial relationship of the great arteries is variable. In approximately 50% of cases the aorta lies to the right of the pulmonary artery and in the remainder the aorta is anterior or to the left of the pulmonary artery. The majority of cases will have associated pulmonary outflow obstruction (in the case of subaortic defects) or coarctation (in the case of subpulmonary defects). Atrioventricular valve abnormalities occur in approximately 30% of patients with this condition.

CONGENITALLY CORRECTED TRANSPOSITION OF THE GREAT ARTERIES

Congenitally corrected transposition of the great arteries is a rare anomaly, being present in approximately 0.5% of children with congenital heart disease. It is a malformation characterised by a discordant atrioventricular connection and a discordant ventriculo-arterial connection. Thus the right atrium connects, via the mitral valve, to the morphological left ventricle, from which the pulmonary artery arises. The left atrium connects, via the tricuspid valve, to the morphological right ventricle, from which the aorta arises. This results in the right ventricle being the systemic pump and the left ventricle being the pulmonary ventricle. This may occur in the context of the usual atrial arrangement or mirror image arrangement. By definition the condition cannot be present when there is right or left atrial isomerism as this results in an ambiguous atrioventricular connection. The ventricular topology will usually be left handed for usual atrial arrangement, and right handed if there is a mirror image arrangement to the atria.

The examination must start as usual by the determination of the atrial situs followed by assessment of the atrioventricular connection from subcostal and apical four chamber views, supplemented by parasternal long and short axis views.[47,48] This approach relies on recognising the characteristics of the mitral and tricuspid valves and the morphology of the two ventricles. The mitral valve has two leaflets with chordal attachments to its two papillary muscles. Conversely the tricuspid valve has three leaflets with chordal attachments to the ventricular septum. The tricuspid septal leaflet attaches to the septum nearer the apex than the corresponding leaflet of the mitral valve (normal 'offsetting' of the mitral and tricuspid valves). Therefore, in atrioventricular discordance the left atrioventricular valve will be a morphological tricuspid valve. There will be reverse 'offsetting' of the atrioventricular valves, with the septal leaflet of the left atrioventricular valve inserting nearer the apex than the right atrioventricular valve (the reverse of normal) (Fig. 17). This may be appreciated from an apical four chamber view or

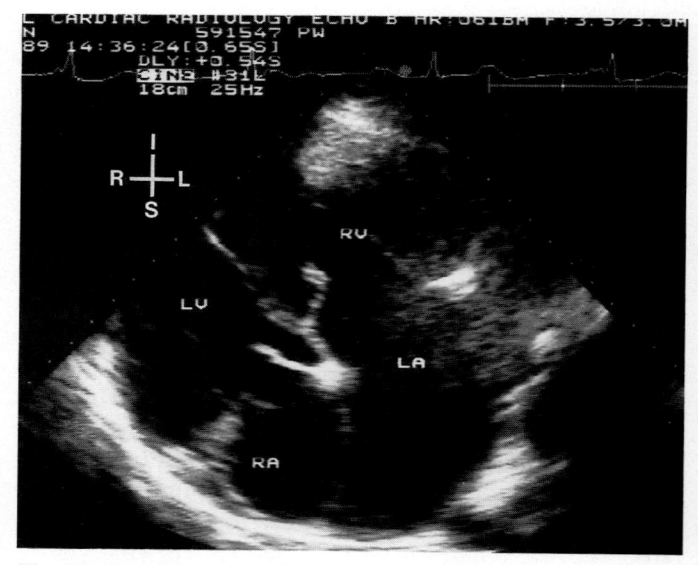

Fig. 17 Apical four chamber view in congenitally corrected transposition of the great arteries. The presence of atrioventricular discordance is demonstrated. There is reverse offsetting of the atrioventricular valves with the septal leaflet of the left atrioventricular (tricuspid) valve being attached to the septum more apically than the attachment of the right atrioventricular (mitral) valve.

from the subcostal four chamber view. This diagnostic feature cannot be used if there is an associated inlet ventricular septal defect, as this will result in the atrioventricular valves being at the same level. The left atrioventricular valve can be examined from a parasternal short axis view to look for the three leaflets of the tricuspid valve (Fig. 18). Similarly, the right atrioventricular valve can be shown to be a mitral valve by its 'fish mouth' appearance in its short axis and the presence of two papillary muscles can be noted. The morphology of the two ventricles can also be determined by examining the trabecular pattern of each. The right ventricle can be recognised by its coarse trabecular pattern and the presence of the moderator band in its apical portion. Conversely the left ventricle has a much finer trabecular pattern.

Having determined the atrioventricular connection, attention should then be directed to the ventriculo-arterial connection. In congenitally corrected transposition the aorta is usually to the left and anterior to the pulmonary artery. This may be appreciated from parasternal long and short axis views (Fig. 19). Other arterial relationships are uncommon though the aorta can be directly anterior, right anterior or side by side and to the left of the pulmonary artery. Therefore rather than relying on the characteristic spatial arrangement of the great arteries to make the diagnosis, the arterial connection should be examined in detail. Examination from the subcostal region, with a moderate amount of anticlockwise rotation of the transducer, will show the aorta arising from the right ventricle and the pulmonary artery from the left ventricle. Similar information can be obtained from subcostal long axis views and serial

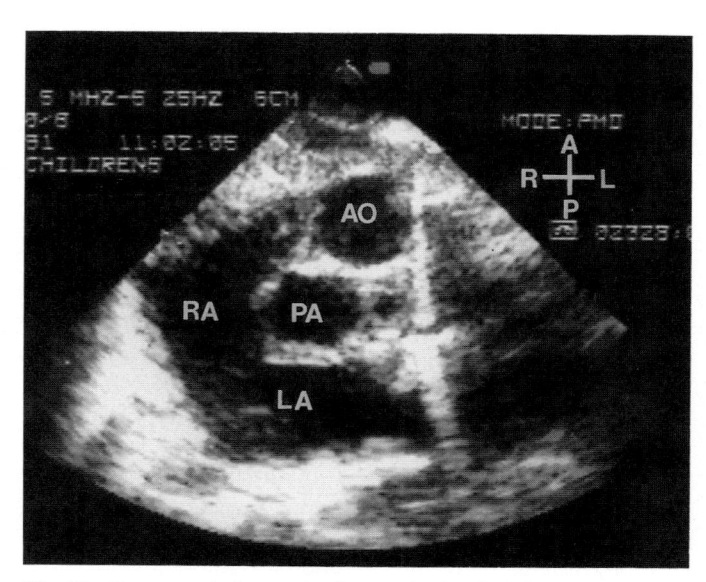

Fig. 19 Parasternal short axis view at the level of the great arteries in congenitally corrected transposition of the arteries. The aorta is anterior and to the left of the pulmonary artery.

parasternal short axis views, scanning from the base down to the apex. It should also be noted that the pulmonary outflow is 'wedged' between the atrioventricular valves and that the pulmonary valve is in fibrous continuity with the mitral valve (in a manner akin to that seen with the aortic valve in the normal heart).

The majority of patients with congenitally corrected transposition have associated defects that will need to be sought. These include ventricular septal defect, abnormalities of left and right atrioventricular valves, aortic and pulmonary outflow obstruction.

Corrected transposition with ventricular septal defect

Ventricular septal defect occurs in approximately 60% of patients with congenitally corrected transposition of the great arteries. The defect is usually perimembranous and may extend into the inlet or the outlet region of the interventricular septum. Inlet extension can best be appreciated from the apical four chamber view. The atrioventricular valves will be in fibrous continuity through the central fibrous body and will appear at the same level. Other features will need to be examined to determine the atrioventricular connection because the offsetting of the valves is lost, as described above. The tension apparatus of the valves should be carefully examined, as straddling may occur.[49]

Extension of a perimembranous defect into the outlet region is the most frequently seen type of ventricular septal defect. This produces a subpulmonary defect and the pulmonary valve frequently overrides the defect. These defects may be seen from subcostal long axis views or parasternal long axis views.

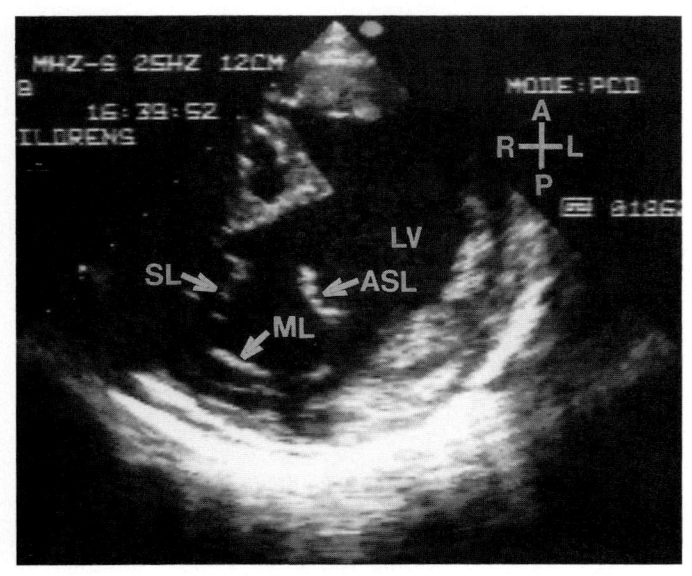

Fig. 18 Short axis parasternal view of the left atrioventricular valve in congenitally corrected transposition of the great arteries. The septal leaflet (SL), antero-superior leaflet (ASL) and mural leaflet (ML) are arrowed. The presence of a three leaflet valve and the coarse septal trabeculations are all features of atrioventricular discordance.

Muscular outlet defects, muscular trabecular defects and doubly committed subarterial defects occur rarely.

Corrected transposition with left ventricular outflow obstruction

Subpulmonary and pulmonary valve stenosis are frequently seen lesions, particularly if there is an associated ventricular septal defect[50] where it may result from rightwards deviation of the outlet septum. Pulmonary valve stenosis may occur, usually associated with subvalve stenosis, and rarely as an isolated lesion. Other forms of stenosis have been described and include hypertrophied muscle bands in the left ventricular outflow, fibrous diaphragmatic obstruction and aneurysmal tissue derived from the membranous septum that projects into the left ventricular outflow. Rarely there may be obstructive tissue tags originating from the pulmonary or atrioventricular valves.

Left ventricular outflow obstruction may be best seen from parasternal and subcostal long axis views. Doppler study can be used to quantitate the resulting pressure gradient. Optimal alignment is likely to be achieved from the subcostal approach.

Corrected transposition with abnormalities of the left atrioventricular valve

Abnormalities of the left atrioventricular valve (morphological tricuspid valve) are frequent and result in tricuspid regurgitation. Post-mortem studies have described valve anomalies in 90% of cases but clinically important valve regurgitation only develops in a third of cases. Minor degrees of valve dysplasia are difficult to diagnose on cross-sectional imaging. The use of colour flow Doppler examination is likely to increase the diagnostic yield (Plate 6). More severe degrees of valve dysplasia cause severe valve regurgitation, resulting in dilatation of the left atrium and right ventricle (Fig. 20). When of long standing there is likely to be pulmonary hypertension with consequent left ventricular hypertrophy.

The septal leaflet of the tricuspid valve may have short chordae and may be 'stuck down' to the septum. Occasionally a more severe malformation similar to Ebstein's anomaly may develop with displacement of the valve leaflets further into the right ventricle, leaving an atrialised portion of the right ventricle.[51]

The tricuspid valve morphology can best be examined from the apical four chamber view, supplemented by parasternal long and short axis views to view the attachments of the anterosuperior leaflet.

Rarely obstruction to the tricuspid valve may develop due to a supravalvar stenosing membrane, morphologically similar to that seen in association with the mitral valve when the atrioventricular connection is normal.[52]

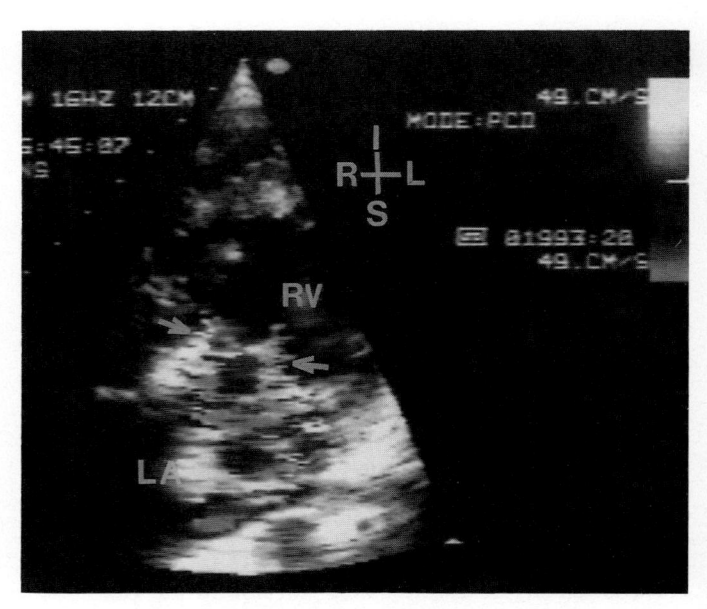

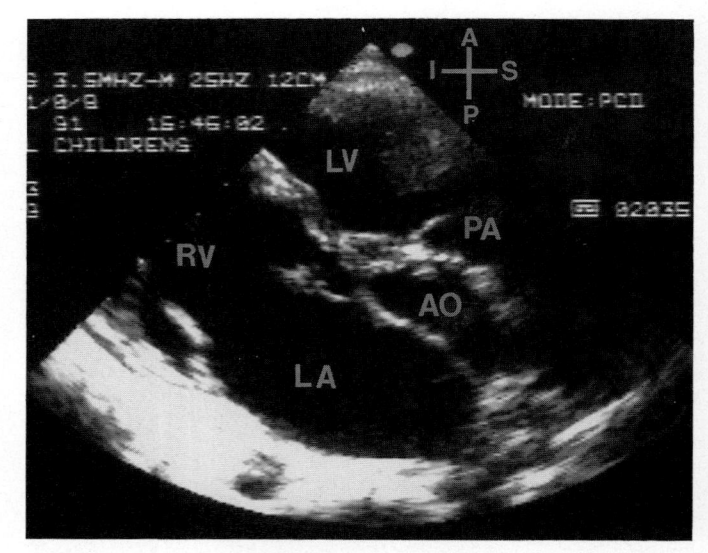

Plate 6 Severe left atrioventricular valve regurgitation in congenitally corrected transposition of the great arteries. Apical view showing two separate regurgitant jets (arrowed). This figure is reproduced in colour in the colour plate section at the front of this volume.

Fig. 20 Severe left atrioventricular valve regurgitation in congenitally corrected transposition of the great arteries. Modified parasternal long axis view showing left atrial and right ventricular dilatation.

Corrected transposition with right ventricular outflow obstruction

Subaortic stenosis may be found in a small number of patients. It usually results from infundibular hypertrophy or abnormal muscle bundles in the subaortic region. Its presence may be recognised from subcostal and parasternal long or short axis views.[52]

Aortic valve atresia, interruption of the aortic arch and coarctation of the aorta have also been described in association with corrected transposition. There is usually also an associated ventricular septal defect and malformation of the tricuspid valve when these associated lesions are present.[53] The aortic arch can be examined from high parasternal and suprasternal views. The course of the aortic arch is different to normal because of the usual left anterior position of the aorta; this requires slight modification of the normal aortic arch views.

DOUBLE OUTLET RIGHT VENTRICLE WITH ATRIOVENTRICULAR DISCORDANCE

The diagnosis of double outlet right ventricle in the setting of atrioventricular discordance, is made in a similar way to when there is a normal atrioventricular connection. The trabecular septum is orientated in a more sagittal plane so subcostal views will allow the relationships of the ventricular septal defect to be identified. The majority of the ventricular septal defects will be subpulmonary, though

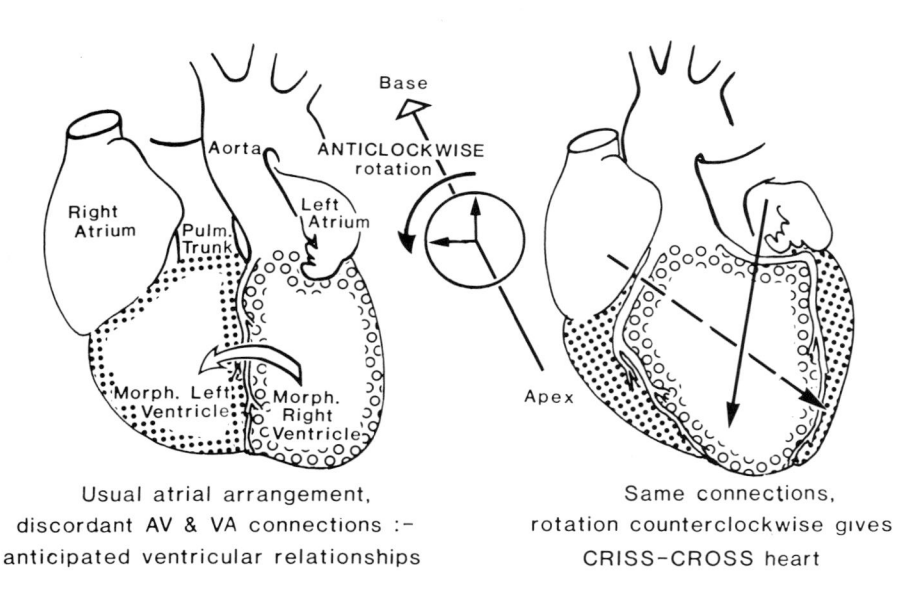

Fig. 21 Diagram illustrating the rotation along the long axis of the ventricular mass which produces a criss-cross arrangement in the setting of congenitally corrected transposition.

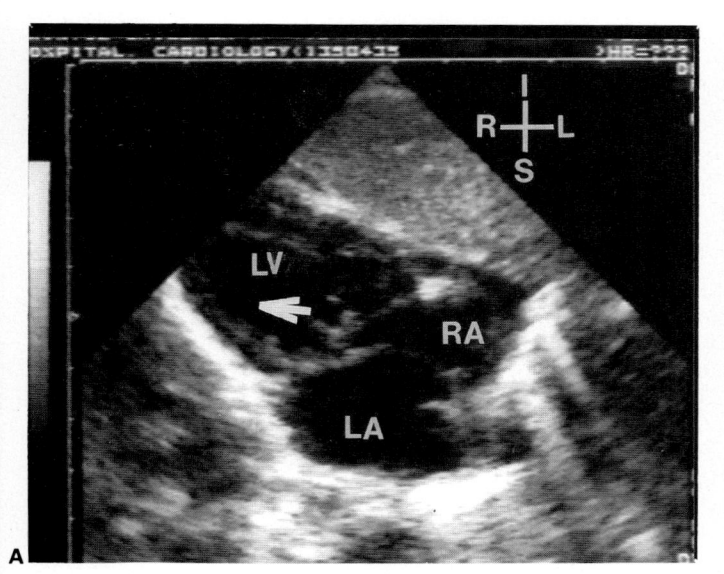

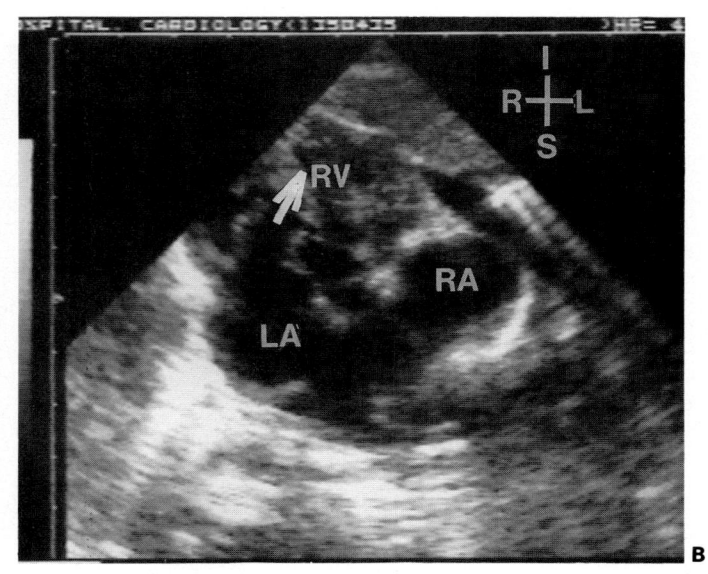

Fig. 22 Criss-cross atrioventricular connection in congenitally corrected transposition of the great arteries with situs inversus.
A: Subcostal 'four' chamber view shows an inverted atrial arrangement. The right atrium connects to the left ventricle and the arrow indicates the place of this connection. **B:** Superior angulation from A shows the left atrium connecting to the right ventricle. The plane of the atrioventricular connection is arrowed and comparison with A shows that it is at approximately 90° to the other atrioventricular connection. This contrasts to the normal heart where the planes of the atrioventricular connection run parallel to each other.

subaortic, non-committed and doubly-committed defects have been described. One well described group that deserves mention is the 'Mayo Clinic syndrome', where there is atrioventricular discordance, double outlet right ventricle, pulmonary stenosis, and dextrocardia.[54]

CRISS-CROSS ATRIOVENTRICULAR CONNECTION AND SUPERIOR-INFERIOR VENTRICLES

A criss-cross atrioventricular connection is characterised by rotation of the ventricular mass around its long axis, such that the line of the inlets cross each other, rather than being parallel to each other. This may occur with concordant or discordant atrioventricular connection. In congenitally corrected transposition with normal atrial arrangement, the morphological left ventricle is a right-sided structure with the morphological right ventricle lying to the left with the apex directed anteriorly. A criss-cross atrioventricular connection is associated with anticlockwise rotation of the ventricular mass such that the left ventricle becomes more left sided and posterior and the right ventricle moves to the right (Fig. 21). These positional changes of the chambers may be recognised on cross sectional imaging[55] (Fig. 22). A criss-cross atrioventricular connection may be seen when the ventricles are in a superior-inferior position.[56] Superior-inferior ventricles are common in congenitally corrected transposition and are produced by tilting of the ventricular mass along its long axis (Fig. 23).

The septum moves to a transverse plane with upwards tilting of the ventricular apex because of the sagittal orientation of the ventricular septum in congenitally corrected transposition. When the heart is left sided, this will leave the right ventricle superior to the left ventricle. There will usually be an associated ventricular septal defect, atrioventricular valve abnormality and pulmonary stenosis or atresia.

ATRIOVENTRICULAR DISCORDANCE WITH A CONCORDANT VENTRICULO-ARTERIAL CONNECTION

This rare anomaly presents with clinical features similar to that of complete transposition. There may be normal or mirror image arrangement of the atria. Echocardiography will show the discordant atrioventricular connection. The aorta will usually be posterior and to the right of the pulmonary trunk, and takes its origin from a right-sided morphological left ventricle (Fig. 24).

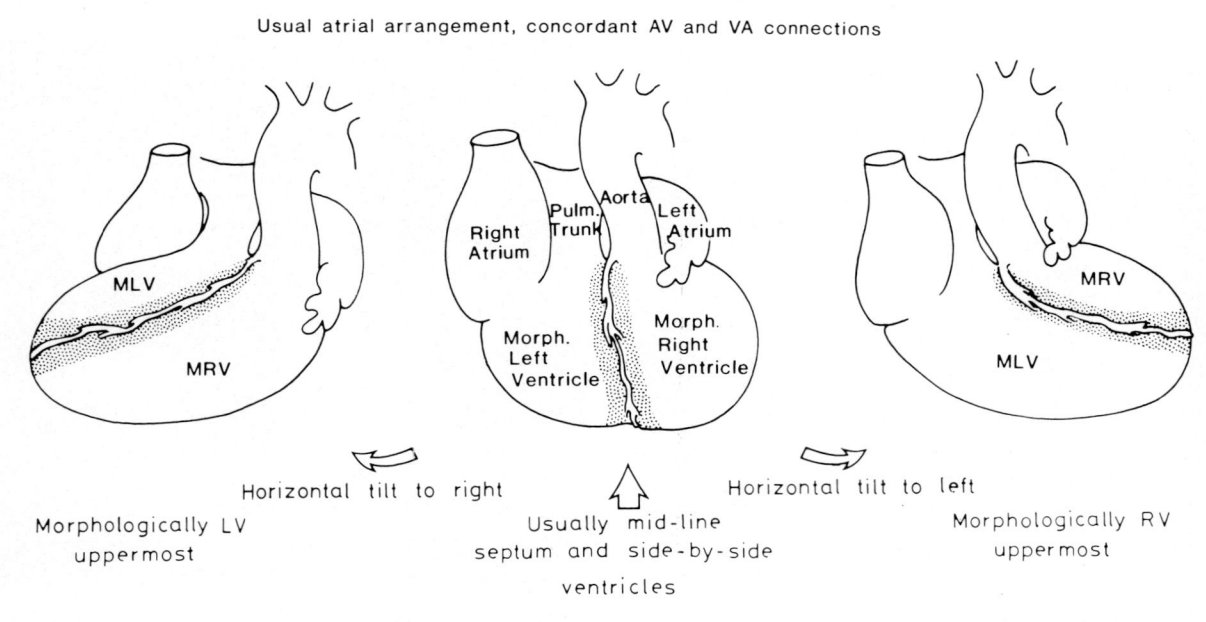

Fig. 23 The mechanisms involved in producing a superior-inferior arrangement of the ventricle in the setting of congenitally corrected transposition.

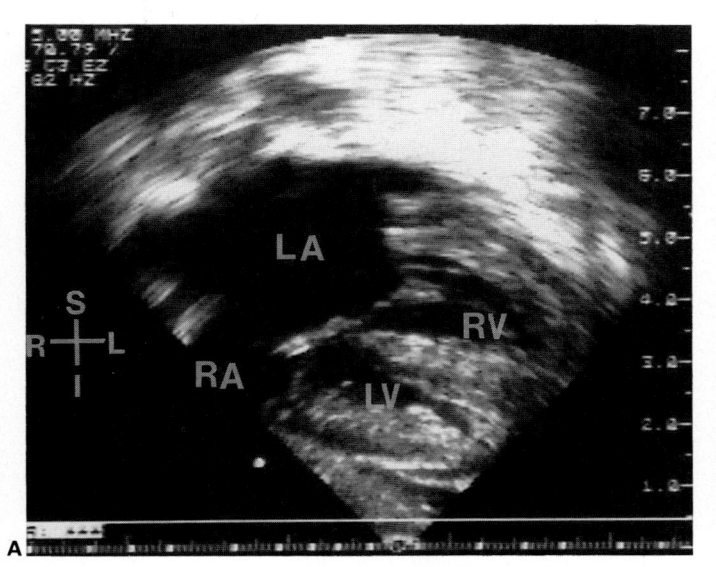

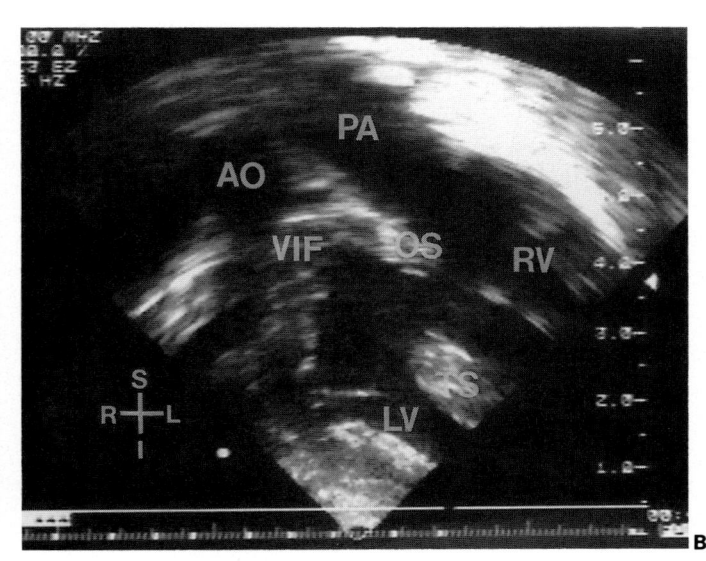

Fig. 24 **Atrioventricular discordance with ventriculo-arterial concordance. A:** Subcostal four chamber view demonstrating atrioventricular discordance. Note the septal attachment of the left atrioventricular valve is nearer the apex than the insertion of the right atrioventricular valve. **B:** Subcostal ventricular outflow view. The pulmonary artery connects to the right ventricle. The aorta overrides the trabecular septum (TS) and there is a malalignment ventricular septal defect with a right sided ventriculo-infundibular fold (VIF). OS – outlet septum.

REFERENCES

1 Dickinson D F, Arnold R, Wilkinson J L. Congenital heart disease among 1648 liveborn children in Liverpool 1960 to 1969. Implications for surgical treatment. Br Heart J 1981; 46: 55–62
2 Tynan M J, Becker A E, Macartney F J, Quero-Jiminez M, Shinebourne E A, Anderson R H. Nomenclature and classification of congenital heart disease. Br Heart J 1979; 41: 544
3 Anderson R H, Macartney F J, Shinebourne E A, Tynan M (eds) Paediatric cardiology. Edinburgh: Churchill Livingstone. 1987: p 831–837
4 Pasquini L, Sanders S P, Parness I A, Colan S D. Diagnosis of coronary artery anatomy by two-dimensional echocardiography in patients with transposition of the great arteries. Circulation 1987; 75: 557–564
5 Yacoub M H, Radley-Smith R. Anatomy of the coronary arteries in transposition of the great arteries and methods for their transfer in anatomical correction. Thorax 1978; 33: 418–424
6 Quaegebeur J M. The arterial switch operation: rationale, results, perspectives. MD thesis. Uitgeverij Rozengaard, Deerlijk (Belgium) 1986
7 Pedroni E, Batisse A, Sidi D, Villain E, Piechaud J F, Auriacombe L, Kachaner J. Estimation de la pression systolique du ventricule droite par l'etude echocardiographique de la geometrie ventriculaire gauche. Arch Mal Coeur 1986; 79: 701–707
8 Silverman N H, Hudson S. Evaluation of right ventricular volume and ejection fraction in children by two-dimensional echocardiography. Pediatr Cardiol 1983; 4: 197–203
9 Lange P E, Seiffert P A, Preis F et al. Value of image enhancement and injection of contrast medium for right ventricular volume determination by two-dimensional echocardiography in congenital heart disease. Am J Cardiol 1985; 55: 152–157
10 Trowitzsch E, Colan S D, Sanders S P. Global and regional right ventricular function in normal infants and infants with transposition of the great arteries after Senning operation. Circulation 1985; 72: 1008–1014
11 Satomi G, Nakazawa M, Takao A, Mori K, Touyama K, Konishi T, Tomimatsu H, Nakamura K. Blood flow pattern of the interatrial communication in patients with complete transposition of the great arteries: a pulsed Doppler echocardiographic study. Circulation 1986; 73: 95–99

12 Allan L D, Leanage R, Wainwright R, Joseph M C, Tynan M. Balloon atrial septostomy under two dimensional echocardiographic control. Br Heart J 1982; 47: 41–43
13 Baker E J, Allan L D, Tynan M J, Jones O D, Joseph M C, Deverall P B. Balloon atrial septostomy in the neonatal intensive care unit. Br Heart J 1984; 51: 377–378
14 Lin A E, Di Sessa T G, Williams R G. Balloon and blade atrial septostomy facilitated by two-dimensional echocardiography. Am J Cardiol 1986; 57: 273–277
15 Marino B, de Simone G, Pasquini L, Giannico S, Marceletti C, Ammirati A, Guccione P, Boldrini R, Ballerini L. Complete transposition of the great arteries: visualisation of left and right outflow tract obstruction by oblique two-dimensional echocardiography. Am J Cardiol 1985; 55: 1140–1145
16 Yacoub M H, Arensman F W, Keck E, Radley-Smith R. Fate of dynamic left ventricular outflow tract obstruction after anatomic correction of transposition of the great arteries. Circulation 1983; 68: 1156–1162
17 Johnson G L, Cottrill C M, Noonan J A. False diagnosis of subpulmonary obstruction by echocardiography in d-transposition of the great arteries. Am J Cardiol 1982; 49: 1984–1989
18 Robinson P J, Wyse R K, Macartney F J. Left ventricular outflow tract obstruction in complete transposition of the great arteries with intact ventricular septum. A cross sectional echocardiography study. Br Heart J 1985; 54: 201–208
19 Rastelli G C, Wallace R B, Ongley P A. Complete repair of transposition of the great arteries with pulmonary stenosis. A review and report of a case corrected by using a new surgical technique. Circulation 1969; 39: 83–95
20 Vogel M, Freedom R M, Smallhorn J F, Williams W G, Trusler G A, Rowe R D. Complete transposition of the great arteries: a review. Pediatr Cardiol 1984; 53: 1627–1632
21 Graham T P Jr. Hemodynamic residuae and sequelae following intra-atrial repair of transposition of the great arteries: a review. Pediatr Cardiol 1982; 2: 203–213
22 Deal B J, Chin A J, Sanders S P, Norwood W I, Casteneda A R. Subxiphoid two-dimensional echocardiographic identification of tricuspid valve abnormalities in transposition of the great arteries with ventricular septal defect. Am J Cardiol 1985; 55: 1146–1151

23 Chin A J, Sanders S P, Williams R G, Lang P, Norwood W I, Casteneda A R. Two-dimensional echocardiographic assessment of caval and pulmonary venous pathways after the Senning operation. Am J Cardiol 1983; 52: 118–126
24 Silverman N H, Snider A R, Colo J, Ebert P A, Turley K. Superior vena caval obstruction after Mustard's operation: detection by two-dimensional contrast echocardiography. Circulation 1981; 64: 392–396
25 Stevenson J G, Kawabori I, Guntheroth W G, Dooley T K, Dillard D. Pulsed Doppler echocardiographic detection of obstruction of systemic venous return after repair of transposition of the great arteries. Circulation 1979; 60: 1091–1096
26 Satomi G, Nakamura K, Takao A, Imai Y. Two-dimensional echocardiographic detection of pulmonary venous channel stenosis after Senning's operation. Circulation 1983; 68: 545–549
27 Smallhorn J F, Gow R, Freedom R M, Trusler G A, Olley P, Pacquet M, Gibbons J, Vlad P. Pulsed Doppler echocardiographic assessment of the pulmonary venous pathway after the Mustard or Senning procedure for transposition of the great arteries. Circulation 1986; 73: 765–774
28 Chin A J, Sanders S P, Norwood W I, Casteneda A R. Two-dimensional echocardiographic localisation of residual atrial shunts after the Senning procedure. Am J Cardiol 1985; 55: 1238–1239
29 Colan S D, Trowitzsch E, Wernovsky G, Sholler G F, Sanders S P, Casteneda A R. Myocardial performance after arterial switch operation for transposition of the great arteries with intact ventricular septum. Circulation 1988; 78: 132–141
30 Borow K M, Arensman F W, Webb C, Radley-Smith R, Yacoub M H. Assessment of left ventricular contractile state after anatomic correction of transposition of the great arteries. Circulation 1984; 69: 106–112
31 Arensman F W, Radley-Smith R, Yacoub M H, Lange P, Bernhard A, Sievers H H, Heintzen P. Catheter evaluation of left ventricular shape and function 1 or more years after anatomic correction of transposition of the great arteries. Am J Cardiol 1983; 52: 1079–1083
32 Gibbs J L, Qureshi S A, Grieve L, Webb C, Smith R R, Yacoub M H. Doppler echocardiography after anatomical correction of transposition of the great arteries. Br Heart J 1986; 56: 67–72
33 Martin M M, Snider A R, Bove E L, Serwer G A, Rosenthal A, Peters J, Pollock P. Two-dimensional and Doppler echocardiographic evaluation after arterial switch repair in infancy for complete transposition of the great arteries. Am J Cardiol 1989; 63: 332–336
34 Gibbs J L, Qureshi S A, Wilson N, Smith R R, Yacoub M H. Doppler echocardiographic comparison of haemodynamic results of one- and two-stage anatomic correction of complete transposition. Int J Cardiol 1988; 18: 85–92
35 Graham T P Jr, Franklin R C, Wyse R K, Gooch V, Deanfield J E. Left ventricular wall stress and contractile function in transposition of the great arteries after the Rastelli operation. J Thorac Cardiovasc Surg 1987; 93: 775–784
36 Wilkinson J L. Double outlet ventricle. In: Anderson R H, Macartney F J, Shinebourne E A, Tynan M. eds. Paediatric cardiology. Edinburgh: Churchill Livingstone. 1987: p 889–991
37 Anderson R H, Becker A E, Wilcox B R, Macartney F J, Wilkinson J L. Surgical anatomy of double outlet right ventricle – a reappraisal. Am J Cardiol 1983; 52: 555–559
38 Macartney F J, Rigby M L, Anderson R H, Stark J, Silverman N H. Double outlet right ventricle. Cross sectional echocardiographic findings, their anatomical explanation and surgical relevance. Br Heart J 1984; 52: 164–177

39 Henry W L, Maron B J, Griffith J M. Cross sectional echocardiography in the diagnosis of congenital heart disease. Identification of the relation of the ventricles and great arteries. Circulation 1977; 56: 267–273
40 Hagler D J, Tajik A J, Seward J B, Mair D D, Ritter D G. Double outlet right ventricle: wide-angle two-dimensional echocardiographic observations. Circulation 1981; 63: 419–428
41 Sanders S P, Bierman F Z, Williams R G. Conotruncal malformations: diagnosis in infancy using subxiphoid two-dimensional echocardiography. Am J Cardiol 1982; 50: 1361–1367
42 Taussig H B, Bing R J. Complete transposition of the aorta and a levoposition of the pulmonary artery. Am Heart J 1949; 37: 551–559
43 Sondheimer H M, Freedom R M, Olley P M. Double inlet right ventricle: clinical spectrum and prognosis. Am J Cardiol 1977; 39: 709–714
44 MacMahon H E, Lipa M. Double outlet right ventricle with intact interventricular septum. Circulation 1964; 30: 745–748
45 Otero-Coto, Quero Jimenez M, Castaneda A R, Rufilanchas J J, Deverall P B. Double outlet from chambers of left ventricular morphology. Br Heart J 1979; 42: 15–21
46 Van Praagh R, Weinberg M D. Double outlet left ventricle. In: Moss A J, Adams F H, Emmanoulides M D. eds. Heart disease in infants, children and adolescents, 2nd Edn. Baltimore: Williams & Wilkins. 1977
47 Hagler D J, Tajik A J, Seward J B, Ritter D G. Atrioventricular and ventriculoarterial discordance (corrected transposition of the great arteries). Wide-angle two-dimensional echocardiographic assessment of ventricular morphology. Mayo Clin Proc 1981; 56: 591–600
48 Sutherland G R, Smallhorn J F, Anderson R H, Rigby M L, Hunter S. Atrioventricular discordance; cross sectional echocardiographic-morphological correlative study. Br Heart J 1983; 50: 8–20
49 Becker A E, Ho S Y, Caruso G, Milo S, Anderson R H. Straddling right atrioventricular valves in atrioventricular discordance. Circulation 1980; 61: 1133–1141
50 Anderson R H, Becker A E, Gerlis L M. The pulmonary outflow tract in classically corrected transposition. J Thorac Cardiovasc Surg 1975; 69: 747–757
51 Anderson K R, Danielson G, McGoon D C, Lie J T. Ebstein's anomaly of the left sided tricuspid valve; pathological anatomy of the valvular malformation. Circulation 1978; 58: 87–91
52 Marino B, Sanders S P, Parness I A, Colan S D. Obstruction of right ventricular inflow and outflow in corrected transposition of the great arteries (S, L, L): two-dimensional echocardiographic diagnosis. J Am Coll Cardiol 1986; 8: 407–411
53 Craig B G, Smallhorn J F, Rowe R D, Williams W G, Trusler G A, Freedom R A. Severe obstruction to systemic blood flow in congenitally corrected transposition (discordant atrioventricular and ventriculo-arterial connexions): an analysis of 14 patients. Int J Cardiol 1986; 11: 209–217
54 Kiser J C, Ongley P A, Kirklin J W, Clarkson P M, McGoon D C. Surgical treatment of dextrocardia with inversion of ventricles and double outlet right ventricle. J Thorac Cardiovasc Surg 1968; 55: 6–15
55 Robinson P J, Kumping V, Macartney F J. Cross sectional echocardiographic correlation in criss-cross hearts. Br Heart J 1985; 54: 61–67
56 Hery E, Jiminez M, Didier D, van Doesburg N H, Guerin R, Fouron J C, Davignon A. Echocardiographic and angiographic findings in superior-inferior cardiac ventricles. Am J Cardiol 1989; 63: 1385–1389

23

Right sided obstructions and malformations

Isolated right ventricular outflow tract obstruction
Pathology
Echocardiography
   Pulmonary valve stenosis
   Isolated subvalve pulmonary stenosis
   Supravalve pulmonary artery stenosis

Tetralogy of Fallot
Pathology
Echocardiography
Pulmonary atresia with ventricular septal defect
Pathology
Echocardiography

Pulmonary atresia with intact ventricular septum
Echocardiographic assessment
Ebstein's malformation
Pathology
Echocardiography

Michael J. Godman

ISOLATED RIGHT VENTRICULAR OUTFLOW TRACT OBSTRUCTION

Pathology

Obstruction to the right ventricular outflow tract may be (1) valvular, (2) subvalvular, (3) supravalvular. Although all three forms can be associated with more complex congenital heart disease this section focuses on isolated varieties.

The typical features of pulmonary valve stenosis are usually the consequence of fusion of three well-developed commissures with thickening of the valve cusps and a dome-like appearance. There is a wide spectrum of abnormality from only partial fusion of the commissures to an imperforate valve with intact ventricular septum.[1] The valve may be unicuspid or bicuspid and rarely can be formed by four leaves. The pulmonary valve annulus and valve sinuses are usually of normal size. In pulmonary valve stenosis there is usually post-stenotic dilatation of the main pulmonary artery and the left pulmonary artery. The left pulmonary artery dilatation is always much more marked than that of the right because of the preferential flow from the main to the left pulmonary artery which takes off at a much more acute angle to the main trunk than the right. An uncommon form of pulmonary valve obstruction is pulmonary valve dysplasia which may be associated with Noonan's syndrome. The valve leaflets are thickened and rigid and myomatous but there is usually no commissural fusion.[2] As a consequence of the pulmonary valve obstruction there is concentric hypertrophy of the right ventricle. In addition, in more marked degrees of valve obstruction there may also be hypertrophy of the infundibular septum, the anterior wall of the right ventricular and of the septo-marginal trabecula (see tetralogy of Fallot) producing severe secondary infundibular stenosis. If the pulmonary valve stenosis is satisfactorily relieved by surgery or balloon dilatation, this secondary infundibular stenosis usually resolves.[3]

Less commonly than valve stenosis, subvalvular infundibular stenosis can exist as an isolated abnormality and may be the consequence either of a discrete obstruction from a fibromuscular ring at the proximal end of the infundibulum or from an anomalous muscle bundle bisecting the right ventricle to produce a double chamber. This anomalous muscle bundle is principally composed of an abnormal hypertrophied moderator band and septo-marginal trabeculations which cross the right ventricle in a perpendicular plane to the septum inserting into the right ventricle. More distally the infundibulum, pulmonary valve annulus and pulmonary valve are normal.

Supravalve pulmonary arterial stenosis may be produced by one or more anomalies producing obstruction of the pulmonary arterial tree at the level of the main pulmonary artery, its two branches or more peripherally within the segments of these branches. Stenosis involving the main pulmonary artery alone is rare and may be caused by a fibrous ring or diaphragm immediately above the pulmonary valve sinuses. More commonly, stenosis of the main pulmonary artery is characterised by tubular hypoplasia and is associated with lesions at the bifurcation of the pulmonary trunk into its right and left branches and more distally in the pulmonary artery segments. Some of these stenoses may be the result of intrauterine infection with the Rubella virus or may be seen with William's Syndrome, which is an association of hypercalcaemia, often transiently in infancy, supravalve aortic stenosis and peripheral pulmonary arterial lesions.

Echocardiography

Pulmonary valve stenosis

The main pulmonary valve annulus and pulmonary valve leaflets are best displayed in the parasternal short axis views at the base of the heart or the parasternal right ventricular long-axis view. It is usually, though not invariably, possible to make some assessment of the pulmonary valve leaflet morphology and identify thickening and characteristic doming of the pulmonary valve leaflets in systole (Fig. 1). The apical four-chamber view allows assessment of the degree of hypertrophy of the right ventricle and in patients with severe valve obstruction this view may also show the right atrium to be dilated and the atrial septum may bulge from right to left as a consequence of the elevated right atrial pressure secondary to the thickened non-compliant right ventricle. Further assessment of right ventricular thickness can be made from parasternal

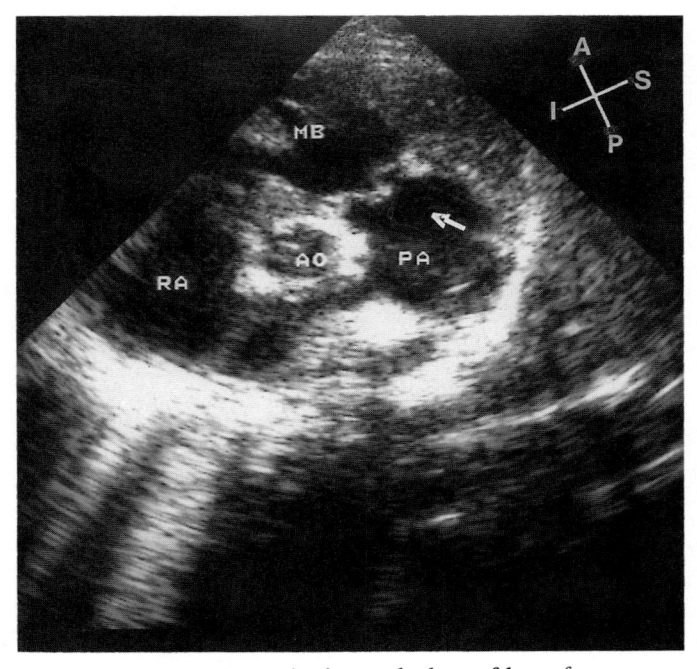

Fig. 1 Parasternal short axis view at the base of heart from a 1 year old with pulmonary valve stenosis and secondary infundibular obstruction. (Moderator band – MB)

short axis views and in the subcostal four-chamber and right coronal and sagittal views of the right ventricle (Figs 2A and B). These views are also helpful in assessing the degree of hypertrophy of the right ventricular outflow tract secondary to the valve stenosis. As indicated it may not be possible in all cases to come to a definitive diagnosis of pulmonary valve stenosis by cross sectional imaging alone, particularly if there are no associated structural changes such as secondary infundibular hypertrophy and post stenotic dilatation. The pattern of motion of the pulmonary valve leaflets in pulmonary valve stenosis has been analysed and compared with normals and the differences in systole and diastole were reported by Weyman and colleagues.[4] In 36% of Weyman's patients there was inadequate visualisation of both leaflets. Others have also emphasised the difficulty in prospectively diagnosing pulmonary valve stenosis using cross-sectional imaging. A false diagnosis occurs with sufficient frequency to make pulmonary valve stenosis amongst the more difficult of the common congenital cardiovascular lesions to predict on the basis of imaging alone.[5]

The accuracy of diagnosis of pulmonary valve stenosis has improved considerably since the development of Doppler echocardiography. Pulsed and continuous wave Doppler techniques have become the principal methods for assessing the severity of obstruction in pulmonary valve and infundibular pulmonary stenosis. Excellent correlations have been found between measurements made in the catheter laboratory of peak-to-peak pressure gradients and the Doppler derived peak instantaneous pressure gradients across the valve. Since the instantaneous gradient is greatest in early systole, peak-to-peak and instantaneous pressure measurements are obviously not directly comparable but this has proved to be less of a problem with pulmonary stenosis than with aortic stenosis: the differences that have been found between the maximum instantaneous and peak-to-peak pressure gradient in pulmonary valve stenosis are less than those in aortic valve stenosis. These good correlations between catheter and Doppler measurements occur not only pre-operatively but also following surgical valvotomy or balloon angioplasty. Doppler sampling can be performed either with a non-imaging continuous wave probe or with a steerable imaging probe. Doppler recordings of the flow velocity across the pulmonary valve are best obtained from the parasternal short axis views, the parasternal long axis views of the right ventricular outflow tract and the subcostal views of the right ventricle. Examination normally begins using the pulsed Doppler mode with the sample volume in the right ventricular outflow tract proximal to the pulmonary valve. The sample volume is then moved distally into the main pulmonary artery and its branches, with care being taken to minimise the angle of incidence between the Doppler signal and the main axis of the pulmonary trunk. This method allows a distinction between increased flow

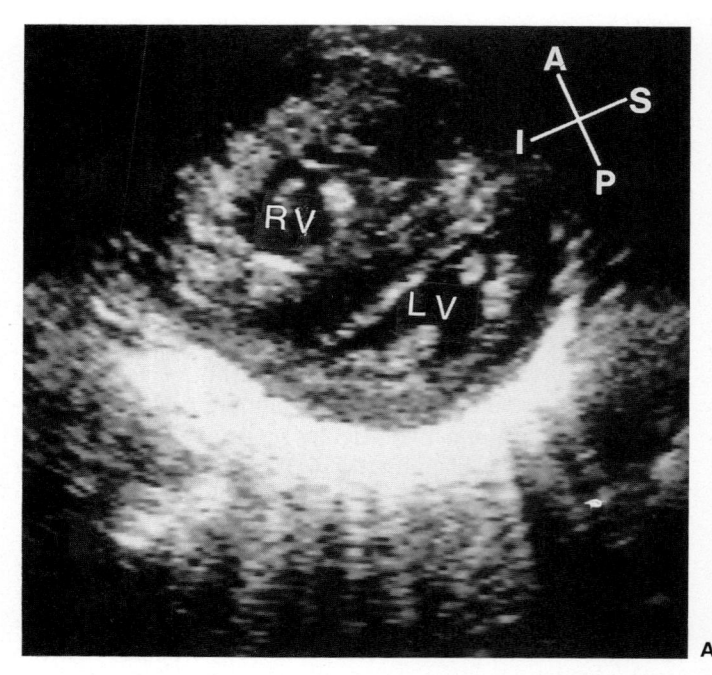

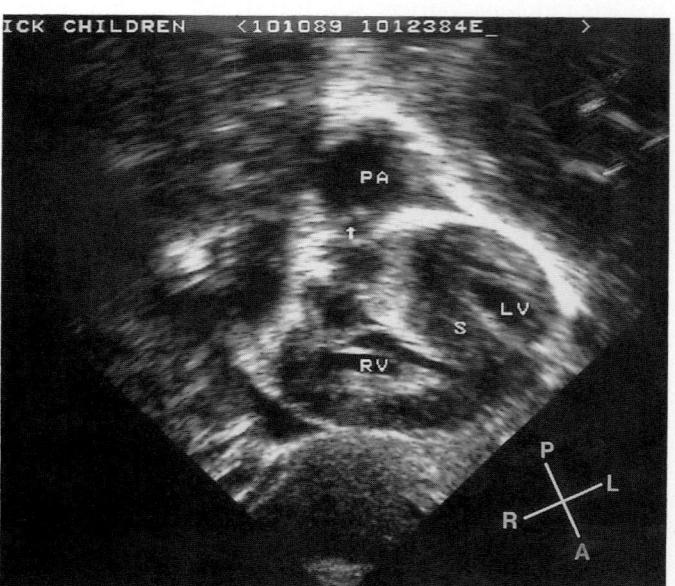

Fig. 2 **A:** Precordial short axis view demonstrating right ventricular hypertrophy. **B:** Subcostal view of right ventricular hypertrophy. S – septum. Arrow points to pulmonary valve.

velocities that may be the consequence of either pulmonary obstruction or increased flow as a consequence of a left to right shunt and also allows determination of the precise level at which the increased flow velocity occurred. Continuous wave Doppler recordings are used to determine the peak velocity of any jets (Fig. 3). The importance of recording the flow velocities from as wide a variety of echocardiographic windows as possible cannot be overemphasised for it is the highest peak velocity which is used to calculate the peak instantaneous pressure gradient across

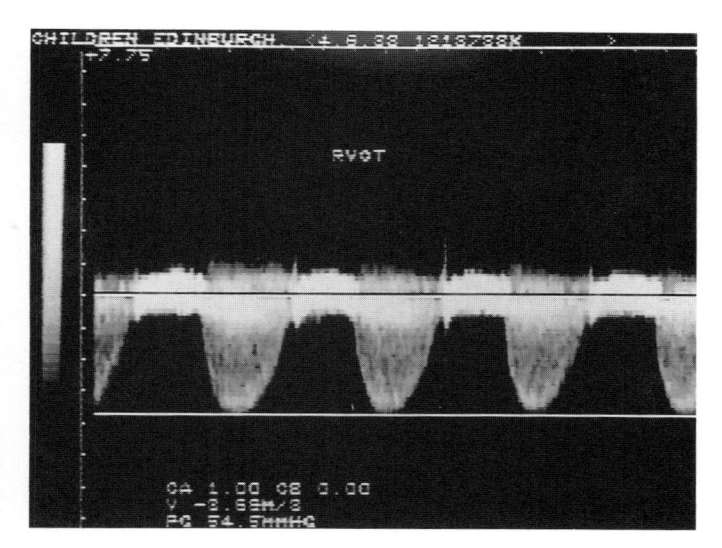

Fig. 3 Continuous wave Doppler examination of the right ventricular outflow tract in a patient with pulmonary valve stenosis. There is a high velocity jet below the base line with a peak velocity of 3.69 m/s and a peak pressure gradient of 54 mmHg.

the pulmonary valve.[6–8] In some patients this may be a high parasternal view and in others a subcostal view. Colour flow mapping may assist in the recognition of maximal flow velocities and again can be performed from the parasternal and subcostal transducer position (Plate 1).

The peak gradient across the valve is calculated by converting the recording of peak flow velocity utilising the modified Bernoulli equation – $PG = 4V^2$ with PG denoting instantaneous pressure gradient in mmHg and V the peak Doppler velocity in m/s. When the velocities proximal to the valve are calculated as greater than 1 m/s then the expanded Bernoulli equation should be used to reduce errors in predicting the peak gradients[6] (see Ch. 6). Under or over estimates of the Doppler derived peak gradient may occur in a number of situations. In the newborn with critical pulmonary stenosis, there may be very poor right ventricular function with reduced right ventricular stroke volume and reduced pulmonary blood flow secondary to shunting at atrial level. In these circumstances flow across the valve is obviously not likely to correlate with the severity of any obstruction. In the newborn this problem may be compounded by flow of a ductus arteriosus resulting in elevation of the pulmonary artery pressure and a further reduction in any pressure gradient between the right ventricle and main pulmonary artery. Over-estimation by the Doppler technique as compared with catheterisation measured peak-to-peak gradient can occur when severe secondary infundibular obstruction occurs secondary to the valve stenosis.

Isolated subvalve pulmonary stenosis

Intracavity obstruction of the right ventricle either from a discrete lesion within the ostium of the infundibulum or from muscle bundles within the right ventricle are best imaged from the subcostal right anterior oblique view complemented by the parasternal short axis and long axis right ventricular views[9] (Fig. 4).

Supravalve pulmonary artery stenosis

Lesions involving the main pulmonary artery and its two artery branches can be assessed by imaging. More peripheral distal lesions within the segmental branches may not

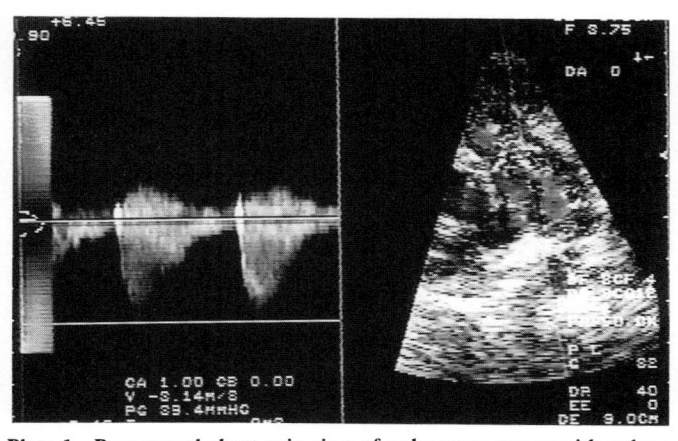

Plate 1 Parasternal short axis view of pulmonary artery with colour flow mapping to guide continuous wave recording and recognition of maximal flow velocities. This figure is reproduced in colour in the colour plate section at the front of this volume.

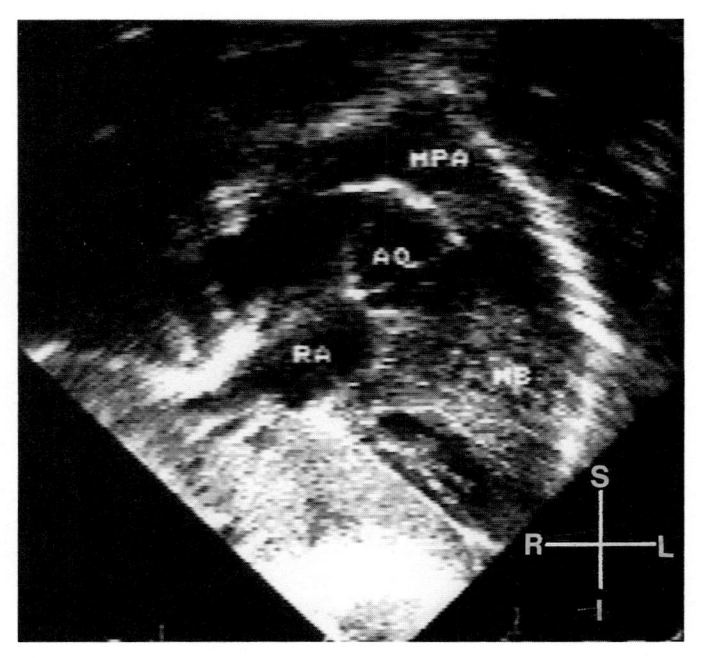

Fig. 4 Subcostal right anterior oblique view illustrating intracavitary obstruction from right muscle bundle. MB – muscle bundle.

be imaged directly although there may be secondary findings such as right ventricular hypertrophy and increased pulsatility of the proximal pulmonary artery branches which may suggest this diagnosis. Discrete lesions within the main pulmonary artery are best seen on the standard subcostal views of the right ventricle, the parasternal short axis planes and the parasternal long axis of the right ventricle. These views also identify more diffuse hypoplasia of the main pulmonary artery and lesions of the origin of the right and left pulmonary artery. From the suprasternal notch the right pulmonary artery can be seen in the long axis view throughout its length whereas only the proximal portion of the left pulmonary artery can be seen. Colour flow mapping may identify localised areas of narrowing.

TETRALOGY OF FALLOT

Pathology

Although the tetralogy of Fallot is characterised by four abnormalities – ventricular septal defect, stenosis of the right ventricular outflow tract, biventricular origin of the aorta and right ventricular hypertrophy, the anatomical hallmark of the condition is the abnormal position of the infundibular septum which is deviated anterosuperiorly.[10] In the normal heart the infundibular septum separates the subaortic and subpulmonary areas and sits between the limbs of the septo-marginal trabecula and is fused with the ventriculo infundibular fold (Fig. 5). In the tetralogy of Fallot the infundibular septum characteristically is deviated anterosuperiorly and lies in a position anterior to the limbs of the septo-marginal trabecula. This deviation separates the infundibular septum from the ventriculo-infundibular fold producing not only narrowing of the right ventricular

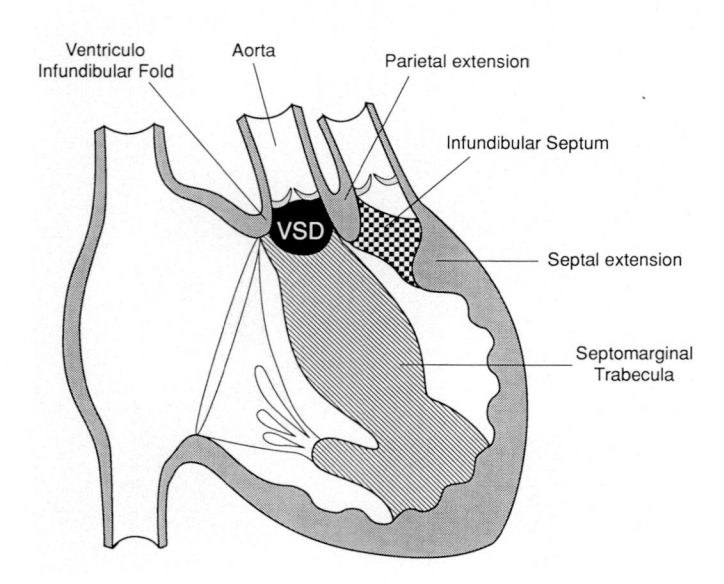

Fig. 5 Anatomy of right ventricular outflow tract and its component parts (see text) in tetralogy of Fallot.

outflow tract but the creation of a ventricular septal defect and anterior and rightward displacement of the aorta with the production of overriding of the aorta.[11] The obstruction in the right ventricular outflow tract produced by the deviation of the infundibular septum is accentuated by hypertrophy of the infundibular septum and by hypertrophy of the anterior wall of the infundibulum. Additionally, in approximately two thirds of cases, there may be stenosis of the pulmonary valve itself, usually on the basis of a bicuspid valve. The ventricular septal defect in tetralogy of Fallot is therefore usually a malalignment defect either of the perimembraneous or muscular infundibular type. More rarely, it may be subarterial. The most common is the perimembraneous ventricular septal defect in which the posterior inferior margin is the area of aortic mitral tricuspid continuity. It is bounded superiorly by the infundibular septum and to the left by the trabecula septum. On the left ventricular side the defect is located directly below the right and non-coronary cusps of the aortic valve. The muscular infundibular/ventricular septal defect associated with tetralogy of Fallot is similar to the perimembraneous type but has a muscular posterior inferior rim which separates the defect from the tricuspid valve. This type of defect is seen in about 20% of cases of tetralogy of Fallot. More rarely, and commoner in the Far East than in the Western World, are subarterial defects in tetralogy of Fallot. In these the defect is roofed by the arterial valves, the muscular boundaries are formed by the trabecula septum and the infundibular septum is usually severely hypoplastic.[12] In addition to subpulmonary stenosis the main pulmonary artery and right and left pulmonary arteries may be hypoplastic or indeed in the most extreme form of tetralogy of Fallot atretic. In particular, generalised hypoplasia of the pulmonary arterial tree is seen frequently. Discrete stenosis may exist at the origin of the right and left pulmonary arteries from the main pulmonary artery, more frequently the left than the right.

There are a number of cardiovascular abnormalities which are commonly found in association with tetralogy of Fallot and it is important to identify them because they may complicate the management.[13] These include atrioventricular septal defects, absence of the pulmonary valve and stenosis of the pulmonary arteries. There may be additional ventricular septal defects in the muscular trabecula or apical muscular septum. There may be persistence of the ductus arteriosus or a left sided superior vena cava. In 5 to 10% of cases there may be an aberrant origin of the left anterior descending coronary artery from the right coronary artery.

Echocardiography

Initial echocardiographic assessment of the tetralogy of Fallot usually begins with examination from the parasternal long axis view which displays the ventricular septal defect

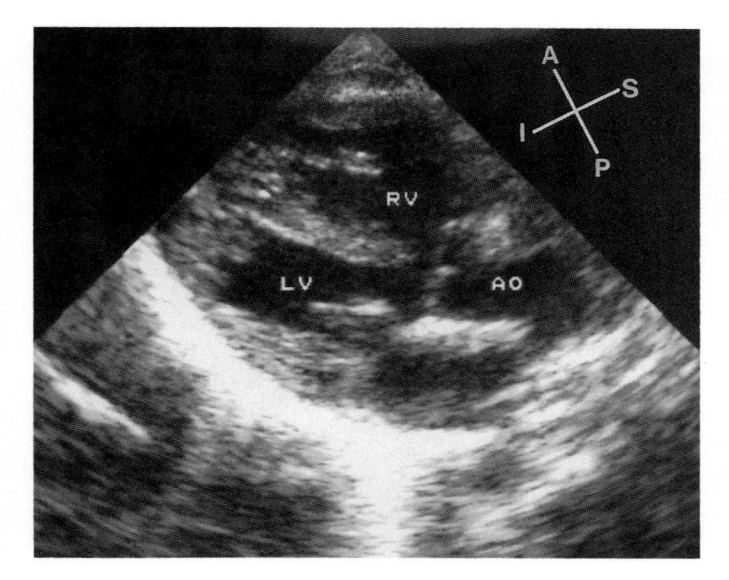

Fig. 6 Parasternal long axis view in tetralogy of Fallot.

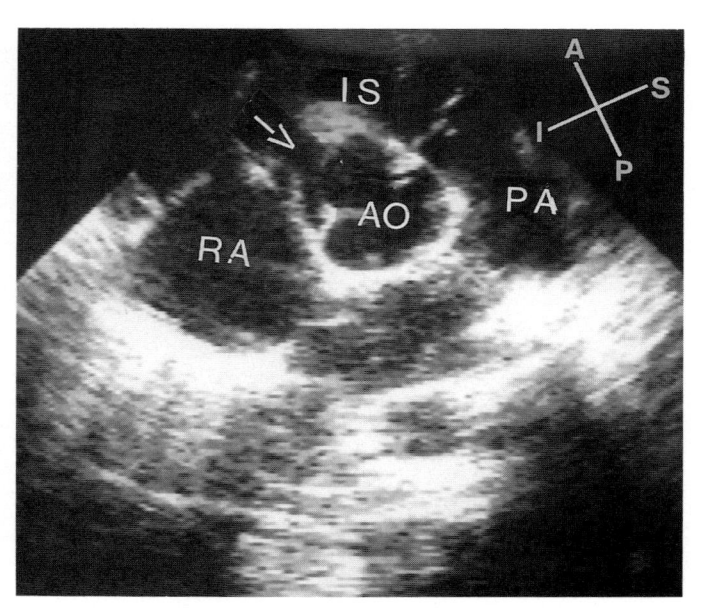

Fig. 7 Parasternal short axis view of perimembranous outlet ventricular septal defect in tetralogy of Fallot. Arrow to ventricular septal defect. IS – infundibular septum.

and the degree of overriding of the ventricular septum by the aorta (Fig. 6). Other views including the four-chamber aortic root and subcostal long axis projections should also be utilised in assessing the degree of overriding but it is important to remember that this feature is not diagnostic for the tetralogy of Fallot.[14,15] It may, for example, also be seen in pulmonary atresia with ventricular septal defect, truncus arteriosus and malalignment forms of ventricular septal defect. In the parasternal long axis views additional defects in the trabecula septum may also be visualised and the presence or absence of aortic mitral continuity can be determined. The morphology of the ventricular septal defect is best seen in the parasternal short axis view which allows differentiation between the usual perimembraneous ventricular septal defect and the rarer infundibular muscular defect or the even more uncommon doubly committed subarterial defect which may be seen in association with the tetralogy of Fallot (Fig. 7). Occasionally in the membraneous ventricular septal defect tricuspid tissue may be identified plugging the margins of the defect resulting in suprasystemic right ventricular pressure.[16] The parasternal short axis view also allows evaluation of the severity of and the extent of right ventricular outflow tract narrowing and obstruction (Fig. 8). Assessment should be made of the relative contribution of infundibular, valvular and arterial narrowing to the obstruction. In some cases the obstruction may be very proximal and the distal infundibulum, pulmonary valve annulus and main pulmonary artery may be well developed. The main pulmonary artery and its bifurcation to the right and left pulmonary arteries are better visualised from a higher parasternal short axis cut (Fig. 9). In this view it is easier to assess the morphology of the pulmonary valve leaflets and the distinction can be made between severe obstruction with antegrade flow and pulmonary valve atresia with and without infundibular atresia. Doppler echocardiography should be performed to assess antegrade systolic and retrograde diastolic flow and this assessment should be augmented by colour flow mapping. This view is valuable in identifying that small number of patients with tetralogy of Fallot who have complete absence of the pulmonary valve leaflets. In this

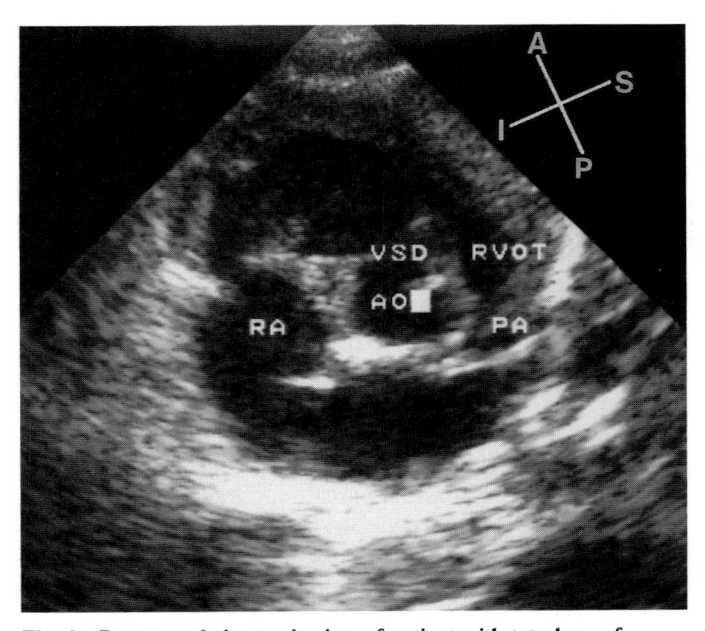

Fig. 8 Parasternal short axis view of patient with tetralogy of Fallot and infundibular muscular ventricular septal defect and narrowing of right ventricular outflow tract. VSD – ventricular septal defect. RVOT – right ventricular outflow tract.

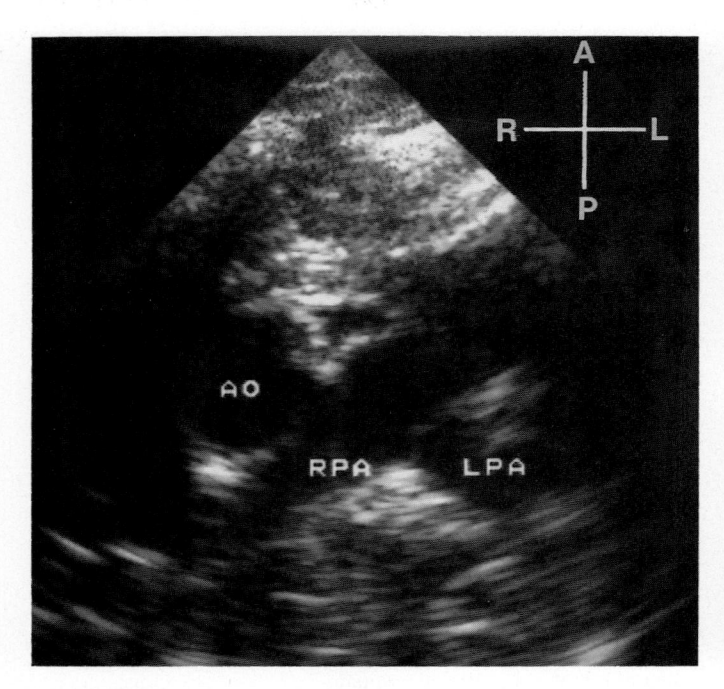

Fig. 9 High parasternal short axis view in patient with tetralogy of Fallot and normal bifurcation of right and left pulmonary arteries.

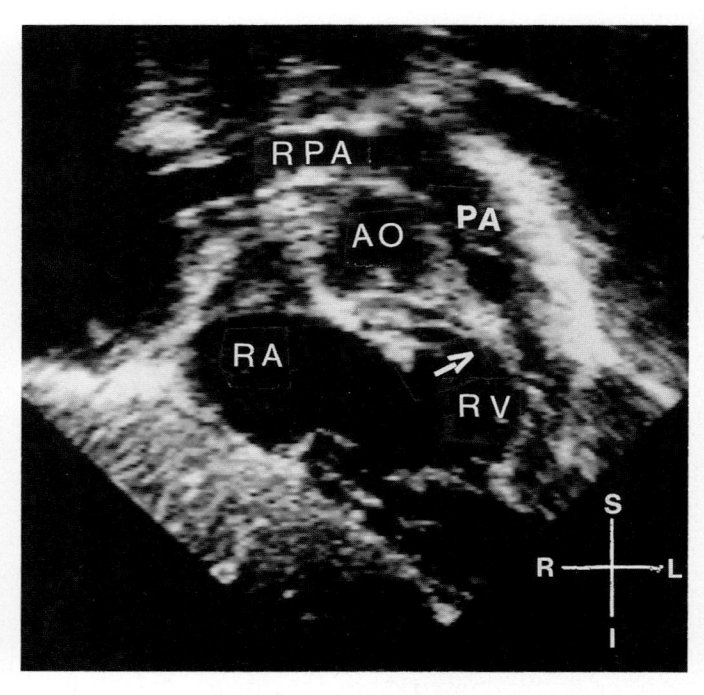

Fig. 10 Subcostal right coronal (anterior oblique view) of right ventricular outflow tract in tetralogy of Fallot. Arrow indicates anterior deviation of outlet septum. RPA – right pulmonary artery.

condition the main and right and left pulmonary arteries are usually grossly dilated as a consequence of the severe pulmonary regurgitation.

In the short axis view the bifurcation of the left main coronary artery may also be seen thus excluding the possibility that the left anterior descending coronary artery arises anomalously from the right coronary artery. This anomalous vessel may occasionally be visualised running anterior to the right ventricular outflow tract or in the parasternal short axis view.

The subcostal right coronal view is also extremely valuable for displaying the anatomy of the right ventricular outflow tract. This projection corresponds closely to what is seen angiographically. The anatomy and severity of infundibular hypoplasia and the anterior deviation of the outlet septum are well visualised in this projection (Fig. 10).

The apical four-chamber aortic root views are of value in assessing the degree of override and the degree of malalignment between the trabecula septum and infundibular septum. With the addition of colour flow mapping the presence of additional apical and trabecula ventricular septal defects may be excluded and colour flow and spectral Doppler interrogation should also be made of the atrioventricular valves in this projection. The presence or absence of any associated left ventricular outflow tract obstruction can be determined.

Following assessment of the morphology of the ventricular septal defect and of the right ventricular outflow tract, it is important to determine as accurately as possible the size of the right and left pulmonary arteries. This information is of prime importance to the surgeon. If he is considering a systemic to pulmonary artery shunt or primary definitive repair, it is important to know whether or not there is selective stenosis at the origin of the right or of the left pulmonary arteries. The most useful information in respect of the pulmonary arteries comes from the suprasternal views both in the short axis and long axis projections (Fig. 11A and B). The short axis view best displays the bifurcation of the main pulmonary artery into the right and left pulmonary branches. In this projection the right pulmonary artery should be followed as far distally as possible, usually to the origin of the right upper lobe branch. The right pulmonary artery should be measured as it passes behind the ascending aorta and then clockwise rotation of the transducer should be made to bring the left pulmonary artery into view. The suprasternal long axis view is better for identifying the left pulmonary artery. The suprasternal view is also of value in the newborn in determining whether or not the ductus arteriosus is still patent and in determining the side of the aortic arch and the pattern of branching of the brachiocephalic vessel. If the position of tracheal air column is noted then the position of the arch relative to the trachea can be determined in order to establish the diagnosis of the right or left aortic arch. The pattern of branching of the innominate artery into subclavian carotid arteries is best seen in the suprasternal short axis cut.

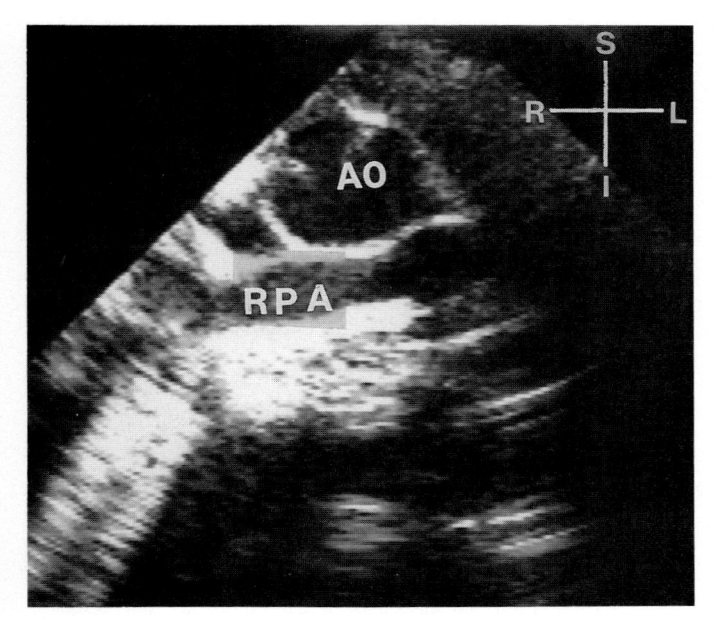

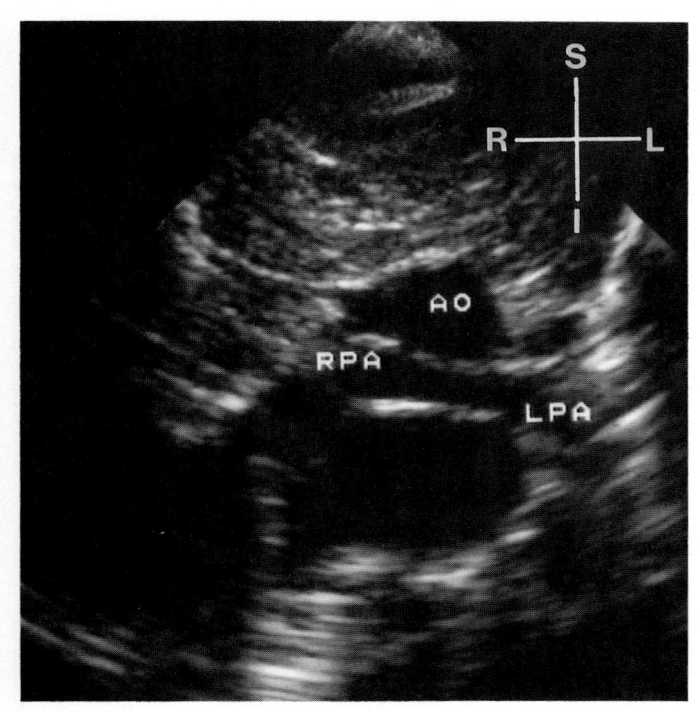

RIGHT SIDED OBSTRUCTIONS AND MALFORMATIONS 437

PULMONARY ATRESIA WITH VENTRICULAR SEPTAL DEFECT

Pathology

Pulmonary atresia with a ventricular septal defect can be considered as the extreme end of the spectrum of tetralogy of Fallot usually with complete infundibular atresia resulting in lack of continuity between the right heart and the pulmonary trunk. The deviation of the infundibular septum which is one of the principal characteristic features of the tetralogy of Fallot is in this condition so marked and severe that the subpulmonary outflow tract is completely occluded.[1,2]

As important as infundibular atresia in characterising this condition are the severe abnormalities found in the pulmonary arterial tree. The assessment of extent of these abnormalities is important in identifying suitability for cardiac surgery. The main pulmonary artery is usually hypoplastic or atretic and is not in continuity with the right ventricular mass. The intrapericardial segments of the right and left pulmonary artery branches can be of normal size but more usually are hypoplastic and on occasion are absent which results in non-confluent central pulmonary arteries. When the intrapulmonary arteries from all portions of both right and left lungs are connected to confluent right and left pulmonary arteries the arrangement which results is termed a unifocal supply.[17] A unifocal supply is most usually via a patent ductus arteriosus. If the ductus arteriosus is absent then the intrapulmonary arterial circulation may be supplied from a variety of different sources – a multifocal supply – but is most usually from major aortopulmonary collateral arteries arising from the descending aorta or less commonly from other branches of the aorta. The aorto pulmonary collateral arteries can co-exist with central confluent pulmonary arteries. Both a patent ductus arteriosus and aortopulmonary collateral arteries can supply the same lung although usually when there is non-confluence of the pulmonary arteries each lung tends to be supplied by one or other source rather than by both. In the most extreme form of non-confluent pulmonary arteries not only is there absence of confluence but there is no evidence of intrapericardial pulmonary arteries at all.

The anatomy of the ventricular septal defect found in pulmonary atresia with ventricular septal defect shows the same variations as seen in tetralogy of Fallot and can be perimembraneous, muscular infundibular, or rarely there may be no subpulmonary infundibulum.

Fig. 11 A: Short axis suprasternal view of right pulmonary artery in tetralogy of Fallot. RPA – right pulmonary artery. B: Short axis suprasternal view showing confluence of right and left pulmonary arteries. RPA – right pulmonary artery; LPA – left pulmonary artery.

Finally, it is important to conclude the assessment of tetralogy of Fallot by excluding any associated abnormalities such as atrioventricular septal defects, a left superior vena cava, additional ventricular septal defects and atrial septal defects.

Echocardiography

The best views for assessing the infundibular atresia and the degree of hypoplasia or absence of the main pulmonary artery are the subcostal right oblique and the standard and high short axis views (Fig. 12).[5,6,18] The subcostal right

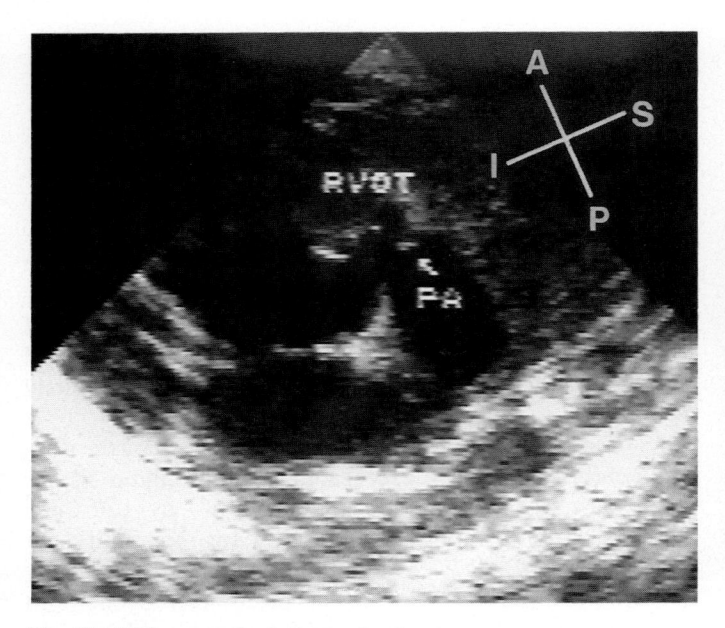

Fig. 12 **High parasternal short axis view** in patient with pulmonary infundibular and valve atresia (arrow) but normal main pulmonary artery (PA).

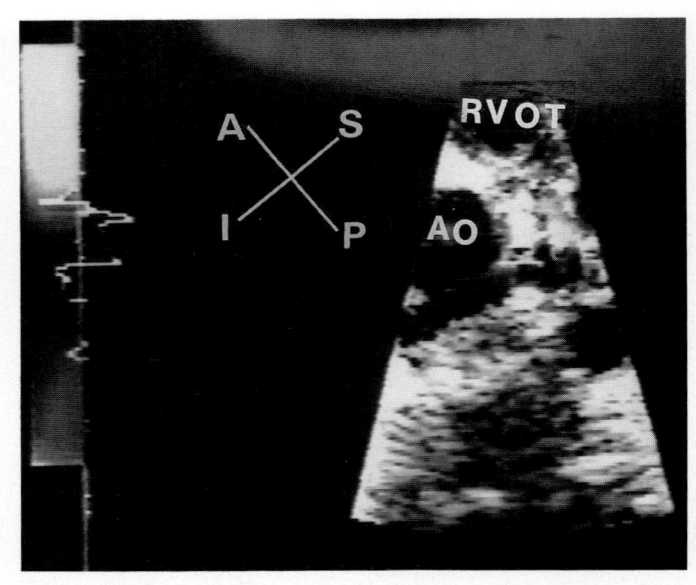

Plate 2 **High precordial short axis view in pulmonary atresia and ventricular septal defect** demonstrating bifurcation of main pulmonary artery. Colour flow mapping documents absence of forward flow through outflow tract but flow from ductus is visualised. This figure is reproduced in colour in the colour plate section at the front of this volume.

oblique view demonstrates the marked deviation of the infundibular septum, valva atresia and the morphology of the main pulmonary artery. The right pulmonary artery and less readily the left pulmonary artery are usually also visualised. Colour flow mapping is helpful in confirming the absence of forward flow across the outflow tract. The precordial short axis views demonstrate the main pulmonary artery and the origin of the right and left pulmonary artery (Plate 2). Doppler and colour flow mapping again will document the absence of forward flow through the outflow tract. From the suprasternal notch in the frontal plane the right pulmonary artery size and origin from the main pulmonary trunk and its confluence with the left pulmonary artery can be assessed (Figs 13 and 14).[19,20] With more clock-wise rotation of the transducer, the left pulmonary artery can then be visualised. The suprasternal cut is also important in determining the presence of a right or left aortic arch and detecting the presence or otherwise of a ductus arteriosus. Cross-sectional echocardiography, however, may not image the aortocollateral vessels well, although the addition of colour flow mapping may improve the sensitivity considerably.[21] Nonetheless, even with the addition of colour flow mapping and Doppler, echocardiography has limitations in defining not only the number and pattern of distribution of the aortopulmonary collateral arteries but also the precise form and type of distribution of the intrapulmonary arterial blood supply: at present angiocardiography or possibly magnetic resonance imaging must be regarded as superior techniques for this information.

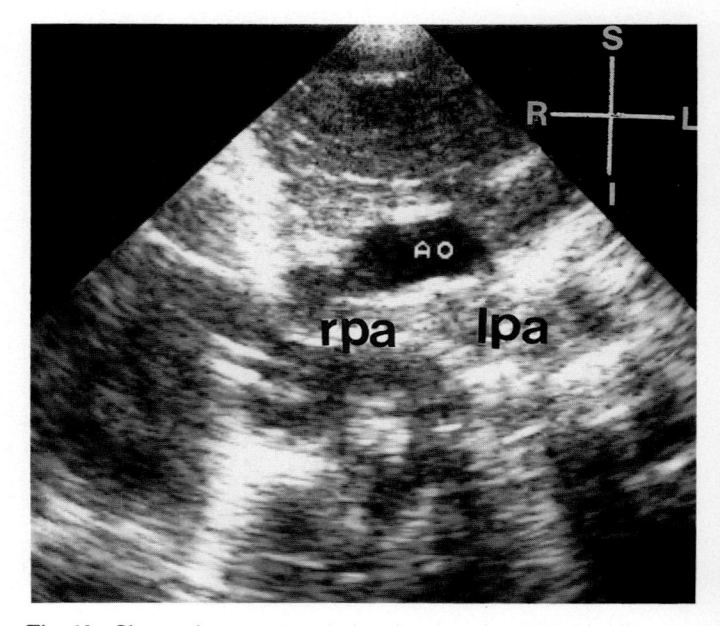

Fig. 13 **Short axis suprasternal view from newborn infant with pulmonary atresia and ventricular septal defect.** The pulmonary arteries are small but confluent. AO – aorta; rpa – right pulmonary artery; lpa – left pulmonary artery.

PULMONARY ATRESIA WITH INTACT VENTRICULAR SEPTUM

Pulmonary atresia with intact ventricular septum is characterised not only by the absence of any communication

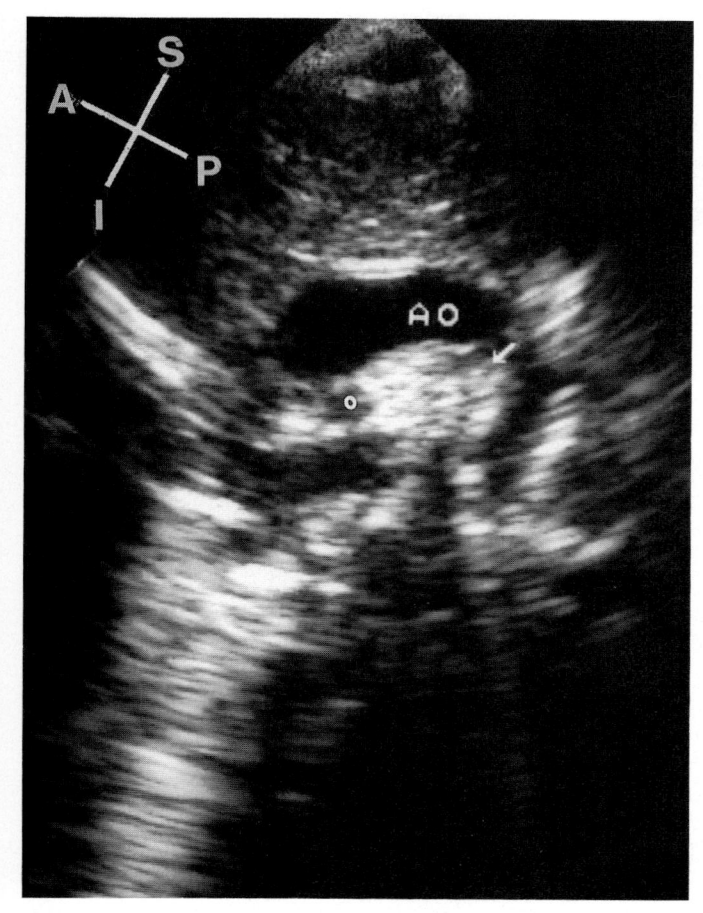

Fig. 14 Long axis suprasternal view in newborn with pulmonary atresia and ventricular septal defect. The left pulmonary artery could not be visualised. The right pulmonary artery (○) was hypoplastic. A small ductus arteriosus (arrow) is visualised.

between the right ventricle and the pulmonary arterial circulation but usually also by hypoplasia of the right ventricular cavity to a variable degree. There is a spectrum of right ventricular cavity size varying from tiny to normal: rarely and exceptionally the right ventricle may be dilated and paper thin.[22,23] It is important to appreciate that there are substantial differences between many of the basic morphological characteristics of pulmonary atresia with an intact ventricular septum and pulmonary atresia with a ventricular septal defect. In pulmonary atresia with an intact ventricular septum:

> The pulmonary arteries are usually of a good size – in contrast to pulmonary atresia with a ventricular septal defect.
> The pulmonary arterial blood supply is nearly always ductus dependent – in pulmonary atresia with a ventricular septal defect the blood supply is more often due to collaterals originating from the aortic arch and descending aorta.
> Tricuspid valve malformation is common in contrast to pulmonary atresia with a ventricular septal defect. The right ventricular cavity is hypoplastic to varying degrees in contrast to pulmonary atresia with a ventricular septal defect.

The systemic venous return must cross the right atrium whereas in pulmonary atresia with a ventricular septal defect right to left shunting occurs at ventricular and/or atrial level.

The right ventricle may be regarded as having three portions, inlet, trabecula and outlet. This tripartite classification when applied to pulmonary atresia with intact septum has value in guiding not only the management of the patient but also is a cornerstone of the echocardiographic assessment with the right ventricle evaluated in terms of the degree of hypoplasia of each component part.[24,25] In just over half of all cases, all three components of the right ventricle are present. In the remainder the trabecula and/or outlet segments are hypoplastic or obliterated. When the outlet portion is atretic its distal part does not end at the pulmonary valve but is occluded by the abnormally positioned infundibular septum and the hypertrophied arterial wall. The inlet part of the right ventricle is only very rarely completely atretic. About 5% of reported cases have a large right ventricle with a thin wall which is usually associated with tricuspid regurgitation. When the infundibulum or outlet portion is patent, only the valve is imperforate and lies in the normal position for the pulmonary valve. This valve may have a domelike appearance similar to that found in critical pulmonary valve stenosis or may be of the 'fixed' type in which it protrudes pouch-like into the right ventricular cavity. The main pulmonary artery and right and left pulmonary arteries are, as emphasised earlier, usually well developed and supplied by a ductus arteriosus and only rarely by aortopulmonary collaterals.

In the vast majority of cases of pulmonary atresia with intact ventricular septum the tricuspid valve is abnormal and dysplastic with short thick chordae. The size of the tricuspid valve annulus is usually related to the degree of cavity obliteration. Measurements of the tricuspid valve annulus may provide a guide to optimal surgical management and outcome. The smallest valves are usually found in those cases with no trabecula or infundibular components.[22] Pulmonary atresia and intact ventricular septum may be associated with Ebstein's anomaly of the tricuspid valve.

Of major significance in the management of pulmonary atresia with intact ventricular septum is the recognition of intramyocardial sinusoids. These are abnormal channels within the right ventricular myocardium which originate in the cavity and end as blind pouches in the myocardium itself. They can connect to the coronary arteries or to the coronary venous system. Their number and size depends on the degree of right ventricular hypertension and they occur most frequently when the right ventricle is severely hypoplastic with only an inlet portion.[26,27]

Echocardiographic assessment

The best views for beginning the assessment of right ventricular morphology are the apical and subcostal four-chamber views.[28] Most commonly, the marked muscular hypertrophy of the apical segment is identified with the inlet region not being so markedly affected (Figs 15 and 16). In these views the size of the tricuspid valve annulus should be assessed for this is important information in planning surgery. The smaller the tricuspid valve annulus the greater usually is the degree of hypoplasia also of the inlet region. The inlet region is defined in essence as that part of the ventricle within which the tricuspid valve apparatus lies, with the apical or trabecula portion being in the zone beyond the insertion of the papillary muscles of the tricuspid valve towards the apex. In these views the tricuspid valve morphology can also be evaluated and the degree of hypoplasia and dysplasia of the valve and/or presence of Ebstein's anomaly can be determined. If on colour flow mapping a jet of tricuspid regurgitation is identified, Doppler recordings can then be used to assess the degree of right ventricular hypertension. Significant right ventricular hypertension should alert one to the possibility that there are myocardial sinusoids connecting the right ventricular cavity to the right coronary arterial system (Fig. 17). During right ventricular systole, blood flows from the right ventricular cavity into the sinusoids, coronary arteries and veins; during diastole blood flows from the aorta into the coronary system. Myocardial ischaemia may result from compromise of perfusion during diastole due to increased resistance from retrograde filling of the coronary arteries as well as the hypertrophy of the right ventricle.[27] The abnormal blood flow in large sinusoids can be identified with colour flow mapping and Doppler interrogation may reveal flow from the right

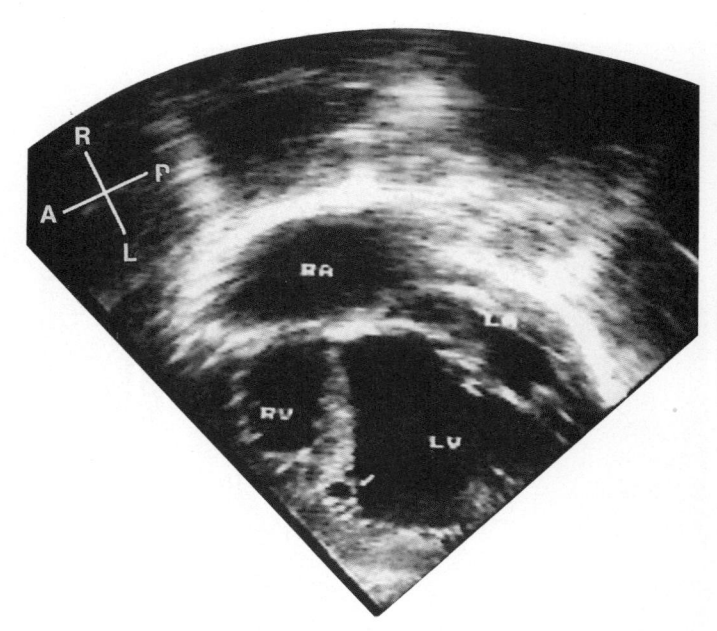

Fig. 16 Apical four-chamber view from same patient as Fig. 15. Arrow indicates myocardial sinusoid.

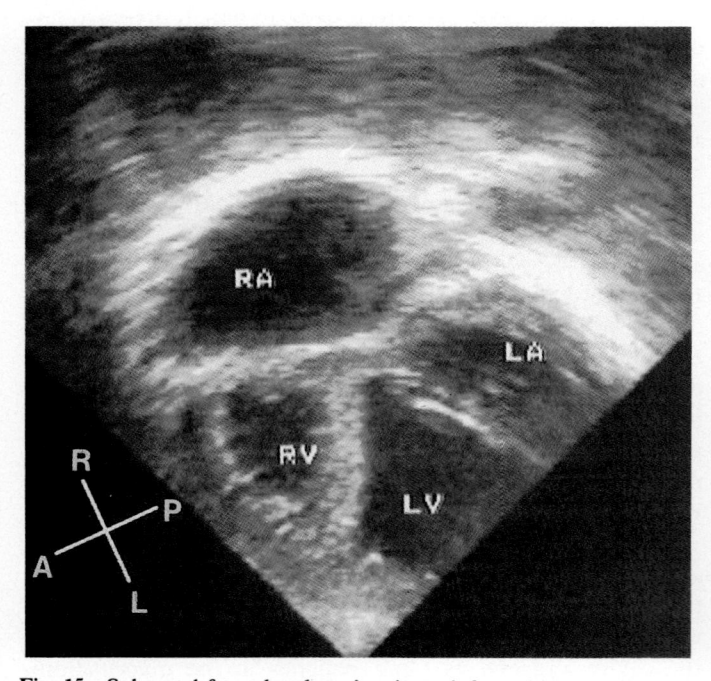

Fig. 15 Subcostal four-chamber view in an infant with pulmonary atresia and intact ventricular septum demonstrating marked apical right ventricular hypertrophy.

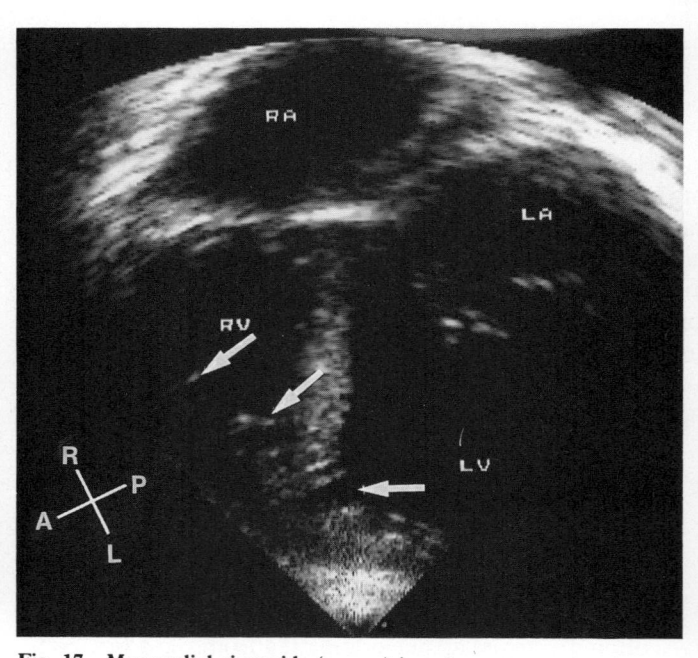

Fig. 17 Myocardial sinusoids (arrows) in pulmonary atresia with intact ventricular septum.

ventricle to the coronary artery during systole with reversed flow in diastole. The myocardial sinusoids are best identified in the cross section in the four-chamber views but are usually only seen when the coronary arteries are dilated due to large non-obstructed fistulous communications. The right ventricular infundibulum is best visualised from the subcostal right oblique view complemented with parasternal long axis parasternal views of the aortic root (Figs 18 and 19). The subcostal right oblique view is helpful not only in evaluating the outlet zone but all parts of the ventricle. It is the best view for determining whether the atresia is confined to the valve or the whole of the infundibulum. The extent of infundibular atresia can be accurately assessed in this view giving valuable information in considering different surgical options for the management of the right ventricular outflow tract.

The distinction between critical pulmonary valve stenosis with an intact septum and pulmonary atresia with an intact septum may be difficult: frequently it is not possible by cross sectional echocardiography alone. Even with Doppler echocardiography the differentiation may still not in practice be easy for it can prove extremely difficult to detect small high velocity jets distal to a pinpoint stenosis. On the other hand, with the addition of colour flow mapping the high velocity jet is usually detected and the differentiation between the two conditions is more readily made.

The pulmonary arterial size can be assessed from the

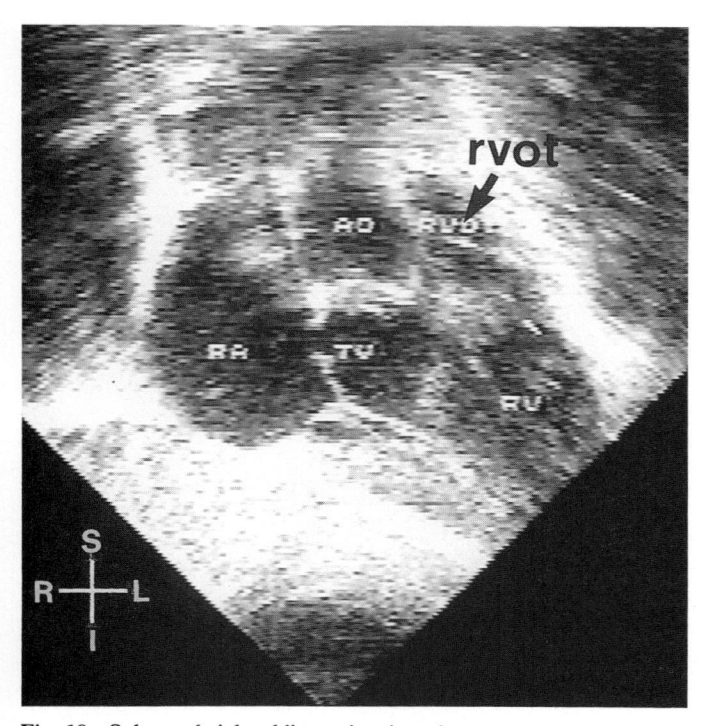

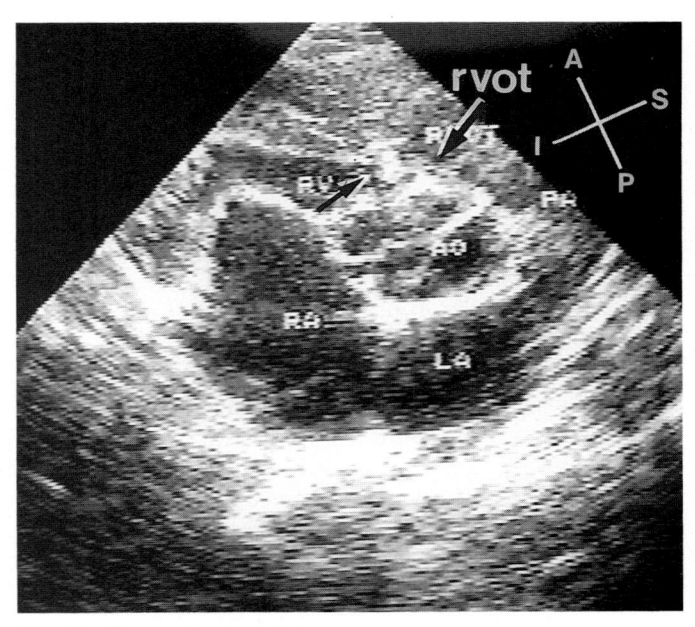

Fig. 19 Short axis precordial view in pulmonary atresia with intact ventricular septum. Infundibular atresia – small arrow. rvot – right ventricular outflow tract.

suprasternal notch. The pulmonary arteries are usually normal or only mildly hypoplastic in contrast to pulmonary atresia with a ventricular septal defect. The aortic arch is almost always left sided again in contrast to pulmonary atresia with a ventricular septal defect in which a right aortic arch occurs more frequently. From the suprasternal notch view the ductus arteriosus can be assessed in terms of its size and flow by Doppler/colour flow mapping interrogation.

EBSTEIN'S MALFORMATION

Pathology

Ebstein's malformation is a congenital defect of the tricuspid valve in which the normal attachments of the septal and posterior (inferior mural) tricuspid valve leaflets are displaced from the atrioventricular junction into the cavity of the right ventricle. The result of this displacement is 'atrialisation' of part of the inlet portion of the right ventricle. The degree to which this occurs is variable and there is, therefore, a spectrum of morphological abnormality and of dysfunction of the valve.[29,30]

In the mildest form only the adjacent parts of the attachment of the septal and posterior leaflets are displaced and the orifice is normal and the valve may be functionally competent. In severe forms the septal leaflet is plastered to the septum and the posterior leaflet to the ventricular wall. The anterosuperior leaflet may be enlarged, elongated and sail like with abnormal attachments from the annulus to a muscular cleft between the ventricular inlet and trabecula partition. The septal and posterior leaflet may be partially

Fig. 18 Subcostal right oblique view in pulmonary atresia with intact ventricular septum. There is marked apical right ventricular hypertrophy and infundibular atresia. rvot – right ventricular outflow tract.

absent and frequently can have multiple short chordae connecting to multiple small papillary muscles. This may also be the case with the sail-like anterior leaflet with multiple short chordae from its free edge binding it close to the septum and/or the free wall. If the entire free margins of the leaflets are adherent and imperforate then a variety of tricuspid atresia is produced. Although important stenosis may be uncommon, severe incompetence may be a result not only of the abnormalities of the valve itself but may also be due to marked dilatation of the true tricuspid annulus.

The result of the displacement of the valve attachments is the division of the right ventricle into a proximal atrialised and a distal ventricularised portion. The atrialised part of the right ventricular wall is dilated and may become so thin that it acquires an aneurysmal appearance: more often, however, the wall of the atrialised portion is thick with variable amounts of muscle. The ventricularised part of the right ventricle is obviously smaller than the normal ventricle but its relative size may be altered by right ventricular dilatation and indeed this is usually present. Anderson & Lie suggest that dilatation of both portions of the ventricle is part of the developmental abnormality rather than essentially related to the haemodynamic disturbance present.[31]

The haemodynamic derangement present is variable and reflects to a considerable degree the associated structural disturbance. In cases with a minor morphological abnormality the valve is functionally normal. In more severe cases a number of factors may produce a higher right atrial than left atrial pressure – tricuspid regurgitation, obstruction or both. With an elevated right atrial pressure right to left shunting occurs at atrial level with cyanosis. This process may be accentuated in the newborn because of the high pulmonary vascular resistance present at this age. If the atrialised portion of the right ventricle is very thin, blood may pool in it during atrial systole and then during right ventricular systole this portion moves, paradoxically backing blood into the true right atrium.

There are a number of important associated defects. Most common is an interatrial communication present in about 60% of cases. This is usually either a patent foramen ovale or an ostium secundum atrial septal defect. In about a third of cases there may be associated pulmonary atresia or severe stenosis with the ventricular septum intact. In congenitally corrected transposition the tricuspid valve or morphologically right ventricle are left sided: tricuspid valve incompetence in this condition is common and may be, but is not always, due to Ebstein's anomaly. Mitral valve prolapse has been reported as have abnormalities of left ventricular contraction. Less commonly there may be ventricular septal defects, tetralogy of Fallot and other abnormalities.

Echocardiography

Echocardiography is the procedure of choice for the diagnostic and morphological assessment of Ebstein's anomaly. Two-dimensional echocardiography provides excellent correlation with direct anatomical inspection and provides the detailed morphological assessment of the tricuspid valve abnormalities and of the right heart structures which is necessary when surgery is being considered.[32-34] Pulsed and continuous wave Doppler with colour flow mapping studies additionally may provide haemodynamic information. Transoesophageal studies may augment the anatomical assessment provided from the standard transthoracic views. The two best views for assessing Ebstein's anomaly are the apical four-chamber and subcostal views which visualise the septal and anterior leaflets and enable assessment of the degree of atrialisation of the right ventricle – important information for the surgeon. In these views the functional size of the right ventricular inflow can also be assessed and the addition of Doppler and colour flow mapping helps to define the degree of regurgitation of stenosis and the pattern of atrial shunting (Figs 20, 21 and Plate 3). Particular attention should be made to the assessment of:

The degree of tricuspid valve displacement.
The degree of tethering of the septal and anterior leaflet.
Dysplasia of the septal and anterior leaflet tissue.
Tricuspid valve regurgitation and stenosis.
Cardiac chamber and annular dimensions.
Ventricular function and dimensions.

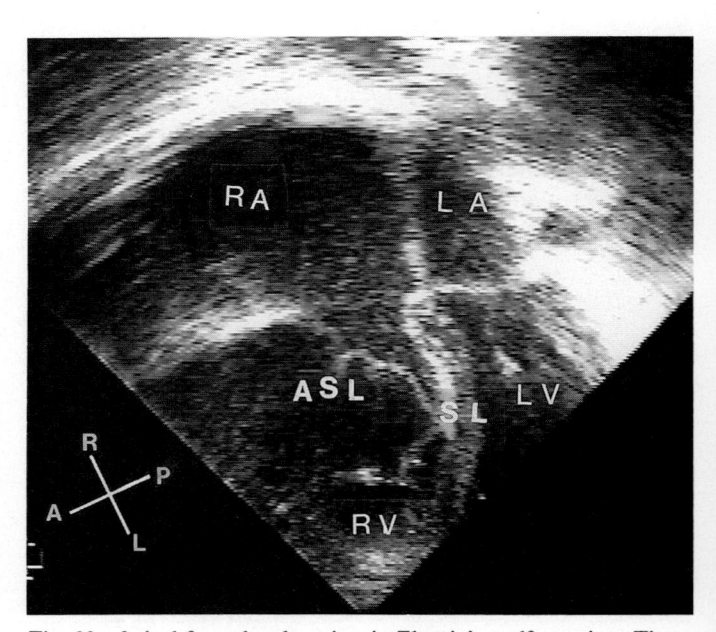

Fig. 20 Apical four-chamber view in Ebstein's malformation. The displacement of the septal leaflet is demonstrated as is the normal attachment to the annulus of the large anterior leaflet. ASL – antero superior leaflet; SL – septal leaflet.

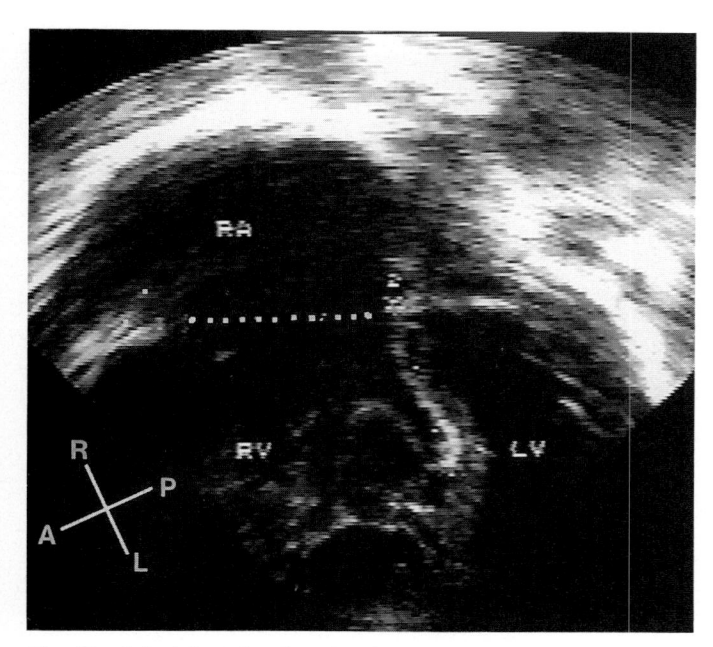

RIGHT SIDED OBSTRUCTIONS AND MALFORMATIONS 443

Fig. 21 Apical four-chamber view in Ebstein's anomaly. Horizontal dots indicate the level of the annulus.

apically on to the ventricular septum. Varying degrees of inferior displacement can be seen in normal hearts and in patients with atrial septal defects or severe tricuspid regurgitation. If the inferior displacement of the septal leaflet is indexed to body area then septal leaflet displacement becomes a very sensitive diagnostic indicator, a value greater than 8 mm/m^2 being conclusive except in small infants and in patients with a very dilated heart.[34] In the assessment of the degree of valve displacement in the apical four-chamber view, it is important to be certain that echoes arising from the true annulus are not mistaken for valve leaflets and that a moderator band also is not mistaken for displaced septal leaflet. A small dysplastic septal tricuspid leaflet is observed in approximately 50% of patients and is associated with a high frequency of tricuspid regurgitation and eccentric coaption of the anterior leaflet.

A large elongated sail like appearance to the anterior leaflet is also characteristic of Ebstein's anomaly. These features are favourable in the surgical assessment for valve repair but if the anterior leaflet is tethered and immobile with short chordae then valve replacement is usually required.

The four-chamber view is also useful in assessing the presence or otherwise of left ventricular contraction abnormalities although the frequency with which this occurs varies between different series.[34-36]

The tricuspid valve annulus is usually significantly dilated though this is not specific to Ebstein's anomaly. The changes in ventricular cavity dimension reflect the anatomic severity with a large atrialised right ventricle and a small functional right ventricle may be seen in the more severe cases.

The displacement and tethering of the tricuspid valve obviously varies from case to case but inferior displacement of the septal leaflet of the tricuspid valve can be regarded as the most useful echocardiographic marker for the recognition of Ebstein's anomaly.

Normally the septal tricuspid leaflet inserts only slightly

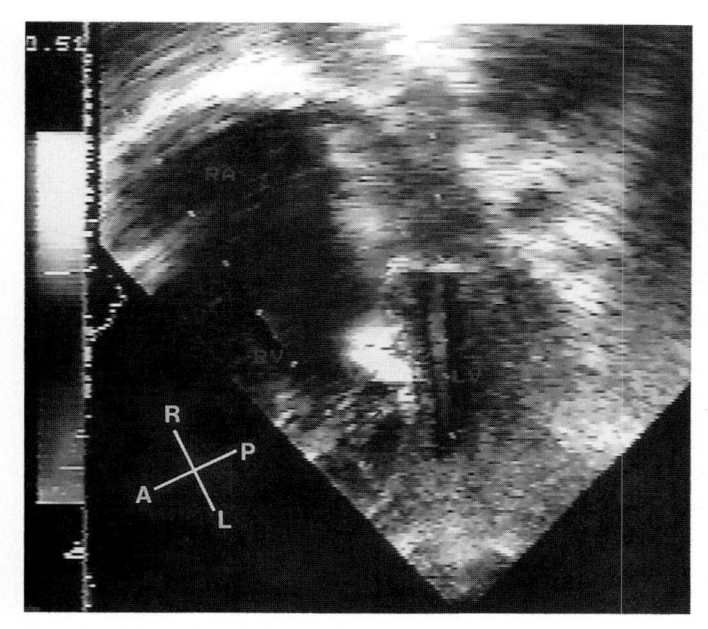

Plate 3 Colour Doppler image from same patient as Fig. 21 showing direction, origin and degree of tricuspid valve regurgitation. This figure is reproduced in colour in the colour plate section at the front of this volume.

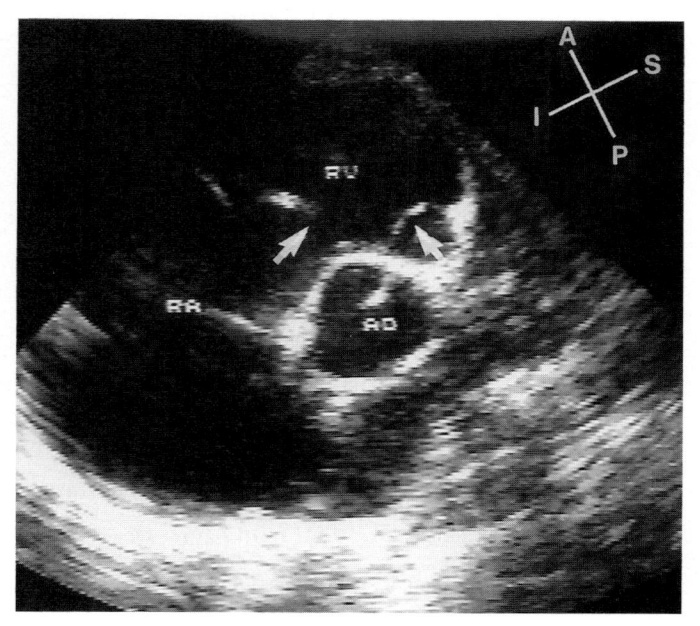

Fig. 22 Parasternal short axis view in Ebstein's malformation. Arrows indicate large antero-superior leaflet and pulmonary valve.

The other transthoracic views, parasternal, long and short axis, complement the information available from the more important apical four-chamber and subcostal views (Fig. 22). In the precordial short axis view it may be possible to image all three leaflets simultaneously. The short axis view also enables an assessment to be made of the right ventricular outflow tract and of the pulmonary valve. In the severest forms of Ebstein's anomaly the anterior tricuspid valve leaflet may obstruct the right ventricular outflow tract and cause a functional/anatomical pulmonary atresia. There may in some cases be true pulmonary atresia or severe pulmonary stenosis. Doppler and colour flow mapping studies may help in this determination. The parasternal long axis view may visualise the anterior leaflet well and identify its attachments very clearly.

Pre and intraoperative transoesophageal echocardiography complement transthoracic views and may help in determining the choice of operative procedure.[37]

Assessment is completed by tabulating any abnormalities associated with the Ebstein's anomaly – atrial septal defect, pulmonary stenosis/pulmonary atresia, mitral valve prolapse, physiologically corrected transposition or ventricular dysfunction.

REFERENCES

1 Becker A E, Anderson R H. Pathology of congenital heart disease. London: Butterworth. 1981
2 Klosetaky E D, Moller J H, Korns M E, Schwartz C J, Edwards J E. Congenital pulmonary stenosis resulting from dysplasia of the valve. Circulation 1969; 60: 43–53
3 Engle M A, Holswade F R, Goldberg H P et al Regression after open valvulotomy of infundibular stenosis accompanying severe valvular pneumonic stenosis. Circulation 1958; 17: 862–868
4 Weyman A E, Hurwitz R A, Girod D A. Cross sectional echocardiographic visualisation of the stenotic pulmonary valve. Circulation 1977; 56: 769–774
5 Gutgesell H P. Accuracy of two-dimensional echocardiography in the diagnosis of congenital heart disease. Am J Cardiol 1985; 55: 514–520
6 Hatle L, Angelson B. Doppler ultrasound in cardiology, ed 2. Philadelphia: Lea & Febriger. 1985
7 Lima C O, Sahn D J, Valdes Cruz L M. Non invasive prediction of transvalvular pressure gradient in patients with pulmonary stenosis by quantitative two dimensional echocardiographic studies. Circulation 1983; 67: 866–871
8 Houston A B, Simpson I A, Sheldon C D et al Doppler ultrasound in the estimation of the severity of pulmonary infundibular stenosis in infants and children. Br Heart J 1986; 55: 381–384
9 Matina D, Van Doesburg N H, Fouron J C, Guerin R, Davignon A. Subxiphoid two dimensional echocardiographic diagnosis of double chambered right ventricles. Circulation 1983; 67: 885–888
10 Becker A E, Connor M, Anderson R H. Tetralogy of Fallot: a morphometric and geometric study. Am J Cardiol. 1975; 35: 402–412
11 Wilcox B R, Anderson R H. In: Surgical anatomy of the heart. Churchill Livingstone 1985
12 Capelli H, Somerville K. Atypical Fallot tetralogy with double committed subarterial ventricular septal defect. Am J Cardiol 1983; 52: 282–286
13 Fellows K E, Smith J, Keane J F. Preoperative angiography in infants with tetrad of Fallot. Am J Cardiol 1981; 9: 1285
14 Henry W L, Maron B J, Griffith J M et al. Differential diagnosis of anomalies of the great arteries by real time two-dimensional echocardiography. Circulation 1975; 51: 283–291
15 Hagler D J, Tajik A J, Seward J B et al Wide-angle two-dimensional echocardiographic profiles of conotruncal abnormalities. Mayo Clin Proc 1980; 55: 73–82
16 Fuggion G, Frescura C, Thiene G, Bortolotti U, Mazzucco A, Anderson R H. Accessory tricuspid valve tissue causing obstruction of the ventricular septal defect. Diagnostic value of two-dimensional echocardiography. Br Heart J 1983; 49: 324–327
17 Haworth S G, McArtney F J. Growth and development of pulmonary circulation in pulmonary atresia with ventricular septal defect and major aortopulmonary collateral arteries. Br Heart J 1980; 44: 14–24
18 Vargas Barron J, Sahn D J, Attie F et al. Two-dimensional echocardiographic study of right ventricular outflow and great artery anatomy and pulmonary atresia with ventricular septal defects and in truncus arteriosus. Am Heart J 1983; 105: 281–286
19 Huhta J C, Piehler J M, Tajik A J et al Two-dimensional echocardiographic detection and measurement of the right pulmonary artery in pulmonary atresia – ventricular septal defect. Angiographic and surgical correlation. Am J Cardiol. 1982; 49: 1235–1240
20 Tinker D D, Nander N C, Harris P J, Manning J A Two-dimensional echocardiographic identification of pulmonary artery branch stenosis. Am J Cardiol 1982; 50: 814–820
21 Smyllie J H, Sutherland G R, Keeton B R The value of colour flow mapping in determining pulmonary blood supply in infants with pulmonary atresia with ventricular septal defect. J Am Coll Cardiol 1989; 14: 1759–1765
22 Zuberbuhler J R, Anderson R H Morphological variations in pulmonary atresia with intact ventricular septum. Br Heart J. 1979; 41: 281–288
23 Davignon A L, Greenwold W E, Du Shane J W, Edwards J E Congenital pulmonary atresia with intact ventricular septum. Clinicopathological correlation of two anatomic types. Am Heart J 1961; 62: 591–602
24 Bull C, de Leval M, Mercanti C, McArtney F J, Anderson R H. Pulmonary atresia and intact ventricular septum, a revised classification. Circulation 1982; 66: 266–272
25 de Leval M, Bull C, Stark J et al Pulmonary atresia and intact ventricular septum: surgical management based on a revised classification. Circulation 1982; 66: 272–280
26 Freedom R M, Harrington D P Contributions of intramyocardial sinusoids in pulmonary atresia and intact ventricular septum to a right-sided circular shunt. Br Heart J 1974; 36: 1061–1065
27 O'Connor W N, Cottrill C M, Johnson C L, Noonan J A, Todd A Pulmonary atresia with intact ventricular septum and ventriculo coronary communications. Circulation 1982; 65: 805–808
28 Mirinob, Franceschini E, Ballerini L et al, Anatomical/echocardiographic correlations in pulmonary atresia with intact ventricular septum. Use of subcostal cross-sectional views. Int J Cardiol 1986; 11: 103–109
29 Anderson K R, Zuberbuhler J R, Anderson R H, Becker A E, Lie J T Morphological spectrum of Ebstein's anomaly of the heart; a review. Mayo Clin Proc 1979; 54: 174–180
30 Zuberbuhler J R, Allwark S P, Anderson R H The spectrum of Ebstein's anomaly of the tricuspid valve. J Thorac Cardiovasc Surg 1979; 77: 202–211
31 Anderson K R, Lie J T Pathologic anatomy of Ebstein's anomaly of the heart revisited. Am J Cardiol 1979; 41: 163–173
32 Gussenhoven W J, Spitaels S E C, Bom N, Becker A E Echocardiographic criteria for Ebstein's anomaly of tricuspid valve. Br Heart J 1980; 43: 31–37
33 Shiina A, Seward J B, Tajik et al Two-dimensional echocardiographic surgical correlation in Ebstein's anomaly:

Pre-operative determination of patients requiring tricuspid valve plication v replacement. Circulation 1983; 68: 534–544
34 Shiina A, Seward J B, Edwards W D Two-dimensional echocardiographic spectrum of Ebstein anomaly. Detailed anatomic assessment. J Am Coll Cardiol 1984; 3: 356–370
35 Monibi A A, Neches W H, Lenox C C Left ventricular anomalies associated with Ebstein's malformation of the tricuspid valve. Circulation 1978; 57: 303–306
36 Benson L N, Child J S, Schwaiger M, Perloff J K, Schelbert H R Left ventricular geometry and function in adults with Ebstein's anomaly of the tricuspid valve. Circulation 1987; 75: 353–359
37 Carpentier A, Chouvaud S, Mace L, Relland J, Mihauleanu S, Mariona J P, Abry B, Guibourt P A new reconstructive operation for Ebstein's anomaly of the tricuspid valve. J Thorac Cardiovasc Surg 1988; 86: 92–101

24

Univentricular atrioventricular connection

Introduction
Echocardiographic appearances

Stewart Hunter

INTRODUCTION

In the last 20 years controversy has raged over the description of hearts in which both atria drain into one ventricle. Paediatric cardiologists have used terms such as 'single ventricle', 'primitive ventricle', and 'univentricular heart'. Anderson et al[1] in 1982 seem to have settled the argument to most people's satisfaction. The univentricular atrioventricular connection is a generic term given to a group of anomalies whose unifying feature is the connection of both atria, directly or potentially, to only one ventricle. Anderson et al stated that it is 'not the heart which is univentricular but the atrioventricular connection.'

Some of the hearts in this group do genuinely have only one ventricle. The majority, however, have a rudimentary ventricle in addition to the large main chamber. Univentricular atrioventricular connection can consist of a double inlet ventricle or an absent right or left atrioventricular connection. The morphology of the main ventricular chamber can be left, right or indeterminate.

The commonest type of heart with univentricular connection is the double inlet left ventricle. In this condition the right ventricle is rudimentary and is usually positioned antero-superiorly on the 'shoulder' of the left ventricle. The next most common form of double inlet ventricle is that in which there is a main chamber of right ventricular morphology and a rudimentary postero-inferior left ventricle. The least common type of double inlet ventricle is one in which there is truly a single ventricle which is of interderminate morphology.

Abnormalities of the atrioventricular junction are supremely well diagnosed by cross sectional echocardiography. In these conditions Doppler ultrasound can be used to assess the degree of regurgitation or stenosis of the individual valves. The echocardiogram can also be used to demonstrate the associated ventriculo-arterial connection which can be concordant, discordant, single outlet from the heart, pulmonary atresia or aortic atresia.

ECHOCARDIOGRAPHIC APPEARANCES

In accordance with sequential chamber localisation technique, the echocardiographer must in the first instance identify whether the heart is in the right chest or the left chest. The atrial arrangement should also be determined either by the use of penetrated films of the bronchi according to the method of Deanfield et al[2] or by the use of abdominal ultrasonography as described by Huhta et al.[3] Once the type and position of the atria has been identified, the atrioventricular junction is examined from subcostal and apical four chamber views and the anatomy of the atrioventricular valves, valve rings, and the subvalvar apparatus is noted.

When the univentricular connection is double inlet type each atrium drains directly or potentially into the same large ventricular chamber be it of left, right or indeterminate morphology. Anderson et al[1] introduced descriptions of the mode of connection and the morphology of the valves at the atrioventricular junction. In cases of double inlet ventricle the two valves are rarely morphologically mitral or tricuspid and they are best described as right and left atrioventricular valves. Sometimes the valves straddle or override the ventricular septum and quite frequently they may be stenotic, hypoplastic or, in 15% of cases, imperforate.[4] Double inlet ventricles may also have one common valve which may in part override or straddle the septum into the rudimentary ventricle.

The echocardiographic appearance of the two inlet valves and a double inlet left ventricle is fairly characteristic. There is continuity of the adjacent leaflets through the central fibrous body which produces a very characteristic movement of diastolic apposition. This is well demonstrated on real time cross sectional views (Fig. 1A) but was appreciated many years ago on M-mode echocardiography (Fig. 1B). Apical and parasternal views are

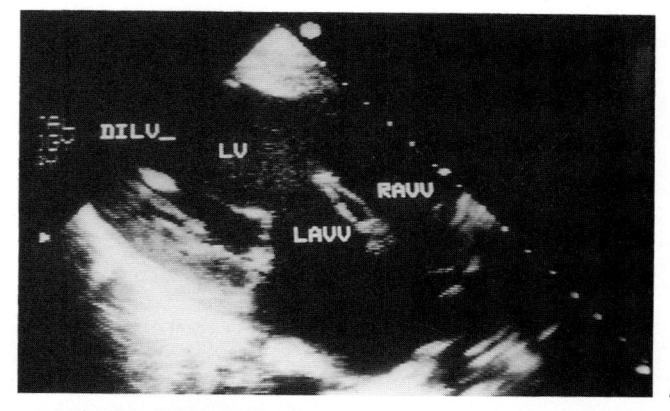

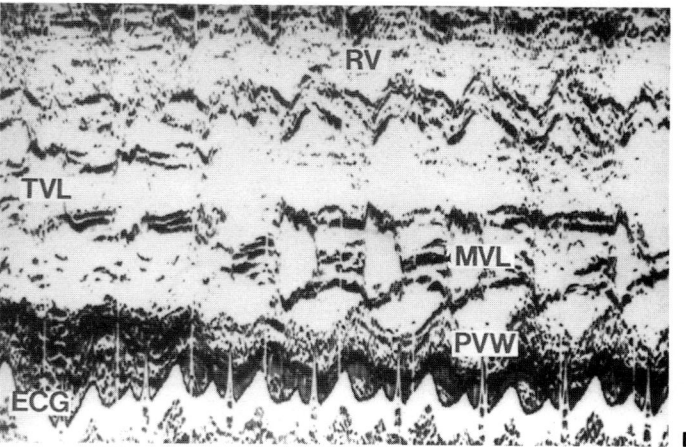

Fig. 1 A: Four chambered view in double inlet ventricle. The apex is facing upwards and the right and left atrioventricular valves are seen fully open and touching. DILV = double inlet left ventricle; LAVV = left atrioventricular valve; RAVV = right atrioventricular valve. **B:** M-mode trace of double inlet left ventricle. PVW = posterior ventricular wall; MVL = left atrioventricular valve; TVL = right atrioventricular valve.

probably the best for studying this relationship. An intermediate view between the four chambered and the short axis view is often the most valuable because of the abnormal positioning of the valves and the ventricles. When two atrioventricular valves are present their planes are often different and minor adjustments of angulation are thus required to confirm the presence of two valves and rule out absent atrioventricular connection (Fig. 2). In some cases of double inlet ventricle, imperforate valves are seen to balloon into the ventricle during atrial systole (Fig. 3). Doppler examination can be very valuable in demonstrating flow, or absence of flow, across such valves. A single atrioventricular valve with a common orifice in a double inlet heart looks very similar, morphologically, to the valve structures seen in a complete atrioventricular septal defect (Fig. 4). The bridging leaflets frequently float freely across

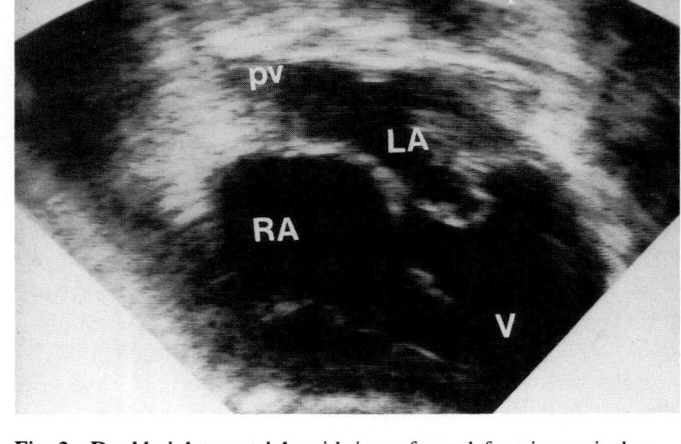

Fig. 3 Double inlet ventricle with imperforate left atrioventricular valve which balloons into the ventricle. The right atrium is enlarged and the interatrial septum appears intact. V = ventricle.

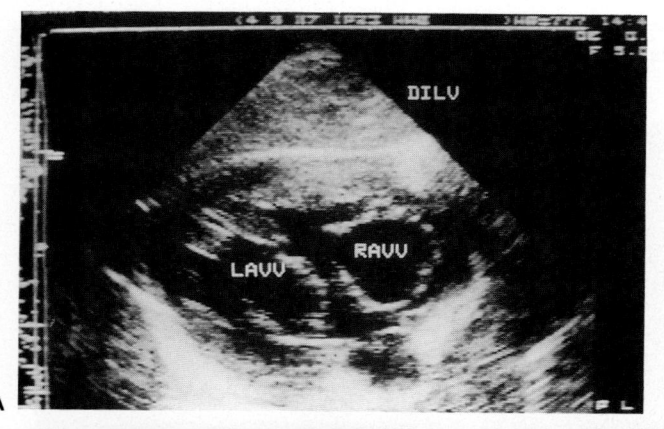

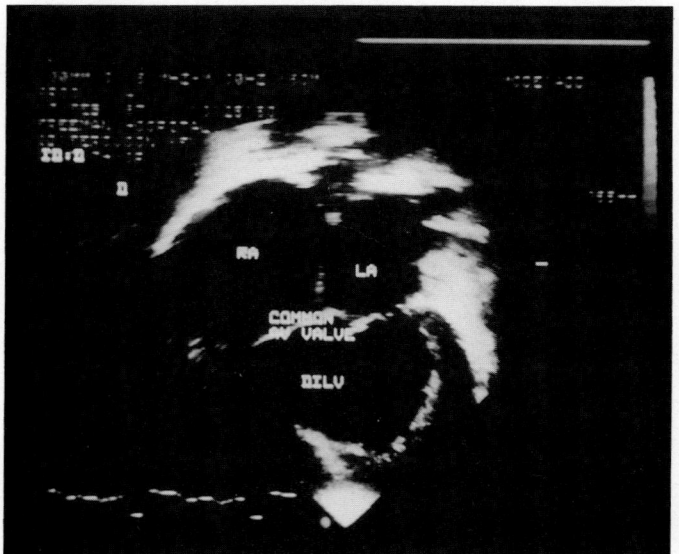

Fig. 2 A: Short axis parasternal view of double inlet left ventricle. The round valve orifices are seen within the main ventricular chamber. DILV = double inlet left ventricle; RAVV = right atrioventricular valve; LAVV = left atrioventricular valve. **B:** Four chambered view of double inlet left ventricle with a common atrioventricular valve. DILV = double inlet left ventricle.

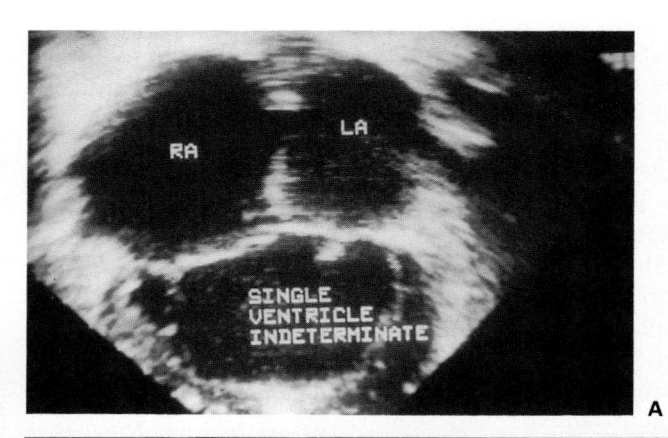

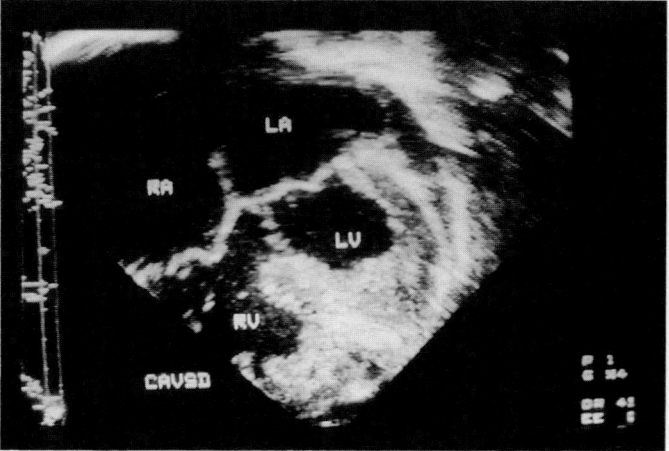

Fig. 4 A: Double inlet ventricle with common atrioventricular valve and no rudimentary chamber – a truly single ventricle with indeterminate morphology. **B:** Complete atrioventricular septal defect with bridging leaflets from the common atrioventricular valve spanning the atrioventricular junction. A nubbin of septum is seen to which some chords and the common valve are attached.

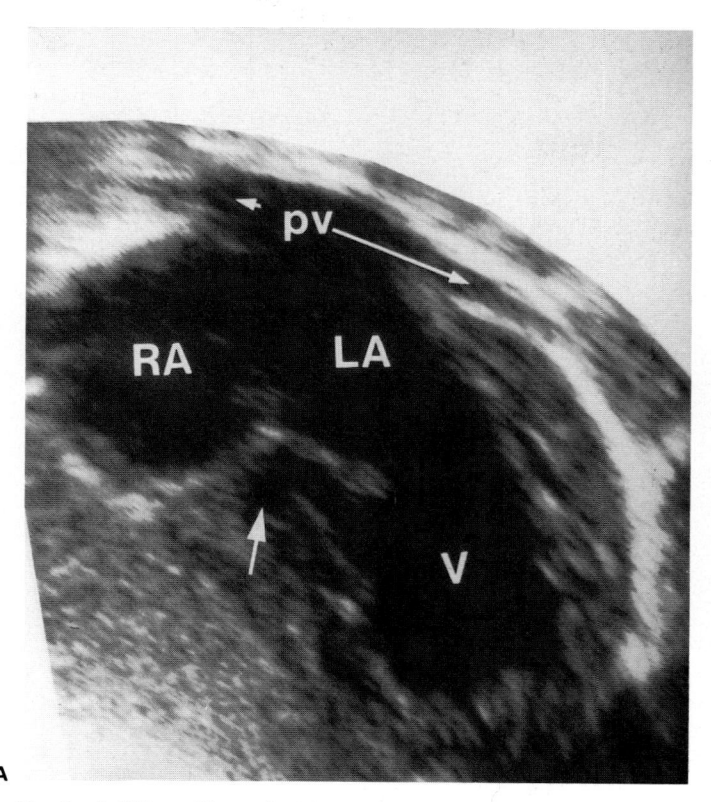

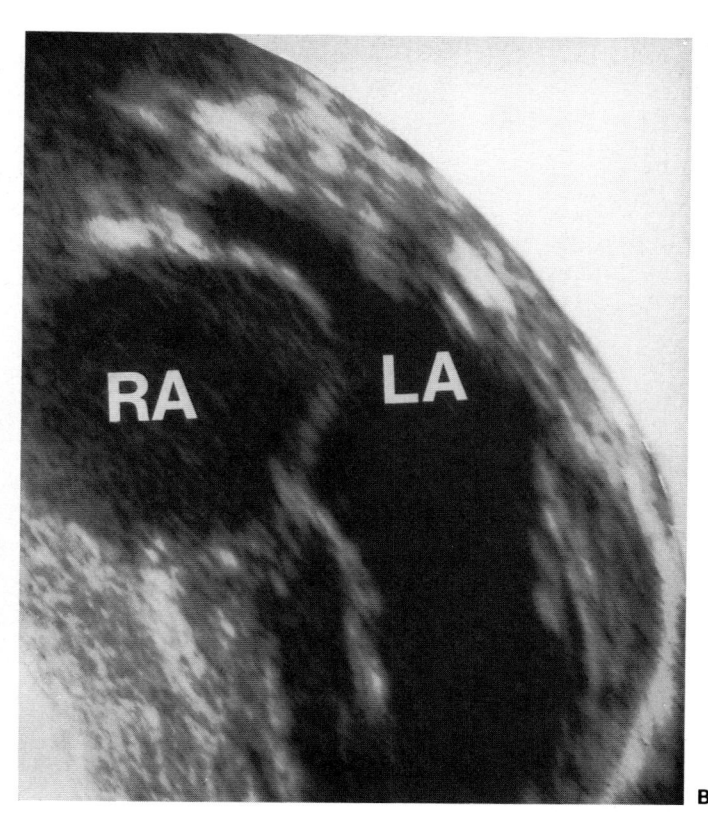

Fig. 5 A: Tricuspid atresia (absent right atrioventricular connection) with atrioventricular sulcus tissue separating the right atrium from the left ventricle (V). There is a good sized atrial septal defect present. **B:** Absent right atrioventricular connections with small atrial septal defect – the right atrium is enlarged and the septum bows to the left.

the ventricular cavity and are supported by two lateral leaflets. The echocardiographic differentiation between these two conditions is thus very difficult. The identification of an interventricular septum and its relationship to the atrioventricular valve is obviously an important differentiator but when the septal remnant is very small in complete atrioventricular septal defect, differentiation is difficult. Rigby et al[4] suggest that malalignment between the atrial septum and the ventricular septum is frequently though not invariably seen in the double inlet group. If there is a common atrium, however, the distinction between the two lesions may be impossible.

The difference between a double inlet ventricle and a concordant atrioventricular connection with a ventricular septal defect and a straddling and overriding valve can be quite subtle. The anatomist's 50% rule suggests that more than 50% of an overriding valve annulus must be assigned to the ventricle which receives this second atrioventricular valve for it to be called a double inlet ventricle. In the case of a common valve, more than 75% of the structure must be committed to one ventricle for the definition of double inlet ventricle to apply. These findings are relatively easy to legislate for but quite difficult to demonstrate echocardiographically in practice.

Absent atrioventricular connections may occur on either right or left sides. The most common anomaly encountered with a dominant left ventricle is tricuspid atresia or right atrioventricular valve absence. No valve structure is seen and there is a wedge of sulcus tissue at the atrioventricular junction in the place of normal valve tissue which separates the right atrium from the ventricular mass (Fig. 5A). There should be a sizeable atrial defect for the patient to

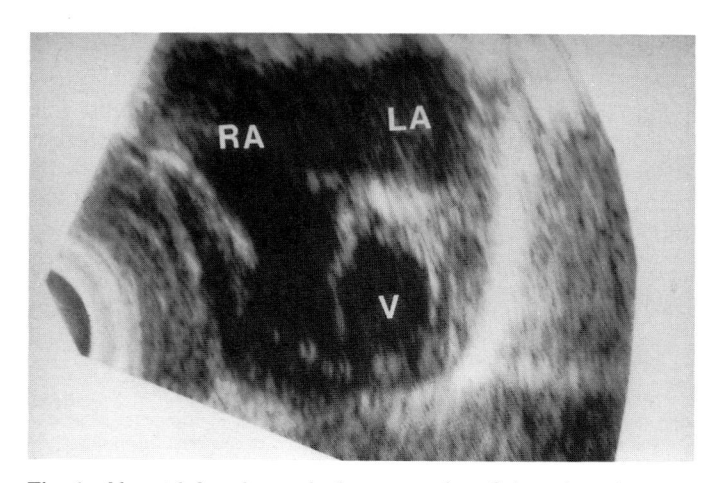

Fig. 6 Absent left atrioventricular connection. Sulcus tissue is seen separating the left atrium from the ventricular cavity (V).

452 CARDIAC ULTRASOUND

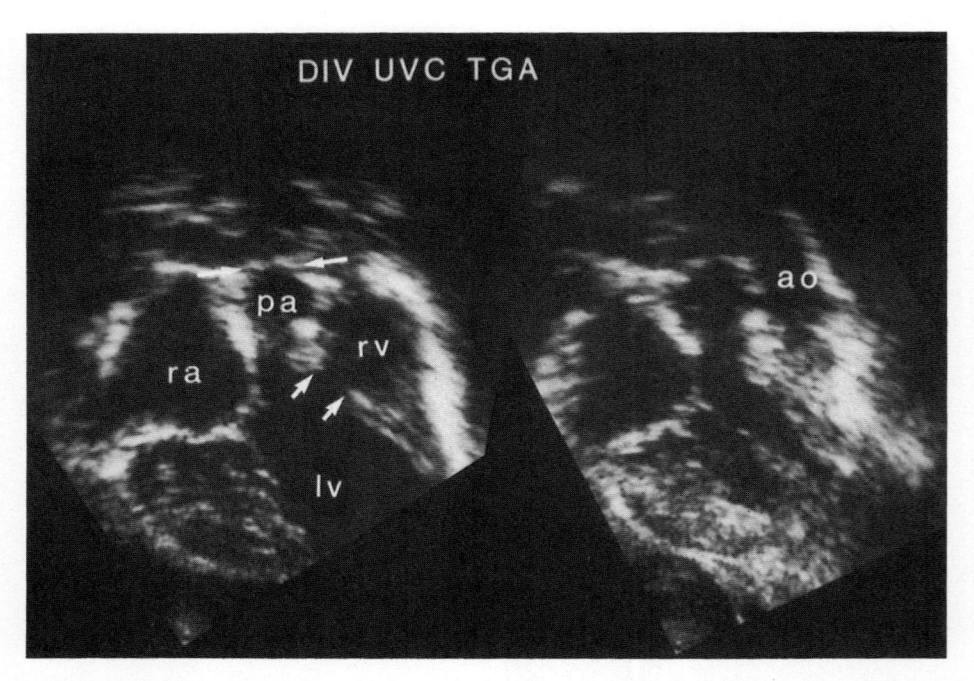

Fig. 7 Double inlet ventricle with transposition of the great arteries (ventriculo-arterial discordance). The small right ventricle is on the left shoulder of the heart and gives off the aorta. The pulmonary artery arises from the left ventricle. The arrows indicate the ventricular septal defect connecting left and right ventricles. Two adjacent sections are shown.

be haemodynamically stable (Fig. 5B) since the whole cardiac outlet goes across the interatrial septum. Usually the dominant chamber is left ventricular in type and the small right ventricle lies to the right and anteriorly. Both concordant and discordant ventriculo-arterial connections are associated with this anomaly. It is very rare to see an imperforate right atrioventricular valve in which valve tissue is recognised but in which leaflets remain fused.

Absence of the left atrioventricular connection is found with a main ventricle of right ventricular morphology and a small posterior left ventricle. Imperforate left atrioventricular valves are more common than absent left atrioventricular valves (Fig. 6).

In a heart with univentricular connection and two ventricular chambers there is always a ventricular septal defect connecting the two cavities (Fig. 7). In double inlet left ventricle with discordant ventriculo atrial connections (transposition of the great arteries) the size of the ventricular septal defect is crucial as the entire cardiac output must pass through it (Fig. 8). Echocardiography readily delineates this defect and provides information about its size, the pressure drop across it and the size of the rudimentary ventricle beyond.

Fig. 8 A: Double inlet ventricle, transposition of the great arteries and a ventricular septal defect. The patient underwent pulmonary artery banding (arrowed). **B:** A similar case to A. The banding is well seen in this long axis view and the ventricular septal defect is small and restrictive.

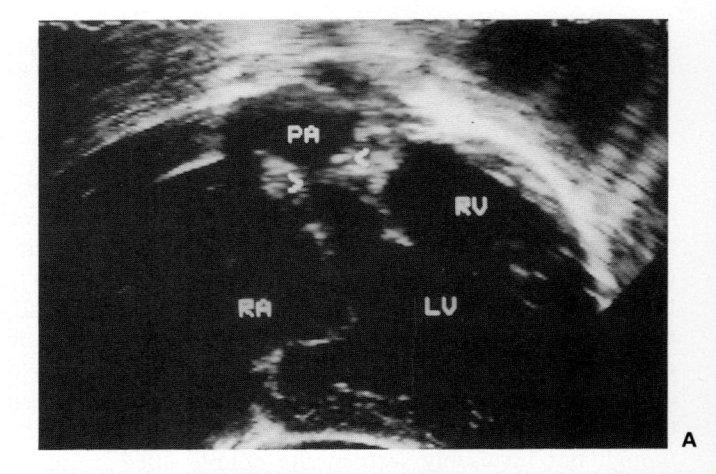

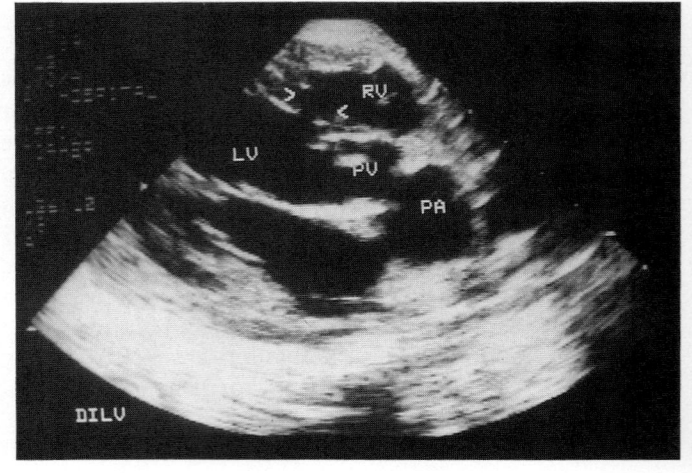

In conclusion cross sectional echocardiography very readily identifies the complex anatomy in hearts with a univentricular atrioventricular connection. Recognition of the individual valve structures, their patency and attachment is better carried out by cross sectional echo than any other technique. The addition of Doppler ultrasound gives an improved appreciation of the degree of regurgitation or stenosis of individual valve structures.

REFERENCES

1 Anderson R H, Macartney F J, Tynan M J et al. Univentricular atrioventricular connection: the single ventricle trap unsprung. Pediatr Cardiol 1983; 4: 273–80.
2 Deanfield J, Leaugge R, Stroobaut J, Chrispin A R, Taylor J F N, Macartney F J. Use of high kilovoltage filtered beam radiography for detection of bronchial situs in infants and young children. Br Heart J 1980; 44: 577–583.
3 Huhta J C, Smallhorn J F, Macartney F J. Two dimensional echocardiography diagnosis of situs. Br Heart J 1982; 48: 97–108.
4 Rigby M L, Gibson D G, Joseph M C, Lincoln J C R, Shinebourne E A, Shore D F, Anderson R H. Recognition of imperforate atrioventricular valves by two dimensional echocardiography. Br Heart J 1982; 47: 326–329.

25

Venous anomalies

Systemic venous drainage
Pulmonary venous drainage
Total anomalous pulmonary venous connection (TAPVC)
    Supracardiac TAPVC
    Cardiac TAPVC
    Infracardiac TAPVC
    Mixed TAPVC
    Common pulmonary vein atresia
Partial anomalous pulmonary venous connection (PAPVC)
Pulmonary venous connections in atrial isomerism
Cor triatriatum
Postoperative assessment

Ian D. Sullivan and Vanda M. Gooch

VENOUS ANOMALIES 457

Systemic venous drainage

Normal systemic venous drainage from below the diaphragm passes into a right sided inferior vena caval vein which receives the hepatic veins and then drains into the morphological right atrium. Abnormalities of this drainage include situs inversus and interruption of the vena caval vein with azygos or hemiazygos connection. The superior systemic venous drainage is to a right sided superior vena caval vein which drains to the morphological right atrium. The commonest abnormality of superior systemic venous drainage is the presence of a second superior vena caval vein on the left side which most commonly drains to the coronary sinus but can drain elsewhere.

Normal and abnormal systemic venous connections are considered in more detail under the headings 'atrial situs' and 'venous connections' in Chapter 19.

Pulmonary venous drainage

Anomalous pulmonary venous connection is the connection of pulmonary veins to sites other than the left atrium. When all pulmonary veins are involved, there is total anomalous pulmonary venous connection (TAPVC). When only some pulmonary veins are connected abnormally, there is partial anomalous pulmonary venous connection (PAPVC). The normal pulmonary venous connection is described and illustrated in Chapter 4.

Total anomalous pulmonary venous connection (TAPVC)

For several years it has been apparent that TAPVC could accurately be assessed by cross-sectional echocardiography.[1,2] This was one of the first major structural cardiac abnormalities to lend itself to surgery without prior cardiac catheterisation,[3] and improved surgical results for correction of this condition may be due to the avoidance of pre-operative invasive investigation.[4,5] TAPVC is usually an isolated abnormality in hearts with normal atrial arrangement although occasionally intracardiac structural abnormalities may coexist. Hearts with an isometric atrial arrangement will be considered separately.

There are three cardinal echocardiographic features which should be sought when TAPVC is suspected. These are: a) volume overload of the right heart, b) right atrial to left atrial flow, c) demonstration of a pulmonary venous confluence which is separate from the left atrium.

The abnormality usually most evident in TAPVC is volume overload of the right heart. The right atrium, right ventricle and pulmonary artery are all enlarged. The left heart looks relatively small in comparison to the dilated right sided structures in most cases (Fig. 1). The absolute

Fig. 1 TAPVC to coronary sinus. Modified apical four chamber view with the transducer angled posteriorly in a patient with TAPVC to the coronary sinus demonstrating volume overload of the right heart. The right ventricle forms the cardiac apex. The separate pulmonary veins are indicated by small arrows. cs – coronary sinus.

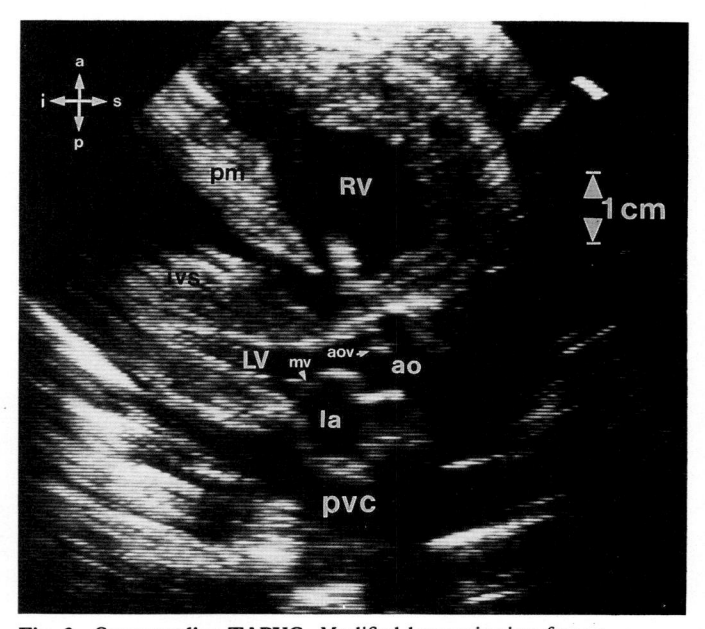

Fig. 2 Supracardiac TAPVC. Modified long axis view from a neonate with supracardiac TAPVC. There is marked discrepancy between the dimensions of left ventricle and right ventricle. This had led to a referral diagnosis of hypoplastic left heart syndrome for this patient. aov – aortic valve, ivs – ventricular septum, pm – papillary muscle of tricuspid valve, pvc – pulmonary venous confluence.

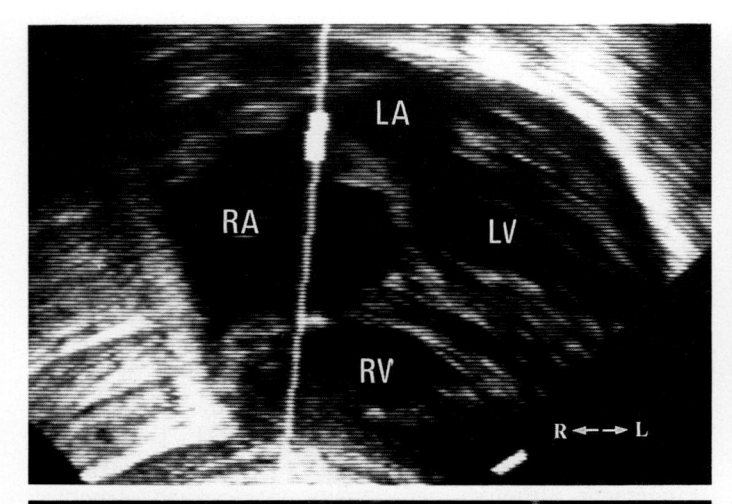

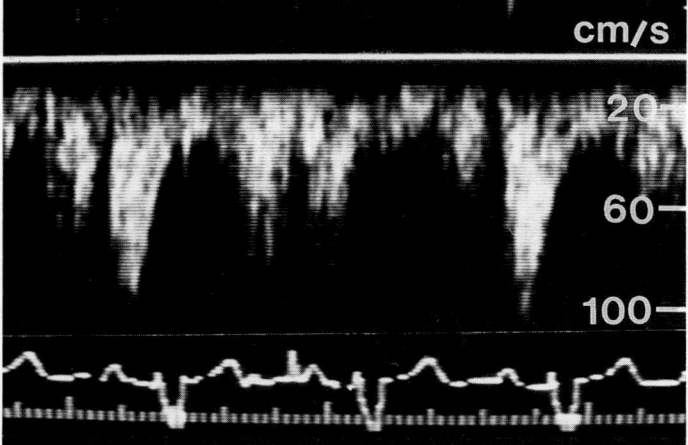

Fig. 3 Doppler in TAPVC. Pulsed Doppler demonstration of the obligatory right atrium to left atrium flow via the atrial septal defect (flow away from the transducer) in a patient with TAPVC.
Top: Sample volume placed in the atrial septal defect. **Bottom:** Pulsed Doppler trace obtained from this position. Note flow below the baseline is away from the transducer position.

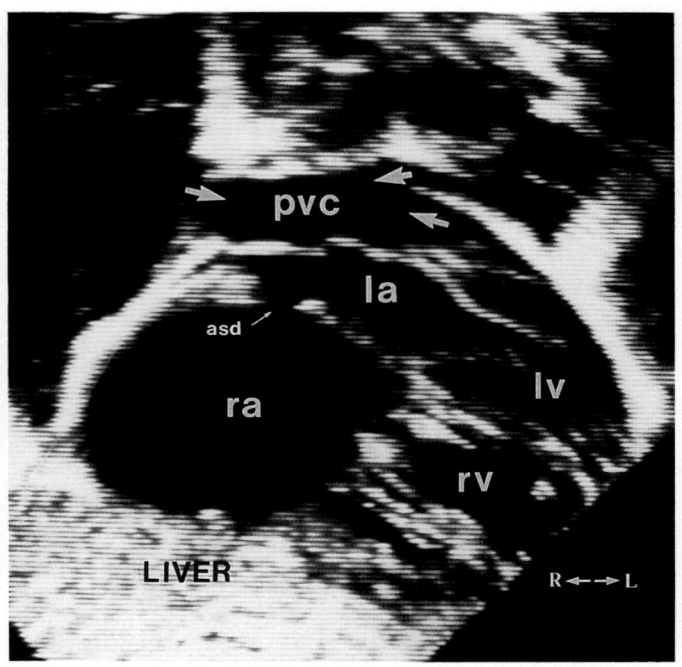

Fig. 4 TAPVC to pulmonary venous confluence. Subcostal oblique four chamber view demonstrating pulmonary veins (arrows) draining to a pulmonary venous confluence behind the left atrium in an infant with TAPVC to a left vertical vein. asd – atrial septal defect. pvc – pulmonary venous confluence.

left ventricular volume is abnormally low in some cases and in these the postoperative course may be less favourable.[6] It is, therefore, important not to diagnose hypoplastic left heart syndrome erroneously (Fig. 2). An atrial communication (patent foramen ovale or atrial septal defect) is invariable, with the exception of two case reports in the literature. Right to left flow at this interatrial communication is obligatory in TAPVC. Conventional pulsed Doppler or colour flow imaging can confirm flow direction at this site (Fig. 3). Flow from left atrium to right atrium excludes TAPVC. In most patients with TAPVC, the confluence of the pulmonary veins can be seen immediately posterior to the left atrium, but separated from it. The confluence can usually be imaged from subcostal (Fig. 4), apical, precordial and suprasternal views. However, this may not be the case in some patients with infradiaphragmatic TAPVC in whom the pulmonary veins converge in a more inferior location. Visualisation of the confluence may also be difficult in patients with TAPVC to the coronary sinus (see below).

When these features are present, the site of the abnormal connection must be sought. Presentation of TAPVC is highly variable, with a population spectrum which ranges from a moribund neonate to an asymptomatic child. The variability is most dependent on whether or not the abnormal pulmonary venous drainage channel is obstructed. The likelihood of important obstruction varies with the site of the anomalous pulmonary venous connection. Obstruction to pulmonary venous drainage is usually apparent from clinical findings and the chest radiograph but echocardiography may be valuable in assessing the site and severity of obstruction from both structural and Doppler features.[7] Obstruction to flow, when present, usually occurs in the abnormal drainage channel 'downstream' to the pulmonary venous confluence, but the pulmonary veins themselves may be hypoplastic, in which case the obstruction is intrapulmonary.

The aim of the echocardiographer should be to identify sites of connection of all four pulmonary veins, as mixed patterns of anomalous pulmonary venous connection exist. Sites of TAPVC may be supracardiac, cardiac or infracardiac as shown in Figure 5.[8] These will be considered in turn.

Supracardiac TAPVC The most common form of TAPVC, about 50% of total cases, is connection of the

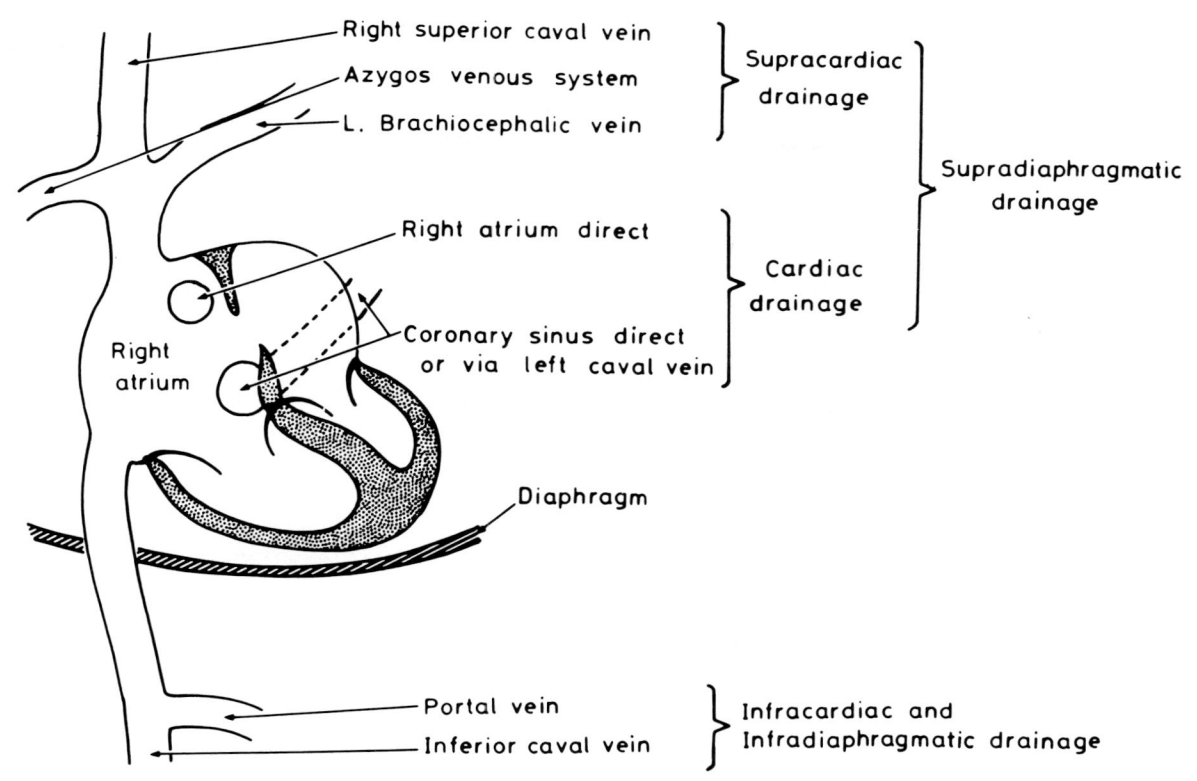

Fig. 5 TAPVC. Diagrammatic representation of the possible sites of anomalous pulmonary venous connection. (Reproduced with permission from Reference 8.)

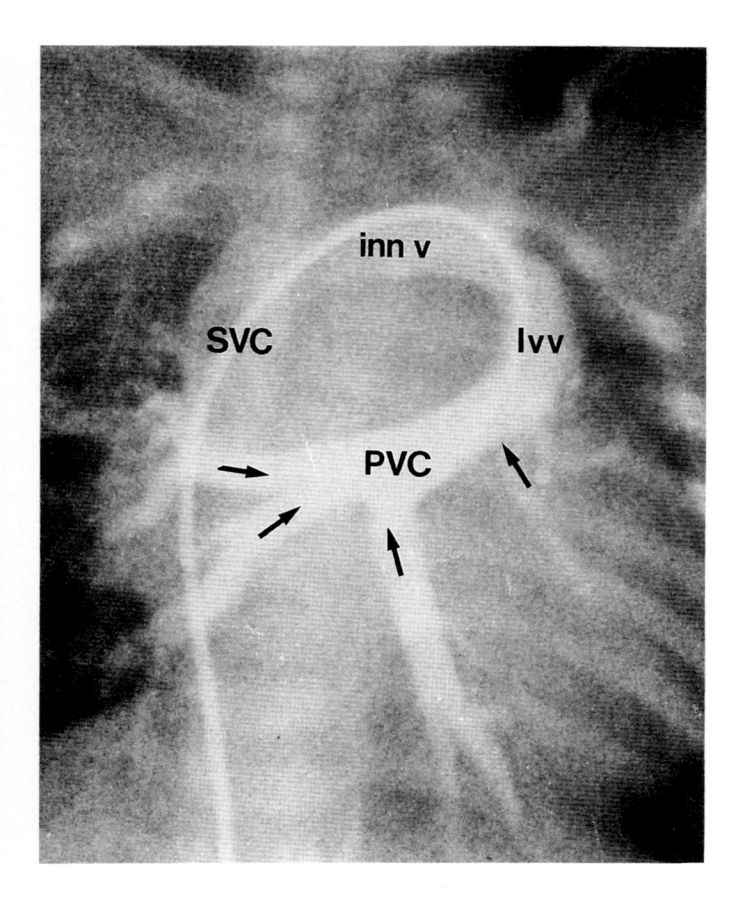

pulmonary venous confluence to a left vertical vein which ascends to join the innominate vein (Fig. 6). Drainage is then via the superior caval vein to the right atrium. The best images to demonstrate the separate pulmonary venous connections to the confluence are generally obtained from a suprasternal paracoronal cut posterior to the left atrium. Whilst it may not be possible to image all four pulmonary veins entering the confluence and the connection of the confluence to the ascending left vertical vein in a single cut, gently rotating the scanhead will usually allow demonstration of these structures (Fig. 7). Commonly, supracardiac pulmonary venous drainage is not obstructed, so that left vertical vein, innominate vein and superior caval vein are all large (Fig. 8). The resulting widening of the superior mediastinum can give rise to the so-called 'snowman' or 'cottage loaf' chest X-ray appearance, although this is rarely present in infancy. The left vertical vein may ascend either anterior or posterior to the left pulmonary artery. When it is posterior, the flow in the left vertical vein may be obstructed by extrinsic compression

Fig. 6 Angiogram in TAPVC. Frontal plane cine-angiogram in an infant with supracardiac TAPVC. The catheter has been introduced into the pulmonary venous confluence via the superior caval vein, innominate vein and left vertical vein. Arrows indicate the four separate pulmonary veins. PVC – pulmonary venous confluence, inn v – innominate vein, lvv – left vertical vein.

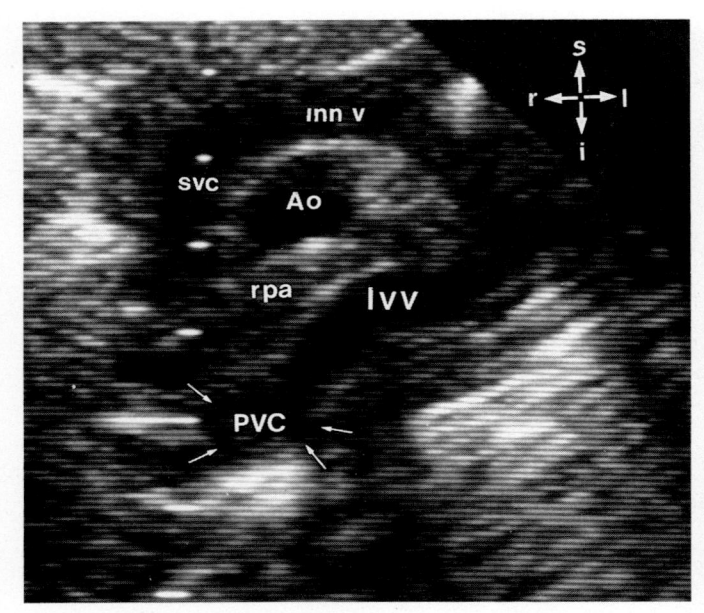

Fig. 7 TAPVC to vertical vein. Suprasternal paracoronal view in a patient with TAPVC to a left vertical vein. The junction of right upper pulmonary vein with pulmonary venous confluence is slightly out of the plane of this cut. The arrows indicate separate pulmonary veins. PVC – pulmonary venous confluence, lvv – left vertical vein, inn v – innominate vein, rpa – right pulmonary artery.

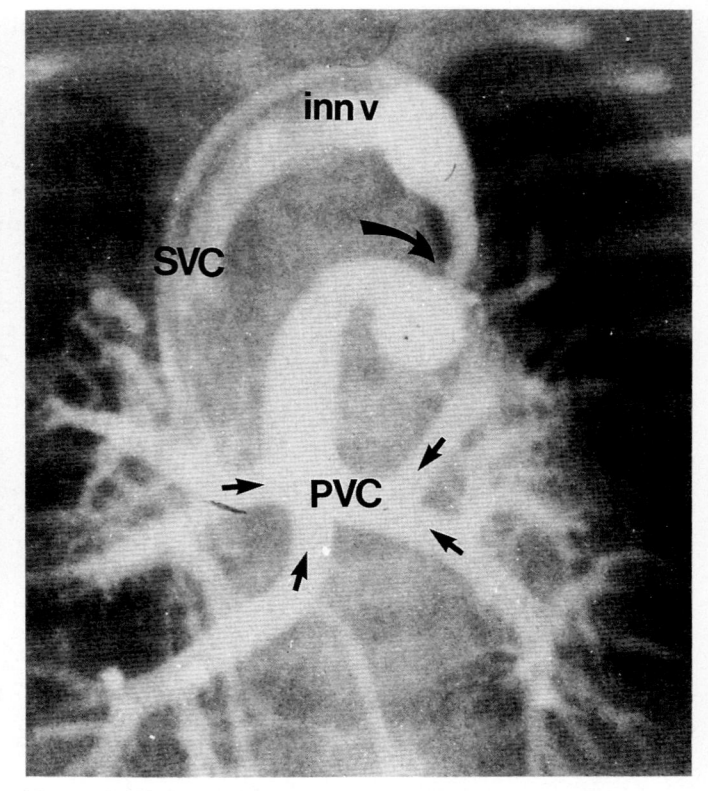

Fig. 9 TAPVC – angiogram. Frontal angiographic view in a patient with TAPVC to left vertical vein. The drainage channel is obstructed by extrinsic compression as it passes between left pulmonary artery and left main bronchus (curved arrow). inn v – innominate vein, PVC – pulmonary venous confluence.

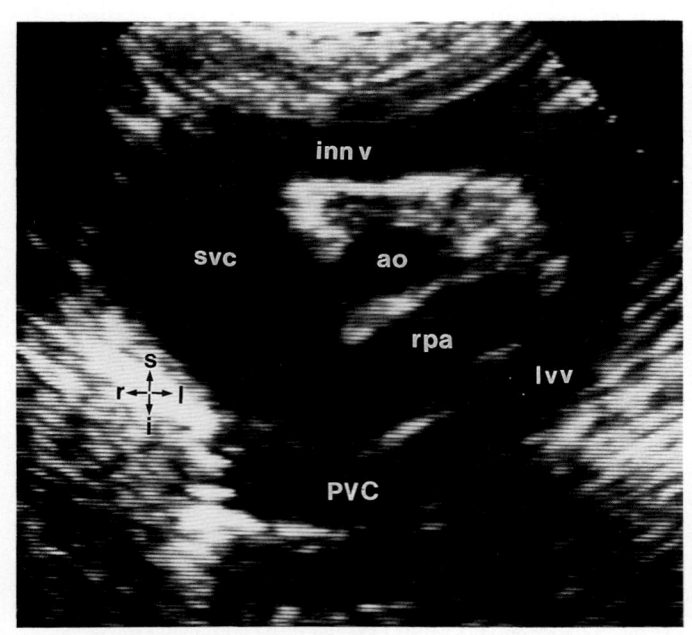

Fig. 8 TAPVC to vertical vein. Suprasternal paracoronal view demonstrating non-obstructed TAPVC to left vertical vein. The pulmonary venous drainage channel is very large. PVC – pulmonary venous confluence, lvv – left vertical vein, inn v – innominate vein, rpa – right pulmonary artery.

between the left pulmonary artery in front and the left main bronchus behind (Fig. 9). Localised obstruction to flow in the left vertical vein may still occur however, when it passes anterior to the left pulmonary artery. The left vertical vein may be differentiated from a left sided superior caval vein by the direction of flow, which will be superiorly directed in the left vertical vein (Fig. 10). Turbulent continuous flow in the left vertical vein, varying only with respiration and not the cardiac cycle, may be useful to confirm obstruction (Fig. 10).[7]

Supracardiac TAPVC to other sites is uncommon. The pulmonary venous confluence may drain to superior caval vein or azygos vein, via a channel which will be seen immediately behind the right atrium. This pattern of drainage may be difficult to differentiate from TAPVC directly to right atrium unless the connection of the pulmonary venous channel is clearly seen (Fig. 11). However, indirect evidence for this site of connection is dilatation of the junction between superior caval vein and right atrium (Fig. 12) with turbulent flow at the site. The innominate vein is also smaller than superior caval vein, rather than more or less uniformly enlarged as is the case when pulmonary venous drainage is via a left vertical vein (Figs 6 to 10).

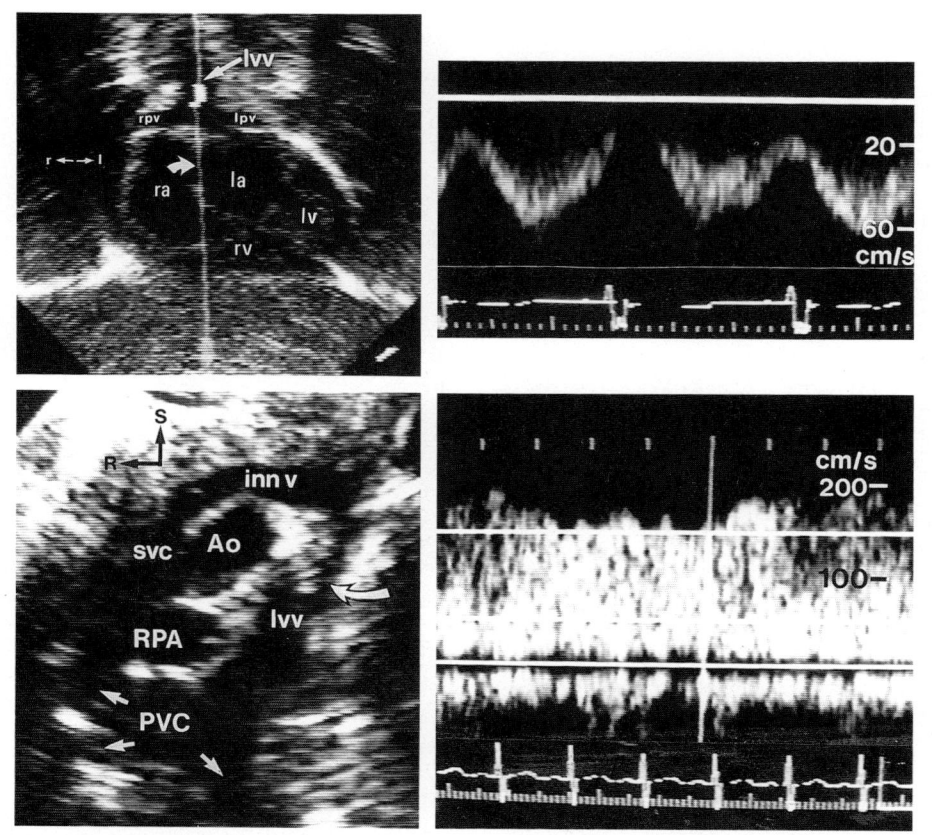

Fig. 10 TAPVC – Doppler. Top left: Subcostal oblique view in an infant with supracardiac TAPVC to left vertical vein. The Doppler sample volume is at the base of the left vertical vein. There is a sinus venosus atrial septal defect (curved arrow). lvv – left vertical vein, rpv – right pulmonary vein, lpv – left pulmonary vein. **Top right:** Doppler signal demonstrates superiorly directed flow (away from the transducer) which is at low velocity (Vmax 0.6 m/s) and phasic with the cardiac cycle. **Lower left:** Suprasternal paracoronal cut in a neonate with obstructed supracardiac TAPVC to left vertical vein which is compressed as it passes between left pulmonary artery and left main bronchus (curved arrow). The pulmonary veins (arrows) are congested. inn v – innominate vein, RPA – right pulmonary artery, PVC – pulmonary venous confluence.
Lower right: Continuous wave Doppler signal from the site of narrowing confirms superiorly directed flow (towards the transducer which is in the suprasternal notch) at high velocity (Vmax 2.0 m/s) varying only with respiration and not the cardiac cycle, indicative of obstruction to flow.

Of course, it is not sufficient to demonstrate enlargement of superior caval vein and innominate vein alone for this diagnosis. Other causes of excessive flow in these vessels such as an intracranial arteriovenous malformation (vein of Galen aneurysm) should be considered. In this situation, the grossly dilated vein of Galen can be demonstrated from a parasagittal or posteriorly directed paracoronal cut with the transducer placed in the anterior fontanelle (Fig. 13).

Cardiac TAPVC The usual site of intracardiac TAPVC is the coronary sinus. In this situation, the pulmonary venous confluence is usually the coronary sinus itself, which is markedly dilated. It is usually possible to demonstrate continuity between the pulmonary veins and the coronary sinus from subcostal (Fig. 14) or apical (Fig. 1) positions. Cardiac TAPVC is rarely obstructed, although this may occur. Again, imaging a large coronary sinus alone is insufficient for diagnosis, as the usual causes of coronary sinus enlargement are persistence of a left sided superior caval vein draining into the coronary sinus, or merely the presence of right heart pressure overload. TAPVC directly to the right atrium (Fig. 15) has been mentioned above. It may be difficult to demonstrate separate pulmonary venous connections when they enter the right atrium separately in this situation but this is rare.

Infracardiac TAPVC Infracardiac, or infradiaphragmatic, TAPVC is usually to the portal venous system but may be occasionally to the inferior caval vein. When the connection is to the portal venous system, pulmonary venous return has to traverse the ductus venosus or the portal system within the liver to get back to right atrium (Fig. 16). While the ductus venosus is widely open, flow may be relatively non-obstructed. Inferior caval venous blood preferentially streams through the foramen ovale in fetal life. The Eustachian valve in the right atrium contributes to this flow pattern (Fig. 17). Consequently, a neonate with relatively non-obstructed infradiaphragmatic

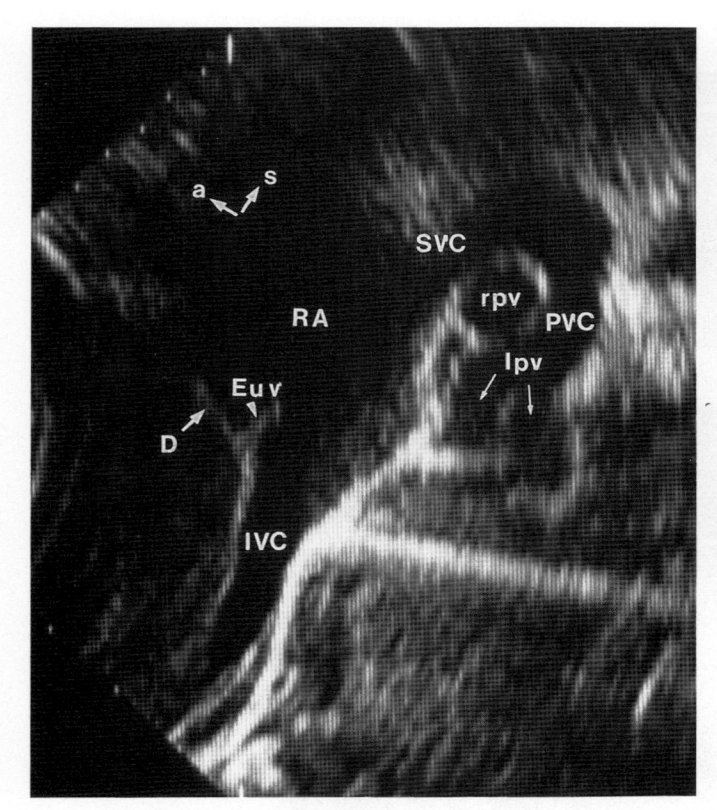

Fig. 11 TAPVC to superior caval vein. Subcostal parasagittal view demonstrating TAPVC to superior caval vein. In this cut, the two left pulmonary veins are seen entering the confluence. The right pulmonary venous channel is perpendicular to the imaging plane, but rotation of the transducer head confirmed non-obstructed right pulmonary venous connection to the confluence. D – diaphragm, Euv – Eustachian valve, lpv – left pulmonary veins, rpv – right pulmonary veins, PVC – pulmonary venous confluence.

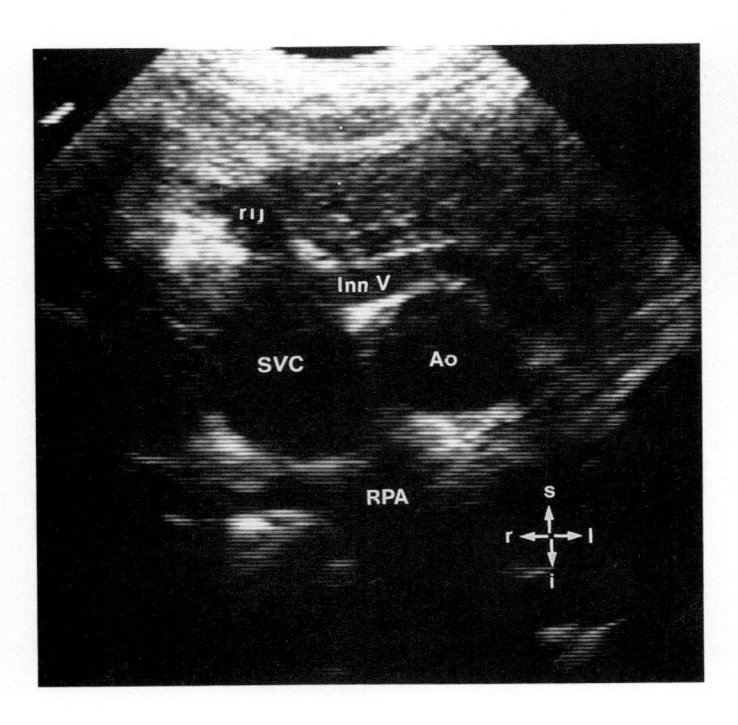

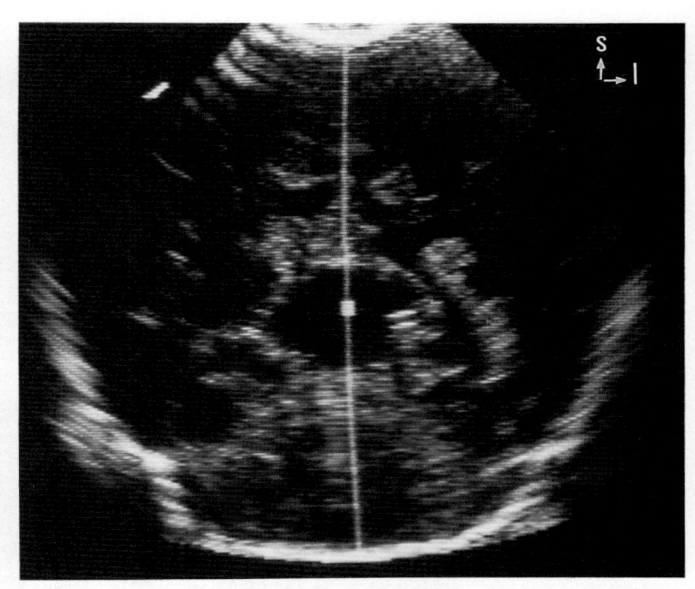

Fig. 13 Vein of Galen aneurysm. Paracoronal slice through the brain with the transducer directed posteriorly from the anterior fontanelle. The Doppler sample volume is placed in the 'vein of Galen aneursym'.

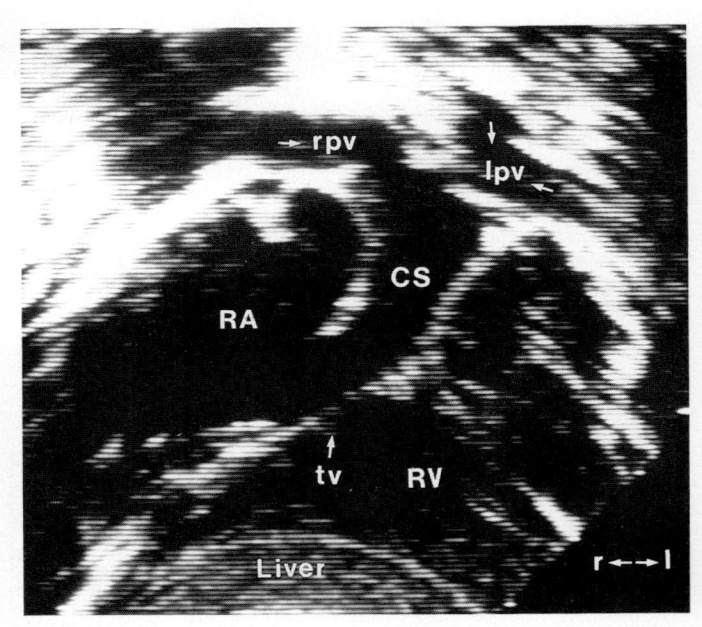

Fig. 14 TAPVC to coronary sinus. Subcostal oblique view with the imaging plane just posterior to the usual four chamber plane demonstrating TAPVC to coronary sinus. rpv – right pulmonary vein, lpv – left pulmonary vein, CS – coronary sinus.

Fig. 12 TAPVC to the superior caval vein. Suprasternal paracoronal cut in a patient with TAPVC to the superior caval vein. The superior caval vein is dilated, so that it is much larger than the innominate or internal jugular vein. rij – right internal jugular vein, Inn V – innominate vein, RPA – right pulmonary artery.

VENOUS ANOMALIES   463

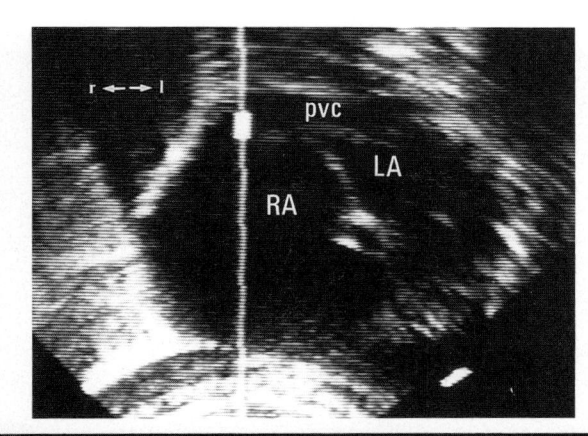

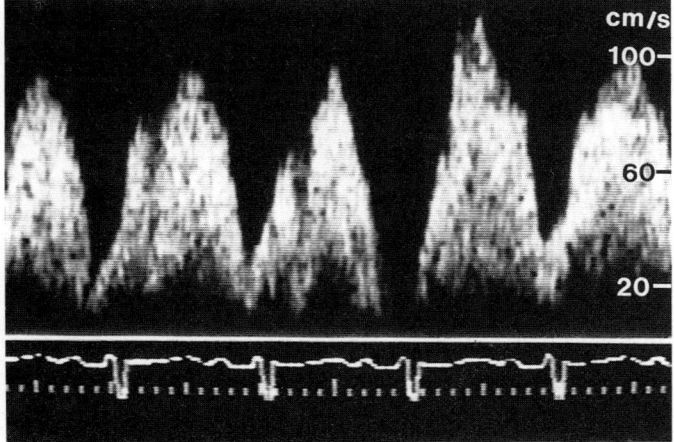

Fig. 15 **TAPVC to right atrium.** Top: Subcostal oblique view demonstrating TAPVC to the right atrium. The Doppler sample volume is at the junction of the pulmonary venous confluence with the right atrium. pvc – pulmonary venous confluence. **Lower:** The Doppler signal from this site demonstrates venous flow towards the transducer which is phasic with the cardiac cycle, indicative of non-obstructed pulmonary venous drainage. Compare the Doppler signal at the atrial septal defect in the same patient (Fig. 3).

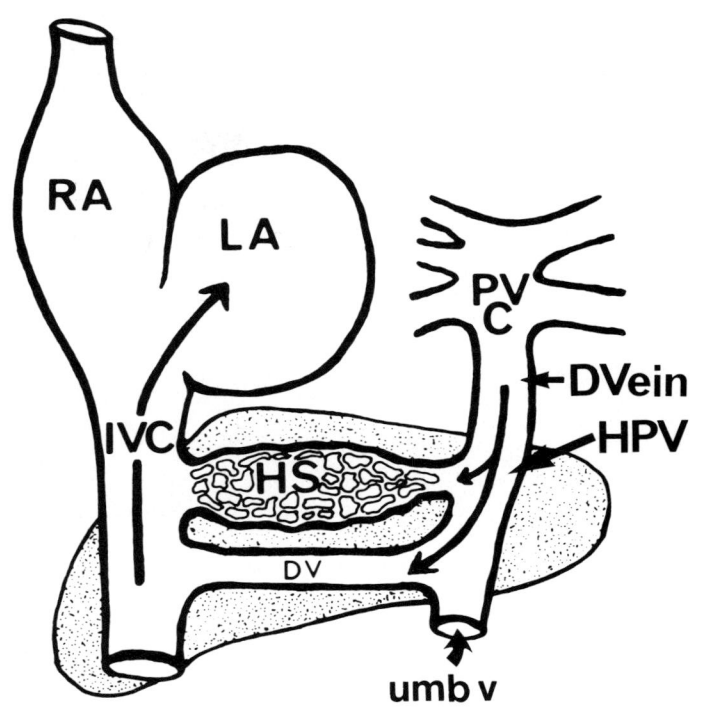

Fig. 16 **TAPVC to hepatic portal vein.** Diagram of infradiaphragmatic TAPVC to the hepatic portal venous system, with a patent ductus venosus. The inferior caval blood may stream preferentially to the left atrium. DV – ductus venosus, D Vein – descending vein, HPV – hepatic portal vein, HS – hepatic sinusoids, umb v – umbilical vein, PVC – pulmonary venous confluence.

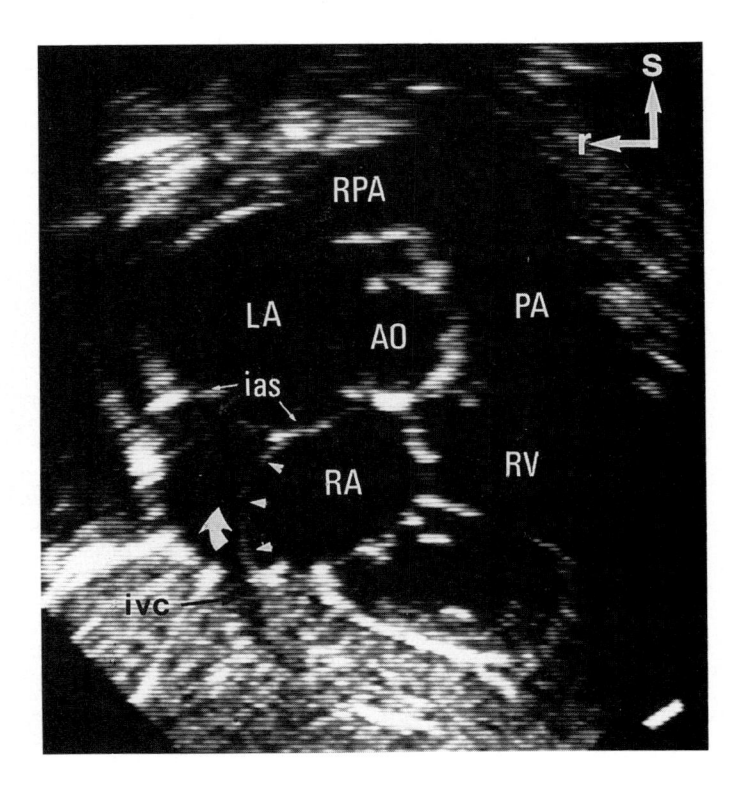

TAPVC may not be cyanosed and, exceptionally, may even have a 'normal' rise in systemic oxygen saturation when breathing oxygen.[9] However, the ductus venosus usually closes soon after birth. Consequently, pulmonary venous flow is 'obstructed' within the hepatic sinusoids and it is not surprising that this form of TAPVC typically presents with severe pulmonary venous congestion in the first week of life. A diagnosis may be apparent as soon as the transducer is placed on the infant's abdomen, as the liver is usually enlarged and the portal venous system is grossly distended giving rise to large echo-free spaces within the

Fig. 17 **Eustachian valve.** Subcostal oblique view in a neonate demonstrating the role of the Eustachian valve (arrowheads) in directing the stream of inferior caval venous blood (curved arrow) through the foramen ovale. ias – interatrial septum, RPA – right pulmonary artery.

464 CARDIAC ULTRASOUND

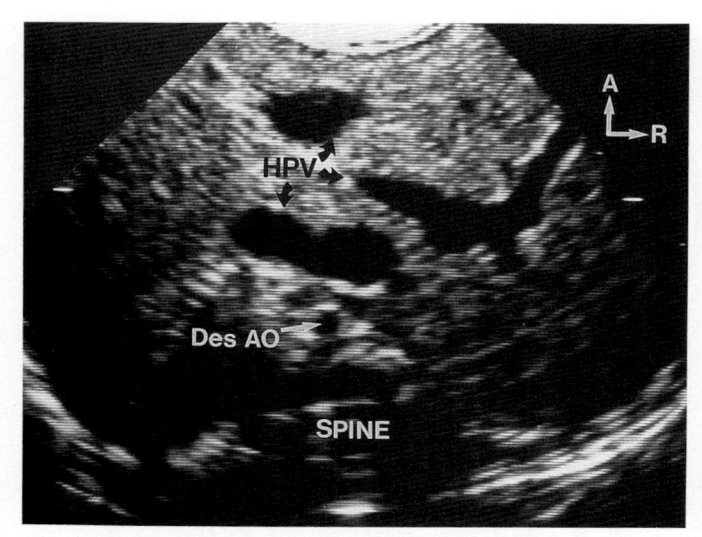

Fig. 18 Infradiaphragmatic TAPVC. Transverse section through the upper abdomen in a neonate with obstructed infradiaphragmatic TAPVC. The portal venous system is grossly distended. Des AO – descending aorta, HPV – hepatic portal veins.

Fig. 19 Infradiaphragmatic TAPVC – angiogram. Frontal cine-angiogram in a neonate with obstructed infradiaphragmatic TAPVC. Pulmonary veins converge just above the diaphragm and a descending vein then drains pulmonary venous blood into the hepatic venous system. Compare the site of the pulmonary venous confluence to the typical location in supracardiac TAPVC depicted in Figure 9. HPV – hepatic portal vein, rpv – right pulmonary vein, lpv – left pulmonary vein.

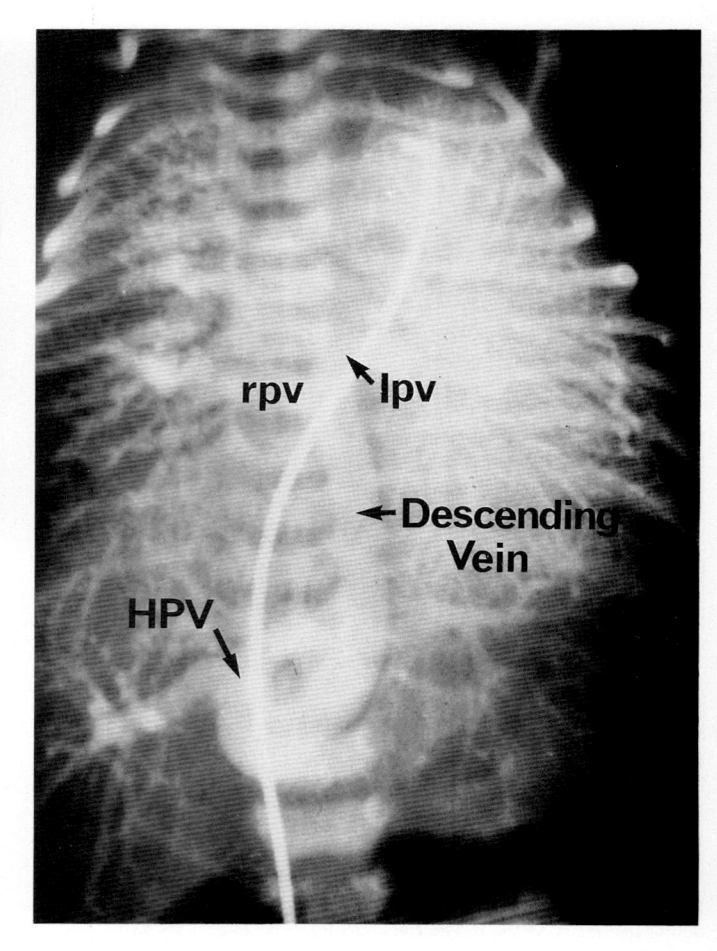

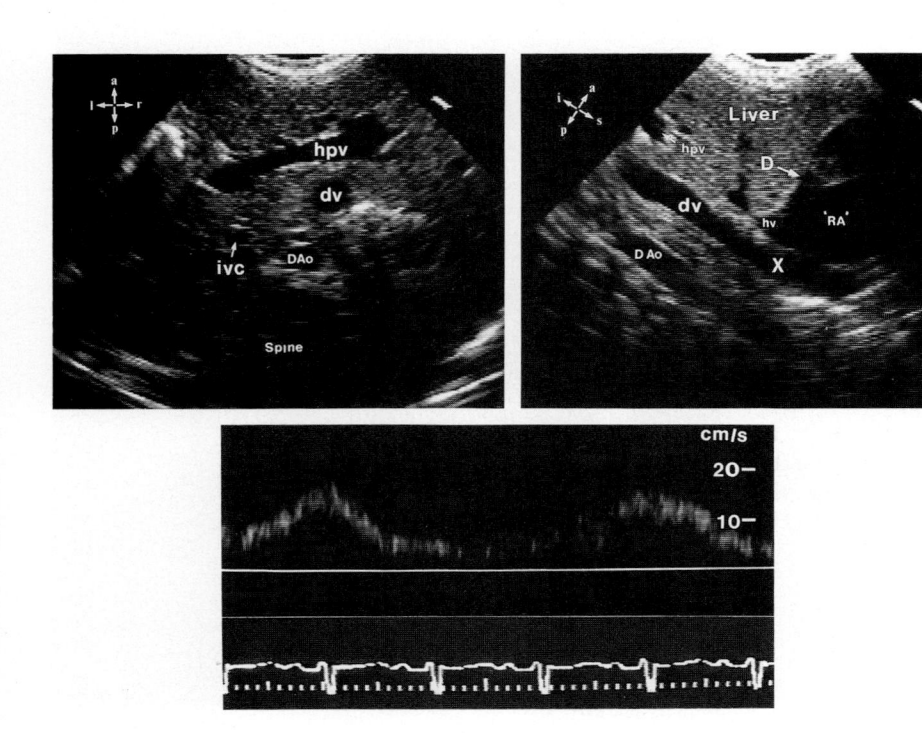

Fig. 20 Infradiaphragmatic TAPVC. Transverse (top left) and parasagittal (top right) views of the upper abdomen demonstrating the descending vein passing through the diaphragm anterior to the descending aorta in a patient with infradiaphragmatic TAPVC. It is evident from the position of the inferior caval vein that this patient also has right atrial isomerism. Pulsed Doppler interrogation of flow (lower panel) in the descending vein (sample volume at site marked X) demonstrates low velocity flow phasic with respiration only and not with the cardiac cycle, indicating obstruction to flow. dv – descending vein, hpv – hepatic portal vein, hv – hepatic vein, D Ao – descending aorta, D – diaphragm.

VENOUS ANOMALIES

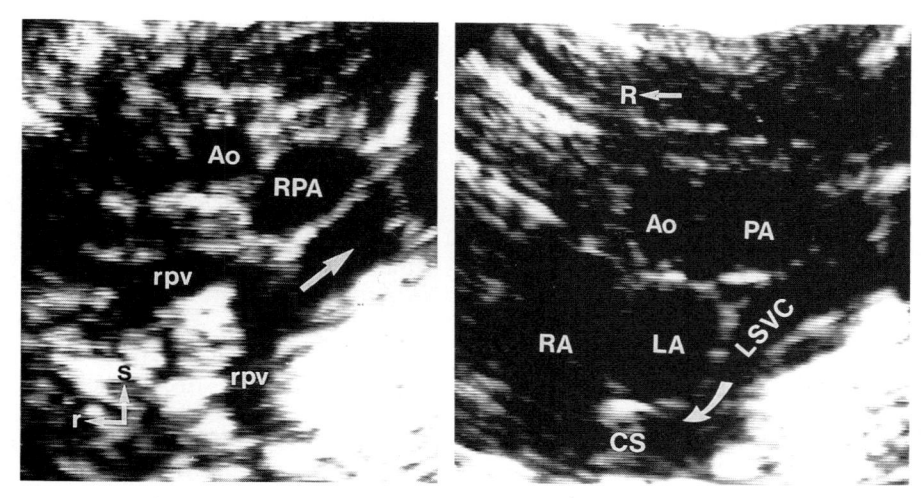

Fig. 21 Anomalous right pulmonary veins. Left: Slightly oblique suprasternal view in an infant with connection of the right pulmonary veins to the left superior caval vein. The left pulmonary veins connected normally. There was also coarctation of the aorta. The confluence of the right pulmonary veins is indicated by an arrow in the direction of flow. rpv – right pulmonary veins, RPA – right pulmonary artery. **Right:** Oblique high parasternal view demonstrating a left sided superior caval vein draining to the coronary sinus. The junction of the pulmonary venous channel and caval vein is between the planes of these two views of the same patient. Pulsed Doppler signal from the caval vein demonstrated non-obstructed venous flow in the direction of the curved arrow. CS – coronary sinus, LSVC – left superior vena cava.

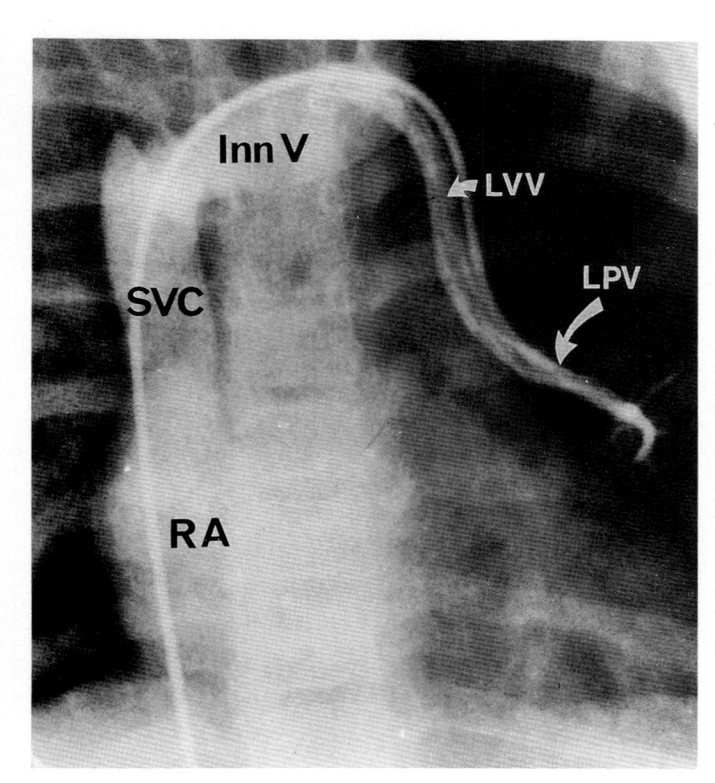

Fig. 22 Anomalous pulmonary vein angiogram. Frontal plane angiogram demonstrating the left lower pulmonary vein draining to left vertical vein. The other pulmonary veins drained normally in this child who otherwise had typical cardiovascular manifestations of William's syndrome. LPV – left pulmonary vein, LVV – left vertical vein, Inn V – innominate vein.

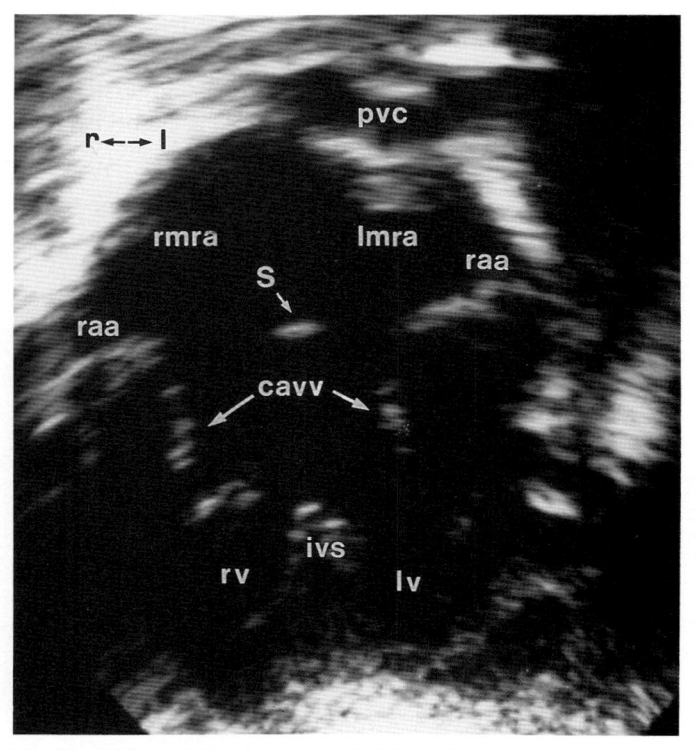

Fig. 23 Right atrial isomerism. Apical four chamber view in a patient with right atrial isomerism. Note the pulmonary venous confluence behind the left sided atrium. The intracardiac anatomy is typical of right isomerism. There are bilateral right atrial appendages, and a complete atrioventricular septal defect with a common atrioventricular orifice. There is virtually a common atrium, with the atrial septum represented by a strand of tissue only. pvc – pulmonary venous confluence, cavv – common atrioventricular valve, rmra – morphological right atrium, lmra – left morphological right atrium, raa – right atrial appendage, S – strand of atrial septum. ivs – inter-ventricular septum.

substance of the liver (Fig. 18). The pulmonary veins typically converge in a more inferior location than is the case with supracardiac TAPVC (Fig. 19) so a pulmonary venous confluence behind the left atrium may not be seen. Moreover, the confluence has a vertical, rather than horizontal orientation. On the other hand, as pulmonary venous flow is usually obstructed to a greater or lesser extent, the pulmonary veins and descending channel are often large. The descending channel passes through the diaphragm just anterior to the oesophagus and descending aorta (Fig. 20). Flow directed inferiorly in this channel may be confirmed by Doppler interrogation from a subcostal transducer position,[10] but it must be remembered that flow velocity is usually very slow at this site, and flow signals may not be detected unless filter settings are low.

Mixed TAPVC While pulmonary veins typically drain to a single confluence in the usual varieties of TAPVC described above, mixed drainage patterns occasionally occur. Virtually any combination of drainage sites for separate pulmonary veins may be found. Consequently, the aim must always be to attempt to identify the site of drainage of each individual pulmonary vein when TAPVC is suspected.

Common pulmonary vein atresia If a pulmonary venous confluence is located behind the left atrium in a newborn with features of severely obstructed TAPVC, but no drainage channel from the confluence is identified, there is probably common pulmonary vein atresia which is usually rapidly fatal.[8]

Partial anomalous pulmonary venous connection (PAPVC)

In PAPVC, some pulmonary veins are connected normally and some are connected anomalously. There is a bewildering array of possible anatomical combinations but some patterns are clearly recognised. The extracardiac interatrial communication characteristically described as a sinus venosus atrial septal defect, for example, typically results in drainage of right upper pulmonary vein blood to the right superior caval vein. Another pattern is the so-called Scimitar syndrome in which PAPVC from part or all of a hypoplastic right lung drains to the inferior caval vein.[11]

Anomalously connected pulmonary veins may drain to any of the sites described for TAPVC. Important structural congenital heart defects may be associated (Figs 21 and 22). More typically, PAPVC is an isolated abnormality and presents with clinical features of an atrial septal defect. The absence of a pulmonary venous confluence and the lack of right to left atrial shunting may make this a very difficult echocardiographic diagnosis, especially as a secundum atrial septal defect with demonstrable left to right shunting on Doppler interrogation often coexists. This is why the separate connection of all pulmonary veins should be

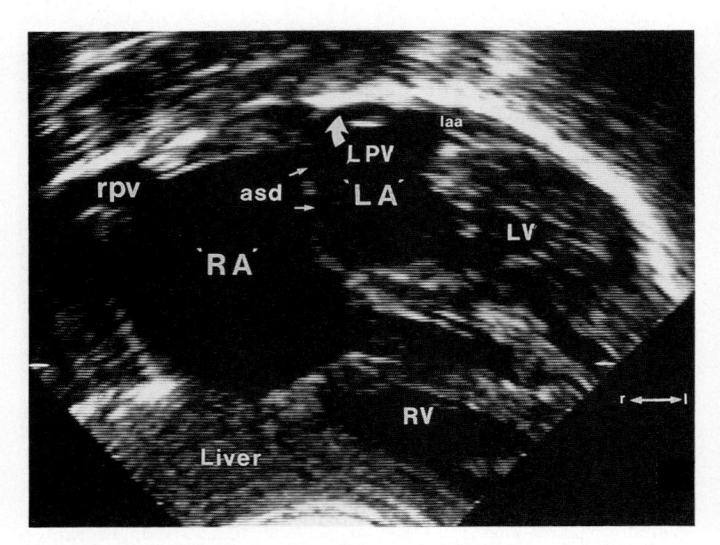

Fig. 24 Left atrial isomerism. Subcostal oblique four chamber view in a patient with left atrial isomerism demonstrating pulmonary venous connection to the ipsilateral atria. There is also a fenestrated atrial septal defect (small arrows). 'LA' – left sided morphological left atrium, 'RA' – right sided morphological left atrium, rpv – right pulmonary vein, asd – atrial septal defect, LPV – left pulmonary vein, laa – left atrial appendage.

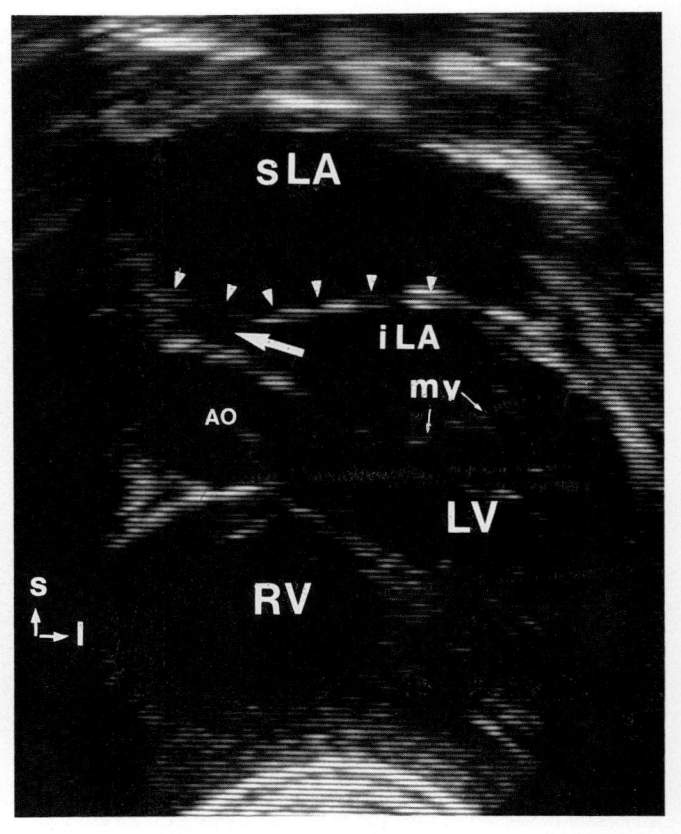

Fig. 25 Cor triatriatum. Subcostal oblique view in a patient with a partition (arrowheads) in the left atrium (cor triatriatum). Note the subaortic recess (arrow). sLA – superior left atrium, iLA – inferior left atrium.

assessed in any patient in whom PAPVC is a possibility. It is also why surgeons should always confirm pulmonary venous connection to the left atrium during closure of a secundum atrial septal defect. Thus, while PAPVC may be confidently diagnosed when an abnormal connection is identified, it may be difficult to exclude confidently an abnormal connection of at least one pulmonary vein.

Pulmonary venous connections in atrial isomerism

TAPVC must exist, by definition, in right atrial isomerism (Fig. 23). Any of the drainage patterns described above may occur (Fig. 5), although in a few cases, pulmonary veins drain to a confluence which then connects to the midline of the atrial mass,[12] which is usually a common atrium. In left atrial isomerism, by far the most common

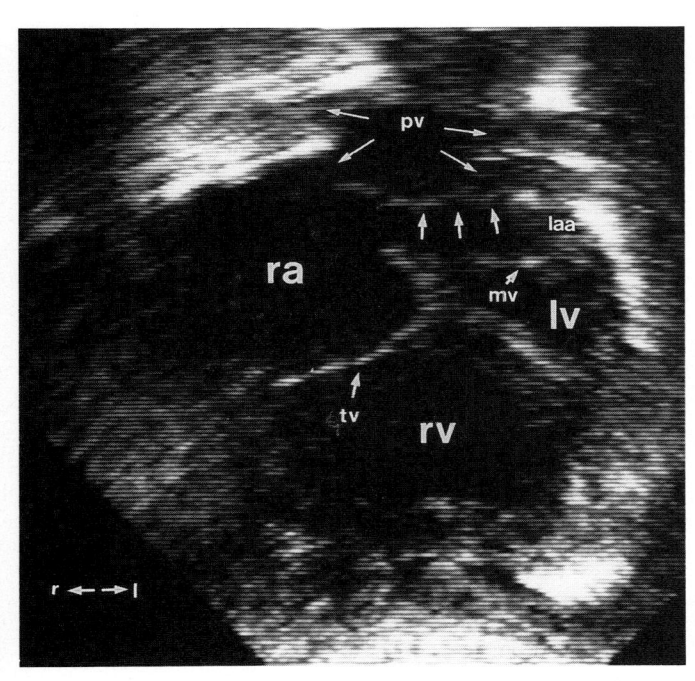

Fig. 26 Cor triatriatum. Modified apical four chamber view in the same patient as Figure 25. Note that the left atrial appendage is 'down stream' from the obstructing partition (arrows) in the left atrium. pv – pulmonary veins, laa – left atrial appendage.

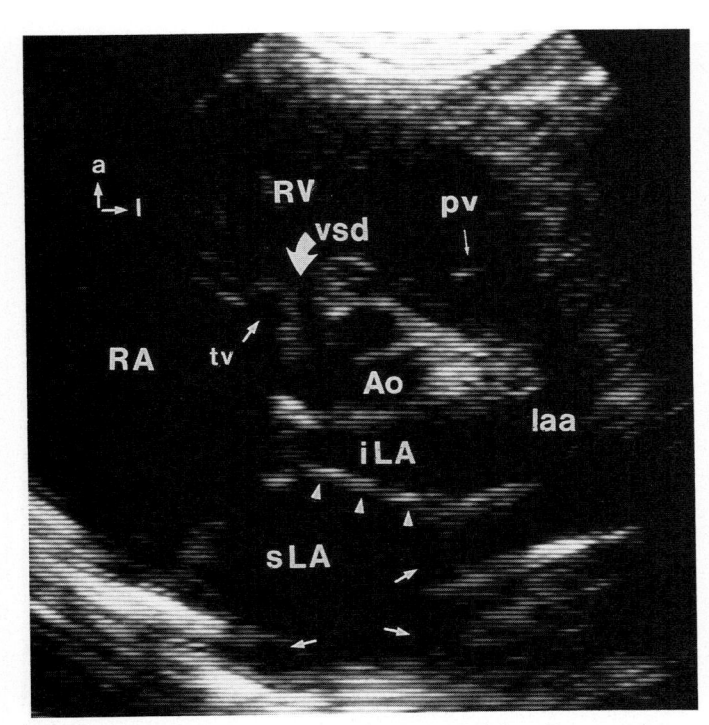

Fig. 27 Cor triatriatum and ventricular septal defect. Parasternal short axis in the same patient as Figures 25 and 26 demonstrating a partition (arrowheads) in the left atrium. Pulmonary veins (arrows) drain to the superior left atrial chamber (sLA) and the left atrial appendage (laa) arises from the inferior left atrial chamber (iLA). There is also a perimembranous ventricular septal defect. Note the fibrous continuity between tricuspid valve and aortic valve at its margin. vsd – ventricular septal defect.

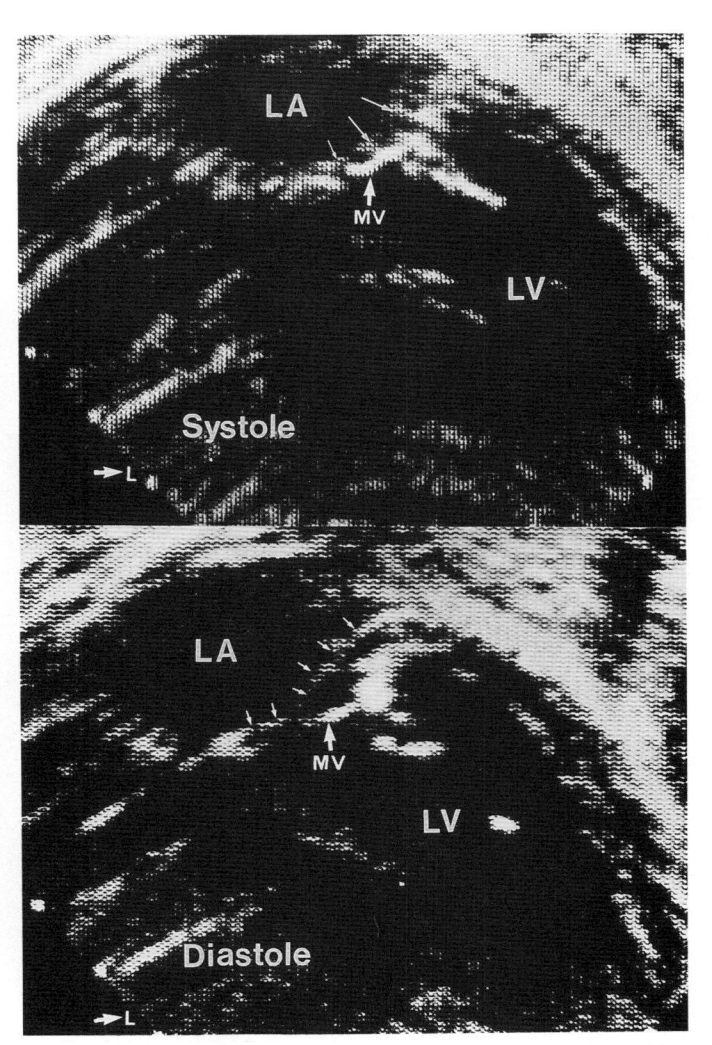

Fig. 28 Mitral membrane. Subcostal oblique views in a patient with a supravalvar mitral membrane. **Top:** In systole, the membrane (small arrows) and mitral valve are in apposition. **Bottom:** In diastole separation between the supravalvar membrane (small arrows) and mitral valve is evident.

pulmonary venous connection is for the ipsilateral paired pulmonary veins to connect to the ipsilateral atrium (Fig. 24).[13] Occasionally, the pulmonary venous connection will be lateralised to one atrium.

The assessment of pulmonary venous connection, together with actual or potential obstruction, is especially important in newborns with right atrial isomerism when severe pulmonary stenosis or pulmonary atresia coexists. The decision must be made as to whether a palliative systemic to pulmonary artery shunt alone should be constructed, whether surgical measures to avoid obstruction to pulmonary venous drainage will be necessary at the same time, or whether no intervention at all is more appropriate. The dextrocardia present in about half of the patients presenting with atrial isomerism[13] makes echocardiographic assessment of pulmonary venous connection even more challenging.

Cor triatriatum

Cor triatriatum, or partitioned left atrium, may be considered a pulmonary venous abnormality in that it occurs because of failure of complete incorporation of the pulmonary veins into the left atrium.[14] The obstructing partition within the left atrium is best assessed by a combination of subcostal (Fig. 25), apical (Fig. 26) and parasternal (Fig. 27) views.[15] Doppler studies show obstruction of flow at the partition. The condition is distinguished from membranous supravalvar mitral stenosis (Fig. 28) by the fact that

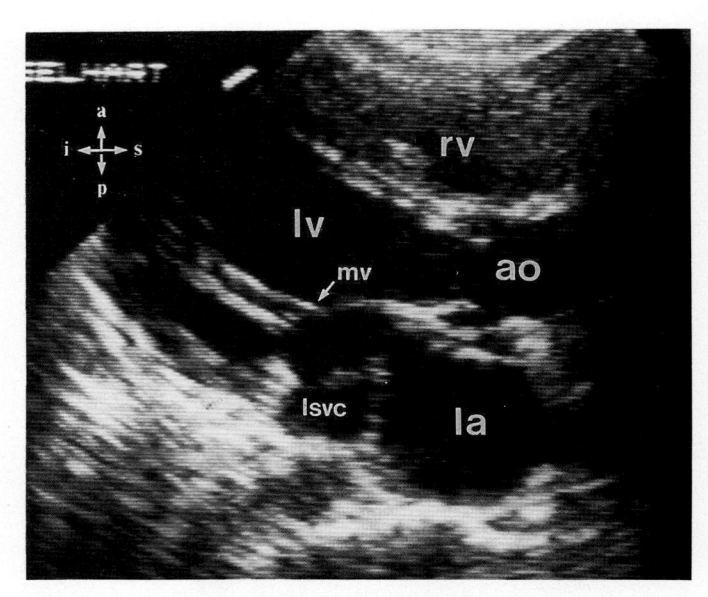

Fig. 30 **Left sided cava**. Modified parasternal long axis view in a patient with a left sided caval vein draining to the coronary sinus. The imaging plane identifies the left superior caval vein (lsvc) just above its entry into coronary sinus.

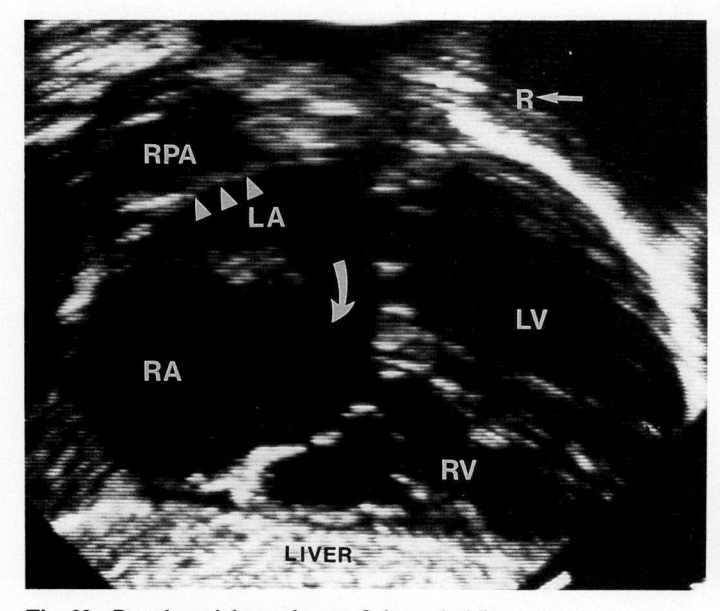

Fig. 29 **Pseudo-atrial membrane**. Subcostal oblique view in a plane just anterior to a four chamber plane. The inferior wall of the right pulmonary artery (arrowheads) may give rise to the impression of a partition in the left atrium. This patient also has an atrioventricular septal defect with a large atrial communication (curved arrow). RPA – right pulmonary artery.

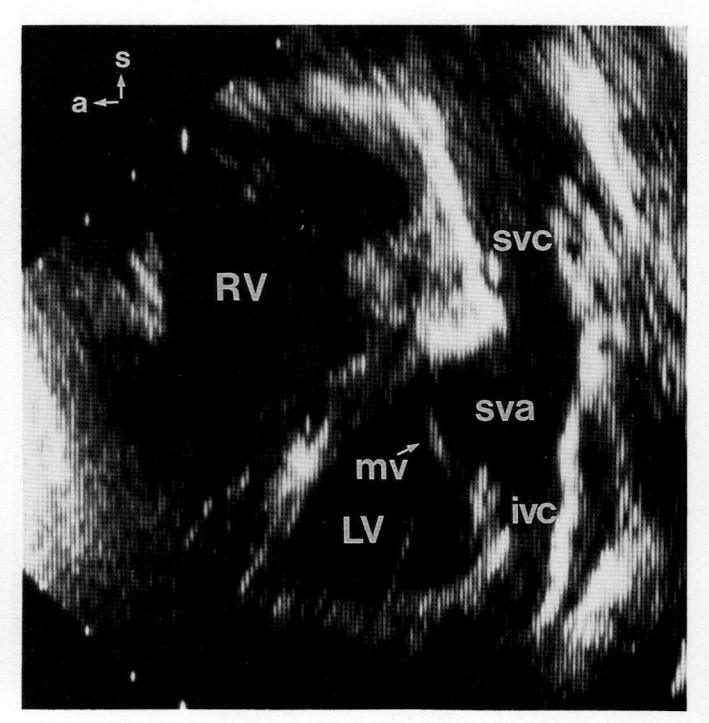

Fig. 31 **Systemic venous pathway in transposition**. Low parasternal parasagittal cut demonstrating both superior and inferior limbs of the systemic venous pathway in a patient who has had a Mustard operation for transposition of the great arteries. sva – systemic venous atrium.

the obstructing partition in cor triatriatum is 'upstream' to the left atrial appendage whereas obstruction is 'downstream' to the left atrial appendage in supravalvar mitral stenosis.[16] A communication with the right atrium may be from either the superior (upstream) or inferior (downstream) portion of the partitioned left atrium. It is important not to be misled by the inferior wall of an enlarged right pulmonary artery which may give rise to a spurious appearance of a partitioned left atrium as the transducer is angled anteriorly from a subcostal four chamber view (Fig. 29) or by coronary sinus enlargement which may give rise to the same incorrect diagnosis when the scanning plane is angled posteriorly (Fig. 30). Connections of individual pulmonary veins must be assessed carefully in cor triatriatum, as PAPVC may coexist.[17] Although a rare abnormality, cor triatriatum is a diagnosis with which all paediatric echocardiographers should be familiar. The condition is potentially lethal as obstruction to flow is often severe and diagnosis at cardiac catheterisation may be difficult, but the condition is readily amenable to surgical 'cure'.[18]

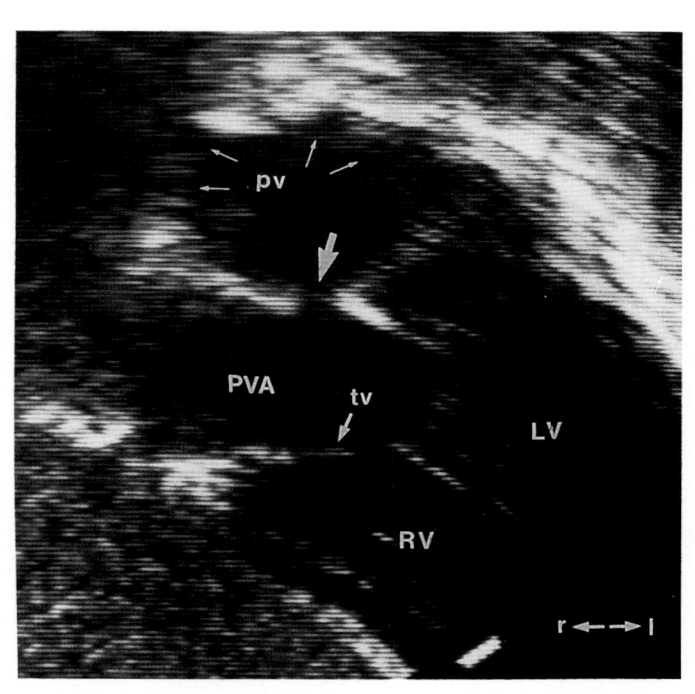

Fig. 33 Mustard operation. Subcostal oblique view in a patient following a Mustard operation, demonstrating severe obstruction in the mid-portion of the pulmonary venous pathway (large arrow). pv – pulmonary veins, PVA – pulmonary venous atrium.

Postoperative assessment

The Mustard and Senning operations for ventriculo-arterial discordance (transposition of the great arteries) redirect systemic venous return to the left ventricle and pulmonary venous return to the right ventricle. Obstruction to flow in the surgically created venous pathways is a potential postoperative complication, especially after the Mustard procedure where prosthetic material is used to fashion the atrial baffle. Beyond infancy, the superior and inferior caval pathways are best seen from a transducer position medial to the cardiac apex. Occasionally both limbs of the systemic venous pathway may be seen in a single cut (Fig. 31), but more commonly it is necessary to rotate the scanning plane from the long axis of one limb of the pathway to that of the other. Obstruction to systemic venous return after the Mustard procedure usually occurs at the site where the superior caval vein and the inferior caval vein respectively enter the heart. Doppler interrogation may confirm narrowing by the demonstration of turbulence in the low velocity venous flow signal at either or both of these sites, more commonly at the upper site. Pulmonary venous pathway obstruction is a more important but less common complication. The pulmonary venous pathway is best imaged either from a subcostal or modified apical position (Fig. 32). Pulmonary venous pathway obstruction usually occurs in the mid-portion of the pathway (Fig. 33).

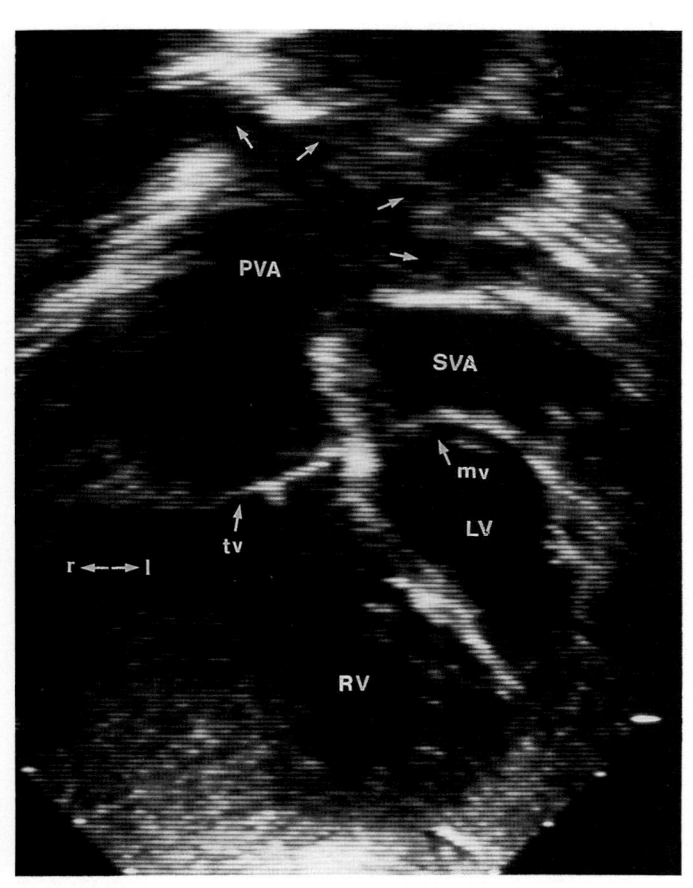

Fig. 32 Pulmonary venous pathway in transposition. Apical view in the same patient as Figure 31 which demonstrates a non-obstructed pulmonary venous pathway. Sites of entry of separate pulmonary veins are seen (arrows). PVA – pulmonary venous atrium, SVA – systemic venous atrium.

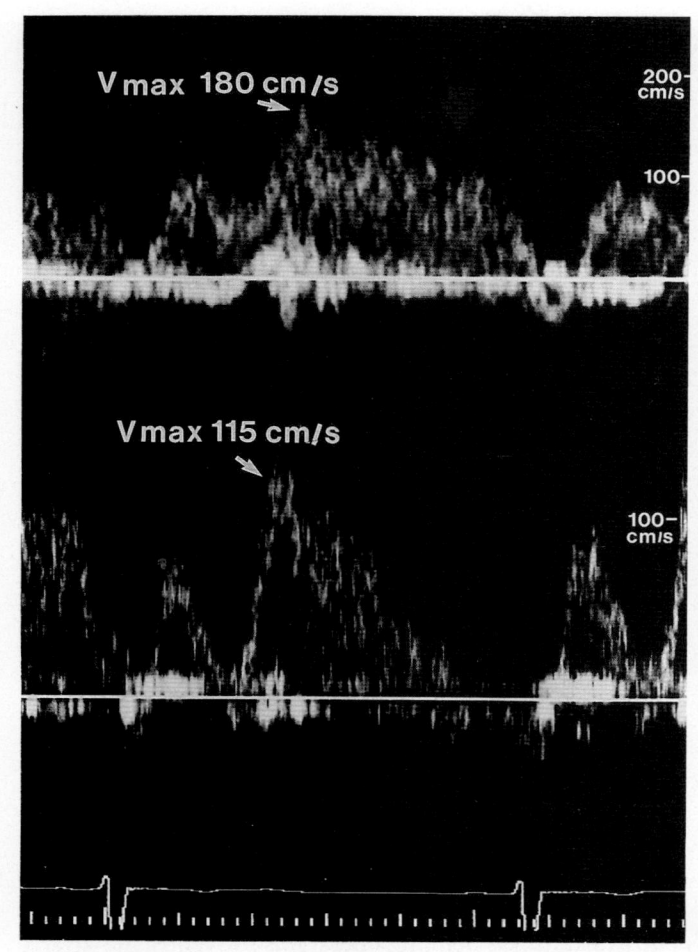

Fig. 34 Pulmonary venous obstruction. Top: Pulsed Doppler signal at the site of pulmonary venous pathway obstruction after a Mustard operation. Maximum flow velocity is increased and remains high throughout diastole. **Bottom:** After balloon dilatation of the obstructed site in the mid-portion of the pulmonary venous pathway, maximal flow velocity is diminished and flow is no longer continuous throughout diastole.

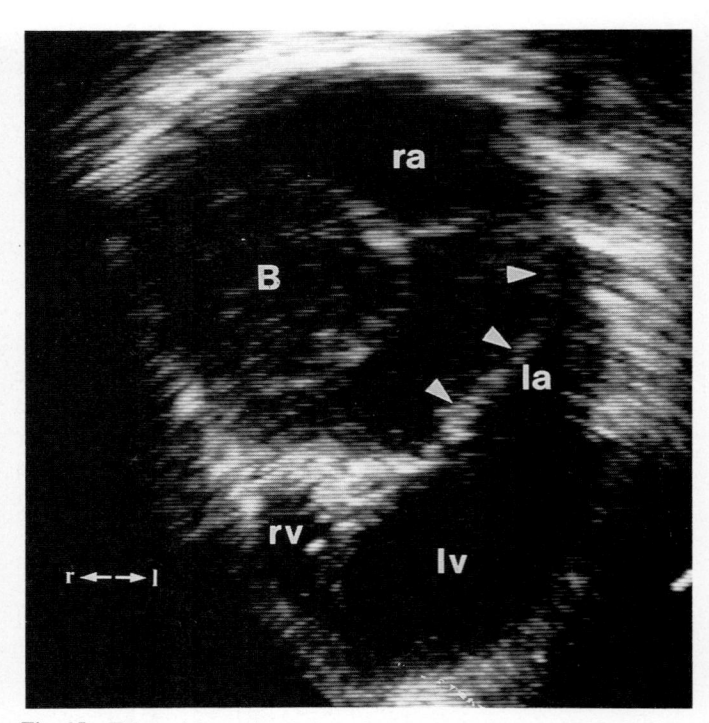

Fig. 35 Tricuspid atresia. Apical view in a patient with tricuspid atresia following a Fontan operation. The right atrium is grossly enlarged, (arrowheads delineate the atrial septum) and is occupied by a large ball of thrombus (B).

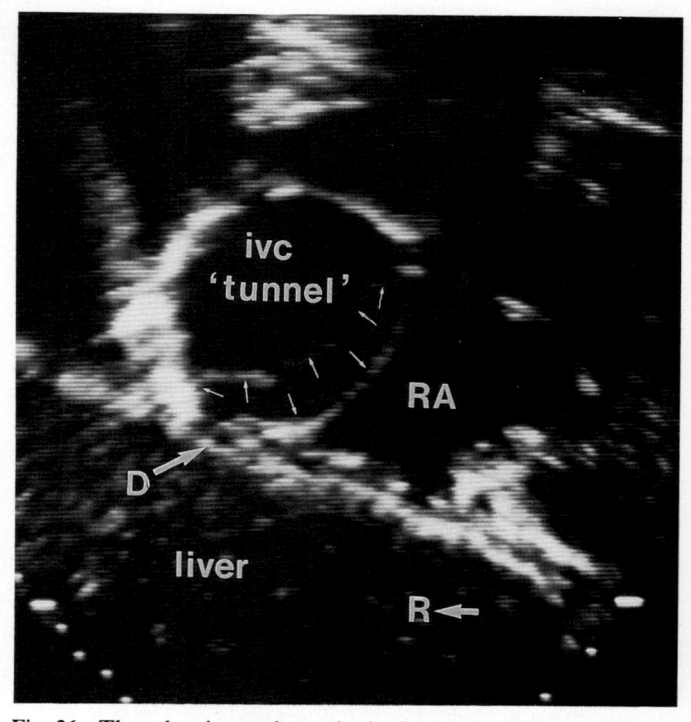

Fig. 36 Thrombus in caval prosthesis. Subcostal oblique view in a patient who has had a total cavopulmonary connection (modified Fontan operation). There is thrombus delineated by small arrows within the inferior caval venous prosthetic tunnel. D – diaphragm.

High velocity turbulent flow at this site confirms obstruction[19] and may be used for serial assessment of severity, as this serious complication may be amenable to balloon dilatation in some patients (Fig. 34).[20]

Modifications of the Fontan operation, in which systemic venous blood is routed directly to the pulmonary arteries, are employed as definitive palliation for some hearts with only one effective ventricle. The low velocity venous flow predisposes to areas of stasis with the attendant risk of thrombosis and pulmonary embolism, which is catastrophic for this fragile circulation. Thrombi may form in the right atrium where there is a right atrial to pulmonary artery conduit or direct anastomosis (Fig. 35), or in surgically constructed venous channels within the heart (Fig. 36).

Finally, a potential complication following surgical re-

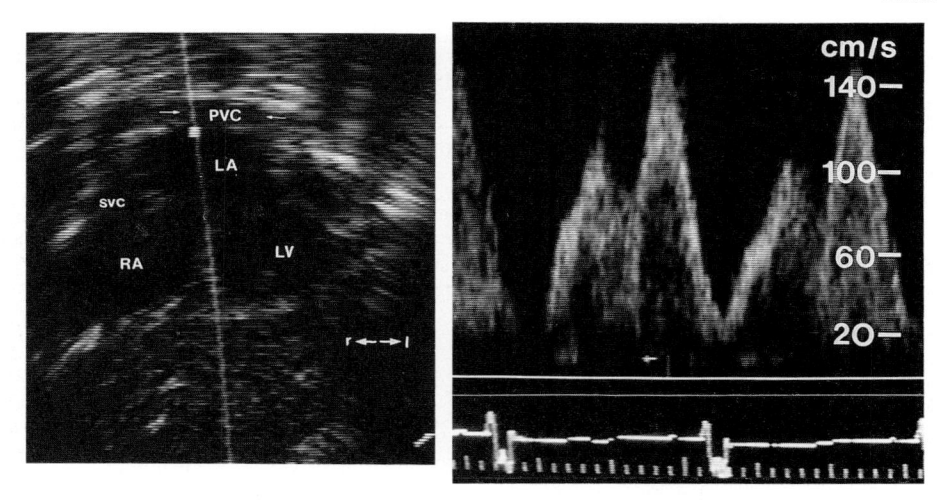

Fig. 37 Repaired TAPVC. Left: Subcostal oblique view in a patient with surgically repaired TAPVC. The Doppler sample volume is positioned in the surgically created opening between the pulmonary venous confluence and left atrium. PVC – pulmonary venous confluence. **Right:** Doppler signal from this site demonstrates phasic flow towards the transducer with peak velocity 1.4 m/sec.

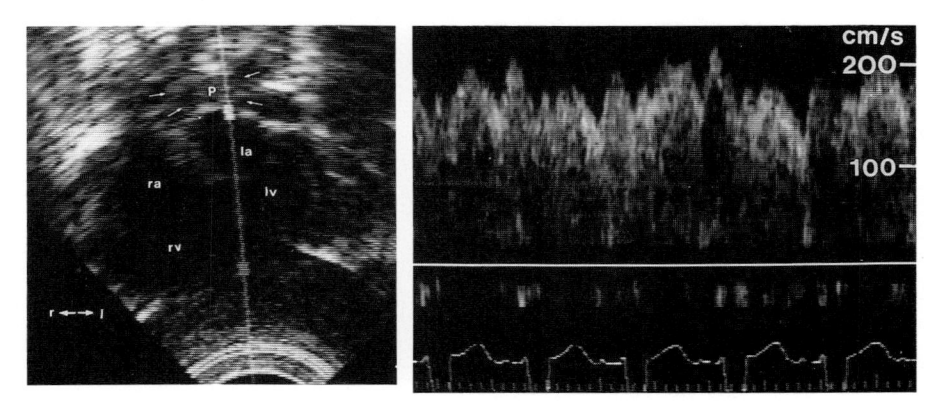

Fig. 38 Repaired TAPVC. Left: Subcostal oblique view in a patient with repaired TAPVC, and obstruction at the site of the anastomosis between the pulmonary venous confluence (P) and left atrium. The Doppler sample volume is located at the anastomosis. **Right:** Doppler signal from this site demonstrates high velocity flow (Vmax 2 m/s), continuous throughout the cardiac cycle. The tricuspid regurgitation signal demonstrated maximal velocity of 4.8 m/sec, indicative of right ventricular systolic pressure in excess of 100 mmHg. P – pulmonary venous confluence.

pair of TAPVC is obstruction to pulmonary venous return at the site of anastomosis of the pulmonary venous confluence to the left atrium. The adequacy of this anastomosis can be assessed by Doppler interrogation. Pulmonary venous flow through an unrestricted anastomosis is phasic with the cardiac cycle (Fig. 37), whereas obstruction to flow is characterised by high velocity turbulent flow continuously throughout the cardiac cycle (Fig. 38).

REFERENCES

1 Smallhorn J F, Sutherland G R, Tommasini G. Hunter S, Anderson R H, Macartney F J. Assessment of total anomalous pulmonary venous connection by two-dimensional echocardiography. Br Heart J 1981; 46: 613–623
2 Huhta J C, Gutgesell H P, Nihill M R. Cross sectional echocardiographic diagnosis of total anomalous pulmonary venous connection. Br Heart J 1985; 53: 525–534
3 Stark J, Smallhorn J, Huhta J, et al. Surgery for congenital heart defects diagnosed with cross-sectional echocardiography. Circulation 1983; 68: (suppl II) 129–138
4 Lincoln C R, Rigby M L, Mercanti C, et al. Surgical risk factors in total anomalous pulmonary venous connection. Am J Cardiol 1988; 61: 609–611
5 Lamb R K, Qureshi S A, Wilkinson J L, Arnold R, West C R, Hamilton D I. Total anomalous pulmonary venous drainage. J Thorac Cardiovasc Surg 1988; 96: 368–375
6 Lima C O, Valdes-Cruz L M, Allen H D, et al. Prognostic value of left ventricular size measured by echocardiography in infants with total anomalous pulmonary venous drainage. Am J Cardiol 1983; 51: 1155–1159

7. Smallhorn J F, Freedom R M. Pulsed Doppler echocardiography in the pre-operative evaluation of total anomalous pulmonary venous connection. J Am Coll Cardiol 1986; 8: 1413–1420
8. Anderson R H, Macartney F J, Shinebourne E A, Tynan M. eds. Pulmonary venous abnormalities. In: Paediatric cardiology. Edinburgh: Churchill Livingstone. 1987: p 509–540
9. Enriques A M C, McKay R, Arnold R M, Wilkinson J L. Misleading hyperoxia test. Arch Dis Child 1986; 61: 604–606
10. Cooper M J, Teitel D F, Silverman N H, et al. Study of the infradiaphragmatic total anomalous pulmonary venous connection with cross-sectional and pulsed Doppler echocardiography. Circulation 1984; 70: 412–416
11. Clements B S, Warner J O, Shinebourne E A. Congenital bronchopulmonary vascular malformations: clinical application of a simple anatomical approach in 25 cases. Thorax 1987; 42: 409–416
12. Sapire D W. Atrial isomerism. In: Anderson R H, Macartney F J, Shinebourne E A, Tynan M. eds. Paediatric cardiology. Edinburgh: Churchill Livingstone. 1987: p 473–496
13. Sapire D W, Yen Ho S, Anderson R H, Rigby M L. Diagnosis and significance of atrial isomerism. Am J Cardiol 1986: 58: 342–346
14. Anderson R H, Macartney F J, Shinebourne E A, Tynan M. eds. Partitioning of atrial chamber ('cor triatriatum'). In: Paediatric cardiology. Edinburgh: Churchill Livingstone. 1987: p 563–570
15. Ostman-Smith I, Silverman N H, Oldershaw P, Lincoln C, Shinebourne E A. Cor triatriatum sinestrum. Diagnostic features on cross sectional echocardiography. Br Heart J 1984; 51: 211–219
16. Sullivan I D, Robinson P J, de Leval M, Graham T P. Membranous supravalvular mitral stenosis: a treatable form of congenital heart disease. J Am Coll Cardiol 1986; 8: 159–164
17. Wolf W J. Diagnostic features and pitfalls in the two-dimensional echocardiographic evauation of a child with cor triatriatum. Pediatr Cardiol 1986; 6: 211–213
18. Sethia B, Sullivan I D, Elliott M J, de Leval M, Stark J. Congenital left ventricular inflow obstruction: is the outcome related to the site of the obstruction? Eur J Cardio Thorac Surg 1988; 2: 312–317
19. Smallhorn J F, Gow R, Freedom R M, et al. Pulsed Doppler echocardiograpic assessment of the pulmonary venous pathway after the Mustard or Senning procedure for transposition of the great arteries. Circulation 1986; 73: 765–774
20. Cooper S G, Sullivan I D, Bull C, Taylor J F N. Balloon dilation of pulmonary venous pathway obstruction after mustard repair for transposition of the great arteries. J Am Coll Cardiol 1989; 14: 194–198

26

Cardiomyopathy in childhood

Hypertrophic cardiomyopathy
Echocardiographic features
Left ventricular outflow obstruction
Other associated abnormalities
Association with other cardiac malformations and systemic diseases
Association with congenital heart disease
Noonan's syndrome
Glycogen storage disease type II (Pompe's disease)
Infants of diabetic mothers
Friedreich's ataxia

Dilated cardiomyopathy
General echocardiographic features
Viral myocarditis
Acute rheumatic fever
Endocardial fibroelastosis
Duchenne muscular dystrophy
Connective tissue disorders
Thalassaemic cardiomyopathy
Anthracycline cardiomyopathy
Restrictive cardiomyopathy
Idiopathic restrictive cardiomyopathy
Endomyocardial fibrosis

Robin P. Martin

INTRODUCTION

Cardiomyopathy is a term used to describe ventricular dysfunction resulting from a myocardial disease of unknown aetiology. Cardiomyopathy is generally subdivided into three groups, namely hypertrophic, dilated, and restrictive cardiomyopathies, each being characterised by differences of chamber morphology and each being associated with abnormalities of systolic and diastolic function. In childhood many features will be similar to those seen in adults with cardiomyopathy but there are important differences that will be described later. The WHO/ICRF report on the definition of cardiomyopathy[1] excluded cardiac muscle abnormalities where the aetiology was known or where there was an associated general system disease. The term specific heart muscle disease was used to describe this group. In practice many clinicians prefer to use the term cardiomyopathy to include all conditions associated with disorders of the myocardium whether the aetiology is known or not. This is the approach that will be used in this chapter.

HYPERTROPHIC CARDIOMYOPATHY

This form of cardiomyopathy is characterised by myocardial hypertrophy with a normal or decreased left ventricular cavity volume. The hypertrophy may be generalised, affecting left and right ventricles and taking on a concentric form that may appear similar to that seen in systemic hypertension. Alternatively it may be asymmetric, affecting any portion of the myocardium with the interventricular septum being most frequently abnormal.

Hypertrophic cardiomyopathy may be found from the prenatal period to adulthood. In the dominantly inherited familial form it has been shown that the echocardiogram may not become abnormal until adolescence.[2] The later presenting hypertrophic cardiomyopathy has similar clinical and echocardiographic features to the adult form. Presentation in infancy is associated with a poor prognosis[3,4] due to the early development of cardiac failure.

Echocardiographic features

The diagnosis depends on the demonstration of the abnormal left ventricular hypertrophy. M-mode echocardiography has been used extensively and a ratio of interventricular septal to posterior left ventricular wall thickness of over 1.3 is generally considered abnormal in adults (Fig. 1). This ratio is unreliable in the newborn period and in patients with congenital heart disease, when values of over 1.3 may be seen in the absence of hypertrophic cardiomyopathy.[5] Difficulties may also occur if the septomarginal trabeculum is prominent, as this may erroneously indicate that the interventricular septum is hypertrophied. The M-mode examination may also show the additional features of systolic anterior motion of the mitral valve (Fig. 2) and mid-systolic closure of the aortic valve.

Cross-sectional imaging can be used more reliably to make the diagnosis because of its ability to evaluate all of the myocardium. It is recognised that M-mode examination alone may miss the abnormal hypertrophy particularly if it is situated towards the left ventricular apex. More commonly there may be hypertrophy affecting the superior portion of the interventricular septum giving the classical appearance that has been called ASH (asymmetric septal hypertrophy) (Fig. 3). Other forms that may be seen in-

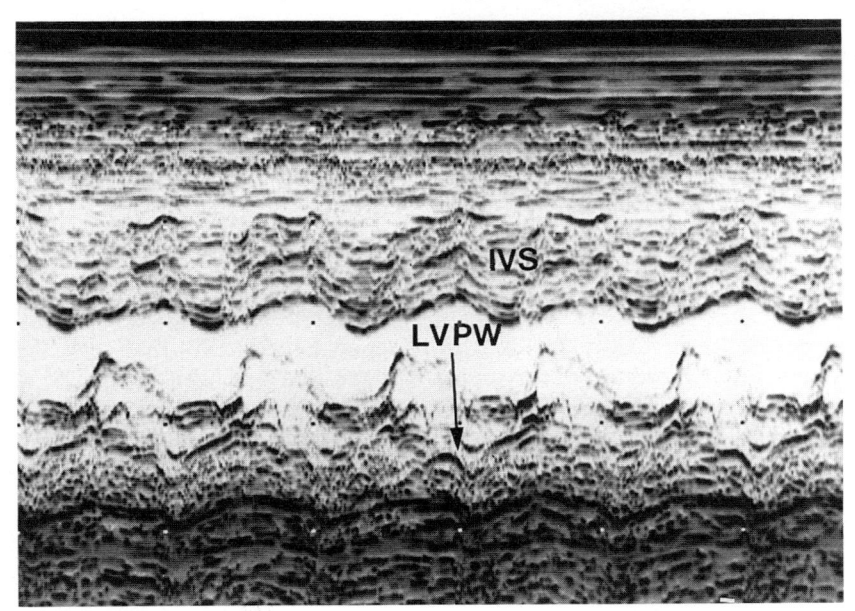

Fig. 1 **M-mode echocardiogram in infant with hypertrophic cardiomyopathy showing moderate septal hypertrophy.** IVS – Interventricular septum; LVPW – Left ventricular posterior wall.

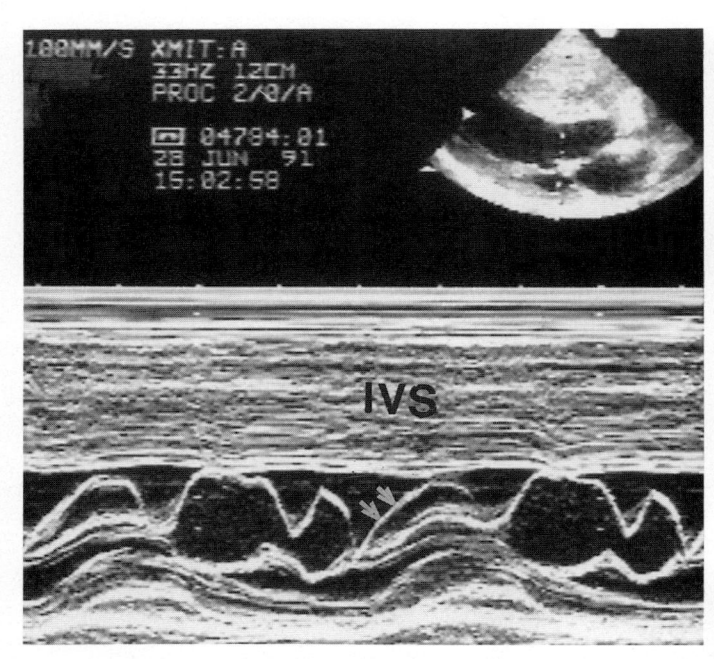

Fig. 2 M-mode echocardiogram showing systolic anterior motion of the mitral valve (arrowed) **in hypertrophic cardiomyopathy.** Note marked septal hypertrophy. IVS – Interventricular septum.

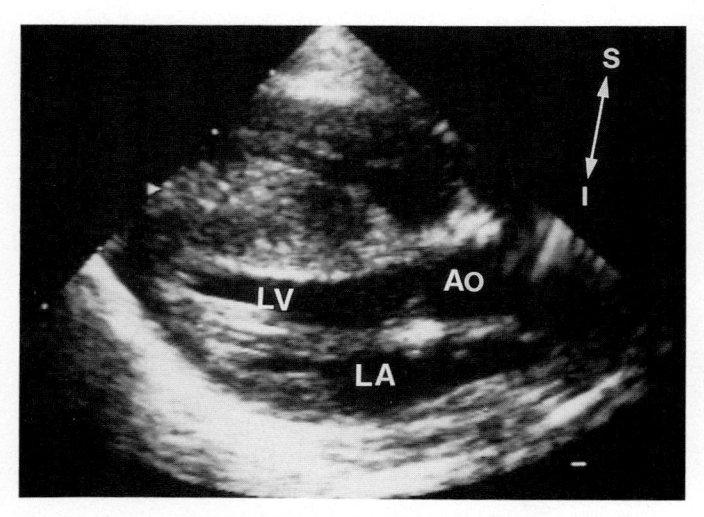

Fig. 3 Parasternal long axis view in an infant with hypertrophic cardiomyopathy. There is prominent septal hypertrophy.

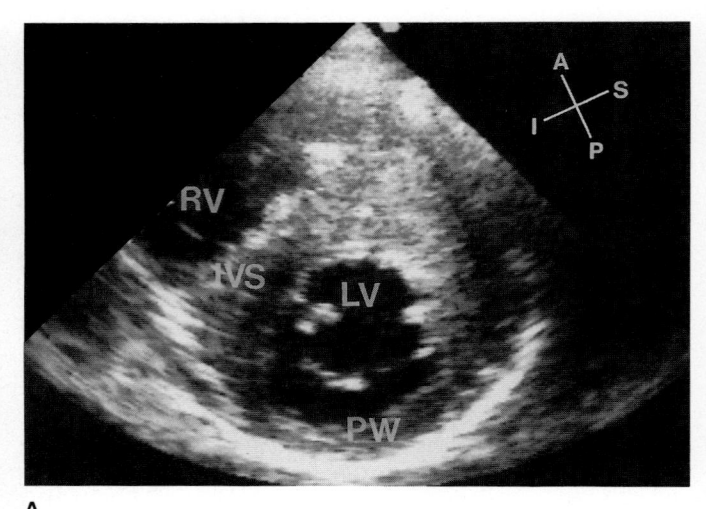

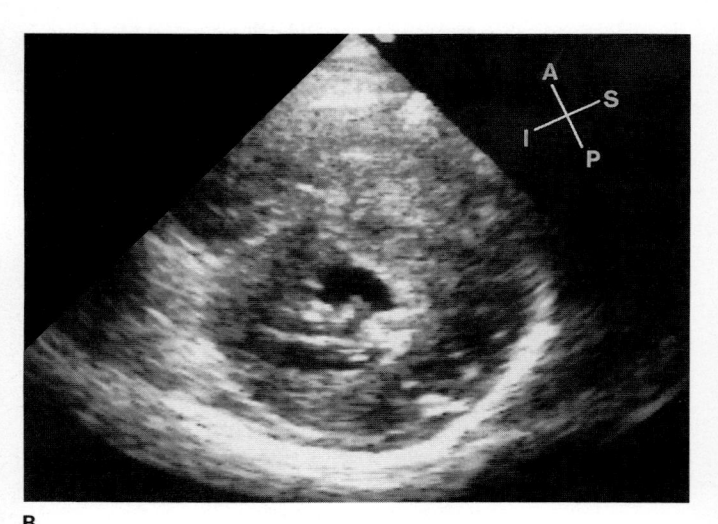

Fig. 4 A: Parasternal short axis view at the level of the mitral valve. End-diastolic frame showing normal cavity dimension with hypertrophy of the interventricular septum and normal left ventricular posterior wall thickness. IVS – Interventricular septum; PW – Left ventricular posterior wall. **B:** End systolic frame in the same patient showing reduced left ventricular volume.

clude those where the hypertrophy is mainly localised in the left ventricular apex and those where the hypertrophy is concentric, affecting all portions of the left ventricle to an equal extent. This latter form may be indistinguishable from the left ventricular hypertrophy seen when afterload is increased as in systemic hypertension, aortic valve stenosis or coarctation of the aorta. In infants the right ventricle may appear more noticeably involved and right ventricular outflow obstruction may be present due to the infundibular hypertrophy.[4]

The left ventricular end diastolic dimension is usually normal. The end systolic dimension of the left ventricle is likely to be decreased as cavity obliteration is common (Fig. 4). The papillary muscles of the mitral valve are often hypertrophied and this in combination with the asymmetric septal hypertrophy may give the left ventricular cavity a shape that has been likened to a 'banana' or a 'ballerina's foot'. It may also be noticed that the myocardium has an increased speckled echogenicity that presumably reflects the underlying abnormal histological appearance of myocardial fibre disarray.[6]

Left ventricular outflow obstruction

Left ventricular outflow obstruction is frequently seen in hypertrophic cardiomyopathy, though it is not a prerequisite for making the diagnosis. There has been much debate regarding its aetiology and pathological importance. The presence of systolic anterior motion (SAM) of the mitral valve has been used as a marker for outflow obstruction and the duration of apposition of the mitral valve apparatus to the septum can be used to predict the outflow gradient.[7] Cross-sectional imaging will show the anterior motion of the mitral valve in early systole. This may affect the mitral valve at the tip of the leaflets or the chordal attachments may be predominantly affected. The mitral valve apparatus usually makes contact with the septum, often resulting in a 'contact lesion' of thickened endocardium at the point of septal contact. At the end of systole the mitral valve moves backwards to its previous position (Fig. 5).

Doppler echocardiography can be used to quantitate and localise the degree and site of obstruction. The site of

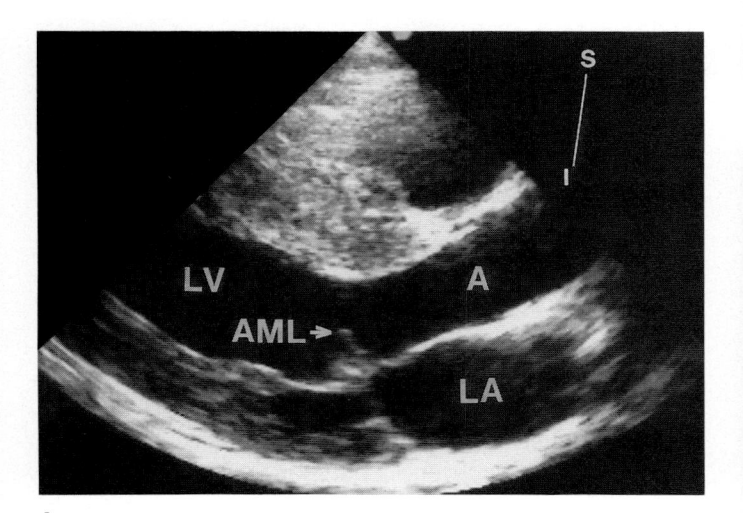

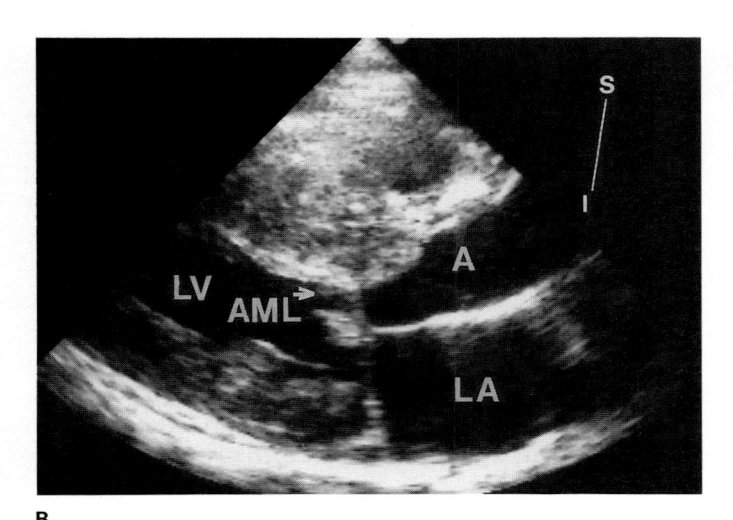

Fig. 5 A: **Parasternal long axis view in hypertrophic cardiomyopathy with systolic anterior motion of the mitral valve.** Early systolic frame showing the anterior mitral leaflet (AML) just starting to move anteriorly. B: Later systolic frame in same patient. The anterior mitral leaflet has contacted the interventricular septum.

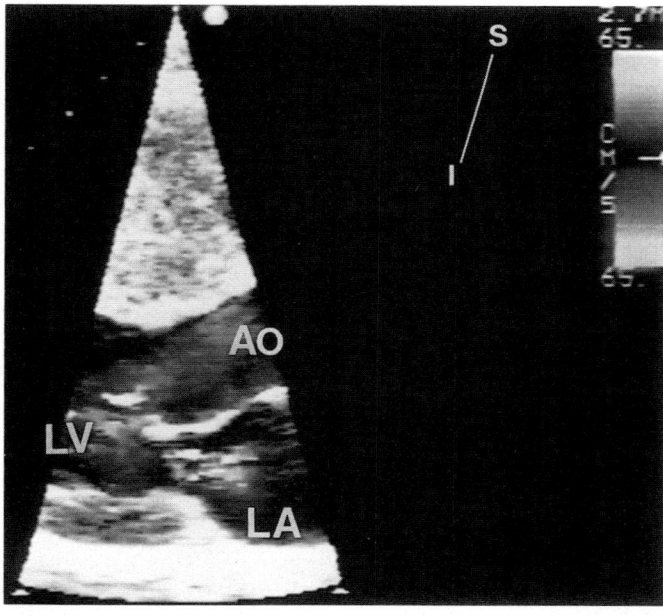

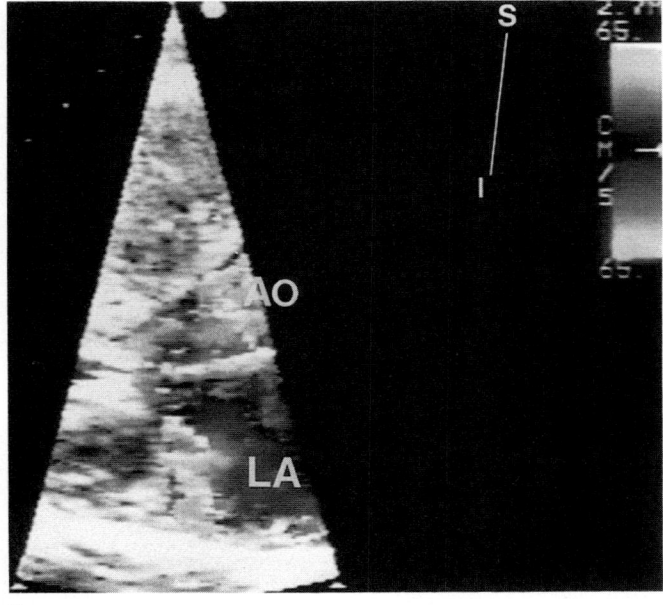

Plate 1 A: **Parasternal long axis colour flow image in hypertrophic cardiomyopathy with left ventricular outflow obstruction.** In early systole there is low velocity (orange) flow in the left ventricular outflow and a mitral regurgitant jet in the left atrium (blue). B: Later systolic frame showing high velocity aliasing flow in the left ventricular outflow due to the development of left ventricular outflow obstruction. There is also a high velocity jet in the left atrium from the mitral regurgitation. This figure is reproduced in colour in the colour plate section at the front of this volume.

obstruction can be localised using pulsed wave sampling from an apical long axis view and this will usually be just beyond the point of contact of the mitral valve apparatus with the ventricular septum. Occasionally increased flow velocities may be encountered in the mid-cavity region, corresponding to intra-cavitary pressure gradients that may be encountered at the time of cardiac catheterisation. The aortic valve should be closely inspected as aortic valve stenosis may coexist, particularly in children with Noonan's syndrome. Colour flow mapping may also be useful in localising the site of obstruction (Plate 1), though it should be appreciated that acceleration of blood flow may start just proximal to the apparent site of obstruction. Continuous wave or high pulse repetition frequency Doppler studies can be used to quantitate the pressure gradient. The velocity spectra will often show the dynamic nature of the stenosis, with the peak velocity being reached later in systole compared to that seen in isolated valve stenosis[8,9] (Fig. 6).

In infants with hypertrophic cardiomyopathy, the right ventricular outflow should be examined in a similar manner, to evaluate the presence and severity of right ventricular outflow obstruction (Fig. 7 and Plate 2). Imaging and Doppler examination is best achieved from subcostal right ventricular outflow views, produced by anticlockwise rotation and superior angulation from the standard subcostal four chamber view.

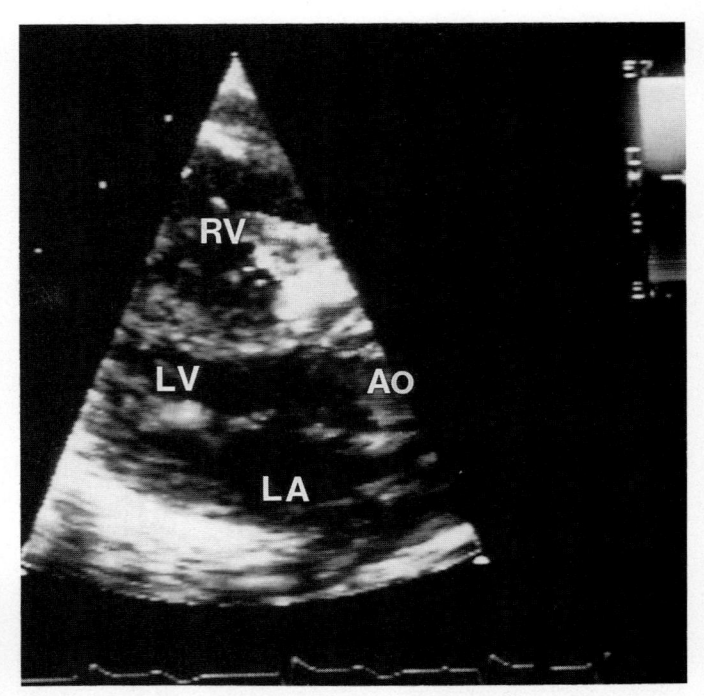

Plate 2 Right ventricular outflow obstruction in an infant with hypertrophic cardiomyopathy. Parasternal long axis colour flow image with normal (blue) velocities in left ventricular outflow and high velocity aliasing flow in the right ventricular outflow. This figure is reproduced in colour in the colour plate section at the front of this volume.

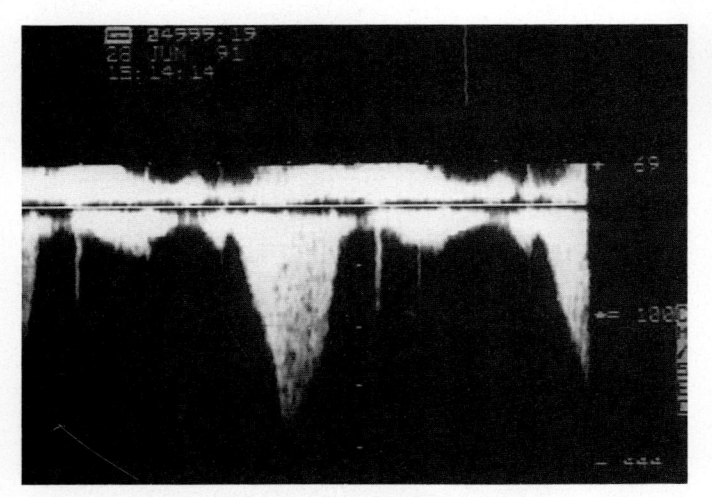

Fig. 6 Continuous wave Doppler recording from the apex in hypertrophic cardiomyopathy with left ventricular outflow obstruction. There is the typical late peaking high velocity jet of dynamic obstruction with a peak velocity of 3.7 m/s (55 mmHg pressure gradient).

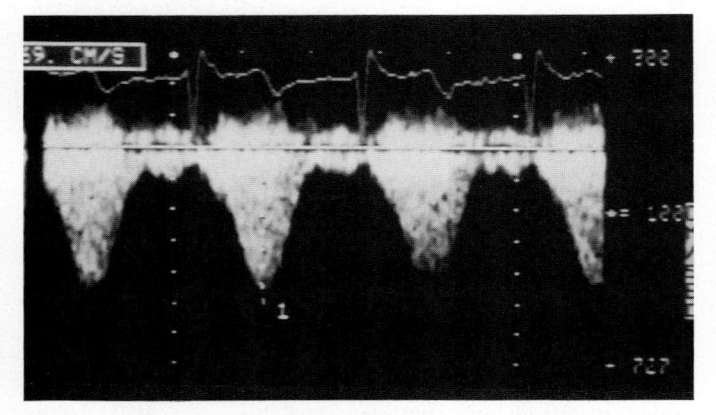

Fig. 7 Continuous wave Doppler recording from the patient in Plate 2 with dynamic right ventricular outflow obstruction. There is a peak velocity of 4.7 m/s (88 mmHg pressure gradient).

Other associated abnormalities

Mild aortic valve regurgitation is relatively common in patients with hypertrophic cardiomyopathy.[10] More often of haemodynamic importance is the presence of mitral regurgitation. This may be seen in approximately 50% of patients with hypertrophic cardiomyopathy[11] and probably results from the distortion of the mitral valve apparatus that results from the abnormal ejection mechanics of the left ventricle and the systolic anterior motion of the mitral valve (Fig. 8). The severity of the mitral regurgitation may vary from mild to severe. Severe regurgitation will be associated with dilatation and increased pulsatility of the left atrium. A mild degree of left atrial dilatation is not unusual in the absence of mitral regurgitation and probably relates to impaired diastolic filling of the left ventricle which produces a rise in the left atrial pressure. Quantitation of the degree of mitral regurgitation by analysis of the Doppler regurgitant jet can be attempted. Jet mapping with

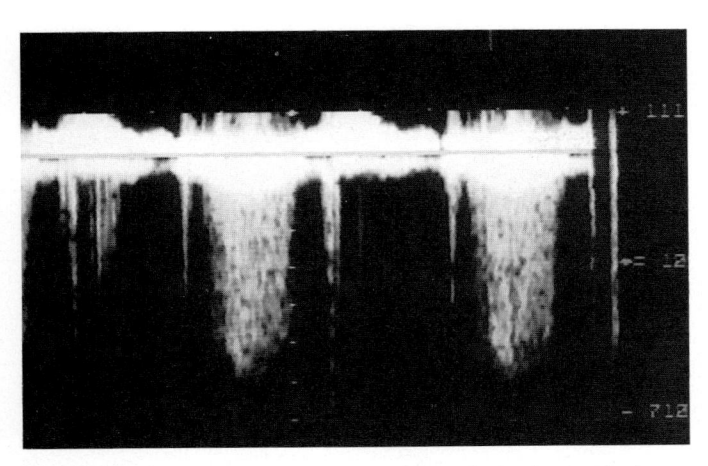

Fig. 8 Continuous wave Doppler recording of mitral regurgitation in hypertrophic cardiomyopathy with left ventricular outflow obstruction. The peak velocity is high (6.1 m/s) predicting that the left ventricular systolic pressure is elevated (>150 mmHg).

pulsed wave Doppler and colour flow mapping may be used to give a semi-quantitative assessment of severity, though Doppler methods are probably not as accurate as left ventricular angiography.

The impaired left ventricular diastolic function that results from the abnormal left ventricular hypertrophy may be detected by Doppler echocardiography. Trans-mitral flow characteristically shows a reduced (and often longer duration) peak early filling (E wave) velocity and an increased peak A wave velocity that corresponds to atrial systole. This results in a reduction of the E/A velocity ratio.[12]

Association with other cardiac malformations and systemic diseases

Hypertrophic cardiomyopathy may occur as an isolated lesion in childhood, as described above. It may also occur with a variety of syndromes, neuromuscular and metabolic abnormalities. Sometimes it is associated with congenital heart disease. In some cases the cardiomyopathy may be the presenting problem, before abnormalities in other areas are apparent. The clinician therefore needs to be aware of these associations and the following section will describe the more frequent associations that need to be considered when a child presents with hypertrophic cardiomyopathy.

Association with congenital heart disease

Hypertrophic cardiomyopathy may be found in patients with a variety of congenital cardiac lesions, such as complete and congenitally corrected transposition, pulmonary valve stenosis and atrial septal defect.[13-16] It may also be seen occasionally in children with fixed left ventricular outflow obstruction. It is possible that abnormal loading conditions result in the development of hypertrophic cardiomyopathy in those with a genetic predisposition.

Noonan's syndrome

This is a dominantly inherited syndrome characterised by a phenotype similar to Turner's syndrome but with a normal complement of chromosomes. A number of cardiac abnormalities have been described, including pulmonary valve stenosis (typically with a dysplastic valve), aortic valve stenosis and atrial septal defect. Hypertrophic cardiomyopathy may also be seen and can be rapidly progressive in infancy[17,18] (Fig. 9). Noonan's syndrome should be considered in any child presenting with pulmonary valve stenosis and hypertrophic cardiomyopathy.

LEOPARD syndrome (an acronym for multiple Lentigines, Electrocardiographic abnormalities, Ocular hypertelorism, Pulmonary stenosis, Abnormal genitalia, Retardation and Deafness) is similar in many respects to Noonan's syndrome and is also associated with hypertrophic cardiomyopathy.[19]

Glycogen storage disease type II (Pompe's disease)

This condition has an autosomal recessive inheritance and results from a deficiency of lysosomal maltase. This results in deposition of glycogen in the myocardium, skeletal muscle and liver. The presentation is with progressive cardiac failure in infancy and echocardiography shows hypertrophic cardiomyopathy[20,21] often with associated left ventricular outflow obstruction (Fig. 10). Most infants will have generalised hypotonia, a large tongue and hepatomegaly. Diagnosis is confirmed by assay of enzyme activity from blood leucocytes or fibroblast culture.

Other metabolic disorders

Various metabolic diseases may produce hypertrophic cardiomyopathy, but the cardiac lesion is rarely the presenting abnormality and the echocardiographic features are non-specific. The possibility of an underlying metabolic disorder should be considered if the cardiomyopathy is associated with neurological abnormalities such as hypotonia, hepato-splenomegaly or ocular abnormalities.

Mucopolysaccharidosis type 1 (Hurler's syndrome) produces generalised ventricular hypertrophy with infiltration of the mitral and aortic valves. The thickening of the valves may be recognised by cross-sectional imaging and there is frequently aortic and mitral valve regurgitation of variable severity. Diagnosis may be suspected by the demonstration of abnormal amounts of urinary mucopolysaccharides and can be confirmed by fibroblast culture. Most children present in the first two years of life and death from cardiac failure usually occurs by ten years of age.

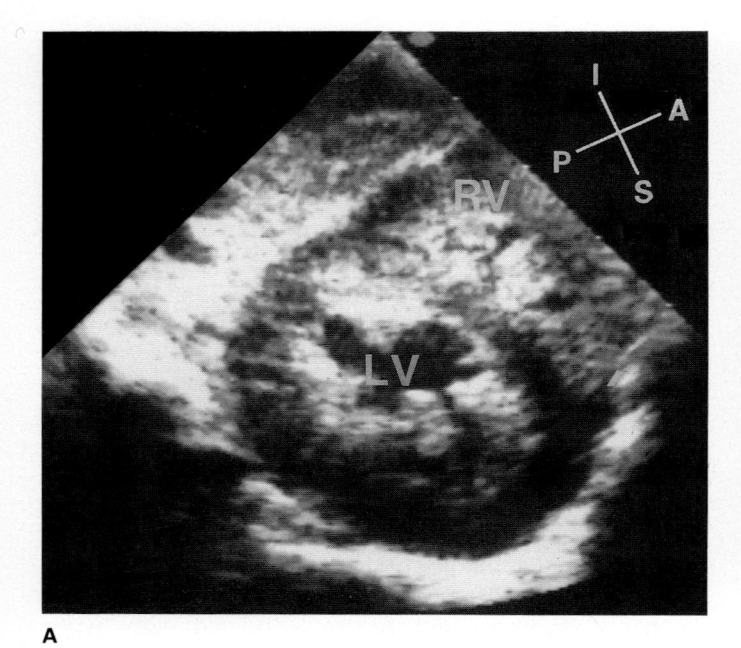

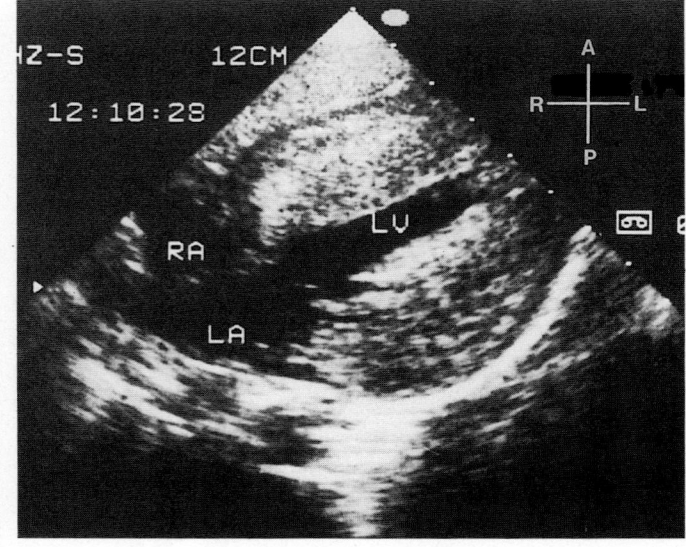

Fig. 10 Hypertrophic cardiomyopathy in Pompe's disease. Subcostal four chamber view showing severe left ventricular hypertrophy.

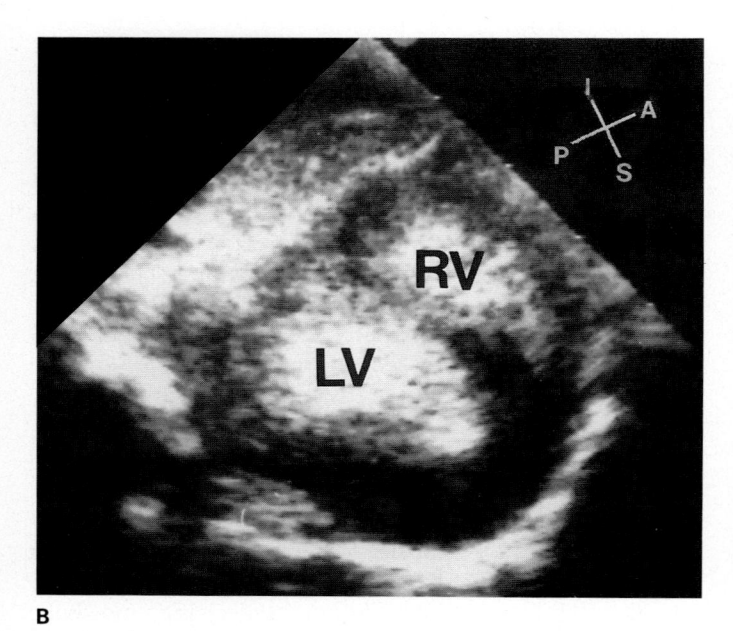

Fig. 9 A: Hypertrophic cardiomyopathy in an infant with Noonan's syndrome. Subcostal short axis view of left and right ventricles. In diastole there are reduced left and right ventricular dimensions with severe concentric hypertrophy of both ventricles. **B:** Systolic frame in same patient showing obliteration of both cavities.

Inclusion cell disease (mucolipidosis II) presents a similar clinical picture to Hurler's syndrome though presentation tends to be earlier and death usually follows before five years of age.

Fabry's disease (alpha-galactosidase-A deficiency) is an X-linked disorder that presents in childhood. There is deposition of phosphosphingolipids that results in generalised myocardial hypertrophy. In adult life there may be early coronary disease and mitral and aortic valve disease.[22,23]

Disorders of fat and carnitine metabolism can produce either a dilated or a hypertrophic cardiomyopathy.[24] Diagnosis can be made by measurement of the serum carnitine level.

Infants of diabetic mothers

Infants born to diabetic mothers may present soon after birth with cardiac failure secondary to hypertrophic cardiomyopathy. The echocardiographic features are similar to those seen in the familial type of hypertrophic cardiomyopathy. There is usually prominent septal hypertrophy (Fig. 11) and there may be left ventricular outflow gradients on Doppler examination. Generally symptoms are rare in such infants and the abnormality may only be found if an echocardiographic examination happens to be performed incidentally. Septal hypertrophy has been found in 25–30% of these infants[25-27] and it usually regresses during the first few months of life. There is evidence to suggest that the hypertrophy results from hyperinsulinism in the foetus and that the severity is greater when the diabetic control in the mother is poor.

Infants with the Beckwith–Wiedemann syndrome may also present with a hypertrophic cardiomyopathy that may be reversible.[28] This rare syndrome is characterised by macrosomia, visceromegaly, exomphalos and neonatal hypoglycaemia.

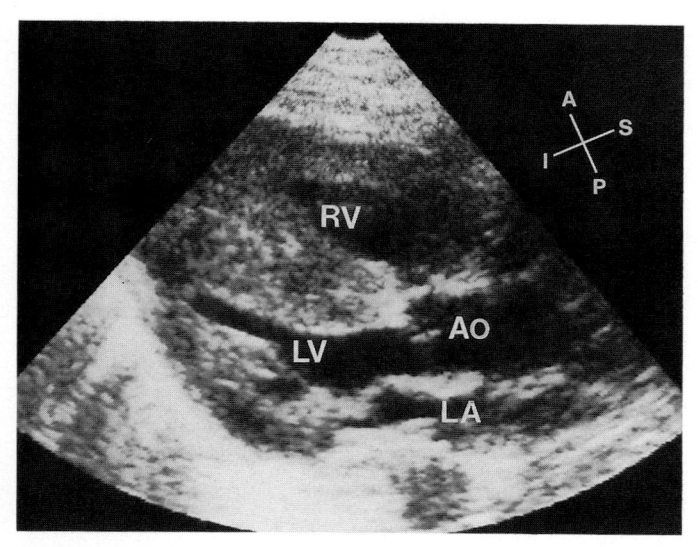

Fig. 11 Hypertrophic cardiomyopathy in an infant of a diabetic mother. Parasternal long axis view showing a small cavity left ventricle and hypertrophy mainly affecting the interventricular septum.

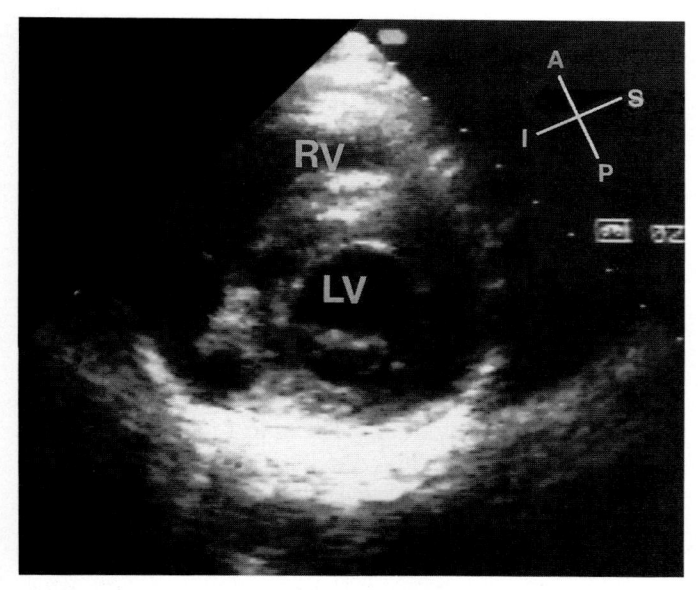

Fig. 12 Concentric left ventricular hypertrophy in child with Friedreich's ataxia. Parasternal short axis view at the level of the mitral valve.

Friedreich's ataxia

This neurological disorder is characterised by progressive cerebellar ataxia, skeletal malformations and hypertrophic cardiomyopathy. The cardiomyopathy may occasionally precede the neurological symptoms. The myocardial hypertrophy is usually concentric and slowly progressive during childhood[29-31] (Fig. 12). Occasionally there may be reduced systolic function or a dilated cardiomyopathy.

The hypertrophic cardiomyopathy is not specific to Friedreich's ataxia so it is not possible to make the neurological diagnosis from the cardiac findings. For instance, Roussy–Lévy hereditary polyneuropathy may produce a similar type of hypertrophic cardiomyopathy.

DILATED CARDIOMYOPATHY

This form of cardiomyopathy is characterised by a global reduction in left, and sometimes right, ventricular function. There are increased end-diastolic and end-systolic volumes with a reduction in left ventricular ejection fraction.

There are numerous causes of dilated cardiomyopathy in children which include viral myocarditis, endocardial fibroelastosis, drug toxicity and ischaemia resulting from anomalous origin of the left coronary artery from the pulmonary trunk. These will be described in later sections. In many children, no specific cause can be identified and this may be called 'idiopathic' dilated cardiomyopathy.

General echocardiographic features

M-mode echocardiography will reveal left ventricular dilatation, with increases in the left ventricular end-diastolic and end-systolic dimensions.[32] There is concomitant reduction in the indices of systolic function, such as shortening fraction and ejection fraction. These changes are secondary to the dilated ventricle and the reduced excursion of the left ventricular posterior wall and the interventricular septum. There will be an increase in the separation of the mitral E point from the septal surface with left ventricular dilatation. When the cardiac output is very reduced there is also reduced excursion of the mitral valve. The left atrium is likely to be dilated due to the raised filling pressure in the left ventricle. The right ventricle may also be dilated if there is pulmonary hypertension secondary to chronic elevation of left atrial pressure. The aortic valve may also show reduced excursion when the cardiac output is low. The left ventricular myocardium may have normal or only mildly increased thickness.

Cross-sectional echocardiography will similarly show the left ventricular dilatation and reduced systolic function[33] (Fig. 13). The left ventricular myocardium may be mildly hypertrophied but the degree of hypertrophy is inadequate to compensate for the increase in end-systolic wall stress associated with the increase in cavity dimension. The tissue character of the myocardium will usually be normal, but when endocardial fibroelastosis is present there will be increased echogenicity and thickness of the endocardial surfaces.

The shape of the left ventricle changes as the chamber becomes more dilated and it eventually assumes a spherical shape. It will be noted that the left ventricular dimension

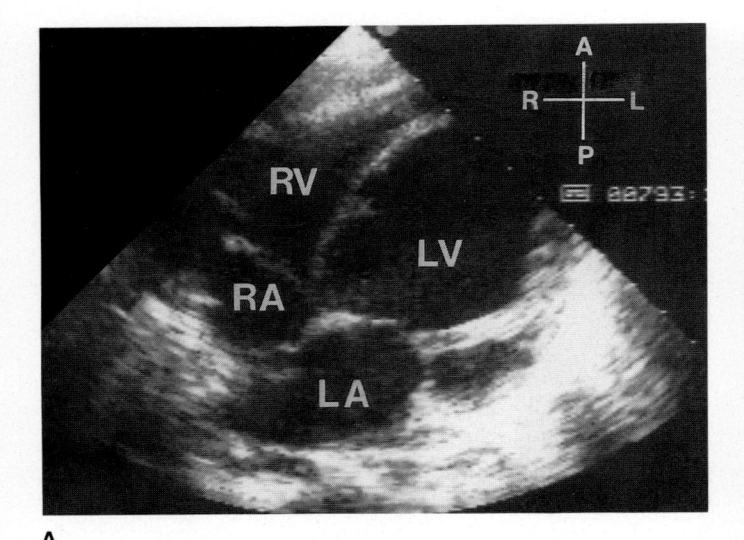

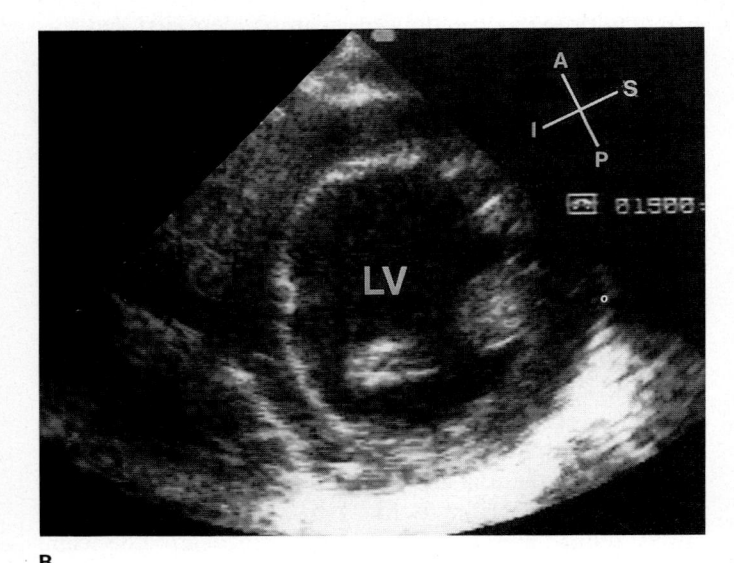

Fig. 13 **A: Child with dilated cardiomyopathy.** Subcostal four chamber view showing left ventricular dilatation. **B:** Short axis parasternal view at the level of the papillary muscles in the same child. End systolic frame shows an increased end systolic diameter.

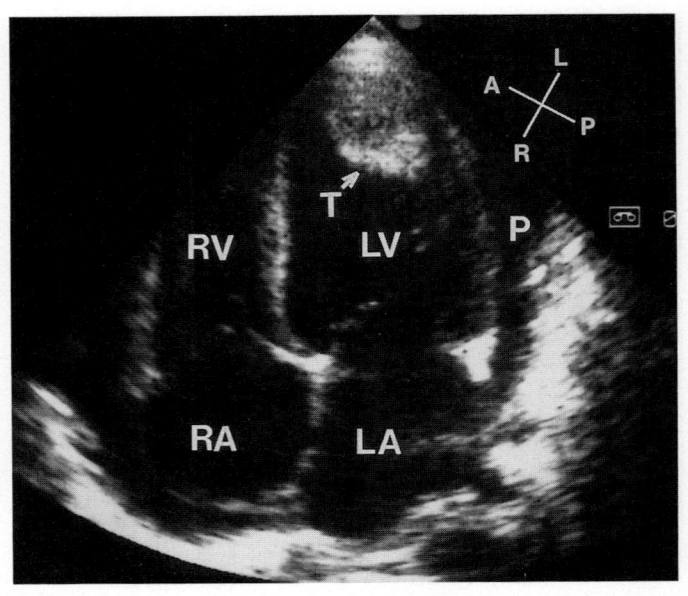

Fig. 14 Dilated cardiomyopathy in a child receiving treatment with an anthracycline drug. There is thrombus (T) at the left ventricular apex and a pericardial effusion (P).

is greater in its midpoint (at the level of the papillary muscles) than it is nearer the mitral valve.

Cross-sectional imaging may also show the presence of dilatation of the left atrium and the reduced movements of the mitral and aortic valves. The right ventricle and pulmonary trunk may become enlarged when there has been chronic elevation of the left atrial pressure with subsequent pulmonary hypertension. The right ventricle may be affected by the myopathic process and this can cause right ventricular dilatation in the absence of pulmonary hypertension. The right atrium is likely to be dilated as are the inferior caval vein and hepatic veins.

When ventricular function is severely compromised, a careful search should be made for intracardiac thrombus (Fig. 14). The cavity dilatation and reduced wall motion result in reduced blood flow within the heart and it is likely that this is the substrate for thrombogenesis. Thrombus formation tends to occur at the left ventricular apex, though the right ventricle and both atria should also be carefully evaluated. Thrombus may be sessile or it may be protuberant and mobile. The left ventricular apex may be difficult to evaluate because it is in the near field and there are often apical trabeculations that can be difficult to differentiate from thrombus. The apical four chamber and long axis views tend to give the most information, but apical angulation of parasternal short axis views may be helpful if near field resolution is a problem.

In infants presenting with dilated cardiomyopathy, the possibility of anomalous origin of the left coronary artery from the pulmonary trunk should be considered (Fig. 15). High resolution short axis parasternal views will usually show the coronary artery origins. In this condition the left main coronary artery will be seen to course anteriorly just before its normal connection with the left aortic sinus of Valsalva where it connects with the pulmonary trunk. Sometimes there is a small pouch in the region where the left coronary would normally originate and this may erroneously give the impression that the coronary origin is normal (Fig. 16).

Further clues to the correct diagnosis such as the increased size of the right coronary artery,[34] and the presence of retrograde flow in the coronary artery on colour flow Doppler examination may be sought. The left ventricle

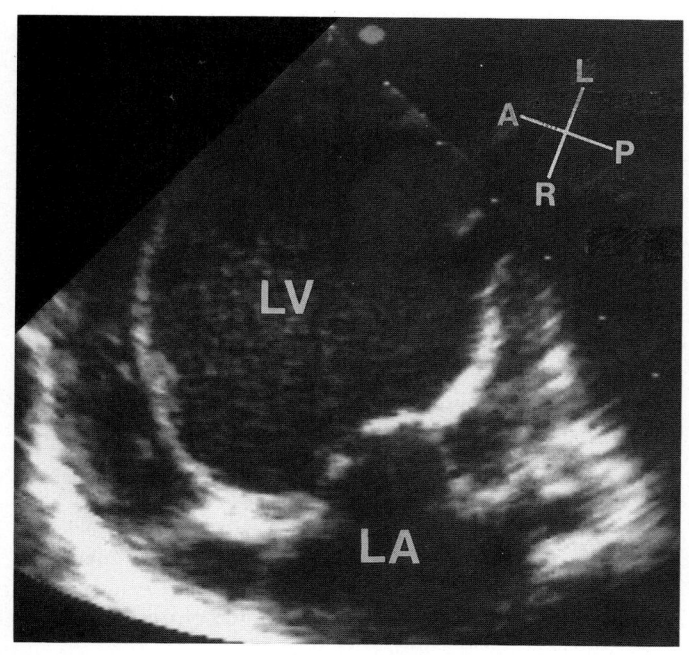

Fig. 15 Apical four chamber view in an infant with anomalous origin of the left coronary artery from the pulmonary trunk. There is a severe dilated cardiomyopathy with the left ventricle taking on a spherical shape.

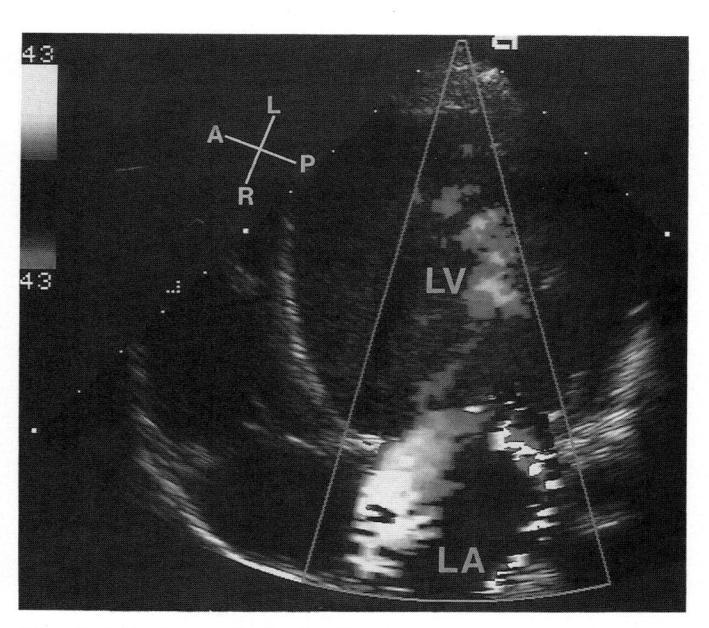

Plate 3 Mitral regurgitation in dilated cardiomyopathy. Apical four chamber colour flow Doppler image. There is a high velocity turbulent jet of mitral regurgitation that hugs the lateral wall of the left atrium. This figure is reproduced in colour in the colour plate section at the front of this volume.

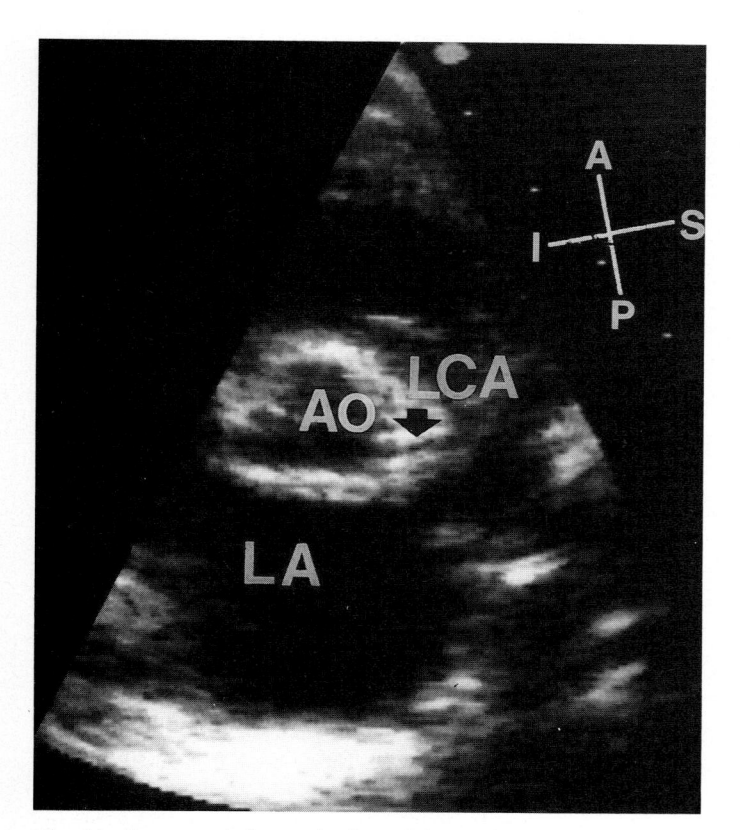

Fig. 16 Parasternal short axis view of the aortic root. In this child with anomalous origin of the coronary artery from the pulmonary trunk, the origin of the left coronary artery erroneously appears to be from the aorta. LCA – Left coronary artery.

may have prominent dyskinetic wall motion abnormalities but this should be interpreted with caution as similar findings may be seen in the dilated cardiomyopathy which follows viral myocarditis.

Dopper echocardiography will usually reveal the presence of mitral valve regurgitation (Plate 3). This results from dilatation of the mitral annulus and from the papillary muscles either being affected in the disease process or being displaced by ventricular dilatation such that there is longer full coaptation of the valve leaflets. There may also be tricuspid valve regurgitation. Measurement of the peak velocity of the tricuspid regurgitant jet may be used to detect the presence of right ventricular hypertension secondary to pulmonary hypertension.

There is little information on mitral inflow velocities in children with dilated cardiomyopathy. Studies in adults suggest that the pattern seen depends on the loading conditions and on the presence and degree of mitral regurgitation.[35,36]

Doppler echocardiography can also be used to estimate the cardiac output and to monitor the effects of therapeutic intervention.[37] A continuous wave Dopper probe is commonly used to record the aortic velocity spectra. Volumetric flow may be estimated if there is concurrent measurement of the aortic annulus dimension from cross-sectional echocardiography. Alternatively, the stroke distance (aortic flow velocity integral) can be measured to monitor changes in an individual patient. This has the advantage of avoiding the error inherent in measuring the

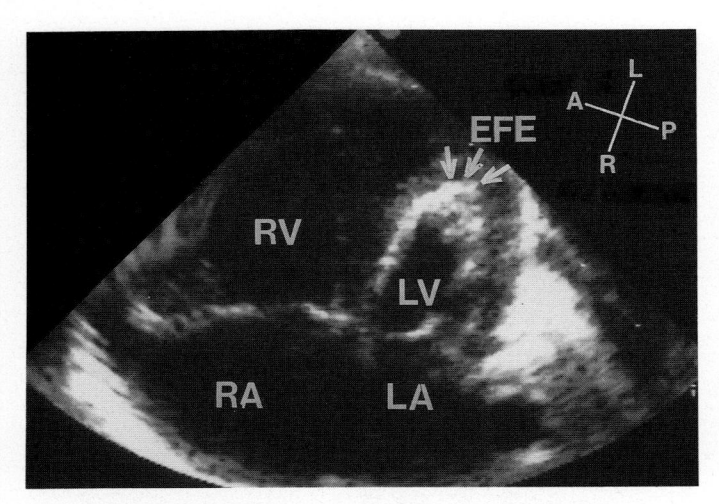

Fig. 17 Apical four chamber view in neonate with contracted endocardial fibroelastosis. There is a small left ventricle with an echogenic endocardial layer characteristic of endocardial fibroelastosis (EFE).

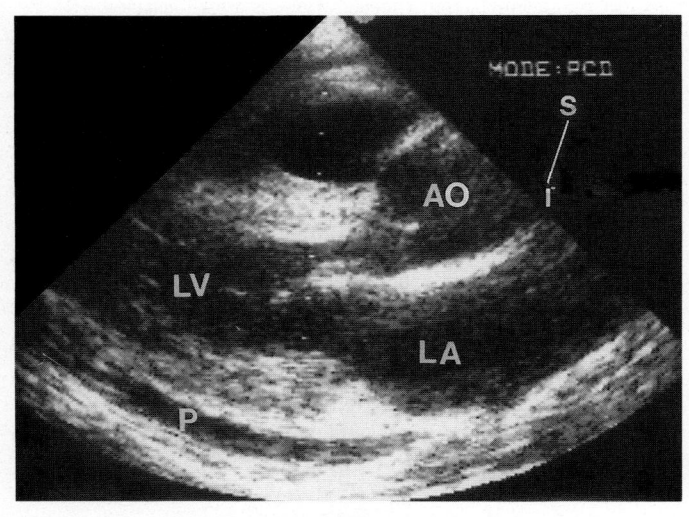

Fig. 18 Severe myocarditis secondary to high dose cyclophosphamide treatment. Parasternal long axis view. The left ventricular myocardium is thicker and more echogenic than normal. There is reduced systolic function and a pericardial effusion (P).

cross-sectional area of flow needed to calculate the cardiac output, as over a short time period there is not likely to be a significant change in the aortic dimensions in an individual.

Viral myocarditis

The echocardiographic features are non-specific, there being a dilated cardiomyopathy of variable severity. The child will usually present with a relatively short history of heart failure, often preceded by a viral illness. The chest X-ray will show an enlarged heart and sometimes pulmonary venous congestion. With this presentation, a pericardial effusion is an important differential diagnosis. Cross-sectional echocardiography can easily resolve matters.

Many viruses can produce a myocarditis, the most common being Coxsackie, influenza, Echo, mumps and rubella. One cause that may become more frequent in the future is the left ventricular dysfunction seen in acquired immunodeficiency syndrome (AIDS).[38]

Serial echocardiography will usually show improvement in left ventricular function with time. The period of recovery takes several months, and whilst these children may become asymptomatic, there are usually persisting abnormalities of left ventricular systolic function at late follow up.[39]

Acute rheumatic fever

This illness is rare in the Western countries but remains common in the developing nations. Recently there have been outbreaks of the illness in parts of North America and Western Europe.[40,41]

The acute phase of the illness is characterised by a carditis often with pericardial, myocardial and endocardial involvement. The endocardial involvement is often most prominent and produces valve thickening and a variable degree of mitral or aortic regurgitation. The myocardial involvement produces a dilated cardiomyopathy and any pericardial involvement may result in a pericardial effusion. The diagnosis is clinical and is based on the revised Duckett Jones criteria.[42]

Endocardial fibroelastosis

The characteristic feature of this condition is thickening of the endocardium due to a dense mass of collagen and elastic tissue. It may occur in association with congenital heart disease, such as aortic atresia or aortic valve stenosis, when it is considered to be 'secondary' to the malformation. It may also occur as a 'primary' disorder, in an otherwise normal heart, and generally presents in the first year of life. It has been divided into two groups, the more common dilated form which presents as a dilated cardiomyopathy and the rarer contracted form which presents as a restrictive cardiomyopathy.

The left ventricle is dilated with reduced systolic function and the endocardial fibroelastosis may be recognised as a bright, thick endocardial surface.[43,44] It may appear most marked in the region of the papillary muscles of the mitral valve and there is frequently associated mitral regurgitation.

The contracted form has the similar dense endocardial surface but there is a small left ventricular cavity with reduced systolic function. Such patients tend to present soon after birth with severe heart failure, akin to patients with aortic atresia. This condition has a high mortality (Fig. 17).

Many children with the dilated form will die from progressive heart failure, but some do appear to make a partial or complete recovery.

Association of dilated cardiomyopathy with other diseases

There are a number of systemic diseases and various drug treatments that may be associated with or produce a dilated cardiomyopathy in childhood.

Duchenne muscular dystrophy

This is an X-linked recessive disorder that usually presents with muscle weakness in the first few years of life. There is progressive muscular wasting resulting in death in late childhood or early adulthood.

Myocardial involvement is common and pathologically there is fibrous and fatty tissue replacement of the myocardium with selective scarring of the posterolateral wall of the left ventricle and of the posterolateral papillary muscle.

The echocardiographic features consist of impaired systolic and diastolic left ventricular function with reduced left ventricular wall thickness.[45-47] Mitral valve regurgitation, secondary to leaflet prolapse, is a frequent finding and presumably results from the papillary muscle involvement.

Dilated cardiomyopathy may also be seen in other muscular dystrophies, such as Becker's muscular dystrophy,[48] scapuloperoneal myopathy,[49] and Emery–Dreifuss muscular dystrophy.[50]

Connective tissue disorders

Cardiac involvement in these disorders may rarely occur in childhood. Juvenile rheumatoid arthritis may produce a myocarditis in the acute phase of the illness[51] and there may be an associated pericarditis that can produce a pericardial effusion.

Systemic lupus erythematosus and dermatomyositis may also be associated with a diffuse myocarditis.[52]

Thalassaemic cardiomyopathy

Whilst idiopathic haemochromatosis is extremely rare in childhood, secondary haemochromatosis is frequently seen in children with beta-thalassaemia major because of the need for frequent blood transfusions and subsequent iron overload.

The echocardiographic features consist of increased left ventricular dimensions with reduced systolic function[53] and serial testing is likely to show deteriorating left ventricular function with time.[54] Iron chelation therapy with desferoxamine has been shown to protect the myocardium[55] and serial echocardiographic monitoring of these patients is accepted practice.

Abnormalities of diastolic left ventricular function have also been described in thalassaemia. Doppler echocardiographic study has shown a restrictive pattern to left ventricular filling,[56] with an increased peak early filling velocity (E wave), rapid deceleration of early filling and increased E/A ratio (ratio of the peak early to peak atrial filling velocities).

Anthracycline cardiomyopathy

The anthracycline group of drugs (doxorubicin, daunorubicin and epirubicin) are widely used to treat childhood malignancies. They produce a cumulative dose-related, dilated cardiomyopathy. There is individual variation in susceptibility but a cumulative dose of greater than 500 mg/m^2 significantly increases the risk of cardiomyopathy.[57]

The echocardiographic findings are non-specific, there being left ventricular dilatation with reduced systolic function indices. Generally, echocardiography has not been a good predictor of impending congestive cardiac failure and myocardial biopsy is considered the best method for assessing the degree of cardiac damage.[58] Many centres monitor left ventricular function, either by echocardiography or radionuclide angiography, curtailing anthracycline treatment if function falls below the normal range.

Diastolic function abnormalities have been described at relatively low cumulative anthracycline dosage,[59] however it is not known whether these are better predictors of impending cardiac decompensation.

Cardiac irradiation, for the treatment of childhood malignancy, may potentiate the cardiotoxic effects of anthracycline chemotherapy and can on its own produce a restrictive cardiomyopathy.[60]

High dose treatment with cyclophosphamide may produce a severe, haemorrhagic myocarditis[61] (Fig. 18).

Miscellaneous causes

A number of nutritional disorders may be associated with a dilated cardiomyopathy and should be considered in areas where they are endemic. Examples include selenium deficiency, kwashiorkor, beriberi and carnitine deficiency.[24]

The possibility of a chronic incessant arrhythmia should also be considered in a child presenting with cardiac failure and a dilated cardiomyopathy.[62]

RESTRICTIVE CARDIOMYOPATHY

This form of cardiomyopathy is rare in childhood, though many of the forms of dilated cardiomyopathy described above may have a restrictive element to their dysfunction (for instance thalassaemic cardiomyopathy). The cardinal features of a restrictive cardiomyopathy are a normal left ventricular end diastolic dimension with preserved systolic function. The left ventricular myocardium may be of normal thickness or there may be mild hypertrophy.

Idiopathic restrictive cardiomyopathy

M-mode echocardiography has been used to evaluate children with this condition.[63] The features present were normal left and right ventricular diastolic dimensions with either a normal left ventricular posterior wall thickness or mild hypertrophy. Whilst systolic function is normal there is evidence of diastolic dysfunction with a prolonged isovolumic relaxation time and slow early filling. There are increased ventricular end-diastolic pressures associated with the relaxation abnormalities which lead to high atrial pressures. This produces dilatation of both atria and when long-standing they may assume enormous proportions.[64,65]

Cross-sectional echocardiography will show the normal dimensions of the left and right ventricles and the dilated atria. When the cardiomyopathy is long-standing, the chronic elevation of left atrial pressure leads to pulmonary hypertension. This will result in dilatation of the pulmonary trunk and right ventricular hypertrophy.

Doppler echocardiography will frequently reveal the presence of mild mitral and tricuspid regurgitation. Measurement of the peak velocity of the tricuspid regurgitant jet can be used to estimate the right ventricular systolic pressure and thus identify those patients with significant pulmonary hypertension.

In adults, Doppler echocardiography has been shown to be a useful method of detecting restrictive physiology. There are characteristic changes in the mitral inflow velocity profile and the flow patterns in the pulmonary and systemic veins.[66,67] The mitral inflow patterns have a normal or increased peak early filling velocity (E wave) with a shortened E wave deceleration time. The atrial filling wave (A wave) has a reduced peak velocity and this, together with the increased E wave velocity, produces an increased E/A ratio. Diastolic mitral or tricuspid regurgitation has also been described in some patients.

The flow velocity patterns in the pulmonary and systemic veins of normal subjects show dominant forward flow in systole. In restrictive physiology there is dominant flow during diastole often with flow reversal during inspiration (usually during systole, occasionally during diastole as well). The sensitivity and specificity of these changes remain to be assessed.

Endomyocardial fibrosis

This disorder is a common cause of cardiomyopathy in tropical regions and is rare in Europe and North America. It has been divided into two types depending on the presence of blood eosinophilia. It is characterised by a restrictive cardiomyopathy with a dense build up of fibrotic material and thrombus in the apical region of the affected ventricle. Either or both ventricles may be affected.

The echocardiographic features are the presence of relatively normal left and right ventricular dimensions at the base of the heart but with obliteration of the apical region with dense echogenic material.[68] Ventricular wall thickness is normal or mildly increased and systolic function is normal or mildly depressed. The atria are enlarged and may become aneurysmal in the more severe cases. The fibrotic process frequently involves the tensor apparatus of the mitral and tricuspid valves and thus may result in valve regurgitation.

Other causes of restrictive cardiomyopathy

Chagas' disease produced by the parasite *Trypanosoma cruzi* is endemic in parts of South America. In the acute phase of parasite infestation there may be an acute myocarditis with a dilated cardiomyopathy. In later life there is a chronic cardiomyopathy characterised by regional wall motion abnormalities, often with apical left ventricular aneurysm formation. The left ventricle may become dilated with reduced systolic function but often diastolic dysfunction predominates.[69]

Other rare causes of restrictive cardiomyopathy in childhood might include amyloidosis, iron overload in thalassaemia major and chronic rejection in cardiac transplant recipients.[70] The latter may become more frequent as cardiac transplantation in childhood increases.

REFERENCES

1 Report of the WHO/ISFC Task Force on the definition and classification of cardiomyopathies. Br Heart J 1980; 44: 672–673
2 Maron B J, Spirito P, Wesley Y, Arce J. Development and progression of left ventricular hypertrophy in children with hypertrophic cardiomyopathy. N Engl J Med 1986; 315: 610–614
3 Goodwin J F. The frontiers of cardiomyopathy. Br Heart J 1982; 48: 1–18
4 Maron B J, Tajik A J, Ruttenberg H G, Graham J P, Atwood G F, Victorica B E, Lie J J, Roberts W C. Hypertrophic cardiomyopathy in infants: clinical features and natural history. Circulation 1982; 65: 7–17
5 Maron B J, Edwards J E, Ferrans V J, Clark C E, Lebowitz E A, Henry W L, Epstein S E. Congenital heart malformations associated with disproportionate ventricular septal thickening. Circulation 1975; 52: 926–932
6 Maron B J, Sato N, Roberts W C, Edwards J E, Chandra R S. Quantitative analysis of cardiac muscle cell disorganization in the ventricular septum. Comparison of fetuses and infants with and

without congenital heart disease and patients with hypertrophic cardiomyopathy. Circulation 1979; 60: 685–696
7 Henry W L, Clark C E, Glancy D L, Epstein S E. Echocardiographic measurement of the left ventricular outflow gradient in idiopathic hypertrophic subaortic stenosis. N Engl J Med 1973; 288: 989–993
8 Maron B J, Gottdiener J S, Arce J, Rosing D R, Wesley Y E, Epstein S E. Dynamic subaortic obstrucon in hypertrophic cardiomyopathy: analysis by pulsed wave echocardiography. J Am Coll Cardiol 1985; 6: 1–15
9 Yock P G, Hatle L, Popp R L. Patterns and timing of Doppler detected intracavitary and aortic flow in hypertrophic cardiomyopathy. J Am Coll Cardiol 1986; 8: 1047–1058
10 Theard M, Bhatia S B, Plappert T, St John Sutton M. Doppler echocardiographic study of the frequency and severity of aortic regurgitation in hypertrophic cardiomyopathy. Am J Cardiol 1987; 60: 1143–1147
11 Kinoshita N, Nimura Y, Okamoto M, Miyatake K, Nagata S, Sakakibara H. Mitral regurgitation in hypertrophic cardiomyopathy. Non-invasive study by two-dimensional Doppler echocardiography. Br Heart J 1983; 49: 574–583
12 Maron B J, Spirito P, Green K J, Westley Y E, Bonow R O, Arce J. Non-invasive assessment of left ventricular diastolic function by pulsed Doppler echocardiography in patients with hypertrophic cardiomyopathy. J Am Coll Cardiol 1987; 10: 733–742
13 Shem-Tov A, Deutsch V, Yahini J H, Neufeld H M. Cardiomyopathy associated with congenital heart disease. Br Heart J 1971; 33: 782–793
14 Somerville J, McDonald L. Congenital anomalies in the heart with hypertrophic cardiomyopathy. Br Heart J 1968; 30: 713–722
15 Honey M, Gold R G. Congenital physiologically corrected transposition with hypertrophic obstructive cardiomyopathy. Br Heart J 1971; 22: 214–219
16 Schneeweiss A, Shem-Tov A, Hegesh J, Blieden L C, Feigel A, Neufeld H N. Severe congestive heart failure in mild pulmonic stenosis due to dysplastic pulmonary valve associated with cardiomyopathy. Eur Heart J 1983; 4: 286–288
17 Ehlers K H, Engle M A, Levin A R, Deeley W J. Eccentric ventricular hypertrophy in familial and sporadic instances of 46 XX, XY Turner phenotype. Circulation 1972; 45: 639–652
18 Hirsch H D, Gelband H, Carcia O, Gottlieb S, Tanner D M. Rapidly progressive obstructive cardiomyopathy in infants with Noonan's syndrome. Circulation 1975; 52: 1161–1165
19 Somerville J, Bonham-Carter R E. The heart in lentigenosis. Br Heart J 1972; 34: 58–66
20 Shapir Y, Roguin N. Echocardiographic findings in Pompe's disease with left ventricular obstruction. Clin Cardiol 1985; 8: 181–185
21 Buckley B H, Hutchins G M. Pompe's disease presenting as hypertrophic cardiomyopathy with Wolff–Parkinson–White syndrome. Am Heart J 1978; 96: 246–252
22 Bass J L, Shrivastava S, Grabowski G A, Desnick R J, Moller J H. The M mode echocardiogram in Fabry's disease. Am Heart J 1980; 100: 807–812
23 Goldman M E, Cantor R, Schwartz M F, et al. Echocardiographic abnormalities and disease severity in Fabry's disease. J Am Coll Cardiol 1986; 7: 1157–1161
24 Ino T, Sherwood W E, Benson L E, Wilson G J, Freedom R M, Rowe R D. Cardiac manifestations in disorders of fat and carnitine metabolism in infancy. J Am Coll Cardiol 1988; 11: 1301–1308
25 Mace S, Hirschfield S S, Riggs T, et al. Echocardiographic abnormalities in infants of diabetic mothers. J Pediatr 1979; 95: 1013–1019
26 Reller M D, Tsang R G, Meyer R A, Baun C P. Relationship of prospective diabetes control in pregnancy to neonatal cardio-respiratory function. J Pediatr 1985; 106: 86–90
27 Deodari A K, Saxena A, Singh M, Shrivastava S. Echocardiographic assessment of infants born to diabetic mothers. Arch Dis Child 1989; 64: 721–724
28 Ryan C A, Boyle M H, Burggraff G W. Reversible obstructive cardiomyopathy in the Beckwith–Wiedermann syndrome. Pediatr Cardiol 1989; 10: 225–228
29 St John Sutton M G, Olukotun A J, Tajik A J, Lovett J L, Giuliani E R. Left ventricular function in Friedreich's ataxia. An echocardiographic study. Br Heart J 1980; 44: 309–316
30 Alboliras E T, Shub C, Gomez M R, et al. Spectrum of cardiac involvement in Friedreich's ataxia: clinical, electrocardiographic and echocardiographic observations. Am J Cardiol 1986; 58: 518–524
31 Child J S, Perloff J K, Bach P M, et al. Cardiac involvement in Friedreich's ataxia: a clinical study of 75 patients. J Am Coll Cardiol 1986; 7: 1370–1378
32 Ghafour A S, Gutgesell H P. Echocardiographic evaluation of left ventricular function in children with congestive cardiomyopathy. Am J Cardiol 1979; 44: 1332–1338
33 Goldberg S J, Valdes-Cruz L M, Sahn D J, Allen H D. Two-dimensional echocardiographic evaluation of dilated cardiomyopathy in children. Am J Cardiol 1983; 52: 1244–1248
34 Koike K, Musewe N N, Smallhorn J F, Freedom R M. Distinguishing between anomalous origin of the left coronary artery from the pulmonary trunk and dilated cardiomyopathy: role of echocardiographic measurement of the right coronary artery. Br Heart J 1989; 61: 192–197
35 Takenaka K, Dabestani A, Gardin J M, et al. Pulsed Doppler echocardiographic study of left ventricular filling in dilated cardiomyopathy. Am J Cardiol 1986; 58: 143–147
36 Appleton C P, Hatle L K, Popp R L. Relation of transmitral flow velocity patterns to left ventricular diastolic function: new insights from a combined hemodynamic and Dopper echocardiographic study. J Am Coll Cardiol 1988; 12: 426–440
37 Morrow W R, Murphy D J, Fisher D J, Huhta J C, Jefferson L S, O'Brian-Smith E. Continuous wave Doppler cardiac output: Use in paediatric patients receiving inotropic support. Pediatr Cardiol 1988; 9: 131–136
38 Cohen I S, Anderson D W, Virmani R, Reen B, Macher A M, Sennesh J. Congestive cardiomyopathy in association with the acquired immunodeficiency syndrome. N Engl J Med 1986; 315: 628–630
39 Weinhouse E, Wanderman K L, Sofer S, Gussarsky Y, Gueron M. Viral myocarditis simulating dilated cardiomyopathy in early childhood: evaluation by serial echocardiography. Br Heart J 1986; 56: 94–97
40 Veasey L G, Wiedmier S E, Orsmund G S, et al. Resurgence of acute rheumatic fever in the intermountain area of the United States. N Engl J Med 1987; 316: 421–427
41 Bonova G, Rogani P, Acerbi L, et al. Outbreak of acute rheumatic fever in Northern Italy. J Pediatr 1988; 114: 334
42 WHO Technical Report Series, No 764, 1988 (Rheumatic fever and rheumatic heart disease).
43 Bjorkhem G, Lundstrom N R, Wallentin I, Carlgren L E. Endocardial fibroelastosis with predominant involvement of left atrium. Possibility of diagnosis by non-invasive means. Br Heart J 1981; 46: 331–337
44 Yoshida Y, Sato T, Kano I, et al. Ultrasonic studies on endocardial fibroelastosis. Tohoku J Exp Med 1977; 123: 329–335
45 Hunsaker R H, Fulkerson P K, Barry F J, Lewis R P, Leier C V, Unverferth D V. Cardiac function in Duchenne's muscular dystrophy. Results of 10 year follow-up study and non-invasive tests. Am J Med 1982; 73: 235–238
46 Goldberg S J, Stern L Z, Feldman L, Sahn D J, Allen H D, Valdes-Cruz L M. Serial left ventricular wall measurements in Duchenne's muscular dystrophy. J Am Coll Cardiol 1983; 2: 136–142
47 D'Orsogna L, O'Shea J P, Miller G. Cardiomyopathy of Duchenne muscular dystrophy. Pediatr Cardiol 1988; 9: 205–213
48 Katiyar B C, Misra S, Somani P N, Chaterji A M. Congestive cardiomyopathy in a family of Becker's x-linked muscular dystrophy. Postgrad Med J 1977; 53: 12–15
49 Chakrabarti A, Pearce J M S. Scapuloperoneal syndrome with cardiomyopathy: report of a family with autosomal dominant inheritance and unusual features. J Neurol Neurosurg Psych 1981; 44: 1146–1152
50 Yoshioka M, Saida K, Itagaki Y, Kamiya T. Follow up study of cardiac involvement in Emery'Dreifuss muscular dystrophy. Arch Dis Child 1989; 64: 713–715
51 Miller J J, French J W. Myocarditis in juvenile rheumatoid arthritis. Am J Dis Child 1977; 131: 205–209

52 Isaeva L A, Deliagin V M, Bazhenova L K. Main manifestations of carditis in diffuse connective tissue diseases in children. Cor Vasa 1988; 30: 211–217
53 Henry W L, Nienhuis A W, Weiner M, Miller D R, Canale V C, Piomelli S. Echocardiographic abnormalities in patients with transfusion-dependent anemia and secondary myocardial iron deposition. Am J Med 1978; 64: 547–555
54 Canale C, Terrachini V, Vallebona A, Bruzzone F, Masperone M A, Caponnetto S. Thalassemic cardiomyopathy: echocardiographic difference between major and intermediate thalassemia at rest and during isometric effort: yearly follow up. Clin Cardiol 1988; 11: 563–571
55 Wolfe L, Olivieri N, Sallan D, Colan S, Rose V, Propper R, Freedman M H, Nathan D G. Prevention of cardiac disease by subcutaneous desferoxamine in patients with thalassemia major. N Engl J Med 1985; 312: 1600–1603
56 Spirito P, Lupi G, Melevendi C, Vecchio C. Restrictive diastolic abnormalities identified by Doppler echocardiography in patients with thalassemia major. Circulation 1990; 82: 88–94
57 Von Hoff D D, Rozencweig M, Layard M, Slavik M, Muggia F M. Daunomycin-induced cardiotoxicity in children and adults. Am J Med 1977; 62: 200–208
58 Mason J W, Bristow M R, Billingham M E, Daniels J R. Invasive and non-invasive tests of assessing adriamycin toxic effects in man: Superiority of histopathologic assessment using endomyocardial biopsy. Cancer Treat Rep 1978; 62: 857–864
59 Bu'Lock F A, Mott M G, Martin R P. Doppler echocardiographic assessment of anthracycline induced ventricular dysfunction in children. Pediatr Cardiol 1990; 11: 239–240
60 Stewart J R, Fajardo L F. Radiation induced heart disease: an update. Prog Cardiovasc Dis 1984; 27: 173–194
61 Mills B A, Roberts R W. Cyclophosphamide-induced cardiomyopathy. A report of two cases and review of the English literature. Cancer 1979; 43: 2223–2226
62 Gladman G, Wilkinson J L, Evans-Jones G. Pseudocardiomyopathy secondary to chronic incessant supraventricular tachycardia. Arch Dis Child 1989; 54: 402–404
63 Mehta A V, Ferrer P L, Pickoff A S, Singh S S, Wolff G S, Tamer D S, Garcia O L, Gelband H. M-mode echocardiographic findings in children with idiopathic restrictive cardiomyopathy. Pediatr Cardiol 1984; 5: 273–279
64 Erath H G, Graham T P Jr, Smith C W, et al. Restrictive cardiomyopathy in an infant with massive biatrial enlargement and normal ventricular size and pump function. Cathet Cardiovasc Diagn 1978; 4: 289–296
65 Siege R J, Shah P K, Fishbein M C. Idiopathic restrictive cardiomyopathy. Circulation 1984; 70: 165–169
66 Appleton C P, Hatle L K, Popp R L. Demonstration of restrictive physiology by Doppler echocardiography. J Am Coll Cardiol 1988; 11: 757–768
67 Schiavone W A, Calafiore P A, Salcedo E E. Transesophageal Doppler echocardiographic demonstration of pulmonary flow velocity in restrictive cardiomyopathy and constrictive pericarditis. Am J Cardiol 1989; 63: 1286–1288
68 Acquatella H, Schiller N B, Puigbo J J, Gomez-Mancebo J R, Suarez C, Acquatella G. Value of two-dimensional echocardiography in endomyocardial disease with and without eosinophila. A clinical and pathologic study. Circulation 1983; 67: 1219–1226
69 Caeiro T, Amuchastegui L M, Moreyra E, Gibson D G. Abnormal left ventricular diastolic function in chronic Chaga's disease: an echocardiographic study. Int J Cardiol 1985; 9: 417–424
70 Valantine H A, Appleton C P, Hatle L K, Hunt S A, Billingham M E, Shumway N E, Stinson E B, Popp R L. A hemodynamic and Doppler echocardiographic study of ventricular function in long-term cardiac allograft recipients. Circulation 1989; 79: 66–75

27

Great arterial anomalies

Introduction
Aortic arch abnormalities
Pulmonary artery sling
Associated abnormalities

John L. Gibbs

INTRODUCTION

A wide variety of abnormalities of the aortic arch and the arterial duct may form a vascular ring.[1,2] Ultrasound may be helpful in the detection of some forms of vascular ring but it cannot reveal complete anatomical detail of the structures involved and thus it rarely allows treatment to be planned without further investigation. Although echocardiography may allow the basic diagnosis in pulmonary artery sling, barium swallow and angiography remain the mainstay of diagnosis in aortic arch abnormalities.

Magnetic resonance imaging is becoming increasingly important in the diagnosis and evaluation of these conditions. There is correspondingly very little available literature on the echocardiography of vascular rings.

Ultrasound may contribute to the diagnosis of vascular rings in four ways: to establish whether the aortic arch is right or left sided, to establish whether the descending aorta is on the left or the right, to detect abnormal branching or duplication of the aortic arch, and to detect abnormal origin of the left pulmonary artery (pulmonary artery sling).

AORTIC ARCH ABNORMALITIES

Double aortic arch may be a relatively straightforward echocardiographic diagnosis when both the right and left arches are well developed and patent.[3] The bifurcation of the ascending aorta may be seen in suprasternal views[3,4] (Fig. 1), but is often best detected using a subcostal approach[5] (Fig. 2). More commonly there is inequality of the sizes of the two arches, which may be marked. One arch can often be atretic distal to the origin of its brachiocephalic branches, the vascular ring being completed by a thin ligamentous remnant of the arch which is invisible to cross-sectional echocardiography. When the latter occurs with a patent left arch and an atretic right arch, images obtained from the suprasternal position may

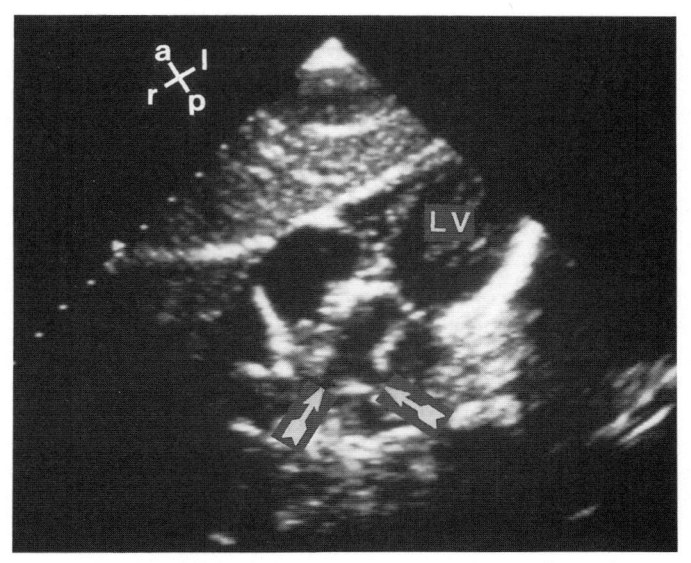

Fig. 2 The bifurcation of the ascending aorta (arrowed) may be better appreciated from a subcostal transducer position, particularly when respiratory difficulties are present as is often the case with vascular rings.

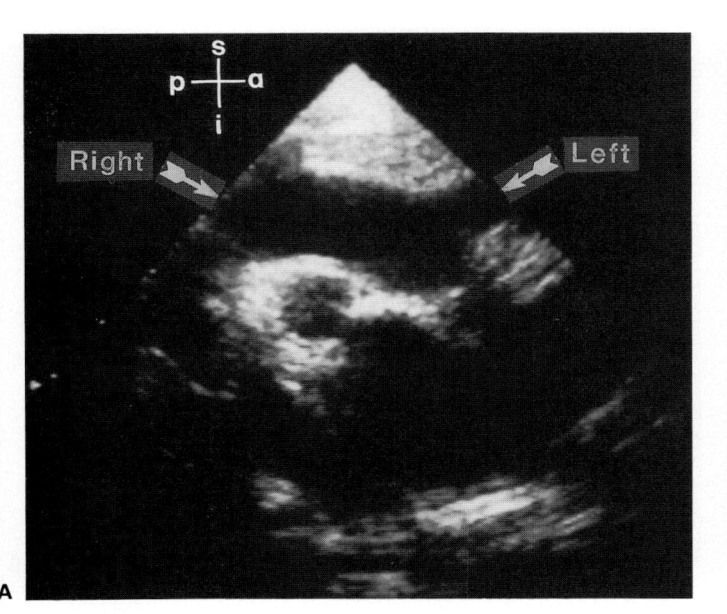

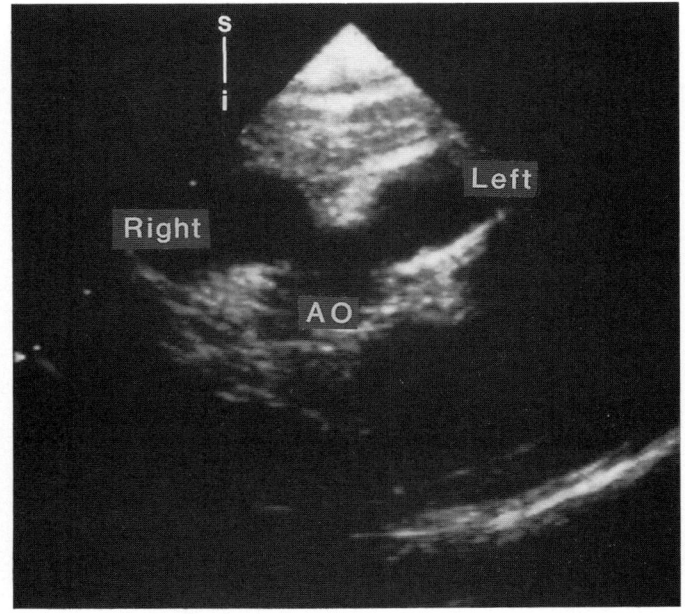

Fig. 1 Double aortic arch. A: The dominant right sided arch is clearly seen in a high left parasternal view and the origin of the left sided arch from the ascending aorta is also visible. **B**: The bifurcation of the ascending aorta may be more readily appreciated from a coronal plane suprasternal view.

be very difficult to distinguish from those of a normal left sided aortic arch with an unusual origin of the innominate artery. Conversely when there is a patent right arch and atretic left arch differentiation from right sided aortic arch with a proximal origin of the left sided innominate artery may be difficult.

Echocardiographic recognition of a right sided aortic arch in a patient with symptoms suggestive of a vascular ring should always prompt further investigation. Visualisation of a right sided aortic arch is usually possible with cross-sectional echocardiography[6] and this variation should be sought when standard views fail to reveal a left sided arch (Fig. 3). In the latter situation an incorrect diagnosis of interruption of the aortic arch should be avoided as the appearances of attempted standard left arch views may be very similar in these two abnormalities.[6] Awareness of the cross-sectional appearances of interruption of the arch is therefore of great importance.[7,8] The finding of a right aortic arch can only raise suspicion of the presence of a vascular ring as it does not in itself form a ring unless it is associated with a left sided arterial duct or ligament, neither of which are readily detectable by ultrasound.

Cross-sectional echocardiography allows detailed anatomical assessment of the aortic arch and will often also reveal the origin of its branches.[9-12] Anomalous origin of the right subclavian artery from the descending aorta with a left sided aortic arch (with or without a left sided arterial duct or ligament) may produce symptoms similar to those of a vascular ring, although it does not constitute a complete ring anatomically. Cross-sectional echocardiography may allow visualisation of the origin of the right subclavian artery but will rarely allow demonstration of the posterior relationship of the aberrant artery to the oesophagus. Similarly, anomalous origin of the innominate artery may be associated with symptoms suggestive of a vascular ring but this is very rare.

A left aortic arch with a right descending aorta and a right arterial duct or ligament together form a complete vascular ring.[13-15] Echocardiographic diagnosis is possible (at least in theory) by establishing that the aortic arch is left sided and by demonstrating that the thoracic descending aorta lies to the right of the spine. The descending aorta, when in its normal position behind the left atrium or atrioventricular groove, is best imaged in the long and short axis parasternal views[17] and its inferior course may be followed by subcostal imaging.

PULMONARY ARTERY SLING

Pulmonary artery sling, being due to anomalous origin of the left pulmonary artery from the right pulmonary artery, may usually be detected by echocardiography.[18] But obtaining high quality images, particularly from the precordium, may be difficult as many patients present with respiratory embarrassment. When obstruction to air flow has caused difficulty in imaging from the chest wall, a subcostal approach will usually allow adequate images to be obtained.[18,19] Anatomical detail of the pulmonary artery bifurcation and of the abnormal early course of the left pulmonary artery may be obtainable, but little if any detail of the more distal pulmonary arteries may be seen. When clear images of the origin of the left pulmonary artery are difficult to obtain, colour flow imaging may be helpful in identifying the origin of blood flow to the left lung[20]

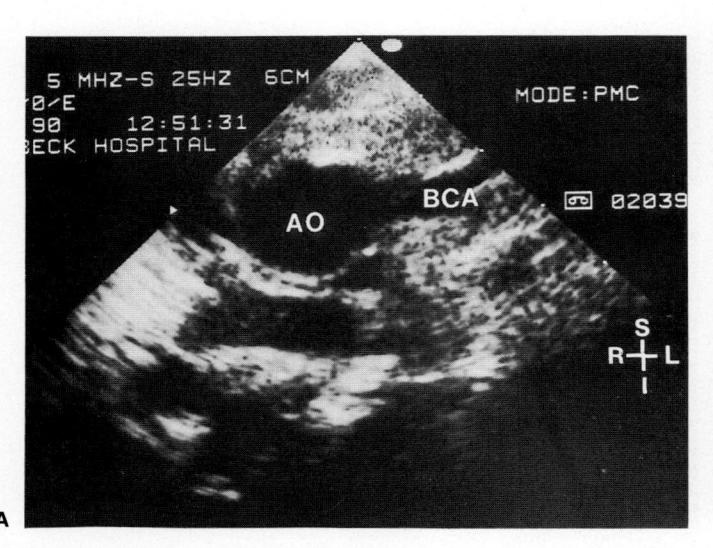

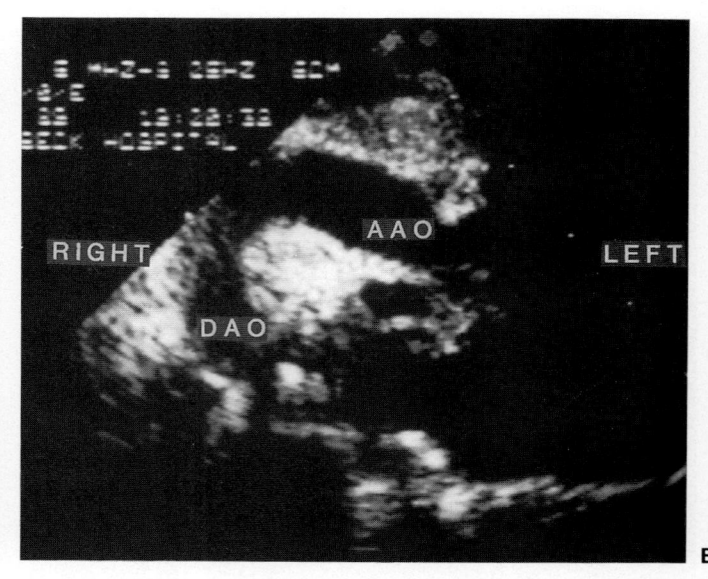

Fig. 3 **Right aortic arch. A**: A standard high left parasternal or suprasternal view in the usual orientation to image a left arch may be confused with the appearance of interrupted aortic arch. This appearance is due to the aorta appearing in short axis, with the brachiocephalic artery (BCA) arising from it. **B**: Anticlockwise rotation of the transducer through 90 degrees will reveal that a normal right sided aortic arch is present. (AAO – ascending acute, DAO – descending aorta.)

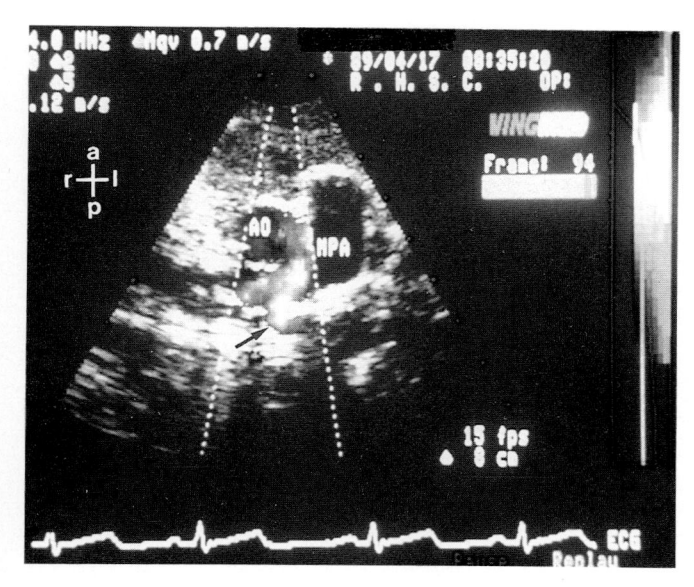

Plate 1 Pulmonary artery sling. In a left parasternal short axis view the left pulmonary artery is seen to arise from the proximal right pulmonary artery (arrowed). The abnormal branching of the pulmonary artery is most easily appreciated using colour flow Doppler. (By courtesy of Dr James Gnanapragasam.) This figure is reproduced in colour in the colour plate section at the front of this volume.

(Plate 1). Branch pulmonary artery anatomy is important to define, as part of the right upper lobe may be supplied by an anomalous branch of the left pulmonary artery but this information is frequently impossible to obtain using ultrasound alone. For this reason, pulmonary angiography is still required in most patients with pulmonary artery sling prior to planning surgical treatment.

ASSOCIATED ABNORMALITIES

Double aortic arch usually occurs in isolation, but may occur in the presence of other congenital heart disease such as ventricular septal defect, atrial septal defect or tetralogy of Fallot. Right aortic arch and anomalous origin of the right subclavian artery may also coexist with congenital heart disease, notably tetralogy of Fallot. The association with cardiac abnormalities is sufficiently frequent to warrant routine echocardiography in all patients with suspected vascular ring. Indeed, it could be argued that the primary indication for echocardiography in these patients is to assess the presence of coexistent congenital heart defects rather than to confirm the diagnosis of vascular ring. Pulmonary artery sling may occasionally be associated with congenital heart disease, notably ventricular septal defect or an arterial duct.[2] Cross-sectional echocardiography and Doppler ultrasound allows detection of these abnormalities as well as being diagnostic of the abnormal origin of the left pulmonary artery.

REFERENCES

1 Park S C, Zuberbuhler J R. Vascular ring and pulmonary sling. In: Tynan M, Anderson R H, Shinebourne E A, Macartney F J (eds) Paediatric cardiology. Edinburgh: Churchill Livingstone 1969: 1123–1136
2 Moes C. Vascular rings and anomalies of the aortic arch. In: Keith J, Rowe R, Vlad P (eds) Heart disease in infancy and childhood. New York: Macmillan Publishing Co. 1979: p. 856–881
3 Enderlein M A, Silverman N H, Stanger P, Heymann M A. Usefulness of suprasternal notch echocardiography for diagnosis of double aortic arch. Am J Cardiol 1986; 57: 359–361
4 Kan M-N, Nanda N C, Stopa A R. Diagnosis of double aortic arch by cross sectional echocardiography with Doppler colour flow mapping. Br Heart J 1987; 58: 248–286
5 Sahn D J, Valdes-Cruz L M, Ovitt T W, Pond G, Mammana R, Goldberg S J, Allen H D, Copeland J G. Two dimensional echocardiography and intravenous digital video subtraction angiography for diagnosis and evaluation of double aortic arch. Am J Cardiol 1982; 50: 342–346
6 Celano V, Pieroni D R, Gingell R L, Roland J-M A. Two-dimensional echocardiographic recognition of the right aortic arch. Am J Cardiol 1983; 51: 1507–1512
7 Smallhorn J F, Anderson R H, Macartney F J. Cross-sectional echocardiographic recognition of interruption of the aortic arch between the left carotid and subclavian arteries. Br Heart J 1982; 48: 229–235
8 Riggs T W, Berry T E, Aziz K U, Paul M H. Two-dimensional echocardiographic features of interruption of the aortic arch. Am J Cardiol 1982; 50: 1385–1390
9 Huhta J C, Gutgesell H P, Latson L A, Huffines F D. Two-dimensional echocardiographic assessment of the aorta in infants and children with congenital heart disease. Circulation 1984; 70: 417–424
10 Snider A R, Silverman N H. Suprasternal notch echocardiography: a two-dimensional technique for evaluating congenital heart disease. Circulation 1981; 63: 165–173
11 George L, Waldman D, Kirkpatrick S E, Turner S W, Pappelbaum S J. Two-dimensional echocardiographic visualization of the aortic arch by right parasternal scanning in neonates and infants. Pediatr Cardiol 1982; 2: 277–280
12 Tajik A J, Seward J B, Hagler D J, Mair D D, Lie J T. Two-dimensional real-time ultrasonic imaging of the heart and great vessels. Technique, image orientation, structure identification and validation. Mayo Clin Proc 1978; 53: 271–303
13 Park S C, Siewers M D, Neches W H, Lenox C C, Zuberbuhler J R. Left aortic arch with right descending aorta and right ligamentum arteriosum. J Thorac Cardiovasc Surg 1976; 71: 779–784
14 Berman W, Yabek S M, Dillon T, Neal J F, Akl B, Burstein J. Vascular ring due to left aortic arch and right descending aorta. Circulation 1981; 63: 458–460
15 McFaul R, Millard P, Nowicki E. Vascular rings necessitating right thoracotomy. J Thorac Cardiovasc Surg 1981; 82: 306–309
16 Ergin M A, Jayaram N, LaCorte M. Left aortic arch and right descending aorta: diagnostic and therapeutic implications of a rare type of vascular ring. Ann Thorac Surg 1981; 31: 82–85
17 Mintz G S, Kotler M N, Segal B L, Parry W R. Two dimensional echocardiographic recognition of the descending thoracic aorta. Am J Cardiol 1979; 44: 232–238
18 Yeager S B, Chin A J, Sanders S P. Two-dimensional echocardiographic diagnosis of pulmonary artery sling in infancy. J Am Coll Cardiol 1986; 7: 625–629
19 Dupuis C, Vaksmann G, Pernot C, Gerard R, Martinez J, Van Egmond H. Asymptomatic form of left pulmonary artery sling. Am J Cardiol 1988; 61: 177–181
20 Gnanapragasam J P, Houston A B, Jamieson M P G. Pulmonary artery sling: definitive diagnosis by colour Doppler flow mapping avoiding cardiac catheterisation. Br Heart J 1990; 63: 251–252

28

Coronary artery anomalies

Normal trans-thoracic ultrasound studies of coronary arteries
Left main coronary artery
Left anterior descending artery
Left circumflex coronary artery
Right coronary artery
Practical difficulties in imaging coronary arteries
Coronary artery disease
Variation in the distribution of the coronary arteries

Transposition of the great arteries
Tetralogy of Fallot
Kawasaki disease
Anomalous origin of a coronary artery from the pulmonary trunk
Anomalous left coronary artery
Anomalous right coronary artery
Coronary artery fistula
Stenosis or atresia of the left coronary artery

Alan Houston

Echocardiographic imaging of the coronary arteries has been less extensively studied than intracardiac anatomy and great vessel abnormalities. This is largely because of the difficulty of imaging curving vessels, which move continuously and change position throughout the cardiac cycle in such a manner that only a relatively small part can be shown in a single image. The requirement for multiple views is even greater for showing coronary artery than for showing other intracardiac anatomy. Furthermore the practical value of echocardiographic images of the coronary arteries is limited since congenital anomalies are rare and most surgeons prefer an angiogram showing the whole vessel with its origin, branches, distribution and any areas of narrowing or dilation. Limited demonstration of the coronary arteries is of clinical importance in some situations however, and the development of high resolution ultrasound systems, colour Doppler flow mapping, and transoesophageal echocardiography have made the ultrasound study of the coronary arteries of potential clinical significance in the following circumstances:

(a) Left main coronary artery disease;
(b) Variation in coronary artery origin and distribution. This is sometimes seen in some normal hearts but is particularly important in tetralogy of Fallot and transposition of the great arteries;
(c) Anomalous origin of a coronary artery from the pulmonary artery;
(d) Kawasaki disease (mucocutaneous lymph node syndrome);
(e) Coronary artery fistula.

NORMAL TRANS–THORACIC ULTRASOUND STUDIES OF CORONARY ARTERIES

Early two-dimensional echocardiography studies showed that it was possible to image the proximal left main coronary artery.[1-3] A systematic approach to the detailed echocardiographic visualisation of coronary artery anatomy was subsequently described in children with coronary artery abnormalities[4] and in adults with non-dilated arteries.[5] It has proved possible in some patients to demonstrate the left main coronary artery and thence the proximal left anterior descending and occasionally the circumflex coronary artery, and also to show parts of the proximal and peripheral right coronary artery. The normal proximal course of the coronary arteries is illustrated diagrammatically in Figure 1.

Left main coronary artery

This vessel is most easily imaged from a parasternal short axis view of the aortic valve (usually from the second or third left intercostal space) by adjusting it to a plane just above the valve cusps and altering the transducer angula-

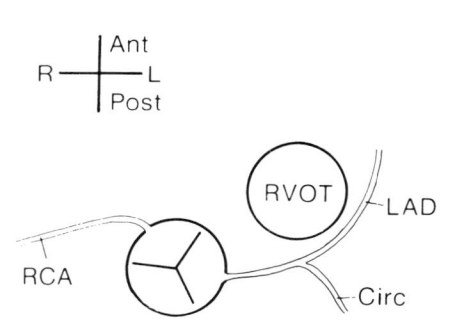

Fig. 1 Diagrammatic representation of the distribution of the coronary arteries in a normal subject. LAD – left anterior descending coronary artery, RVOT – right ventricular outflow tract, Circ – circumflex coronary artery, RCA – right coronary artery.

tion and position to demonstrate the tissue between the left ventricular outflow tract and the main pulmonary artery. This may involve clockwise rotation up to 30° and an inferior tilt from the view showing the aortic valve. In a proportion of cases the pulmonary valve annulus may be seen in cross-section.

In suitable subjects the left coronary artery can then be seen in the position of 3 to 4 o'clock to the aortic root, arising from the left coronary cusp and, as the left anterior descending artery, coursing in an anterior leftward direction behind the right ventricular outflow tract and main pulmonary artery, usually through a relatively dense mass of echoes (Fig. 2). The investigator must be aware of the potential for error in this study in that the transverse sinus of the pericardium between the great arteries and veins

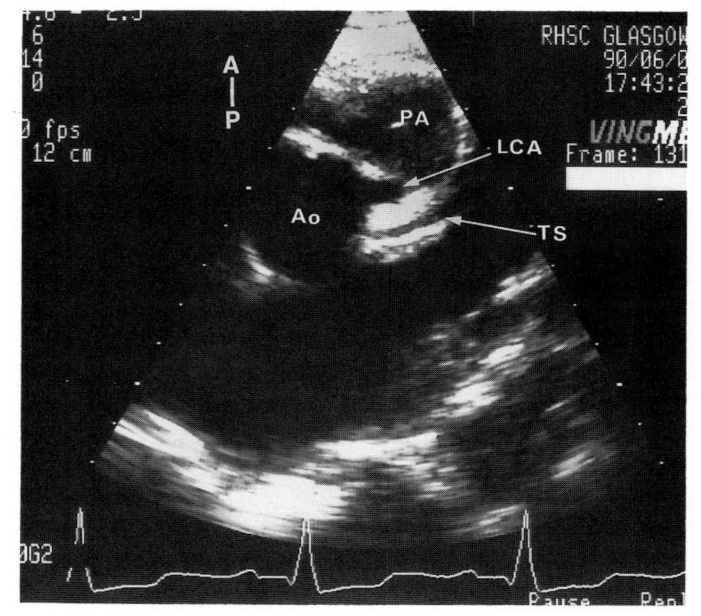

Fig. 2 Short axis view just above the aortic valve demonstrating the normal left coronary artery (LCA) arising from the aortic root. The transverse sinus (TS) lies posterior to the left coronary artery.

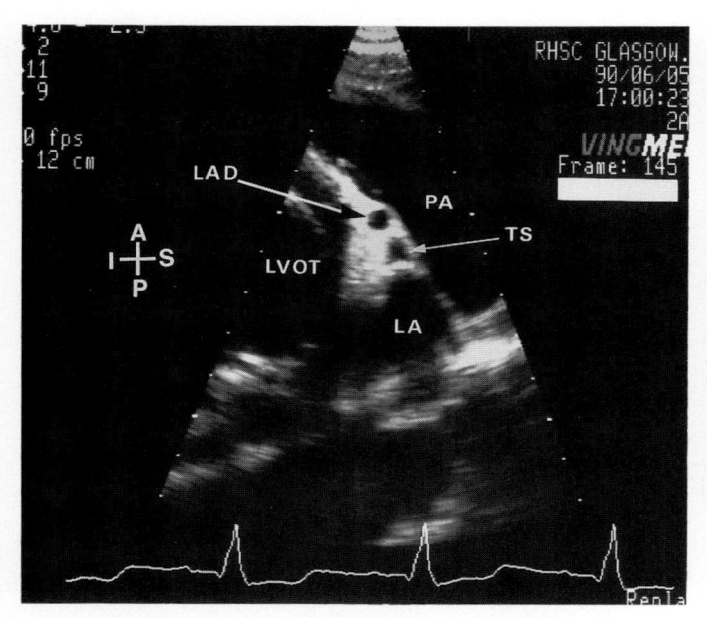

Fig. 3 Modified short axis view showing the left anterior descending coronary artery (LAD) as a circular structure behind the pulmonary artery and just anterior to the left ventricular outflow tract (LVOT) and left atrium. The transverse sinus (TS) lies posterior to the coronary artery.

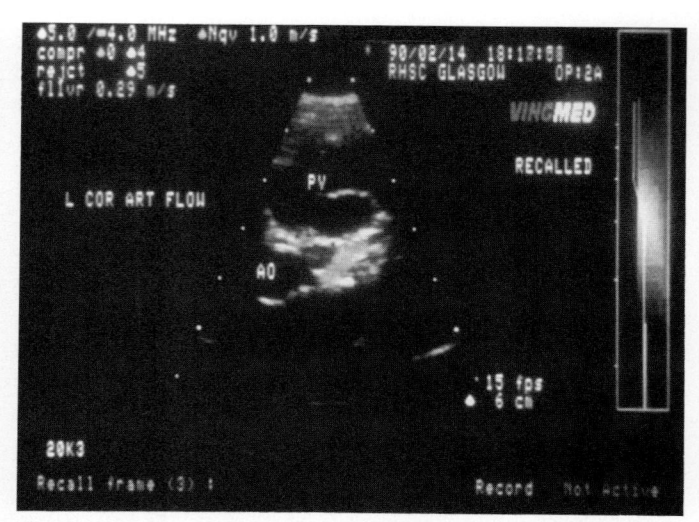

Plate 1 Short axis view showing the aortic root and left coronary artery. Flow in the artery is shown in red, towards the transducer. This figure is reproduced in colour in the colour plate section at the front of this volume.

may be misinterpreted as the left coronary artery.[6] Careful study should ensure that this mistake is not made; the transverse sinus appears to pass directly laterally behind the pulmonary artery while the left coronary and its continuation as the anterior descending artery follow an anterior and leftward course behind the pulmonary artery before turning anteriorly and to the left. Where there is uncertainty it is useful to turn the transducer through 90° to a plane showing both the mitral and pulmonary valves simultaneously; this should demonstrate that the structure has a circular shape confirming that it is a vessel (Fig. 3).[7] Colour Doppler flow mapping can be of use in ensuring that the left main coronary artery and its continuation have been correctly identified; flow within the lumen of the vessel will be shown passing from aorta in a distal (anterior) direction (i.e. red) (Plate 1). This blood flow may be of relatively low velocity and at an angle to the beam and therefore its demonstration may require that the colour algorithm is adjusted to show flow with a low mean velocity.

The width of the normal left main coronary artery at its widest diameter (as leading edge to leading edge measurement) has been measured as 4.4 ± 0.9 mm in adults.[8] Studies on children show both left and right proximal coronary arteries to be about the same size with a small but progressive increase in size with increasing age. From the ostia to 1 cm distally there is little alteration in the diameter of the vessels which have been reported as being 2 to 4 mm in infants increasing to 3 to 5 mm in teenagers.[9]

Left anterior descending artery

The continuation of the left main coronary artery as the proximal left anterior descending artery, coursing to the left of the main pulmonary artery and then anteriorly, is usually apparent in the modified short axis view. A cross-sectional view of the more distal continuation of this vessel may on occasion be traced inferiorly in a standard left parasternal short axis view. Alternatively it may be possible to show it in longitudinal section in a modified parasternal long axis view, often from the third left interspace with the transducer angled 10 to 30° superiorly and laterally towards the pulmonary artery and then rotated slightly (about 10°) clockwise.

Left circumflex coronary artery

Good quality images of the circumflex coronary artery are seldom obtained although the very proximal part may be shown to arise from the left main coronary artery (Fig. 4) by slightly modifying the view described above, often by slight anticlockwise rotation and superior angulation. The more distal part of the circumflex coronary artery may be seen in the left atrioventricular groove just lateral to the mitral valve in an apical four chamber view.

Right coronary artery

The proximal right coronary artery can be shown to arise from the right coronary cusp from a short axis view of the aortic valve by superior angulation and slight clockwise[5] or anticlockwise[10] rotation. The orifice is usually seen in a position from 11 to 1 o'clock (Figs 5 and 6). The more

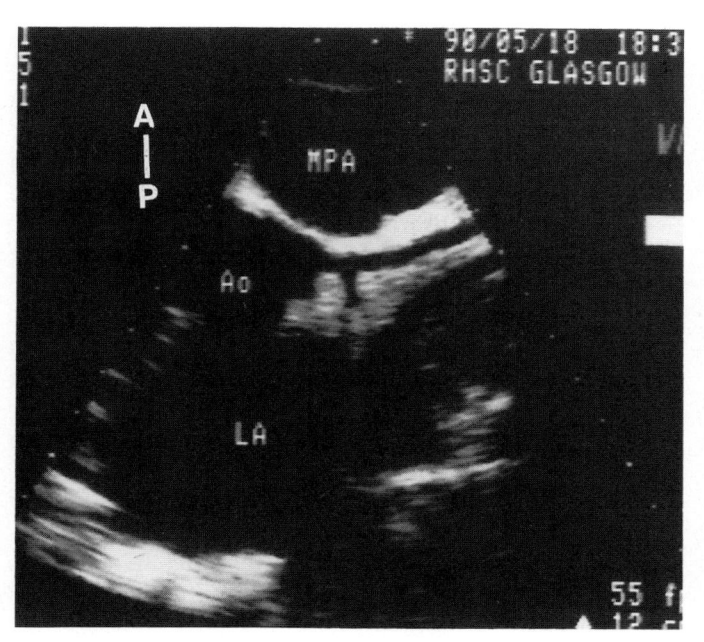

Fig. 4 Modification of the view shown in Fig. 2 to demonstrate the circumflex coronary artery arising from the left main coronary artery before it gives rise to the left anterior descending branch. MPA – main pulmonary artery.

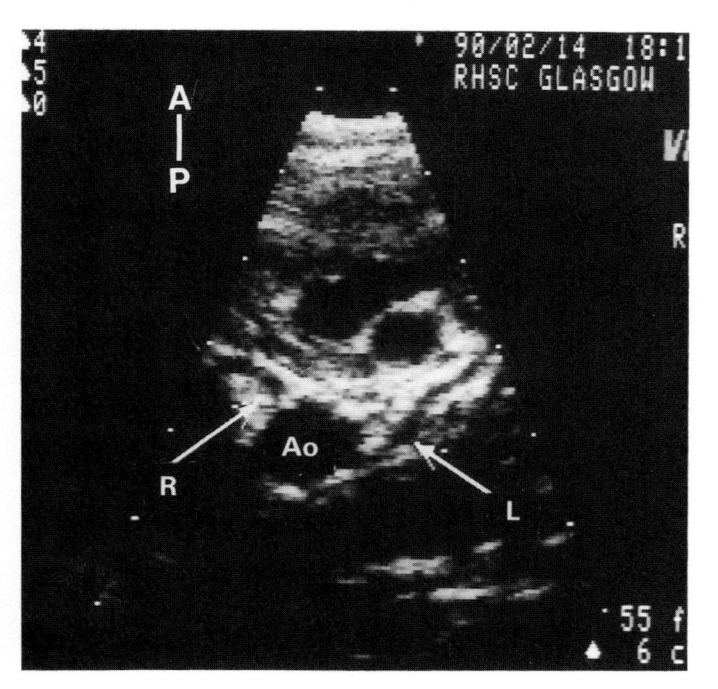

Fig. 5 Short axis view adjusted to show the right coronary artery (**R**) and the left coronary artery (L) arising from the aorta.

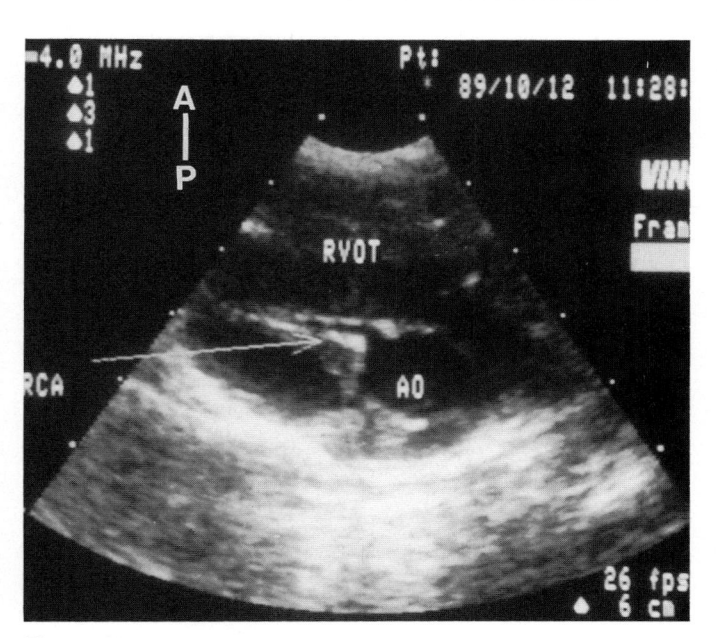

Fig. 6 Short axis view showing the origin of the right coronary artery (**RCA**). RVOT – right ventricular outflow tract.

distal parts of the right coronary artery are more easily shown from a subxiphoid or apical four chamber view with slight clockwise rotation and posterior angulation of the transducer. It is not common to obtain good images of both coronary arteries in a single view.

Part of the proximal right vessel in the right anterior atrioventricular groove and distal vessel in the posterior atrioventricular groove can be shown in relation to the upper and lower parts of the tricuspid ring if, from a long axis view, the plane is tilted rightward with some clockwise rotation to show the area next to the tricuspid ring.[4] A similar view of the proximal third of the right coronary artery is obtained from a short axis view of the great arteries by adjusting it to show the aortic and tricuspid leaflets then tilting it superiorly till the tricuspid leaflets are lost.[9] A dilated part of the distal right coronary artery may be shown in cross-section just lateral to the tricuspid valve in an apical four chamber view.[4,11]

The peripheral portion of the right coronary artery can be seen in longitudinal section in the posterior atrioventricular groove by tilting a subxiphoid or apical four chamber view posteriorly to show the tissue just posterior to the tricuspid valve ring (Fig. 7).

An artefact similar to that of the transverse sinus, but to the right side of the aorta, has been reported in patients with dilated cardiomyopathy and marked left atrial enlargement where a tubular structure apparently arising from the aorta at about 8 o'clock has been found. It was suggested that it might be due to displacement of the atrial septum with anterior and superior bowing bringing it into juxtaposition to the Eustachian valve and producing an apparent tubular structure.[12]

Practical difficulties in imaging coronary arteries

Full demonstration of these coronary vessels can be dif-

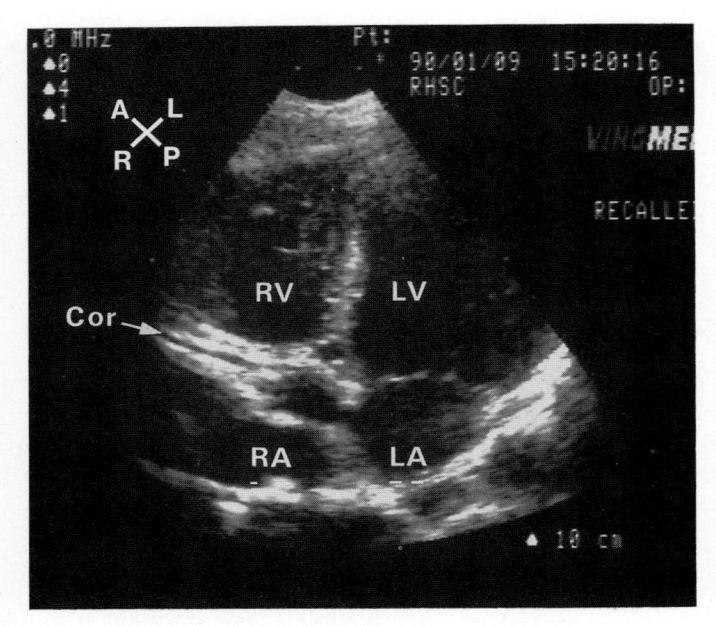

Fig. 7 Modification of a four chamber view to show the distal extension of the right coronary artery (Cor) posterior to the tricuspid valve ring.

ficult and is often not achieved. The only detailed reported study of attempted full assessment of coronary artery anatomy in adults contains only 35 patients.[5] This study reported that the proximal left main, left anterior descending and right coronary arteries could be visualised in over 80% of the adult patients studied and concurs with a previous one of imaging the left main coronary artery[8] in which it was demonstrated in 80% of 100 subjects with angina. The bifurcation of the left main coronary artery and thus the proximal circumflex coronary artery (Fig. 4) is less frequently apparent and was shown in only about one third of subjects. In routine clinical studies it is to be expected that satisfactory images will be obtained less frequently.

As with other echocardiographic studies there is no uniform approach to imaging the coronary arteries and different views may show better images of the same structure in different subjects. In addition different positions of the patient, such as left or right lateral decubitus, may be useful. It should be borne in mind that when a coronary artery is dilated it is more likely that it will be possible to identify the affected segment with ultrasound.

CORONARY ARTERY DISEASE

Echocardiography is not an accepted technique for the demonstration of coronary artery obstruction in ischaemic heart disease. Although there are some reports that it is sometimes possible to show lesions in the left main coronary artery,[1,8] and descending or right coronary artery[5] echocardiography is not a reliable screening technique for left main coronary artery stenosis. In addition to the difficulty in deciding that apparent narrowing is not due to alteration in the vessel orientation as it moves to a position outside the scanning plane, there is also the potential for false positive diagnosis with apparently dense echoes within a normal lumen being misinterpreted as an arteriosclerotic plaque.[8] It is doubtful if improved ultrasonic resolution or colour Doppler flow mapping will markedly improve the accuracy and thus clinical value of trans-thoracic echocardiography.

Transoesophageal echocardiography provides a much clearer image of the left main coronary artery than can be achieved from a trans-thoracic site. The left main coronary artery can be shown in most subjects, the circumflex in about half, and the anterior descending in about 15%.[13] The anterior descending artery can be followed inferiorly but when using a transducer with a single transverse scanning plane it is shown in cross-section and its course is only appreciated by studying a large number of frames as the transducer is moved more inferiorly towards the stomach. This is of limited value but the introduction of transducers which can image in a longitudinal or variable plane have the potential to improve the clinical usefulness of this in the future. However with the present systems stenosis of the left main and circumflex coronary arteries can be seen in some patients[13] and the clinical value of this will become apparent as further studies are undertaken.

Variation in the distribution of the coronary arteries

The coronary arteries in hearts which are normal or nearly normal usually have a normal origin and distribution. There can be minor anatomical variations which are usually of no clinical importance. An aberrant coronary artery passing between the aorta and right ventricular outflow tract may be of significance if it is compressed between

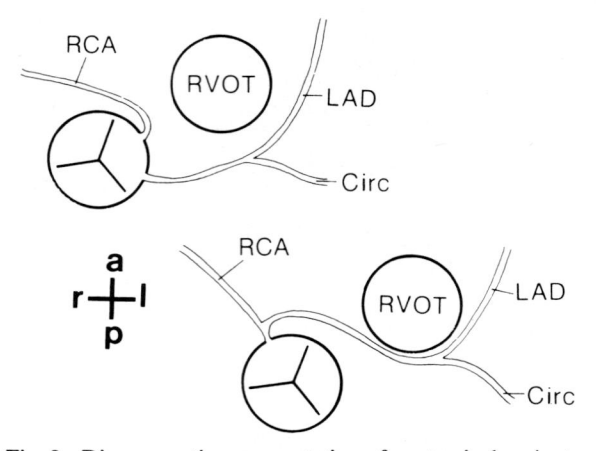

Fig. 8 Diagrammatic representation of anatomical variants which may cause coronary compression between the aorta and the pulmonary artery. RCA – right coronary artery, LAD – left anterior descending artery, Circ – circumflex artery.

them with resultant sudden death (usually with proximal left coronary artery stenosis), syncope or angina.[14] The common anatomical arrangements in which this may occur are illustrated in Figure 8. Thus in young subjects with symptoms of cardiac ischaemia echocardiographic examination for an abnormal coronary vessel between the great arteries is worthwhile, though reports of the clinical value of this are still awaited.

Variations in the coronary artery distribution occur in some congenital heart defects. In most congenital lesions knowledge of such a variation is unnecessary for the surgeon. In infants and young children the distribution will usually be visible through the visceral pericardium on inspection at surgery, but this is not possible in older subjects where they can be buried in fat. Prior knowledge of abnormalities which may demand modification of the proposed surgical procedure is useful to the surgeon before thoracotomy is undertaken. This is important in tetralogy of Fallot, where the presence of a major vessel crossing in front of the right ventricular outflow tract would prevent a standard operation with a right ventricular outflow tract patch. In patients with transposition of the great arteries undergoing an arterial switch procedure the coronary arteries can be reimplanted in virtually all situations, but if the surgeon wishes information before surgery echocardiographic demonstration of this may decrease the requirement for catheterisation and aortic root angiography.

Transposition of the great arteries

In subjects with transposition of the great arteries the anatomy of the coronary arteries is extremely variable.[15,16] Performance and interpretation of ultrasound studies of the coronary arteries in transposition of the great arteries is facilitated by knowledge of the more common variations in the coronary artery anatomy, illustrated in Figure 9.

Most commonly the left and right coronary arteries arise from the left and right posterior sinuses (Figs 10 and 11); the left divides into the anterior descending artery, which courses anteriorly, and the circumflex coronary artery, which passes in front of the main pulmonary artery before turning posteriorly to its left.

Echocardiographic views similar to those for imaging the coronary arteries in the normal heart should be used and have been described in detail.[17] The coronary artery origins are usually shown in a short axis view of the aortic root, but the right may be better shown in a modified long axis view through it. If the bifurcation of the left main coronary artery is not shown in this view a parasternal long axis view may be used and tilted leftward; the left main coronary artery may appear as a circle and further leftward angulation may show its bifurcation into the left anterior descending artery and circumflex arteries. The origin of the left circumflex coronary artery from either the left or right coronary artery can be difficult to demonstrate and this may not be shown. In this situation it is important to look

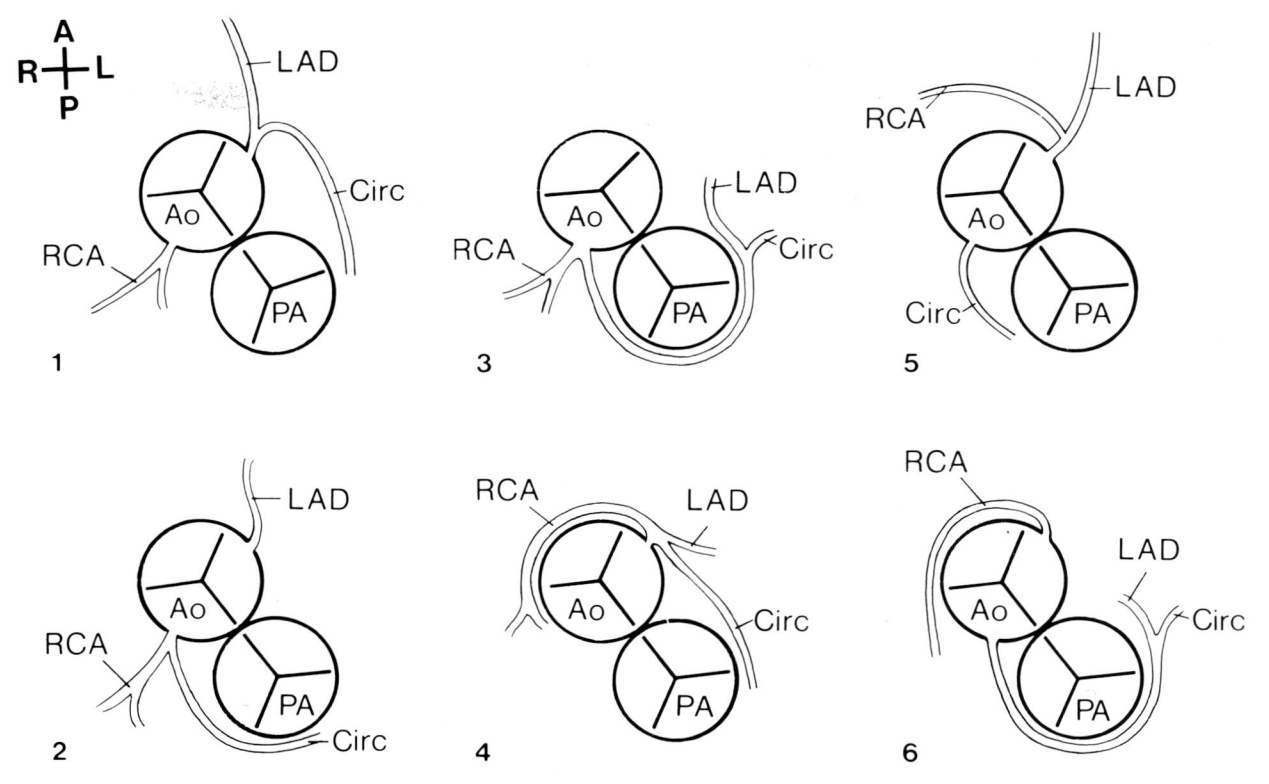

Fig. 9 Diagrammatic representation of the common anatomical variations in the distribution of the coronary arteries in patients with transposition of the great arteries. RCA – right coronary artery, LAD – left anterior descending artery, Circ – circumflex artery.

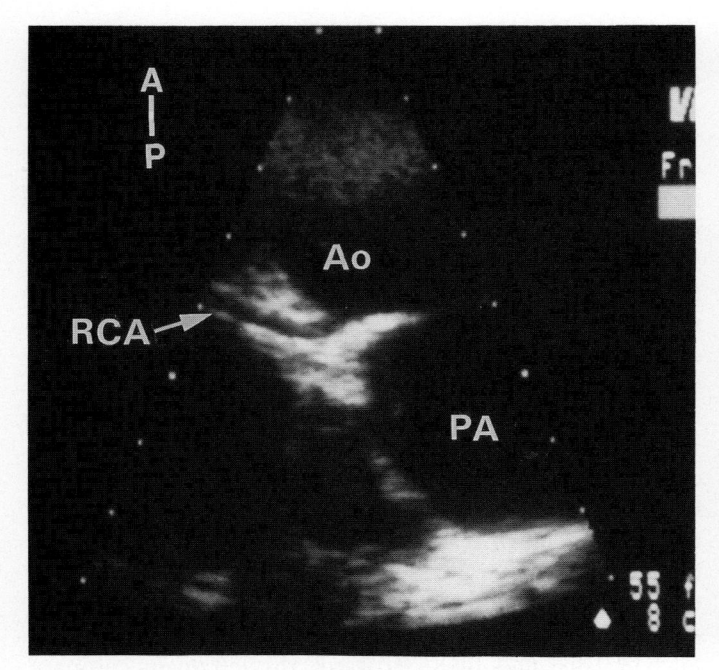

Fig. 10 Short axis view of the great arteries in a case of transposition of the great arteries showing the origin of the right coronary artery (RCA) from the posterior aspect of the aorta.

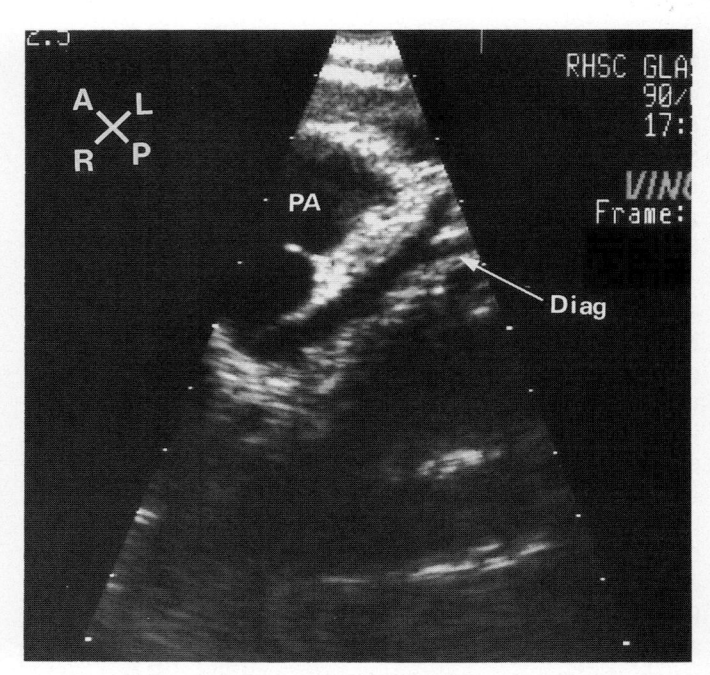

Fig. 12 Modified short axis view showing the acute angle of origin of a normal diagonal branch (Diag) of the anterior descending artery.

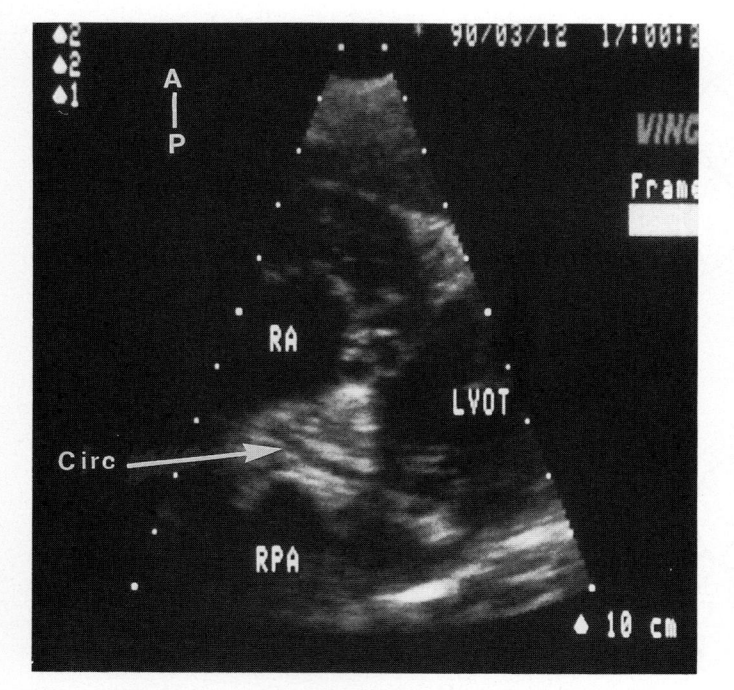

Fig. 11 Modification of a subxyphoid short axis view in a patient with transposition of the great arteries to show an aberrant circumflex coronary artery (Circ) passing anterior to the right pulmonary artery (RPA). LVOT – left ventricular outflow tract.

for the presence or absence of a vessel posterior to the main pulmonary artery; this is often best demonstrated in an apical four chamber or subxiphoid left oblique view. Its presence would support origin of the left circumflex coronary artery from the right coronary artery, and its absence origin from the left. A similar vessel is found where there is a single right coronary artery or inverted origins of the coronary arteries, but it is absent with a single left coronary artery. There is potential for error if a diagonal branch arising from the left anterior descending artery is mistaken for the left circumflex coronary artery. The former comes off at an acute angle (Fig. 12) and runs nearly parallel to the left anterior descending artery while the latter arises at almost right angles to it. With this technique it has proved possible to image the coronary arteries in 90% of infants in a single study with a correct assessment being made in 86% of them.[17]

There are problems inherent in imaging the small coronary arteries in infants where co-operation may be sub-optimal and sedation inadvisable. However with modern high resolution equipment a basic assessment should be possible in most cases, and this should give sufficient information for an arterial switch procedure to be performed without aortic root angiography.

Tetralogy of Fallot

As with transposition of the great arteries the likely anatomical variations should be known (Fig. 13); the left

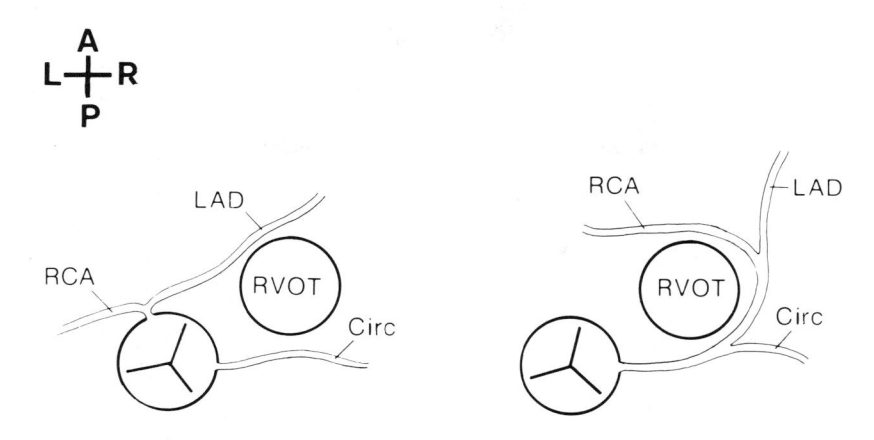

Fig. 13 Diagrammatic representation of the common anatomical variations of the coronary arteries in tetralogy of Fallot. RCA – right coronary artery, LAD – left anterior descending artery, Circ – circumflex artery.

anterior descending artery may arise from the right coronary artery; the right coronary artery may arise from the left anterior descending artery; there may be a normal left coronary artery and left anterior descending artery with a separate right anterior descending artery from the right coronary artery; there may be a large conal branch; the right and left coronary artery may arise together from the left coronary cusp. The clinical importance of imaging the coronary arteries in tetralogy of Fallot is to ensure that the anterior right ventricular outflow tract is not crossed by a major coronary branch which would preclude a right ventricular outflow tract or transannular patch. Thus echocardiographic study of the coronary arteries should be directed at excluding or confirming the presence of such an abnormality.

For practical purposes the most valuable image is that of the right ventricular outflow tract and pulmonary artery to look for any anterior vascular structure (Fig. 14).[7] Such an image is much less easy to obtain where the right ventricular outflow tract and main pulmonary artery are severely hypoplastic. The use of a stand-off medium may be helpful in some cases. Standard views for imaging the coronary arteries can then be used in an attempt to confirm normal distribution of coronary arteries or to determine the origin of an abnormal anterior vessel.

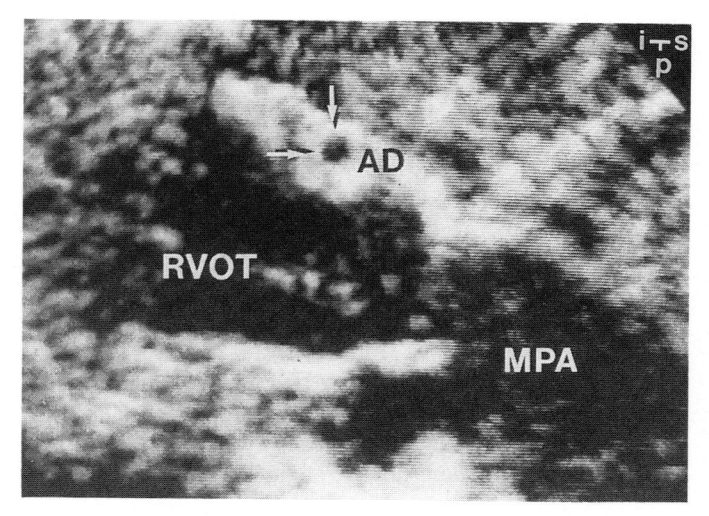

Fig. 14 Short axis view from a patient with tetralogy of Fallot, showing an aberrant anterior descending artery (AD), anterior to the right ventricular outflow tract (RVOT).

Kawasaki disease

The only serious consequence of Kawasaki disease is the development of an aneurysm or stenosis of a coronary artery with the subsequent development of the potentially fatal complication of thrombosis and myocardial infarction. Echocardiography provides a simple, routine means of determining the presence of aneurysms.

The technique for imaging the coronary arteries is similar to that described for normal arteries. Since dilated vessels are more readily demonstrated than normal ones the most detailed report of the technique for imaging the coronary arteries is in relation to its use in the demonstration of aneurysms in Kawasaki disease.[4] Although the distal parts of normal coronary arteries can be difficult to image, dilated aneurysmal areas are more readily recognised and the investigation should include the use of all the views which may show the distal arteries. Echocardiography has proved to be an extremely sensitive means of detecting an aneurysm of the right or left main coronary artery (Figs 15 and 16). It is less reliable in showing an aneurysm in the left anterior descending or circumflex coronary artery, and shows only about half of those positioned more distally.

The majority of coronary artery aneurysms occur in the proximal coronary arteries including the left anterior descending and circumflex, and an isolated distal aneurysm

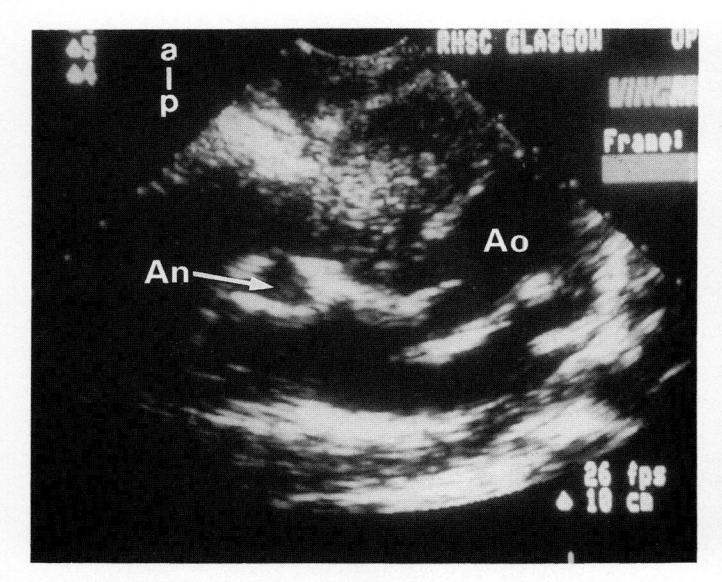

Fig. 15 **Modification of a high parasternal view** showing a dilated aneurysm (An) of the right coronary artery in cross-section.

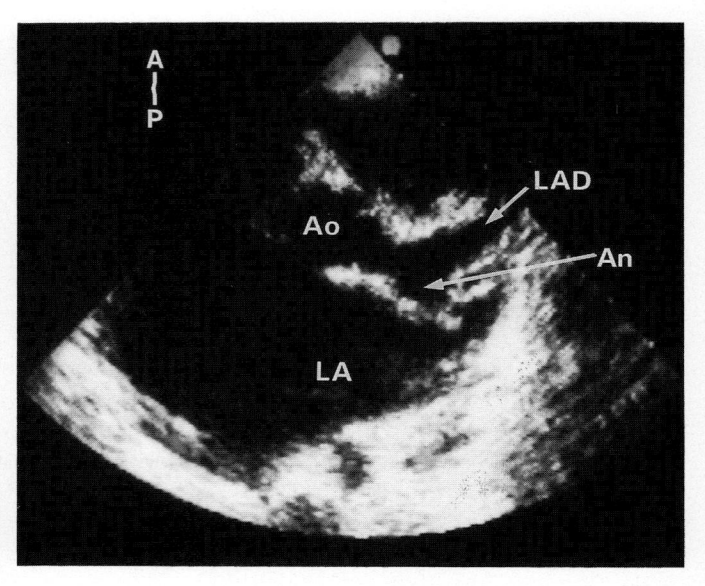

Fig. 16 **Short axis view of the aortic root** in an infant with dilatation and aneurysm (An) of the left anterior descending coronary artery (LAD) and its branches.

rarely occurs.[18] Thus most aneurysms will be demonstrated by echocardiography and in the presence of a normal ultrasound study of the coronary arteries there is a low probability that the patient will have a coronary artery aneurysm.[19] Echocardiography can be used to determine the appropriate treatment and the need for coronary angiography. Even in the presence of an echographically demonstrated aneurysm, angiography may he appropriate to look for distal aneurysms which have been missed and to demonstrate stenotic lesions.

A problem can sometimes arise in deciding if an artery is dilated or in distinguishing a large normal coronary artery from one with a proximal aneurysm. Reported studies indicate that the left and right arteries do not change in calibre in the first 1.0 cm and are of a similar internal dimension which increases from 2 to 4 mm in infants to 3 to 5 mm in teenagers.[9] Other investigations have suggested the internal diameter is normally somewhat less with values of 1 to 2 mm in newborns rising to 2 to 3 mm at 12 years.[20] The ratio of the internal diameter of the coronary artery to aorta can also be used to assess the size: there is no change in this ratio with age, the normal being 0.05 to 0.20 and an aneurysm can be considered to exist when the ratio is 0.3 or more.[21] The morphology of the dilated area is also important: a large normal artery will be of uniform calibre along its length whereas a proximal aneurysm will narrow suddenly or taper gradually depending on the morphology of the aneurysm.

Echocardiography can occasionally show mural thrombi within an aneurysm. Experience is still awaited as to the value of colour Doppler flow mapping in demonstrating areas of abnormal flow and thus stenosis or thrombosis.

Although transoesophageal echocardiography has been used to demonstrate coronary aneurysms in an adult,[22] studies in children are still awaited. It may be that the use of small transoesophageal probes will prove that this can increase the diagnostic ability of echocardiography.

ANOMALOUS ORIGIN OF A CORONARY ARTERY FROM THE PULMONARY TRUNK

Anomalous left coronary artery

Anomalous origin of the left coronary artery from the pulmonary trunk is a relatively uncommon lesion. Patients present either in infancy with heart failure, dilated cardiomyopathy and evidence of cardiac ischaemia, or later in life, with mitral regurgitation or ischaemic symptoms.

The definitive diagnosis of this abnormality requires unequivocal demonstration of the anomalous origin of the left coronary artery but a variety of other echocardiographic features are found and should raise suspicion as to the diagnosis. In the infant with cardiac failure, M-mode or two-dimensional echocardiography will show a large left atrium and a dilated, poorly contracting left ventricle. The hypokinesia of the left ventricle is likely to be asymmetrical with diminished excursion of the posterior wall. In addition M-mode echocardiography has shown characteristic septal motion with abrupt posterior motion soon after the QRS complex on the electrocardiogram, followed by rapid return to its initial position and continued anterior motion throughout the rest of systole.[23] Long or short axis views of the papillary muscles often show that the postero-lateral one, or both, are of increased echo density, presumably the result of ischaemia and fibrosis. Dilation of the proximal part of the right coronary artery was recognised early as an echocardiographic feature.[24] A detailed evaluation of this has suggested that it can be recognised in almost all cases.[20] In the latter study it was found that the ratio of the diameter of the right coronary artery origin to the aorta was greater than 0.2, as opposed to the normal value of 0.05 to 0.20. This feature cannot be used as a single diagnostic criterion since it can also occur in other situations such as right coronary artery fistula or aneurysm. However its presence is strong evidence for the diagnosis in the context of the clinical presentation and a dilated cardiomyopathy.

The coronary artery origins and distal course must be sought since firm echocardiographic diagnosis requires unequivocal demonstration that the left coronary artery arises from the pulmonary artery and not the aorta. Standard views are used to demonstrate the origin of the left coronary artery. Although it is possible to show this vessel in the majority of infants with normal coronary arteries, failure to do so is not sufficient to make the diagnosis since the origin may have been missed. In this context there is potential for error when the ultrasound study is difficult to perform and of suboptimal quality. The incorrect assessment of normal left coronary artery origin may also be reached when a false impression of an echo-free space communicating with the aorta can be obtained. This seems to be due to drop out of echoes along the posterior aortic wall which appears to connect to an echo-free space which has been identified as the transverse sinus of the pericardium lying between the great arteries and the pulmonary and systemic veins. There should be no confusion if the scanning plane is adjusted to provide images of the distal course and demonstrate that this apparent vessel continues as the anterior descending artery. Alternatively the transducer can be rotated through 90° to show the vessel in cross-section or colour Doppler can be used to confirm flow in the vessel.

The anomalous vessel often follows a virtually normal course, but takes origin from the pulmonary artery near the position from which it would usually arise from the aorta. Careful study is then necessary to try unequivocally to ascertain its origin.[25] In this respect colour Doppler examination should be used when available to demonstrate the direction of flow within the artery, with normal connection this being from proximal to distal but within anomalous connection to the pulmonary artery it will be reversed, flowing towards the pulmonary artery. To demonstrate such flow optimally requires the adjustment of the colour algorithm to show low flow velocities and this may necessitate a lower scanning rate with the resulting lower velocity flow appearing as colour and movement artefacts, but nevertheless coronary flow can be picked out from this.

Flow from the anomalous coronary artery into the

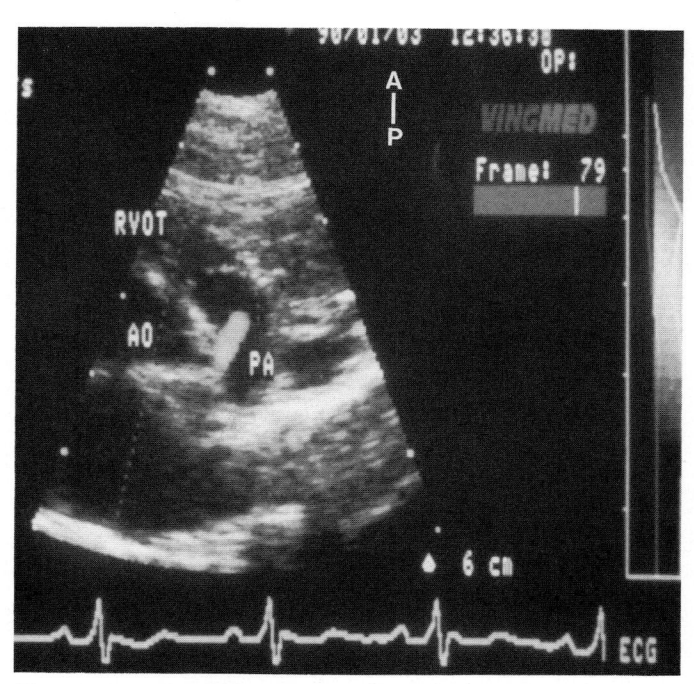

Plate 2 Diastolic short axis view of the great arteries in diastole using colour flow mapping. Flow from the anomalous left coronary artery into the pulmonary artery is clearly shown in red. (RVOT – right ventricular outflow tract). This figure is reproduced in colour in the colour plate section at the front of this volume.

pulmonary artery can be demonstrated with Doppler examination. Although it is theoretically possible to pick up this flow with pulsed Doppler[26] examination it is much more simply performed with colour Doppler which can be used to guide the sample volume if required. The scanning plane with colour Doppler is adjusted to show all parts of the main pulmonary artery and proximal branches. With pulsed Doppler studies the flow can be either systolic or continuous biphasic.[27] Flow from the anomalous vessel into the artery is usually shown,[27-29] most clearly in diastole when other flow signals are not apparent (Plate 2). This allows the left coronary artery orifice to be unequivocally located and the distal part of the vessel may be more clearly followed subsequently. Echocardiographic localisation of the artery is important since the exact point of communication with the pulmonary artery can be difficult to locate even with catheterisation and angiography. Although in most patients the anomalous artery arises from the posterior sinus of the pulmonary trunk this is not always the case and very rarely it will be from the right pulmonary artery.[30] Colour Doppler will clearly show this and allow the appropriate surgical approach. Where colour Doppler flow mapping is not available the site may be localised similarly by the use of contrast echocardiography. Echo contrast from an aortic root injection at catheterisation will pass from the left coronary through the collaterals into the right coronary artery and thence into the pulmonary artery.[31] Flow into the pulmonary artery will not be apparent when the pulmonary artery pressure is high and in one patient seen by the author it was not apparent on the day an 8 week infant presented with severe congestive cardiac failure but it became so the following day when the infant's condition had improved with anti-failure therapy. Another striking feature on colour Doppler examination is the demonstration of prominent flow signals in the septum and ventricular walls, probably in dilated intraseptal and epicardial vessels respectively.[29]

There is some uncertainty as to when such echocardiographic abnormalities become apparent and it seems that the only feature which may be missed is flow into the pulmonary artery when an infant is in severe heart failure with markedly raised pulmonary artery pressure. Collateral flow may also be less easily recognised at this stage.

Rarely there can be origin of the circumflex and right coronary arteries from the aorta with the anterior descending arising directly from the pulmonary artery.[32] Providing the pulmonary artery is studied for abnormal flow it is likely that in this rare situation colour Doppler will show the abnormal flow into the pulmonary artery. It is also to be expected that there will be dilated septal and epicardial vessels but direction of flow in them will be different from that in the patient with classical abnormal origin of the left coronary artery.

A flow signal into the pulmonary artery can be found in normal subjects who have normal origins and distributions of the coronary arteries. This is likely to be due to flow from a small coronary artery to pulmonary artery communication which is only rarely recognised by other means.[33] These show similar colour Doppler signals to those seen in anomalously arising coronary arteries but are difficult to record with spectral Doppler and are not associated with any other clinical, electrocardiographic or echocardiographic abnormalities and thus should simply be considered as normal variants.

Anomalous right coronary artery

Anomalous origin of the right coronary artery is a less frequently recognised entity. Although patients are often asymptomatic reports of cardiorespiratory arrest have led to the acceptance of the need for surgical correction.

Standard views are used to show, where possible, the vessel arising from the pulmonary artery and passing anterior to the aorta.[34] Flow in the vessel is more readily demonstrated using colour Doppler and flow from the ostium into the pulmonary artery has been recognised in a way similar to that found with anomalous left coronary artery.[35]

CORONARY ARTERY FISTULA

A coronary artery fistula usually arises from the right coronary artery and can drain into any of the cardiac chambers or large vessels, most frequently the systemic venous side, and in particular the right ventricle. The connection can be a simple direct one from the coronary artery lumen to the chamber or vessel or through a tortuous dilated communication.

The coronary artery affected becomes dilated and the wide proximal part should be easily shown on standard views.[36,37] In addition the more distal dilated vessel may be shown,[38] but this will depend on its course and size and may be difficult to show. When the left coronary artery is affected the dilated origin is often apparent on the initial long axis view as an echo-free space posterior to the aortic root (Fig. 17).

Spectral Doppler will often show a low velocity continuous signal of flow in the dilated vessel.[39] Thus although imaging and spectral Doppler will help confirm the diagnosis they are of limited value in establishing the site of drainage of the fistula. Colour Doppler can demonstrate flow from the fistula into the receiving chamber and is thus useful in determining the site of communication.[40] Where colour Doppler is not diagnostic or is unavailable contrast echocardiography with injection into the aortic root at catheterisation may also demonstrate the communication and may be more accurate than angiocardiography in making this assessment.

A potential error has been reported in a patient with dilated cardiomyopathy where it was considered that a dilated vessel arose from the aorta at a position of 8 o'clock and seemed, on colour Doppler, to drain into the right atrium. This tubular structure was subsequently considered to be an artefact due to gross left atrial dilation and anterior and superior displacement of the atrial septum with its juxtaposition to the Eustachian valve and the flow signal to be due to flow through the foremen ovale or atrial septal defect.

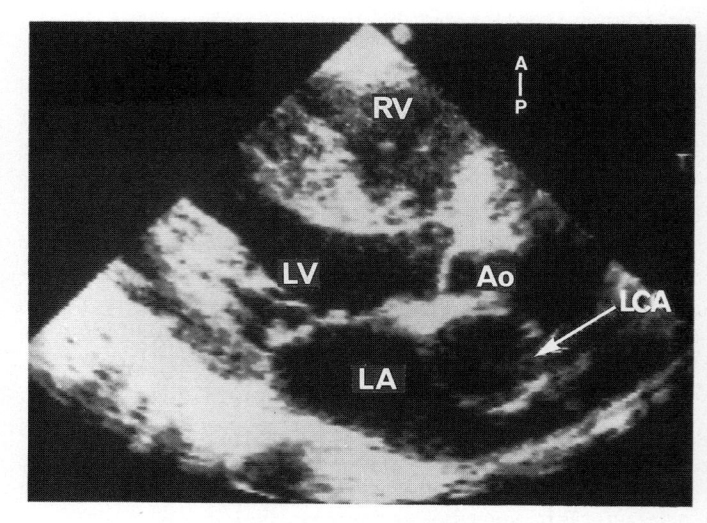

Fig. 17 Parasternal long axis view in a patient with a fistula from the left coronary artery. The very dilated left coronary artery (LCA) is shown as a circular structure posterior to the aortic root.

Stenosis or atresia of the left coronary artery

There are no published results of the application of ultrasound studies in this situation. Imaging echocardiography is unlikely to be diagnostic but a small left coronary artery may be shown and there is likely to be a dilated right coronary artery. Colour Doppler demonstration of increased velocity through a stenotic orifice or retrograde flow where the orifice is atretic may prove to be useful. Unlike anomalous origin of the left coronary artery there will be no flow into the pulmonary artery. In some normal subjects colour Doppler may show small areas of apparently turbulent flow at the edge of the aortic root. They do not seem to be related to ostial obstruction and may be a movement artefact.

REFERENCES

1 Weyman A E, Feigenbaum H, Dillon J C, et al. Noninvasive visualization of the left main coronary artery by cross-sectional echocardiography. Circulation 1976; 54: 169–174
2 Rogers E W, Feigenbaum H, Weyman A E, et al. Evaluation of coronary artery anatomy in vitro by cross-sectional echocardiography. Am J Cardiol 1979; 43: 386
3 Ogawa S, Chen C C, Hubbard F E, et al. A new approach to visualize the left main coronary artery using apical cross-sectional echocardiography. Am J Cardiol 1980; 45: 301–304
4 Satomi G, Nakamura K, Narai S, et al. Systematic visualization of coronary arteries by two-dimensional echocardiography in children and infants: evaluation in Kawasaki's disease and coronary arteriovenous fistulas. Am Heart J 1984; 107: 497–505
5 Douglas P S, Fiolkoski J, Berko B, Reichek N. Echocardiographic visualization of coronary artery anatomy in the adult. J Am Coll Cardiol 1988; 11: 565–571
6 Robinson P J, Sullivan I D, Kumpeng V, et al. Anomalous origin of the left coronary artery from the pulmonary trunk. Potential for false negative diagnosis with cross sectional echocardiography. Br Heart J 1980; 52: 272–277
7 Berry J M, Einzig S, Krabill K A, Bass J L. Evaluation of coronary artery anatomy in patients with tetralogy of Fallot by two-dimensional echocardiography. Circulation 1988; 78: 149–156
8 Vered Z, Katz M, Rath S, et al. Two-dimensional echocardiographic analysis of proximal left main coronary artery in humans. Am Heart J 1986; 112: 972–976
9 Arjunan K, Daniels S R, Meyer R A, et al. Coronary artery caliber in normal children and patients with Kawasaki disease but without aneurysms: an echocardiographic and angiographic study. J Am Coll Cardiol 1986; 8: 1119–1124
10 Oberhoffer R, Lang D, Feilen K. The diameter of coronary arteries in infants and children without heart disease. Eur J Pediatr 1989; 148: 389–399
11 Reeder G S, Tajik A J, Smith H C. Visualization of coronary artery fistula by two-dimensional echocardiography. Mayo Clin Proc 1980; 55: 185–189
12 Kimball T R, Daniels S R, Meyer R A, et al. Colour flow mapping in the diagnosis of coronary artery fistula in the neonate: benefits and limitations. Am Heart J 1989; 117: 968–971
13 Tamms M A, Gussenhoven E J, Cornel J H, et al. Detection of left coronary artery stenosis by transoesophageal echocardiography. Eur Heart J 1988; 9: 1162–1166
14 Liberthson R R, Dinsmore R E, Fallon J T. Aberrant coronary artery origin from the aorta. Report of 18 patients, review of literature and delineation of natural history and management. Circulation 1979; 59: 748–754
15 Elliot L P, Amplatz K, Edwards E. Coronary arterial patterns in transposition complexes. Anatomic and angiocardiographic studies. Am J Cardiol 1966; 17: 362–372
16 Hvass U. Coronary arteries in d-transposition. A necropsy study of reimplantation. Br Heart J 1977; 39: 1234–1238
17 Pasquini L, Sanders S P, Parness I A, Colan S D. Diagnosis of coronary artery anatomy by two-dimensional echocardiography in patients with transposition of the great arteries. Circulation 1987; 75: 557–564
18 Kato H, Ichinose E, Yoshioka F, et al. Fate of coronary aneurysms in Kawasaki disease: serial coronary angiography and long-term follow up study. Am J Cardiol 1982; 49: 1758–1766
19 Capannari T E, Daniels S R, Meyer R A, et al. Sensitivity, specificity and predictive value of two-dimensional echocardiography in detecting coronary artery aneurysms in patients with Kawasaki disease. J Am Coll Cardiol 1986; 73: 55–60
20 Koike K, Musewe N N, Smallhorn J F, Freedom R M. Distinguishing between anomalous origin of the left coronary artery from the pulmonary trunk and dilated cardiomyopathy: role of echocardiographic measurement of the right artery diameter. Br Heart J 1989; 61: 192–197
21 Yanagisawa M, Yano S, Shiraishi K, et al. Coronary aneurysms in Kawasaki disease: follow-up observation by two-dimensional echocardiography. Pediatr Cardiol 1985; 6: 11–16
22 Tunick P A, Slater J, Pasternack P, Kronzon I. Coronary artery aneurysms: a transoesophageal echocardiographic study. Am Heart J 1989; 118: 176–179
23 Shapiro J, Boxer R, Krongrad E. Echocardiography in infants with anomalous origin of the left coronary artery. Pediatr Cardiol 1979; 1: 23
24 Yosikawa J, Owaki T, Kato H, et al. Ultrasonic features of anomalous origin of the left coronary artery from the pulmonary artery. Jpn Heart J 1978; 19: 46–57
25 Fisher E A, Sepehri B, Lendrum B, et al. Two-dimensional echocardiographic visualization of the left coronary artery in anomalous origin of the left coronary artery from the pulmonary artery. Pre- and postoperative studies. Circulation 1981; 63: 698–704
26 King D H, Danford D A, Huhta J C, Gutgesell H P. Noninvasive detection of anomalous origin of the left main coronary artery from the pulmonary trunk by pulsed Doppler echocardiography. Am J Cardiol 1985; 55: 608–609
27 Voksmann G, Mauran P, Rey C, et al. Visualization of anomalous origin of the left main coronary artery from the pulmonary trunk by pulsed Doppler and color Doppler echocardiography. Am Heart J 1988; 116: 181–182
28 Schmidt K G, Cooper M J, Silverman N H, Stanger P. Pulmonary artery origin of the left coronary artery: diagnosis by two-dimensional echocardiography, pulsed Doppler ultrasound and color flow mapping. J Am Coll Cardiol 1988; 11: 396–402
29 Houston A B, Pollock J C S, Doig W B, et al. Anomalous origin of the left coronary artery from the pulmonary trunk; elucidation with colour Doppler flow mapping. Br Heart J 1990; 63: 50–54
30 Hamilton J R L, Mulholland H C, O'Kane H O J. Origin of the left coronary artery from the right pulmonary artery: a report of successful surgery in a 3-month-old child. Ann Thorac Surg 1986; 41: 446–448
31 Martin G R, Cooper M J, Silverman N H, Soifer S J. Contrast echocardiography in the diagnosis of anomalous left coronary artery arising from the pulmonary artery. Pediatr Cardiol 1986; 4: 203–205
32 El Habbal M M, de Laval M, Somerville J. Anomalous origin of the left anterior descending coronary artery from the pulmonary trunk; recognition in life and successful surgical treatment. Br Heart J 1988; 60: 90–92
33 Lee G B, Gobel F L, Lillehei C W, et al. Correction of shunt from right conal artery to pulmonary trunk with relief of symptoms. Circulation 1968; 37: 244–248
34 Worsham C, Sanders S P, Burger B M. Origin of the right coronary artery from the pulmonary trunk: diagnosis by two-dimensional echocardiography. Am J Cardiol 1985; 55: 232–233

35 Shah R M, Nanda N C, Hsuing M C, et al. Identification of anomalous origin of the right coronary artery from pulmonary trunk by Doppler color flow mapping. Am J Cardiol 1986; 57: 366–367
36 Rodgers D M, Wolf N M, Barrett M J, et al. Two-dimension echocardiographic features of coronary arteriovenous fistula. Am Heart J 1982; 104: 872–874
37 Yoshikawa J, Katao H, Yanagihara K, et al. Noninvasive visualization of the dilated main coronary arteries in coronary artery fistulas by cross-sectional echocardiography. Circulation 1982; 65: 600–603
38 Barton C W, Snider A R, Rosenthal A. Two-dimensional and Doppler echocardiographic features of left circumflex coronary artery to right ventricle fistulas: case report and literature review. Pediatr Cardiol 1986; 7: 167–170
39 Miyatake K, Olamoto M, Kinoshita N, et al. Doppler echocardiographic features of coronary arteriovenous fistulas. Complementary roles of cross-sectional echocardiography and the Doppler technique. Br Heart J 1984; 51: 508–518
40 Ke W L, Wang N K, Lin Y M, et al. Right coronary artery fistula into right atrium: diagnosis by color Doppler echocardiography. Am Heart J 1988; 886–889

SECTION 4

Echocardiography in perspective

29

The clinical view

Valvular disease
Ventricular function
Congenital heart disease
Limitations of cross-sectional
echocardiography in congenital heart disease
The contribution of other noninvasive
methods to the diagnosis of congenital heart
disease
Summary

Andrew N. Redington and Derek G. Gibson

A major achievement of the 1940s and 1950s was to introduce and adopt cardiac catheterisation as a diagnostic method. Intracardiac pressures and flows could be measured and valvular stenosis and regurgitation could be assessed for the first time. The presence and nature of ventricular disease could be detected and shunts and pulmonary resistance could be quantified. The accurate diagnosis it provided was one of the foundations of modern cardiac surgery, and it led to the correction of congenital defects and valve lesions, initially by valvotomy, and later, in the early 1960s, by valve replacement. Though the early results of noninvasive investigation were viewed with tolerance and sometimes even with interest, cardiac catheterisation was regarded as the only way in which the 'actual' haemodynamics were determined, allowing the 'correct' diagnosis to be established.

Cardiac catheterisation, however, has disadvantages. It is an expensive investigation compared with noninvasive diagnostic methods and it requires specialised equipment which may be difficult to maintain in less developed countries. It is unpleasant for patients and in the ill it carries an element of risk and measurable mortality. It is also difficult to repeat cardiac catheterisation frequently. There would therefore seem to be advantages in avoiding its use if this can be done without loss of diagnostic accuracy. Ten years ago, it had already become apparent that a combination of clinical findings and M-mode echocardiography could be used to give an accurate preoperative diagnosis[1-3] in most patients with valvular heart disease. It was suggested that it was possible to dispense with cardiac catheterisation in at least two thirds of such patients. When this was put to the test, no unexpected lesions were encountered at surgery and postoperative survival was not affected. Operative mortality was lower in a subgroup of seriously ill patients when catheterisation was avoided.[1] Since then, two dimensional and Doppler methods have become widely available which further enhance the capabilities of noninvasive methods. At the same time, with the rise in interventional cardiology, interest in purely diagnostic cardiac catheterisation has waned. Cardiac output, when measured at all, is usually estimated by thermodilution rather than by the 'gold standard' of the direct Fick method. Valve areas are seldom calculated and the effect of exercise is frequently not documented.

Invasive and noninvasive methods may disagree because they do not measure the same thing. Doppler techniques, for example, detect the peak pressure difference across the aortic valve, which bears no constant relation to the 'peak to peak' values obtained by catheter pull-back at cardiac catheterisation. Had Doppler echocardiography appeared before catheterisation, it would probably be taught that the so-called 'peak to peak' gradient has no existence, since the two peaks occur at different times; such values could not thus be relevant to determining possible effects of the valve lesion on the pattern of ejection or the development of left ventricular disease. The only reason for the opposite point of view still being viable is that cardiac catheterisation preceded Doppler as a method of measuring pressure differences, so that clinical experience is based on peak to peak rather than peak gradients.

Angiographic methods of assessing valvular regurgitation are semiquantitative at best, poorly reproducible, and are without any clearly defined physical or physiological basis. Nevertheless, they, rather than regurgitant fraction or any other defined index of regurgitation, are used as the basis for decision making. It is therefore against this rather unsatisfactory background that the relative place of noninvasive methods, and in particular those based on ultrasound, must be compared with cardiac catheterisation.

VALVULAR DISEASE

Echocardiography is now the major means of investigating valvular heart disease, whatever its severity or type, whether right or left sided. Valve anatomy can be studied in detail. This implies the ring, the cusps, the chordae and the papillary muscles for the atrioventricular valves, and the cusps, the ring and the adjoining regions, both below and above the valve for the semilunar valves. This is a major advance on information obtainable at cardiac catheterisation. On the right side of the heart, doming on cross-sectional echocardiography is undoubtedly the method of choice in detecting organic tricuspid valve disease, which was frequently missed invasively unless it was suspected clinically. On both sides of the heart, vegetations can be detected. Cusp thickening, fibrosis, retraction, and their associated disturbances of motion are clearly seen and documented. The mitral subvalve apparatus cannot be imaged by angiography, yet chordal rupture is a major cause of acquired valve disease, particularly in populations in whom the incidence of rheumatic disease is low. The information is of practical importance since patients with rupture of the posterior mitral chordae do particularly well with repair rather than replacement and have correspondingly improved long-term survival.

Continuous wave Doppler examination has proved remarkably successful in the detection and quantitation of valvular stenosis.[4,5] The simplified Bernoulli equation is at least as satisfactory for detecting mitral gradients as the comparison of simultaneous pulmonary artery wedge to left ventricular pressures: indeed, in our experience, a value derived from a satisfactory Doppler record can only be overturned by simultaneous left atrial and left ventricular pressures. Unfortunately, it may be difficult to record adequate signals from valves inserted into conduits on the anterior surface of the heart, which are difficult of access from both the transthoracic and transoesophageal approaches. Limitations of the Bernoulli equation itself may give rise to problems. The equation is frequently and inappropriately used in the absence of obstruction to describe flow across normally functioning prostheses or even across the normal mitral valve. In general, high velocities proximal to obstructions do not usually cause difficulty, though errors do occur with a long narrowed segment or with obstruction at two sites anatomically close together, such as the right or left ventricular outflow tract. As with cardiac catheterisation, a pressure drop must be combined with a flow estimate to derive a valve area; either alone may be misleading in assessing stenosis.

It is much more difficult to assess the severity of regurgitation than stenosis.[6] In part, this is because the problem has not been as clearly defined. All modes of Doppler examination are very sensitive in detecting regurgitation, even across otherwise normal valves. The problem is to assess the significance of the leak, which is not necessarily the same thing as its severity measured in absolute terms or as regurgitant fraction. A small stoke volume regurgitating into a noncompliant chamber can cause a striking pressure rise which leads to pulmonary oedema when it occurs on the left side of the heart or fluid retention when it occurs on the right side. Interrelations between regurgitation and ventricular disease are poorly understood. Finally, regurgitation may be secondary to a destructive lesion whose mere presence may be an indication for surgery, as with a failing xenograft or aortic valve regurgitation due to dissection of the aortic wall.

The rise and fall of colour Doppler in quantifying regurgitation has been instructive, demonstrating that the superficial similarity of the new method to angiography was misleading.[7,8] Disagreement between the two techniques could only be resolved when mechanisms of image generation were more fully understood. Colour Doppler examination thus contrasts with magnetic resonance imaging whose flow images are based much more directly on bulk motion of liquid rather than pressure differences. Simpler methods have stood the test of time. Significant regurgitation is likely to be accompanied by a large ventricular stroke volume. Very severe regurgitation is associated with equalisation or near equalisation of pressure across the valve towards the end of the period over which regurgitant flow occurs, while effective absence of the valve is associated with laminar flow across it. High ventricular end-diastolic pressures can often be estimated indirectly from isovolumic relaxation time or apexcardiography. The simple criterion of premature mitral closure on the M-mode examination remains an invaluable indication for recommending early surgery in acute aortic regurgitation.

Echocardiographic methods have proved particularly satisfactory in studying patients who have undergone valve surgery. Valve anatomy can be clearly documented after repair and for those in whom the valve has been replaced, ventricular function, a major determinant of postoperative survival, can be studied in detail. Malfunction, regurgitation or stenosis can be detected, and additional valve disease or deteriorating ventricular function can be clearly documented for clinical deterioration. Perivalvular abscess, multiple sites of regurgitation or abnormal shunts can be identified using the transoesophageal route. Echocardiography thus provides a practical method of following up these patients much more satisfactorily than would ever be possible invasively or by the use of other currently available noninvasive imaging methods.

VENTRICULAR FUNCTION

The detection and analysis of abnormal left ventricular function has been a second field where methods based on echocardiography have had a major clinical impact. Left ventricular cavity size and shape can be determined by cross sectional echocardiography and image quality is high enough in the majority of patients to allow regional abnormalities in the amplitude of motion to be localised by simple inspection, even if they cannot adequately be analysed quantitatively. The clinical implications of these relatively simple methods have been very considerable. The extent to which left ventricular function is impaired determines prognosis, operative risk, and functional status in many common forms of heart disease, particularly those associated with valve or coronary artery disease.

It is usually possible to determine the nature of the underlying disturbance in most cases that are diagnosed clinically as 'heart failure'. Left ventricular wall thickness can be measured, and the anatomy and function of the septum can be studied in a way that is virtually impossible using contrast angiography. The high repetition rate of M-mode examination makes it possible to detect rates of wall motion, and thus study disturbances of early diastolic function for the first time. The latter are common, particularly in hypertrophy and coronary artery disease. These results have subsequently been reproduced by nuclear and contrast angiography and more recently by Doppler examination.[9,10] Methods based on E/A ratio have been used particularly widely since they are felt to be simple to record, in contrast to the M-mode, which is now considered by some to be technically more difficult. All these methods confirm the presence of abnormalities of ventricular function during diastole in a number of different types of heart disease. Exact interrelations between the information provided by these different approaches has been less carefully considered and discrepancies are coming to light which may undermine some of the rather simplistic ideas about ventricular function in the current literature.

Other recent developments have included increasing experience with echocardiographic tissue characterisation, the myocardium being particularly suitable for such studies.[11] In the clinical field, semiquantitative estimates of myocardial echo amplitude or total backscatter can be made. These values are characteristically increased with fibrosis or oedema of the myocardium, while loss or blunting of the normal phasic variation during the cardiac cycle appears to be nonspecific evidence of disease.

Echo-Doppler methods have proved particularly fruitful in the evaluation of hypertrophic cardiomyopathy. M-mode techniques demonstrate the extent of the hypertrophy and disturbances of mitral and aortic valve motion. Cross-sectional studies enable variation in the anatomy between cases to be documented, and Doppler examination permits the extent and localisation of gradients as well as atrioventricular regurgitation to be evaluated. Other methods have confirmed this information, often at much greater cost for each individual study, but have added little to it.

In patients with coronary artery disease, nuclear cardiology has a major role. Blood pool scanning gives information similar to cross-sectional echocardiography in measuring ejection fraction and in detecting regional disturbances in wall motion and abnormalities of diastole. Exercise studies appear to be easier than with echocardiography. A major advantage of nuclear cardiography follows from the digitisation of the results which allows objective analysis of wall motion by regional ejection fraction and phase mapping. This contrasts with subjective methods used by echocardiographers, and their relative lack of interest in disturbances of timing rather than amplitude of motion. At present echocardiography cannot compete with thallium scanning in displaying myocardial perfusion. The likely development of new and improved radionuclides suggests that this advantage will persist in the future, although myocardial contrast imaging has shown promise in experimental animals.

In acute myocardial infarction, the balance of advantage in determining the extent to which the function of the left ventricle is affected seems to lie with echocardiography. Early screening of wall motion gives an excellent impression of the severity of involvement and thus of prognosis; aneurysm formation can be detected by echocardiography or blood pool scanning, but for pseudoaneurysm, acquired ventricular septal defect, and mitral regurgitation, echo-Doppler methods are superior.

Echo-Doppler methods should thus be regarded as the primary means of studying left ventricular function and its modification by drugs or surgery. Nuclear methods are of value in the special setting of coronary artery disease. Magnetic resonance imaging allows ventricular anatomy to be delineated in rather more detail than echocardiography and avoids problems of integrating different cuts. Neither allows rapid and repeated screening of ventricular function, nor do they have the frequency response that allows wall motion to be documented in detail.

Further specific applications of echocardiography are well known. It remains the investigation of first choice for detecting and quantifying pericardial effusion and intracardiac masses. Transoesphageal echocardiography has proved extremely effective in visualising the thoracic aorta and thus in diagnosing the site and extent of dissection. Its potential in surgery and intensive care is only now being explored.

CONGENITAL HEART DISEASE

There can be no doubt that diagnostic cross sectional echocardiography has been the most important single advance in paediatric cardiology since the introduction of prostaglandins to maintain duct patency in neonates with duct-dependent systemic or pulmonary blood flow. So dramatic has been its influence that one might question the place of more conventional diagnostic techniques. The images obtained in children of 10 kg or less are generally outstanding in their clarity. Indeed, it is possible to establish a full sequential diagnosis in most neonates using cross sectional echocardiography alone,[12,13] describing the abdominal and atrial situs,[14] the type and mode of atrioventricular and ventriculoarterial connections,[15,16] as well as demonstrating the detailed anatomy or any associated intracardiac anomalies.

All neonates referred with a diagnosis of possible complex congenital heart disease require a detailed cross sectional echocardiogram and for most the decision to perform palliative or corrective surgery is based on the echocardiogram alone, without cardiac catheterisation. It could be argued that even the electrocardiogram and chest radiograph are largely redundant in these circumstances though as screening tests they are often useful and their value as 'baseline' data for later comparison cannot be underestimated.

The role of cardiac catheterisation is even less certain. The two palliative procedures most commonly required in young children are banding of the pulmonary artery, usually performed when there is complex congenital heart disease and unrestricted pulmonary blood flow, and systemic to pulmonary shunting (modified Blalock–Taussig shunt), performed when pulmonary blood flow is reduced. Cardiac catheterisation is rarely required before these procedures in the neonatal period. The patient with pulmonary atresia and intact septum is an exception since there is commonly an abnormal coronary artery supply, with right ventricular to coronary artery sinusoids, anomalous origin of one or other coronary from the pulmonary artery, or occasionally right ventricular dependent coronary circulation. These patients would normally undergo a systemic to pulmonary shunt procedure with either pulmonary valvotomy or right ventricular outflow tract patching to decompress the right ventricle. Decompressing the right ventricle when there is a right ventricular dependent coronary blood flow would clearly be disastrous. So while the cross-sectional echocardiogram will demonstrate the intracardiac anatomy and pulmonary artery size adequately, the details of coronary artery supply, with very few exceptions, can only be demonstrated adequately by angiography.

Corrective surgery can also be performed in most neonates and infants without the need for cardiac catheterisation. Coarctation of the aorta, interrupted aortic arch, common arterial trunk, transposition of the great arteries, double outlet right ventricle with subaortic or subpulmonary ventricular septal defect and atrioventricular septal defect are examples of complex lesions which are routinely corrected without prior cardiac catheterisation.[17-20] Intuitively, the benefits of avoiding an invasive procedure in a critically ill neonate are obvious, although these are difficult to demonstrate objectively. An example where these benefits are amply demonstrated, however, is seen in the group of patients with totally anomalous pulmonary venous drainage.[21] These patients, particularly when they present in the first few days of life with obstructed pulmonary venous return, are often in extremely poor condition before surgical correction. Cardiac catheterisation can only worsen the situation. In our series of 83 patients the overall mortality from cardiac catheterisation was 14%. There were no deaths amongst the last 28 patients in this series, in whom the full sequential diagnosis had been established by echocardiography alone, cardiac catheterisation being performed in only 4. Indeed, using multivariate analysis, the use of echocardiography alone was the only significant factor shown to improve survival in these patients.

Limitations of cross-sectional echocardiography in congenital heart disease

Cross-sectional echocardiography is an exquisitely operator- and equipment-dependent technique. Published results on the high diagnostic specificity of cross-sectional echocardiography in demonstrating abnormalities of coronary artery anatomy in tetralogy of Fallot, for instance,[22] are of no immediate relevance to the inexperienced operator or to those limited by the performance of their equipment. Recognising one's own limitations is the key to a sensible approach to noninvasive diagnosis. There can be no place for avoiding cardiac catheterisation in a situation where to do so would be an admission of personal failure, or failure of the noninvasive study.

Cardiac catheterisation will be required whenever there is uncertainty or disagreement between clinical signs and the echocardiogram. It is here that other techniques most often play an important role. Thus if a ventricular septal defect looks small on the cross-sectional echocardiogram yet the patient is failing to thrive, with florid pulmonary oedema and cardiomegaly on the chest radiograph, further investigations are required. It may be that repeat echocardiogram will demonstrate a previously unrecognised aortopulmonary window, for example, but if not, cardiac catheterisation is mandatory.

There are more specific areas where cross sectional echocardiography cannot provide all the answers. We have already alluded to the problem of demonstrating the precise anatomy of the coronary arteries. A much more commonly encountered area of uncertainty concerns the pulmonary vascular tree. The size and anatomy of the main, right and left pulmonary arteries can usually be demonstrated adequately in neonates. In older children, particularly after palliative surgery, cross-sectional echocardiography lacks the precision required to plan surgical management. Most children who have undergone pulmonary artery banding or systemic to pulmonary artery shunt procedures will require cardiac catheterisation and angiography before surgical correction to evaluate pulmonary artery anatomy.

The functional characteristics of the pulmonary vascular bed, that is the pulmonary vascular resistance and its response to therapeutic intervention is another noninvasive 'blind spot'. The decision to catheterise is usually based on a clinical suspicion of a raised pulmonary vascular resistance (the power of the stethoscope in determining the intensity of the pulmonary component of the second sound, which in turn reflects pulmonary diastolic pressure, cannot be underestimated). Noninvasive clues to the presence or absence of pulmonary vascular disease may be obtained by Doppler examination but the final arbiter in terms of assessing pulmonary vascular resistance must remain the measurement made at catheterisation.

The contribution of other noninvasive methods to the diagnosis of congenital heart disease

Pulsed and continuous wave Doppler techniques have become part of the routine assessment of the patient with congenital heart disease. As in adult cardiology, it is not usually necessary to catheterise in order to measure valve gradients. Furthermore, paediatric cardiologists routinely use Doppler techniques to assess the haemodynamic consequences of other pathologies. The literature is replete with studies demonstrating the accuracy of the modified Bernoulli equation in determining the pressure drop across ventricular septal defects,[23] the arterial duct,[24] and systemic to pulmonary shunts.[25] What is not clear from these studies is the extent to which the information obtained from these methods truly adds to our assessment of the patients. The clinician does not need a Doppler measurement to confirm the presence of a restrictive ventricular septal defect in an asymptomatic patient with a loud pansystolic murmur, a normal pulmonary component of the second sound and a normal electrocardiogram, and is thus unlikely to act on any Doppler measurement which erroneously suggests a nonrestrictive defect in such a patient.

One can raise the same caveat regarding the use of colour-flow mapping. There can be no doubt that in some circumstances, colour-flow mapping will allow normal and abnormal flow patterns within the heart to be identified rapidly. Small ventricular septal defects, the small arterial duct, and atrial septal defects will all 'light up' dramatically with colour-flow imaging. But does the technique really add to our diagnostic sensitivity? We have all discovered small additional muscular defects which surely would have been missed otherwise, but these are rarely of any clinical significance. The discovery of additional major defects is clearly much more important,[26] but whether the technique is specific and sensitive enough to justify abandoning ventriculography in patients with multiple defects remains to be determined.

Magnetic resonance imaging is the newest of the noninvasive imaging techniques. Its ability to produce dramatic images of the heart and great vessels is unquestioned, but its place in the routine assessment of patients is not. Cross-sectional echocardiography is at its weakest in the adolescent and young adult with complex congenital heart disease. It is here that magnetic resonance is strongest. Magnetic resonance imaging will provide details of the atrioventricular junction, ventricular outlets, and great vessels which cannot be obtained in any other way.[27] Its place in the younger child is uncertain, however. Even if real-time magnetic resonance imaging becomes available, it is uncertain if it will replace cross-sectional echocardiography in assessing neonates with complex anomalies. The question as to whether the technique will further reduce the need for cardiac catheterisation in older children is unanswered. However, it is likely that it will be possible to demonstrate the gross anatomy of the pulmonary arteries, for example, in patients with tetralogy of Fallot[28] and so avoid the need for angiography before correction.

The information obtained in neonates and young children with cross-sectional echocardiography is thus unsurpassed. The newer techniques such as Doppler examination with colour-flow mapping and magnetic resonance imaging may well be useful adjuncts but only rarely contribute to clinical decision making when high quality cross-sectional echocardiographic images are obtained.

Thus, echocardiography cannot reproduce all the results of invasive investigation. Pressures cannot be measured directly. From time to time unexplained discrepancies occur between cardiac catheter and Doppler and in this setting, for the present time, invasive measurement must remain the standard. Though proximal coronary arteries can often be imaged by 2-D echocardiography, there is no prospect of replacing the coronary arteriogram yet by any noninvasive method. Echocardiography remains poor in detecting extracardiac masses, and in delineating pericardial anatomy in the absence of effusion. It also has the major disadvantage of image quality being subject to thoracic deformity, lung disease, and obesity. In such cases, the transoesophageal route can, of course, be used, though this requires a higher threshold for performing the investigation. Fortunately, magnetic resonance imaging has been shown to demonstrate pericardial disease and other extracardiac abnormalities very clearly.

SUMMARY

There are thus many qualities which have contributed to the widespread use of echocardiography both in paediatric and adult patients. Clearly, its ability to give diagnostic images of intracardiac structures in the large majority of patients is a major one, but certainly not the only attribute of the method which has led to its being so generally accepted. Other techniques such as magnetic resonance imaging, high speed computerised tomography or even angiography may give superior ones, particularly in selected groups of patients, while some areas, such as myocardial perfusion or coronary artery anatomy are effectively inaccessible to it. Rather, the wide appeal of echocardiograpy seems to depend on a series of additional qualities which make it particularly attractive in the 'least squares fit' environment of clinical medicine. Unlike ionising radiation, diagnostic ultrasound can be considered safe. Any danger from echocardiography comes from misleading information: an underestimated aortic gradient, an erroneously diagnosed pericardial effusion or inappropriate use of the Bernoulli equation in children with high-flow lesions. Like cardiac catheterisation, the technique strikingly combines anatomy with physiology, but at much faster sampling rates of up to 1000 cycles per second. Transthoracic echocardiography can be performed rapidly, informally, and repeatedly, lending itself to follow-up studies, and its use in seriously ill patients without the risk of the haemodynamic deterioration associated with angiography. At the other end of the scale, its safety means that its indications need not be as clearly defined as for more expensive or hazardous methods, giving it an additional quality of serendipity in its use. Even the moderate increase in formality associated with the transoesophageal route loses these qualities.

Finally, the echocardiographic examination is frequently undertaken by the clinician caring for the case. This implies a much closer relation to the clinical process than one where the patient is simply referred to a department of imaging with a 'request'. Indeed, it is perhaps this last, our possession of a powerful imaging and physiological tool which can be assimilated into clinical work, and which becomes, effectively, an extension of the stethoscope, that epitomises the appeal of echocardiography. Using it, we manage our patients better, refine our clinical judgement, and extend our knowledge of the fascinating patterns of disturbed anatomy and physiology seen in disease. We must, however, always be careful to use it skillfully, objectively and in the context of other available techniques.

REFERENCES

1. St John Sutton M G, St John Sutton M, Oldershaw P, Sacchetti R, Paneth M, Lennox S C, Gibson R V, Gibson D G. Valve replacement without cardiac catheterisation. N Engl J Med 1981; 305: 1233–1238.
2. Hall R J C, Kadushi O A, Evemy K. Need for cardiac catheterisation in assessment of patients for valve surgery. Br Heart J 1983; 49: 268–275.
3. Alpert J S, Sloss L J, Cohn P F, Grossman W. The diagnostic accuracy of combined clinical and noninvasive evaluation: comparison with findings at cardiac catheterisation. Cath Cardiovasc Diag 1980; 6: 359–370.
4. Hatle L, Brubakk A, Tromsdal A, Angelsen B. Noninvasive assessment of pressure drop in mitral stenosis by Doppler ultrasound. Br Heart J 1978; 40: 131–140.
5. Hatle L, Angelsen B A, Tromsdal A. Noninvasive assessment of aortic stenosis by Doppler ultrasound. Br Heart J 1980; 43: 284–292.
6. Lopez J F, Hanson S, Orchard R C, Tan L. Quantification of mitral valvular incompetence. Cath Cardiovasc Diagn 1985; 11: 139–152.
7. Adhar G C, Nanda N C. Doppler Echocardiography, Part II. Adult valvular heart disease. Echocardiogr 1984; 1: 219–241.
8. Miyatake K, Izumi S, Okamoto M. Semiquantitative grading of severity of mitral regurgitation by real-time two-dimensional Doppler flow imaging technique. J Am Coll Cardiol 1986; 7: 82–88.
9. Nishimura R A, Housmans P R, Hatle L K, Tajik A J. Assessment of diastolic function of the heart: background and current applications of Doppler echocardiography. Part I. Mayo Clin Proc 1989; 64: 71–81.
10. Nishimura R A, Abel M D, Hatle L K, Tajik A J. Assessment of diastolic function of the heart: background and current applications of Doppler echocardiography. Part II. Clinical Studies. Mayo Clin Proc 1989; 64: 181–204.
11. Miller J G, Perez J E, Sobel B E. Ultrasonic characterisation of myocardium. Progr Cardiovasc Dis 1985; 28: 85–110.
12. Shinebourne E A, Macartney F J, Anderson R H. Sequential chamber localisation — logical approach in diagnosis in congenital heart disease. Br Heart J 1976; 38: 327–340.
13. Rigby M L, Redington A N. Cross sectional echocardiography. Br Med Bull 1989; 45: 1036–1060.
14. Huhta J C, Smallhorn J F, Macartney F J. Cross sectional echocardiographic diagnosis of situs. Br Heart J 1982; 48: 97–108.
15. Berman F Z, Williams R G. Prospective diagnosis of d-transposition of the great arteries in neonates by subxiphoid, two dimensional echocardiography. Circulation 1979; 60: 1496–1502.
16. Disessa T G, Hagan A D, Pope C, Samtoy L, Friedman W F. Two dimensional echocardiographic characteristics of double outlet right ventricle. Am J Cardiol 1979; 44: 1146–1154.
17. Stark J, Smallhorn J, Huhta J et al. Surgery for heart defects diagnosed with real time echocardiography. Circulation 1982; 66: 11–30.
18. Huhta J C, Glasow P, Murphy D J et al. Surgery without catheterisation for congenital heart defects: management of 100 patients. J Am Coll Cardiol 1987; 9: 823–829.
19. Silverman N H, Zuberbuhler J R, Anderson R H. Atrioventricular septal defects — cross sectional echocardiographic and morphologic comparisons. Int J Cardiol 1986; 13: 309–332.
20. Smallhorn J F, Anderson R H, Macartney F J. Cross sectional echocardiographic recognition of interruption of the aortic arch between left carotid and subclavian arteries. Br Heart J 1982; 48: 229–235.
21. Lincoln C R, Rigby M L, Mercanti C, Al-Faigih M, Joseph M C, Miller G A, Shinebourne E A. Surgical risk factors in total anomalous pulmonary venous connexion. Am J Cardiol 1988; 61: 608–611.
22. Jureidini S B, Appleton R S, Nouri S, Crawford C J. Detection of coronary artery abnormalities in tetralogy of Fallot by two dimensional echocardiography. J Am Coll Cardiol 1989; 14: 960–967.
23. Marx G R, Allan H D, Goldberg S J. Doppler echocardiographic estimation of systolic pulmonary artery pressure in pediatric patients with interventricular communications. J Am Coll Cardiol 1985; 6: 1132–1137.
24. Musawe N N, Smallhorn J F, Benson L N, Burows P E, Freedom R M. Validation of Doppler-derived pulmonary artery pressure in patients with ductus arteriosus under different hemodynamic states. Circulation 1987; 76: 1081–1091.
25. Marx G R, Allen H D, Goldberg S J. Doppler echocardiographic estimation of systemic pulmonary artery pressure in patients with aortico-pulmonary shunts. J Am Coll Cardiol 1986; 7: 880–885.
26. Sutherland G R, Smyllie J H, Ogilvie B C, Keeton B R. Colour flow imaging in the diagnosis of multiple ventricular septal defects. Br Heart J 1989; 62: 43–49.
27. Smith M A, Baker E J, Ayton V T, Parsons J M, Ladusans E J, Maisey M N. Magnetic resonance imaging of the infant heart at 1.5T. Br J Radiol 1989; 62: 327–370.
28. Hayes A N, Parsons J M, Baker E J et al. Evaluation of the pulmonary arteries in right heart obstruction (abstract). Br Heart J 1990; 64: 94

30

Recent advances

Developments in conventional ultrasound modalities
Imaging resolution
Analysis of left ventricular function
Colour flow mapping
Developments in transoesophageal echocardiography
Intraoperative echocardiography

Stress echocardiography
Exercise echocardiography
Atrial pacing and echocardiography
Pharmacological stress echocardiography
Doppler studies during stress
Contrast echocardiography
Ultrasonic tissue characterisation

Intravascular ultrasound
Intravascular Doppler
Intravascular ultrasonic imaging
Intracardiac ultrasound
Three dimensional reconstruction
Therapeutic applications of ultrasound
Conclusion

Robert L. Parry and Alan G. Fraser

INTRODUCTION

The range and scope of ultrasonic investigations in cardiology are expanding rapidly. It is difficult to keep up to date with all developments and so any account of new techniques and of new applications of old ones is likely to be selective. Nevertheless, we shall try to review the major fields of current enquiry or development, while concentrating on those which appear to have major clinical relevance.

Most cardiovascular diagnoses can now be evaluated by echocardiography. Analysis is becoming less qualitative and subjective and more accurate and reproducible. Quantitative measurement of cardiac function is an integral part of a full echocardiographic examination, complementing the visual recognition of abnormal morphology, and enhancing the diagnostic value of the study. A modern, fully-equipped echocardiographic laboratory should thus have facilities for reviewing, analysing and quantifying images stored on videotape.

The full range of techniques in cardiovascular ultrasound includes transoesophageal, intraoperative, intravascular, and even intracardiac imaging, in addition to established precordial methods. These have blurred traditional distinctions between invasive and non-invasive investigations for assessing cardiac structure and function. If an invasive test is one which carries some risk to the patient, however small, then transoesophageal echocardiography becomes invasive, and intravascular ultrasound is certainly so. These developments are forcing clinicians to re-examine the diagnostic value and accuracy of all techniques, whether 'invasive' or 'non-invasive'.

It is recognised that in certain circumstances, cardiac catheterisation is no longer the 'gold standard'. Direct comparisons of data from catheterisation and angiography with those obtained from ultrasound studies are difficult, because in many instances the techniques measure different things. Obviously, the choice of investigation in a patient with heart disease should be the most appropriate for the suspected diagnosis. If that choice is an echocardiographic study, then as much care, attention and expertise should be applied to its execution and interpretation, as would be expected in a complex invasive study. This is essential when important clinical decisions, such as whether or not to refer a patient for surgery, are taken on the basis of echocardiographic data.

Since echocardiographic studies are only as good as the echocardiographer, who should do them? Recent guidelines on educational requirements in the USA[1] suggested minimum levels of training and proposed that when non-medical personnel perform echocardiography, an appropriately trained doctor should be available at all times. As equipment becomes more easy to use, it is tempting for inexperienced operators to believe that they are competent simply because they can obtain reasonable cross-sectional images. Inappropriate conclusions may be made, and serious disease may be missed. It is also possible that 'non-disease' may be diagnosed when minor variations from normal are detected by a very sensitive technique. These dangers should be recognised, so that the technique is not blamed for what may well be operator error or inexperience. The guidelines also suggest that continuing competence in echocardiography should be assessed by peer group review within the hospital, or by a qualified expert from outside the hospital. To satisfy these requirements and use cardiac ultrasound to its full potential, it is necessary to keep abreast of technological developments and new applications.

DEVELOPMENTS IN CONVENTIONAL ULTRASOUND MODALITIES

Imaging resolution

The resolution of cross-sectional echocardiography has been improved by increasing the number of elements in phased array transducers (now up to 128), and by using electronic methods to focus the ultrasonic beam. The scope for further improvements in the lateral resolution of images produced by phased array transducers is limited, because increasing the dimensions of transducers to allow more elements to be incorporated would make them too large for most precordial echocardiographic windows. Axial resolution is enhanced by using higher-frequency transducers but in many adults these are impractical because the associated loss of penetration means that distant structures cannot be imaged. Thus, lower frequencies will still be used and this will continue to limit axial resolution, for example to 1 mm for a 3 MHz transducer.

The frame rate of cross-sectional imaging is limited by the pulse repetition frequency, which in turn depends on the depth of the field and the width of the sector which are being examined. There is always a compromise between these features, and also the scan line density. Optimising any one parameter causes an unavoidable reduction in the others. The temporal resolution of cardiac events is always greatest with M-mode echocardiography, because of its much faster sampling rate. This simple technique remains an integral part of ultrasonic studies, especially when accurate measurements of valve motion, myocardial function, wall thickness or chamber dimensions are required.

With conventional scanning, the transmission of a second ultrasound pulse cannot occur until the first pulse has returned from the deepest structure being examined. It is possible, however, to transmit several pulses in different directions simultaneously, and to process the returning echoes in parallel using independent receivers. This obviates the necessity to wait for the first pulse to return before transmitting a second one. One system allows the insonation of the complete plane of imaging with a single echo pulse which is transmitted in all directions.[2] It can be used to increase the pulse repetition frequency and give a faster frame rate. However, this system has not been incorporated into a commercially available machine.

Analysis of left ventricular function

Detailed echocardiographic assessment of left ventricular function is possible, using either qualitative or quantitative techniques. If precordial images are of poor quality, then transoesophageal echocardiography can be used.

If standard precordial and apical imaging planes are studied, it is recommended that the left ventricle is divided into a total of 16 segments of myocardium.[3] These correspond to regions supplied by all major branches of the coronary arteries. Each segment is assessed qualitatively, to determine if motion is normal, hypokinetic, akinetic, or dyskinetic. A score is assigned to each segment, ranging from 1 for a normally functioning segment to 4 for a dyskinetic segment. When the total score is divided by the number of segments studied, a wall motion score index is obtained. This approach has been used in many studies.[4] After myocardial infarction, the wall motion score index provides a good estimate of left ventricular damage,[5] and it can be used to estimate prognosis.[6]

Left ventricular function can be analysed quantitatively, by digitising cross-sectional echocardiographic images and analysing these with microcomputer programmes. Many different methods have been developed, including estimates of area ejection fraction from cross-sectional images of the short axis of the left ventricle, and also single plane and biplane methods of calculating left ventricular volumes and function from orthogonal apical long-axis images. All these techniques have potential technical difficulties, in part due to movement and rotation of the heart with normal systole and during respiration. To compensate for such movement, the centre of reference may need to be changed when each successive image is analysed. A 'floating centroid' within the left ventricle overcomes many problems but does not eliminate artefacts completely. It is probably best to measure images which are recorded at end-expiration.[7]

One method of analysis which has been developed provides estimates of regional function of the left ventricle, as well as global function (Fig. 1).[8] It has been extensively validated (coefficient of variation for measurements of left ventricular volumes = 8–10%), and it has been used in multicentre pharmacological trials to assess changes in left ventricular function.[9] With appropriate standardisation, it seems likely that these or similar techniques will be used increasingly in the future. Ideally, all echocardiographic laboratories should use comparable methods.

Echocardiographic measurements of left ventricular function are at least as accurate and reproducible as those derived from left ventricular angiograms.[10] The main difficulty using echocardiography is that it is sometimes difficult to define the contour of the left ventricular cavity, if poor or incomplete echoes are obtained from the endocardial surface. In addition, qualitative visual inspection is not sensitive enough to detect temporal dyskinesia, or the early changes in diastolic function which occur during ischaemia and precede the onset of systolic dysfunction. New methods have been developed for computerised detection of the edge of the left ventricular cavity, thus enhancing visual recognition of the endocardium. The first system to be available commercially uses acoustic quantification based on an analysis of backscatter, for automatic detection of boundaries. It displays the endocardial border in real time, and provides an analysis of rate of change of the cross-sectional area of the ventricle.[11] Ultimately, it is hoped that accurate on-line automated detection of contours will be available, so that left ventricular function can be quantitated rapidly and reproducibly, and repeatedly.

Colour flow mapping

The introduction of colour flow mapping was a major advance in echocardiography and it is now an integral part of almost all studies. The images which are produced are often visually very impressive, but they are easily overinterpreted. Since colour flow mapping is a pulsed Doppler technique, aliasing remains a problem. The multiple gating technique employed imposes temporal constraints on the computing power of the ultrasound machine, which has to process all the information returning to the transducer before obtaining the next flow map. The time required to interrogate each scan line limits the scan speed and hence the frame rate. In practice, colour flow maps do not display actual velocities. Instead, a process called autocorrelation is used to compute the change in velocity in each gated sample from one scan to the next, and the flow map displays the difference.[12] Instead of displaying absolute velocities, colour flow maps therefore display changes in mean velocity and superimposed patterns of turbulence. The technique is best used to identify abnormal patterns of flow, which can then be studied in detail with pulsed or continuous wave Doppler.

The initial promise of colour Doppler flow mapping, which was that it would provide accurate quantification of regurgitant volumes, has not yet been fulfilled. Only semiquantitative information has been derived from colour flow jets and their dimensions.[13,14] Other parameters such as the time to maximum jet area have been incorporated in equations which link the Doppler findings to volumetric flow.[15] Improved correlations are obtained, but they are still inadequate for clinical applications. Such attempts are too simplistic, because colour flow maps reflect turbulence rather than flow. The pattern of turbulence is significantly influenced by the size and shape of the orifice, the geometry of the jet, and the haemodynamic conditions in

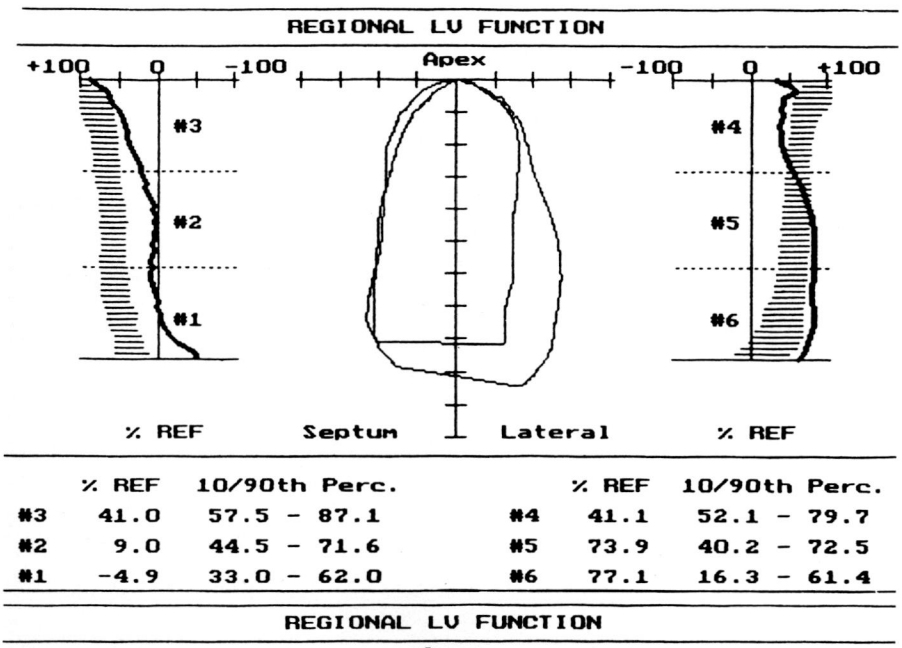

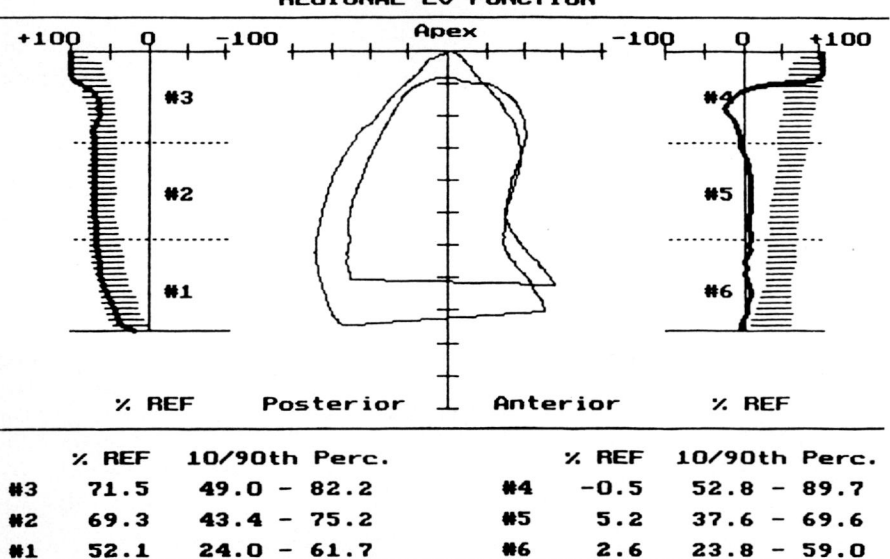

Fig. 1 End systolic and end diastolic contours produced by digitising frames obtained on precordial echocardiography in apical four chamber (above) and long axis (below) planes in a patient with anteroseptal myocardial infarction. The analytic programme divides each side of each contour into 50 divisions and 3 regions. The horizontal bars show normal ranges (10th–90th percentiles) of regional function in 44 normal subjects. The dense black lines demonstrate the measured regional ejection fractions in this patient. There is akinesis of the infarcted septum and anterior wall, mild compensatory hyperkinesis of the basal lateral wall and a normal posterior wall. These digitised images can be used to calculate left ventricular volumes and ejection fraction using a biplane disc method. In this example end diastolic volume is 128 ml, end systolic volume is 82 ml, ejection fraction is 36%, cardiac output is 4.4 l/min and stroke volume is 46 ml. (Courtesy of S. G. van der Borden, Thorax centre, Rotterdam.)

the regurgitant and receiving chambers. A high velocity jet creates lateral eddies around it which amplify the region of turbulence far beyond the central core of the jet. A 'freestanding' jet within the middle of a cardiac chamber is greatly amplified, whereas an eccentric jet which adheres to the wall of a chamber becomes flattened out over that surface, rather than amplified. It is not surprising, therefore, that areas of turbulence on colour flow maps do not correlate particularly well with volumetric flow.

New methods of assessing flow and regurgitant volumes are being developed. The ability of conventional colour flow maps to display true velocities is limited by the phenomenon of aliasing, as observed also with pulsed Doppler. Aliasing occurs when the velocity being encoded exceeds the Nyquist limit, which is half of the pulse repetition frequency. Tracking along the spatial axis of the real time flow velocity profile allows corrections of the display at harmonic transitions of the Nyquist frequency.[16] Alternatively, a fast Fourier transform analysis can be used to unravel the frequency shifts, thereby allowing ultrasound pulsed Doppler analysis of higher frequency velocities.[17] Systems which 'unwrap' aliasing in this way improve the ability of the echocardiographic machine to display high velocities in an unambiguous way.

Alternative methods of displaying colour flow maps can be used. The power mode display is particularly useful for detecting low velocities of flow, for example in the great veins.[18] It has also been reported that estimates of regurgitant volumes obtained using power mode displays correlate better with 'real' regurgitant volumes, than do estimates which are derived from conventional colour flow maps.[19] Another approach is to analyse the colour flow Doppler data to detect the high velocity central core of a jet.

The sampling rate of colour flow mapping is often rather slow. This makes it difficult, especially in children with rapid heart rates, to time flow events accurately while using a real-time display or while reviewing a cine loop. These difficulties can be overcome by using the colour M-mode display, which is extremely helpful for discriminating between systolic and diastolic events (Plate 1). It is also valuable for timing 'flow events' which are very short in duration, and for improving the spatial resolution of regions of turbulent flow (Plate 2).

An alternative approach has been to ignore the turbulent jet through a valve, and instead analyse the pattern of flow into a stenotic or regurgitant orifice. As flow accelerates into a small orifice, the velocity increases. This is displayed on the colour flow map as lines of aliasing (Plate 3). The distance from the first line of aliasing in this so-called convergence zone, to the orifice, can be measured, and the surface area of a hemisphere at this radius can be calculated. The velocity of flow across this surface is given by the Nyquist limit. If the peak velocity of flow across the orifice is measured, then the continuity equation can be used to calculate the size of the stenotic or regurgitant orifice. This method has also been used to provide estimates of regurgitant volume[20] and is also known as the proximal isovelocity surface area (PISA) method.

Yet another method of quantitating blood flow within the heart has been developed, which dispenses with colour

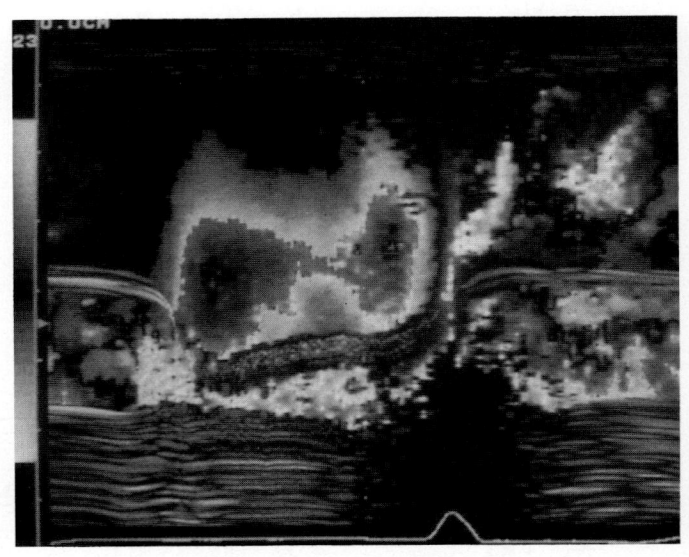

Plate 2 Colour M-mode recording obtained during a trans-oesophageal study showing flow events within the left atrium (upper part of trace) and left ventricular outflow tract (lower part of trace). During diastole there is aortic regurgitation which occupied almost the whole width of the outflow tract at this level. In systole the colour M-mode confirms that there is mitral regurgitation and shows its duration and depth. This figure is reproduced in colour in the colour plate section at the front of this volume.

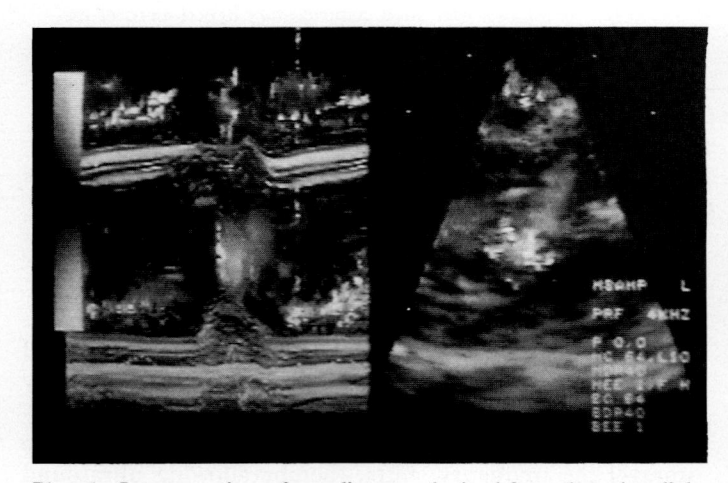

Plate 1 Intraoperative echocardiogram obtained from the epicardial approach after bypass in a child who had undergone repair of a ventricular septal defect. On colour flow mapping in real time (right panel) turbulence was visible within the right ventricle. This was interpreted as systolic turbulence, possibly indicating a residual ventricular septal defect. The colour M-mode recording (left panel) however, demonstrates that the turbulence within the right ventricle is mostly diastolic and therefore due to turbulent inflow over the ventricular septal patch rather than to a residual defect. This figure is reproduced in colour in the colour plate section at the front of this volume.

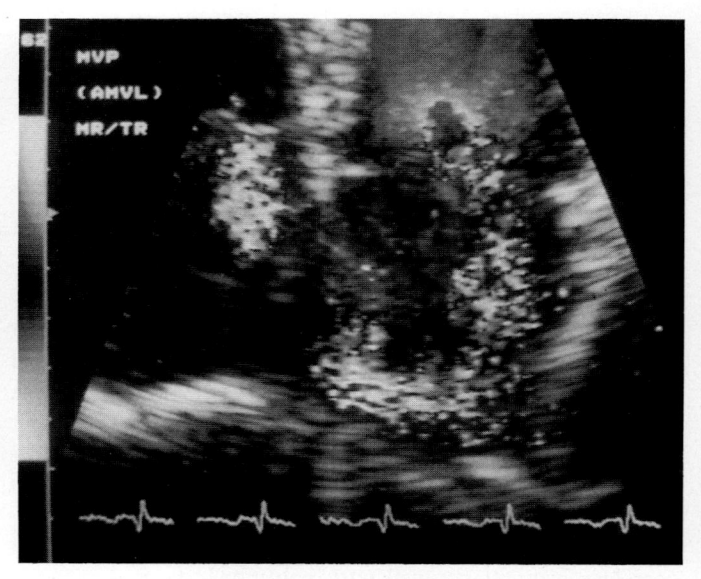

Plate 3 Apical four chamber view obtained from the precordium. There is a central mitral regurgitant jet directed into the middle of the left atrium and then around the posterior wall. The convergence zone within the left ventricle (of blood accelerating into the regurgitant orifice) is clearly demonstrated. This patient also has some tricuspid regurgitation. This figure is reproduced in colour in the colour plate section at the front of this volume.

flow mapping altogether. Direct echocardiographic imaging of the red blood cells is possible if very high gain is used. Red cells tend to act as groups of cells, or 'ensembles', when reflecting the ultrasonic beam and these echoes can be visualised directly. Red cell 'tracking' in this manner eliminates the problem of aliasing which afflicts measurements obtained with pulsed Doppler techniques. Early work suggests that this may be a feasible method for cardiac studies in the future;[21] at present, however, such 'colour velocity imaging' is being used for non-cardiac applications.

DEVELOPMENTS IN TRANSOESOPHAGEAL ECHOCARDIOGRAPHY

Within less than ten years, transoesophageal echocardiography has developed into an essential part of the ultrasonic armamentarium.[22] This process was accelerated by the incorporation of colour flow mapping into oesophageal transducers. Recently, facilities for continuous wave Doppler have been added by some manufacturers.

Basic transoesophageal probes consist of a single transducer which is mounted to produce images which are orientated in transverse planes to the shaft of the probe. This limitation has proved to be relatively unimportant, as transoesophageal echocardiography has become established as the investigative technique of choice in many important clinical circumstances, such as suspected aortic dissection,[23] infective endocarditis,[24] or assessment of prosthetic valve function (Plate 4).[25] Nevertheless, there are regions of the heart and great vessels such as the right ventricular outflow tract and the upper ascending aorta, which are relatively inaccessible to imaging in transverse planes. There are also structures such as the mitral and tricuspid valves which are difficult to assess fully in three dimensions, without being able to display structure and flow in multiple planes.[26] To overcome these problems and extend the capacity of transoesophageal echocardiographic systems, biplane probes have been developed. These incorporate a second transducer which is orientated to image in longitudinal planes, orthogonal to conventional transverse ones.

Several accounts of the anatomical basis of longitudinal imaging have been published.[27,28] These have confirmed that biplane transoesophageal echocardiography has considerable theoretical advantages over imaging in the transverse axis alone. Structures which are demonstrated more clearly with the longitudinal transducer include the superior vena cava, the flap of the oval fossa (helpful when trying to assess patency of the oval foramen), the lateral aspect of the tricuspid valve, the medial aspect of the mitral valve and its subvalvar apparatus (Fig. 2), the right ventricular outflow tract and pulmonary trunk (Figs 3 and 4), the upper ascending aorta, and the apical, inferior and anterior segments of the left ventricular myocardium (Fig. 5). The quality of images obtained with biplane

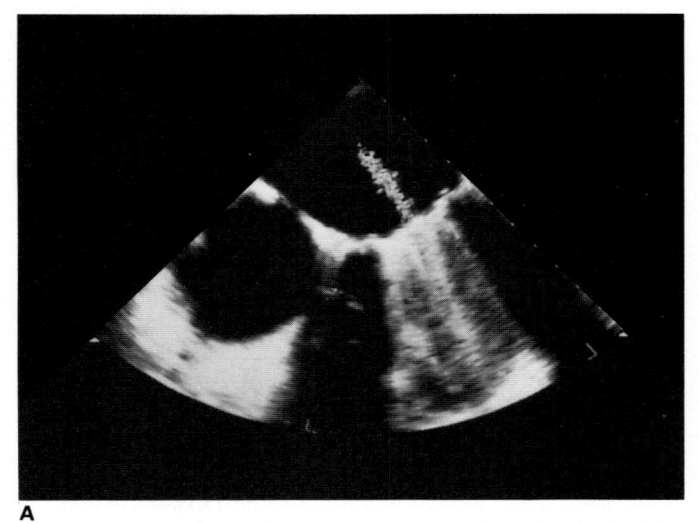

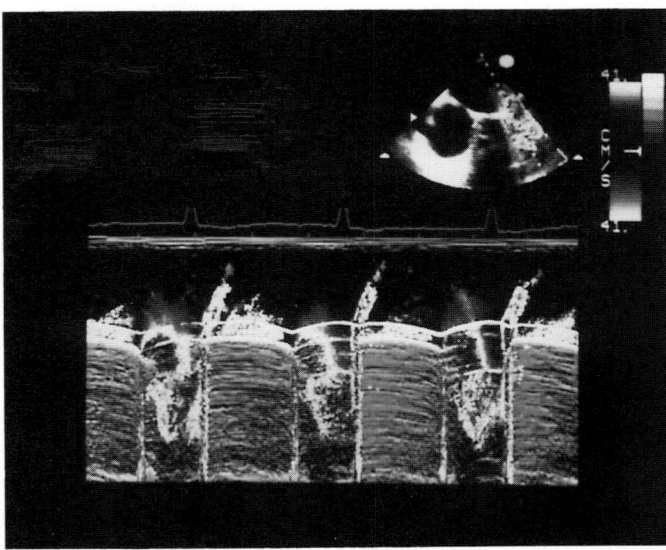

Plate 4 A: Trans-oesophageal cross-sectional image and colour flow map and B: colour M-mode recording of a normally functioning Medtronic Hall tilting disc mitral prosthesis. There is a long jet of mitral regurgitation in the left atrium but it is present only at the start of systole and is therefore a normal closure jet. The colour M-mode recording also shows mild persistent regurgitation adjacent to the valve ring during the remainder of systole. This is also a normal phenomenon for this valve. This figure is reproduced in colour in the colour plate section at the front of this volume.

probes improved rapidly so that they are already standard equipment in many centres. Initial clinical reports have demonstrated that biplane transoesophageal echocardiography has greater sensitivity than single plane transoesophageal echocardiography for detecting paraprosthetic leaks around prosthetic mitral valves.[29] It also allows eccentric regurgitant jets to be mapped in orthogonal planes (Plate 5). Biplane transoesophageal echocardiography has also been used for sizing atrial septal defects,

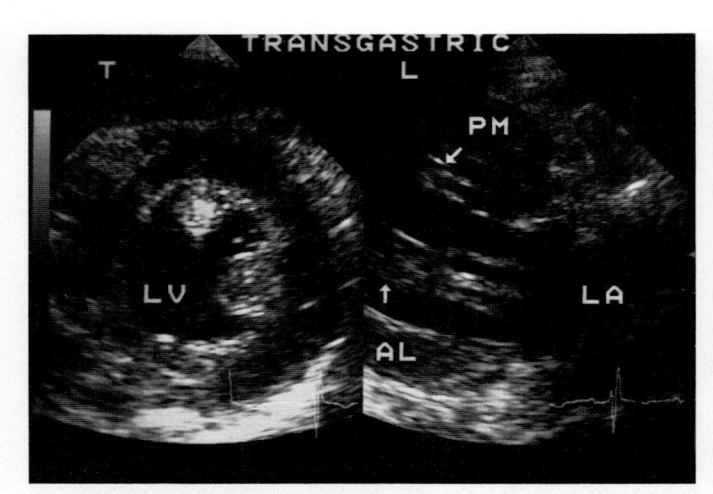

Fig. 2 Biplane trans-oesophageal images of the subvalvar apparatus of the mitral valve, obtained with the ultrasound transducer in the stomach. The cross-sectional image obtained with the transverse transducer shows the papillary muscles in cross section (left). The corresponding longitudinal image demonstrates both papillary muscles in their long axis and also the primary and secondary tendinous cords attached to the mitral leaflets (right). Anterolateral papillary muscle – AL, postero-medial papillary muscle – PM.

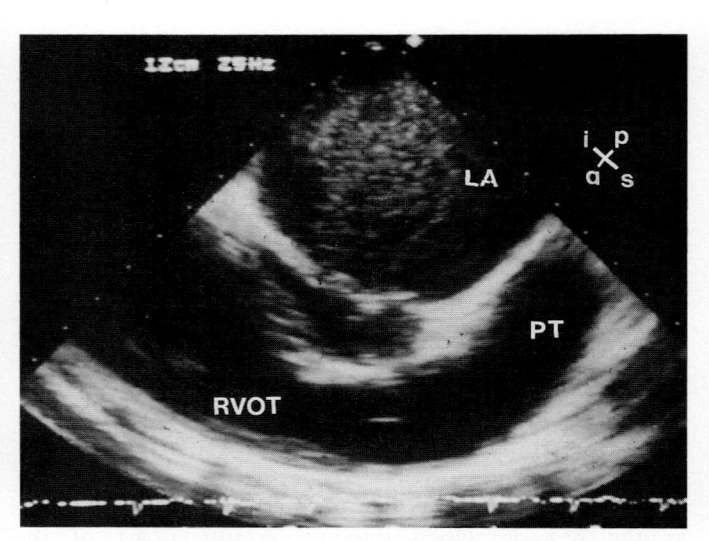

Fig. 4 Longitudinal image through the right ventricular outflow tract (RVOT), the pulmonary valve and the pulmonary trunk (PT). This patient (not the same as in Fig. 3) also has spontaneous echocardiographic contrast in the left atrium.

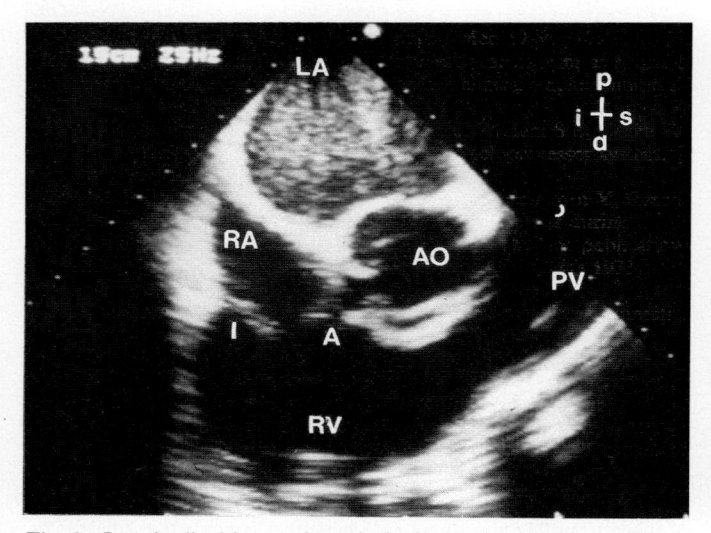

Fig. 3 Longitudinal image through the body of the right ventricle, also demonstrating the anterosuperior (A) and inferior (I) leaflets of the tricuspid valve. There is spontaneous echocardiographic contrast within the left atrium.

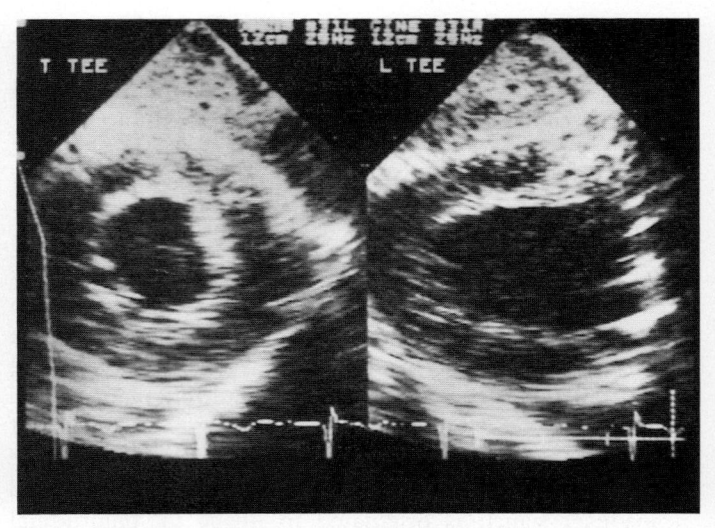

Fig. 5 Biplane trans-oesophageal images of the left ventricle obtained from the fundus of the stomach. The transverse image (left) shows a cross section of the ventricle at the level of the mid-papillary muscles. The longitudinal axis image (right) demonstrates the inferior (diaphragmatic) and anterior surfaces of the left ventricle. It may also demonstrate the true apex although foreshortening of the long axis of the ventricle is possible in this orientation.

and for guiding the placement of umbrella closure devices at cardiac catheterisation.[30]

In biplane probes, the centres of the two transducers are positioned about one centimetre apart on the tip of the probe. Thus the transducers image from slightly different points, and when switching from one transducer to the other, the tip of the probe sometimes has to be repositioned to maintain contact with the oesophageal mucosa. To overcome these problems, and to provide optimal quality of images by not dividing the elements between two transducers, multiplane transoesophageal probes are being developed. These have two basic designs – either a two-dimensional matrix of elements in a phased array transducer, in which the direction of imaging can be switched electronically, or more commonly a single element which can be rotated to direct the plane of imaging in any orientation between 0° and 360°. Early clinical experience with prototypes has been very promising[31]

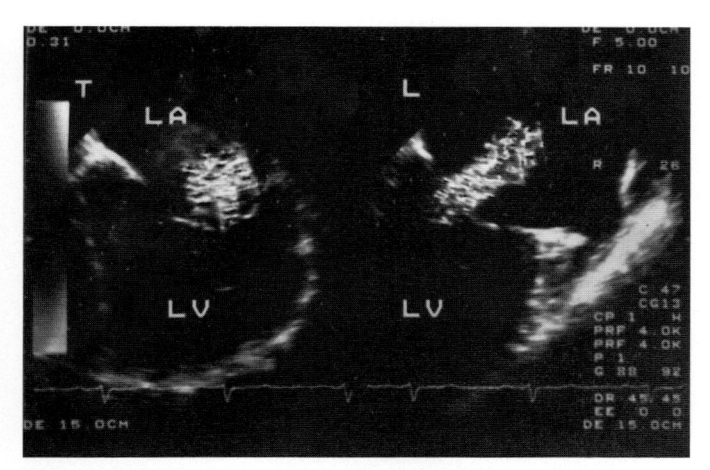

Plate 5 Biplane trans-oesophageal colour flow maps of a mitral regurgitant jet. The transverse image (left panel) shows a broad jet just above the mitral valve. The longitudinal image (right panel) demonstrates that the jet is quite long but is directed superiorly within the left atrium. This figure is reproduced in colour in the colour plate section at the front of this volume.

suggesting that multiplane probes may supersede biplane probes.

The other major technical development in trans-oesophageal echocardiography has been the miniaturisation of transducers so that they can be incorporated into the shafts of adapted paediatric fibreoptic bronchoscopes, in order to perform transoesophageal echocardiography in children and babies. With these probes, diagnostic information can be obtained in babies weighing as little as 2.5 kg. Major benefits are anticipated, especially in children with complex congenital heart disease, or with abnormalities of the venous connections, atria, and atrioventricular junctions.[32] In older children and adolescents or adults who have had previous surgery for congenital heart disease, transoesophageal echocardiography is especially valuable, because these patients are often difficult to image from the precordium. Examples of conditions in which there is a particular benefit include survivors of atrial correction procedures (Mustard or Senning operations) for complete transposition of the great arteries,[33] patients who have had a Fontan operation,[34] and patients with obstruction of the left ventricular outflow tract.[35]

As worldwide experience with transoesophageal echocardiography grows, new indications and applications are being reported. For example, the technique makes it easy to obtain pulsed Doppler signals of flow within the extraparenchymal portions of the pulmonary veins.[36] Retrograde flow into the pulmonary veins during ventricular systole is a good indicator of severe mitral regurgitation, irrespective of the size or eccentricity of the turbulent jet within the left atrium.[37] It has also been demonstrated, in patients who have no mitral regurgitation, that reduced emptying of the pulmonary veins during ventricular systole is a sign of an elevated left atrial pressure.[38] The combined analysis of flow within the pulmonary veins and across the mitral valve can be used to distinguish between normal and pseudonormal Doppler traces at the mitral orifice, and to study filling of the left ventricle in constriction and restriction.[39]

Transoesophageal echocardiography can also be used to obtain pulsed Doppler recordings of flow within the left anterior descending coronary artery. This technique will never supplant coronary arteriography for diagnosing obstructive coronary atheroma and it is not possible to measure absolute levels of flow. Nevertheless, it has been possible to show changes in coronary blood flow after drug treatment.[40]

INTRAOPERATIVE ECHOCARDIOGRAPHY

The complexity of cardiac surgery is increasing, so that surgeons now tackle more ambitious and intricate operations in sicker patients than before. The trend in surgery for congenital heart disease is towards more total corrections rather than palliative or staged procedures. In adults with valvar disease, reconstructive surgery is preferred to valve replacement. These developments mean that surgeons may be uncertain after cardiopulmonary bypass whether or not they have achieved the desired outcome. Significant residual lesions produce postoperative morbidity, and patients with suboptimal results may need late reoperation. Traditional methods of assessing the quality of a repair, before coming off bypass or before closing the chest, have relied on direct visual inspection, non-physiological tests of valve competence, and direct pressure recordings. Clearly, there is a need for more sophisticated intraoperative methods of assessing the outcome of surgery before the chest is closed, which would allow surgeons to revise the repair when necessary. Intraoperative echocardiography has evolved to meet these needs.

All of the standard echocardiographic modalities can be used in patients of all ages. Direct epicardial imaging and Doppler studies (mostly colour flow mapping) are performed using standard precordial transducers packed inside sterile plastic sleeves containing some ultrasonic gel at their tips.[41,42] High frequency transducers can be used, and images of excellent quality are obtained. The epicardial approach is extremely versatile, and unconventional imaging planes can be studied, as well as planes equivalent to precordial views. In neonates, the relatively large size of the transducers relative to the size of the sternotomy may restrict the views which can be obtained. In children and in adults, intraoperative studies can also be performed using a transoesophageal probe. A single plane transducer is less useful than epicardial imaging, but the biplane probe probably provides information equivalent to that available from the epicardial approach, and it has the advantage that it does not involve invading the sterile operative field.

Specialised small epicardial transducers are being developed for use solely in the operating room. These allow access to more structures within the chest,[43] but they can cause arrhythmias.

The choice of approach and technique depends on the type of operation being performed. In patients with congenital heart disease, a pre-bypass study should be performed to confirm the preoperative diagnosis; the diagnosis may be refined in as many as 30% of patients.[44] This information can also be used by the cardiac surgeon to plan the operative approach. For example, echocardiography can be used to determine if an inlet ventricular septal defect can be closed through the tricuspid valve, rather than via a right ventriculotomy. After bypass, the choice of approach is influenced by the presence of prosthetic materials such as dacron patches used to repair septal defects, or conduits or prosthetic valves, because these all block the transmission of ultrasound. Thus, in many circumstances a complete echocardiographic evaluation can be undertaken only by combining the oesophageal and epicardial approaches.[45] In babies or small children with rapid heart rates it may be very difficult to interpret colour flow maps quickly, and so contrast echocardiographic studies can be very helpful, for example to demonstrate whether or not there is a residual intracardiac shunt after closure of a ventricular septal defect.[46]

Intraoperative echocardiography is also very useful in adults with acquired heart disease. After mitral valve reconstruction, transoesophageal echocardiography is the best technique for studying residual mitral regurgitation. In many other circumstances, epicardial echocardiography is preferred because it is more versatile than transoesophageal imaging in transverse planes. For example, it can be used to define the extent of septal damage in a patient with a post-infarction ventricular septal defect (Plate 6), or to pinpoint the site of attachment of a myxoma (Fig. 6). In patients with acute aortic dissection, epivascular imaging (with the probe placed directly on the aorta) may define the sites of entry or re-entry tears (Plate 7).

Immediately after cardiopulmonary bypass, the haemodynamic condition of the patient may be unstable, and it can change quickly. It is not surprising, therefore, that the echocardiographic findings can change significantly from the immediate post-bypass study to a repeat study performed a few days later. The incidence of some residual lesions is underestimated at the initial study.[47] Nevertheless, if residual abnormalities are detected immediately after cardiopulmonary bypass they are likely to remain significant, and patients who leave the operating room with echocardiographic evidence of a suboptimal surgical result have a worse prognosis and a higher postoperative mortality rate than patients who have an echocardiographically perfect result.[48] Some paediatric cardiac surgeons now use intraoperative echocardiography routinely.

Echocardiography can be invaluable in the differential diagnosis of patients who become acutely unwell either after coming off cardiopulmonary bypass in the operating theatre or in the intensive care unit. Transoesophageal studies will rapidly distinguish between causes of profound hypotension such as pericardial effusion with tamponade, hypovolaemia, or left ventricular failure from myocardial dysfunction.

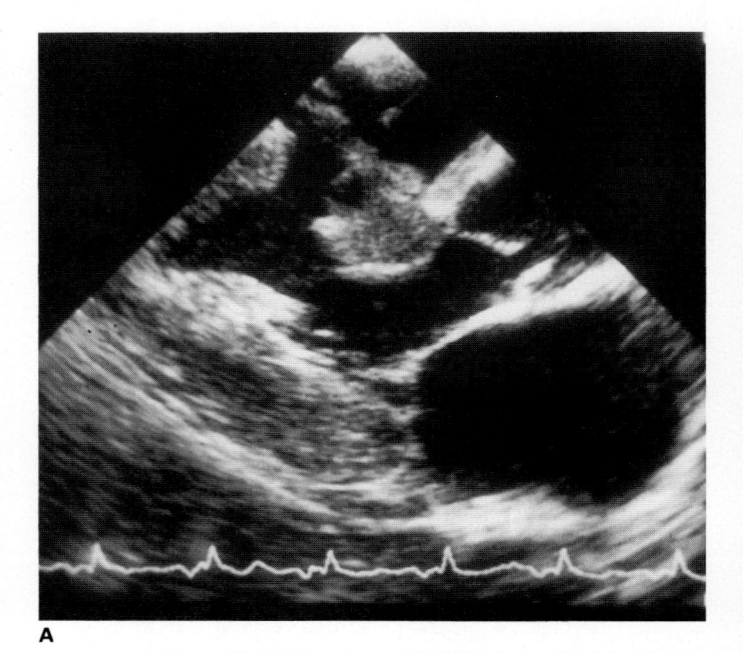

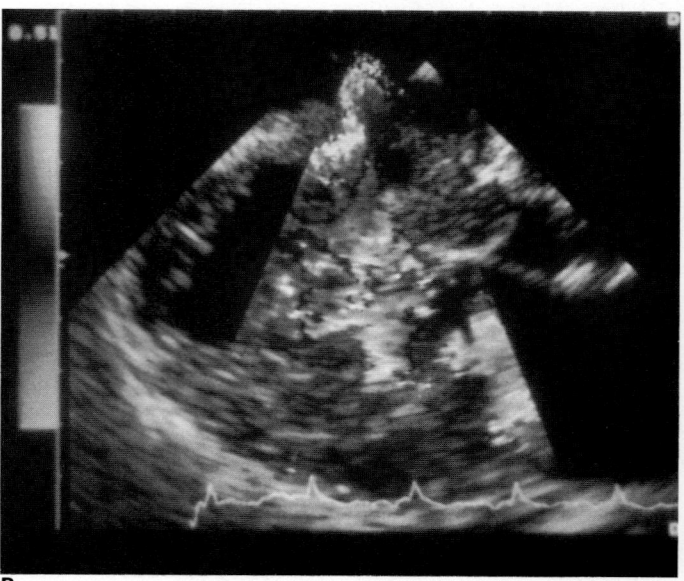

Plate 6 A: Intraoperative epicardial cross-sectional image in the longitudinal axis in a patient with acute ventricular septal rupture. The margins of the defect within the mid-ventricular septum are clearly defined. There is little undermining of the adjacent edges of the septum. **B**: The corresponding colour flow map confirms a left to right shunt. This figure is reproduced in colour in the colour plate section at the front of this volume.

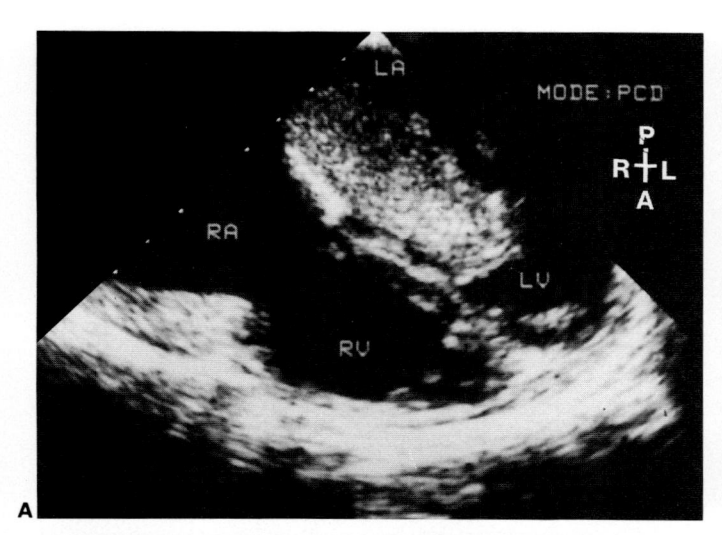

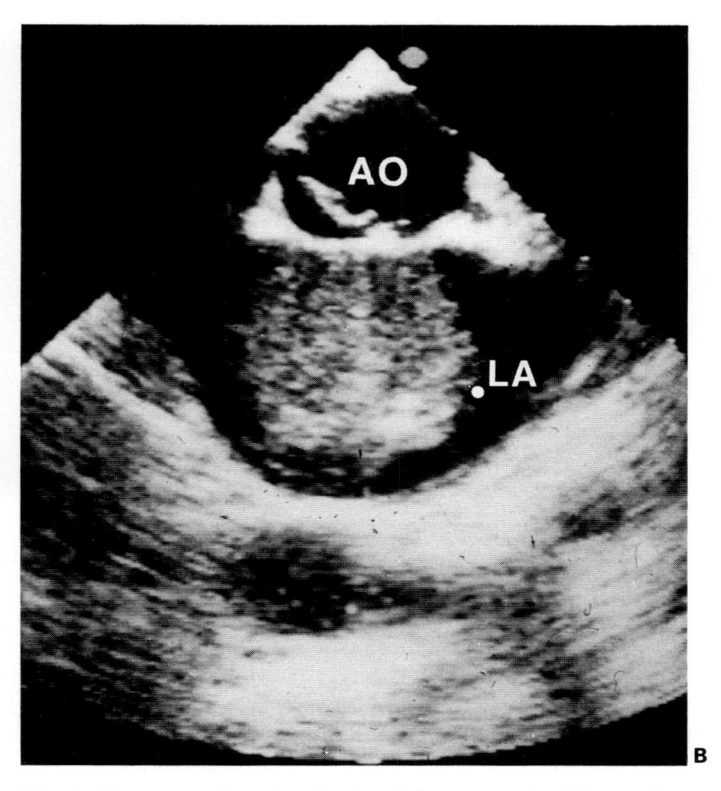

Fig. 6 Trans-oesophageal and epicardial cross-sectional images in a patient with an atrial myxoma. A: The trans-oesophageal echocardiogram in this four chamber view was interpreted as showing clear evidence of attachment of the myxoma to the middle of the atrial septum. B and C: Epicardial echocardiography in short axis views demonstrated that the myxoma was free of the atrial septum and attached to the roof of the left atrium posterior to the aortic valve.

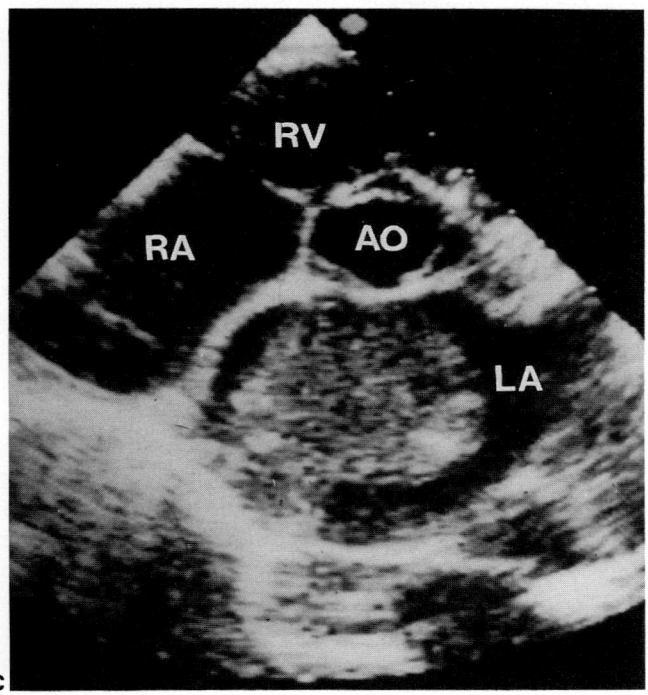

Intraoperative transoesophageal echocardiography can also be performed during non-cardiac operations. For example, elderly patients with extensive vascular disease have a significant chance of developing perioperative myocardial infarction if they undergo a prolonged general anaesthetic. Transoesophageal monitoring of left ventricular function allows any new abnormalities of wall motion to be detected quickly and treated promptly. This technique is significantly better than either electrocardiographic monitoring or the recording of pulmonary capillary wedge pressures with a Swan Ganz catheter,[49] and it is used increasingly by anaesthetists.[50]

STRESS ECHOCARDIOGRAPHY

Precordial echocardiography is a simple non-invasive technique which can be repeated as often as required. Both cross-sectional imaging and Doppler studies can be performed after a variety of stresses to the circulation, including exercise, atrial pacing, and the infusion of drugs.

Exercise echocardiography

Exercise *electro*cardiography (ECG stress test) is an excellent technique for demonstrating ischaemia, but its overall sensitivity and specificity are limited (to 68% and 77% respectively, in a meta-analysis of 24 074 patients).[51] Many patients are unable to perform sufficient exercise on a treadmill to provoke ischaemia, and in young patients the incidence of false positive diagnoses may be high. When ischaemia occurs, reductions in myocardial contractility develop before the surface electrocardiogram changes.[52] *Echo*cardiography during or immediately after peak exercise can therefore be used to detect abnormalities of ventricular wall motion, in order to enhance the diagnostic

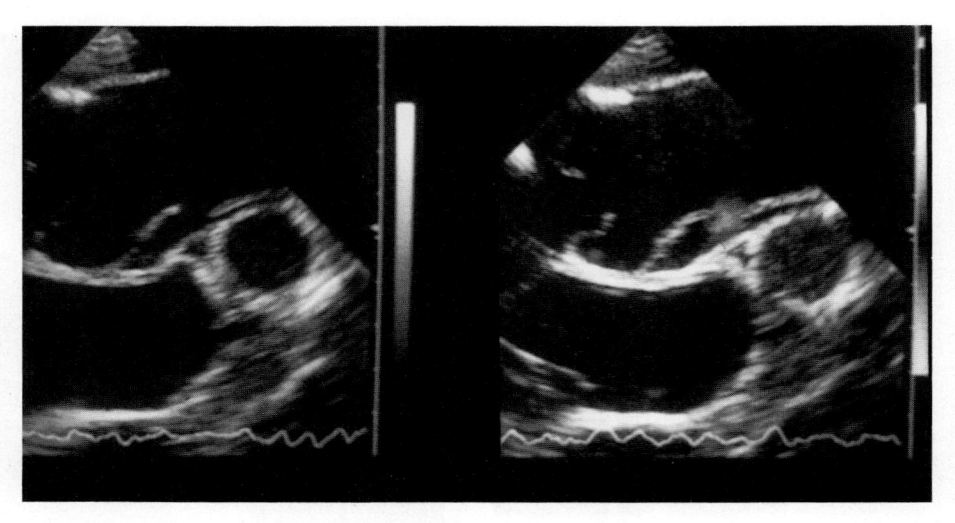

Plate 7 Epivascular image and colour flow map obtained during cardiopulmonary bypass in a patient with aortic dissection. The aorta is imaged along its long axis. The cross-sectional image (left) shows the site of the intimal tear. This is confirmed on colour flow mapping (right). This figure is reproduced in colour in the colour plate section at the front of this volume.

sensitivity of the test. There is a close correlation between the development of new abnormalities of regional wall motion, and the presence of ischaemia or the finding of significant coronary stenoses at angiography.[53–55]

An echocardiographic study should be performed before the patient exercises on the treadmill or bicycle, in order to document function at rest and to establish the optimal positions for the transducer. Thus no time is wasted in obtaining standardised parasternal long and short axis images, and apical 2 and 4 chamber views, immediately after exercise. Considerable experience is required to perform such studies rapidly, and to obtain accurate and reproducible images in the majority of patients.[56]

In healthy patients, stress echocardiograms show preserved systolic thickening of the ventricular wall, and hyperdynamic or normal contraction with inward motion of the endocardium. In patients with ischaemia, there may be absent thickening of the ventricular wall in systole, and abnormal motion of the wall such as hypokinesis, akinesis or dyskinesis. The interpretation of images may be affected by marked respiratory variation in the position of the heart, and difficulties also arise in distinguishing between hypokinetic and dyskinetic segments, in patients who have abnormal function at rest but become more abnormal on exercise. Nevertheless, exercise echocardiography appears to have very high sensitivity, especially in patients with cross-sectional coronary stenoses of greater than 90%.[55] The sensitivity falls considerably in patients with lesser degrees of coronary obstruction, but it still compares favourably with that obtained on exercise electrocardiography alone.[57] When performed by experienced observers, exercise echocardiography is as sensitive as isotopic studies using single photon emission computed tomography.[58,59] Interobserver agreement is high.[60]

Atrial pacing and echocardiography

When patients are unable to perform dynamic exercise, alternative methods of stressing the heart are required. Echocardiography can be performed during atrial pacing in patients with angina pectoris or myocardial infarction,[61,62] and this approach has the advantage that the patient can remain still while imaging is performed. Atrial pacing is achieved either by a transvenous pacing electrode in the right atrium, or more commonly by atrial pacing from a pill electrode within the oesophagus. The initial approach was to combine pacing with precordial echocardiography. More recently, a technique has been developed for pacing the heart with an electrode attached to the surface of a transoesophageal probe, while simultaneously recording transgastric short axis images of the left ventricle.[63] The standard transgastric image of the left ventricle includes regions of myocardium supplied by all three major coronary arteries. Lambertz et al reported extremely high sensitivities and specificities with the combined transoesophageal pacing and imaging technique (Fig. 7).

Pharmacological stress echocardiography

Dipyridamole, an analogue of adenosine, provokes regional disparities in myocardial blood flow and ischaemia by causing a coronary steal syndrome. It selectively dilates normal blood vessels, thereby diverting flow from the region supplied by stenosed coronary arteries. Dipyridamole can be administered as an alternative to exercise electrocardiography since it provokes electrocardiographic changes in about 50% of patients with angiographically proven coronary disease, and either ECG changes or angina in about 80% of patients.[64] When echocardiography is com-

Diagnostic sensitivities	Bicycle exercise	Atrial pacing	Stress TEE
1VD	44%	25%	85% *
2VD	50%	64%	100% *
3VD	83%	86%	100%

20 + 14 + 7 = 41 pts.   Lambertz, JACC 1990

Fig. 7 **Comparison of the sensitivity of stress trans-oesophageal echocardiography with atrial pacing to that of stress electrocardiography** in the diagnosis of single (IVD), double (2VD), and triple (3VD) vessel coronary artery disease. Data adapted from Lambertz et al.[63]

bined with dipyridamole ECG stress testing, the sensitivity varies from 52% to 89%, depending on the types of patients who are studied and the number of echocardiographic cross sections which are analysed.[65,66] Picano et al have shown that dipyridamole echocardiography has a similar sensitivity but a higher specificity for angiographically proven coronary artery disease, than has exercise electrocardiography.[67] Recently, adenosine itself has also been used as an agent for pharmacological stress echocardiography, but this test appears to be relatively insensitive.[68]

Dobutamine may be infused during echocardiography, and it has proven to be valuable in detecting some latent or residual myocardial function in myocardial segments which are hypokinetic or akinetic at rest. This technique appears promising for the detection of stunned myocardium. It has been used to identify viable myocardium immediately after myocardial infarction and following thrombolysis. Myocardial wall thickening during dobutamine implies that early reperfusion has occurred, and it is associated with good recovery of myocardial function.[69]

Pharmacological stress echocardiography is also being used after coronary angioplasty, to demonstrate changes in regional ischaemia. After successful treatment, most patients show improved regional and global left ventricular function.[70,71]

Doppler studies during stress

Doppler studies can be performed during interventions. For example, the development of obstruction within the left ventricular outflow tract may be provoked by inhaling amyl nitrite, as a diagnostic test for hypertrophic obstructive cardiomyopathy. Changes in aortic valvar or mitral Doppler profiles may be recorded while a patient exercises on a supine bicycle ergometer.

Colour flow mapping during exercise may demonstrate the development of mitral regurgitation. Dynamic regurgitation is difficult to diagnose, but it may cause significant morbidity in patients who develop papillary muscle dysfunction or increasing dilatation of the mitral annulus on exercise, due to ischaemia.[72]

CONTRAST ECHOCARDIOGRAPHY

Contrast echocardiography was first described in 1968.[73] During the seventies, contrast effects obtained after the venous injection of hand-agitated saline were studied during M-mode echocardiography to detect intracardiac shunts. This application has been largely superseded by cross-sectional imaging and colour flow mapping, but contrast echocardiography has remained useful in certain special circumstances. Its applications are now expanding once more, because of the development of special ultrasonic contrast agents.

Contrast techniques are still more suited than is colour flow mapping, to the detection of a small low-velocity shunt such as that across a patent oval foramen. The most sensitive technique for detecting a patent oval foramen is to inject contrast during a Valsalva manoeuvre, while imaging the left atrium and the atrial septum with a trans-oesophageal transducer (Fig. 8). In patients with complex

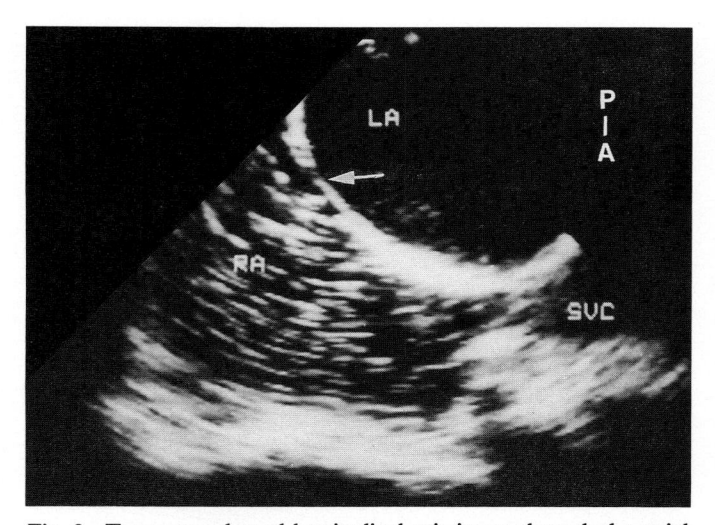

Fig. 8 **Trans-oesophageal longitudinal axis image through the atrial septum and the right side of the heart** following a peripheral venous injection of echocardiographic contrast and during a Valsalva manoeuvre. The thin septum primum within the oval fossa is well demonstrated (arrow). There is no evidence of a patent oval foramen.

congenital heart disease, contrast injected into an upper limb vein during precordial echocardiography can delineate the site of anomalous systemic venous connections. Contrast echocardiography can also help to distinguish between critical stenosis and true atresia of a valve, and the time of appearance of contrast within the left heart can differentiate between intracardiac and pulmonary shunts. Injected contrast also amplifies the intensity of signals obtained with colour flow mapping, which may be useful when identifying small regurgitant jets prior to continuous wave Doppler interrogation.

The safety of hand-agitated mixtures of blood and saline is uncertain, and the intensity of the contrast effect cannot be controlled. To overcome these problems, methods were developed using sonicated radiological contrast media, but more recently specific echocardiographic contrast agents such as sonicated albumin, and saccharide molecules, have become available.[74,75] Since the dose of contrast can now be controlled, it can be used to measure blood flow. The efficacy and safety of one of these new agents, albunex (sonicated albumin), has been reported.[74] The particles are uniform in size, and after a peripheral venous injection they pass through the pulmonary circulation and appear in the left heart (Fig. 9). Contrast accurately outlines the endocardial surface of the left ventricle (Fig. 10), thereby improving the accuracy of echocardiographic estimates of left ventricular systolic function and ejection fraction.

Echocardiographic contrast which reaches the aorta causes a measurable contrast effect in the myocardium. However, the application of peripheral venous contrast injections for the study of myocardial blood flow is still hindered by technical problems. Instead, echocardiographic contrast agents have been injected directly into

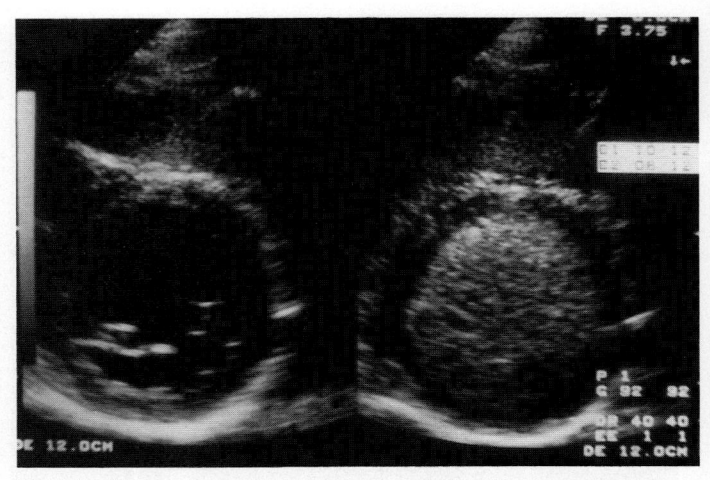

Fig. 10 Short axis images from the precordium demonstrating the use of echocardiographic contrast to improve the recognition of the endocardial border of the cavity of the left ventricle. (Courtesy of Dr Folkert Ten Cate, Thoraxcentre, Rotterdam.)

the orifices of the coronary arteries during cardiac catheterisation, or down vein grafts during coronary artery surgery. Sharply demarcated distributions of coronary blood supply are observed, and time intensity curves, or the time to the appearance of the peak contrast effect, can be used to measure perfusion.[76,77] Changes in perfusion, indicated by an increase in the intensity of the myocardial contrast effect, have been observed after successful coronary angioplasty or surgical revascularisation.[76,78]

Much experimental development of echocardiographic contrast agents is still required, but it is likely that their clinical applications will continue to expand over the next few years.

ULTRASONIC TISSUE CHARACTERISATION

When an ultrasonic beam meets the myocardium, the brightest echoes are returned to the transducer from the interfaces between blood and muscle. As the ultrasonic beam traverses the muscle it is reflected in all directions, but a small proportion of the transmitted ultrasonic signals (in fact, < 1%) is reflected back to the transducer, even when the angle of incidence is 90°. At present, these signals are not analysed in detail by most ultrasound machines. However, if the digitally-coded information from each pixel within the cross-sectional image is processed and analysed in a special way (such as 'rational gain compensation'),[79] before it is converted to analogue inputs for the video screen, then the echoes from the myocardium are displayed in a manner which carries information about its structure. So-called 'integrated backscatter' signals can be used to characterise properties of soft tissue.

In both animals and man, it has been shown that the integrated backscatter signal from the myocardium is less

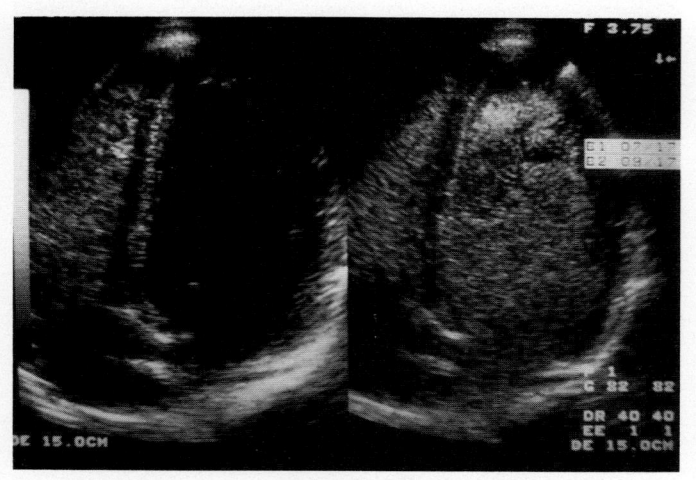

Fig. 9 Apical four chamber images obtained following the injection of Albunex in a normal subject. The echocardiographic contrast is visible first within the right ventricle (left panel) and then crosses the pulmonary circulation to opacify the cavity of the left ventricle (right panel). (Courtesy of Dr Folkert Ten Cate, Thoraxcentre, Rotterdam.)

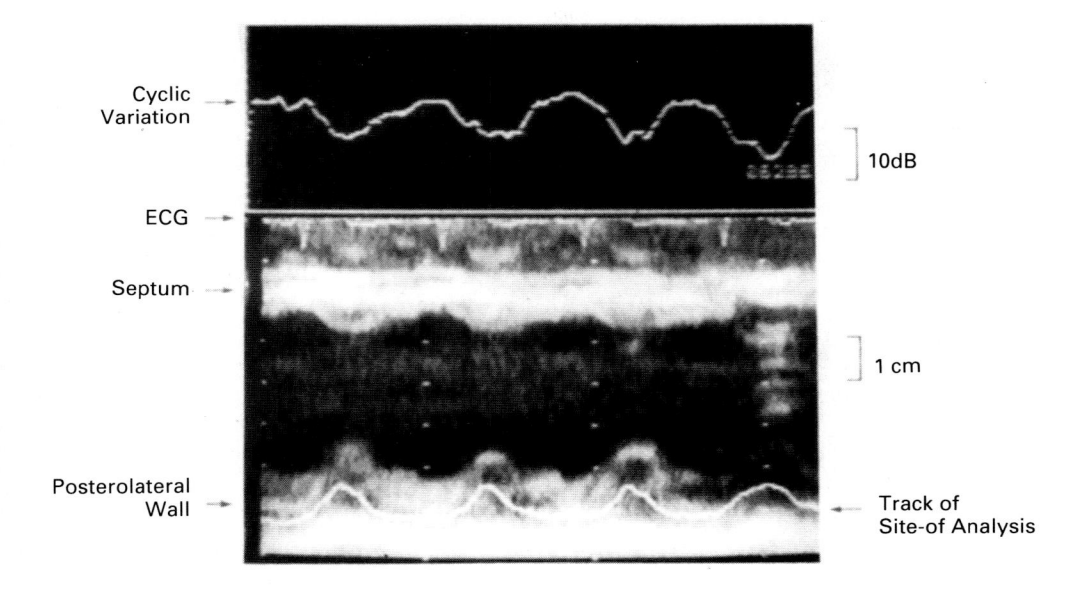

Fig. 11 Tissue characterisation in a normal left ventricle. The M-mode echocardiogram demonstrates variation in integrated back scatter, with relatively bright echoes being returned from the left ventricular posterior wall during diastole compared with a relatively echolucent appearance during systole. The upper panel shows the cyclic variation in back scatter with a normal range of about 8 decibels between systole and diastole. (Reproduced with permission from Milunski et al.)[80]

during systole than diastole (Fig. 11).[80] This cyclic variation of backscatter reflects myocardial contractile performance, and it is reduced significantly with both ischaemia and infarction.[81] After reperfusion, integrated backscatter returns to normal very quickly,[82] so that it is restored before contractile function recovers. Thus detectable variation in integrated backscatter suggests that myocardium is viable.[83]

The precise histological or physiological correlate of backscatter is unknown. Variation in backscatter occurs in perfused contracting muscles in the absence of blood flow, and restoration of blood flow to myocardium which has been ischaemic for 1 hour produces no immediate recovery of cyclic variation.[84] Thus changes in backscatter are not due primarily to the loss or the restoration, of blood flow per se.[85] Equally, the variation in backscatter from a myocardial segment may increase even when there is no detectable improvement in its contraction. Thus, neither is backscatter due to myocardial cell contraction alone.

The second major application of tissue characterisation is to detect abnormalities of the myocardium due to infiltration or hypertrophy. Tissue characterisation is capable of distinguishing between thickened myocardium caused by hypertrophic cardiomyopathy, and that due to infiltration of amyloid.[86] However, it may be difficult to distinguish between normal myocardium and hypertrophic myocardium in hypertension.[87]

At present, tissue characterisation is not widely available, because most machines need to be modified before they can analyse and display backscatter. Once these systems are incorporated into commercially available machines, however, there seems little doubt that tissue characterisation will be of considerable clinical value. In addition to encoding abnormalities of myocardial structure and function, it may be able to distinguish thrombus from muscle.

INTRAVASCULAR ULTRASOUND

Intravascular Doppler

It has been recognised for some time that there may be considerable disparity between the angiographic appearance of a stenosis and its functional significance. Patients with anatomically similar stenoses may have differing symptoms and dissimilar long-term prognoses. Objective assessment of the importance of recurrent stenoses after angioplasty or bypass grafting requires measurement of their functional significance. Several studies have suggested that this can be done with intra-arterial Doppler.

The use of intra-arterial Doppler in coronary artery disease was described in 1986,[88] when it was shown in animals that intracoronary flow measured by Doppler techniques correlated well with values obtained from external, validated flow meters. Thereafter, intracoronary Doppler catheters were used to measure coronary flow reserve in patients undergoing cardiac catheterisation.[89] The Doppler catheters presently in use have a distal diameter of about 1 mm (3F), and a central lumen through which a guidewire may be inserted (usually 0.014 inches). The ultrasonic crystal is mounted on the tip of the catheter, facing forwards.

Intravascular Doppler techniques have been used to investigate coronary blood flow in response to drug treatment[90] and coronary angioplasty.[91] Examples of the traces obtained when using intracoronary Doppler to estimate coronary flow reserve following the injection of

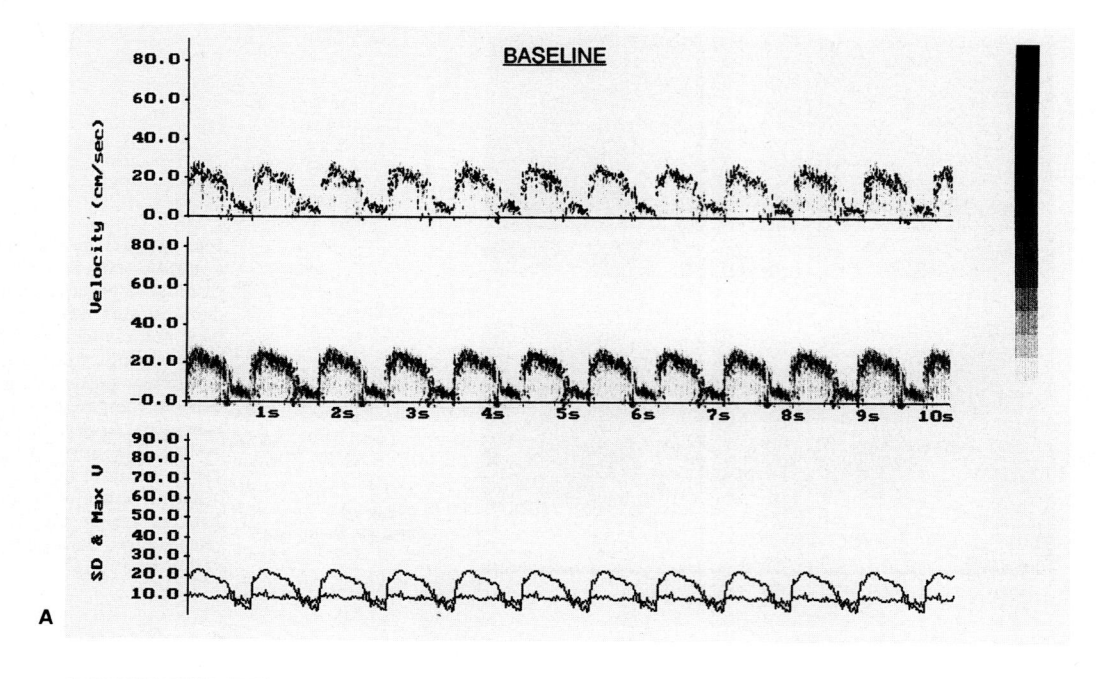

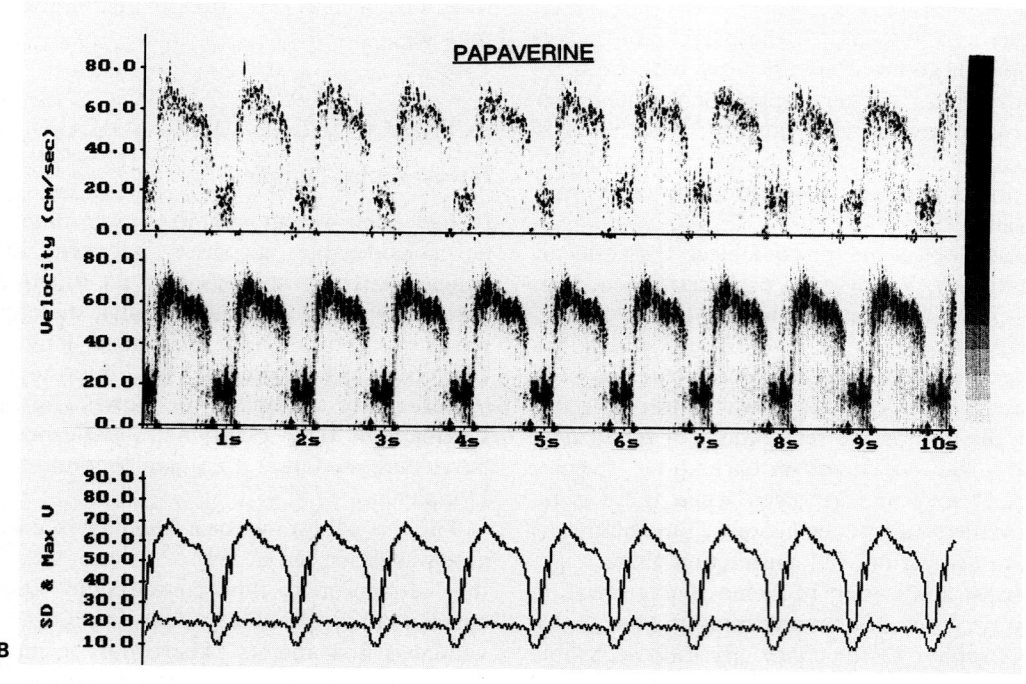

Fig. 12 Intracoronary Doppler recordings of the velocity of blood flow A: at rest (baseline) and B: after the injection of papaverine to assess coronary flow reserve. The velocity increases by more than 20%. (Courtesy of Dr Carlo di Maria and Professor Patrick Serruys, Thoraxcentre, Rotterdam.)

papaverine, are shown in Figure 12. Initial studies reported simple parameters such as the Doppler frequency shift, and related them to the volume of flow. More recently, fast Fourier transform analysis has been used to assess coronary flow after vasodilation[92] and angioplasty.[93] More sophisticated analyses of intra-arterial flow, employing indices such as resistance index, pulsatility index and spectral broadening index, can now be performed, and these may prove to be of more clinical value.

Measurements obtained with intracoronary Doppler catheters reflect changes in coronary blood flow only. The inability to measure the intracoronary diameter, changes

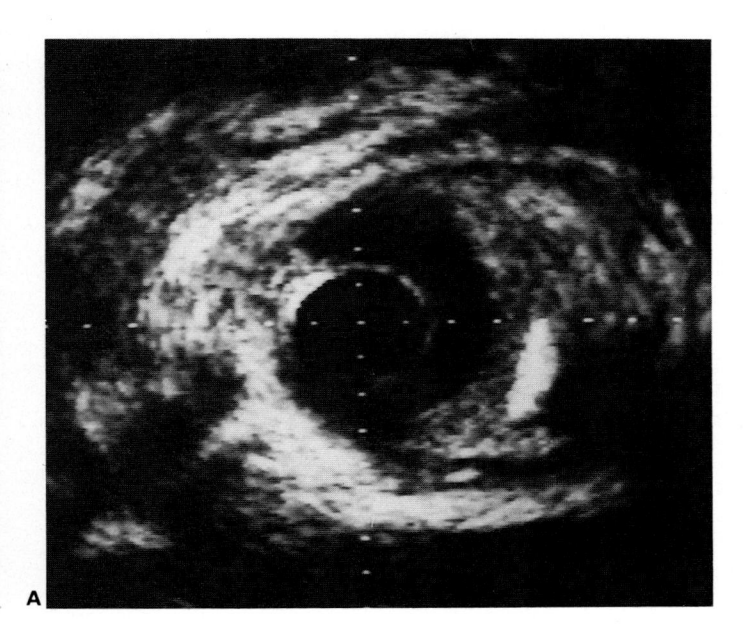

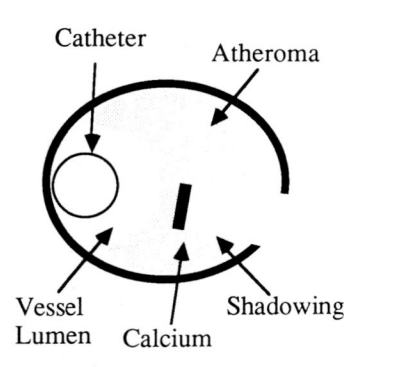

Fig. 13 **Intravascular ultrasonic image in a patient with peripheral vascular disease.** This intraoperative image demonstrates a large crescentic atheromatous lesion, occupying most of the lumen of the iliac artery. Calcification within the atheromatous plaque causes acoustic shadowing. There are also regional variations in the brightness of the echoes within the plaque which are thought to represent variations in its composition and increased fibrosis. (Reproduced with permission from; Surgical use of intra-arterial ultrasound, Linker D T, Saether O D, Myhre H O, Angelsen B A J. European Journal of Surgery, 1991, in press.)

during systole and diastole, and non-linear patterns of flow, currently preclude the determination of absolute flow.

Intravascular ultrasonic imaging

Intravascular ultrasonic imaging is currently the subject of considerable research and enthusiasm.[94,95] Systems have been developed and are commercially available which provide intravascular images of excellent quality. These use catheters which incorporate a single element and a rotating mirror which sweeps the ultrasonic beam around the circumference of the lumen, or else a catheter with a circular array of elements around its tip.

Correlations of intravascular imaging in vitro with subsequent histology have shown that there is a close relationship between the images obtained and the distribution and composition of atheromatous plaques. Nevertheless, controversy exists about the relationship of intravascular ultrasound images to the histological structure of the vessel wall. The usual cross-sectional appearance of muscular arteries shows three layers: an echogenic intimal interface, an echolucent midzone, and a second echogenic outer region. Originally, these appearances were thought to correspond to the intima, media and adventitia respectively. The triple-layer appearance is frequent but not universal,[96] however, and the echoes may relate to differences in the flexibility of structures rather than to their composition or histological findings.[97]

Intravascular imaging demonstrates many details of atheromatous lesions, as was shown first in *peripheral* vascular disease. An example of an intravascular image in a human peripheral artery is shown in Figure 13. Calcified plaques are readily identified, but they cast strong acoustic shadows and so more distal structures cannot be imaged. There may be associated lack of movement of the overlying vessel wall. The distensibility of the arterial wall is related to the composition of a plaque, with fibrous atheroma having a more adverse effect than fatty atheroma. Tissue characterisation is also being used to study the composition of atherosclerotic lesions although there are many technical problems to be overcome. There is considerable angle-dependence and frequency-dependence of echo intensity when performing intravascular imaging.

Intravascular imaging is being used in *coronary* arteries and vein grafts in the cardiac catheterisation laboratory, as a research technique. The cost of imaging catheters, which are disposable, and the current lack of controlled trials proving clinical benefit as a consequence of intracoronary ultrasound, mean that it cannot yet be recommended for routine clinical work.

In patients undergoing angioplasty, good matching of the size of the balloon to the size of the vessel is crucial. Mismatching is an important predictor of residual stenosis, acute closure and restenosis. Sometimes it is difficult to select the size of the angioplasty balloon, when the outline of the lumen of the coronary artery is irregular or dilated, and it appears that angiographic assessment consistently undersizes the required balloon.[98] Measurements of the true diameter of the vessel lumen are best made with intravascular imaging, which can discriminate between normal, remodelled, and concentrically narrowed segments. After angioplasty or another interventional procedure, intracoronary imaging may show a localised dissection (Fig. 14) or other complication. Prospective studies are being performed to try to determine how such findings

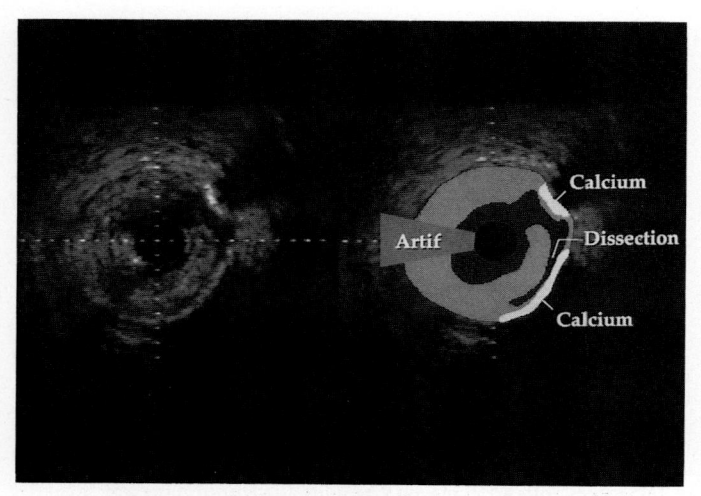

Fig. 14 Intravascular ultrasonic image of a human coronary artery. Following angioplasty there is a localised dissection with undermining of the atheromatous plaque. (Reproduced with permission from Dr Paul Yock and Dr Peter Fitzgerald, University of California, San Francisco.)

relate to the outcome of angioplasty. Catheters are available in which the ultrasonic imaging is combined with a balloon.

Three-dimensional reconstructions of coronary arteries can be assembled from serial cross-sectional images obtained during a systematic timed pullback of the imaging catheter. The subsequent display makes it easier to appreciate the pattern of stenoses, atheroma, and dissections. Intracoronary imaging can also be used to follow the progression or regression of atherosclerosis in response to diet or other treatment,[99,100] but it is difficult to perform repeat studies because the orientation and precise relocation of the catheter within the coronary artery are hard to control.

Intracardiac ultrasound

It is about 20 years since the first multi-element, real-time intracardiac scanner was developed.[101] Interest lapsed because of technical difficulties and concurrent advances in non-invasing imaging. Now, 'invasive' intracardiac echocardiography is again being evaluated.[102] The 12.5 MHz catheters which have been tested, provide excellent visualisation of all intracardiac structures, but clear clinical applications have yet to emerge.

THREE-DIMENSIONAL RECONSTRUCTION

The ultimate goal for echocardiography is perhaps a three-dimensional reconstruction of the heart, upon which blood flow could be superimposed. This could be used to study ventricular function, or anatomical relationships in congenital heart disease. The major obstacle in achieving this goal is difficulty in recording precisely the spatial location of each cross-sectional image. The possibility of transmitting both the two-dimensional image, and the information from the system which locates the transducer, simultaneously to one computer has been explored.[103] It is then able to locate the signals in three dimensions. Initial experience[104] suggests that excellent measurement of volumes can be obtained with a three-dimensional reconstruction of two-dimensional images. This opens the way for accurate assessment of left ventricular function in humans. Rapid progress may be made in three-dimensional reconstruction, especially when experts in computed tomography and magnetic resonance imaging combine their efforts to solve the computational problems.

THERAPEUTIC APPLICATIONS OF ULTRASOUND

Sound energy itself may be applied as a tool with potential therapeutic applications.[105] Ultrasonic energy delivered from a catheter can cause the dissolution of thrombi both in vitro and in vivo.[106] The usual dose of pulsed wave energy is between 11 and 25 Watts (compared with a power of 0.1 Watts during a normal examination). Since it appears that thrombi may be disrupted without causing thermal injury to the endothelial lining, this technique raises the prospect of using one catheter in acute infarction, first to assess stenoses in the coronary arteries (by Doppler and imaging) and then to perform an angioplasty.

It has been reported that ultrasound can be used at operation to decalcify stenotic aortic valve leaflets. However, the procedure has not gained acceptance, because the post-operative incidence of aortic regurgitation appears to be very high.[107-108]

CONCLUSIONS

During the past ten years, there have been many exciting developments in the field of cardiovascular ultrasound. New techniques such as colour flow mapping and transoesophageal echocardiography have had a great impact on clinical practice. Now, cardiac ultrasound in its various modalities can make most cardiac diagnoses apart from providing coronary angiograms. The pre-eminent role of cardiac ultrasound will not remain unchallenged, however, since other diagnostic techniques such as magnetic resonance imaging may prove to be superior in certain circumstances. Always, echocardiographic results should be interpreted in their clinical context, and all non-invasive and invasive imaging techniques should be considered when investigating a patient.

Every year, the technology involved in echocardiographic investigations becomes more complex, and the need for communication between clinicians and physicists, engineers, and systems analysts increases. Developments should be led by the need to find solutions to basic scientific and clinical problems; it is inappropriate for technological advances to be pursued in isolation, before determining whether or not they have clinical applications.

Given continued collaboration between clinicians, scientists and engineers, however, there is every reason to believe that the dramatic pace of recent developments will be maintained.

REFERENCES

1 ACP/ACC/AHA Taskforce on clinical privileges in cardiology: clinical competence in adult echocardiography. J Am Coll Cardiol 1991; 15: 1465-1468
2 Shattock D P, Weishenker M D, Smith S W, Von Ramm O T. Explososcan: a parallel processing technique for high speed ultrasonic imaging with linear phased arrays. J Acoust Soc Am 1987; 75: 1273-1282
3 Schiller N B, Shah P M, Crawford M, et al. Recommendations for quantitation of the left ventricle by two-dimensional echocardiography. J Am Soc Echo 1989; 2: 358-367
4 Fraser A G, Smyllie J H, Assmann P E, Sutherland G R, Roelandt J R T C. Analysis of left ventricular function in patients with myocardial infarction. Methodological problems and possible solutions. In: Iliceto S, Rizzon P, Roelandt J R T C (eds). Ultrasound in coronary artery disease. Dordrecht: Kluwer Academic Publishers. 1991: pp. 213-229.
5 Heger J J, Weyman A E, Wann L S, Rogers E W, Dillon J C, Feigenbaum H. Cross-sectional echocardiographic analysis of the extent of left ventricular asynergy in acute myocardial infarction. Circulation 1980: 61: 1113-1118
6 Nishimura R A, Reeder G S, Miller F A, et al. Prognostic value of predischarge 2-dimensional echocardiogram after acute myocardial infarction. Am J Cardiol 1984; 53: 429-432
7 Assmann P E, Slager C J, van der Borden S G, et al. Quantitative echocardiographic analysis of global and regional left ventricular function: a problem revisited. J Am Soc Echocardiog 1990; 3: 478-487
8 Assmann P E, Slager C J, Dreysse S T, Borden S G van der, Oomen J A, Roelandt J R. Two-dimensional echocardiographic analysis of the dynamic geometry of the left ventricle: the basis for an improved model of wall motion. J Am Soc Echo 1988; 1: 393-405
9 Smyllie J, MacNeill A B, Vos J, Borden S vd, Roelandt J. Is two-dimensional echocardiography a reliable tool for assessing left ventricular function? Reproducibility data from DEFIANT, a multicentre European trial. Eur Heart J 1991; (Abstract Suppl): 71
10 Gordon E P, Schnittger I, Fitzgerald P J, Williams P, Popp R L. Reproducibility of left ventricular volumes by 2D echocardiography. J Am Coll Cardiol 1983; 2: 506-513
11 Perez J E, Waggoner A D, Barzilai B, Melton H E, Miller J G, Sobel B E. New edge detection algorithm facilitates 2D echocardiographic on line analysis of left ventricular performance. J Am Coll Cardiol 1991; 17: 291A (Abstract)
12 Omoto R, Kasai C. Basic principles of Doppler color flow imaging. Echocardiography 1986; 3: 463-473
13 Miyatake K, Izumi S, Okamoto M, et al. Semiquantitative grading of severity of mitral regurgitation by real time two dimensional Doppler flow imaging techniques. J Am Coll Cardiol 1986; 7: 82-88
14 Perry G J, Helmcke F, Nanda N C, Dyard C, Soto B. Evaluation of aortic insufficiency by Doppler flow mapping. J Am Coll Cardiol 1987; 9: 952-959
15 Ohman E M, Helmy S, Shaughnessy E, Adams D B, Kisslo J. In vitro analysis of jets by Doppler colour flow imaging. The importance of time to maximum jet area. Eur Heart J 1990; 11: 361-367
16 Baek K M, Bae M H, Parks B. A new aliasing extension method for ultrasonic 2 dimensional pulsed Doppler systems. Ultrasonic Imaging 1989; 11: 233-244
17 Tortolli P, Valgimigli F, Guida G. Clinical evaluation of a new anti-aliasing technique for pulsed Doppler ultrasonic analysis. Ultrasound Med Biol 1989; 15: 749-756

18 Sahn D J. Instrumentation and physical factors related to visualisation of stenotic and regurgitant jets by Doppler color flow mapping. J Am Coll Cardiol 1988; 12: 254-265
19 Simpson I A, Tamura T, Valdes-Cruz L, Murillo A, Sahn D J. Color flow mapping Doppler studies of regurgitant jets. Effect of hemodynamic variables in a pulsatile flow model. Circulation 1987; 76: IV-139 (abstract)
20 Recusani F, Bargiggia G S, Yoganathan A P, et al. A new method of quantification of regurgitant flow rate using color Doppler flow imaging of the flow convergence region proximal to a discrete orifice. An in vitro study. Circulation 1991; 83: 594-604
21 Gardiner M W, Fox M D. Colour flow ultrasound imaging through the analysis of speckle motion. Radiology 1989; 172: 866-868
22 Sutherland G R, Roelandt J R T C, Fraser A G, Anderson R H (eds). Transesophageal echocardiography in clinical practice. London: Gower Medical Publishing. 1991
23 Erbel R, Engberding R, Daniel W, et al. Echocardiography in diagnosis of aortic dissection. Lancet 1989; i: 457-461
24 Taams M A, Gussenhoven W J, Bos E, et al. Enhanced morphological diagnosis in infective endocarditis by transesophageal echocardiography. Br Heart J 1990; 63: 109-113
25 Brink R B A van den, Visser C A, Basart D C G, Dren D R, de Jong A P, Dunning A J. Comparison of transthoracic and transesophageal color Doppler flow imaging in patients with mechanical prostheses in the mitral valve position. Am J Cardiol 1989; 63: 1471-1474
26 Fraser A G, Stmper O F W, van Herwerden L A, et al. Anatomy of imaging planes used to study the mitral valve: advantages of biplane transesophageal echocardiography. Circulation 1990; 82: III-668 (abstract)
27 Stmper O, Fraser A G, Ho S Y, et al. Transoesophageal echocardiography in the longitudinal axis: correlation between anatomy and images and its clinical implications. Br Heart J 1990; 64: 282-288
28 Seward J B, Khandheria B K, Edwards W D, Oh J K, Freeman W K, Tajik A J. Biplanar transesophageal echocardiography: anatomic correlations, image orientation, and clinical applications. Mayo Clin Proc 1990; 65: 1193-1213
29 Sutherland G R, Stmper O F W, Statuch C, Ikram S, Fraser A G. Biplane transoesophageal echocardiography: valuable new diagnostic information or simply more of the same? Br Heart J 1991; 66: 74 (abstract)
30 Van de Velde M E, Sanders S P, Stanton B P. Transesophageal echocardiographic guidance for transcatheter device closure of ventricular septal defects. J Am Coll Cardiol 1991; 17: 19A (abstract)
31 Flachskampf F, Hoffman R, Hanrath P. Experience with a transoesophageal echo transducer allowing full rotation of the viewing plane – the omniplane probe. J Am Coll Cardiol 1991; 17: 34A (abstract)
32 Stmper O, Elzenga N J, Hess J, Sutherland G R. Transesophageal echocardiography in children with congenital heart disease – an initial experience. J Am Coll Cardiol 1990; 16: 433-441
33 Kaulitz R, Stmper O F W, Geuskens R, et al. Comparative values of the precordial and transesophageal approaches in the echocardiographic evaluation of atrial baffle function after an atrial correction procedure. J Am Coll Cardiol 1990; 16: 686-694
34 Stmper O, Sutherland G R, Geuskens R, Roelandt J R T C, Bos E, Hess J. Transoesophageal echocardiography in evaluation and management after a Fontan procedure. J Am Coll Cardiol 1991; 17: 1152-1160

35 Sutherland G R, Schneider B, Smyllie J H, et al. Transesophageal echocardiography – an improved diagnostic technique for 'discrete' fibromuscular subaortic obstruction in the adolescent and adult population. Circulation (in press)
36 Tuccillo B, Fraser A G. Pulmonary venous flow. In: Sutherland G R, Roelandt J R T C, Fraser A G, Anderson R H. eds. Transesophageal echocardiography in clinical practice. London, Gower Academic Publishers, 1991; 5.1–5.18
37 Dennig K, Henneke K H, Dacian S, Rudolph W. Estimation of the severity of mitral regurgitation by parameters derived from the velocity profile of pulmonary venous flow using transeosophageal Doppler technique. J Am Coll Cardiol 1990; 15: 91a (abstract)
38 Kuecherer H F, Muhiudeen I A, Kusumoto F M, et al. Estimation of mean left atrial pressure from transesophageal pulsed Doppler echocardiography of pulmonary venous flow. Circulation 1990; 82: 1127–1139
39 Appleton C P, Hatle L K, Popp R L. Relation of transmitral flow velocity patterns to left ventricular diastolic function: new insights from a combined hemodynamic and Doppler echocardiographic study. J Am Coll Cardiol 1988; 12: 426–440
40 Iliceto S, Marangelli V, Memmola C, Rizzon P. Transesophageal Doppler echocardiography evaluation of coronary blood flow velocity in baseline conditions and during dipyridamole-induced coronary vasodilation. Circulation 1991; 83: 61–69
41 Herwerden L A van, Gussenhoven W J, Roelandt J, et al. Intraoperative epicardial two-dimensional echocardiography. Eur Heart J 1986; 7: 386–395
42 Takamoto S, Kyo S, Adachi H, et al. Intraoperative color flow mapping by real-time two-dimensional Doppler echocardiography for evaluation of valvular and congenital heart disease and vascular disease. J Thorac Cardiovasc Surg 1985; 90: 802–812
43 Brommersma P, Smyllie J H, van Herwerden L A, de Jong N, Bom N, Bos E, Gussenhoven E, Roelandt J, Sutherland G R. The design, construction and clinical evaluation of small phased array transducer for intraoperative echocardiography. Med Prog Technol 1990; 16(4): 213–218
44 Sheikh K H, de Bruijn N P, Rankin J S, et al. The utility of transesophageal echocardiography and Doppler color flow imaging in patients undergoing cardiac surgery. J Am Coll Cardiol 1990; 15: 363–372
45 Stmper O, Kaulitz R, Sreeram N, et al. Intraoperative transesophageal versus epicardial ultrasound in surgery for congenital heart disease. J Am Soc Echocardiog 1990; 3: 392–401
46 Stmper O, Fraser A G, Elzenga N, et al. Assessment of ventricular septal defect closure by intraoperative epicardial ultrasound. J Am Coll Cardiol 1990; 16: 1672–1679
47 Sreeram N, Kaulitz R, Stmper O F W, Hess J, Quaegebeur J M, Sutherland G R. Comparative roles of intraoperative epicardial and early postoperative transthoracic echocardiography in the assessment of surgical repair of congenital heart defects. J Am Coll Cardiol 1990; 16: 913–920
48 Ungerleider R M, Greeley W J, Sheikh K H, et al. Routine use of intraoperative epicardial echocardiography and Doppler color flow imaging to guide and evaluate repair of congenital heart lesions. A prospective study. J Thorac Cardiovasc Surg 1990; 100: 297–309
49 van Daele M, Sutherland G R, Mitchell M M, et al. Do changes in pulmonary capillary wedge pressure adequately reflect myocardial ischemia during anesthesia? A correlative hemodynamic, electrocardiographic and transesophageal echocardiographic study. Circulation 1990; 81: 865–871
50 Smith J S, Cahalan M K, Benefiel D J, et al. Intraoperative detection of myocardial ischemia in high risk patients: electrocardiography versus two-dimensional transesophageal echocardiography. Circulation 1985; 72: 1015–1021
51 Gianrossi R, Detrano R, Mulvihill D, et al. Exercise-induced ST depression in the diagnosis of coronary artery disease. A metanalysis. Circulation 1989; 80: 87–98
52 Tennant R, Wiggers C J. The effect of coronary occlusion on myocardial contraction. Am J Physiol 1935; 112: 351–361
53 Ryan T, Vasey C G, Presti C F, O'Donnell J A, Feigenbaum H, Armstrong W F. Exercise echocardiography: detection of coronary artery disease in patients with normal left ventricular wall motion at rest. J Am Coll Cardiol 1988; 11: 993–999

54 Armstrong W F, O'Donnell J, Ryan T, Feigenbaum H. Effect of prior myocardial infarction and extent and location of coronary disease on the accuracy of exercise echocardiography. J Am Coll Cardiol 1987; 10: 531–538
55 Sheikh K H, Bengston J R, Helmy S. Relation of quantitative coronary lesion measurements to the development of exercise induced ischaemia assessed by exercise echocardiography. J Am Coll Cardiol 1990; 15: 1043–1051
56 Picano E, Lattanzi F, Orlandini A, Marini C, L'Abbate A. Stress echocardiography and the human factor: the importance of being expert. J Am Coll Cardiol 1991; 17: 666–669
57 McHenry P L, Phillips J S, Knoebel S B. Correlation of computer quantitated treadmill exercise electrocardiogram with arteriographic location of coronary artery disease. Am J Cardiol 1972; 30: 747–782
58 Rigo P, Bailey I K, Griffith L S C et al. Value and limitations of segmental analysis of stress thallium myocardial imaging for localisation of coronary artery disease. Circulation 1980; 61: 973–981
59 Pozzoli M M, Fioretti P M, Salustri A, Reijs A E, Roelandt J R. Exercise echocardiography and technetium-99m MIBI single-photon emission computed tomography in the detection of coronary artery disease. Am J Cardiol 1991; 67: 350–355
60 Oberman A, Fan P H, Nanda N C et al. Reproducibility of two dimensional exercise echocardiography. J Am Coll Cardiol 1989; 14: 923–928
61 Iliceto S, Amico A F, Tota F, et al. Echocardiography during transesophageal atrial pacing. In: Iliceto S, Rizzon P, Roelandt J R T C eds. Ultrasound in coronary artery disease. Dordrecht, Kluwer Academic Publishers, 1991: 37–48
62 Iliceto S, Sorino M, D'Ambrosio G, et al. Detection of coronary artery disease by two-dimensional echocardiography and transesophageal atrial pacing. J Am Coll Cardiol 1985; 5: 1188–1197
63 Lambertz H, Kreis A, Trmper H, Hanrath P. Simultaneous transesophageal atrial pacing and transesophageal two-dimensional echocardiography: a new method of stress echocardiography. J Am Coll Cardiol 1990; 16: 1143–1153
64 DeGraff A C, Lyon A F. Evaluation of dipyridamole. Am Heart J 1963; 64: 423–424
65 Margonato O A, Chierchia S, Cianflane D et al. Limitations of dipyridamole echocardiography in effort angina pectoris. Am J Cardiol 1987; 59: 225–230
66 Josephson R A, Weiss J L, Flaherty J T, Ouyang P, Shapiro E P. Dipyridamole echocardiography detects vulnerable myocardium in the early post infarct period. Circulation 1986; 74: II, 469
67 Picano E. Dipyridamole echocardiography test: historical background and physiologic basis. Eur Heart J 1989; 10: 366–376
68 Nguyen T, Jaekyeong H, Ogilby D, et al. Single photon emission computed tomography with thallium 201 during adenosine induced coronary hyperaemia. Correlation with coronary arteriography exercise thallium imaging and two dimensional echocardiography. J Am Coll Cardiol 1990; 16: 1375–1383
69 Pierard L A, De Landsheere C M, Berthe C. Identification of viable myocardium by echocardiography during dobutamine infusions in patients with myocardial infarction after thrombolytic therapy. Comparison with positron emission tomography. J Am Coll Cardiol 1990; 15: 1021–1031
70 Labovitz A J, Lewen M, Kern M J, et al. The effects of successful PTCA on left ventricular function. Assessment by exercise echocardiography. Am Heart J 1989; 117: 1003
71 Broderick T, Sawada S, Armstrong W F, et al. Improvement in rest and exercise induced wall motion abnormalities after coronary angioplasty. An exercise echocardiographic study. J Am Coll Cardiol 1990; 15: 591–599
72 Keren G, Katz S, Strom J, Sonnenblick E H, LeJemtel T H. Dynamic mitral regurgitation. An important determinant of the hemodynamic response to load alterations and inotropic therapy in severe heart failure. Circulation 1989; 80: 306–313
73 Gramiak R, Shah P M. Echocardiography of the aortic root. Invest Radiol 1968; 3: 356–358
74 Feinstein S B, Cheirif J, Ten Cate F J, et al. Safety and efficacy of a new transpulmonary ultrasound contrast agent: initial multicenter clinical results. J Am Coll Cardiol 1990; 16: 316–324
75 Smith M D, Elion S L, McLure R R, Kwan O C, Demaria A N.

Left heart opacification with peripheral venous injection of a new saccaride echo contrast agent in dogs. J Am Coll Cardiol 1989; 13: 1622–1628

76 Keller M W, Glasheen W, Smucker M L, Burwell L R, Watson D D, Kaul S. Myocardial contrast echocardiography in humans. Assessment of coronary blood flow reserve. J Am Coll Cardiol 1988; 12: 925–934

77 Cheirif J, Zoghbi W A, Minor S T et al. Assessment of myocardial perfusion in humans by contrast echocardiography. Evaluation of regional coronary reserve by peak contrast intensity. J Am Coll Cardiol 1988; 11: 735–743

78 Reisner S A, Ong L S, Lichtenberg G S, et al. Quantitative assessment of the immediate results of coronary angioplasty by myocardial contrast echocardiography. J Am Coll Cardiol 1989; 13: 852–856

79 Vered Z, Barzilai B, Mohr G A, et al. Quantitative ultrasonic tissue characterisation with real-time integrated backscatter imaging in normal human subjects and patients with dilated cardiomyopathy. Circulation 1987; 76: 1067–1073

80 Milunski M R, Mohr G A, Perez J E, et al. Ultrasonic tissue characterisation with integrated backscatter. Circulation 1989; 80: 491–503

81 Vered Z, Mohr G A, Gessler C J. Ultrasound integrated backscatter tissue characterisation of remote myocardial infarction in human subjects. J Am Coll Cardiol 1989; 13: 84–91

82 Wickline S A, Thomas L J, Miller J G, Sobel B E, Perez J E. Sensitive detection of the effects of reperfusion on myocardium by ultrasonic tissue characterisation with integrated backscatter. Circulation 1986; 74: 389–400

83 Milunski W C, Mohr G A, Wear K A, Sobel B E, Perez J E, Wickline S A. Early detection with integrated ultrasonic backscatter of viable but stunned myocardium in dogs. J Am Coll Cardiol 1989; 14: 462–471

84 Wickline S A, Thomas L S, Miller J G, Sobel B E, Perez J E. The dependence of myocardial ultrasonic backscatter on contractile performance. Circulation 1985; 72: 183–192

85 Glueck R M, Mottley J G, Sobel B E, Miller J G, Perez J E. Changes in ultrasonic attenuation and backscatter of muscle with the state of contraction. Ultrasound Med Biol 1985; 11: 605–610

86 Krishnaswamy C, Aylward P E, Fleagle S R, et al. Feasibility of identifying amyloid and hypertrophic cardiomyopathy with the use of computerised quantitative texture analysis of clinical echocardiographic data. J Am Coll Cardiol 1989; 13: 832–840

87 Tanaka M, Fujiwara H, Onodera T, et al. Quantitative analysis of myocardial fibrosis in normals, hypertensive hearts and hypertrophic cardiomyopathy. Br Heart J 1986; 55: 575–581

88 Sibley D H, Millar H D, Hartley C J, Whitlow P L. Subselective measurement of coronary blood flow velocity using a steerable Doppler catheter. J Am Coll Cardiol 1986; 8: 1332–1340

89 Hartley C J, Millar H D. Ultrasonic sensors for measuring coronary blood flow. Society of Photo Optical Engineers Symposium, Los Angeles, 1988

90 Hodgson J M C B, Cohen M D, Szentpetery S, Thames M D. Effects of regional a and b blockade on resting and hyperaemic coronary blood flow in conscious unstressed humans. Circulation 1989; 79: 797–809

91 Eichorn E J, Grayburn P A, Anderson H V, Bedotto J B, Carry M M, Willerson J J. Cyclic coronary artery flow variations before and after percutaneous transluminal coronary angioplasty in man. Circulation 1989; 80: II, 371. (abstract)

92 Tanouchi J, Kitabatake A, Ischihara K, et al. Experimental validation of Doppler catheter technique using fast fourier spectrum analysis for measuring coronary flow velocity. Circulation 1989; 80: II, 566

93 Denardo S J, Yock P G, Srebro J P, et al. Measurement of coronary blood flow turbulence post PTCA and coronary atherectomy. Circulation 1989; 80: II, 371 (abstract)

94 Bom N, Roelandt J (eds). Intravascular ultrasound. Techniques, developments, clinical perspectives. Dordrecht: Kluwer Academic Publishers, 1989

95 Gussenhoven W J, Bom N, Roelandt J (eds). Intravascular ultrasound 1991. Dordrecht: Kluwer Academic Publishers, 1991

96 Gurley J C, Nissen S E, Diaz C, et al. Is the trilayer arterial appearance an artifact? Differences between in vivo and in vitro intravascular ultrasound. J Am Coll Cardiol 1991; 17: 112A (abstract)

97 Junbo G, Erbel R, Seidel I. Controversial conclusion of the wall structure in intravascular ultrasound imaging. J Am Coll Cardiol 1991; 17: 112A (abstract)

98 Cacchione J, Nair R, Hodgson J McB. Intracoronary ultrasound better than conventional methods for determining optimal PTCA balloon size. J Am Coll Cardiol 1991; 17: 112A (abstract)

99 Chandrasekeran K, Seligal C M, Hsu T, et al. Three dimensional intravascular ultrasound imaging of arterial atherosclerosis and its complications. J Am Coll Cardiol 1991; 17: 233A (abstract)

100 Rosenfield K, Harding M, Pieczek A. 3 dimensional reconstruction of balloon dilated coronary renal and femoro-popliteal arteries from 2D intravascular ultrasound images. J Am Coll Cardiol 1991; 17: 234A (abstract).

101 Bom N, Lancee C T, Van Egmond F C, et al. An ultrasonic intracardiac scanner. Ultrasonics 1972; 10: 72–76

102 Schwartz S, Weintraub A, Pandian N, et al. Percutaneous and intraoperative intracardiac echocardiography in humans with the use of a small size (6F) low frequency (12.5 MHz) ultrasound catheter with expanded depth of field. J Am Coll Cardiol 1991; 17: 94A (abstract)

103 Handschumacher M D, Weyman A E, Lethor J P, Levine R A. Three dimensional echocardiography. A new method for real time integration and computer storage of images and positional data in high volume. J Am Coll Cardiol 1991; 17: 3A (abstract)

104 Mensah G A, Pini R, Monnini E, et al. Three dimensional echocardiographic reconstruction. Experimental validation of volume measurement. J Am Coll Cardiol 1991; 17: 291A (abstract)

105 Meltzer R S, Schwarz K Q, Mottley J G, Everbach E C. Therapeutic cardiac ultrasound. Am J Cardiol 1991; 67: 422–424

106 Ariani M, Fishbein M C, Siegel R S. Angioscopically guided dissolution of arterial thrombi by ultrasound. J Am Coll Cardiol 1991; 17: 178 (abstract)

107 Schwinger M E, Colvin S, Harty S, Feiner H, Opitz L, Kronzon K. Clinical evaluation of high-frequency (ultrasonic) mechanical debridement in the surgical treatment of calcific aortic stenosis. Am Heart J 1990; 120: 1320–1325

108 Leithe M E, Harrison J K, Davidson C J, Jones R H, Kisslo K, Bashore T M. Surgical aortic valvuloplasty and decalcification using the Cavitron Ultrasonic Surgical Aspirator: long-term hemodynamic and angiographic follow-up. J Am Coll Cardiol 1990; 15: 179A (abstract)

Index

Page numbers in **bold type** indicate main discussions; those in *italics* indicate figures.

Abdominal cysts, 337, *339*
Abdominal views
 congenital heart disease, 309, 311, 312
 sagittal, *311*, 312
 transverse upper, 50, *51*, 311, *312*
Abscess
 amoebic liver, 292–293
 aortic root, see Aortic root, abscess
 perivalvular, 216–218, *219*, *220*, 221
Acceleration
 convective, 82, 85, 99
 proximal flow, colour flow mapping, 99–100, *101*
 spatial flow, colour flow mapping, 100, *101*
 temporal or local, 82
Acceleration slope, coarctation of aorta, 401
Acceleration time (AT)
 corrected, coarctation of aorta, 401
 pulmonary artery, 111, 174
Acceleration time/ejection time (AT/ET) ratio, pulmonary artery, 111
Acoustic dynamic range, 36
Acquired immunodeficiency syndrome (AIDS), myocarditis, 484
Adenosine, 531
Afterload, 67
Age
 cardiac output and, 122
 left ventricular function and, 75
Air emboli, intracardiac, intraoperative detection, **143–144**
Albunex (sonicated albumin), 532
Aliasing, **21–22**, 32, 63–64
 aortic regurgitation, *168*, 169
 colour flow mapping and, 23, 37–38, 99, *100*
 mitral regurgitation, *159*, 161
 mitral stenosis, 157, *159*
 pressure drop estimation and, 85
 'unwrapping', quantitative colour flow mapping, 99–100, 523
Alpha-galactosidase A deficiency (Fabry's disease), 480
A-mode display, **16–17**
Amoebic liver abscess, 292–293
Amplitude, ultrasound waves, 11
Amyl nitrite inhalation, 531
Amyloidosis, cardiac, **204–205**, 301, *302*, 486
 Doppler findings, 207
 tissue characterisation, 183, 533
 vs. hypertrophic cardiomyopathy, 199
Aneurysms
 aortic, 137, 167, **278**, *279*, 285–286
 atrial septum, 347–348
 congenital sub-mitral, 299
 coronary arteries, *335*, 336, 503–504
 false, see Pseudo-aneurysms
 left ventricle, 181, **184**
 mycotic, **285**
 sinus of Valsalva, 217, 220, *282*, **286**
 vein of Galen, 461, *462*
 ventricular septal defects, 361–362
Angiography, 513
 coarctation of aorta, 402
 coronary artery, 516
 valvular regurgitation, 102
Angioplasty, coronary, 531, **535–536**
Angiosarcoma, cardiac, 251–252
Angle of beam incidence, 19, *20*, 24, 37, 53
 colour flow mapping, 23

correction, 86–87, 392
 mitral pressure half-time estimation and, 93
 pressure drop estimation, 86–87
Ankylosing spondylitis, 167
Annular phased array scanheads, **31**
Annuloaortic ectasia, **285–286**
Anthracycline cardiomyopathy, *482*, **485**
Antibiotic prophylaxis, 133
Anticoagulation, 297
Aorta, **275–286**, 318, *319*
 abdominal
  coarctation, 399–400
  dissection, 278, *280*
 ascending, 136, 277
  aortic arch interruption, 403
  diameter, 116–117, 277
  dissection, 278, 279, 280–283
  Doppler examination, 56–57, *58*, 59
  flow velocities, 182–183
  hypoplastic left heart syndrome, 328, *329*, 395, 396–397
  pulmonary arteries arising from, 331, *332*, 377–378
  right parasternal view, 52–53
  suprasternal view, 51, 52
  supravalve aortic stenosis, 394
 coarctation, see Coarctation of aorta
 descending, 277
  atrial arrangement and, 311
  Doppler examination, 56–57, *58*
  flow reversal, 169, 170, 372
  flow velocities in coarctation, 400, 401
  right, with left aortic arch, 492
  suprasternal view, 51, 52
  transverse upper abdominal view, 50, *51*
 diameters, 116–117, 277
  dissection, 280
  Marfan's syndrome, 285–286
 dilatation, **278**
  annuloaortic ectasia, 285–286
  dissection, 280
  post-stenotic, coarctation, 399
 flow patterns, *116*, 117
 hypoplastic, hypoplastic left heart syndrome, 328, *329*, 395
 overriding
  double outlet right ventricle, 420
  tetralogy of Fallot, 319, *320*, 434, 435
  ventricular septal defects, 365, *366*
 parasternal views, 46
 surgically repaired transposition, 419
 transoesophageal imaging, 136, **137–138**, 277
 transposition of great arteries, 409–410, 423
 volumetric flow estimation, **115–119**
Aortic aneurysms, 137, 167, **278**, *279*
 annuloaortic ectasia, 285–286
 mycotic, **285**
 traumatic, **285**
Aortic arch, 277
 congenital anomalies, 328–330, **491–492**
 Doppler examination, 56–57, *58*
 double, 332, *333*, 491–492, 493
 hypoplasia, 403
 interruption, 96, 330, **403**, 492
  associated abnormalities, 377, 425
  classification, 403
 left, 328, *329*
  with right descending aorta, 492
  pulmonary atresia with intact ventricular septum, 441
 right, 328–330, 492, 493
  with truncus arteriosus, 376, *378*
 suprasternal view, 51, 52

tetralogy of Fallot, 436
 transposition of great arteries, 416–417, 425
 velocity profiles, 117
Aortic dissection, **278–285**
 annuloaortic ectasia, 285
 conditions associated with, 279
 haemopericardium, 269, 284
 intraoperative epivascular imaging, 528, *530*
 transoesophageal imaging, 137–138, 284–285
 type A (De Bakey types 1 and 2), 279
 type B (De Bakey type 3), 279
Aortic regurgitation, **166–170**, 175
 aortic aneurysms, 278
 aortic dissection, 284
 developing countries, 297
 Doppler examination, 57
 hypertrophic cardiomyopathy, 478
 infective endocarditis, 167, 219, 301
 physiological, *160*, 164
 prosthetic valves, 234–235
 quantitative colour flow mapping, 101
 surgically repaired transposition, 419
 ventricular septal defects, 360, 362–363
 volumetric flow estimation, 125
Aortic root
 abscess, 216–218, *219*, *220*, 300, 301, *339*
 aneurysms, 167, 278
 calcification, 163, 164
 cross-sectional area, 73, 116
 diameter, 63, 116, 277
 dissection, 278
 parasternal views, 46–47, *48*
 post-stenotic dilatation, 164
 supravalve aortic stenosis, 394
Aortic rupture
 annuloaortic ectasia, 285
 traumatic, 269, **285**
Aortic stenosis
 acquired, **164–166**, 175
 aortic valve area estimation, **90–91**
 calcific, 164, 299, *300*
 congenital, 164, **389–394**
 congenital valvular, 389, **390–392**
 Doppler examination, 56, 57, *59*, 391–392
 flow jets, 83
 hypertrophic cardiomyopathy, 478
 pressure drops, 82, 86, **88–90**, 97, 166, 391
 quantitative Doppler, **88–91**, 123–124
 subvalve, see Subaortic stenosis
 supravalve, 389, **394**
 ultrasonic therapy, 536
 volumetric flow estimation, 123–124
Aortic valve, **162–170**
 annulus, diameter, 117–118, 277
 aortic dissection involving, 280–283
 atresia
  hypoplastic left heart syndrome, 395
  transposition of great arteries, 425
 balloon valvuloplasty, 143
 bicuspid, 163, 164, 167, **389–390**
 calcification, 164
 coarctation of aorta, 398
 Doppler examination, 53, **56–57**
 flow patterns, *116*, 117
 flow velocities, 116, 118–119
  aortic regurgitation, 169–170
  aortic stenosis, 166, 391
  bicuspid valve, 390
  cardiac tamponade, 267
  left ventricular function and, 73–75
 prosthetic valves, 233–234

Aortic valve (contd)
    hypoplastic left heart syndrome, 395
    infective endocarditis, 211–214, 219, 301
    normal, 162–164
    orifice area
        aortic stenosis, **90–91**, 123–124, 391
        prosthetic valves, 232–233
        transoesophageal echocardiography, 141
    orifice dimension, 116, **117–118**
        aortic stenosis, 390–391
    parasternal views, 46–47, 48
    premature closure
        aortic dissection, 280
        dilated cardiomyopathy, 202
        hypertrophic cardiomyopathy, 193, 194
        mitral regurgitation, 161
    prolapse of right coronary cusp, 327, *328*, 362
    subcostal four chamber view, 51, *52*
    transoesophageal imaging, 134, 135
    volumetric flow estimation, **115–119**
Aortic valve prostheses
    area estimation, 233
    developing countries, 301
    Doppler evaluation, 232, **233–235**
    infective endocarditis, 221
    transoesophageal studies, 142, *143*
Aortopulmonary collateral arteries, 437, 438
Aortopulmonary window, 331–332, **378–379**, *380*
Apex, cardiac
    cardiac position and, 312
    parasternal long axis view, 46
Apex cardiogram
    digitised, 73, 75
    synchronous M-mode echocardiogram, 181
Apex cardiogram/left ventricular dimension loop, *72*, 73
Apical views
    'five chamber', 49, *50*, 56, 62
    four chamber, 48–49, *50*, 53–56, 62
    two chamber (long axis), 50, 56, 62
Apical window, 45, **48–50**, 277
Area measurements, 33
Artefacts, **24–26**, 37
Arterial duct, patent, *see* Patent ductus arteriosus
Arterial switch operations, transposition, 419
Arterial trunk
    common, *see* Truncus arteriosus
    solitary, 319, 321
Arteries
    great, *see* Great arteries
    intravascular Doppler, 533–535
    intravascular imaging, 535–536
Arteriovenous malformations, 337, 345, 461, *462*
Ascites, 337
Asplenia, 314
Atheromatous plaques, intravascular imaging, 535, 536
Atherosclerosis, 140–141, 278
Athletes, 76, 199
Atrial appendages, 310
Atrial arrangement, *see* Atrial situs
Atrial dominance, atrioventricular septal defects, 358
Atrial enlargement
    endomyocardial fibrosis, 205
    restrictive cardiomyopathy, 204, 486
Atrial fibrillation
    mitral pressure half-time estimation, 94
    mitral stenosis, 156, 297

thrombus formation, 255
Atrial isomerism, 310
    atrioventricular septal defects, 359
    left, 311–312, *466*, 467–468
    pulmonary venous connections, *465*, *466*, 467–468
    right, 312, *465*, 467, 468
    systemic venous connections and, 313, 314
Atrial pacing, echocardiography and, 39, **530**, *531*
Atrial redirection operations, transposition of great arteries, 355, **417–419**
Atrial septal defects, 321–322, 343, **344–355**
    assessing shunt size, 125, 355
    associated abnormalities, 352–354
    coronary sinus, 343, *349*, 352, *353*
    Ebstein's anomaly, 442
    foramen ovale (secundum), 301, 322, *323*, 343, **347–349**, *350*, 354–355
    iatrogenic, **352**, *354*, 412–413
    postoperative appearances, 354–355
    primum, 323–324, 343, 356
    right heart volume overload, 344–347
    sinus venosus, 322, *323*, 343, *349*, *351*, 466
    total anomalous pulmonary venous drainage, 458
    transoesophageal imaging, 141, 352
    univentricular atrioventricular connection, 451–452
Atrial septectomy, 352
Atrial septostomy, balloon, 352, *354*, **412–413**
Atrial septum, 322, **343–344**
    aneurysms, 347–348
    apical four chamber view, 49
    hypoplastic left heart syndrome, 396
    normal, 343–344
    subcostal four chamber view, 50–51
Atrial situs (arrangement), **310–312**
    ambiguous, *see* Atrial isomerism
    corrected transposition of great arteries, 422
    mirror image (inversus), 310, 311
    usual (solitus), 310, 311
Atrioventricular connection, **315–317**
    absent, 451–452
    ambiguous, 315–317
    concordant, 315, *316*, *317*
    criss-cross, and superior-inferior ventricles, *425*, *426*
    discordant, 315, *316*, *317*
        concordant ventriculo-arterial connection, 426, *427*
        corrected transposition of great arteries, 422–425
        double outlet right ventricle, 425–426
    univentricular, 317, *318*, *319*, **447–453**
Atrioventricular septal defects, 323–324, *325*, **355–360**
    assessing shunt size/pulmonary artery pressure, 360
    associated abnormalities, 359
    atrioventricular junction abnormalities, 356–357
    complete, 323, 356, 450–451
    haemodynamics, 359
    partial, 323–324, 356
    postoperative appearances, 359–360
    transposition of great arteries, 417
    ventricular abnormalities, 357–359
Atrioventricular septum, **322–324**, 355
Atrioventricular valves
    atresias, 317, *319*

atrioventricular septal defects, 324, *325*, 356, 357
    common, 357, 449, 450, 451
    overriding, 363, 414, 451
    regurgitant, atrioventricular septal defects, 359
    straddling, 363, **414**, *415*
    transposition of great arteries, 422–423, 424
    univentricular atrioventricular connection, 317, *318*, *319*, 449–451
    ventricular septal defects and, 327–328, 363
    see also Mitral valve; Tricuspid valve
Atrium
    double outlet, 358
    superior vena cava draining into, 313, *314*
    thrombus formation, *254*, 255–256
    see also Left atrium; Right atrium
Attenuation, **15–16**
Audio Doppler signal, 21
    patent ductus arteriosus, 372
    regurgitant mitral prosthetic valves, 236
Autocorrelation, colour flow mapping, 22–23
A wave, hypertrophic cardiomyopathy, 199, *200*
Azygos vein, 311
    pulmonary venous drainage to, 460

Backscatter, integrated, 532–533
Bacterial endocarditis, *see* Endocarditis, infective
Bacterial infections, post-infarction, 188
Balloon atrial septostomy, 352, *354*, **412–413**
Balloon valvuloplasty, aortic, 143
Basal short axis view, **134**, *135*
Baseline shift, Doppler systems, 63
Beam, ultrasound
    angle, *see* Angle of beam incidence
    shapes, 13
    sweeping/steering methods, 18
    width effects, 26
Becker's muscular dystrophy, 485
Beckwith–Wiedemann syndrome, 480
Beriberi, 485
Bernoulli equation, 82
    extended, **82**
    modified (simplified), **85**, 124
        pitfalls, 97, 513–514
    prosthetic heart valves and, 231, 232
Bioprosthetic heart valves, 225
    causes of failure, 226
    Doppler evaluation, 231, 232, 235–236
    M-mode and cross-sectional imaging, 227, *228*, 229
Biopsy, right atrium, 143
Biplane transoesophageal echocardiography, 39, **145–146**, 525–526
Bjork–Shiley prosthetic valve, 225
    Doppler evaluation, 232, 237–239
    M-mode and cross-sectional imaging, 226, 227, 229–230
Blalock Hanlon procedure, 352
Blalock–Taussig shunt, modified, 515
Blood flow
    beam angle and, *see* Angle of beam incidence
    patterns, **19–20**
    velocity, *see* Velocity, flow
Brachiocephalic (innominate) arteries, 51, *52*
    anomalous origin, 492
    aortic dissection involving, 278, *280*

Brachiocephalic (innominate) arteries (contd)
  ductus arteriosus arising from, 331
Brachiocephalic (innominate) veins, *52*, 313
  retro-aortic, 313–314
  total anomalous pulmonary venous
    drainage, 459, *460*
Breast carcinoma, 252
Bronchogenic carcinoma, 252
Bullet formula, 33
Burstin nomogram, 368

Calcification
  aortic root, 163, 164
  aortic valve, 164
  constrictive pericarditis, 293
  mitral valve annulus, 155, 197, *198*, 201
Carcinoid disease, **253**
  pulmonary valve, 174, 253
  tricuspid valve, 171, 172, 253
Cardiac arrhythmias/dysrhythmias
  cardiac tumours, 250
  dilated cardiomyopathy, 202, 485
  ischaemic heart disease, 184
Cardiac catheterisation
  aortic stenosis, 166, 391
  atrioventricular septal defects, 359
  congenital heart disease, 515–516
  disadvantages, 513
  pressure drop estimation, 87–88, 90, 92, 95, 97
  prosthetic heart valve assessment, 232
  pulmonary artery pressure measurement, 110
Cardiac chambers, congenital heart disease, **321–322**
Cardiac index, 122
Cardiac masses, **243–257**
  differential diagnosis, 216, 256–257
  transoesophageal imaging, **138–140**
Cardiac output (CO), 68, 115, **122–123**
  aortic orifice flow and, 73, 91, 115–119
  mitral orifice flow and, 73, 119–122
  transoesophageal measurement, 145
Cardiac position, 312
Cardiac surgery
  developing countries, 291
  intraoperative echocardiography, 143–145, 527–528
  pericardial effusions, 269
  septal motion after, 228–229
Cardiac tamponade, **263–267**
  amoebic liver abscess, 292–293
  aortic disease, 269
  developing countries, 292–293, *294*
  post-traumatic/post-surgical, 269
  pyopericardium, 268
Cardiac transplantation, chronic rejection, 486
Cardiac tumours, **245–253**, 337, *338*
  benign, 245–251
  differential diagnosis, 257
  malignant, 245, 251–252
  primary, 245–252
  secondary, 245, 252–253
  transoesophageal imaging, 138–139, 246–247, *248*, 249
Cardiac valves
  Doppler examination technique, 53–56
  infective endocarditis, 211–214
  reconstructive surgery, transoesophageal echocardiography, 144
  regurgitant, see Regurgitation, valvular
  stenosed, see Stenoses, valvular
  see also Atrioventricular valves; Valvular heart disease; specific valves
Cardiomyopathy, **191–207**
  childhood, 336–337, **473–486**
  definition, 475
  developing countries, 291
  dilated (congestive), 193, **201–204**
    causes in childhood, 484–485
    children, 336–337, **481–485**
    developing countries, **299–300**
    differential diagnosis, 202–203
    echocardiographic findings, 202, 481–484
    intracardiac flow and embolisation, 203
    mitral regurgitation, 157, 201, 483
    prognostic indicators, 203–204
    thrombus formation, 203, 254, 299–300, 482
  hypertrophic, 166, *167*, **193–201**
    associated abnormalities in children, 478–479
    association with cardiac malformations/systemic diseases, 479–481
    children, *337*, **475–481**
    differential diagnosis, 198–199, 250
    Doppler findings, 199–201, 477–478, 515
    elderly, 197, *198*
    familial, 475
    mitral apparatus, 197–198
    myocardial features, 193–197
    subaortic stenosis, 164, 165
    tissue characterisation, 533
  restrictive, 193, **204–207**
    children, **485–486**
    Doppler echocardiography, 205–207, 486
    idiopathic, 486
    vs. pericardial constriction, 270, 295
Cardiopulmonary bypass, 527, 528
Carnitine deficiency, 337, 485
Carnitine metabolism, disorders in infancy, 480
Carotid artery, common
  right, aortic dissection involving, *280*
  suprasternal view, 51, *52*
Carpentier–Edwards prosthetic valve, *225*, 231, *236*
Catheter embolus, intracardiac, 143
Central venous pressure, cardiac tamponade, 266
Chagas' disease, 203, 486
Chart recorders, 35
Chest trauma, see Trauma
Children, 515
  acquired abnormalities, **336–340**
  aortic orifice diameter, 116–117
  cardiac tumours, 249–251
  cardiomyopathy, 336–337, **473–486**
  examination technique, 309–310
  transoesophageal imaging, 141, 527
Chloral hydrate, 309
Cineloop (cine review), 34, 309
Circumferential fibre shortening, left ventricular, see Left ventricle, circumferential fibre shortening
Clarity, image, 24
Clinical view, **511–517**
Coarctation of aorta, 330, **398–403**
  annuloaortic ectasia, 285
  associated abnormalities, 377, 421, 425
  classification, 398
  Doppler examination, 56–57, **400–403**
  hypoplastic left heart syndrome, 396–397
  imaging, 398–400
  pressure drop estimation, **96–97**, 400–401
  quantitative colour flow mapping, 97–98
Coefficient of orifice contraction, 83
Colour flow mapping, 153
  aortic dissection, 280, *281*, *282*
  aortic stenosis, 391, 393–394
  aortic valve, 164, 165–166, *168*, 169
  atrial septal defects, 349
  autocorrelation method, 22–23
  coarctation of aorta, 96–97, 402
  congenital heart disease, 517
  determination of jet direction, 86, *87*
  dilated cardiomyopathy, 203, 482–483
  equipment, 29, **32–33**
  examination technique, 55, 56, 57–58
  history, 7
  hypertrophic cardiomyopathy, 199, 200–201, *477*, 478
  image recordings, 35
  mitral valve, 154, 156, 157, *159*, *160*, 161
  patent ductus arteriosus, 372–373
  practical aspects, 37–38
  principles, **22–24**
  prosthetic heart valves, 231, 234–235, 236, *237*, 239
  pulmonary valve, *173*, 174, 175
  quantitative, 86, **97–102**, 514, **522–523**
    basic principles, 98–101
    clinical applications, 101–102
  recent advances, **522–525**
  transoesophageal echocardiography, 137, *138*, 142
  tricuspid valve, 171–172, *173*
  ventricular septal defects, 366
Colour M-mode imaging, 524
'Colour velocity imaging', 525
Common arterial trunk, see Truncus arteriosus
Computer disks, image storage, 34, 35
Computerised tomography, aortic dissection, 283
Congenital heart disease
  clinical aspects, **515–517**
  contrast echocardiography, 531–532
  coronary artery anomalies, 333–336, **500–506**
  Doppler echocardiography, 309–310, 340, 516–517
  examination technique, 309–310
  great arterial anomalies, **489–493**
  hypertrophic cardiomyopathy and, 479
  image orientation, 310
  intraoperative echocardiography, 527, 528
  left sided obstructions, **387–403**
  left to right shunts, 321, 322, **341–379**
  right sided obstructions and malformations, **429–444**
  sequential segmental approach, **307–340**
  transoesophageal imaging, 141, 527
  univentricular atrioventricular connection, **447–453**
  venous anomalies, **455–471**
  ventriculo-arterial discordance, **407–426**
Connective tissue disorders, dilated cardiomyopathy, 485
Continuity principle (equation), 81, 123
  aortic valve area estimation, 91, **123–124**
  prosthetic heart valves, 232–233
  subaortic stenosis, 394

Continuous wave (CW) Doppler
  aortic stenosis, 391
  aortic valve, 164, 166, 167, 170
  congenital heart disease, 516
  equipment, 29, **32**
  examination technique, 55, 56
  hypertrophic cardiomyopathy, 200
  mitral valve, 154, 157, 162
  patent ductus arteriosus, 372, *373*
  physics and principles, 20–21
  practical aspects, 37
  pressure drop estimation, 85, 86, 88–90, 95–96, 513
  prosthetic heart valves, 231, 233–234, 235–239
  pulmonary valve, 175
  'stand-alone', 32, 55
  'steerable', 32, 55
  tricuspid valve, 171, 172
  ventricular septal defects, 369
  volumetric flow estimation, 118
Contrast echocardiography
  atrial septal defects, 349
  coronary arteries, 184, 505–506, 532
  developing countries, 291, 301
  intraoperative, 528
  ischaemic heart disease, **183–184**
  recent advances, **531–532**
  sinus of Valsalva aneurysms, 286
  surgical repair of transposition, 418–419
  tricuspid regurgitation, 109, 301
Contrast media, echocardiographic, 532
Contrast resolution, 24, 36
Control optimisation, **59–64**
Convective acceleration, 82, 85, 99–100
Coronary angioplasty, 531, 535–536
Coronary artery(ies), **495–507**
  anatomical variations, 500–501
  aneurysms, *335, 336,* 503–504
  congenital anomalies, 333–336, **500–506**
    tetralogy of Fallot, 336, 436, 501, **502–503**
    transposition of great arteries, 334–336, 410, **501–502**
  contrast echocardiography, 184, 505–506, 532
  dilatation, *334, 335,* 505
    coronary artery fistula, 506
    Kawasaki disease, 336, 504
    supravalve aortic stenosis, 394
  embolism, infective endocarditis, 214–215
  fistula, **506**
  intravascular Doppler, 533–535
  intravascular imaging, 40, 535–536
  ischaemic heart disease, 140–141, 181, 500
  left, 333, **497–498,** 500
    arising from pulmonary trunk, 334, *335,* 482–483, **504–506**
    stenosis/atresia, 507
    transposition of great arteries, 501
  left anterior descending, 333, *497,* **498,** 500
    arising from pulmonary trunk, 506
    arising from right coronary artery, 436
    Doppler recordings, 527
  left circumflex, 333, *497,* **498,** *499,* 500
    transposition of great arteries, 501–502
  normal appearances, **497–500**
  problems in imaging, 499–500, 516
  right, 333, *334, 497,* **498–499**
    arising from pulmonary trunk, 506
    transposition of great arteries, 502
  stress echocardiography, 529–531
  three-dimensional reconstruction, 536

transoesophageal imaging, 134, 140–141, 500, 504
transposition of great arteries, 410
Coronary artery bypass grafting, 144–145
Coronary artery disease, *see* Ischaemic heart disease
Coronary blood flow
  contrast echocardiography, 184, 532
  intravascular Doppler, 534–536
Coronary-cameral fistulae, 334
Coronary sinus
  dilatation, 349, *352, 353, 468,* 469
  fistula, 349
  left superior vena cava draining into, 313
  pulmonary venous drainage to, *457,* 461, *462*
Cor pulmonale, 301, 302
Cor triatriatum, 354, *466, 467,* **468–469**
Cross-sectional imaging (real-time, two-dimensional imaging), 29
  anomalous pulmonary venous drainage, 457–458
  aorta, 277
  aortic dissection, 280–283
  aortic stenosis, 390–391, 392–393
  aortic valve, 162–163
  bicuspid aortic valve, 390
  cardiac tumours, 246, 248–249
  cardiomyopathy, 193–197, 202
  coarctation of aorta, 398–400
  combined with M-mode imaging, 18–19
  congenital heart disease, 309–310, 515–516
  control optimisation, 59–61
  developing countries, 291
  digitised images, 522, *523*
  dilated cardiomyopathy, 202, 481–482
  examination technique, **46–53**
  history, 5, 6
  hypertrophic cardiomyopathy, 193–198, 475–476
  hypoplastic left heart syndrome, 395
  imaging resolution, 521–522
  infective endocarditis, 211, 214
  intracardiac thrombi, 253–254, 255, 256
  mitral stenosis, 155
  patent ductus arteriosus, 370–371
  pericardial disease, 261–262, 270, 292
  principles, **17–19**
  prosthetic heart valves, **226–231**
  pulmonary stenosis, 431–432
  restrictive cardiomyopathy, 204–205, 486
  transoesophageal echocardiography, 131, **134–136**
  transposition of great arteries, 409–411
  truncus arteriosus, 375
  univentricular atrioventricular connection, 449–453
  ventricular septal defects, 361, 368–369
  volume calculations, 33
Crosstalk, 37, 63
Cyclophosphamide-induced myocarditis, *484,* 485
Cystic medial necrosis, 285
Cysts
  abdominal, 337, *339*
  pancreatic, *339*
  pericardial, 272

Depth gain compensation (DGC), 15, 60–61
Dermatomyositis, 485
Developing world, **289–302**
  applications of echocardiography, 292–302

instruments, 291
Dextrocardia, 312, 468
Diabetic mothers, infants of, 337, **480,** *481*
Diaphragmatic palsy, 337
Diastole
  hypertrophic cardiomyopathy, **199,** 479
  left ventricular function, 75–76
  restrictive cardiomyopathy, 204, 486
Diastolic compliance, 75
Diastolic filling, 75
  hypertrophic cardiomyopathy, 199
  ischaemic heart disease, 181, *182*
  restrictive cardiomyopathy, 204
DiGeorge syndrome, 377
Digital echocardiography, **38–39**
  further applications, 39
  stress tests, 38–39
Digital image storage, **34–35**
Digital velocity map, 99
Dipyridamole stress echocardiography, 39, 530–531
Distance measurements, **33**
Dobutamine, 531
Doppler echocardiography, 153, 372–373
  analysis methods, **34**
  aortic dissection, 284
  aortic stenosis, 56, 57, *59,* 391–392
  atrial septal defects, 349, *350*
  atrioventricular septal defects, 359
  cardiac tamponade, 266–267
  coarctation of aorta, 56–57, 400–403
  colour flow mapping, *see* Colour flow mapping
  congenital heart disease, 309–310, 340, 516–517
  continuous wave, *see* Continuous wave Doppler
  control optimisation, 61–64
  coronary artery anomalies, 505
  developing countries, 291
  dilated cardiomyopathy, 203, 483–484
  display techniques, 21
  equipment, 20–22, 29, **32–33,** 44
  examination technique, **53–59**
  high pulse repetition frequency, *see* High pulse repetition frequency (HPRF) Doppler
  history, **5–7**
  hypertrophic cardiomyopathy, 199–201, 477–478, 515
  hypoplastic left heart syndrome, 397
  infective endocarditis, 219–220
  intravascular, **533–535**
  ischaemic heart disease, 182–183
  physics and principles, **19–24**
  prosthetic heart valves, 231–240
  pulmonary stenosis, 432–433
  pulsed, *see* Pulsed wave Doppler
  quantitative
    pressure drop estimation, **79–102**
    pulmonary artery pressure estimation, **105–112**
    volumetric flow estimation, **113–125**
  restrictive cardiomyopathies, 205–207, 486
  scanhead frequency, 31
  stress tests, 531
  transoesophageal, 142–143, 527
  truncus arteriosus, 376, *377*
  ventricular septal defects, 361
Doppler effect, **19–20**
Double inlet left ventricle, *318,* 449–450, 451–452
Double inlet right ventricle, *318,* 452

Double inlet ventricle, 363, 449–453
Double outlet atrium, 358
Double outlet left ventricle, 319, *320*, **422**
Double outlet right ventricle (DORV), 318–319, 365, **419–422**
  associated lesions, 421–422
  with atrioventricular discordance, 425–426
  double committed VSD, 420, 421
  intact ventricular septum, 422
  non-committed VSD, 421
  subaortic VSD, 319, *320*, 420–421
  subpulmonary VSD (Taussig-Bing anomaly), 319, *320*, 414, 421
Double outlet ventricle, 318
Dressler's syndrome, **187–188**, 268–269
Drug abuse, intravenous, 214
Duchenne muscular dystrophy, **485**
Ductus arteriosus, 370
  patent, *see* Patent ductus arteriosus
Ductus venosus, patent, 461–463
Duplex scanning
  equipment, 32
  history, 6–7
  pressure drop estimation, 85
Dynamic range
  acoustic, 36
  Doppler signals, 37
Dyskinesia, ventricular wall, 181

E/A ratio, 75, 514
  hypertrophic cardiomyopathy, 199, *200*
  restrictive cardiomyopathy, 486
Ebstein's anomaly, 172, 315, *317*, 439, **441–444**
  echocardiography, 442–444
  pathology, 441–442
Eccentricity index, bicuspid aortic valve, 389
Echocardiographic windows, 35, 44–46, 309
Echocardiography
  clinical view, **511–517**
  control optimisation, **57–61**
  developing world, **289–302**
  equipment, **27–40**
  examination technique, **41–64**
  history, **3–7**
  measurement and analysis packages, 33–34
  physics and principles, **9–26**
  recent advances, **519–537**
  standard examination, **62**
  three-dimensional reconstruction, 536
Echoes, ultrasound, 14–15
Ehlers Danlos syndrome, 278
Ejection fraction (EF), 68
  Doppler determination, 123
  parasternal long axis view, 47
Ejection period, systolic (SEP), 91
Ejection time, left ventricular (LVET), 68, 75
Elderly, hypertrophic cardiomyopathy, 197, *198*
Electrocardiography (ECG)
  electrode placement, 44
  exercise, 529
  simultaneous recordings, 63
Embolisation
  intracardiac thrombi, 187, *188*, 203, 254
  myxomas, 247
  vegetations of infective endocarditis, **214–215**
Emery–Dreifuss muscular dystrophy, 485
Endocardial cushion defect (complete atrioventricular septal defect), 323, 356, 450–451

Endocardial fibroelastosis, **484–485**
Endocarditis, infective, 175, **209–222**
  aortic regurgitation, 167, 219, 301
  children, 337, *338*
  developing countries, **300–301**
  differential diagnosis, 215–216
  embolisation risks, 214–215
  follow-up, 221–222
  haemodynamic effects, 219–220
  mitral regurgitation, 157, *158*, 219–220
  mycotic aortic aneurysms, 285
  native valves, 211–220
  pericardial effusion, 218–219
  perivalvular damage, 216–218, *219*, *220*, 221
  prosthetic valves, 137, 211, **220–221**, 229, 230–231
  right-sided, 172, 174, 214, *215*, 216
  role of echocardiography, 211
  sinus of Valsalva aneurysms, 217, 220, 286
  transoesophageal imaging, **136–137**, 211–214, 220–221, 231
  underlying heart disease, 211
  valvular damage, 211–214
Endomyocardial fibrosis, **205**, *206*
  childhood, **486**
  Doppler findings, 207
Endoscopic imaging, *see* Transoesophageal imaging
Enhancement artefacts, 25, 26
Environment, echocardiographic examination, 43–44
Epicardial echocardiography, 527–528
Epivascular scanning, intraoperative, 528, *530*
Equipment, **27–40**
  transoesophageal echocardiography, 131–132
Eustachian valve, prominent, 256
E wave, hypertrophic cardiomyopathy, 199, *200*
Examination technique, **41–64**
  congenital heart disease, 309–310
  standard, **62**
Exercise
  digital echocardiography, 38–39
  Doppler studies during, 531
  echocardiography, **529–530**
  electrocardiography, 529
  left ventricular function and, 76
  recovery times, coronary artery disease, 181

Fabry's disease, 480
Fast Fourier Transform (FFT) method, 21, 32–33
Fat metabolism, disorders in infancy, 480
Fetal circulation, persistent, 343, *344*
Fibroelastomas, papillary, 251
Fibromas, cardiac, 245, **250–251**
Fidelity, image, 24
'Five chamber' view, apical, 49, *50*, 56, 62
Flow
  across prosthetic valves, 231
  laminar, 20, 23
  parabolic, 20
  patterns, **19–20**
  plug, 20
  turbulent, *see* Turbulent flow
  velocity, *see* Velocity, flow
  volume estimation, *see* Volumetric flow estimation
Focal ranges, 31
Focusing, 13, **31**

phased array scanheads, 30
Fontan operation, 470
'Footprint', transducer, 18, 44
Foramen ovale (oval foramen), 322, 343
  patent, 343–344, *345*
    contrast echocardiography, 531
    Ebstein's anomaly, 442
    total anomalous pulmonary venous drainage, 458
    transoesophageal imaging, 525
Four chamber plane, 45
Four chamber views
  apical, 48–49, *50*, 53–56, 62
  subcostal, 50–51
  transoesophageal, *134*, **135**
Fourier transformation, fast, 21, 32–33
Fractional shortening (FS), left ventricular, 68, 69, 355
Frame grabbers, 34
Frame rate, colour flow Doppler, 38
Frequency
  filtering, Doppler systems, 63
  scanhead, **31**
  ultrasound waves, 11
Friedreich's ataxia, **481**

Gain control, 15, 60–61
  Doppler systems, 61–63
Gel, ultrasound, 44
Gerbode defect, 357
Glycogen storage disease, *336*, 337
  type II (Pompe's disease), **479**, *480*
'Goose neck' appearance, atrioventricular septal defects, 324, *325*, 358
Gorlin equation, 91, 124
  prosthetic heart valves, 232
Grating lobes, 37
Great arteries, 318, *319*, *320*, **328–333**
  congenital anomalies, **489–493**
  position of ventricular septal defect and, 318–319, *320*
  transposition, *see* Transposition of great arteries
  see also Aorta; Pulmonary artery(ies), main trunk
Grey scale processing, 36

Haemochromatosis, 485
Haemopericardium
  aortic disease, 269, 284
  pericardial thickening, 269
  post-infarction, 269
  post-traumatic/post-surgical, 269
Hancock bioprosthetic valve, 232
Heart
  imaging planes, 45, *134*
  single outlet, 318, 319
Heart failure
  anomalous coronary artery arising from pulmonary trunk, 506
  coronary artery disease, 203
  developing countries, 292, 299
  dilated cardiomyopathy, 201–202
  left ventricular function, 514
  pericardial effusion, 268
  prosthetic heart valve failure, 225, 226
  right, 109
  right atrial myxomas, 247
Hemiazygos vein, 311, *312*
Hemitruncus (pulmonary artery arising from ascending aorta), 331, *332*, 377–378

Hepatic veins, 311
  atrial isomerism, 311, 312
  Doppler examination, 58
High pulse repetition frequency (HPRF) Doppler, 22, **32**, **63–64**
  pressure drop estimation, 86
History of echocardiography, **3–7**
Hurler's syndrome, 479
Hyperkinesia, ventricular wall, 181
Hypertension
  annuloaortic ectasia, 285
  aortic aneurysms, 278
  aortic dissection, 278
  pulmonary arterial, *see* Pulmonary hypertension
Hypertensive heart disease, developing countries, 291
Hypokinesia, ventricular wall, 181
Hypoplastic left heart syndrome, 328, *329*, **394–398**
Hypotension, post-operative, transoesophageal echocardiography, 144

Image
  aesthetics (presentation), **36**
  clarity, 24
  factors affecting quality, 35–36
  fidelity, 24
  orientation, **310**
  processing, 36
  recordings, **35**, 62
  resolution, *see* Resolution, image
  storage, **34–35**
  uniformity, 36
Imaging planes, 45–46, *134*
Inclusion cell disease, 480
Infants
  of diabetic mothers, 337, **480**, *481*
  examination technique, 309–310
  transoesophageal imaging, 527
Infective endocarditis, *see* Endocarditis, infective
Inferior vena cava
  atrial isomerism, 311–312
  dilatation, constrictive pericarditis, 293, 295
  Doppler examination technique, 58
  mirror image atrial arrangement, 311
  obstruction, surgically repaired transposition, 418–419, 469
  plethora, cardiac tamponade, 266
  pulmonary venous drainage into, 461, 466
  respiratory variations in diameter
    cardiac tamponade, 266
    right atrial pressure estimation, 109
  transverse upper abdominal view, 50, *51*
Infundibular atresia, 437–438, 441
Infundibular septum, tetralogy of Fallot, 434
Infundibular stenosis, *see* Pulmonary stenosis, infundibular
Innominate arteries, *see* Brachiocephalic arteries
Innominate veins, *see* Brachiocephalic veins
Instruments
  developing countries, 291
  factors affecting performance, 35–36
  technologies, 29
Integrated backscatter, 532–533
Intensity
  spatial average, time average (Isata), 13
  ultrasound, 12–13

Intensive care, transoesophageal echocardiography, 132–133, **143–145**
Interatrial septum, *see* Atrial septum
Interventional procedures, transoesophageal echocardiography during, **143**
Interventricular septum (IVS), **324–328**
  angulation, 198–199
  apical four chamber view, 49
  asymmetrical hypertrophy (ASH), 193–194, 195, 198–199, 250, 390, 475–476
  infants of diabetic mothers, 480, *481*
  infective endocarditis, 217–218
  localised thickening, 197
  morphological areas, 360, *361*
  movements
    absence of pericardium and, 272
    arrhythmias, 184
    cardiac tamponade, 293, *294*
    constrictive pericarditis, 293, *295*
    digitised images, *68, 69*
    ischaemic heart disease, 181, *183*
    normal amplitude, 67
    paradoxical, atrial septal defects, 321, 344, 345–347, 355
    prosthetic heart valves and, 228–229
  normal thickness, 63, 67
  parasternal long axis view, 47
  transposition of great arteries, 411–412
  see also Ventricular septal defects
Intracardiac air, detection during surgery, **143–144**
Intracardiac catheter embolus, 143
Intracardiac thrombi, *see* Thrombi, intracardiac
Intracardiac ultrasound, 7, 536
Intrahepatic veins, constrictive pericarditis, 293
Intramyocardial sinusoids, 439–441
Intraoperative echocardiography, 40, **527–529**
  atrioventricular septal defects, 359–360
  transoesophageal imaging, 132–133, **143–145**, 527, 529
Intravascular ultrasound, 7, 40, **533–536**
  Doppler studies, 533–535
  imaging, 535–536
Intravenous drug abuse, 214
Ionescu–Shiley prosthetic valves, 225
Iron overload, thalassaemia, 485, 486
Ischaemic heart disease, **179–188**
  complications, 184–188
  contrast echocardiography, 183–184
  coronary artery imaging, 140–141, 181, 500
  developing countries, 291
  intraoperative transoesophageal monitoring, 144–145
  left ventricular function, *68, 69*, 181–183, 515
  mitral regurgitation, 157, 158
  pathological effects of ischaemia and infarction, 181–183
  stress echocardiography, 38, 529–531
  tissue characterisation, 183
  transoesophageal imaging, **140–141**
  vs. dilated cardiomyopathy, 203
  see also Myocardial infarction
Isomerism, atrial, *see* Atrial isomerism
Isovolumic contraction phase, left ventricle, 73
Isovolumic relaxation phase, left ventricle, 75
Isovolumic relaxation time, right ventricle (RIRT), **111–112**

Jets
  confined, **83–84**
  direction, ultrasound beam alignment and, 86–87
  free, 83, **84–85**
  measurement, colour flow mapping, 97–98
  regurgitant, colour flow mapping, 102
Jugular vein, right internal, 313
Jugular venous pressure, clinical estimation, 108, 109

Kawasaki disease, *334, 335*, 336, **503–504**
Kwashiorkor, 485

Laminar flow, 20, 23
Laryngeal nerve palsy, recurrent, 134
Left atrial appendage, 134, *135*, 310
  thrombus, 139–140
Left atrial dilatation
  aortopulmonary window, 378, *379*
  dilated cardiomyopathy, 202, 481, 482
  hypertrophic cardiomyopathy, 478
  mitral stenosis, 155, 156
  patent ductus arteriosus, 373, *374*
  pericardial constriction, 270
  ventricular septal defects, 361
Left atrial isomerism, 311–312, 466, 467–468
Left atrium
  apical four chamber view, 49, *50*
  compression, cardiac tamponade, 264–265
  dimensions, 63
  dominance, atrioventricular septal defects, 358
  hypoplastic left heart syndrome, 395
  masses, 257
  myxomas, 245–247, *248, 249*, 302, 528, *529*
  parasternal views, 46
  partitioned (cor triatriatum), 354, *466, 467*, **468–469**
  pulmonary venous drainage, 314, *315*
  thrombi, *254*, 255
  transoesophageal imaging, 134, 135
Left atrium:aortic root diameter (LA/AO) ratio
  patent ductus arteriosus, 373, *374*
  ventricular septal defects, 361, 367–368
Left bundle branch block, 184
Left heart
  hypoplasia, atrioventricular septal defects, 358
  hypoplasia syndrome, 328, *329*, **394–398**
  volume overload, patent ductus arteriosus, 373
Left sided obstructions, congenital, **387–403**
Left to right shunts
  congenital, 321, 322, **341–379**
  infective endocarditis, 217
Left ventricle
  aneurysms, 181, **184**
  apical four chamber view, 49, *50*
  atrioventricular septal defects, 357, 358
  circumferential fibre shortening (Vcf), 68
    ischaemic heart disease, 182
    variation across ventricle, 73, *74*
  coarctation of aorta, 398
  diastolic filling, 75, 181, *182*
  double inlet, *318*, 449–450, 451–452
  double outlet, 319, *320*, **422**
  ejection time (LVET), 68, 75
  fractional shortening (FS), *68, 69*, 355
  hypoplastic left heart syndrome, 395–396

Left ventricle (contd)
  identification, 423
  ischaemia/infarction, **181–183**
  parasternal views, 46, 47, 48, *49*
  shape, size and function, 67–69
  'stiffness' (elasticity), 75
  stress indices, **70–71**
  thrombi, 186–187, *188*, 254
  total anomalous pulmonary venous
      drainage, 458
  trabeculations, vs. intracardiac masses, 257
  transoesophageal imaging, 135, 525, *526*
  transposition of great arteries, 411–412
  volume overload
      aortopulmonary window, 378, *379*
      childhood, 321–322
Left ventricular dilatation
  aortic orifice measurement, *117*, 118
  aortic regurgitation, 167, 169
  aortic stenosis, 164
  dilated cardiomyopathy, 202, 299, 481
  mitral regurgitation, 157, 158
  patent ductus arteriosus, 373
  working guidelines, 63
Left ventricular dimensions, 63, 67, 68–69, 123
  digitised plots, *68*, *69*, 73, 181, *182*
  end diastolic (EDD), 63, *67*
  end systolic (ESD), 63, *67*
  hypertrophic cardiomyopathy, 476
  hypoplastic left heart syndrome, 395
  intraoperative transoesophageal
      echocardiography, 144
  ischaemic heart disease, 69, 181, *182*, 183
Left ventricular function, **65–76**
  age effects, 75
  aortic dissection, 284
  aortic stenosis, 390
  cardiac amyloidosis, 207
  cardiac tamponade, 266
  clinical aspects, **514–515**
  diastolic, 75–76
  dilated cardiomyopathy, 202
  exercise and, 76
  hypertrophic cardiomyopathy, 193,
      199–201, 478
  infective endocarditis, 221
  intraoperative transoesophageal
      monitoring, 144–145, 529
  ischaemic heart disease, *68*, *69*, 181–183, 515
  mitral regurgitation, 161
  prosthetic heart valves, 226, 228
  recent advances, **522**, *523*
  regional, 522, *523*
  right ventricle relationship, 76
  surgically repaired transposition, 419
  systolic, 71–75
  transposition of great arteries, 411
Left ventricular hypertrophy
  aortic stenosis, 164, 389, 390
  appropriate, 71
  asymmetrical (ASH), 193–194, 195,
      198–199, 250, 390, 475–476
  athletes, 76, 199
  concentric/symmetrical, 195, *196*
  distal (apical), 195–197
  hypertrophic cardiomyopathy, 193–197,
      475–476
  inadequate, 71
  inappropriate, 71
  left ventricular mass, 70
Left ventricular mass, **70**
  dilated cardiomyopathy, 202
  index, 70

Left ventricular outflow tract (LVOT)
  apical 'five chamber' view, 49, *50*
  area, 91
  atrioventricular septal defects, 357, 358,
      360
  diameter measurement, 117–118
  flow velocities
      aortic stenosis, 91
      hypertrophic cardiomyopathy, 200
      infective endocarditis, 217–218
  obstruction
      congenital, **389–394**
      hypertrophic cardiomyopathy, **476–478**
      transposition of great arteries, **414–415**,
          424
Left ventricular pressures
  aortic stenosis, 390
  diastole, 75
  systole, 73
  transposition of great arteries, 411–412
Left ventricular volumes, 33, 67–68, 123
Left ventricular (posterior) wall
  amplitude, 67
  thickness, 63, *67*, **70**
      dilated cardiomyopathy, 202
  see also Wall motion analysis
Left vertical vein, 459–460, *465*
Levocardia, 312
Libman–Sacks vegetations, 216, *218*
Lighting, 43
Lignocaine, topical anaesthesia, 133
Lipomas, cardiac, 251
Liver
  obstructed anomalous pulmonary venous
      drainage, 466
  position, 312
Liver abscess, amoebic, 292–293
Löffler's syndrome, *see* Endomyocardial
      fibrosis
Long axis plane, 45
Long axis views
  apical, 50, 56, 62
  parasternal, 46–47, 62
Low frequency filter, Doppler systems, 60
Lupus erythematosus, systemic, 216, *218*, 485
Lutembacher's syndrome, 354
Lymphoma, pericardial, *271*, 272

Magnetic resonance imaging, 515
  aortic dissection, 283–284
  congenital heart disease, 517
  great arterial anomalies, 491
  Marfan's syndrome, 285–286
  aortic aneurysms, 278
  aortic regurgitation, 167
  haemopericardium, 269
  mitral regurgitation, 158, 285
  pulmonary regurgitation, 174
  tricuspid regurgitation, 172
'Mayo Clinic' syndrome, 426
Mechanical sector scanheads (probes), **29–30**
  oscillatory, 30
  rotating, 29
Melanoma, 252–253
Mesocardia, 312
Mesothelioma, pericardial, 252, 271
Metabolic disorders, hypertrophic
      cardiomyopathy, 479–480
Metastatic tumours
  cardiac, 245, 252–253
  pericardium, 271
Mitral atresia, 317, *319*

Mitral pressure half-time, **92–94**, 156–157
  prosthetic valves, 93, 235, *238*
Mitral regurgitation, **157–162**, 175
  congenital sub-mitral aneurysm, 299
  dilated cardiomyopathy, 157, 201, 483
  Doppler examination, 55, 57, *59*
  dynamic, 531
  endomyocardial fibrosis, 205, *206*, 207, 486
  hypertrophic cardiomyopathy, 157, 201,
      478–479
  infective endocarditis, 157, *158*, 219–220
  Marfan's syndrome, 158, 285
  mitral pressure half-time, *93*, 94
  post-myocardial infarction, 158, 184,
      185–186
  pressure drop estimation, 84–85
  prosthetic valves, 221, 228, 235–239
  quantitative colour flow mapping, 101–102
  transoesophageal imaging, 139, 142, *160*,
      162, 525, 527
  volumetric flow estimation, 124–125
Mitral stenosis, **155–157**, *159*, 161
  atrial septal defects, 354
  developing countries, 296–297, *298*
  Doppler examination, 55
  membranous supravalvular, *467*, 468–469
  mitral pressure half-time, **92–94**, 156–157
  pressure drops, 91–92, 156
  quantitative Doppler, **91–94**
  recurrent, after closed valvotomy, 297
Mitral valve, **153–162**
  annulus
      calcification, 155, 197, *198*, 201
      dilatation, 186
      hypoplastic left heart syndrome, 395
      measurement, **119–120**
  apical four chamber view, 49, *50*
  'cleft', atrioventricular septal defects, 324,
      325, 357
  doming, 155
  Doppler examination technique, **53–55**
  flail cusps, 158, 185, *186*
  floppy, vs. infective endocarditis, 216, *218*
  flow velocities
      aortopulmonary window, 378, *379*
      cardiac tamponade, 266
      mitral regurgitation, 161, 162
      mitral stenosis, 156
      patent ductus arteriosus, 373
      prosthetic valves, 235, 236, 237, *238*
      restrictive cardiomyopathy, 486
  hypertrophic cardiomyopathy, 197–198,
      477
  hypoplastic left heart syndrome, 395
  infective endocarditis, 211–214, 219–220
  leaflets
      left atrial myxomas and, 247, *248*
      measurement at tip, 120–122
  morphological recognition, 315, *316*
  normal, 153–154
  obstruction, left atrial myxomas, 247
  orifice area
      cardiac output estimation, 73, **119–122**
      mitral stenosis, 92, 157
      prosthetic valves, 232–233, 235
  parasternal views, 46, *47*, 48
  perivalvular abscess, 216, *218*
  premature closure, infective endocarditis,
      301
  prolapse, 157, *158*, 161
      atrial septal defects, 352–354
      post-infarction, 185, *186*
  reconstructive surgery, 144, 528

INDEX

Mitral valve (contd)
  straddling, 414, 421
  subvalve apparatus, 513, 525, *526*
  systolic anterior motion (SAM), 165, 193–195, **197–198**, 201, *476*, 477
  transoesophageal imaging, 135, 525
  transposition of great arteries, 414, 422–423
  ventricular septal defects, 363
  volumetric flow estimation, **119–122**
Mitral valve prostheses
  area, 232–233
  assessment of function, 227, 228, 229, 230
  developing countries, 297
  Doppler evaluation, 232–233, **235–239**
    abnormal function, 235–239
    normal function, 235
  infective endocarditis, 221
  mitral pressure half-time, 93, 235, *238*
  thrombus formation, 255
  transoesophageal studies, 142
Mitral valvotomy, closed, 296–297
M-mode echocardiography, 153, 521
  aorta, 277
  aortic dissection, 280–283
  aortic regurgitation, 167–169
  aortic stenosis, 164–165, 390, 392
  aortic valve, 163, *164*
  bicuspid aortic valve, 389
  cardiac tumours, 246
  combined with real-time imaging, 18–19
  control optimisation, 59–61
  developing countries, 291
  digitised, 270
  dilated cardiomyopathy, 202, 481
  examination technique, **46–53**
  history, 5
  hypertrophic cardiomyopathy, 193–198, 475
  hypoplastic left heart syndrome, 395
  infective endocarditis, 211
  left ventricular indices, *67*
  mitral regurgitation, 161
  mitral stenosis, 155–156
  mitral valve, 154
  mitral valve orifice area, 120–121
  normal dimensions, 63
  pericardial effusion, 261–262
  pericardial thickening/constriction, 270
  principles, **17**
  prosthetic heart valves, **226–231**
  restrictive cardiomyopathy, 204, 486
  tricuspid valve, 171
  truncus arteriosus, 375–376
  volume calculations, 33, 123
Momentum conservation, 84
Moving target indicator, colour flow mapping, 23
Mucolipidosis II (inclusion cell disease), 480
Mucopolysaccharidosis, *336*, 337
  type I (Hurler's), 479
Multiplane transoesophageal transducers, 39–40, 526–527
Muscular dystrophy, dilated cardiomyopathy, **485**
Mustard's operation, 417–419, *468*, 469–470
Mycotic aortic aneurysms, **285**
Myocardial infarction
  complications, **184–188**
  infective endocarditis, 214–215
  intraoperative transoesophageal monitoring, 144
  left ventricular function, 515, 522
  mitral regurgitation complicating, 158, 184, **185–186**
  pathological effects, **181–183**
  pericardial effusion, 268–269
  stress echocardiography, 38, 531
  thrombus formation, **186–187**, *188*, 254
  tissue characterisation, 183
  transoesophageal imaging, *140*, 141
  vs. dilated cardiomyopathy, 203
  vs. hypertrophic cardiomyopathy, 199
Myocardial ischaemia, 144, **181–183**
Myocardial necrosis, 182
Myocardial rupture, **184–185**
  into pericardium, 185, 269
Myocardial sinusoids, 439–441
Myocardial wall motion analysis, *see* Wall motion analysis
Myocarditis, 203
  connective tissue disorders, 485
  cyclophosphamide-induced, *484*, 485
  viral, **484**
Myocardium
  false aneurysms, 184–185
  hypertrophic cardiomyopathy, 193–197
  'thick walled', children, 337
  tissue characterisation, **183**, 203, 514–515, 532–533
Myxomas, **245–249**
  left atrial, 245–247, *248*, *249*, 302, 528, *529*
  right atrial, 171, 246, 247–249
  syndrome, 245
  transoesophageal imaging, 138–139
  ventricular, 246, 249

Neonates, 44, 515
  atrial septum, 343–344, *345*
  pulmonary stenosis, 433
Neurological damage, air emboli and, 143–144
Neurosurgical procedures, 143
Noonan's syndrome, 337, 431, 478, *479*, *480*
Nuclear cardiology, 515
Nyquist frequency, **22**, 32, 63–64
  quantitative colour flow mapping and, 98, 99

Obstructions
  colour flow mapping, 99–100
  congenital left sided, **387–403**
  congenital right sided, **429–444**
  discrete, pressure drop estimation, **83–85**
  non-discrete (tunnel-like and multiple) pressure drop estimation, **94–97**
  quantitative colour flow mapping, 101
Operators
  position, 44
  training, transoesophageal echocardiography, 132
  variability between, 35
Orifice contraction, coefficient of, 83
Oval foramen, oval fossa, *see* Foramen ovale

Pancreatic cyst, *339*
Papaverine, 534
Papillary fibroelastomas, 251
Papillary muscles
  hypertrophic cardiomyopathy, 476
  parasternal short axis view, 48, *49*
  post-infarction damage, 158, 185–186
  vs. intracardiac masses, *256*, 257

Parabolic flow, 20
Parasternal views
  long axis, 46–47, 62
  short axis, 47–48, *49*, 57–58, 62
Parasternal window
  left, 45, **46–48**, 277
  right, 45, **52–53**, 277
Patent ductus arteriosus (PDA, arterial duct), *321*, 331, *332*, **370–375**
  assessing shunt size, 373–374
  coarctation of aorta, 399
  Doppler examination, 372–373
  hypoplastic left heart syndrome, 397
  imaging, 370–371
  pulmonary artery pressure estimation, 374–375
  pulmonary atresia with intact ventricular septum, 439, 441
  pulmonary atresia with ventricular septal defect, 437
  transposition of great arteries, *330*, 410–411
  volumetric flow estimation, 125, 373–374
Patients
  positioning, 35, 43–44, 309
  preparation, **43–44**, 133
  transducer selection and, 44
Pericardectomy, 271, 272, 296
Pericardial aspiration (pericardiocentesis), **267**, 292, 293
Pericardial cysts, 272
Pericardial effusion, **261–269**, 270–271
  aortic disease, 269, 284
  causes, 261
  children, 337–340
  constrictive pericarditis with, **295–296**
  developing countries, **292–293**, *294*
  diagnosis, 261–263
  Dressler's syndrome, 187–188, 268–269
  echo free spaces mimicking, 261–262
  heart failure, 268
  idiopathic, 263
  infective endocarditis, **218–219**
  inflammatory, 263
  malignant, 251–252, 263, *264*, 271, 272
  myocardial infarction, 268–269
  pericardial aspiration, 267
  post-traumatic/post-surgical, 269
  quantitation of size, 262–263
  tuberculosis, 267–268
  types, 267–269
  see also Cardiac tamponade
Pericardial knock, constrictive pericarditis, 293, 295, *296*
Pericardial thickening/constriction, **269–271**
  developing countries, **293–296**
  effusive constrictive pericarditis, 295–296
  pericardial tumours, 271, 272
  pyopericardium, 268
  tuberculosis, 268
Pericardial tumours, **271–272**
  benign, 271
  malignant, 263, *264*, 271–272
Pericarditis
  amoebic, 292–293
  connective tissue disorders, 485
  constrictive, 207, 269–270, **293–295**
    chronic calcific, 293
    sub-acute, 293–295
  developing countries, **292–296**
  effusive constrictive, **295–296**
  infective endocarditis, 219
  myocardial infarction, 268–269
  tuberculous, *see* Tuberculous pericarditis

Pericardium, **259–272**
  absence, 272
  congenital abnormalities, 272
  myocardial rupture into, 185, 269
  normal appearances, 261
  transverse sinus, 334, 497–498, 505
Perimeter measurements, 33
Peripheral vascular disease, intravascular imaging, 535
Perivalvular damage, infective endocarditis, 216–218, *219*, *220*, 221
Pharmacological stress echocardiography, 39, 530–531
Phased annular array scanheads, **31**
Phased array scanheads (probes), **30–31**
Phonocardiography, prosthetic heart valve assessment, 229
Photographic slides, 35
Physics, **9–26**
Planes, imaging, 45–46, *134*
Pleural effusions, 262, 337, *339*
Plug flow, 20
Polysplenia, 314
Pompe's disease, **479**, *480*
Portal venous system, pulmonary venous connection, 461–466
Positioning
  patients, 35, 43–44, 309
  transducers, **44–46**
Post-myocardial infarction (Dressler's) syndrome, **187–188**, 268–269
Power, ultrasound beam, 12
Power coding, colour flow mapping, 23, 523–524
Power output
  Doppler systems, 58
  real-time and M-mode imaging, 60
Pre-ejection phase, 71–73
Preload, 67
Premature babies, 309
  patent ductus arteriosus, 370, 371
  shunts across foramen ovale, 344
Pressure, ultrasound, 11
Pressure drops (gradients), **79–102**, 513–514, 516
  aortic stenosis, 82, 86, **88–91**, 97, 166, 391
  aortic valve prostheses, 233, 234
  clinical applications, 87–97
  coarctation of aorta, 96–97, 400–401
  discrete obstructions, 83–85
  Doppler techniques used in estimation, 85–86
  hypertrophic cardiomyopathy, 193, 200
  mean, 34, 91–92
  mitral prostheses, 235
  mitral stenosis, 91–94, 156
  non-discrete, tunnel-like and multiple obstructions, 94–97
  peak instantaneous, 34, 88, 513
  peak-to-peak, 88, 513
  practical aspects of estimation, 86–87
  problems and pitfalls in estimation, 97
  prosthetic heart valves, 94, 231–232
  pulmonary artery-to-right ventricle, 110
  pulmonary stenosis, 94, 95–96, 432–433
  right ventricle-to-right atrium, 107, **108**, 109
  right ventricular outflow tract obstruction, 95–96, 432–433
  septal, ventricular septal defects, 369
  subaortic stenosis, 393–394
  theory of Doppler estimation, 81–82
  tricuspid stenosis, 94, 171

Pressure gradients, *see* Pressure drops
Pressure half-time, 34
  aortic valve prostheses, 235
  mitral valve, *see* Mitral pressure half-time
  tricuspid valve, 94
  tricuspid valve prostheses, 240
Pressure recovery, 83–84, 88
Probes, *see* Scanheads
Prosthetic heart valves, **223–240**
  biological, *see* Bioprosthetic heart valves
  Doppler evaluation, **231–240**
    aortic prostheses, 232, 233–235
    mitral prosthesis, 232–233, 235–239
    technical problems and limitations, 231
    theoretical basis, 231
    tricuspid prostheses, 240
    in vitro studies, 231–232
    in vivo studies, 232–233
  infective endocarditis, 137, 211, **220–221**, 229, 230–231
  mechanisms of failure, 225–226
  mitral pressure half-time, 93, 235, *238*
  M-mode and cross-sectional imaging, 226–231
    abnormal function, 227–230
    normal function, 226–227
  pressure drop estimation, 94, 231–232
  transoesophageal imaging, 142, *143*, 231, 239, 240
  types, 225
Proximal isovelocity surface area (PISA), 524
Pseudo-aneurysms
  aorta, 278
  myocardium, 184–185
Pulmonary arterial hypertension, *see* Pulmonary hypertension
Pulmonary artery(ies), 330–331
  arising from ascending aorta (hemitruncus), 331, *332*, 377–378
  atretic/hypoplastic, 437–438, *439*
  atrioventricular septal defects, 358
  banding, *101*, 515
  bifurcation, 48, *49*, 375, *376*
  confluent, 331
  dilatation
    atrial septal defects, 344, *346*
    atrioventricular septal defects, 359
    pulmonary valve stenosis, 431
    ventricular septal defects, 365–366
  flow patterns
    patent ductus arteriosus, 372, *373*
    pulmonary artery pressure and, **110–111**, 174
  flow velocities
    cardiac tamponade, 267
    pulmonary stenosis, 174
    ventricular septal defects, 368
  hypoplastic, 437
    hypoplastic left heart syndrome, 397
    tetralogy of Fallot, 434
    truncus arteriosus, 321
  left, 330–331
    patent ductus arteriosus, 370
    stenosis, 434
    tetralogy of Fallot, 436
  main trunk, 318, *319*, 330–331
    Doppler examination, 58, *60*
    hypoplastic left heart syndrome, 328, *329*
    identification, 375, *376*
    left coronary artery arising from, 334, *335*, 482–483, **504–506**
    parasternal short axis view, 48, *49*
    right coronary artery arising from, 506

    stenosis, 431, 433–434
    transoesophageal imaging, 525, *526*
  non-confluent, 331, 437
  overriding, 319, *320*, 414, 420, 421
  problems of imaging, 516
  right, 330
    stenosis, 434
    suprasternal view, 52
    tetralogy of Fallot, 436, *437*
  stenosis, 431, **433–434**
  surgically repaired transposition, 419
  transoesophageal imaging, 134
  transposition of great arteries, 409, 410, 423
Pulmonary artery pressure, **105–112**
  atrioventricular septal defects, 360
  patent ductus arteriosus, 374–375
  pulmonary forward flow method, 110–111
  pulmonary regurgitation method, 110
  right ventricular isovolumic relaxation method, 111–112
  tricuspid regurgitation method, 107–110, 172
  ventricular septal defects, 368–370
Pulmonary artery sling, 332–333, **492–493**
Pulmonary artery-to-right ventricle pressure drop, 110
Pulmonary atresia
  Ebstein's anomaly, 442, 444
  intact ventricular septum, **438–441**, 515
  ventricular septal defect, 319–321, 331, **437–438**, *439*
Pulmonary embolism
  infective endocarditis, 214
  transoesophageal imaging, 140
Pulmonary hypertension
  mitral stenosis, 155
  patent ductus arteriosus, 374–375
  pulmonary artery flow patterns, 111, 174
  pulmonary artery pressure measurement, 107, 109, 110, 172, 175
  pulmonary regurgitation, 174
  restrictive cardiomyopathy, 486
  tricuspid regurgitation, 170, 172
  ventricular septal defects, 368–369
  vs. hypertrophic cardiomyopathy, 199
Pulmonary regurgitation, *173*, **174–175**
  physiological, 58, *61*, 174
  pulmonary arterial hypertension, 174
  pulmonary artery pressure measurement, **110**
Pulmonary stenosis
  acquired, **174**
  congenital, 174, **431–434**
  Ebstein's anomaly, 442, 444
  infundibular (subpulmonary), 174
    congenital, 431, 433
    double outlet right ventricle, 420, 422
    pressure drop estimation, 95–96
    secondary, 431, 433
    tetralogy of Fallot, 434
    transposition of great arteries, 415, *417*, 424
  supravalvular, 431, **433–434**
  surgically repaired transposition, 419
  valvular
    acquired, **174**
    confined jets, 83
    congenital, **431–433**
    Noonan's syndrome, 479
    pressure drop estimation, **94**, 95–96, 432–433
    tetralogy of Fallot, 434, 435–436
    transposition of great arteries, 415, 424
    vs. hypertrophic cardiomyopathy, 199

Pulmonary:systemic flow ratio, 125
   atrial septal defects, 355
   ventricular septal defects, 361, 367–368
Pulmonary trunk, *see* Pulmonary artery(ies), main trunk
Pulmonary valve, **174–175**
   annulus, measurement, 122
   atresia, tetralogy of Fallot, 435–436
   carcinoid disease, 174, 253
   closure:tricuspid valve opening time, 368
   Doppler examination technique, **57–58**, *60*, *61*
   dysplasia, 431
   flow velocities
      atrial septal defects, 345
      valvular stenosis, 174, 432–433
   infective endocarditis, 214, *216*
   parasternal short axis view, 48
   stenosis, *see* Pulmonary stenosis, valvular
   tetralogy of Fallot, 435–436
   transposition of great arteries, 414–415
   volumetric flow, **122**
Pulmonary vascular disease, surgically repaired transposition, 419
Pulmonary vascular resistance, 516
Pulmonary vascular tree, 516
Pulmonary veins, 314, *315*
   common, atresia, 466
   dilatation, patent ductus arteriosus, 373
   Doppler examination, 59
   flow velocities, restrictive cardiomyopathy, 486
   left
      anomalous drainage, *465*
      apical four chamber view, 49, *50*
   right
      anomalous drainage, 349, *351*, *354*, *465*, 466
      apical four chamber view, 49, *50*
   transoesophageal echocardiography, 143, 527
Pulmonary venous drainage (connection)
   anomalous, **457–471**
      atrial isomerism, *465*, 466, 467–468
      obstructed
         postoperative assessment, 469–471
         surgically repaired transposition, 419, 469–470
         total anomalous pulmonary venous connections, 458, 460, 463–466
      partial anomalous (PAPVC), 314, 457, *465*, **466–467**
      sinus venosus atrial septal defects and, 349, *351*, *354*, 466
      postoperative appearances, 469–471
      total anomalous (TAPVC), 314, **457–466**, 516
         cardiac, *459*, 461, *462*, *463*
         infracardiac (infradiaphragmatic), *459*, 461–466
         mixed, 466
         supracardiac, *457*, *458*–461, *462*
         surgically repaired, 471
Pulsed wave (PW) Doppler
   aortic regurgitation, *168*, 169, 170
   aortic stenosis, 165
   aortic valve, 163, *164*
   cardiac tamponade, 266–267
   congenital heart disease, 516
   equipment, 29, **32**
   examination technique, 55–56
   hypertrophic cardiomyopathy, 199
   mitral regurgitation, 161

   mitral stenosis, 156–157
   mitral valve, 154
   patent ductus arteriosus, 372
   physics and principles, 21
   practical aspects, 37
   pressure drop estimation, 85
   pulmonary valve, 174–175
   tricuspid valve, 171, 172
   volumetric flow estimation, 118–119
Pulse echo technique, **14–16**
Pulse repetition frequency (PRF), 17
   high, *see* High pulse repetition frequency (HPRF) Doppler
   pulsed wave Doppler, 32
Pulses, ultrasound, 14
Pulsus paradoxus
   cardiac tamponade, 266, 293, *294*
   constrictive pericarditis, 293
Pyopericardium, 262, **268**

'Quad screen' format, 38, *39*

Radioisotope scanning, 515
Range measurement, 15
Rashkind double umbrella, patent ductus arteriosus, 375
Rashkind procedure (balloon atrial septostomy), 352, *354*
Rastelli operation, 415–416, 419
Real-time imaging, *see* Cross-sectional imaging
Reconstruction, three-dimensional, **536**
Recordings, image, **35**, 62
Records, echocardiographic examination, 43
Recurrent laryngeal nerve palsy, 134
Red blood cell 'tracking', 525
Reflection
   non-specular, 14–15
   specular, 14
Refraction artefacts, 25
Regurgitant fraction, 124–125
Regurgitation, valvular, 514
   dilated cardiomyopathy, 203
   infective endocarditis, 219–220, 221
   pressure drop estimation, 83, 84–85, 86
   prosthetic valves, 228–229, 234–239
   quantitative colour flow mapping, 98, 101–102, 522–523
   volumetric flow estimation, 115, **124–125**, 524
   see also specific types
Renal abnormalities, 337
Renal failure, chronic, 199
Resolution, image, **24**
   contrast, 24, 36
   phased array scanheads, 30
   recent advances, 521–522
   spatial, 24, 35–36
   temporal, 24
   wavelength and, 12
Respiratory disease, tricuspid regurgitation, 109
Reverberation artefacts, 24–25, 37
   prosthetic heart valves, 225, 229
Rhabdomyomas, cardiac, 245, **249–250**, 337
Rheumatic fever, acute, **484**
Rheumatic heart disease
   aortic regurgitation, 167
   aortic stenosis, 164
   developing countries, 291, **296–299**
   infective endocarditis, 211

   mitral regurgitation, 157, 161
   mitral stenosis, 155, 161
   pulmonary stenosis, 174
   tricuspid regurgitation, 172
   tricuspid stenosis, 171
   vs. infective endocarditis, 215, *217*
Rheumatoid arthritis, juvenile, 485
Right atrial appendage, 256
Right atrial dilatation
   pulmonary valve stenosis, 431
   total anomalous pulmonary venous drainage, 457
Right atrial isomerism, 312, *465*, 467, 468
Right atrial pressure
   alternative methods of assessing, **109**
   cardiac tamponade, 264
   clinical estimation, **108**
   shape of atrial septum and, 343, *344*
Right atrium
   apical four chamber view, 49, *50*
   biopsy, 143
   compression/collapse, cardiac tamponade, 264–265
   dominance, atrioventricular septal defects, 358
   enlargement, atrial septal defects, 321, *322*
   myxomas, 171, 246, *247*–249
   parasternal long axis view, 47
   pulmonary venous drainage to, 460, 461, *463*
   secondary tumours, 253
   thrombi, 255–256
   transoesophageal imaging, 134, *135*
Right heart
   hypoplasia, atrioventricular septal defects, 358
   transoesophageal imaging, 135
   volume overload
      atrial septal defects, **344–347**, 349
      differential diagnosis, 345
      total anomalous pulmonary venous drainage, 457–458
Right heart failure, 109
Right sided obstructions and malformations, **429–444**
Right to left shunts
   atrial septal defects, 321, *322*
   Ebstein's anomaly, 442
   persistent fetal circulation, 343, *344*
   total anomalous pulmonary venous drainage, 458
Right ventricle
   apical four chamber view, 49, *50*
   atrioventricular septal defects, 358
   coarctation of aorta, 398
   compression/collapse, cardiac tamponade, 265–266
   congenital absence of pericardium, 272
   dilated cardiomyopathy, 202
   dimensions, 63, *67*
   double inlet, *318*, 452
   double outlet, *see* Double outlet right ventricle
   Ebstein's anomaly, 442, 443
   hypoplastic
      pulmonary atresia with intact ventricular septum, 439, 440
      transposition of great arteries, 417
   hypoplastic left heart syndrome, 396
   identification, 315, *316*, 425
   infarction, **187**
   isovolumic relaxation time (RIRT), **111–112**

Right ventricle (contd)
 left ventricular diastolic function and, 76
 parasternal long axis view, 47
 thrombi, 253–254
 transoesophageal imaging, 135
 transposition of great arteries, 411, 412
 volume overload
  atrial septal defects, 344–347, 349, 355
  atrioventricular septal defects, 359
  differential diagnosis, 345
Right ventricle-to-right atrium pressure drop, 107, *108*, 109
Right ventricular dilatation
 atrial septal defects, 321, *322*, 344, 345, *346*, 355
 differential diagnosis, 345
 dilated cardiomyopathy, 202, 481, 482
 Ebstein's anomaly, 442
 total anomalous pulmonary venous drainage, 457
Right ventricular function
 surgically repaired transposition, 418
 transposition of great arteries, 412
Right ventricular hypertrophy
 atrioventricular septal defects, 359
 hypertrophic cardiomyopathy, 197, *198*, 476
 pulmonary stenosis, 431–432
Right ventricular outflow tract
 atretic, 319–321
 Doppler examination, 57–58, *60*, *61*
 flow patterns, pulmonary artery pressure and, **110–111**
 narrowing, tetralogy of Fallot, 434, 435–436
 obstruction
  hypertrophic cardiomyopathy, 476, 477
  isolated, **431–434**
  pressure drop estimation, **95–96**, 432–433
  tetralogy of Fallot, 434, 435–436
  transposition of great arteries, 424–425
  ventricular septal defects, 360
 transoesophageal imaging, 134, 135, 525, *526*
Right ventricular pressure
 systolic, 107, 109
 ventricular septal defects, 369
Roussy–Lévy hereditary polyneuropathy, 481
Rubella, intrauterine infection, 431

St Jude prosthetic valve, 225, 230, 231
Sample volume size, Doppler systems, 64
Sampling, 16–17
Sampling rate (frequency), aliasing and, 21–22
Sarcoidosis, myocardial, 203
Sarcomas, cardiac, 245, 251–252
Scanheads (probes), **29–31**
 frequency and focus, **31**
 infants and children, 309
 intravascular, 40
 mechanical sector, 29–30
 phased annular array, 31
 phased array, 30–31
 transoesophageal, 31, 131–132
 see also Transducers
Scapuloperoneal muscular dystrophy, 485
Scimitar syndrome, 466
Screening, Marfan's disease, 285–286
Sector scan, 18, 29

Sedation
 infants and children, 309
 transoesophageal echocardiography, 133
Selenium deficiency, 485
Senning's operation, 417–419, 469–470
Sequential segmental approach, congenital heart disease, **307–340**
Shadowing, acoustic, 25–26, 37
 prosthetic heart valves, 225, 231, 236, *238*, 239
Short axis plane, 45
Short axis views
 basal, **134**, *135*
 parasternal, 47–48, *49*, 57–58, 62
 subcostal, 51, *52*
 ventricular, *134*, **135**, *136*
Shunts
 cardiac, volumetric flow estimation, **125**
 see also Left to right shunts; Right to left shunts
Side lobes, 37
Simpson's rule, 33
Single outlet heart, 318, 319
Sinusoidal waves, 11
Sinusoids, intramyocardial, 439–441
Sinus of Valsalva aneurysms, 217, 220, **286**
 ruptured, *282*, 286
Slice thickness, 18, 36
'Sonospirometry', 109
Sound, physical properties, **12–13**
Spatial average, time average intensity (Isata), 13
Spatial resolution, 24, 35–36
Spatial smoothing, 36
Speckle, 14, 36
Spectrum analyser, 21
Specular reflection, 14
Speed, ultrasound, 12
Standard echocardiographic examination, **62**
Starr–Edwards prosthetic valve, 225, *235*, 236
Stenoses, valvular, 513–514
 pressure drop estimation, 83–84
 prosthetic valves, 234, 235
 volumetric flow estimation, 115, 123–124, 524
 see also specific types
Storage disorders, *336*, 337
Stress echocardiography, **529–531**
 atrial pacing, 530, *531*
 digital echocardiography, 38–39
 Doppler studies, 531
 exercise, 529–530
 pharmacological, 39, 530–531
Stroke distance, aortic, *115*, 116
Stroke volume (SV), 68, 115, 116, 119
 aortic valve area and, 73, 124
 ejection fraction determination, 123
 mitral orifice flow and, 121
Subaortic stenosis, 389, **392–394**
 atrioventricular septal defects, 358, 359, 360
 double outlet right ventricle, 422
 hypertrophic cardiomyopathy, 164, 165
 transposition of great arteries, 416–417, 424
Subclavian arteries
 left
  aortic arch interruption, 403
  aortic dissection and, 279, 284
  coarctation of aorta, 398
 right
  anomalous origin, 332, 492, 493
  coarctation of aorta, 398–399

 suprasternal view, 51, *52*
Subcostal views
 four chamber, 50–51
 short axis, 51, *52*
Subcostal window, 45, **50–51**, 62, 277
 children and infants, 309
Sub-mitral aneurysms, congenital, 299
Subpulmonary stenosis, see Pulmonary stenosis, infundibular
Subxiphoid window, see Subcostal window
Sudden death, cardiac fibromas, 250–251
Superior vena cava, 313
 abnormal connection, 354
 Doppler examination, 57, 58, *59*
 left, 313, 314, *468*
  hypoplastic left heart syndrome, 397
  right pulmonary vein draining into, *465*
 obstruction, surgically repaired transposition, 418, 469
 pulmonary venous drainage to, 460, *462*
 total anomalous pulmonary venous drainage, 459
 transoesophageal imaging, 525
Supraclavicular fossae, 277
Suprasternal window, 45, **51–52**, 56–57, 62, 277
 children, 309
'Swan (goose) neck' appearance, atrioventricular septal defects, 324, *325*, 358
Sweep speed, Doppler systems, 63
Swept gain (SG), 15
Syphilis, tertiary, 278
Systemic lupus erythematosus, 216, *218*, 485
Systemic to pulmonary shunts, 515
Systemic venous drainage
 congenital abnormalities, 313–314, 457
 obstructed, surgically repaired transposition, 418, 469
 surgically repaired transposition, *468*
Systole
 dilated cardiomyopathy, 481
 hypertrophic cardiomyopathy, **199–201**
 left ventricular function, 71–75
Systolic velocity time integrals, 73, *115*, 116

Tachycardia, ischaemic heart disease, 184
'T' artefacts, secundum atrial septal defect, *322*, *323*
Taussig-Bing anomaly, 319, *320*, 414, **421**
Teichholz formula, 123
Temporal resolution, 24
Temporal smoothing, 36
Tetralogy of Fallot, 319, *320*, 359, 420, **434–437**
 coronary artery anomalies, 336, 436, 501, **502–503**
 echocardiography, 434–437
 pathology, 434
 pulmonary arteries, 331, 436, *437*
Thalassaemic cardiomyopathy, **485**, 486
Therapeutic applications of ultrasound, 536
Thermocouples, transoesophageal instruments, 132
Three-dimensional reconstruction, **536**
Thrombi
 aortic aneurysms, 278, *279*
 coronary artery aneurysms, 504
 intracardiac, **253–257**
  atrial, *254*, 255–256
  children, 337
  differential diagnosis, 216, 256–257

Thrombi (contd)
  dilated cardiomyopathy, 203, 254, 299–300, 482
  endomyocardial fibrosis, 205
  Fontan operation, 470
  mitral stenosis, 155, 297, *298*
  post-infarction, **186–187**, *188*, 254
  prosthetic heart valves, 225, 230, 255
  transoesophageal imaging, **139–140**
  ventricular, 186–187, 253–254
  ultrasonic dissolution, 536
Thymic aplasia, 377
Thymus
  inferior extension, 340
  neonates, 377
Time gain compensation (TGC), 15
Tissue characterisation
  myocardial, **183**, 203, 514–515, 532–533
  recent advances, **532–533**
Topical anaesthesia, transoesophageal echocardiography, 133
Transaortic pressure gradient, mean (MTP), 91
Transducers
  beam shapes, 13
  biplane transoesophageal, 39, 145–146, 525–526
  'footprint', 18, 44
  future developments, 39–40
  multiplane transoesophageal, 39–40, 526–527
  positioning, **44–46**
  selection, **44**
  see also Scanheads
Transoesophageal echocardiography, **129–146**
  aorta, 136, **137–138**, 277
  aortic dissection, 137–138, 284–285
  aortic stenosis, 393
  atrial pacing and, 530
  atrial septal defects, 141, 352
  biplane, 39, **145–146**, 525–526
  cardiac tumours, 138–139, 246–247, *248*, 249
  coarctation of aorta, 402
  complications, 134
  congenital heart disease, **141**, 527
  contra-indications, 134
  coronary arteries, 134, 140–141, 500, 504
  cross-sectional anatomy, 134–136
  endoscopic technique, 133–134
  equipment, 131–132
  history, 7, 131
  indications, 136–145, 146
  infective endocarditis, **136–137**, 211–214, 220–221, 231
  intensive care patients, 132–133, **143–145**
  interpretation, 132
  interventional procedures, 143
  intraoperative, 132–133, **143–145**, 527, 529
  mitral regurgitation, 139, 142, *160*, 162, 525, 527
  multiplane, 39–40, 526–527
  outpatient examination, 133
  patent ductus arteriosus, 375
  physician training, 132
  prosthetic heart valves, 142, *143*, 231, 239, 240
  recent developments, **525–527**
  scanheads (probes), **31**, 131–132
  technique, 132–134
Transposition of great arteries, 315, 318
  arterial switch operations, 419

atrial redirection operations, 355, 417–419
complete, **409–419**
  aortic arch abnormalities and subaortic stenosis, 330, 416–417, 425
  intact ventricular septum, 409–413
  left ventricular outflow obstruction, 414–416
  postoperative appearances, 417–419, *468*, 469–470
  ventricular septal defect, 413–414, *415*
congenitally corrected, **422–425**
  Ebstein's anomaly, 442
  left atrioventricular valve abnormalities, 424
  left ventricular outflow obstruction, 424
  right ventricular outflow obstruction, 424–425
  superior-inferior ventricles, 426
  ventricular septal defect, 423–424
coronary artery anomalies, 334–336, 410, **501–502**
double inlet ventricle with, 452
Rastelli operation, 415–416, 419
Transverse sinus of pericardium, 334, 497–498, 505
Transverse upper abdominal view, 50, *51*, 311, *312*
Trauma
  aortic aneurysms and aortic rupture, 285
  haemopericardium, 269
  ventricular septal defect, 301, *302*
Tricuspid atresia
  Fontan operation, *470*
  univentricular atrioventricular connection, 317, 319, 451–452
Tricuspid pressure half-time, 94
Tricuspid regurgitation, 170, 172, *173*
  contrast echocardiography, 109, 301
  dilated cardiomyopathy, 483
  failure to detect, 109–110
  flow velocities, 107–108, 172, *173*
  hypoplastic left heart syndrome, 397
  physiological (functional), 55–56, 170, 172
  pressure drop estimation, 84–85
  pulmonary artery pressure measurement, **107–110**, 172
  pulmonary hypertension, 170, 172
  restrictive cardiomyopathy, 207, 486
  surgically repaired transposition, 418
  transposition of great arteries, 424
  ventricular septal defects, 369
Tricuspid stenosis, 170, **171–172**
  pressure drops, **94**, 171
Tricuspid valve, **170–172**
  apical four chamber view, 49
  carcinoid disease, 171, 172, 253
  Doppler examination technique, **55–56**
  Ebstein's anomaly, *see* Ebstein's anomaly
  flow velocities
    atrial septal defects, 345, *347*
    cardiac tamponade, 266
    prosthetic valves, 240
    tricuspid regurgitation, 107–108, 172, *173*
    tricuspid stenosis, 171
  infective endocarditis, 214, *215*
  morphological recognition, 315, *316*
  normal, 170–171
  parasternal short axis view, 48, *49*
  prostheses, Doppler evaluation, 240
  pulmonary atresia with intact ventricular septum, 439, 440
  straddling, *328*, 414, *415*
  transoesophageal imaging, 525, *526*

transposition of great arteries, 414, *415*, 422–423, 424
traumatic rupture, 172
ventricular septal attachment, *323*, 324
ventricular septal defects, 361–362, 363
volumetric flow estimation, **122**
Truncal valve, 319, *321*, 375, *377*
Truncus arteriosus (common arterial trunk), 319, *321*, **375–378**
  associated abnormalities, 376–377
  differential diagnosis, 377–378
  overriding, 375
  postoperative findings, 378
Tuberculosis, developing countries, 291
Tuberculous pericarditis, 263, **267–268**, 270
  developing countries, 291, *292–296*
Tuberous sclerosis, 245, 337
Turbulent flow, 20
  colour flow mapping, 23, 522–523
  free jets, 84
  mitral prostheses, 235, *236*
  mitral regurgitation, *159*, *160*, 161
  tricuspid stenosis, 171–172
  velocity-variance colour flow map algorithms, 100–101
T-waves, giant negative, 195–197
Two chamber (long axis) view, apical, 50, 56, 62
Two-dimensional imaging, *see* Cross-sectional imaging

Ultrasound
  cardiac, *see* Echocardiography
  intravascular, 7, 40, **533–536**
  physical properties, 12–13
  physics and principles, **9–26**
  recent advances, **519–537**
  therapeutic applications, 536
Uniformity, image, 36
Univentricular atrioventricular connection, 317, *318*, 319, **447–453**

Valves, *see* Cardiac valves
Valvular heart disease, **513–514**
  acquired, **151–176**
  infective endocarditis, 211
  intraoperative echocardiography, 527, 528
  transoesophageal imaging, **141–143**
  vs. infective endocarditis, 215–216
  see also specific disorders
Valvuloplasty, aortic balloon, 143
Variance, colour flow mapping, 23
Vascular rings, 332–333, **491–493**
Vegetations, 175, 211–214, 337, *338*
  aortic regurgitation, 167
  differential diagnosis, 215–216, 257
  embolisation, 214–215
  Libman-Sacks, 216, *218*
  mitral regurgitation, 157, *158*
  non-valvular, 215
  prosthetic valves, 220, 221, 229, 230–231
  pulmonary regurgitation, 174
  serial assessment, 221–222
  transoesophageal imaging, 136–137
Vein of Galen aneurysms, 461, *462*
Velocity, flow
  accurate Doppler estimation, 86
  aortic valve, *see* Aortic valve, flow velocities
  coding, colour flow mapping, 23
  determination, colour flow mapping, 98–100

Velocity, flow (contd)
  dilated cardiomyopathy, 203
  hypertrophic cardiomyopathy, 199, 200
  low, detection by colour flow mapping, 23
  mitral valve, see Mitral valve, flow velocities
  patent ductus arteriosus, 374–375
  pressure drop relationship, 81–82
  pulmonary, see Pulmonary artery(ies), flow velocities; Pulmonary valve, flow velocities
  tricuspid valve, see Tricuspid valve, flow velocities
Velocity map, digital, 99
Velocity profiles, aorta, *116*, 117
Velocity time integrals (VTI), 34
  systolic, 73, *115*, 116
Velocity-variance colour flow map algorithms, 100–101
Vena contracta, 83
Venous anomalies, **455–471**
Venous connections
  congenital heart disease, **313–317**
  pulmonary, see Pulmonary venous drainage
  systemic, see Systemic venous drainage
Ventilation, assisted, transoesophageal echocardiography, 144
Ventricle(s)
  atrioventricular septal defects, 357–359
  double inlet, 363, 449–453
  double outlet, 318
  myxomas, 246, 249
  single indeterminate, 317, *318*, 449, *450*
  superior-inferior
    corrected transposition, 426
    and criss-cross atrioventricular connection, *425*, **426**
  thrombi, 253–254
  see also Left Ventricle; Right ventricle
Ventricular dominance, atrioventricular septal defects, 357–358, 359
Ventricular septal defects (VSD), **324–328**, **360–370**

apical, 326, *327*, 364, 366, *367*
classification, 360
colour flow mapping, 366
confluent, 360
double outlet right ventricle, 319, 419–420
doubly committed, 326–327, *328*, 364, 365–366, 420, 421
examination, 361
fibrous tissue near, 328
infective endocarditis, 214, *215*
inlet muscular, 356–357, **363**
membranous, 324
mid muscular, 364, *365*
multiple, 326, 363, 364, 421–422
muscular, 326, **363–366**
muscular outlet, 364–366
non-committed, double outlet right ventricle, 421
perimembranous, 324–326, **361–363**
position of great arteries and, 318–319, *320*
post-infarction, *140*, 141, **185**, 528
pulmonary atresia with, 319–321, 331, **437–438**, *439*
quantitation, 367–370
  pulmonary artery pressure, 368–370
  shunt size, 367–368
  size of defect, 367
quantitative colour flow mapping, 97–98
subaortic, 364–365, *366*, 420–421
subpulmonary, 364, 365–366, 421
tetralogy of Fallot, 434–435
transposition of great arteries, 413–414, *415*, 423–424
traumatic, 301, *302*
univentricular atrioventricular connection, 452
volumetric flow estimation, 125, 368
Ventricular septum, see Interventricular septum
Ventricular short axis view, *134*, **135**, *136*
Ventricular topology (looping), 317
Ventricular wall motion analysis, see Wall motion analysis

Ventriculo-arterial connection, **317–321**
  concordant, 318
  discordant, 318, 326, *327*, **407–426**
  see also Transposition of great arteries
Vertical vein, left, 459–460, *465*
Video printers, 35
Video recorders, **34**
Video review, 34, 309
Viral myocarditis, **484**
Viscous friction, 82, 85
Volume calculations, **33**
Volumetric flow estimation, **113–125**
  aorta, 115–119
  cardiac shunts, 125
  mitral valve, 119–122
  patent ductus arteriosus, 373–374
  pulmonary, 122
  tricuspid valve, 122
  valvular regurgitation, 115, 124–125, 522–523
  valvular stenosis, 115, 123–124, 524
  ventricular septal defects, 368
  see also Cardiac output; Stroke volume

Wall motion analysis, 33, *68*, 69
  intraoperative transoesophageal, 144–145
  left ventricular ischaemia/infarction, 181–182, *183*, 522
  right ventricular infarction, 187
  stress tests, 529–530
  transoesophageal imaging, 141
Wall motion score index, 181, 522
Warfarin, 297
Wavelength, ultrasound, 12
Waves, ultrasound, **11–12**
Wessex bioprosthetic valve, 229
William's syndrome, 431, *465*
Wilms' tumour, 337, *338*
Windows, echocardiographic, 35, 44–46, 309

Xiphisternal window, see Subcostal window